AAOS Atlas of Orthoses and Assistive Devices

Fourth Edition

AAOS Atlas of Orthoses and Assistive Devices

Fourth Edition

John D. Hsu, MD, CM, FACS
Chairman
Department of Surgery
Chief of Orthopaedics
Rancho Los Amigos National Medical Center
Emeritus Clinical Professor, Orthopaedics
University of Southern California
Keck School of Medicine
Downey, California

John W. Michael, MEd, CPO
Adjunct Faculty, MSPO Program
Applied Physiology
Georgia Institute of Technology
Atlanta, Georgia

John R. Fisk, MD
Professor Emeritus
Department of Surgery
Southern Illinois University School of Medicine
Springfield, Illinois

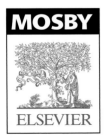

MOSBY

ELSEVIER

MOSBY
ELSEVIER

1600 John F. Kennedy Blvd.
Ste 1800
Philadelphia, PA 19103-2899

AAOS ATLAS OF ORTHOSES AND ASSISTIVE DEVICES, FOURTH EDITION

ISBN: 978-0-323-03931-4

Notice

Knowledge and best practice in this field are constantly changing. As new research and experience broaden our knowledge, changes in practice, treatment and drug therapy may become necessary or appropriate. Readers are advised to check the most current information provided (i) on procedures featured or (ii) by the manufacturer of each product to be administered, to verify the recommended dose or formula, the method and duration of administration, and contraindications. It is the responsibility of the practitioner, relying on their own experience and knowledge of the patient, to make diagnoses, to determine dosages and the best treatment for each individual patient, and to take all appropriate safety precautions. To the fullest extent of the law, neither the Publisher nor the Editors assume any liability for any injury and/or damage to persons or property arising out of or related to any use of the material contained in this book.

The Publisher

Library of Congress Cataloging-in-Publication Data

AAOS atlas of orthoses and assistive devices / [edited by] John D. Hsu, John W. Michael, John R. Fisk.—4th ed.
        p. ; cm.
    Rev. ed. of: Atlas of orthoses and assistive devices / editors, Bertram Goldberg, John D. Hsu. 3rd ed. c1997.
    Includes bibliographical references and index.
    ISBN-13: 978-0-323-03931-4.
1. Orthopedic apparatus.
    [DNLM: 1. Orthotic Devices. 2. Biomechanics. 3. Orthopedic Fixation Devices. 4. Self-Help Devices. WE 26 A111 2008] I. Title: Atlas of orthoses and assistive devices. II. Hsu, John D. III. Michael, John W. IV. Fisk, John R., 1943 V. American Academy of Orthopaedic Surgeons. VI. Atlas of orthoses and assistive devices.
RD755.A85 2008
617'.9—dc22

                                                                        2007026936

Acquisitions Editor: Emily Christie
Developmental Editor: Adrianne Brigido
Project Manager: Bryan Hayward
Design Direction: Lou Forgione

Printed in China

Last digit is the print number: 9 8 7 6 5 4 3 2

Contents

v

Contents

Section 5
Pediatric orthoses
Introduction by John D. Hsu

Section 6
Assistive devices
Introduction by Shubhra Mukherjee, Deborah J. Gaebler-Spira, and John R. Fisk

Contributors

Kai-Nan An, PhD
John and Posy Krehbiel Professor of Orthopedics
Department of Orthopedic Surgery
Mayo Clinic College of Medicine
Rochester, Minnesota

Samuel Andrews, BS
Director of Volunteer Services
Craig Hospital
Englewood, Colorado

John Anschutz, BS, ATP
Visiting Scholar
ECE, HCI
Georgia Institute of Technology
Manager of Assistive Technology Center
Assistive Technology Center
Atlanta, Georgia

David F. Apple, Jr., MD
Associate Clinical Professor of Orthopaedic Surgery
Clinical Associate Professor in Rehabilitative Medicine
Orthopaedic Surgery
Rehabilitation Medicine
Emory University School of Medicine
Medical Director Emeritus
Shepherd Center
Atlanta, Georgia

Keith A. Bengtson, MD
Assistant Professor
Department of Physical Medicine and Rehabilitation
Mayo Clinic
Rochester, Minnesota

Richard A. Berger, MD, PhD
Professor of Orthopedics
Department of Orphopaedic Surgery
Mayo Clinic
Rochester, Minnesota

Robert James Bowers
Senior Lecturer
National Centre for Prosthetics and Orthotics
University of Strathclyde
Glasgow, Scotland
United Kingdom

John H. Bowker, MD
Professor Emeritus
Department of Orthopaedics
Miller School of Medicine
University of Miami
Co-Director
Diabetic Foot and Amputee Clinics
Rehabilitation Center
Jackson Memorial Hospital
Miami, Florida

Wilton H. Bunch, MD, PhD
Professor of Divinity
Beeson Divinity School
Samford University
Birmingham, Alabama

Mary C. Burns, OTR/L, CHT
Assistant Professor, Senior Hand Therapist
Department of Surgery
Southern Illinois University School of Medicine
Springfield, Illinois

Christina L. Calhoun, MSPT
Department of Rehabilitation
Shriners Hospital for Children
Philadelphia, Pennsylvania

Ross S. Chafetz DPT, MPH
Clinical Research Associate
Clinical Research Department
Shriners Hospital for Children
Philadelphia, Pennsylvania

Richard B. Chambers, MD
Associate Clinical Professor of Orthopaedic Surgery
University of Southern California
Rancho Los Amigos Medical Center
Downey, California

David N. Condie, BSc, MI Mech E, C Eng
Consultant Clinical Engineer
Glasgow, Scotland
United Kingdom

Elizabeth Condie, FCSP Grad.Dip.Phys
Reader
National Centre for Prosthetics and Orthotics
University of Strathclyde
Glasgow, Scotland
United Kingdom

David Constantine
Co-Founder and Executive Director
Motivation Charitable Trust
Brockley Academy
Bristol, United Kingdom

Bill Contoyannis
Manager, Monash Rehabilitation Technology
 Research Unit
Department of Electrical and Computer Systems
 Engineering
Monash University
Caulfield, Victoria
Australia

Damon Cooney, MD, PhD
Department of Plastic Surgery
Southern Illinois University School of Medicine
Springfield, Illinois

Patricia P. Daviou, OTR/L, ATP, CORS
Assistive Technology Coordinator
Assistive Technology Center
Shepherd Center
Atlanta, Georgia

Thomas V. DiBello, BS
President
Dynamic Orthotics and Prosthetics Ltd.
Houston, Texas

Honor Duderstadt-Galloway, BS, OTR/L
Occupational Therapist II
Occupational Therapy
Rancho Los Amigos National Rehabiliation Center
Downey, California

Joan E. Edelstein, MA, PT, FISPO
Senior Lecturer
Program in Physical Therapy
Columbia University
New York, New York

Patrick Matthew Edens, CTRS
Sports Team Coordinator
Therapeutic Recreation
Shepherd Center
Atlanta, Georgia

Nancy Elftman, BA, BSCO, BPed
Orthotic Department
Ranco Los Amigos Medical Center
Downey, California

Alberto Esquenazi, MD
Director, Gait and Motion Analysis Laboratory
Director, Regional Amputee Center
Chair and Professor
Department of Physical Medicine and Rehabilitation
Chief Medical Officer
MossRehab and Albert Einstein Medical Center
Phialdelphia, Pennsylvania

Laura Fenwick, CO
Instructor
Northwestern University Medical Center
Consulting Orthotist
Rehabilitation Institute of Chicago
Chicago, Illinois

Deanna J. Fish, MS, CPO
Director of Clinical Support
Innovative Neurotronics, Inc.
Austin, Texas

John R. Fisk, MD
Professor Emeritus
Department of Surgery
Southern Illinois University School of Medicine
Springfield, Illinois

Jan Furumasu
Physical Therapy Instructor
Physical Therapy
Rancho Los Amigos National Rehabilitation Center
Downey, California

Keith Gabriel
Associate Professor
Department of Surgery
Division of Orthopaedics and Rehabilitation
Southern Illinois University School of Medicine
Springfield, Illinois

Deborah J. Gaebler-Spira, MD, FAAP, FAACPDM
Professor of Pediatrics, and Physical Medicine and
 Rehabilitation
Northwestern University Feinberg School of Medicine
Rehabilitation Institute of Chicago
Chicago, Illinois

Donna Q. Gavin, CO
Director of Orthotics
Bioconcepts, Inc.
Orthotic-Prosthetic Center
Burr Ridge, Illinois

Thomas M. Gavin, CO
President and Director of Clinical Services
BioConcepts, Inc.
Burr Ridge, Illinois

Dr. Prof. Hans Jürgen Gerner
Department of Orthopaedics II-Rehabilitation Medicine
Orthopaedic University Hospital
Heidelberg, Germany

Monica R. Godinez, MA, OTR/L
Occupational Therapist II
Occupational Therapy
Rancho Los Amigos National Rehabiliation Center
Downey, California

Joeseph Gomez, MCTRS
Director of Therapeutic Recreation
Craig Hospital
Englewood, Colorado

Letha Y. Griffin, MD, PhD
Adjunct Professor
Department of Kinesiology and Health
Georgia State University
Atlanta, Georgia

Andrew Haskell, MD
Assistant Clinical Professor
Department of Orthopaedic Surgery
University of California, San Francisco
San Francisco, California

Marjorie Johnson Hilliard, PT, MS
Assistant Professor
Department of Physical Therapy and Human Movement
  Sciences
Northwestern University, Feinberg School of Medicine
Chicago, Illinois

Edward C. Hitchcock, OTR/L
Occupational Therapist
Technology Center
Rehabilitation Institute of Chicago
Chicago, Illinois

Gregory D. Horneber, CTRS
Clinical Supervisor
Therapeutic Recreation
Shepherd Center
Atlanta, Georgia

John D. Hsu, MD, CM, FACS
Chairman
Department of Surgery
Chief of Orthopaedics
Rancho Los Amigos National Medical Center
Emeritus Clinical Professor, Orthopaedics
University of Southern California
Keck School of Medicine
Downey, California

Carol Huserik
Department of Therapeutic Recreation
Craig Hospital
Englewood, Colorado

Dennis J. Janisse, C. Ped.
Assistant Clinical Professor
Department of Physical Medicine and Rehabilitation
Medical College of Wisconsin
Milwaukee, Wisconsin

Therese E. Johnston, PT, PhD, MBA
Clinical Assistant Professor
Physical Therapy
Temple University
Research Associate
Shriners Hospitals for Children
Philadelphia, Pennsylvania

Teresa D. Kaldis, MD
Program Director
Specialty Rehabilitation
The Institute for Rehabilitation and Research
Houston, Texas

Donald E. Katz, CO, LO, FAAOP
Administrative Director
Orthotics and Prosthetics Departments
Texas Scottish Rite Hospital for Children
Dallas, Texas

Mary Ann E. Keenan, MD
Chief, Neuro-Orthopaedics Service
Professor and Vice Chair for Graduate Medical Education
Department of Orthopaedic Surgery
University of Pennsylvania
Philadelphia, Pennsylvania

Carolyn Kelley, PT, MS, NCS
Associate Clinical Professor
School of Physical Therapy
Texas Woman's University
Physical Therapist Consultant
Memorial Hermann—The Institute for Rehabilitation and
  Research
Houston, Texas

James Kennedy, CDRS, CDI
Driver Rehabilitation Specialist
Assistive Technology Center
Shepherd Center
Atlanta, Georgia

James Kercher, MD
Medical House Staff
Emory University School of Medicine
Atlanta, Georgia

Loren L. Latta, PhD, PE
Director, Max Biedermann Institute for Biomechanics
Professor and Director of Research
Department of Orthopaedics
University of Miami School of Medicine
Miami, Florida

Judy Leonard, OTR, OHT
Director
Regional Hand Rehabilitation Services, Inc.
Grand Rapids, Michigan

Phyllis D. Levine, PT
Chicagoland Orthopaedic Rehabilitation Services
Palos Heights, Illinois

Dulcey Lima, CO, OTR/L
Adjunct Faculty
Orthotics Program
Northwestern University
Chicago, Illinois

Anna Lindström, BA
Project Coordinator
International Secretariat
Hjälpmedelsinstitutet/
Swedish Institute for Assistive Technology
Vällingby, Sweden

Thomas R. Lunsford, MSE, CO
Assistant Professor
Baylor College of Medicine
Certified Orthotist
Lone Star Orthotics
The Institute for Rehabilitation and Research
Houston, Texas

Michele Luther-Krug, COTA/L, AP, CDRS, CDT
Driver Rehabilation Specialist
Assistive Technology Center
Shepherd Center
Atlanta, Georgia

Bryan S. Malas, MHPE, CO
Instructor
Prosthetics-Orthotics Center
Northwestern University Feinberg School of Medicine
Director
Orthotics-Prosthetics Department
Children's Memorial Hospital
Chicago, Illinois

Roger A. Mann, MD
Private Practice of Orthopaedic Surgery
Director of Foot Fellowship Program
Oakland, California
Associate Clinical Professor
Department of Orthopaedic Surgery
University of California, San Francisco
San Francisco, California

Chiara Mariani, MD
Neuro-Orthopaedics Fellow
Department of Orthopaedic Surgery
University of Pennsylvania
Philadelphia, Pennsylvania

Shannon K. McClure, MD
Children's National Medical Center
Division of Orthopaedic Surgery and Sports Medicine
Clinical Instructor of Orthopaedic Surgery
Washington, DC

Kevin P. Meade, PhD
Professor of Mechanical Engineering
Mechanical, Materials and Aerospace Engineering
Illinois Institute of Technology
Chicago, Illinois

Barry Meadows, BSc, PhD, CEng, MIMechE, CSci, MIPEM, FISPO
Visiting Professor
National Centre for Prosthetics and Orthotics
University of Strathclyde
Head of Neurobiomechanics
Westmarc
Southern General Hospital
Glasgow, United Kingdom

Joseph A. Metzger, BS
Outdoor Specialist
Therapeutic Recreation
Shepherd Center
Atlanta, Georgia

John W. Michael, MEd, CPO
Adjunct Faculty, MSPO Program
Applied Physiology
Georgia Institute of Technology
Atlanta, Georgia

Kelly Mixon, MS, CTRS
Sports Specialist
Therapuetic Recreation
Shepherd Center
Atlanta, Georgia

Miguel Mojica, CP, CO
Instructor
Department of Orthotics and Prosthetics
UT Southwestern Medical Center at Dallas
Dallas, Texas

Steven L. Moran, MD
Associate Professor of Plastic and Orthopedic Surgery
Division of Hand and Microvascular Surgery
Mayo Clinic
Staff Surgeon
Shriner's Hospital for Sick Children
Rochester, Minnesota

Shubhra Mukherjee, MD
Instructor
Northwestern University Feinberg School of Medicine
Attending Physician
Department of Pediatric Rehabilitation
Rehabilitation Institute of Chicago
Chicago, Illinois

M.J. Mulcahey, PhD, OTR/L
Director of Rehabilitation and Clinical Research
Shriners Hospitals for Children
Philadelphia, Pennsylvania

Michael W. Neumeister, MD
Professor
Division of Plastic Surgery
Program Director
Plastic Surgery Residency Program
Department of Surgery
Southern Illinois University School of Medicine
Springfield, Illinois

Frans Nollet, MD, PhD
Department of Rehabilitation
Academic Medical Center
University of Amsterdam
Amsterdam, The Netherlands

Cornelis Th. Noppe, CPO
Director, Noppe Orthopedietechniek
Noordwijkerhout, The Netherlands

Tom F. Novacheck, MD
Associate Professor
Department of Orthopaedic Surgery
University of Minnesota
Minneapolis, Minnesota
Director, Center for Gait and Motion Analysis
Gillette Children's Specialty Healthcare
St. Paul, Minnesota

Elaine Owen, MSc, MCSP, SRP
Clinical Specialist
Superintendent Paediatric Physiotherapist
Child Development Centre
Bangor, North Wales, United Kingdom

Avinash G. Patwardhan, PhD
Professor
Department of Orthopaedic Surgery and
    Rehabilitation
Loyola University School of Medicine
Maywood, Illinois
Director
Musculoskeletal Biomechanics Laboratory
Veterans Administration Hospital
Hines, Illinois

Jacquelin Perry, MD
Emeritus Chief, Polio and Gait Clinic
Emeritus Chief, Pathokinesiology
Rancho Los Amigos National Rehabilitation Center
Downey, California

Troy D. Pierce, MD
Private Practice
The Bone and Joint Center
Bismark, North Dakota

H. Duane Romo, CPO
Ossur North America, Inc.
Aliso Viejo, California

Dipl.-Ing. Rüdiger Rupp
Department II
Orthopaedic University Hospital
Heidelberg, Germany

Augusto Sarmiento, MD
Professor
Department of Orthopaedics and Rehabilitation
University of Miami School of Medicine
Miami, Florida

John F. Sarwark, MD
Martha Washington Professor of Orthopaedic Surgery
Northwestern University School of Medicine
Head, Division of Pediatric Orthopaedic Surgery
Children's Memorial Hospital
Chicago, Illinois

Alexander Y. Shin, MD
Associate Professor
Department of Orthopaedic Surgery
Division of Hand Surgery
Mayo Clinic
Rochester, Minnesota

James L. Shoop, ATC
Director of Sports Medicine
Georgia Institute of Technology
Atlanta, Georgia

Susan A. Skolnick, MS, CTRS
Manager
Therapeutic Recreation
Shepherd Center
Atlanta, Georgia

K. Brandon Strenge, MD
Resident
Division of Orthopaedics and Rehabilitation
Department of Surgery
Southern Illinois University
Springfield, Illinois

Terry J. Supan, CPO, FAAOP, FISPO
Clinical Professor
Department of Surgery
Southern Illinois University School of Medicine
Clinical Associate
Orthotic & Prosthetic Associates of Central Illinois
Springfield, Illinois

Alfred B. Swanson, MD
Professor of Surgery
Michigan State University
East Lansing, Michigan
Director of Orthopaedic Surgery Residency Training
    Program of the Grand Rapids Hospitals
Director of Hand Surgery Fellowship and Orthopaedic
    Research
Blodgett Memorial Medical Center
Grand Rapids, Michigan

Geneviève de Groot Swanson, MD
Assistant Clinical Professor of Surgery
Michigan State University
East Lansing, Michigan
Coordinator
Orthopaedic Research Department
Blodgett Memorial Medical Center
Grand Rapids, Michigan

Mukul C. Talaty, PhD
Visiting Faculty
School of Biomedical Engineering and Health Systems
Drexel University
Philadelphia, Pennsylvania
Research Scientist
Gait & Motion Analysis Laboratory
MossRehab
Elkins Park, Pennsylvania

Susan Johnson Taylor, BS, OTR/L
Wheelchair and Seating Center
Rehabiltation Institute of Chicago
Chicago, Illinois

Laura L. Tosi, MD
Associate Professor of Orthopaedic Surgery
George Washington University
Children's National Medical Center
Washington, DC

Heikki Uustal, MD
Associate Professor
Department of Medicine
University of Medicine and Dentistry of New Jersey
New Brunswick, New Jersey
Attending Psychiatrist
Director, Prosthetic/Orthotic Team
Department of Rehabilitation Medicine
JFK Medical Center
Edison, New Jersey

Carlos Vallbona, MD
Professor
Department of Family and Community Medicine
Baylor College of Medicine
Houston, Texas

Jill Stelley Virden
Department of Therapeutic Recreation
Craig Hospital
Englewood, Colorado

Bradon J. Wilhelmi, MD
Associate Professor
Director Hand
Director of Burn Unit
Plastic Sugery
Southern Illinois University
Springfield, Illinois

Brett William Wolters, MD
Orthopaedic Surgery and Sports Medicine
Department of Orthopaedics
Memorial Medical Center
Springfield, Illinois

Preface

The development and application of orthoses to reduce the impact of physical disability is an ancient art. Two of the devices discussed in this text as contemporary interventions have been documented as being in use more than 4500 years ago: the crutch depicted in a bas relief carving on the entrance to Hirkouf's tomb executed in 2830 B.C. and the fracture splint unearthed from the 5th Egyptian Dynasty (2750–2625 B.C.).

Vernon L. Nickel, MD, former Medical Director and founder of the Orthopaedic Rehabilitation Services at Rancho Los Amigos Hospital, defines *rehabilitation* as the care of patients with chronic diseases involving the neuromuscular skeletal system. Nicholas Andry in the 1740s laid down the principles of care for chronic disability. Sir Robert Jones after the first World War established rehabilitation units for the war wounded. The multidisciplinary approach grew out of necessity as the complex medical, social, and psychological problems and equipment needs for the disabled required professionals knowlegeable in these areas to provide input and assistance in treatment and management.

This edition of the *Atlas* is the direct descendant of the 1952 classic *Orthopaedic Appliances Atlas*, which was published at the behest of Dr. M.E.M. Thompson, President of the American Academy of Orthopaedic Surgeons (AAOS) in 1947. Its purpose was to "...familiarize orthotists, brace makers ... [and] orthopaedic surgeons with the development of standards and technical production of orthopaedic appliances...." This project was supported by the Surgeon-General, the Veterans Administration, and the National Research Council together with many industrial manufacturers. Its aim was to clarify, standardize the nomenclature, and classify the use and production of such disease-specific devices.

Almost a quarter century elapsed before the *Atlas of Orthotics* was published by C. V. Mosby under the auspices of the AAOS Committee on Prosthetics and Orthotics in 1975. The primary focus of this edition was the application of the growing body of bioengineering knowledge to provide "... a rational and generic basis for the prescription of an orthosis best suited for a particular patient's needs." This has now become one of the hallmarks of quality care, rendering disease-specific application of orthoses obsolete. A newly adopted nomenclature using terminology to describe orthoses, "... by the joints they encompass and ... their effect on the control of anatomic joint motions" has been adopted by the International Standards Organization (ISO) and is accepted worldwide as the proper nomenclature for prostheses and orthoses.

Within a decade, advances in material science and in the application of orthoses led the American Academy of Orthopaedic Surgeons to sponsor the publication of the *Atlas of Orthoses*, a volume intended to "bridge the gap between a rote therapeutic approach and the frontiers of science." This edition emphasized consideration of the orthosis as one of many treatment options, including pharmacologic, medical, and surgical interventions. The conceptual organization from that text continues to this day, beginning with a summary of the "basic science" of orthoses from such fields as biomechanics, materials engineering, and kinesiology. After a discussion of representative components and examples of commonly used upper limb, lower limb and spinal orthoses, specific biomechanical applications organized by the presenting musculoskeletal disorder are illustrated, along with treatment alternatives.

The 1997 *AAOS Atlas of Orthoses and Assistive Devices* built upon this heritage by assembling "a cross section of experts from multiple fields-orthopedists, orthotists, occupational therapists, and physical therapists-to gain a broad perspective in the usage of orthoses ... [that] reflects present clinical practices." A concerted effort was made to cite available controlled studies to provide scientifically valid justification for the opinions expressed.

This Fourth Edition of *AAOS Atlas of Orthoses and Assistive Devices* continues the tradition of its predecessors by providing an up-to-date overview of the clinical application of contemporary orthoses, which include increasingly sophisticated technology and more specific applications to achieve measurable results. It reflects the evolution of the role of the orthotist from passively filling a doctor's order to serving as an active consultant in the development and implementation of the most effective treatment plan for each individual. New to this edition is material reflecting the unique needs of developing countries. Technology and materials used in the industrialized nations are not always suitable for nonindustralized countries. The information in this volume will be of value not only to readers who actively care for patients but also to students and to those persons interested in a better understanding of this rapidly evolving discipline.

The Key Points boxes at the beginning of each chapter highlight the authors' primary message, including "practice pearls" and key evidence. The literature is filled with expert recommendations but contains only limited controlled studies. Fortunately, there is considerable interest in advancing this field with support given for additional research to be carried out. Results from such well-designed studies on the use of orthoses will enhance the current foundation for evidence-based practice, and in addition, the new information developed will require publication of future revisions of this tome.

John D. Hsu, MD

John W. Michael, MEd, CPO

John R. Fisk, MD   xiii

Dedication

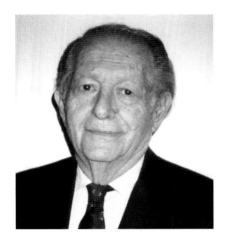

In Memoriam

SIDNEY FISHMAN, PhD
1919–2005

The Editors wish to dedicate this volume to Sidney Fishman, PhD, an esteemed educator and leader in prosthetics and orthotics, in recognition of his lifelong dedication to the field. In 1989, Dr. Newton McCollough III, then 1st Vice President of the American Academy of Orthopaedic Surgeons, nominated Dr. Fishman as an Associate Member of the organization because of his admiration for Dr. Fishman and his numerous contributions to prosthetic and orthotic education and to the development of practice principles guiding the provision of care to persons with disabilities. Sid served faithfully as an advisor to the AAOS Committee on Rehabilitation, Prosthetics and Orthotics, completing a 7-year term. He has been recognized for his contributions to past editions of the *AAOS Atlas of Orthotics and Assistive Devices* as well as its companion volume, the *AAOS Atlas of Limb Prosthetics*. From 2002 until the time of his death after a brief bout with cancer, Sid served as an alternate delegate to Drs. John Hsu and Alan Morris, who represented the American Academy of Orthopaedic Surgeons at a series of Medicare Negotiated Rulemaking hearings in Baltimore, Maryland. Whenever Sid expressed an opinion, the clarity and insightfulness of his comments commanded the respect and admiration of all present.

Dr. Fishman earned his PhD degree from Columbia University, New York, in 1949 and became affiliated with New York University School of Medicine and Post-Graduate Medical School, where he inaugurated and directed the world's first bachelor's degree and post-graduate certificate program in prosthetics and orthotics. In addition, he supervised a series of related interdisciplinary research studies concerned with prosthetic and orthotic rehabilitation of children and adults. He played a primary role in the development and direction of continuing education programs in prosthetics and orthotics. As a consummate multidisciplinary collaborator, Sid worked closely with a Who's Who of physicians and surgeons, nurses, psychologists, physical and occupational therapists, prosthetists, orthotists, engineers, rehabilitation counsellors, psychologists, patient advocates, physiologists, and other interested clinicians, researchers and scientists.

Sidney Fishman was a staunch advocate for optimizing care provided to persons with skeletal or neuromuscular disorders or defects. He devoted his career to advancing the quality and scope of formal education available to the prosthetist-orthotist, arguing for increasing the entry-level academic requirements to ensure evolution of the field parallel to that of other allied health professions. Dr. Fishman's work was recognized internationally. The educational model and curriculum that he developed at New York University have been utilized in many countries around the world, including Colombia, Israel, Portugal, Spain, India, Finland, Australia, Mexico, and Peru. At the time of his death, Dr. Fishman was recognized by Professor Harold Shangali, President of the International Society of Prosthetics and Orthotics (ISPO), as the person most responsible for making educational issues in prosthetics and orthotics one of the cornerstones of this multidisciplinary group. Sid served as a consultant to the Untied Nations, the Pan American Health Organization, the World Health Organization, Project HOPE, the World Rehabilitation Fund, and the International Divisions of the Rehabilitation Services Administration.

Dr. Fishman's impact on this nascent profession is embodied within the contributions to this text by the many authors who enjoyed the privilege of studying and collaborating with him during his long and distinguished career. Publication of this Fourth Edition of the *AAOS Atlas of Orthoses and Assistive Devices* is a fitting way to honor his legacy.

J.D.H.

J.W.M.

J.R.F.

Foreword

This is the fourth edition of this atlas published by the American Academy of Orthopedic Surgeons. The title of the volume has been changed to reflect the additional information that is included. Previous editions limited the information to amputations, prosthetics, and rehabilitation principles. This edition has included assistive devices for the spine and treatments for other deformities.

The art and science of amputations and the fitting of prosthetic devices has continually improved. Because of the body armor worn by our soldiers in Iraq, which protects the head and thorax (and as a result, vital organs), and because of improved resuscitation and rapid availability of medical care, many soldiers are surviving devastating wounds to the extremities that previously would have been fatal. As a result, soldiers are returning home with multiple limb amputations, many with grossly deformed stumps. Heterotopic ossification is also frequent. In addition, new pedicle and free flap techniques have allowed us to significantly alter amputation stumps in a way not previously possible. This has led to unique and innovative ways to design and fit prosthetics and orthotics. In addition, myoelectric technology and computerization of prostheses has led to innovative prosthetics.

This edition also includes a chapter on the technologies for assistive devices available in low-income countries, which will serve as a resource for surgeons, prosthetists, and therapists who venture to third-world countries for humanitarian endeavors.

A thorough knowledge of the new technologies by the surgeon is extremely important. Although in trauma situations surgeons frequently have limited opportunities to vary the result of amputations, it is incumbent on the operating surgeon to understand the technology so that he or she can utilize the latest techniques to get the best result from amputations and the reconstruction of amputation stumps. Cooperation among the surgeon, prosthetist, and physical therapist is essential for optimal results. Many physicians have relegated much of the selection and fitting of prostheses to prosthetists, and although this is often successful, more involvement from the surgeon is desired. This volume describes the latest science of prosthetics, orthotics, and other assistive devices and will be an essential part of the reconstructive surgeon's library.

Robert H. Haralson III, MD, MBA
Medical Director
American Academy of Orthopaedic Surgeons

Section 1 of this fourth edition of the *Atlas* introduces basic concepts and information essential for the effective provision of custom-fitted orthoses. The authors, all recognized experts in the application of this knowledge to orthotic management, reflect the interdisciplinary and international nature of the field. This section will be of particular interest to the orthotist or student who wants an overview of fundamentals, but the information provided will offer any interested reader a better understanding about the underpinnings of this form of non-operative treatment.

Chapter 1 gives a concise overview of the internationally agreed-upon terminology used to describe and prescribe orthoses. In today's global health care environment, it is more important than ever to use a common language that facilitates accurate and effective communication among all members of the treatment team. The terms developed by the International Standards Organization supersede the colloquial phrases ("cock-up splint") and historic eponyms ("Knight-Taylor brace") of yesteryear.

Writing a clear, concise, and complete prescription for an orthosis is one of the most crucial tasks in the rehabilitation process. Chapter 2 emphasizes the required interdisciplinary communication, describing a systematic approach in which the certified orthotist serves as a consultant in formulation of prescription specifics, in addition to having primary responsibility for the design, creation, fitting, and adjustments of orthoses.

Materials Science is the branch of engineering that has the greatest impact on the design and manufacturing of modern thin, lightweight, and durable orthoses. Chapter 3, derived in large part from the classic text *Strength of Materials in Orthotic and Prosthetic Design,*[1] highlights key considerations essential to the provision of durable, functional, and comfortable orthoses. Chapter 4 reviews available measurement and fabrication methods, illustrating the current technical application of these scientific principles.

Section 1 concludes with Chapter 5, which gives a thorough review of normal and pathologic gait. Extensive figures drawn from patient cases are used to illustrate the clinical presentation with, and without, proper management with an orthosis. Collectively these chapters provide a cohesive and up-to-date review of the basic scientific, clinical, and technical principles that form the conceptual foundation for effective application of orthoses and assistive devices in the rehabilitation of patients with neuromuscular disorders.

John W. Michael

---

[1]Lundsford TR: *Strength of materials in orthotic and prosthetic design.* Alexandria, Va, 1996, American Academy of Orthotists & Prosthetists.

Chapter

1

International Organization for Standardization (ISO) terminology

David N. Condie

Key Points

- International terminology standards have been established to facilitate communication and research regarding orthoses and their uses.
- The method of describing orthoses by reference to the body segments they encompass is widely accepted worldwide and now has been complemented by proposals for the classification and description of orthotic components.
- A recently approved international standard describing the methods and the terminology to be used to define the clinical objectives and functional requirements of orthoses fosters the development of evidence-based practice worldwide.

International organization for standardization

The International Organization for Standardization (ISO) is a worldwide federation of national standards organizations, known as ISO member bodies, that has its headquarters in Geneva, Switzerland. The organization is involved in a wide range of standardization activities embracing virtually every aspect of manufacturing, scientific, and commercial activity.

ISO derives its income from two sources: the fees paid by member bodies and the sales of documents, primarily standards, that it publishes. Because of this latter funding stream, all ISO documents are protected by copyright, and no part of them can be reproduced without the permission of the publisher. This consideration limits the detail of the relevant ISO standards that can be given in this chapter.

Technical committees and working Groups

The task of developing ISO standards is performed by Technical Committees (TCs) and their Working Groups (WGs). Every member body that expresses an interest in the work of a TC is entitled to be represented on that TC and its WGs. The process whereby a new international standard is developed and eventually published is complex and lengthy. A proposal must go through a series of stages, first as a New Work Item Proposal (NWIP), then as a Committee Draft (CD), then as Draft International Standards (DIS), and finally as Final Draft International Standards (FDIS), with opportunities for comment or revision at all stages by the participating member bodies. The complete process, from the adoption of a new work item until publication, typically takes a minimum of 5 years.

The purpose of describing the ISO committee structure and its method of operation is to make clear that ISO standards development is a closely regulated and controlled process. The resulting standards genuinely reflect the consensual view of the relevant professional groups.

ISO/TC 168: Prosthetics and Orthotics

ISO/TC 168 was formed in 1979. The Secretariat for the TC and its WGs has been held throughout its entire existence by the German national standards organization Deutsches Institut für Normung (DIN), which is based in Pforzheim.

The TC operates through three WGs:

- WG 1: Nomenclature and terminology
- WG 2: Medical aspects
- WG 3: Physical testing

3

This chapter focuses on the coordinated work of WGs 1 and 2 in the development of ISO standards for terminology in the field of orthotics.

Before describing the content of the current ISO standards, it is perhaps appropriate both to pose and to attempt to answer the question, "Why do we need international terminology standards in orthotics?" An answer might be provided by citing the sentiments expressed in the introductions to some of the more recently published standards.

In the absence of an internationally accepted method of describing either patients being treated (orthotically) or the orthoses and their components being employed, the members of the clinic teams in different countries have tended to develop their own terminology for this purpose.

This situation creates difficulties for practitioners prescribing orthoses and for manufacturers describing their products and has made the reporting of the treatment of particular patient groups and in particular the comparison of the outcomes of orthotic treatment in different centres almost impossible.

After ISO 8551 and ISO 13404

The standards described in this chapter permit the systematic and unambiguous description of the patient being treated with an orthosis, the objectives of the treatment, and both the functional characteristics and the components from which the orthoses has been assembled.

The standards

One of the first tasks undertaken by WGs 1 and 2 at their inaugural meeting in St. Andrews, Scotland, in 1980 was an attempt to define the scope of their future work. This exercise resulted in the model shown in Fig. 1-1.

The initial work program of the WGs included two standards of relevance to the field of orthotics:

- ISO 8549-1:1989 Prosthetics and Orthotics—Vocabulary

  General terms for external limb prostheses and external orthoses[1]

- ISO 8549-3:1989 Prosthetics and Orthotics—Vocabulary

  Terms relating to external orthoses[2]

The majority of the work performed by the WGs in the succeeding 10 years of the TC's existence was directed at the field of prosthetics; however, the past 5 years has seen the focus of the WG 1 and 2 program shift in the direction of orthotics, with the resulting publication of two further important standards:

- ISO 8551:2003 Prosthetics and Orthotics—Functional Deficiencies

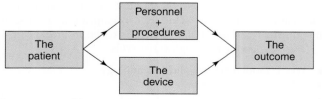

Fig. 1-1 Scope of future work.

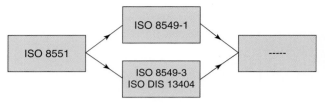

Fig. 1-2 Original scope model.

Description of the person to be treated with an orthosis, clinical objectives of treatment, and functional requirements of the orthosis[3]

- ISO 13404:2005 Prosthetics and Orthotics

  Classification and description of external orthoses and orthotic components[4]

The entire currently existing "family" of ISO orthotic terminology standards is illustrated, as they relate to the original "scope" model, in Fig. 1-2.

ISO 8549-1:1989 Prosthetics and Orthotics—Vocabulary
General terms for external limb prostheses and external orthoses

This first basic step into the world of ISO standardization attempts to define the fields of prosthetics and orthotics, the general terms used to describe prostheses and orthoses, the anatomy of those parts of the body most commonly fitted with these devices, and the personnel and procedures involved in their supply.

The orthotic terms included in this standard are listed in Box 1-1. An *orthosis* is defined as "an externally applied device used to modify the structural and functional characteristics of the neuromuscular and skeletal systems." *Orthotics* is defined as "the science and art involved in treating patients by the use of an orthosis." An *orthotist* is defined as "a person who, having completed an approved course of education and training, is authorised by an appropriate national authority to design measure and fit orthoses."

BOX 1-1
General terms, personnel and procedures

Orthosis; orthotic device	Orthotic assessment
Orthotics	Orthotic casting and measurement
Upper limb orthosis	Cast modification
Lower limb orthosis	Tracing modification
Spinal orthosis	Alignment
Orthotist	Bench assembly and alignment
Orthotic technician	Static and dynamic alignment
	Finishing and check-out

BOX 1-2
Categories of orthoses

Foot orthosis (FO)	Finger orthosis (FO)	Sacroiliac orthosis (SIO)
Ankle–foot orthosis (AFO)	Hand orthosis (HdO)	Lumbosacral orthosis (LSO)
Knee orthosis (KO)	Wrist–hand orthosis (WHO)	Thoracolumbosacral orthosis (TLSO)
Knee–ankle–foot orthosis (KAFO)	Wrist–hand–finger orthosis (WHFO)	Cervical orthosis (CO)
Hip orthosis (HpO)	Elbow orthosis (EO)	Cervicothoracic orthosis (CTO)
Hip–knee orthosis (HKO)	Elbow–wrist–hand orthosis (EWHO)	Cervicothoracolumbosacral orthosis (CTLSO)
Hip–knee–ankle–foot orthosis (HKAFO)	Shoulder orthosis (SO)	
	Shoulder–elbow orthosis (SEO)	
	Shoulder–elbow–wrist–hand orthosis (SEWHO)	

ISO 8549-3:1989 Prosthetics and Orthotics—Vocabulary

Terms relating to external orthoses

This important standard, based on the pioneering work of Dr. E.E. Harris while working for the Committee for Prosthetic Research and Development (CPRD) in Washington, DC, under the direction of A. Bennett Wilson, categorizes orthoses by reference to the anatomical segments and joints they encompass and establishes a system of abbreviations derived from the initial letters of the English terms for each category.

The full range of devices defined in this manner is listed in Box 1-2. For example, an *ankle–foot orthosis* is defined as "an orthosis which encompasses the ankle joint and the whole or part of the foot" and is referred to by the abbreviation "AFO." A *wrist–hand–finger orthosis* is defined as "an orthosis that encompasses the wrist joint, the hand, and one or more fingers" and is referred to by the abbreviation "WHFO." A *lumbosacral orthosis* is defined as "an orthosis that encompasses the whole or part of the lumbar and sacro-iliac regions of the trunk" and is referred to by the abbreviation "LSO."

The degree of acceptance of the system of abbreviations internationally, even by non–English-speaking orthotic practitioners, has been remarkable.

ISO 8551:2003 Prosthetics and Orthotics—Functional Deficiencies

Description of the person to be treated with an orthosis, clinical objectives of treatment, and functional requirements of the orthosis

This ambitious standard, published in 2003, is intended to provide clinicians with a method of describing in a consistent and unambiguous manner the persons they are treating orthotically, their reasons for doing so, and the conditions the orthosis must create. It does not include the description of the complete orthosis or the components from which it is constructed, which are covered by another standard, described later.

The first of the three defined objectives of the standard—the description of the person being treated—is achieved by specifying the method and the terminology to be used to describe the clinical characteristics listed in Box 1-3.

It should be emphasized that the clinician using this standard would not routinely record all this information, but rather would select those items considered relevant to the particular type of patient and the intended use of the information.

The second goal of the standard is to establish a consistent method of defining what are referred to in the standard as "the clinical objectives" of the orthotic treatment. Nine basic objectives (some of which have more than one variant) are identified in Box 1-4.

For each of these objectives, the information that it recommended to be recorded is specified. For example, if the objective is to relieve pain, the clinician should record which joints or segments are involved and what induces the pain.

If the objective is to manage a deformity, the information required includes the joints or segments involved and whether the deformity is "preventable," "reducible," or "irreducible." Where terms like these, which do not already have a generally accepted meaning, are used in the standard, definitions are included that make their meaning absolutely clear.

BOX 1-3
Description of the person to be treated with an orthosis

Personal (e.g., age, height, significant medical history)
Clinical condition to be treated, including diagnosis and
  ICD-10 codes
Other clinical conditions present
Motivation and personal needs
Functional abilities

The final segment of the standard describes the method and the terms to be used to describe the "functional requirements of the orthosis" necessary to achieve the previously defined clinical objectives. The five categories identified are listed in Box 1-5.

The reason adoption of this two-stage approach was considered necessary to the development of what is in effect the orthotic prescription is best illustrated by looking at an example of the use of the standard.

One of the clinical objectives of the orthotic treatment of a person who suffers from a degenerative joint disease might be to relieve pain. Depending on the location and severity of the condition, the *functional requirements* of the orthosis used to achieve this objective might be to prevent, reduce, or stabilize a deformity; to limit the range of a joint; or to reduce or redistribute the load on particular tissues.

A second clinical objective for treatment of this person might be to manage a deformity. Again depending on the severity of the condition, the functional requirements for the orthosis to achieve this objective might be simply to stabilize the deformity (i.e., prevent it from increasing) or alternatively to reduce the external loading on the involved joint.

As with the previous section of this standard, for each of the categories of functional requirement, the information recommended to be recorded is specified. Thus for the first clinical objective just discussed, the information regarding the functional requirements of the orthosis would include (in addition to defining the joint or segment it is to affect) (1) the way in which the deformity is to be controlled, that is, prevented, reduced, or stabilized; (2) the range of joint motion to be imposed; and (3) the type of loading to be reduced.

This standard also contains as an appendix some details of the different "biomechanical effects" that orthoses use to achieve their functional requirements.

ISO 13404:2005 Prosthetics and Orthotics
Classification and description of orthoses and orthotic components

This final element of the existing body of ISO orthotic terminology standards is designed to complement ISO 8551 by providing a means of actually describing the functions and construction of the orthosis used to achieve a particular set of clinical objectives and functional requirements.

The first section of the standard describes the method to be used to classify and describe the complete orthosis. This in turn comprises three elements. The first element is termed the *general description* and recommends the use of the terminology contained in the previously published ISO 8549-3, that is, AFO, WHO, SO, and so on, whereas the second element is termed the *function of the orthosis* and logically uses the same terminology as used in ISO 8551 to describe functional requirements—for example, to prevent, reduce, or stabilize a deformity; to reduce or redistribute the load on tissues; and so on. The final element of this section simply requires the description of the "type of fabrication" as being either custom fabricated or prefabricated.

The second section of the standard specifies the method to be used to classify and describe the components used in the construction of an orthosis.

Four categories of component are identified:

- Interface components
- Articulating components
- Structural components
- Cosmetic components

The standard proceeds to define each category, list the range of components that belong in each category, and specify what information is required to describe them. For example, *interface components* are defined as "those components which are in direct contact with the user and are responsible for transmitting the forces which result in its function and may retain it in place" and are considered as including the following:

- Shells
- Pads
- Straps
- Foot orthoses
- Shoes (used with an orthosis)

Articulating components, which are defined as "components of orthoses used to allow or control the motion of anatomical joints," are to be described by specifying the following:

- The anatomical joint whose motions they are intended to allow or control
- The *permissible motions* of the joint when assembled in the finished orthosis
- The *form of articulation*, either motion between parts of the joint or deformation of a part of the joint
- The *axis of rotation*, either monocentric or polycentric

- The *type of controls* that the joint incorporates (e.g., locks, limiting mechanisms, assist/resist mechanisms)

Structural components are defined as "components which connect the interface and articulating components and maintain the alignment of the orthosis" and include both uprights and shells.

Finally, *cosmetic components* are defined as "the means of providing shape, colour and texture to orthoses" and include fillers, covers, and sleeves.

Conclusion

The publication of ISO 13404 completes the current program of orthotically linked terminology standards of the ISO/TC 168 WGs. It probably is too soon to assess the degree of acceptance and the impact of the methods and the terms contained in the two most recently published standards.

Other current work of the WGs that will be of interest to orthotic practitioners includes an NWIP on which some preliminary work has already taken place to develop a standard for "the description of normal, prosthetic and other pathological gait." Obviously the third element of this proposed standard would be of considerable value when describing patients' functional abilities both before and after orthotic treatment.

It should be reiterated that the principal reason for institution of the program of orthotic terminology development described in this chapter was to facilitate communication among all the parties involved in both the manufacturing and the clinical aspects of the field of orthotics. Therefore it is strongly recommended that all those persons who share this objective should obtain copies of these standards and endeavor to use the methods and the terms they describe in an appropriate manner in their day-to-day professional activity.

References

ISO 8549-1:1989 Prosthetics and Orthotics—Vocabulary. General terms for external limb prostheses and external orthoses. Geneva, Switzerland, International Organization for Standardization.

ISO 8549-3:1989 Prosthetics and Orthotics—Vocabulary. Terms relating to external orthoses. Geneva, Switzerland, International Organization for Standardization.

ISO 8551:2003 Prosthetics and Orthotics—Functional deficiencies. Description of the person to be treated with an orthosis, clinical objectives of treatment, and functional requirements of the orthosis. Geneva, Switzerland, International Organization for Standardization.

ISO 13404:2005 Prosthetics and Orthotics. Classification and description of orthoses and orthotic components. Geneva, Switzerland, International Organization for Standardization.

The orthotic prescription

Heikki Uustal

Key Points

- Writing a prescription for an orthosis is one element of the larger process of rehabilitation to improve patient function. It includes evaluation, assessment, and formulation of the specific treatment plan described in the prescription.

- Optimal communication and transdisciplinary education occur when the patient, physician, orthotist, and therapist all are present for both patient evaluation and long-term follow-up. Maintaining this level of collaboration outside of the formal clinic team setting is difficult.

- The certified orthotist functions as a consultant to the clinic team with regard to orthotic management and provides fitting and follow-up of the indicated device.

- A clear understanding of the patient's disease process, based on a comprehensive history and physical examination, is the foundation for generating the appropriate prescription.

- An effective prescription for orthotic care summarizes the medical issues related to the patient, details the biomechanical functions desired, and specifies key technical attributes of the desired orthosis.

Writing a prescription for an orthosis is a small part of the much larger process of rehabilitation to improve patient function. To understand this larger process, one must understand the roles of the different individuals involved and the goals set for each of those individuals. In the ideal setting, the patient is evaluated and managed by a team of professionals called the *orthotic team*. The team approach has been used for decades, both in the field of rehabilitation and in the practice of orthotics and prosthetics. The orthotic team at minimum should include the following members: the patient, the physician, the certified orthotist, the physical therapist or occupational therapist, and, when appropriate, the certified pedorthist. The best communication and the best transdisciplinary education among the team members occur if all the team members can be present for both the evaluation and the long-term follow-up of the patient. This ongoing face-to-face interaction fosters a thorough understanding of the disease process and, ultimately, the overall treatment plan. Goals of each component of the treatment plan then can be understood by each member of the team. Contemporary health care cost-containment pressures encourage isolated treatment in the outpatient offices of individual team members, but achieving and maintaining the same level of interdisciplinary understanding as in the formal clinic team setting is difficult.

The overall process of formulating the prescription consists of three distinct phases. *Phase 1* involves evaluation of the patient to identify the underlying problems, disease, and disability and to establish a prognosis for future expectations. *Phase 2* includes the actual treatment plan of writing prescriptions for the orthosis, therapy, and medication that may be appropriate for the underlying disease process. This phase also includes consideration of alternative measures, such as surgery or injections, to improve the patient's underlying condition prior to fabrication and fitting of the orthosis. Education of the patient, and of each team member, also occurs in this phase. *Phase 3* includes follow-up to assess for functional outcome. Functional outcome can be measured as the patient's improved mobility, self-care, and reintegration into the community or as improved quality of life for the patient and caregivers. The orthotic team works best if a good balance of medical knowledge from the physician is combined with a good understanding of biomechanics and materials from the orthotist. The cooperative effort of these two key individuals from the orthotic team, and the sharing of knowledge among the other team members, ultimately will provide the most appropriate prescription for the orthosis and the treatment plan. The orthotic prescription then becomes a part of the road map to achieve the final endpoint of improved patient function.

Orthotic team member roles

The role of each individual team member can be precisely defined, but overlap occurs in several areas. These areas of overlap should enhance discussion and communication among team members to generate the most appropriate treatment plan.

Role of the physician

- Perform the medical evaluation, including chart review, history, and physical examination
- Explain the diagnosis and prognosis to other team members
- Alert the team to special considerations, including skin issues, weight-bearing limitations, vascular disease, and spasticity
- Establish restrictions of the treatment program to prevent complications or danger to the patient
- Assess and manage the patient's pain control regimen
- Assess and manage the patient's psychological status
- Justify the treatment program to the insurance carrier
- Write prescriptions for the orthotic device, therapy program, and medications
- Regular monitoring and long-term follow-up of all components of the treatment program
- Share knowledge with other team members

Role of the certified orthotist

- Participate in patient evaluation and generation of the orthotic prescription
- Act in a consulting role to provide information on device design and materials options
- Educate the patient regarding the device
- Fabricate the device to prescription specifications
- Deliver and check device fit and function
- Modify and repair the orthosis if, and when, appropriate
- Follow up with the patient and team members
- Share knowledge with other team members

Role of the physical therapist and/or occupational therapist

- Participate in patient evaluation, particularly as related to functional ability, such as transfers, ambulation, stair climbing, and assistive devices, in addition to assessment of other durable medical equipment, such as wheelchairs and bathroom equipment
- Participate in generation of the therapy prescription
- Provide the therapy program, which may include strengthening, range of motion, ambulation, wheelchair mobility, self-care activities, proper use of orthotic device, therapeutic modalities, and home program
- Share knowledge with other team members

Role of the certified pedorthist

- Participate in patient evaluation, with particular attention to the patient's feet and footwear
- Participate in generating the prescription for appropriate footwear
- Work cooperatively with the orthotist to provide the footwear and appropriate modifications to the footwear
- Educate the patient, especially the diabetic patient, on footwear and foot care
- Share knowledge with other team members

Role of the patient

- Convey appropriate information to the team members
- Listen, learn, and follow the team recommendations
- Comply with the treatment program and proper use of the orthotic device
- Follow up with the team, particularly if complications or problems related to the orthosis or function occur

Through open discussion and mutual respect, members of the orthotic team can function effectively and efficiently to provide the appropriate services and improve the patient's functional outcome. Communication is the cornerstone of this process.

Definition of orthosis

The simplest definition of an orthosis is any externally applied device to an existing body part that improves function. Common goals for orthotic devices include the following:

1. Stabilize weak or paralyzed segments or joints
2. Support damaged or diseased segments or joints
3. Limit or augment motion across joints
4. Control abnormal or spastic movements
5. Unload distal segments

As we attempt to achieve these fundamental goals, special attention must be given to issues such as the biomechanics of the device, durability of the materials used, and, most importantly, tissue tolerance to pressures exerted by the device. Finally, let us use the term orthosis correctly in our discussions. *Orthosis* or *orthotic device* refers to the actual item delivered to the patient. The term *orthotics* refers to the field of assessment and fabrication of orthoses.

Terminology of orthoses

Universal terminology that is agreed upon by the International Organization for Standardization (ISO) should always be used to describe the basic device. All orthoses should be designated using ISO acronyms according to the joints or body segments involved, such as AFO for ankle–foot orthosis or WHO for wrist–hand orthosis. This is simply the starting point for defining the device and generating the appropriate prescription. The prescription should also include specifics about materials and special designs, such as control features at each joint or segment, to ensure that the orthotist clearly understands the functional goals of the device for this particular individual. Locally accepted eponyms may be useful as adjectives to further describe the design, such as a "Miami J-style" cervical orthosis. Using eponyms alone should be avoided, however, because they do not provide a complete and accurate description of the device. Eponym prescriptions may lead to errors in device fabrication and compromise the treatment goal of improving function. Other general descriptive terms, such as the terms *static*, *dynamic*, and *progressive*, may be helpful in clarifying the orthotic goals. The term *static* implies that there is no motion across the joint or segment involved; therefore, stabilization is the primary goal. The term *dynamic* indicates there is motion across the joint. Specific motion can be further described as follows:

1. No motion in one plane and unlimited in other planes
2. Limited motion with fixed endpoints in one or more planes
3. Free motion in one or more planes
4. Augmented motion using an external source, such as rubber bands, springs, or cables
5. Resistance to motion using an external source, such as rubber bands, springs, or cables

Note that many orthoses have static features at one joint and dynamic features at another joint.

The orthosis can be designed to have different biomechanical functions as the disease process or disability changes. This type of device is sometimes called a *progressive orthosis* because of anticipated modifications or changes to accommodate improvement or deterioration of the disease. An example of a progressive orthotic device is a wrist–hand–finger orthosis, which will be modified at fixed intervals during recovery after finger flexor tendon surgery. A second example is the ankle joint on a metal ankle–foot orthosis, which will be adjusted to accommodate a plantar flexion contracture as it slowly resolves from a stretching program in physical therapy.

Special features of the orthosis should be explicitly described using functional or descriptive terminology. For example, off-loading distal segments in the lower extremity is commonly performed when plantar ulceration, fracture, or Charcot joint deformity exists. The foot and ankle can be partially off-loaded using an unweighting orthosis of the calf corset lacer design or the plastic clamshell design. The choice from among these designs may depend on medical issues such as fluctuating edema in the leg, skin tolerance, or arthritis in the knee. The physician and the orthotist should carefully discuss these special features prior to fabrication and fitting of the orthosis.

Evaluation of the patient

A clear understanding of the patient's disease process is the foundation for generating the appropriate prescription for the orthotic device. Ideally, the patient would be seen in the orthotic team format, with both physician and orthotist present to evaluate the patient. However, if this is not available, both the physician and the orthotist should spend some time evaluating both the history and the physical examination of the patient. Key components of the history include the initial presentation of the disease, trauma, or problem, the course of the disease to date, and other treatments applied. The impact of the disease on the patient's current functional status and the patient's expectations or functional goals should be discussed in detail. A review of comorbid conditions that may impact orthotic management should be addressed, specifically diabetes, neurologic disease, vascular disease, visual impairment, or hand dysfunction.

Physical examination of the patient should include assessment of strength, range of motion, sensation, tone, skin integrity, and presence of edema. Physical examination should include all of these components in the involved limb but also in uninvolved limbs to obtain a better understanding of the patient's current function and potential function. An overall description of the patient's body size and habitus, including specific body weight, should be documented. It is imperative to actually observe the patient involved in functional tasks such as transfers, ambulation, and self-care tasks. This observation is critical because certain medical conditions, such as ataxia and apraxia, may alter the patient's ability to use his or her existing strength and range of motion during functional tasks. *Ataxia* is a dysfunction of the cerebellar system that impairs coordination of muscular activities during functional tasks. *Apraxia* is a failure of sequencing and timing of existing muscle activity that may impair functional activity, such as ambulation and self-care tasks. In addition, significant changes in the patient's tone may occur during a static sitting examination compared to a dynamic task such as ambulation.

Finally, the patient's cognitive status should be assessed to determine whether he or she can follow through with education and instructions regarding the orthotic device. If the patient is unable to do so, then social support systems must be in place to assist the patient to don and doff the device appropriately and to monitor for complications or skin problems from the device. A patient who lacks sensation in the involved body part must be aware that visual feedback can be used to assess for skin irritation or problems. A patient with visual impairment must rely on other individuals to inspect his or her skin on a daily basis.

Writing the prescription

The *orthotic prescription* is the actual document that clearly defines and summarizes the medical issues related to the patient and the specifics of the orthotic device. The patient's name, date of birth, and other identifying information should be clearly printed at the top of the prescription. The medical information should be specific and directly related to the functional deficit or reason for the orthosis. The resulting disability or handicap should be clearly stated, and the prognosis related to the disease should be included. An example of a typical disease process is diabetes with peripheral neuropathy, and the associated disability may be footdrop with gait dysfunction. The name of the orthotic practitioner or orthotic company should be clearly marked on the prescription for both the patient's information and for the physician's documentation purposes. The main body of the prescription should include details of the orthosis, starting with the basic ISO acronyms using universal terminology. Each segment or component of the orthosis ideally should be described in a preprinted menu format to avoid any concerns about illegible handwriting. These descriptors should include generic materials specification, such as thermoplastics, metals, or carbon fiber, and specific descriptions of joint controls to be used. The range of motion or limitation at each joint should be indicated clearly on the prescription. Any corrective straps, flanges, or wedges should be included for complete specification of the desired configuration. Special features, such as tone-reducing contours or inversion control extensions, should be included. The final prescription should be sufficiently detailed that all certified orthotists could create a custom orthosis offering the same biomechanical functions. Each prescription should include the physician's name, signature, and handwritten date, in addition to identifying information such as office phone number, address, or medical provider number, to avoid treatment delays until third-party requirements have been met.

If the physician assesses the patient independently and is uncertain of the best orthotic design to accomplish the orthotic goals, then the physician should send the patient to the orthotist for consultation and evaluation. The consultation request should include as much information as possible, including medical diagnosis, prognosis, orthotic goals, and the request to "evaluate for orthotic management and call to discuss the alternatives." Based on this discussion, a detailed prescription is written.

A *certificate of medical necessity* sometimes is required to justify the orthotic device as a covered benefit. A statement to this effect can be included in the orthotic prescription for simple cases but is best accomplished with a separate letter for more elaborate explanation of the patient's underlying condition and the functional improvement anticipated with the orthotic device. A letter of medical necessity may include specifics regarding the patient's current functional status and how the orthotic device may lead to improvement in the patient's function or greater independence. The letter also may discuss prevention of falls or deterioration of the condition because safety in patient mobility and independence in self-care tasks often are primary goals of the treatment program. The letter should clearly state the risks to the patient if the device is not supplied because many third-party reviewers are not familiar with rehabilitation or the critical role of orthoses in functional activities.

One example of a detailed lower extremity orthotic prescription template is included as an addendum to this chapter. Similar prescriptions can be generated for upper limb and spinal orthoses. The physician and orthotist should review these prescriptions in detail and update them regularly to accommodate changing materials and designs.

Patient case presentations and orthotic prescriptions

Case 1

A 34-year-old white woman recently diagnosed with multiple sclerosis reports an approximately 1-year history of progressive weakness of the left leg. She reports difficulty walking longer distances and on uneven terrain, with recurrent falls due to left leg weakness. She reports at least three events over the last year when she noticed in her left leg sudden weakness that stabilized over the course of several weeks. The patient has undergone no orthotic management to date but does use a cane for ambulation. She lives with her husband and two young children in a two-story house with five steps to enter from the outside. The patient is primarily a homemaker and caretaker for the children. Up to 1 year ago, she was totally independent and safe in ambulation, self-care, and even recreational sports such as tennis and golf. At this time her functional goals are safe ambulation both indoors and outdoors, especially when she must carry her young child. On examination, she is alert and oriented, with cognition intact. She has a medium frame and stature. Examination of the upper extremities reveals normal strength, sensation, and tone in both right and left limbs. Her fine motor skills in both hands are intact. The right lower extremity shows normal strength, sensation, and tone. However, the left lower extremity shows some weakness throughout. The hip flexors, extensors, and abductors are only 4/5. Knee flexors and extensors are 4−/5. Ankle plantar flexion is 3/5, but dorsiflexion, inversion, and eversion are only 1/5 for strength. Ankle passive range of motion is five degrees of dorsiflexion and normal plantar flexion. Tone is increased throughout the left lower extremity in an extensor pattern. Sensation is impaired throughout the limb and nearly absent on the plantar surface of the left foot. Proprioception is absent at the left big toe. The skin is intact, but the patient reports moderate fluctuating edema that worsens as the day progresses. Assessment of the patient's gait reveals left foot drop in swing phase and a tendency to maintain the left knee in full extension throughout stance phase. The patient reports that her gait pattern changes depending on her overall tone on any particular day. On days when she is rested and relaxed, she can use a steppage gait pattern to clear the left foot, but on days when the tone is significantly increased she uses a stiff knee gait pattern throughout swing phase with circumduction on the left and vaulting on the right.

In this case, the disease process is progressive-type multiple sclerosis causing a disability of left leg weakness with footdrop. The patient has a gait disorder causing recurrent falls that make safety a significant concern for the patient and her young child when the patient is carrying the child. The prognosis indicates that the conditioning is worsening, and further weakness of the left leg or other extremities can be anticipated in the future.

The orthotic prescription for this patient is written as a left metal AFO with aluminum calf band, hook-and-loop closure, aluminum uprights, and dual-channel ankle joints articulating with a solid stirrup to be attached to an orthopedic shoe with lace closure. The rationale for this orthotic prescription hinges on several components of the history and physical examination. Foot drop alone can be controlled with metal or plastic AFOs; however, the intermittent edema of the leg and foot is most easily accommodated by limited skin contact of the metal AFO attached to an orthopedic shoe with removable insole. The fluctuating nature of the disease and the overall worsening prognosis also make the dual-channel ankle joints the best choice because of the adjustability and biomechanical versatility of this component. The dual-channel ankle joint allows dorsiflexion assist for the footdrop as well as the option of adding an anterior pin to prevent excessive dorsiflexion in late stance, thereby providing indirect stability to the knee should the quadriceps become weaker in the future. A hinged plastic AFO with a similar dual-channel ankle joint also could have been provided, but then particular attention would be necessary to control or accommodate the edema and ensure skin integrity with this more intimately fitting orthosis. With either type of orthosis, this patient must be taught to inspect the insensate skin areas regularly to avoid breakdowns.

Case 2

An 18-year-old man who suffered a traumatic brain injury in a motor vehicle accident 3 months ago is evaluated for an orthosis to assist in reducing a flexion contracture at the right knee and to assist in ambulation. He has significant cognitive impairment and spastic right hemiparesis. He currently is hospitalized at a rehabilitation facility and is dependent in most self-care activities. He is able to use his left arm and leg to assist in transfers to a wheelchair, but he is not able to proceed with ambulation training or standing because of 60-degree flexion contracture at the right knee. Attempts by physical therapy to reduce the contracture with stretching and serial casting have been slow because of the patient's issues with skin tolerance and pain. The patient has no other underlying diseases and was completely independent prior to the injury. On examination, he is a slender man with little or no verbalizations. He follows simple verbal or gestural commands. He conveys indication of pain with grimaces or groans. His left upper extremity strength and sensation are intact with good hand dexterity. His right upper extremity is held in a flexed posture with the hand clenched tight. Tone is increased in the hand, but there is no contracture of the fingers, wrist, or elbow at this time. There is no voluntary movement of the right upper extremity, and sensation is impaired. There is mild edema of the hand. The left lower extremity is normal for strength and sensation. Range of motion is well preserved at the left hip, knee, and ankle. The right lower extremity is held in a flexed posture. Hip passive range of motion is normal for flexion, but no extension is achieved. The right knee has 60-degree flexion contracture with strong flexor tone. The ankle is held in 5 degrees dorsiflexion position but can be ranged to 20 degrees plantarflexion. The skin on the right leg and foot is intact, but sensation is impaired. No edema is noted or is reported by staff.

In this case, the disease process is traumatic brain injury with disabilities of spastic right hemiparesis and cognitive dysfunction. The subsequent complication of right knee flexion contracture contributes to the handicap of gait inability and dependence in self-care. The prognosis is more challenging to establish because young patients with brain injury may show slow improvement over 12 months or longer. The treatment plan for reducing the flexion contracture may include an orthosis, medications for tone reduction, botulinum toxin injections, nerve blocks, or surgical releases. The outcome will depend on appropriate and aggressive use of all these components. Future ambulation training can occur only if tone reduction is achieved and the flexion contracture is reduced. Aggressive physical therapy must continue throughout the treatment program.

The orthotic prescription could include a right knee–ankle–foot orthosis (KAFO) with plastic thigh shell, hook-and-loop closure, ratchet lock knee joints, plastic ankle–foot shell using rigid trim lines, and full footplate extending beyond the toes. The ankle should be positioned in neutral or slight dorsiflexion. The footplate should incorporate tone-reducing contours and should have a padded figure-of-eight strap to hold the foot in the footplate if a laced shoe or sneaker will not be used. Additional infrapatellar and suprapatellar straps likely will be needed to prevent the knee from coming forward in the brace during stretching. The rationale for this brace is based on the primary goal of stretching the knee and progressively adjusting the orthotic knee joint to accommodate the new position. The ratchet joint starts at a comfortable position of flexion and is slowly extended to a position of strong stretch for several hours. The ratchet joint locks every few degrees to maintain the stretch that has been gained during active therapy. The ratchet lock is easily released for a period of rest every 3 hours. The plastic thigh and calf shells provide a wide area of contact to minimize the risk of excessive pressure and skin breakdown. Because this orthosis is custom-made, it can be used 24 hours per day and removed on a regular basis to inspect the skin and provide hygiene. This approach has a great advantage over serial casting because of its inherent adjustability and easy removal. As the patient's knee contracture resolves, the same orthosis can be used as an ambulatory KAFO to stabilize the knee and ankle during the stance phase of gait.

In this case, the orthotic team should also recommend a static positioning orthosis for the right wrist, hand, and fingers to prevent flexion contracture. This upper limb orthosis can be fabricated from thermoplastic, with padding at all contact areas and hook-and-loop straps to maintain position. The wrist should be placed in neutral or slight extension, and the metacarpophalangeal (MCP) joints and interphalangeal (IP) joints should be in slight flexion. The thumb should always be opposite the fingers. A compression glove should be placed on the right hand to control edema and further protect the skin.

Conclusion

The responsibility of writing the orthotic prescription falls upon the physician, but the process of evaluating the patient, establishing orthotic goals, and fitting the appropriate orthotic device requires critical input from other team members. The orthotist should be considered the consultant or expert on orthotic biomechanical designs and materials, and discussion between the physician and orthotist can only improve the functional outcome for the patient. Each member of the orthotic team should recognize his or her unique role and responsibility and should foster the sharing of knowledge. Follow-up and long-term monitoring of the patient and his or her use of the orthosis is essential to prevent complications and ensure the best long-term outcome.

Addendum

Figure 2-1 is a sample lower extremity orthotic prescription template.

LOWER LIMB ORTHOTIC PRESCRIPTION

NAME: _____ AGE: _____ DOB: _____ SEX: _____ PT.#: _____

REFERRING M.D.: _____ PRESCRIBING M.D.: _____

DIAGNOSIS: _____ DISABILITY: _____

PROGNOSIS: _____ PRACTITIONER: _____

TYPE OF ORTHOSIS: HKAFO: R__ L__ KAFO: R__ L__ AFO: R__ L__ FOOT: R__ L__ SHOES: R__ L__

Specialty Orthosis: Craig-Scott: _____ Floor Reaction Orthosis: _____ Patellar-Tendon Bearing Orthosis: _____

TRUNK COMPONENTS:

Corset: _____
Pelvic Band: _____
Other: _____

HIP JOINTS:

Free: _____
Drop Lock: _____
Adjustable: _____
Other: _____

THIGH COMPONENTS:

Metal Uprights: _____
Steel: _____
Aluminum: _____
Thigh Bands: _____
Aluminum: _____
Carbon: _____
Plastic Shell: _____
Gluteal Bearing: _____
Ischial Bearing: _____
Velcro Strap Closure: _____
Laced Leather Closure: _____

KNEE JOINT:

Offset: _____
Dial Lock: _____
Drop Lock: _____
Retention Buttons: _____
Bail Lock: _____
Trigger Lock: _____
Rachet Lock: _____
Trick Knee: _____
Other: _____

CORRECTIVE STRAPS:

Valgum: _____
Varum: _____
Recurvatum: _____
Knee Cap: _____
Suprapatellar: _____
Infrapatellar: _____

CALF COMPONENTS:

Plastic Calf Shell: _____
Metal Uprights: _____
Aluminum: _____
Steel: _____
Calf Bands: _____
Aluminum: _____
Carbon: _____
Pre-Tibial Shell: _____
Velcro Strap Closure: _____
Calf Corset Design: _____

TRIM LINES:

Ant. Mall: _____
Mid. Mall: _____
Just Behind Mall: _____
Flexible PLS: _____
3 Point Inv. Control: _____

PLASTIC FOOTPLATE:

Full Length: _____
Standard ¾ Length: _____
Padding: _____
Tone Reducing Design: _____

ANKLE JOINT:

Post Channel: _____
Dual Channel: _____
Plastic Hinge: _____
Free Motion: _____
Rigid Stop: _____
Dorsiflexion Angle: _____

CORRECTIVE STRAPS:

Medial T-Strap: _____
Lateral T-Strap: _____
Ankle Strap: _____

SHOE/FOOT CONNECTION:

Solid Stirrup: _____
Split Stirrup: _____
Caliper Box: _____
Long Steel Shank: _____
Heel to Toe: _____
Heel to Met Heads: _____

SHOES:

Orthopedic/Blucher: _____
Sneaker Style: _____
Surgical: _____
High Top: _____
Extra Depth: _____
High Toe Box: _____
Bunion Lasts: _____
Deer Skin: _____
Heel/Sole Lift: _____
Type of Sole: _____
Other: _____

CLOSURE TYPE:

Laces: _____
Velcro Patch: _____
Velcro D-Ring: _____

CUSTOM FOOT ORTHOTICS:

Left: _____
Right: _____
Accommodative: _____
Corrective: _____

MATERIAL:

Plastazote: _____
PPT: _____
Neoprene: _____
Polypropylene: _____
Other: _____

Special Features/Instructions: _____

The above prescribed devices are a medical necessity to increase the patient's safety and functional status.

Duration of Necessity: _____

Date: _____ Physician Signature: _____

Fig. 2-1 Sample prescription template.

Chapter

3

Materials science

Thomas R. Lunsford and Bill Contoyannis

Key Points

- A thorough knowledge of the principles summarized in this chapter is prerequisite to ensuring that the orthosis provided will be durable, safe, and unobtrusive and perform the required function for as long as necessary. Understanding these fundamentals enables the practitioner to assess designs, materials, and failures and to clearly justify the decisions, practices, and techniques used in the creation of each orthosis.

- Despite publicity for exotic materials, no single material is a panacea. Selection of the correct material for a specific orthosis requires an understanding of the elementary principles of mechanics and materials; concepts of forces; deformation and failure of structures under load; improvement in mechanical properties by heat treatment, work (strain) hardening, and similar means; and design of structures.

- To ensure clear and precise communication, international standards for terminology should be used to describe orthoses, prostheses, properties of materials, units of measure (whether imperial or metric) as well as the engineering principles for describing the various effects of loading on these materials.

- The practitioner must have a thorough understanding of the specific application of a device and the biomechanical forces to be applied by the device in order to choose the proper plastic and the proper methods of fabrication. The service success of any orthosis depends as much on the design and fabrication process as on the material itself.

- The range of elasticity, yield, and ultimate stress points are sufficiently high in most commonly used materials to prevent orthosis failure. Fatigue stresses, which are the result of repeatedly applied small loads rather than application of any single large load, are generally responsible when structural failure occurs in orthoses or prostheses.

Metals and plastics are the basic principal materials used in orthotics and prosthetics. To understand recommended design and fabrication procedures, a basic knowledge of the properties of the various available materials is necessary. The practitioner must be familiar with these materials in order to cope with both standard and difficult designs and fabrication problems and have the ability to prevent structural or functional failures of device due to the material.

Selection of the correct material for a given design depends partially on understanding the elementary principles of mechanics and materials, concepts of forces, deformation and failure of structures under load, improvement in mechanical properties by heat treatment, work (strain) hardening or other means, and design of structures. For example, the choices for a knee–ankle–foot orthosis (KAFO) may include several types of steels, numerous alloys of aluminium, and titanium and its alloys. Important but minor uses of other metals include copper or brass rivets and successive platings of copper, nickel, and chromium. Plastics, fabrics, rubbers, and leathers have wide indications, and composite structures (plastic matrix with reinforcing fibers) are beginning to be used. Often complex combinations of materials are used in manners that are not appropriate from the material point of view but are appropriate for the particular clinical application. Understanding these properties not only assists with the selection, manufacture, and management of the device but extends to the management of the patient and the information that the practitioner will instill into patients. A simple example is the combination of flexible materials such as a strap and thermoplastic, using an alloy rivet.

Despite publicity for exotic materials, no single material is a panacea. One reason is that a single design frequently requires divergent mechanical properties (e.g., stiffness and flexibility required in an ankle–foot orthosis [AFO] for dorsiflexion restraint and free plantar flexion). In addition, practitioners rarely are presented with situations where they will use only one material or with single-design situations that will not require modification, customization, or variation over time.

In general, understanding by the practitioner of the mechanics and strength of materials, even if intuitive, is important during the design stage. A general understanding of stresses arising from loading of structures, particularly from the bending of beams, is needed. The practitioner then can appreciate the importance of simple methods that allow controlled deformation during fitting, provide stiffness or resiliency as prescribed, and reduce breakage whether from impact or repeated loading. A general discussion of materials and specific theory related to design, fabrication, riveting guidelines, troubleshooting, and failure considerations follows.

Consideration should be given to the international standards of terminology that are used to describe orthotics, prosthetics, properties of materials, and units of measure (whether imperial or metric) as well as the engineering principles for describing the various effects of loading upon these materials. Unless they are familiar with the particular definitions of the terms used, practitioners should generally avoid using specific terminology in favor of more objective descriptive language.

Strength and stress

One of the practitioner's main considerations is the strength of the material selected for fabrication of orthoses or prostheses. *Strength* is defined as the ability of a material to resist forces. When comparative studies are made of the strength of materials, the concept of stress must be introduced.

Stress relates to both the magnitude of the applied forces and the amount of the material's internal resistance to the forces. *Stress* is defined as force per unit cross-sectional area of material and usually is expressed in pounds per square inch (psi, imperial) or megapascals (MPa, Newtons per square meter, metric). The amount of stress (σ) is computed using the equation:

$$\sigma = \frac{F}{A}, \qquad (3-1)$$

Where F = applied force (pounds or Newtons), and A = cross-sectional area (square inches or square meters).

The same amount of force applied over different areas causes radically different stresses. For example, a 1-lb weight is placed on a cylindrical test bar having a cross-sectional area of 1 in.[2]. According to Equation 3-1, the compressive stress σ_c in the cylindrical test bar is 1 lb/in.[2] (Fig. 3-1). When the same 1-lb weight is placed on a needle having a cross-sectional area of 0.001 in.[2], the compressive stress σ_c in the needle is 1000 psi (Fig. 3-2).

A force exerted on a small area always causes more stress than the same force acting on a larger area. When a woman wears high-heeled shoes, her weight is supported by the narrow heels, which have an area of only a fraction of a square inch. With flat shoes, the same weight or force is spread over a heel having a larger cross-sectional area.

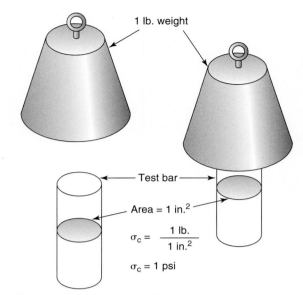

Fig. 3-1 Compressive stress on a cylinder.

The stress in the heel of the shoe is much greater when high-heeled shoes are worn because less material is resisting the applied forces.

Similar problems are encountered in orthoses and prostheses. A child weighing 100 lb and wearing a weight-bearing orthosis with a 90-degree posterior stop (Fig. 3-3) can exert forces at initial contact that create stresses of thousands of pounds per square inch. If the child jumps, the force would increase with the height of the jump. The stress at the stop or on the rivet could be great enough to cause failure.

Tensile, compressive, shear, and flexural stresses

Materials are subject to several types of stresses depending on the way that the forces are applied: tensile, compressive, shear, and flexural.

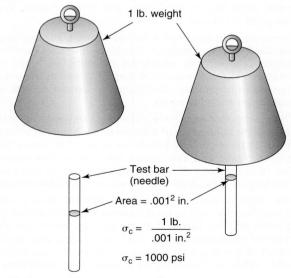

Fig. 3-2 Compressive stress on a needle.

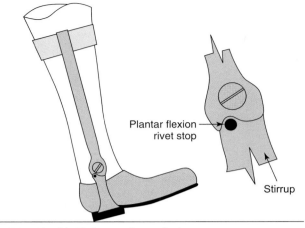

Fig. 3-3 AFO with 90-degree plantar flexion stop.

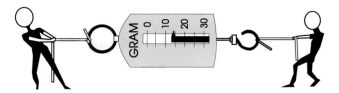

Fig. 3-5 Spring scale can be used to demonstrate tension.

Tensile stresses

Tensile stresses act to pull apart an object or cause it to be in tension. Tensile stresses occur parallel to the line of force but perpendicular to the area in question (Fig. 3-4). If an object is pulled at both ends, it is in tension, and sufficient force will pull it apart. Two children fighting over a fish scale and exerting opposing forces put it in tension, as shown by the indicator on the scale (Fig. 3-5).

Compressive stresses

Compressive stresses act to squeeze or compress objects. They also occur parallel to the line of force and perpendicular to the cross-sectional area (Fig. 3-6).

A blacksmith shapes metal by hitting the material with a hammer to squeeze or compress the metal into the desired shape. In the same manner, clay yields to low compressive stress. Clay is distorted and squeezed out of shape by comparatively small forces.

Shear stresses

Shear stresses act to scissor or shear the object, causing the planes of the material to slide over each other. Shear stresses occur parallel to the applied forces. Consider two blocks (Fig. 3-7, *A*) with their surfaces bonded together. If forces acting in opposite directions are applied to these blocks, they tend to slide over each other. If these forces are great enough, the bond between the blocks will break (Fig. 3-7, *B*). If the area of the bonded surfaces were increased, however, the effect of the forces would be distributed over a greater area. The average stress would be decreased, and there would be increased resistance to shear stress.

A common lap joint and clevis joint are examples of a shear pin used as the axis of the joint (Fig. 3-8). The lap joint has one shear area of the rivet resisting the forces applied to the lap joint (Fig. 3-8, *A*), and the rivet in the box joint (clevis) has an area resisting the applied forces that is twice as great as the area in the lap joint (assuming that the rivets in both joints are the same size; Fig. 3-8, *B*). Consequently the clevis joint will withstand twice as much shear force as the lap joint. The lap joint also has less resistance to fatigue (fluctuating stress of relatively low magnitude, which results in failure) because it is more susceptible to flexing stresses.

Flexural stress

Flexural stress (bending) is a combination of tension and compression stresses. Beams are subject to flexural stresses. When a beam is loaded transversely, it will sag. The top fibers of a beam are in maximum compression while the bottom side is in maximum tension (Fig. 3-9). The term *fiber*, as used here, means the geometric lines that compose the prismatic beam. The exact nature of these compressive and tensile stresses are discussed later.

Yield stress

The yield stress or yield point is the point at which the material begins to maintain a deformational change due to the load and therefore the internal stresses under which it has been exposed.

Ultimate stress

Ultimate stress is the stress at which a material ruptures. The strength of the material before it ruptures also depends on the type of stress to which it is subjected. For example, ultimate shear stresses usually are lower than ultimate tensile stresses (i.e., less shear stress must be applied before the material ruptures than in the case of tensile or compressive stress).

Strain

Materials subjected to any stress will deform or change their shape, even at very small levels of stress. If a material lengthens or shortens in response to stress, it is said to experience *strain*. Strain is denoted by ϵ and can be found by dividing the total elongation (or contraction) ΔL by the original length L_O of the structure being loaded:

$$\epsilon = \frac{\Delta L}{-L_O} \tag{3-2}$$

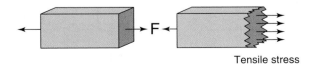

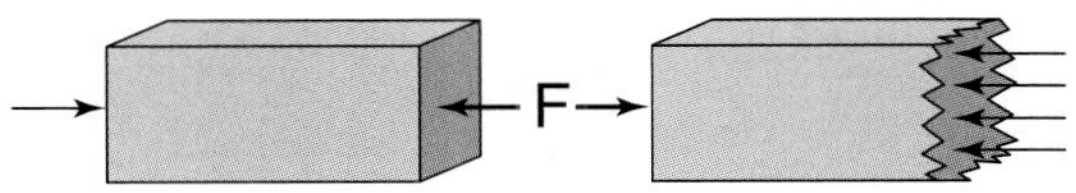

Tensile stress

Fig. 3-4 Tension.

Compressive stress

Fig. 3-6 Compression.

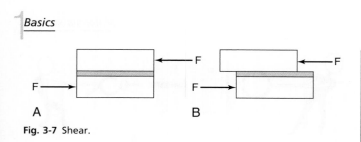

Fig. 3-7 Shear.

Consider a change in length ΔL of a wire or rod caused by a change in stretching force F (Fig. 3-10). The amount of stretch is proportional to the original length of wire. A wire 5 inches long stretches twice as much as a wire 3 to 5 inches long, other things being equal.

Stress–strain curve

The most widely used means of determining the mechanical properties of materials is the tension test. Much can be learned from observing the data collected from such a test. In the tension test, the dimensions of the specimen coupon are fixed by standardization so that the results can be universally understood, no matter where or by whom the test is conducted. The specimen coupon is mounted between the jaws of a tensile testing machine, which is simply a device for stretching the specimen at a controlled rate. As defined by standards, the cross-sectional area of the coupon is smaller in the center to prevent failures where the coupon is gripped. The specimen's resistance to being stretched and the linear deformations are measured by sensitive instrumentation (Fig. 3-11).

The force of resistance divided by the cross-sectional area of the specimen is the *stress* in the specimen (Equation 3-1). The *strain* is the total deformation divided by the original length (Equation 3-2). If the stresses in the specimen are plotted as ordinates of a graph, with the accompanying strains as abscissae, a number of mechanical properties are graphically revealed. Figure 3-12 shows such a stress–strain diagram for a mild steel specimen.

The shape and magnitude of the stress–strain curve of a metal depend on its composition; heat treatment; history of plastic deformation; and strain rate, temperature, and state of stress imposed during testing. The parameters used to describe the stress–strain curve of a metal are tensile strength, yield strength or yield point, percent elongation, and reduction in area. The first two are strength parameters; the last two indicate ductility.

The general shape of the stress–strain curve (Fig. 3-12) requires further explanation. In the region from a to b, the stress is linearly proportional to strain and the strain is elastic (i.e., the stressed part returns to its original shape when the load is removed). When the applied stress exceeds the yield strength, b the specimen undergoes plastic deformation. If the load is subsequently reduced to zero, the part remains permanently deformed. The stress required to produce continued plastic deformation increases with increasing plastic

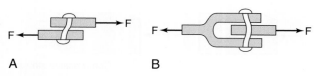

Fig. 3-8 Joint shear.

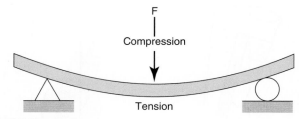

Fig. 3-9 Flexure.

strain (points c, d, and e on Fig. 3-12), that is, the metal strain hardens. The volume of the part remains constant during plastic deformation, and as the part elongates, its cross-sectional area decreases uniformly along its length until point e is reached. The ordinate of point e is the tensile strength of the material. After point e, further elongation requires less applied stress until the part ruptures at point f (breaking or fracture strength). Although this seems counter-intuitive, it actually occurs and is best sensed when bolts are overtorqued. Correct torque settings should always be complied with, but practitioners commonly torque bolts using the "as hard as possible" technique, assuming that this method somehow secures the bolt more appropriately than the correct torque and a thread locking solution. When excessive torque has been applied, the bolt first feels like it has loosened prior to failing. This simply reflects the fact that the yield point of the material has been surpassed and the bolt is plastically deforming under a decreasing load to failure.

Stress–strain diagrams assume widely differing forms for various materials. Figure 3-13, A shows the stress–strain diagram for a medium-carbon structural steel. The ordinates of points p, u, and b are the yield point, tensile strength, and breaking strength, respectively. The lower curve of Fig. 3-13, B is for an alloy steel and the higher curve is for hard steels. Nonferrous alloys and cast iron have the form shown in Fig. 3-13, C. The plot shown in Fig. 3-13, D is typical for rubber.

For any material having a stress–strain curve of the form shown in Figs. 3-13, A–D, it is evident that the relation between stress and strain is linear for comparatively small values of the strain. This linear relationship between elongation and the axial force causing it was first reported by Sir Robert Hooke in 1678 and is called *Hooke's law*. Expressed as an equation, Hooke's law becomes:

$$\sigma = \epsilon_E \qquad (3\text{-}3)$$

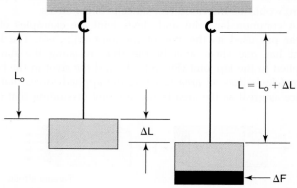

Fig. 3-10 Strain.

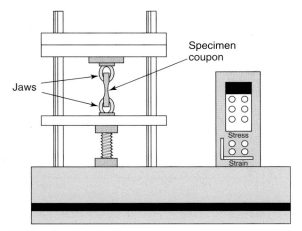

Fig. 3-11 Tension test.

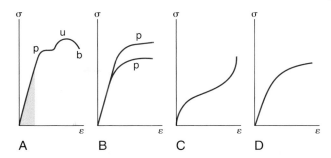

Fig. 3-13 Stress–strain diagrams for different materials.

where σ = stress (psi), ε = strain (inch/inch), and E = constant of proportionality between stress and strain. This constant is also called *Young's modulus* or the *modulus of elasticity*.

The slope of the stress–strain curve from the origin to point p (Figs. 3-13, *A* and *B*) is the modulus of elasticity of that particular material E. The region where the slope is a straight line is called the *elastic region*, where the material behaves in what we typically associate as an elastic manner, that is, it is loaded and stretched, and upon releasing the load the material returns to its original position. The ordinate of a point coincident with p is known as the *elastic limit* (i.e., the maximum stress that may develop during a simple tension test such that no permanent or residual deformation occurs when the load is entirely removed). Values for E are given in Table 3-1.

In a routine tension test (Fig. 3-14), which illustrates Hooke's law, a bar of area A is placed between two jaws of a vise, and a force F is applied to compress the bar. Combining Equations 3-1, 3-2, and 3-3 and solving for the shortening ΔL gives:

$$\Delta L = \frac{FL_O}{AE}. \tag{3-4}$$

Because the original length L_0, cross-sectional area A, and modulus of elasticity E are constants, the shortening ΔL depends solely on F. As F doubles, so does ΔL.

The operation of a steel spring scale is another practical illustration of Hooke's law (Fig. 3-15). The amount of deflection of the spring for every pound of force of the load remains constant. In Fig. 3-15, *A*, the scale indicates three units (pounds, ounces, grams). With one weight added (Fig. 3-15, *B*), the scale indicates 5, or two additional units. A second weight added (Fig. 3-15, *C*) causes the scale to indicate 7, or a total of four additional units, and a third weight stretches the spring two more units (Fig. 3-15, *D*). Therefore, it is possible to make uniform gradations for every unit of force to the point beyond the range of elasticity where the spring would distort or break. Scales are manufactured with springs strong enough to bear predetermined maximum loads. A compression spring scale designed to remain within the elastic range, recording weights to about 250 lb (100 kg) and then returning back to 0, is the common type used for weighing people.

Plastic range

Plastic range is beyond the elastic range (*b* to past *e* on the stress–strain diagram of Fig. 3-12), and the material behaves plastically. That is, the material has a set or permanent deformation when externally applied loads are removed—it has "flowed" or become plastic. In the case of the steel spring scale, if the weight did not actually break the spring, it would stretch it permanently so that the readings on the scale would be no longer accurate.

When forming orthotic bars, the practitioner must bend the bar beyond the elastic limit and into a range of plastic deformation with some associated elastic return. With experience and some basic experiments, the practitioner will be able to accurately predict the range of deformation and return for

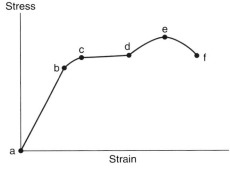

Fig. 3-12 Stress–strain.

Table 3-1 Modulus of elasticity

Material	$E\ (\times 10^6\ \text{psi})$	Material	$E\ (\times 10^6\ \text{psi})$
Steel	30	Magnesium	6.5
Carbon composite	18.5	Bone	2.85
Copper	16	Polyester–Dacron	2
Brass	15	Polyester (4110)	0.65
Bronze	12	Surlyn	0.34
Aluminum	10.3	Polypropylene	0.23
Kevlar	9	High-density Polypropylene	0.113
Glass	8.4	Low-density Polypropylene	0.018

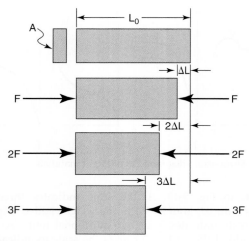

Fig. 3-14 Linearity.

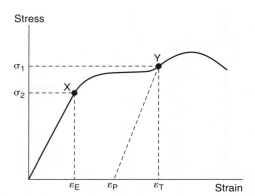

Fig. 3-16 Plastic strain.

particular bends. An advisable strategy is to chart this elastic return for the regular bends and commonly used sidebars.

For most materials, the stress–strain curve has an initial linear elastic region in which deformation is reversible. Note the load σ_2 in Fig. 3-16. This load will cause strain ϵ_E. When the load is removed, the strain disappears, that is, point X (σ_2, ϵ_E) moves linearly down the proportional portion of the curve to the origin. Similarly, when load σ_1 is applied, strain ϵ_T results. However, when load σ_1 is removed, point Y does not move back along the original curve to the origin but moves to the strain axis along a line parallel to the original linear region intersecting the strain axis at ϵ_P Therefore, with no load, the material has a residual or permanent strain of ϵ_P Plastic deformation is difficult to judge because of elastic and plastic deformation but can be predicted for sidebars and charted as previously mentioned. The quantity of permanent strain ϵ_P is the plastic strain, and ($\epsilon_T - \epsilon_P$) is the elastic strain ϵ_E or:

$$\epsilon_T - \epsilon_p = \epsilon_E, \qquad (3\text{-}5)$$

where ϵ_T = total strain under load, ϵ_P = plastic (or permanent) strain, and ϵ_E = elastic strain.

Yield point

Yield point (point b on the stress–strain diagram of Fig. 3-12) refers to that point at which a marked increase in strain occurs without a corresponding increase in stress. The horizontal portion of the stress–strain curve (b-c-d in Fig. 3-12) indicates the yield stress corresponding to this yield point.

The yield point is the "knee" in the stress–strain curve for a material and separates the elastic from the plastic portions of the curve.

Tensile strength

The tensile strength of a material is obtained by dividing the maximum tensile force reached during the test (e on the stress–strain diagram in Fig. 3-12) by the original cross-sectional area of the test specimen. Practical application of the maximal tensile force is minimal because devices are never designed to be loaded to this value.

Toughness and ductility

The area under the curve to the point of maximum stress (a-b-c-d-e in Fig. 3-12) indicates the *toughness* of the material, or its ability to withstand shock loads before rupturing. The supporting arms of a car bumper are an example of where toughness is of great value as a mechanical property. *Ductility* is the ability of a material to sustain large permanent deformations in tension, as drawing a rod into a wire. The distinction between ductility and toughness is that ductility deals only with the ability to deform, whereas toughness considers both the ability to deform and the stress developed during the deformation. The requirement for plastic deformation in sidebars is weighed against the ability of the sidebars to resist large rapid loads and even the forces required by the practitioner to be able to deform them.

Thermal stress

When a material is subjected to a change in temperature, its dimensions increase or decrease as the temperature rises or falls. If the material is constrained by neighboring structures, stress is produced.

The influence of temperature change is noted through the medium of the coefficient of thermal expansion α, which is defined as the unit strain produced by a temperature change of one degree. This physical constant is a mechanical property of each material. Values of α for several materials are given in Table 3-3.

If the temperature of a bar of length L_O inches is increased $\Delta T°$F (or °C, *note*: α indicates which measure of temperature it relates to), the elongation ΔL in inches of the unrestrained bar is given by:

$$\Delta L = \alpha L_O \Delta T. \qquad (3\text{-}6)$$

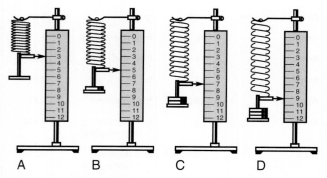

| A | B | C | D |

Fig. 3-15 Linear relationship between stretch and weight.

Table 3-2 Coefficient of thermal expansion

Material	Coefficient α (X 10^{-6} in/in -°F)	Material	Coefficient α (X 10^{-6} in/in -°F)
Steel	6.5	Brass	10.4
Cast iron	6.0	Bronze	10.0
Wrought iron	6.7	Aluminum	12.5
Copper	9.3	Magnesium	14.5

If the heated rod is compressed back to its original length, then it will experience compression as given by Equation 3-4:

$$\Delta L = \frac{FL_O}{AE.} \quad (3\text{-}7)$$

Combining Equations 3-6 and 3-7 and solving for stress, $\sigma = F/A$, gives:

$$\sigma = \alpha \Delta T E. \quad (3\text{-}8)$$

Equation 3-8 allows the calculation of stress in a rod as a function of the increase in temperature ΔT, the modulus of elasticity E (Table 3-1), and the coefficient of thermal expansion α (Table 3-2). The concept of change in dimension as the result of temperature rise is illustrated in Example 1 in the Appendix.

Centroids and center of gravity

The centroid and center of gravity of objects play important roles in their mechanical properties. The center of gravity and centroid of two identically shaped objects are the same if the density is uniform in each object. The centroid is a geometric factor, and center of gravity depends on mass.

For an object of uniform density, the term *center of gravity* is replaced by the *centroid of the area*. The *centroid of an area* is defined as the point of application of the resultant of a uniformly distributed force acting on the area. An irregularly shaped plate of material of uniform thickness t is shown in Fig. 3-17. Two elemental areas (a and b>) are shown with centroids (x_1,y_1) and (x_2,y_2), respectively. If the large, irregularly shaped plate is divided into small elemental areas, each having its own centroid, then the centroid for the irregularly shaped plate is (x,y), where:

$$\bar{x} = \frac{\bar{x}_i, \bar{a}_i}{\Sigma_i A}$$

$$\bar{y} = \frac{\bar{y}_i, \bar{a}_i}{\Sigma_i A}$$

and

$$\bar{x} = \frac{\bar{x}_i, \bar{a}_i + \bar{x}_2, \bar{a}_2 + \dots}{\Sigma_i A}$$

$$\bar{y} = \frac{\bar{y}_i, \bar{a}_i + \bar{y}_2, \bar{a}_2 + \dots}{A.}$$

The y-centroids for several common geometric shapes are given in Table 3-3. The general equations for the x- and y-components of the centroid are given in Example 2 in the Appendix.

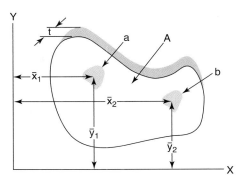

Fig. 3-17 Centroids.

Moment of inertia

The moment of inertia of a finite area about an axis in the plane of the area is given by the summation of the moments of inertia about the same axis of all elements of the area contained in the finite area. In general, the *moment of inertia* is defined as the product of the area and the square of the distance between the area and the given axis. The moments of inertia about the centroidal axes I_{cc} of a few simple but important geometric shapes are determined by integral calculus and are given in Table 3-3. Although Young's modulus is an indication of the strength of the material, the moment of inertia is an indicator of the strength of a particular shape about the aspect in which it will be loaded. This is a highly important parameter for the practitioner to know because he or she often will be able to influence the shape.

Parallel axis theorem

When the moment of inertia has been determined with respect to a given axis, such as the centroidal axis, the

Table 3-3 Geometric factors for common shapes

	Rectangle	Triangle	Circle	Semicircle
$\bar{y}_c$	$h/2$	$h/3$	r	$0.425r$
I_{cc}	$bh^3/12$	$bh^3/36$	$0.785r^4$	$0.11r^4$
I_{xx}	$bh^3/3$	$bh^3/12$	$3.93r^4$	$0.393r^4$
Z	$bh^2/6$	$bh^3/24$	$0.785r^3$	$0.19r^3$
C	$h/2$	$2h/3$ (top)	r	$0.575r$ (top)
		$h/3$ (bottom)		$0.425r$ (bottom)

21

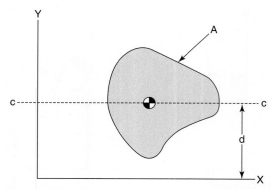

Fig. 3-18 Parallel axis theorem.

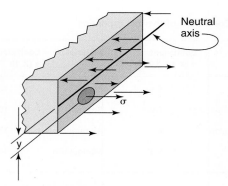

Fig. 3-20 Neutral axis (zero stress).

moment of inertia with respect to a parallel axis can be obtained by the *parallel axis theorem,* provided one of the axes passes through the centroid of the area. The parallel axis theorem states that *the moment of inertia with respect to any axis is equal to the moment of inertia with respect to a parallel axis through the centroid added to the product of the area and the square of the distance between the two axes* (Fig. 3-18):

$$I_{xx} = I_{cc} + Ad^2$$

or

$$I_{cc} = I_{xx} - Ad^2 \qquad (3\text{-}9)$$

where I_{xx} = moment of inertia about *x*-axis, I_{cc} = moment of inertia about centroid, A = area, and d = distance between axes.

An illustration of the moment of inertia concept using the parallel axis theorem is given in Example 3 in the Appendix.

Stresses in beams

If forces are applied to a beam as shown in Fig. 3-19, downward bending of the beam occurs. Imagine a beam is composed of an infinite number of thin longitudinal rods or fibers. Each longitudinal fiber is assumed to act independently of every other fiber (i.e., there are no lateral stresses [shear] between fibers). The beam of Fig. 3-19 will deflect downward and the fibers in the lower part of the beam undergo extension, whereas those in the upper part shorten. The changes in the lengths of the fibers set up stresses in the fibers. Those that are extended have tensile stresses acting on the fibers in the direction of the longitudinal axis of the beam, whereas those that are shortened are subject to compression stresses.

One surface in the beams always contains fibers that do not undergo any extension or compression and thus are not subject to any tensile or compressive stress. This surface is

called the *neutral surface* of the beam. The intersection of the neutral surface with any cross-section of the beam perpendicular to its longitudinal axis is called the *neutral axis*. All fibers on one side of the neutral axis are in a state of tension, whereas those on the opposite side are in compression.

For any beam having a longitudinal plane of symmetry and subject to a bending torque T at a certain cross-section, the normal stress σ, acting on a longitudinal fiber at a distance y from the neutral axis of the beam (Fig. 3-20), is given by:

$$\sigma = \frac{Ty}{I,} \qquad (3\text{-}10)$$

where I = moment of inertia of the cross-sectional area about the neutral or centroidal axis in inches[4].

These stresses vary from zero at the neutral axis of the beam ($y = 0$) to a maximum at the outer fibers (Fig. 3-20). These stresses are called *bending, flexure,* or *fiber stresses.*

Section modulus

The value of y at the outer fibers of the beam is frequently denoted by c. At these fibers, the bending stress is a maximum and is given by:

$$\sigma = \frac{Tc}{I} = \frac{Tc}{I/c.} \qquad (3\text{-}11)$$

The ratio I/c is called the *section modulus* and usually is denoted by the symbol Z. The section moduli for the shapes given in Table 3-3 are obtained by dividing the moment of inertia about the centroidal axis by the length of the centroid. For example, the moment of inertia for a rectangle about its centroidal axis is $bh^3/12$ and the length of the centroid is $h/2$; therefore, the section modulus is $bh^2/6$. Section moduli are given in Table 3-3.

Beam torque

Most structural elements in orthoses can be represented by either a cantilever beam loaded transversely with a perpendicular force at the end (e.g., a stirrup in terminal stance; Fig. 3-21) or a beam freely supported at the ends and centrally loaded (e.g., KAFO prescribed to control valgum; Fig. 3-22).

The maximum *torque* in cantilevered (Fig. 3-21) and freely supported (Fig. 3-22) *beams* is given by:

$$T_{max} = FL \qquad (3\text{-}12)$$

$$T_{max} = \frac{FL}{4.} \qquad (3\text{-}13)$$

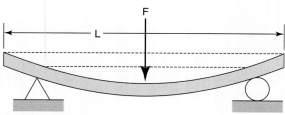

Fig. 3-19 Beam stress.

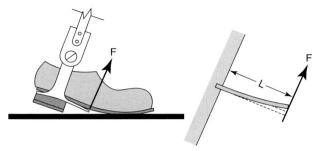

Fig. 3-21 Free body diagram of cantilevered beam.

Figure 3-23 gives the maximum torque for a few simple beams. If more than one external force acts on a beam, the bending torque is the sum of the torques caused by all the external forces acting on either side of the beam. Subsequently and not surprisingly, device failures commonly occur at the corresponding point of maximum torque (bending moment).

Beam stress

The *stress* in a cantilevered or freely supported *beam* now can be determined by substituting Equation 3-12 or 3-13 into Equation 3-11, which gives:

$$\sigma = \frac{FL_c}{I} \text{ (cantilevered beam).} \tag{3-14}$$

and

$$\sigma = \frac{FL_c}{4I} \text{ (freely supported beam).} \tag{3-15}$$

If these beams have rectangular cross-sections with height *h* and base *b* (i.e., $ch/2$ and $I = bh^3/12$), then the expressions for stress can be rewritten as:

$$\sigma = \frac{6FL}{bh^2} \text{(cantilevered beam),} \tag{3-16}$$

and

$$\sigma = \frac{3FL}{2bh^2} \text{(freely supported beam).} \tag{3-17}$$

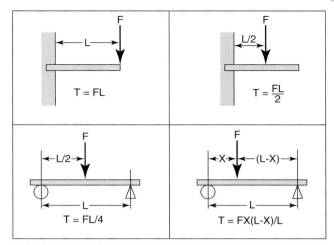

Fig. 3-23 Maximum bending torques of common beams.

As the cross-sectional area of the beam changes shape, so does the expression for the moment of inertia *I* and the outer fiber-to-neutral axis distance *c*.

Beam deflection

The maximum *deflection* of *beams* (sidebars, stirrups) is important to practitioners because the biomechanical objective of a prescribed device frequently depends on the ability of the device either to not deflect or to deflect a given amount. Excessive deflection (bending) of a device may either disturb alignment or prevent successful operation.

Deflection theory provides a technique of analysis for evaluating the nature and magnitude of deformations in beams. The cantilevered beam (Fig. 3-24) carries a concentrated downward load *F* at the free end. A cantilevered beam is, by definition, rigidly supported at the other end. The general expression for the downward deflection *y*, anywhere along the length (*x*-axis) of the beam, is given by:

$$y(x) = \frac{Fx^3}{-6EI} + \frac{FxL^2}{2EI} - \frac{FL^3}{3EI} \tag{3-18}$$

The maximum deflection of the cantilevered beam (y_{max}) occurs at the free end when $x = 0$:

$$y_{max} = -\frac{FL^3}{3EI.} \tag{3-19}$$

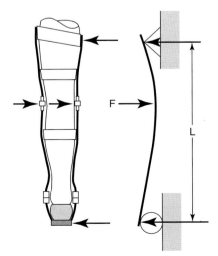

Fig. 3-22 Free body diagram of freely supported beam.

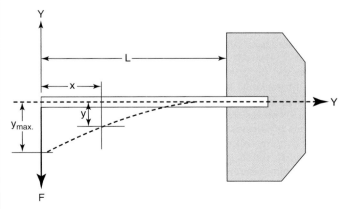

Fig. 3-24 Cantilevered beam.

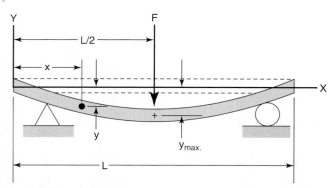

Fig. 3-25 Freely supported beam.

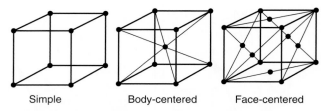

Fig. 3-26 Space lattices for cubes.

The general expression for the deflection of the freely supported beam with the midspan load (Fig. 3-25) is given by:

$$y(x) = \frac{Fx^3}{12EI} - \frac{FxL^2}{16EI} \quad (3\text{-}20)$$

The maximum deflection of the freely supported beam (y_{max}) occurs at the midspan when $x = L/2$:

$$y_{max} = \frac{FL^3}{-48EI} \quad (3\text{-}21)$$

The negative sign in Equations 3-19 and 3-21 indicates that the maximum deflection is downward from the unloaded position. Example 4 in the Appendix provides an illustration of calculating KAFO stress and deflection using the concepts of moment of inertia and centroid.

Metals

A *metal* is defined as a chemical element that is lustrous, hard, malleable, heavy, ductile, and tenacious and usually is a good conductor of heat and electricity. Of the 93 elements, 73 are classified as metals. The elements oxygen, chlorine, iodine, bromine, and hydrogen and the inert gases helium, neon, argon, krypton, xenon, and radon are considered nonmetallic. There is, however, a group of elements, such as carbon, sulfur, silicon, and phosphorus, that is intermediate between the metals and nonmetals. These elements portray the characteristics of metals under certain circumstances and the characteristics of nonmetals under other circumstances. They are referred to as *metalloids*.

The most widely used metallic elements include iron, copper, lead, zinc, aluminum (or aluminium), tin, nickel, and magnesium. Some of these elements are used extensively in the pure state, but by far the largest amount is used in the form of alloys. An *alloy* is a combination of elements that exhibits the properties of a metal. The properties of alloys differ appreciably from those of the constituent elements. Improvement of strength, ductility, hardness, wear resistance, and corrosion resistance may be obtained in an alloy by combinations of various elements. Orthotics and prosthetics typically contain alloys of aluminum and carbon steels, particularly stainless steel. Titanium also is frequently used, and, despite references to "pure titanium" (particularly in applications such as *osseointegration*), it is the alloy that is being referenced. Although these alloys (steel, aluminum, titanium) can be categorized as similar depending on the

base metal and some of the contributing alloy metal, they are potentially infinitely variable.

Crystallinity

One of the important characteristics of all metals is their crystallinity. A *crystalline substance* is one in which the atoms are arranged in definite and repeating order in a three-dimensional pattern. This regular arrangement of atoms is called a *space lattice*. Space lattices are characteristic of all crystalline materials. Most metals crystallize in one of three types of space lattices:

- *Cubic system*: Three contiguous edges of equal length and at right angles—simple lattice, body-centered lattice, and face-centered lattice (Fig. 3-26)
- *Tetragonal system*: Three contiguous edges, two of equal length, all at right angles—simple lattice and body-centered lattice (Fig. 3-27)
- *Hexagonal system*: Three parallel sets of equal length horizontal axes at 120 degrees and a vertical axis—close-packed hexagonal (Fig. 3-28)

This orderly state also is described as balanced, unstrained, or annealed. Some metals can exist in several lattice forms, depending on the temperature. Examples of metals that normally exist in only one form are as follows:

- *Face-centered cubic:* Ca, Ni, Cu, Ag, Au, Pb, Al
- *Body-centered cubic:* Li, Na, K, V, W
- *Face-centered tetragonal:* In
- *Close-packed hexagonal:* Be, Mg, Zn, Cd

Common iron is an example of one of many metals that may exist in more than one lattice form:

- Body-centered cubic: Below 1663 °F
- Face-centered cubic: 1663 °F to 2557 °F
- Body-centered cubic: 2557 °F to 2795 °F

A metal in the liquid state is noncrystalline, and the atoms move freely among one another without regard to interspatial distances. The internal energy possessed by these atoms

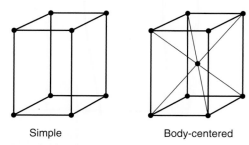

Fig. 3-27 Space lattices for tetragonals.

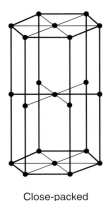

Close-packed

Fig. 3-28 Space lattice for a hexagon.

prevents them from approaching one another closely enough to come under the control of their attractive electrostatic fields. However, as the liquid cools and loses energy, the atoms move more sluggishly. At a certain temperature, for a particular pure metal, certain atoms are arranged in the proper position to form a single lattice typical of metal. The temperature at which atoms begin to arrange themselves in a regular geometric pattern (lattice) is called the *freezing point*. As heat is removed from metal, crystallization continues, and the lattices grow about each center. This growth continues at the expense of the liquid, with the lattice structure expanding in all directions until development is stopped by interference with other space lattices or with the walls of the container. If a space lattice is permitted to grow freely without interference, a single crystal is produced that has an external shape typical of the system in which it crystallizes.

Crystallization centers form at random throughout the liquid mass by the aggregation of a proper number of atoms to form a space lattice. Each of these centers of crystallization enlarges as more atoms are added, until interference is encountered. A diagrammatic representation of the process of solidification is shown in Fig. 3-29. In this diagram, the squares represent space lattices. In *A*, crystallization has begun at four centers.

As crystallization continues, more centers appear and develop with space lattices of random orientation. Successive stages in the crystallization are shown by *B, C, D, E,* and *F*. Small crystals join large ones, provided they have about the same orientation (i.e., their axes are nearly aligned). During the last stages of formation, crystals meet, but there are places at the surface of intersections where development of other space lattices is impossible. Such interference accounts for the irregular appearance of crystals in a piece of metal that is polished and etched (Fig. 3-30).

Grain structure

During the growth process, the development of external features, such as regular faces, may be prevented by interference from the growth of other centers. In this case, each unit is called a *grain* rather than a crystal. The term *crystal* usually is applied to a group of space lattices of the same orientation that show symmetry by the development of regular faces. Each grain is essentially a single crystal. The size of the grain depends on the temperature from which the metal is cast, the cooling rate, and the nature of the metal. In general,

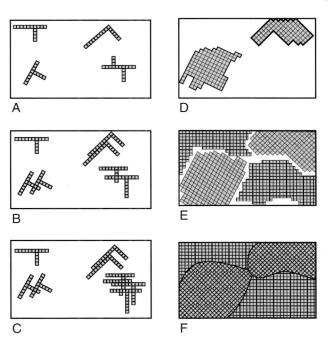

Fig. 3-29 Stages in the process of solidification of metals.

slow cooling leads to coarse grain and rapid cooling to fine grain metals.

Slip planes

When a force is applied to a crystal, the space lattice is distorted as evidenced by a change in the crystal's dimensions. This distortion causes some atoms in the lattice to be closer together and others to be farther apart. The magnitude of the applied force necessary to cause the distortion depends on the forces that act between the atoms in the lattice and tends to restore it to its normal configuration. If the applied force is removed, the atomic forces return the atoms to their normal

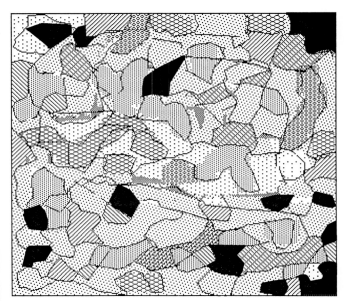

Fig. 3-30 Microscopic schematic of iron grain structure.

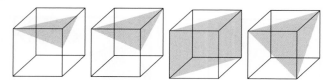

Fig. 3-31 Typical planes of slip in a cubic lattice.

positions in the lattice. Cubic patterns (lattices) characterize the more ductile or workable materials. Hexagonal and more complex patterns tend to be more brittle or more rigid. The force required to bring about the first permanent displacement corresponds to the elastic limit. This permanent displacement, or slip, occurs in the lattice on specified planes called *slip planes*. The ability of a crystal to slip in this manner without separation is the criterion of plasticity. Practically all metals are plastic to a certain degree. During plastic deformations, the lattice undergoes distortion, thus becoming highly stressed and hardened.

Slip, or plastic deformation, can occur more easily along certain planes with a space lattice than along other planes. The planes that have the greatest population of atoms and, likewise, the greatest separation of atoms on each side of the planes under consideration are usually the planes of easiest slip. Therefore, slip takes place along these planes first when the elastic limit is exceeded. Sliding movements tend to take place at 45-degree angles to the direction of the applied load because much higher stresses are required to pull atoms directly apart or to push them straight together.

A particular characteristic of crystalline materials is that slip is not necessarily confined to one set of planes during the process of deformation. Some common planes of slip in the simple cubic system are shown in Fig. 3-31.

Mechanical properties

The mechanical properties of metals depend on their lattice structures. In general, metals that exist with the face-centered cubic structure are ductile throughout a wide range of temperatures. Metals with the close-packed hexagonal type of lattice (Fig. 3-28) are appreciably hardened by cold working, and plastic deformation takes place most easily on planes parallel to the base of the lattice.

Of the many qualities of metals, the most significant are the related properties of elasticity and plasticity. Plasticity depends on the ability to shape and contour aluminum and stainless steel to match body contours; elasticity governs their safe and economical use as load-bearing members. The demand on the material used often is compromised depending on the consideration and prioritization of the manufacturing requirement or the clinical application.

As discussed in the section on Strength and Stress, a body is said to be *elastic* if it returns to its original shape upon removal of an external load. The *elastic limit* is the maximum stress at which the body behaves elastically. The *proportional limit* is the stress at which strain ceases to be proportional to applied stress; it is practically equal to elastic limit.

Plasticity

Plasticity is the term used to express a metal's ability to be deformed beyond the range of elasticity without fracture,

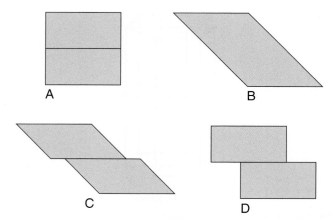

Fig. 3-32 Deformation of a cubic crystal lattice. **A,** Unstrained condition. **B,** Elastic deformation. **C,** Plastic deformation. **D,** Permanent set as a result of slip.

resulting in permanent change in shape. Characteristically the ratio of plastic-to-elastic deformation in metals is high, on the order of 100:1 or 1000:1. Although this is rarely a consideration for commercially designed structural components because they are designed to behave within the elastic range, it is crucial to components such as sidebars, which must be plastically deformed (bent) before they are used clinically.

A simple two-dimensional representation of a cubic crystal lattice in an unstrained condition is represented by *A* in Fig. 3-32. If a shearing force within the elastic range is applied, the lattice is uniformly distorted as in *B*, with the extent of distortion proportional to the applied force.

When the force is removed, the lattice springs back to its original shape (*A*). However, when the force exceeds the elastic (or proportional) limit, a sudden change in the mode of deformation occurs. Without further increase in the amount of elastic strain, the lattice shears along a crystallographic plane (or slip plane). One block of the lattice makes a long glide past the other and stops (*C*). On release of load, the lattice in the two displaced blocks resumes its original shape (*D*). If the applied force is continued, slip does not continue indefinitely along the original slip plane, which on the contrary appears to acquire resistance to further motion; however, some parallel plane comes into action. Both the extent of slip per plane and the distance between active slip planes are large in comparison to the unit lattice dimensions. As slip shifts from one slip plane to another, progressively higher forces are required to accomplish it (i.e., the metal has been *work hardened*). At some stage, resistance to further slip along the primitive set of planes exceeds the resistance offered by some other set of differently directed slip planes, which then come into action. This process elaborates as plastic deformation progresses.

The actual strength of metals as ordinarily measured is but a small fraction of theoretical strength. Some significant comparisons for pure copper are as follows:

- Calculated (theoretical) tensile strength = 1,300,000 psi.
- Measured breaking strength = 62,000 psi.

Similar relations exist for other pure metals.

Imperfections of many kinds, such as flaws in the regularity of the crystal lattice, microcracks within a grain, shrinkage voids, nonmetallic inclusions, rough surfaces, and notches of all kinds, may localize and intensify stresses. Many impurities owe their potency to a high degree of insolubility in the solid matrix coupled with high solubility in the fusion. This permits their freezing out relatively late in the solidification process, as concentrates or films between the grains, thus serving as effective internal notches. The great weakening effect of graphite flakes in cast iron is an example.

Notches act not only as stress raisers but also as stress complicators, frequently inducing stress in many directions. The deeper the notch and the sharper its root, the more effective it is in this respect. Notches are great weakeners, and practitioners do well to recognize their prevalence under many disguises (i.e., from either contouring instruments or grain boundaries). Most importantly, every care should be taken to minimize the contribution to these weakeners by not adding further notches, cracks, scratches, or rough surfaces.

Steel and aluminum alloys
Commercial name for metals

Before the stress–strain diagram is used as a basis for comparing the properties of various metals, it is necessary to discuss the types of steel and aluminum commercially available and used in orthotic and prosthetic applications.

The terms *surgical steel, stainless steel, tool steel,* and *heat treated* along with other general designations are freely used by manufacturers of orthotic and prosthetic components. The chemical content of these products is not identical from vendor to vendor. For example, the term *spring steel,* used by many manufacturers, refers to a group of steels ranging in chemical composition from medium- to high-carbon steel and is used to designate some alloy steels. The term *tool steel* also covers a wide variety of steels that are capable of attaining a high degree of hardness after heat treatment. More care is exercised in manufacturing tool steel to ensure maximum uniformity of desirable properties.

These general designations do not assure the orthotist or prosthetist of obtaining the exact material that is needed. Because the mechanical properties of a material and subsequent fabrication procedures depend on the material's chemical analysis and subsequent heat treatment or working, the practice of using general descriptions for metals is seriously inadequate. In addition, reliance on these categories is not necessary because specific designations already exist for each type of steel and processing treatment. The following sections give a clearer picture of the available steel and aluminum alloys and their specific properties.

Carbon steel

Iron as a pure metal does not possess sufficient strength or hardness to be useful for many applications. By adding as little as a fraction of 1% carbon by weight, however, the properties of the base metal are significantly altered. Iron with added carbon is called *carbon steel.* Within certain limits, the strength and hardness of carbon steel are directly proportionate to the amount of carbon added. In addition to carbon, carbon steel contains manganese and traces of sulfur and phosphorus.

Alloy steel

To achieve desirable physical or chemical properties, other chemicals are added to carbon steel. The resultant product is known as *alloy steel.* In presenting some general characteristics distinguishing these alloys, it is necessary to define some terms commonly used to express them:

- *Toughness:* Ability to withstand shock force
- *Hardness:* Resistance to penetration and abrasion
- *Ductility:* Ability to undergo permanent changes of shape without rupturing
- *Corrosion resistance:* Resistance to chemical attack of a metal under the influence of a moist atmosphere

The addition of elements can increase elasticity and tensile strength as well as improve surface finish and machinability.

Characteristics of specified alloys

Using some of these definitions, the important characteristics distinguishing some alloy steels are described as follows. Nickel steels are characterized by improved toughness, simplified heat treating, less distortion in quenching, and improved corrosion resistance. Nickel chromium steels exhibit increased depth hardenability and improved abrasion resistance. Molybdenum steels rank with manganese and chromium as having the greatest hardenability, increased high-temperature strength, and increased corrosion resistance. Chromium steels have increased hardening effect. (It is possible to decrease the amount of carbon content and obtain a steel with both high strength and satisfactory ductility.) Vanadium steels have increased refinement of the internal structure of the alloy, making them suitable for spring steels and construction steels. Silicon manganese steels possess increased strength and hardness. Double and triple alloys are a combination of two or more of these alloys and produce a steel having some of the characteristic properties of each. For example, chromium molybdenum steels have excellent hardenability and satisfactory ductility. Chromium nickel steels have good hardenability and satisfactory ductility. The effect of combining three alloys produces a material superior in specific characteristic performance to the sum of each alloy used separately.

Stainless steels

Steel alloys containing a large amount of chromium (>3.99%) are called *stainless steels.* The American Iron and Steel Institute (AISI) uses a three-digit system to identify each type of stainless steel. The various grades are separated into three general categories according to their metallurgical structure and properties: austenitic, martinsitic, and ferritic.

Each category has special heat treatment and cold working properties. For example, the well-known "18-8" stainless steel used in orthopedic instruments are austenitic steels containing 18% chromium and 8% nickel. These chromium nickel stainless steels cannot be hardened by heat treatment and attain mechanical properties higher than the annealed (heat-treated) condition resulting from cold working. *Cold working* refers to plastic deformation of a metal at temperatures that substantially increase its strength and hardness.

The tensile strength of the austenitic steel in the softened or annealed condition is more than that of mild steel. By cold working, ultimate strengths of 250,000 psi can be achieved.

Because these steels rapidly work harden, sharp drills and tools are used to work them quickly before they get too hard. These steels have the highest corrosion resistance of the stainless steel family.

Martinsitic stainless steel is the only category of the three stainless steels subject to heat treatment. Ferritic stainless steel is nonhardenable by heat treatment and only slightly hardenable by cold working.

SAE number

The Society of Automotive Engineers (SAE) has assigned a specific number, known as an *SAE number*, to identify each steel according to its chemical analysis. There is an equivalent AISI number, but for simplicity one means of identification is sufficient. Four digits are used in the SAE description as follows.

Digit one refers to the type of steel. Digit two refers to the approximate percentage of the predominating alloy element in a simple alloy steel. Digits three and four refer to the approximate percentage of carbon by weight in $\frac{1}{100}$ of 1%.

List of digit one is as follows:

1XXX = Carbon steel
2XXX = Nickel steel
3XXX = Nickel chromium
4XXX = Chromium molybdenum (cro-moly)
5XXX = Chromium
6XXX = Chromium vanadium
7XXX = Heat-resistant alloy steel castings
8XXX = Nickel cro-moly
9XXX = Silicon manganese

For example, SAE 1020 is carbon steel (first digit 1) with no added element (second digit 0) and 0.20% carbon (third and fourth digits 20). Using the same method, SAE 4012 is chromium molybdenum steel with 0.12% carbon content. SAE 4130 is cro-moly steel with 1% chromium and 0.30% carbon. SAE 4130 is an airplane part alloy used in orthoses.

Comparison of steel and aluminum

Stress–strain diagram

Figure 3-33 is a comparative stress–stain diagram plotting one type of steel and one type of soft aluminum. The straight-line portion of both curves on the diagram indicates the elastic range and stiffness of the material. The dotted lines on the diagram indicate the increased stresses that the material can tolerate before it reaches the yield and ultimate stress phase as the strength of the material is increased. In the case of steel, the modulus of elasticity is 30 million psi. For aluminum the modulus of elasticity is 10 million psi, one third that of steel.

Size, weight, and strength comparisons

For an equal amount of stress, steel strains (deflects) one third as much as aluminum (shown by ϵ and 3ϵ in Fig. 3-33), but aluminum weighs only approximately one third as much as steel. This means that if a rectangular cross-section of steel undergoing bending stresses is duplicated in aluminum, then one dimension of the aluminum rectangle must be increased by 70% to achieve the same stiffness (resistance to bending).

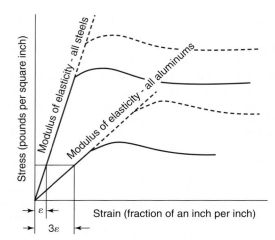

Fig. 3-33 Comparative stress–strain diagram.

Thus, an aluminum orthosis must be made 70% larger in one dimension to be as rigid in this direction as a steel orthosis of the same general shape. Although bulkier, the aluminum orthosis would be only 60% the weight of the steel orthosis.

Aluminum has the advantage of being not only lighter in weight but also easier to work with than steel. Where bulkiness is not critical, it is possible to construct an aluminum device just as rigid as steel and yet lighter in weight. Although the bulk can be limited by maximizing the moment of inertia in the planes of maximum bending moments (typically anteroposterior), the aluminum device is more subject to fatigue failure than steel.

Strengthening aluminum and steel

Although the yield stress and ultimate stress of the aluminum alloy shown in Fig. 3-33 is below that of the steel, all aluminums are not weaker than all steels. By adding certain alloying elements, proper heat treatment, or cold working, some aluminums can be increased in strength to an ultimate stress tolerance of 90,000 psi (7178-T6), which is above the strength of some steels. However, the aluminum still will be more subject to fatigue failure than the steel. Increasing the strength of steel also is possible using similar processes. A practitioner likely will not be required to apply these techniques to metals as commonly needed in the past. A familiarity with the principles and theory of these methods is appropriate and applicable to other materials. This section describes and discusses some of these methods.

Heat treatment

Purposes

Chemical analysis of a metal indicates only its potential properties. For example, alloy steels from the rolling mills are still in a semiprocessed condition, and their mechanical properties are not realized until after heat treatment. Heat treatment can accomplish many purposes: increase or decrease hardness and tensile strength, relieve internal stresses because of hot or cold working, improve machinability, and increase toughness.

Techniques

All of these qualities are desirable at different times and for different applications. They are achieved using varying techniques in the heat treatment processes as follows:

- If steel is heated above its critical temperature range, it undergoes definite internal changes.
- If the steel is slowly cooled from this elevated temperature, the internal changes have time to reverse themselves.
- If the steel is cooled more rapidly than the internal changes can reverse themselves, the structure of the steel is modified and its mechanical characteristics are altered.

Example A specimen of carbon steel (0.30% carbon content) is composed of microscopic grains of ferrite and pearlite. Ferrite is almost pure iron. Pearlite looks like mother-of-pearl and is composed of alternate layers of ferrite and cementite, which is an iron carbide or hard chemical combination of iron and carbon.

As the steel is heated through its critical range, a transformation occurs. The iron changes its form and can no longer remain chemically combined with the carbon. The hard carbides are broken up, and the carbon goes into solution in the iron. This is called a *solid solution* because the material is in a solid state (i.e., it is not molten). This material is now *austenite*.

When the steel is quenched, that is, rapidly cooled from above its critical range, the austenite does not have sufficient time to transform to ferrite and pearlite. Instead, *martinsite*, another iron carbide that is hard and brittle, is formed. Adding other alloying elements affects the formation of the martinsite, and the resultant properties are changed.

Heat-treat cycle

To reduce residual stresses formed as a result of cold working or nonuniform heating and cooling, two similar processes are used that achieve somewhat different results. The material is either *normalized* or *annealed*.

Normalizing the steel returns the steel to its original or normal internal structure. The metal is heated above its critical range (Fig. 3-34, *A*), which is slightly higher than in the annealing process, and then is cooled in air. A piece of normalized steel has higher strength and hardness but less ductility than the same piece of steel annealed.

Annealing the steel (Fig. 3-34, *B*) relieves internal stresses and lowers the yield point to obtain maximum ductility. As a result, the metal can be plastically deformed with minimum force. The steel is heated to a temperature above the critical range and then is slowly cooled in the furnace.

Tempering or drawing (Fig. 3-34, *C*) usually follows quenching. Steel that has been heat treated is fully hardened and is too brittle and hard for use in most applications. To make the steel softer, more ductile, and tougher, it is tempered. In tempering, the steel is heated again to a point below the critical range and then cooled at a controlled rate. The higher the temperature during the tempering process, the lower the strength and hardness and the higher the ductility.

Heat treatment influencing shop practices

The mechanical properties of the metal are influenced by the rate of heating, the heat treatment temperature, the time held at this temperature, the atmosphere surrounding the work, and the rate of cooling. This is a critical process that requires special skills and equipment, so it usually is performed by the manufacturer. Improper shop practices that influence the conditions mentioned can nullify the desired results of the heat treatment and produce substandard metals.

Most fabrication techniques call for use of as little heat as possible on heat-treated alloys unless the material is to be heat treated again.

Aluminum heat treatment

Tempering of an aluminum alloy is the major determinant of its strength, hardness, ductility, and other properties. Some aluminum alloys can be heat treated to improve their properties; others must be strengthened and hardened by cold working. Aluminum alloys are assigned temper designations that are added to the end of the four identifying digits. These figures indicate the type of treatment undergone by the alloy as follows:

XXXX-0: Annealed condition of wrought alloys
XXXX-T2: Annealed condition of cast alloys
XXXX-F: For wrought alloys, no control is exercised over the temper of the alloy; for cast alloys, the term means "as cast" (e.g., 43-F)
XXXX-T (followed by one or more numbers): Heat-treated alloy, where the numbers refer to the type of heat treatment
XXXX-H: Cold work temper of a wrought alloy

Example 2024-T4 refers to aluminum of chemical composition defined by 2024, heat treated and aged at room temperature to a stable condition.

Stress–strain diagram

The stress–strain diagram (Fig. 3-35) compares several steels and aluminums that have been heat treated and/or tempered in a variety of ways. Because all of the aluminums have the same chemical composition (AISI 2024), the effect on the mechanical properties of differing types of heat treatment is clearly demonstrated by the aluminum curves. For instance, the yield and ultimate strength of the annealed alloy (2024-0) were raised from 11,000 psi and 27,000 psi to 71,000 psi and 75,000 psi, respectively, when heat treated (2024-T86).

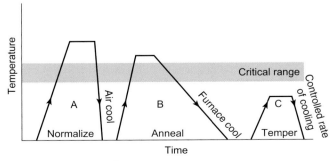

Fig. 3-34 Heat treat cycle.

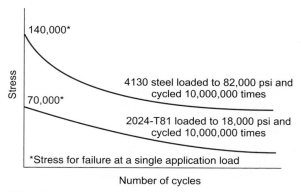

Fig. 3-36 Fatigue.

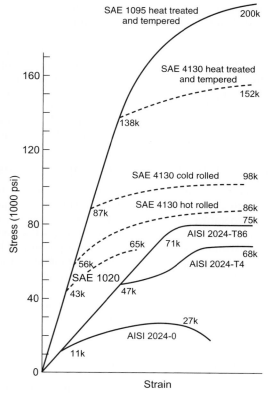

Fig. 3-35 Stress–strain diagram.

The effect of hot and cold working on steel is shown by the SAE 4130 curves. The yield point and ultimate strength point of this alloy were raised from 87,000 psi and 98,000 psi to 138,000 psi and 152,000 psi, respectively, demonstrating the increased strength obtained by heat treating this alloy.

The high-carbon steel curve (SAE 1095) shows the effect of heat treatment on this material, raising the ultimate strength to 200,000 psi.

Preventing failure

Fatigue

The range of elasticity, the yield, and ultimate stress points are high enough in most metals to prevent orthosis failure. Fatigue stresses, which are the result of repeated applications of small loads rather than the application of a large load, are the main cause of breakage.

Fatigue stresses can be partially compared with the physiologic stresses experienced by a normal individual when walking. When a person is walking, the effort required for each step is only a fraction of his or her available energy. After a while, however, the person reaches a point at which even the relatively small expenditure of energy necessary for lifting his or her limbs requires too much effort.

Fatigue stresses are fluctuating stresses of a magnitude less than the ultimate stress of the material. Although the ultimate stress would immediately cause immediate breakage, fatigue stress causes failure after a number of cycles. In physiologic stress, if a person rests for a period, the fatigue lessens or is completely alleviated. However, in fatigue stress, rest from stressing the material has no effect on the number of cycles before breakage occurs. Figure 3-36 illustrates the phenomenon of fatigue failure. Critically the ultimate stress required for failure is reduced to the point where it coincides with the stresses associated with a single step. This means that fatigue failure will occur with no visible signs of yielding and at stresses well below the yield or design stress of the device.

Steel and aluminum fatigue compared

The curves in Fig. 3-36 are obtained by plotting the stresses on a material against the number of applications of such stresses before breakage. In the case of steel, repeated stresses below a certain level do not cause fatigue failure. The steel curve levels off at a value approximately 50% of its ultimate stress. Theoretically, this is the fatigue strength of the material, and any number of stresses at or below this level of 70,000 psi is not expected to cause fatigue failure.

The aluminum curve is quite different. Aluminum does not level off as steel does and therefore is more subject to fatigue failure. Although the addition of alloying elements raises the ultimate strength and yield point of aluminum, it does not appreciably change the fatigue strength. Table 3-4 illustrates this point. Heat treatment also has only a small effect on aluminum fatigue.

Stress concentration

The average value of stress on a given object is obtained by dividing the amount of applied force by the size of the resisting area (Fig. 3-37). However, stress is concentrated at points of nicks, notches, drilled holes, sharply bent corners, or name

Table 3-4 Material strength (psi)*

Alloy	Yield Strength	Ultimate Strength	Fatigue Strength
2024-0	11,000	27,000	13,000
2024-T3	50,000	70,000	20,000
2024-T4	47,000	68,000	20,000
2024-T86	71,000	75,000	18,000
7075-T6	73,000	83,000	22,000

*Based on 50,000,000 cycles of completely reversed stress.
Adapted from *Alcoa Aluminum Handbook*.

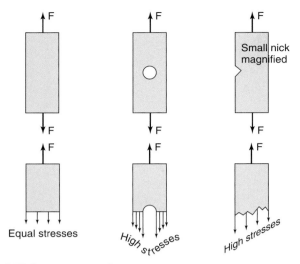

Fig. 3-37 Stress concentration.

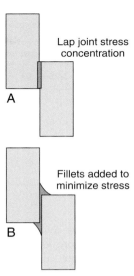

Fig. 3-38 Minimizing stress.

stampings, and its value at these points may be several times the average stress (Fig. 3-37). In fact, a stress concentration can best be described as any change in the material, design, or device. Stress concentration occurs at joints, holes, bends, and even within the same material if it changes cross-sectional area or shape. The increased stress lowers the resistance of the material to impact and fatigue loadings and is one of the more important factors contributing to orthosis failures. In reality, there are few clinical applications where the practitioner is not required to contribute stress concentrations to the design of the device. Therefore, the aim is to minimize the amount of stress concentrations contributed by the practitioner to those that are absolutely necessary.

It is easiest to see the effect of stress concentrations on a brittle material such as glass.

Example A man wants to break a piece of glass in half. If he simply applies force to both ends and bends the glass, it shatters into a mass of splinters. However, if he scribes a line on the surface of the glass with a glazer's cutter and then applies bending forces, the glass is neatly broken into two parts. The material is stressed the highest at the scribed line, concentrating the applied force at that location. Similarly, orthoses will fail when being bent into position, about a drilled hole or a joint.

Although the effects of stress concentration on ductile materials, including some metals, are not as dramatic as with brittle materials, the same phenomenon occurs. With this in mind, it is possible to minimize the points of stress concentration and increase the strength of the material. This is accomplished in orthoses by using certain fabrication procedures that minimize stress.

Minimizing stress concentration

The following recommendations help to minimize the points of stress concentration, thereby increasing the strength of orthoses:

1. Remove nicks and scratches from the material by polishing. (In this instance, material is removed to distribute the stress equally and thereby strengthen the material.)

2. Cap the checkered jaws of the vise before clamping the work into the vise.
3. Ensure that contouring instruments have smooth, curved surfaces.
4. Plan all cuts and bends to ensure smooth transitions and minimal changes.
5. Do not shape the orthosis stirrups with a metal hammer.
6. Avoid abrupt changes in cross-section. When two sections are being joined together, the stress may be concentrated on the joint area depending on the type of joint (Fig. 3-38). However, if extra material is added to form a fillet (Fig. 3-38), the stress concentration is minimized.

Minimizing stress concentration as a result of bending

Table 3-5 lists the minimum radii for bending aluminum alloys. The values given are for a 90-degree cold bend. Bending an orthosis part below the minimum radii causes excess stress concentration and increases the possibility of breakage at the bend.

Shape of orthotic parts

Many orthotic parts act in the same manner as beams. The upper sidebars of an orthosis are subjected to lateral forces causing bending stresses (Fig. 3-39). Bending stresses on a member acting as a beam are not the same as pure tension, compression, or shear stresses, in which the strain depends on the amount of the area and not on the shape of the cross-sectional area. The magnitude of the bending stresses depends on the cross-sectional area of the member.

In the case of a beam, the top fibers of the beam are in maximum compression, whereas the bottom fibers are in maximum tension (Fig. 3-40, *A*). The stresses are in opposite directions and decrease toward the center of the area. In this location, called the *neutral axis*, the stress is zero. Distributing

Table 3-5 Approximate radii for 90-degree cold bend

Radii for Various Thicknesses (inch) Expressed in Terms of Thickness *T*						
Aluminum Alloys	1/16	1/8	3/16	1/4	3/8	1/2
2024-0	0	0	0-1T	0-1T	1.5T-3T	3T-5T
2024-T3	3T-5T	4T-6T	4T-6T	5T-7T	6T-8T	6T-9T
2024-T36	4T-6T	5T-7T	5T-7T	6T-10T	7T-10T	8T-11T
2024-T4	3T-5T	4T-6T	4T-6T	5T-7T	6T-8T	6T-9T

Adapted from *Alcoa Aluminum Handbook.*

as much material as possible away from the neutral axis lowers the stress and therefore lowers the resulting strain on the member. This change in the moment of inertia contributing to the shape strength of the device is a major strength influencing factor that the practitioner can control. Figure 3-40, *B*, illustrates this phenomenon.

Distribution of materials in beams

It is possible and advisable to distribute the same amount of material in different shapes in order to lower stresses. The familiar shape of a structural I beam illustrates this principle (Fig. 3-41).

Instead of rectangular cross-sections, these beams are made in the shape of an I. The material in the rectangular beam, as represented by the hatched areas in the diagram, is removed from the sides and placed on the top and bottom. Thus, the rigidity of the beam is increased with reference to bending in this direction. However, resistance to bending about the sides is diminished. Proper design considers the anticipated direction of maximum bending and orients the structural member accordingly.

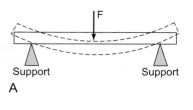

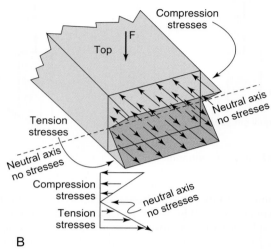

Fig. 3-40 Beam stresses.

Designs in orthoses

In fabricating an orthosis, the certified orthotist positions the sidebars of a lower limb orthosis having rectangular cross-sectional areas so that the long dimension of the rectangle is parallel to the anteroposterior direction (Fig. 3-42). In this position, the bars are able to resist larger forces and are more rigid than in the mediolateral direction. This design and the attachment of cuffs are correct if the maximum anticipated forces are generated by a knee lock preventing flexion for which increased rigidity with reference to mediolateral bending moments is desirable.

Other designing problems

When the direction of maximum stress is not known, the material should be distributed in the form of a ring. The ring shape resists bending equally well in all directions (Fig. 3-43, *A*).

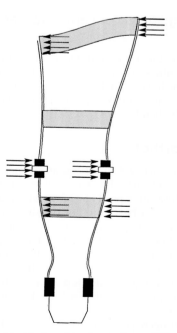

Fig. 3-39 KAFO subject to bending stresses in mediolateral direction.

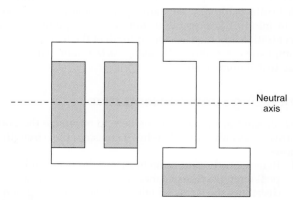

Fig. 3-41 Beam shape.

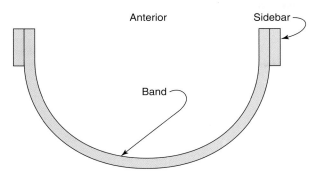

Fig. 3-42 Band design.

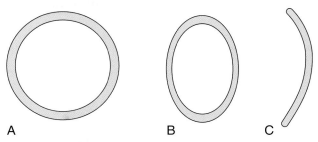

Fig. 3-43 Geometric shapes.

When there are significant moments in two known directions and one is known to be larger than the other, tubular areas can be used to obtain effective resistance to bending (Fig. 3-43, *B*). The contouring of tubular cross-sections is somewhat difficult. An orthotic example is the case of a heavy individual who is bowlegged and therefore has large mediolateral bending moments and anteroposterior bending moments.

European orthotists have used a bar having the shape illustrated in Fig. 3-43, *C*. This shape increases resistance to bending in both directions with a minimum of material.

Fastening components

Riveting aluminum

Several advantages make riveting the most common method of joining aluminum. Welding, brazing, and soldering require the application of heat to material. If the material depends on prior heat treatment for strength, the additional application of heat in fabrication may alter the desired mechanical properties that have been achieved. Rivets can be visually inspected, whereas an x-ray film of a weld usually is necessary to determine its strength. Rivets also can contribute some cold work hardening benefits to the material in which they are placed.

Rivet materials

Aluminum is the preferred material for fastening aluminum. When dissimilar metals are in contact with each other in a moist atmosphere, galvanic corrosion takes place, which lowers service life. In orthoses and certain other instances, however, stainless steel, hot-dipped aluminized or cadmium-plated steel rivets can be used. Because aluminum rivets must be larger than steel rivets to achieve the same strength, larger holes are needed to accommodate the aluminum rivets. In orthoses, the larger holes with respect to the dimensions of the components weaken the material.

Rivet size

When joining different size members, the diameter of the rivet should not be less than the thickness of the thickest part through which the rivet is driven but not greater than three times the thickness of the thinnest part.

Rivet spacing

The recommended minimum spacing between rivets is three times the nominal rivet diameter. As a general rule, the maximum distance should not be greater than two to four times the thickness of the thickest member.

Edge distance

The edge distance from the center of the hole to the end of the member should be at least twice the diameter of the rivet. This yields a joint with maximum bearing strength. Figure 3-44 illustrates these requirements.

Rivet holes

Recommended hole sizes for cold driven aluminum alloy rivets are listed in Table 3-6. Consideration should be given to the fact that holes may wear and elongate in high-stress areas. It may be desirable to apply a hole slightly smaller than optimum and then use a newer slightly larger hole and rivet after some time in service, thus extending the life of the joint.

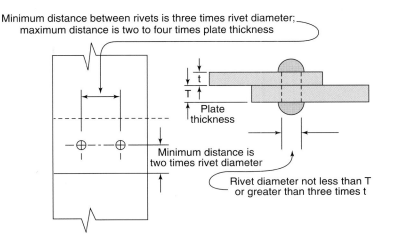

Fig. 3-44 Edge distance.

Table 3-6 Rivet hole size

Nominal Rivet Diameter (inch)	1/8	5/32	3/16	1/4	5/16
Recommended hole diameter	0.1285	0.159	0.191	0.257	0.323
Drill size	30	21	11	F	P

Adapted from *Alcoa Structural Handbook.*

Rivet sets and bucking tools

Rivet sets should have smooth, polished surfaces to allow the metal to flow readily during the forming operation. The bucking tool should have sufficient mass and be of the shape illustrated in Fig. 3-45.

Using the bucking-up set

The cup of the bucking-up set initially should be in contact with the top of the rivet so that the shank is not driven into the head during forming. Proper upsetting of the rivet fills the rivet hole and increases fatigue strength.

Rivet length

The length of rivet necessary for proper forming of a head depends on the total thickness of metal through which the rivet is driven, the clearance between the rivet and the rivet hole, and the form of the head. Because of variations in driving conditions, manufacturers recommend trying various lengths to determine the optimum length. Erring on the long side is preferable. A short rivet may allow the rivet set to contact the member and damage it. Good practice with respect to countersunk rivets requires a unit length that leaves some material above the surface after riveting is completed. This ensures complete filling of the countersunk hole and prevents damage to the surrounding member. The excess can be ground off at a later time. For purposes of comparison, the strengths of some aluminium alloys frequently used for rivets are listed in Fig 3-7.

Aluminum rivet material

Aluminum rivets are produced in the following alloys: 1100-H14, 2017-T4, 2024-T4, 2117-T4, 6053-T61, and 7277-T4 (Table 3-7). All of these rivets, except for 2024-T4 and 7277-T4, can be driven cold in the condition received from the manufacturer. Rivets 2024 and 7277 are strong but must be heated before driving.

A strong rivet should not be used in a weak plate because the plate may become distorted. In addition, the strength of

Table 3-7 Aluminum alloys

Alloys	Shear Strength (psi)
1100-H14	11,000
2017-T4	39,000
2024-T4	42,000
2117-T4	33,000
5056-H32	30,000
6053-T61	23,000
6061-T6	30,000
7244-T4	38,000

Adapted from *Riveting Alcoa Aluminum.*

the rivet may be superfluous because the plate will fail before the rivet does. For aluminum members made of 2024, 2017-T4 rivets can be used; the 6000 series rivets are compatible with 3000 series members.

Riveting stainless steels

Advances in welding techniques have made this type of joining operation suitable for stainless steels. However, riveting still offers many advantages. It is a quick method of joining and requires a minimum of accessory equipment. Also, as in the case of aluminum, cold riveting is not associated with the hazards involved in the intense heat applications of the welding process. The possible loss of corrosion resistance and the danger of warping are eliminated by riveting.

Recommended procedures

- Rivet holes should be drilled and all burrs removed. For steels that rapidly work harden, avoid center punching before drilling because the material will prove too hard to drill.
- Rivet stock should be in the annealed condition. By work hardening the rivet in the forming operation, its physical properties are improved.
- Austenitic rivets up to ¼-inch diameter can be driven cold. Because these rivets work harden rapidly, however, the head should be formed with as few blows as possible.
- Ferritic and martinsitic rivets up to ⅜-inch diameter can be driven cold, preferably with a hydraulic riveter.

Plastics and composites

Plastics are the result of humankind's ability to innovate, to create new materials by combining organic building blocks—carbon, oxygen, hydrogen, nitrogen, chlorine, and other organic and inorganic elements—into new and useful forms (Table 3-8). A plastic is a solid in its finished state. However, at some stage in its manufacture, it approaches a liquid condition and is formed into useful shapes. The name refers to the large plastic range of deformation associated with these materials.

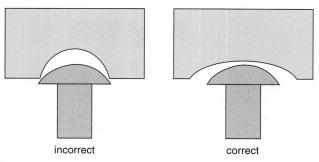

incorrect   correct

Fig. 3-45 Rivet sets.

Table 3-8 Building blocks

Element	Atomic Weight	Energy Bonds	
Hydrogen	1	—H	(1)
Carbon	12	—C—	(4)
Nitrogen	14	—N—	(3)
Oxygen	16	—O—	(2)
Fluorine	19	—F	(1)
Silicone	28	—Si—	(4)
Sulfur	32	—S—	(2)
Chlorine	35	—Cl	(1)

Table 3-9 Typical monomers and their repeating polymer units

Monomer	Polymer
Ethylene	**Polyethylene**
Propylene	**Polypropylene**
Tetrafluoro-ethylene	**Polytetra-fluoroethylene**

Building polymers

Plastics are synthetic materials made from raw chemical materials called *monomers*. A monomer (one chemical unit) such as ethylene is reacted with other monomer molecules into long chains of repeating ethylene units, forming the polymer polyethylene (Table 3-9). In a similar manner, polystyrene is formed from styrene monomer, polypropylene from propylene monomer, and other thermoplastic polymers from their respective monomers.

Polymers consist of atoms of carbon in combination with other elements. Polymer chemists use only eight (Table 3-8) of the more than 100 known elements to create thousands of different plastics.

Combining these atoms in various ways produces extremely large, complex molecules. Each atom has a limited capacity (energy bonds; Table 3-8) for joining to other atoms, and the energy bonds for all atoms within a molecule must be satisfied for the compound to be stable. For example, hydrogen can bond to only one other atom, whereas carbon or silicon must attach to four other atoms to satisfy its four

Forming usually is done through the application of heat and pressure, either singly or together.

The number of permutations possible when combining the many chemical elements is virtually endless. This diversity has made plastics applicable to a broad range of consumer and industrial products. It also has made the job of selecting the best material from such a huge array of candidate plastics quite difficult.

energy bonds. Thus, H—H and H—F are stable molecules, but C—H and Si—Cl are not stable.

For example, consider the simple organic compound methane (CH_4), the main component of natural gas. The carbon in methane is attached to four atoms of hydrogen, and each hydrogen atom is attached to the simple atom of carbon. The molecular weight of methane, 16, is the total of the individual atomic weights of its constituent atoms.

Adding more carbon atoms in a chain and more hydrogen atoms to each new carbon creates heavier molecules. For example, ethane gas (C_2H_6) is heavier than methane because it contains an additional carbon and two additional hydrogen atoms. Its molecular weight is 30. In a similar manner, molecular weight can be increased in increments of 14 (1 C, 2 H) until the compound pentane (C_5H_{12}) is reached. Pentane is too heavy to be a gas; instead it is a liquid at room temperature. Further addition of CH_2 groups makes progressively heavier liquids until $C_{18}H_{38}$ is reached. This is the solid, paraffin wax.

Thermoplastics

As molecules are made longer and become heavier, the polymer wax becomes harder and tougher. At approximately $C_{100}H_{202}$, the material, with a molecular weight of 1402, is tough enough to be useful as a plastic (Table 3-10). This is low-molecular-weight polyethylene, the simplest of the thermoplastics.

Continuing to add CH_2 groups to the chain increases strength and toughness even more. The toughest polyethylene contains more than one quarter million CH_2 groups and is called *ultra-high-molecular-weight polyethylene*.

Although the example of polymer chain growth given in Table 3-10 implies the addition of one CH_2 group at a time, in reality a simple CH_2 group cannot be added easily because it

Table 3-10 Building by adding CH_2 groups

Common Name	Chemical Formula	Molecular Weight
Methane	CH_4	16
Ethane	C_2H_6	30
Propane	C_3H_8	44
Butane	C_4H_{10}	58
Pentane	C_5H_{12}	72
Kerosene	$C_{17}H_{36}$	240
Paraffin	$C_{18}H_{38}$	254
Hard wax	$C_{50}H_{102}$	702
Polyethylene (LMW)	$C_{100}H_{202}$	1402

LMW, Low molecular weight.

does not exist as a stable compound. Instead, groups of organic compounds, called *monomers*, are used.

The structure of these monomers seems to conflict with the rule that carbon must be attached to four other atoms in order to be stable. But, like all rules, there are exceptions. In certain cases, a double bond, which is stable, can form between atoms. As illustrated in Fig. 3-46, ethylene monomer CH_2CH_2 is made by removing (under heat and pressure) two hydrogens from ethane, CH_3CH_3. A redistribution of electrons occurs, and a double bond is formed. The double bond plus the two single bonds satisfy the four energy bonds of the carbon atom, forming a stable monomer.

Starting with billions of molecules of monomers in a reactor, heat and pressure are applied in the presence of catalysts, causing one of the monomer double bonds to rearrange into *half bonds*, one at each end (Fig. 3-47). These half bonds combine with half bonds of other rearranged monomer molecules, forming stable *whole bonds* between them. As each monomer joins (primary bonds) with others, the chain length grows until it meets a stray hydrogen, which combines with the reactive end, stopping chain growth at that point.

During the polymerization reaction, millions of separate polymer chains simultaneously grow in length until all the monomers are exhausted. By adding predetermined amounts of hydrogen (or other chain stoppers), chemists can produce polymers having a fairly consistent average chain length. Chain length is important because it determines many properties of a plastic; it also affects its processing characteristics. The major effects of increasing chain length are greater toughness, creep resistance, stress-crack resistance, melt temperature, melt viscosity, and processing difficulty.

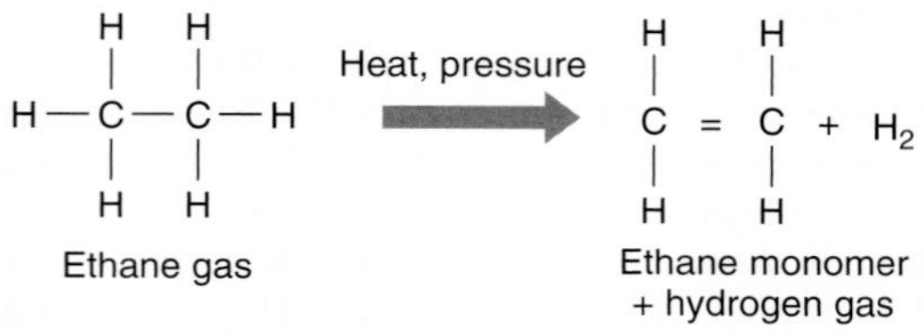

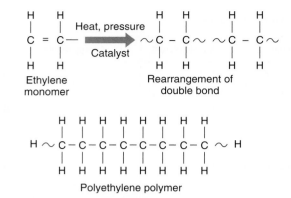

Fig. 3-47 Polymerization of polyethylene.

All polymer molecules cannot be manufactured to an exact specified length; however, each batch has an average molecular weight distribution. There can be either a broad or a narrow spread between molecular weights of the largest and smallest molecules, and the polymer still could have the same average. A narrow distribution provides more uniform properties; a broad distribution makes a plastic easier to process.

After polymerization is completed, the finished polymer chains resemble long, intertwined bundles of spaghetti, with no physical connections between chains. Such a polymer is called a *thermoplastic (heat-moldable) polymer*.

Although there is no direct physical connection between individual thermoplastic chains, there is a weak electrostatic attraction (secondary bonds) between polymer chains that lie close together. This intermolecular force, which tends to prevent chain movement, is heat sensitive, becoming stronger when the plastic is cold and weaker when it is hot. Heating a thermoplastic weakens the intermolecular forces of the secondary bonds, allowing the polymer molecules to slide over each other freely during the forming process. On cooling, the forces become strong again and "freeze" the molecules together in the new shape.

Forming a thermoplastic is similar to molding candle wax. If too much heat is applied or the plastic is heated for too long, the molecular chains' primary bonds break, causing permanent damage, particularly material toughness. Continuous bending or deforming stress on a formed part also causes the chains to slide over each other, resulting in creep, or cold flow, which can seriously affect part shape.

Strength of the intermolecular attractive force (secondary bond) varies inversely with the sixth power of the distance between chains. Thus, as the distance is halved, the attractive force increases by a factor of 64. For this reason, chain shape is as important as chain length. If a polymer molecule has a symmetrical shape that can pack closely, the intermolecular forces are large compared with a molecule having a nonsymmetrical shape.

Two kinds of polyethylene can have different physical properties because of the difference in their density, which depends on their ability to pack together (Fig. 3-48).

Molecules of high-density polyethylene have few side branches to upset their symmetry, so they can approach adjacent molecules quite closely, resulting in high intermolecular attractive forces (secondary bonds). Low-density polyethylene, on the other hand, contains many more side branches, which create asymmetrical areas of low density and, therefore, low intermolecular attraction.

Fig. 3-46 Creating an ethane monomer.

Typical chain structure

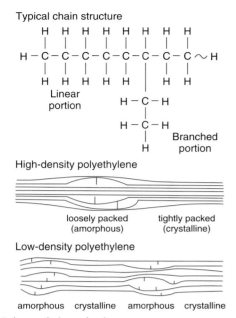

Fig. 3-48 Polymer chain packaging.

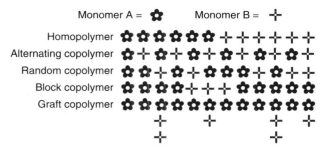

Fig. 3-49 Various copolymer arrangements.

Another consequence of denser molecular packing is higher crystallinity. As symmetrical molecules approach within a critical distance, crystals begin to form in the areas of densest packing. A crystallized area is stiffer and stronger; a noncrystallized (amorphous) area is tougher and more flexible. Other effects of increased crystallinity in a polyethylene polymer are increased resistance to creep, heat, stress cracking, and increased shrinkage after forming.

In general, crystalline polymers are more difficult to process than amorphous polymers. They have higher forming temperatures and melt viscosities, and they tend to shrink and warp more. They have a relatively sharp melting point, that is, they do not soften gradually with an increase in temperature. Furthermore, they remain hard until a given quantity of heat is absorbed, then they rapidly change into a low-viscosity liquid. Reinforcement of crystalline polymers with fibers of glass or other materials improves their load-bearing capabilities significantly.

Amorphous polymers soften gradually as they are heated, but they do not flow as easily (in forming) as crystalline materials. Reinforcing fibers do not significantly improve the strength of amorphous materials at higher temperatures. Examples of amorphous thermoplastics are acrylonitrile-butadiene-styrene (ABS), polystyrene, polycarbonate, polysulfone, and polyetherimide. Crystalline plastics include polyethylene, polypropylene, and polyetheretherketone.

Another method for altering molecular symmetry is combining two different monomers in the polymerization reaction so that each polymer chain is composed partly of monomer A and partly of monomer B. A polymer made from two different monomers is called a *copolymer;* one made from three different monomers is called a *terpolymer.*

All long repeating chains are polymers, regardless of how many monomers are used. However, when a polymer family includes copolymers, the term *homopolymer* is used to identify the single monomer type. An example is the acetal family; acetal resins are available in both homopolymer and copolymer types. Final properties of a copolymer depend on the percentage of monomer A to monomer B, the properties of each, and how they are arranged along the chain. As shown in Fig. 3-49, the arrangement may alternate equally between the two monomers, producing a symmetrical shape capable of a high degree of crystallization. Or the arrangement may be random, creating areas of high crystallinity separated by flexible, amorphous areas. Such a copolymer usually has good rigidity and impact strength.

Block copolymers have large areas of polymerized monomer A alternating with large areas of polymerized monomer B. In general, a block copolymer is similar to an alternating copolymer except that it has stronger crystalline areas and tougher amorphous areas. If both types of blocks are crystalline or both are amorphous, a wide variety of end properties is possible, with characteristics ranging from hard brittle plastics to soft flexible elastomers.

A graft copolymer is made by attaching side groups of monomer B to a main chain of monomer A. A copolymer having a flexible polymer for the main chain and grafted rigid side chains is stiff yet has excellent resistance to impact, a combination of properties not usually found in the same plastic. Copolymers always have different properties from those of a homopolymer made from either monomer.

Compounds of plastics modify the properties of a thermoplastic material by many other methods. For example, fibers are added to increase strength and stiffness, plasticizers for flexibility, lubricants for easier molding or for increasing lubricity of the molded parts, antioxidants for higher temperature stability, ultraviolet (UV) stabilizers for resistance to sunlight, and fillers for economy. Other additives, such as flame retardants, smoke suppressants, and conductive fibers or flakes, provide special properties for certain applications.

Thermosets

Thermoset plastics are made quite differently from thermoplastics. Polymerization (curing) of thermoset plastics is done in two stages, partly by the material supplier and partly by the molder. As illustrated in Fig. 3-50, phenolic (a typical thermoset plastic) is first partially polymerized by reacting phenol with formaldehyde under heat and pressure. The reaction is stopped at the point at which mostly linear chains have formed. The linear chains still contain unreacted portions that are capable of flowing under heat and pressure. The chemical structure of phenol indicates three possible sites (Fig. 3-50) for cross-linking. The hydrogens of two adjacent phenols are replaced by a CH_2 group from formaldehyde. The remaining oxygen combines with the two replaced

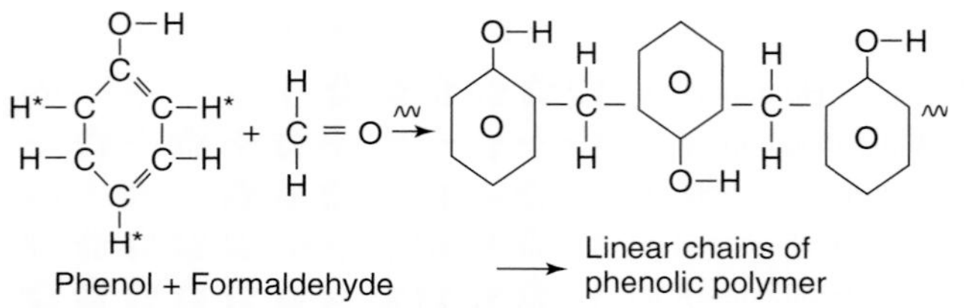

Fig. 3-50 Condensation polymerization of phenolic.

hydrogens to form water, which must be removed. The phenolic structure is shown in simplified form at the right. During molding, the CH_2 groups form cross-links in all planes, creating a single giant molecule.

The final stage of polymerization is completed in the molding press, when the partially reacted phenolic is liquefied under pressure, producing a cross-linking reaction between molecular chains. Unlike a thermoplastic monomer, which has only two reactive ends for linear chain growth, a thermoset monomer must have three or more reactive ends so that its molecular chains cross-link in three dimensions. Rigid thermosets have short chains with many cross-links; flexible thermosets have longer chains with fewer cross-links.

After a thermoset plastic has been molded, virtually all of its molecules are interconnected with strong, permanent, physical bonds that are not heat reversible. Theoretically the entire molded thermoset part could be a single giant molecule. In a sense, curing a thermoset is like cooking an egg. Once the egg is cooked, reheating does not cause remelting, so the egg cannot be remolded. However, if a thermoset is heated too much or too long, the chains break and properties are degraded.

Besides the condensation thermosets for which a byproduct (e.g., water) is created during the reaction in the mold, there are *addition-cured* thermoset plastics. These include epoxy and polyester, which cure by an addition reaction, resulting in no volatile byproducts and fewer molding problems. Most addition-cured thermoset plastics are liquid at room temperature; the two ingredients can simply be mixed and poured into molds where they cross-link (cure) at room temperature into permanent form, much like casting concrete. Molds are often heated, however, to speed the curing process.

In general, thermoset plastics, because of their tightly cross-linked structure, resist higher temperatures and provide greater dimensional stability than do most thermoplastics.

Thermoplastic composites

Thermoplastics that are reinforced with high-strength, high-modulus fibers provide dramatic increases in strength and stiffness, toughness, or dimensional stability. The performance gain of the composites usually more than compensates for their higher cost. Processing usually involves the same methods used for unreinforced resins.

Molded products may contain as little as 5% and as much as 60% fiber by weight. Practically all thermoplastic resins are available in glass-reinforced compounds. Those used in largest volumes are nylon, polypropylene, and polystyrene. Glass-fiber reinforcement improves most mechanical properties of plastics by a factor of two or more. For example, the tensile strength of nylon can be increased from about 10,000 psi to >30,000 psi. A 40% glass-fortified acetal has a flexural

modulus of 1.8×10^6 (up from 0.4×10^6) and a tensile strength of 21,500 psi (up from 8800 psi). Reinforced polyester has double the tensile and impact strength and four times the flexural modulus of the unreinforced resin. Tensile modulus, dimensional stability, and fatigue endurance in reinforced compounds also are improved. Deformation under load of these stiffer materials is reduced significantly.

Carbon-fiber reinforced compounds are available in a number of thermoplastics, including nylon 6/6, polysulfone, polyester, polyphenylene sulfide, polyetherimide, and polyetheretherketone. The carbon-fiber reinforced material, at two to four times the cost of comparable glass-reinforced thermoplastics, offers the ultimate in tensile strength (to 35,000 psi), stiffness, and other mechanical properties.

Aramid fibers, which have greater specific strengths than steel or aluminum, would seem to be an ideal fiber reinforcement for thermoplastic resins. However, chopped aramid fibers do not compound as well as conventional glass or carbon-fiber reinforcements, so the advantages of the theoretical material can be quickly lost due to the limitations of fabrication available to the practitioner.

Thermoset composites

Advanced thermoset composites consist of a resin-matrix material reinforced with high-strength, high-modulus fibers of glass, carbon, aramid (Kevlar), or even boron, usually laid up in layers. An example is epoxy-resin-matrix material reinforced with oriented continuous fibers of carbon or a combination of carbon and glass fibers, laid up in multilayer fashion to form extremely rigid, strong structures.

Most thermoset composites are based on polyester and epoxy resins; of the two, polyester systems predominate. Both can be molded by any process used for thermosetting resins. They can be cured at room temperature and atmospheric pressure. These resins balance low cost and ease of handling along with good mechanical properties and dimensional stability.

Epoxies are low-molecular-weight, syruplike liquids that are cured with hardeners to cross-link thermoset structures that are hard and tough. Because the hardeners or curing agents become part of the finished structure, they are chosen to provide desired properties in the molding part. Epoxies also can be formulated for room temperature curing, but heat curing produces higher properties.

Glass is the reinforcing material most widely used in thermoset composites. Glass fiber, with a tensile strength of 500,000 psi, accounts for almost 90% of the reinforcement in thermosetting resins. Other reinforcements used are carbon, boron, and aramid (Kevlar). Glass fibers are available in several forms: roving (continuous strand), chopped strand, woven fabrics, tubular weaves, continuous-strand mat, chopped-strand mat, and milled fibers. Longer fibers provide the greater strength; continuous fibers, set in tension are the strongest.

Carbon fibers in thermosetting composites can be long and continuous or short and fragmented, and they can be directionally or randomly oriented. In general, short fibers cost less, with lower fabrication costs. However, as with glass, the properties of resulting composites are lower than those obtained with longer or continuous fibers. The outstanding design properties of carbon-fiber/resin-matrix composites are their high strength-to-weight and stiffness-to-weight ratios. With proper selection and placement of fibers, the composites can be stronger and stiffer than equivalent-thickness steel parts and weigh 40% to 70% less. Fatigue resistance of continuous-fiber composites theoretically is excellent. Similar to most rigid materials, however, carbon-fiber composites are relatively brittle and very susceptible to stress concentrations in the form of nicks or scratches. The composites have no yield behavior, and resistance to impact is low.

Mechanical properties

When forces are continuously applied, plastics are subjected to both elastic (springlike) and viscous (slow-flow) behavior. When forces are applied to a plastic, the total resulting deformation is not instantaneous but increases with time, and the deformation most usually is fully recoverable. Because the properties are time dependent, some of the most useful tests for deducing the mechanical behavior of plastics are creep tests. Creep tests are commonly performed by observing the deformation with time of tensile-type or bending specimens.

In the tensile-type creep test, a plastic specimen is clamped on its ends on the tensile tester, and the distance between gauge marks on the specimen is measured. A steady tensile force is applied to the specimen. The magnitude of the force divided by the original cross-sectional area of the specimen is the tensile stress in the material. After the load has been applied, the distance between the gauge marks is measured. The increase in length between the gauge marks divided by the original length is the *strain*. At the particular, constant, controlled, environmental condition of temperature, the strain is regularly observed over a long period of time for a given level of applied stress. The results often are plotted as shown in Fig. 3-51.

The results typically show that the plastic immediately undergoes an elastic strain when the load is applied, followed by a period of further but retarded elastic strain and finally a period of steady viscous flow (Fig. 3-52). The elastic portion of the deformation is deduced by removing the load from the specimen and observing its recovery. Usually the material contracts instantaneously and continues at a slowing rate until it clearly will contract no longer and has suffered some permanent extension.

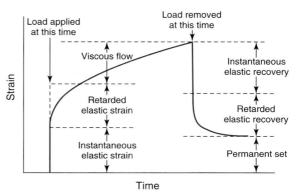

Fig. 3-52 Typical strain "path" a plastic tensile specimen might follow during a loading cycle.

The various sections of the strain path shown in Fig. 3-52 are associated with different types of atomic and molecular motions in the polymer. The instantaneous strain is the result of elastic action of interatomic bond angles and lengths. For all practical purposes, these deformations occur instantaneously. The retarded elastic strain region is thought to result from the cooperative motion of polymer chain segments that cannot occur instantaneously but need time for the necessary coiling or uncoiling and wriggling and jumping of mechanically entangled polymer. The material flow of the polymer is associated with the slipping of one molecule past another.

For example, a polypropylene AFO that has been designed and fabricated to restrain dorsiflexion yields into dorsiflexion as an anteriorly directed force is applied to the calf section with the foot section stabilized. The force required to collapse the AFO to a given angle gradually decreases over time. This *softening* illustrates the creep mechanism.

Changes in the structure of the individual polymer molecule likely will alter the ability of atoms and molecules to move relative to one another and therefore are changes that would alter the deformational characteristics of the plastic. Increasing the molecular weight of the polymer (by increasing the chain length) increases the viscosity of the polymer and the slope of the equilibrium flow region changes (Fig. 3-53). When all the chains are hooked together by cross-links and the molecular weight effectively reaches infinity, the chains cannot slip past one another, so viscous flow is eliminated.

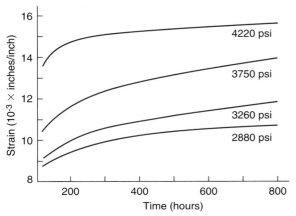

Fig. 3-51 Tensile creep of polycarbonate (at 73°F).

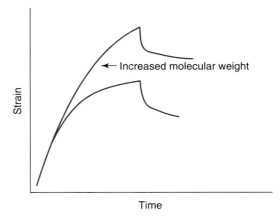

Fig. 3-53 Effect on strain "path" of molecular size.

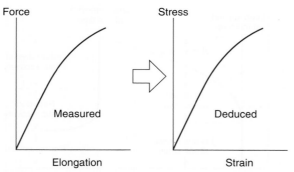

Fig. 3-54 Deduction of short-term stress–strain characteristics.

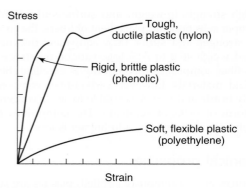

Fig. 3-56 Stress–strain curves for plastics.

The amount of time any material takes to reach a particular level of strain depends on the applied stress and on the temperature; increasing either causes the creeping to accelerate.

Short-term tensile tests

In the short-term tensile test, a specimen of plastic is elongated at a steady rate, and the force applied to the specimen that results in steady elongation is recorded. From these observations, the plastic's short-term tensile stress–strain characteristic is deduced (Fig. 3-54).

For metallic materials, this stress–strain curve is extremely useful. The typical characteristic of a common ductile steel is illustrated in Fig. 3-55. Such materials are considered perfectly elastic if they can be strained to the yield point even if the force is applied for a long time before it is removed. The same is not true for plastics, which are viscoelastic in nature. However, because of the extremely common and appropriate usage of short-term tensile tests for metallic materials and because of their convenience, the natural inclination has been to use the same type of tests for plastics. Typical characteristics results are shown in Fig. 3-56. For these results to have meaning, the temperature and the rate of elongation at which these tests were conducted must be known.

Isochronous stress–strain curve

Isochronous stress–strain curves show the strain that would result if a particular stress were imposed for a particular period of time. The form of this plot is similar to that conventionally used to plot short-term tensile tests, but remember that the types of tests are quite different. However, if the

particular time chosen for obtaining isochronous stress–strain data is reasonably short (e.g., 100 seconds), then the form of the isochronous stress–strain curve will be very similar to short-term stress–strain data derived from test with constant elongation rates (Fig. 3-57).

These curves suggest that if a plastic is strained and the strain is held constant with time, the stress in the plastic reduces with time. Thus, the viscoelastic nature of plastics can cause not only elongation creep under constant stress but also stress relaxation at constant strain.

Stiffness and moduli

Elastic materials are most often used in situations where the stress levels imposed are lower than the material's yield point. The plastic's stiffness is measured by the stress that must be applied to cause strain. This can be viewed graphically on a short-term tensile stress–strain curve as the slope of the elastic portion of the curve. Stiffness for plastics is the same as the modulus of elasticity for metals. The results of short-term tensile tests are often presented in this way (Table 3-11). These nonreinforced plastics have stiffness and strength much lower than those of metals. However, unlike moduli of simple elastic materials such as metals, the moduli of plastics are not single-valued constants but vary with time, temperature, stress, and strain. In general, plastics become less stiff with time and at unexpected rates (Fig. 3-58).

Strain recovery

Although all plastics creep, upon removal of the applied force the strain in the plastic decreases with time as though the

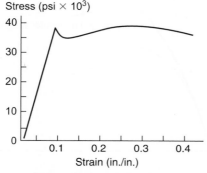

Fig. 3-55 Stress–strain curve for low-carbon steel.

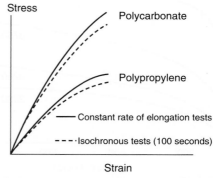

Fig. 3-57 Similarity of stress–strain curves at constant temperature.

Table 3-11 Short-term mechanical properties of some plastics and metals

Material	Specific Gravity	Tensile Strength*	Stiffness in Tensions*
Thermoplastic			
Nylon	1.09–1.14	8–12	200–400
Polyethylene	0.92–0.97	1–6	20–200
Polyester	1.31–1.38	8–10	—
Polypropylene	0.90–0.91	4–6	200
PVC	1.15–1.40	5–9	300–600
Thermosets			
Epoxy	1.11–1.40	4–13	300
Polyester	1.10–1.46	6–13	300–600
Metals			
Aluminum alloys	2.80	11–83	10,000
Steel alloys	7.85–7.92	73–230	28,000

*psi $X10^3$

material had a memory. When the loading on a plastic is intermittent, as occurs during the stance phase of walking in a person with a polypropylene AFO, there is not enough time in the swing phase for the material's memory to return the plastic to its strain-free shape. When the plastic AFO is not worn, however, the creep strain that set in during walking tends to disappear. Creep strain accumulates from loading cycle to cycle (Fig. 3-59).

Plastics may experience a variety of changes under the action of loads continuously applied for long periods of time. The susceptibility of plastics to creep is important. The strength of plastics, like creep, is dependent on time and temperature. Long-term strength data may be derived from creep-type tests in which tensile specimens are subject to steady loads at constant temperature. Tensile specimens eventually fail by either rupture or onset of necking (a phenomenon where the loaded tensile specimen begins to elongate rapidly because of the occurrence of a local area of thinning down). The stress levels that cause failure by rupture or necking are presented as envelopes over creep data (Fig. 3-60). The fact that plastics weaken with age even under steady loads is called *static fatigue*.

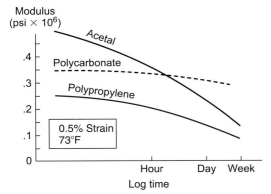

Fig. 3-58 Variation of tensile creep with time.

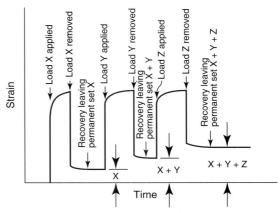

Fig. 3-59 Deforming and recovery with intermittent loading.

Effects of temperature

Temperature has a major effect on the mechanical behavior of plastics. The effects of temperature on the creep of a thermoplastic are shown in Fig. 3-61. Increasing temperature tends to cause softening of a plastic, with consequent reduction in strength. Lowering the temperature below the glass transition temperature can cause the plastic to become brittle.

Impact loading

The performance of plastics under impact loads can be compared by experimentally determining the amount of energy required to break specimens in impact pendulum tests. In the Izod impact test, a cantilevered beam specimen of fixed dimensions with a carefully machined notch is placed in a clamp and a pendulum of known mass swung against it. The energy consumed in breaking the specimen is calculated by measuring the pendulum swing-through height and comparing it with the starting height. The impact strength of the plastic then is calculated as energy units per unit of specimen (ft-lb/in). The results of impact tests show that many plastics have high impact strengths and that some are sensitive to the sharpness of the notch radius and the temperature of testing (Fig. 3-62).

In view of the inherent limitations of the Izod test as a result of the specimen notch, other forms of impact tests have become more commonly used. One tensile-type test involves a tensile specimen mounted between a pendulum head and a cross-head clamp. When the pendulum is released and swings past a fixed anvil, the cross-head clamp is arrested but the pendulum head continues forward, thus loading the specimen. The energy required to cause failure then can be measured without influence of the notch sensitivity.

Hardness

In general, plastics are much softer than many other materials. The hardness of plastics is gauged by indentation tests of the Rockwell type. A steel ball under a minor load is applied to the surface of the specimen. This action slightly indents the surface and ensures good contact. The gauge then is set to zero. The major load is applied for 15 seconds and removed, leaving the minor load still applied. After 15 seconds, the diameter of the indentation remaining is measured and

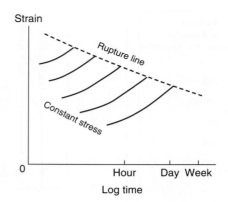

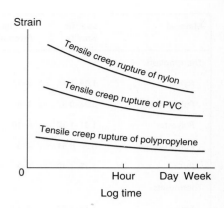

Fig. 3-60 Example of long-term strength data derived from tensile tests at constant loads and temperature.

related to a hardness number. Rockwell hardness can differentiate the relative hardness of different plastics but is not valid for comparing the hardness of plastics based entirely on this test because elastic recovery as well as hardness is involved.

Thermosetting plastics

A thermosetting resin is a synthetic organic polymer that cures to a solid infusible mass by forming a three-dimensional network of covalent chemical bonds.

Thermoset plastics compete with metals, ceramics, and thermoplastics. Compared to metals, they possess corrosion resistance, lighter weight, and insulating properties, and they can be processed at lower pressures and temperatures. The flow characteristics of uncured thermoset plastics can be used to form complex anatomic shapes, allowing low-cost production.

Compared to ceramics, thermoset plastics offer lighter weight, more toughness, and easier processing. The principal advantage of ceramics is high-temperature performance. Thermosets offer advantages over thermoplastics in terms of reduced creep and improved crack resistance. The three-dimensional polymer network in thermosets also leads to improved machinability, low shrinkage, and improved high-temperature performance. The low initial viscosity of thermoset plastics permits incorporation of large amounts of fillers or fibers and has led to the development of many low-cost fabrication processes.

One limitation of many thermoset plastics is poor impact resistance. Consequently, devices requiring enhanced toughness are best served by thermoplastics.

Polyester thermoset plastics are popular because of their relative ease of fabrication and relatively low cost. Epoxy thermoset plastics are only slightly more difficult to fabricate but are much higher in cost. Acrylic thermoset plastics also are popular because of their low viscosity and ease of fabrication.

Acrylic, epoxy, and polyester thermosets cure by an "addition" reaction that results in no volatile byproducts and fewer fabrication problems. These plastics are liquid at room temperature. The two ingredients can simply be mixed and poured where they cross-link (cure) into permanent form at room temperature.

Most thermosetting plastics can be cured, or set, permanently into shape by the heat to which they are subjected during forming. Once thermosetting plastics have hardened, reheating does not soften them. A simplified comparison of the two classifications of plastics is that thermoplastic materials are softened by heat, whereas thermosetting materials are hardened by heat. Paraffin wax, in a sense, is a thermoplastic material that softens when heated and hardens or solidifies when cooled. The principle of thermosetting material can be demonstrated by hard boiling an egg. The egg originally is soft and fluid; however, once hardened by heating, the egg remains hard, and no amount of reheating can return the egg to a fluid state.

Thermosetting plastics exhibit little cold flow and therefore can be subjected to continuous loads. Permissible loads

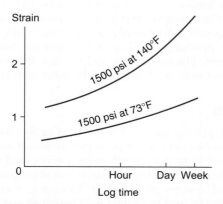

Fig. 3-61 Variation of tensile creep with temperature for a thermoplastic polyester.

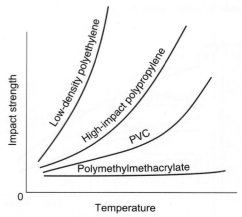

Fig. 3-62 Effect of temperature on impact strength.

must be determined from cold-flow measurements and not from ultimate strengths.

Some thermosetting resins are cured, or hardened, by heat alone. Others are cured by catalysts and promoters. Catalysts are materials that trigger the curing process. Promoters primarily control the rate of cure. An important factor in their use is providing ample working time for the practitioner to form the shape before the plastic hardens. Some plastics give off a heat of reaction once the catalyst starts the cure. The heat speeds the rate of hardening and must be taken into account when determining the amount of catalyst and promoter to be used.

The terms *thermoplastic* and *thermosetting* can be considered chemical classifications of plastics. Plastics also can be divided into the following three physical classifications:

1. *Rigid:* Relatively nondeforming under loads
2. *Flexible:* Deforming under loads
3. *Elastomeric:* Having high elongation

Condensation reactions

Plastic resins are formed by condensation reactions in which two or more *unlike* molecules are combined to form a larger molecule, accompanied by the loss of water or a gas.

After condensation is complete, there is a noticeable separation between the resin and the water; this water must be removed. In certain condensation reactions, the byproduct is a gas, which is carried off while the reaction is taking place.

The raw materials for some plastic products show no disposition toward reacting when mixed together. It then becomes necessary to add a catalyst to start the reaction. Although the catalyst takes no part in the reaction, it has a direct influence on the outcome.

Polymerization

Polymerization is the stage or reaction that follows condensation. The resin formed in the condensation reaction, known as the *monomer*, is not suitable as a molding material but can be used as the base for lacquers. The monomer is converted into the polymer, and this usually takes place during molding or fabricating processes, when the monomer is subjected to the action of a catalyst and varying conditions of heat and pressure. The resin in the monomeric stage has a known molecular weight; the polymer is an unknown multiple of this weight.

By varying the amount of catalyst and the conditions of heat and pressure on a monomer, the degree of polymerization and the molecular weight of the resulting polymer can be increased or decreased. The higher the molecular weight, the harder the material becomes. Prolonged heating at a high temperature produces a polymer with a large molecular weight. High pressure causes the same result.

In general, a monomer is a liquid, whereas a polymer is a solid. Synthetic resins usually are amorphous—that is, noncrystalline—and have no definite melting point. They do, however, have a definite temperature range in which they soften. Because the transformation from monomer to polymer is the change from liquid to solid, there is an increase in viscosity during the polymerization process. Also, as polymerization progresses, the softening point, or temperature at which the material begins to soften, increases. The

practitioner must keep all these factors in mind when choosing and using a thermosetting plastic.

It may seem strange that polymerized synthetic resins are found in both thermoplastic and thermosetting types of molding compounds. This can be explained by the fact that a synthetic resin in the thermoplastic class is fully polymerized when it is used as a molding compound, whereas a synthetic resin in a thermosetting molding material is only partially polymerized. Complete polymerization occurs in the actual molding or laminating operation.

Controlling the rate of polymerization of thermosetting plastics

When fabricating plastics of the thermosetting type, usually the rate of polymerization must be adjusted. The plastic may be polymerizing too fast, or it may not be polymerizing fast enough. The rate adjustment can be made by adding an accelerator or an inhibitor as the need dictates. An accelerator, or promoter, chemically activates the resin so that subsequent operation brings the resin to the desired polymerized state at a faster rate. The inhibitor holds back, or slows up, the rate of polymerization. The percentage of promoter or inhibitor used depends on the storage temperature of the resin, the temperature of the working area, and the amount of working time required by the operator. It has become common practice to use a catalyst that also performs the role of the promoter or inhibitor, so careful consideration must be given to accurate rates and mixing of appropriate materials.

Laminated plastics

Laminates consist of base materials impregnated with a plastic resin that is allowed to harden under pressure. The plastic resins used are thermosetting and are hardened by polymerization. The base materials provide mechanical strength, and the resin provides rigidity and dimensional stability. Some base materials used are nylon, Dacron fabrics, fiberglass, boron, and aramid (Kevlar).

Laminated plastics are divided into three groups, depending on the pressure used in their formation. The first group is *high-pressure laminates*. These laminates are formed from thermosetting materials under pressures ranging from 1000 to 2000 psi. They are strong, are lightweight, and have high-impact resistance. They are suitable for uses such as paneling, countertops, and safety helmets.

The second group is *low-pressure laminates*. These laminates are formed using pressures ranging from 15 to 1000 psi. Vacuum bag molding falls in this group. Layers of resin-impregnated, reinforcing fabric material is placed over the mold, and the layers are covered with a flexible rubber sheeting or bag. The sheeting is sealed along the edges of the mold. Air between the mold and the sheeting is withdrawn, which causes atmospheric pressure (14.7 psi) to press the sheeting uniformly against the entire surface of the mold. With some changes in mold design, the same bag molding principle can be used with positive air pressure considerably in excess of atmospheric pressure.

The third and final group is *contact pressure laminates*. These laminates are formed under pressures as low as 0.25 to 15 psi. This type of lamination is used in situations where each piece must be custom-made using hand pressure. Contact pressure laminates usually are made from thermosetting materials. They are economical, possess high strength, are lightweight, and can be formed in flat or three-dimensional shapes.

Cellular structures

Cellular plastics, or foamed plastics, consist of plastic resins that have been "foamed" or filled with bubbles of gas before the resin hardens. The gas bubbles in the resin can be generated in numerous ways, but a discussion of them is beyond the scope of this chapter. Basically, both thermoplastic and thermosetting resins can be used, and the resulting foam structures can be rigid, semirigid, or flexible as desired.

Sandwich constructions

Sandwich constructions are used where maximum stiffness is required for a given weight of material. They are made by laminating a cellular core between skins of metal or thin plastic fabric laminates. Cellular cores can be resin-impregnated paper honeycombs, balsa wood, or cellular plastics.

Miscellaneous structures

Miscellaneous structures involving plastics that are of interest to the practitioner include glass and cotton fabrics coated with thermoplastic resins and fabrics of glass and plastic fibers woven together. After brief immersion in a solvent, these structures can be easily shaped to a form. When the solvent evaporates, a light, rigid-formed article remains.

The service success of any plastic article depends as much on the design and fabrication process as on the material itself. Frequently, good materials fail when the same materials, if properly engineered, would have been quite satisfactory.

The type and amount of material (reinforcement) also plays a part in the service of the article. The practitioner must have a thorough understanding of the application for a device so that he or she can choose the proper plastic and the proper methods of fabrication.

Polyesters

Polyesters are versatile because they can be molded, cast, and laminated with contact pressure sleeves over inexpensive molds of plaster, rubber, or low-melting metals. Polyesters can range from rubberlike materials to hard, rigid substances. They are rapidly achieving great popularity for small-scale work. They do not liberate moisture in the curing process. Coloring possibilities are unlimited, and special grades that are resistant to flame or to outdoor weathering are available. The chemical resistance of the different grades varies a great deal, but in general polyesters are swollen by ketones and esters and attacked by caustics. Polyesters are quite resistant to common substances such as gasoline, alcohol, acids, and moisture.

Unsaturated polyester resins range in color from clear (water) to white to light tan. Because of this color range, some are used in optical assemblies. However, one of their greatest uses is in fabric laminates, which, on a weight basis, are comparable in strength to steel and are extremely shock resistant.

Using very low pressures, this fabric–resin combination can easily be formed into a large variety of shapes. The working time available before hardening can be controlled by adjusting temperature, catalyst, and promoter. The cured laminate is chemically stable and practically insoluble, so it forms a durable product.

Mixtures of polyesters and other resins are used in prostheses and orthoses to make laminated parts by contact lamination. A lamination made from 100% polyester resin is too brittle, so mixtures of rigid and flexible resins are used. Flexible resins contain about 50% styrene by volume; the remainder is polyester. The composition of mixtures ranges from 60% rigid and 40% flexible resin to 75% rigid and 25% flexible resin.

With special mixtures of resins, catalyst, and promoter, laminates can be formulated that bench cure without the use of external heating. The internal heat of reaction during polymerization is adequate to complete the cure. However, because a toxic gas is given off during the curing process, the recommendation is to heat cure all polyester laminates to drive off all of the gas. Any gas remaining in the laminate is believed to pose a risk of toxic reaction to the patient. Toxic gas can originate from the use of certain plasticizers, such as tricresyl phosphate, which are vaporized by the heat given off during the curing process. Heat curing usually is performed in an oven at a temperature of about 250°F (120°C).

Two types of polyester resins can be used for making laminates: the air-inhibited type and the non–air-inhibited type. Inhibition is the slowing down of polymerization or curing of the resin because of the presence of atmospheric oxygen. Usually a wax additive is used as a seal. It acts by migrating to the surface of the resin and forming a protective coating.

Air-inhibited resins require careful control of the air seal and manual mixing to control the flexibility. The flexibility can range from 100% rigid to 100% flexible. Non–air-inhibited types have a preformulated flexibility. An air seal for these types is advisable but not required.

Uses for polyester laminates include sockets, cuffs, and artificial hands. Other devices used are mentioned in the instruction on lamination given later in this chapter.

Laminating plastic parts

Laminated plastic parts for orthoses and prostheses are best prepared over plaster of Paris forms. After the plaster has dried completely, it should be coated with a lubricant. A polyvinyl alcohol (PVA) bag also can be used to form the first layer against the plaster. In one laminating method, the fabric is next placed in contact with the plaster form (or bag), and a thin coating of resin, sufficient to saturate the fabric, is applied to the exposed surface. Then a dry piece of fabric is smoothed into place in such a way as to provide intimate contact between the two layers of fabric and to force any excess resin to the surface. Another coat of resin and another piece of fabric are alternately added until the desired thickness is obtained. The whole assembly then is surrounded by a PVA bag, excess resin is squeezed out, and the laminate is oven cured.

In another plastic lamination method, fiberglass, tubular nylon, or cotton stockinette is used as a slight resin reinforcement. Normally, three or four layers of the material are placed on the inner PVA bag on the cast to which a release agent has been applied. If extra strength requirements are indicated,

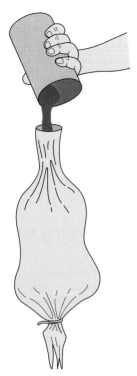

Fig. 3-63 Pouring polyester resin.

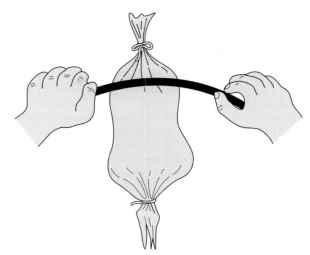

Fig. 3-64 Uniformly distributing resin.

stronger materials such as glass cloth or special metal reinforcements can be used in particularly critical areas.

After the stockinette has been pulled over the plaster cast and tied, a snug-fitting PVA bag is pulled over the stockinette to form a tight and smooth outer surface. Prepared polyester resin is poured into the outer PVA sleeve as shown in Fig. 3-63 and made to impregnate the reinforcing stockinette. When the resin has been poured, the tapered, outer PVA sleeve is pulled down farther to increase the mold pressure, force the resin to impregnate the stockinette more effectively, and force air from the resin. The resin itself acts as a lubricant to facilitate the additional downward movement of the PVA sleeve. The sleeve provides a necessary airtight seal to ensure airless cure of the polyester.

It is necessary to tie the end of the PVA bag and proceed with the *stringing* process using a light but strong cord. As shown in Fig. 3-64, a length of this cord, held between the hands, is pressed against the outside PVA bag and moved up and down to distribute the resin uniformly and to eliminate air pockets.

The plastic laminate is bench cured for about 45 minutes. An oven cure at 180°F to 200°F (80°C–90°C) for about 45 minutes completes the curing and solidification of the plastic. When curing has been completed, the PVA is stripped away, and excess cured plastic is removed.

Thermoforming plastics

Thermoplastic materials can be repeatedly softened by elevated heating and hardened by cooling. Thermoplastics make up 88% to 90% of all plastics processed.

Any thermoplastic resin that can be extruded or calendared into sheet or film can be thermoformed. However, those with low strength at forming temperature may be difficult to form. Sheet and film are produced by extrusion, coextrusion, continuous casting, extrusion casting, calendaring, compression molding, autoclave, and press laminating. Although an infinite range with variable properties of thermoforming plastics is possible, there are two types of thermoplastics.

Amorphous

Amorphous materials are devoid of crystallization (no definite order) and have a randomly ordered molecular structure. Their behavior is similar to a viscous, inelastic liquid. On heating, an amorphous sheet gradually softens and eventually acquires the characteristics of a liquid but without a definite point of transition from solid to liquid state. Amorphous materials normally have better hot strength characteristics than crystalline ones. Amorphous plastics are never as easy flowing as crystalline resins. When cooled, they do not reach a totally *nonflowing* solid state. Therefore, they have a tendency toward creep or movement with age when a load is applied. Examples of amorphous plastics are ABS, styrene, vinyl, acrylic, the cellulosics, and polycarbonates.

Crystalline

Crystalline thermoplastic molecules are an orderly group of molecules that have a tendency to align in rigid, precise, highly ordered structures such as a chainlink fence. This gives them good stiffness and low creep. Most of the crystalline materials used in thermoforming are also partly amorphous (e.g., polypropylene normally is about 65% crystalline and 35% amorphous). Unlike amorphous plastics, crystalline sheet, when heated, remains stiff until it reaches the glass transition temperature (Tg). At the Tg, the crystalline material softens. In the case of high-density polyethylene (HDPE), this temperature is above 257°F (at the Tg, a natural HDPE sheet turns from translucent to transparent). This is also the minimum forming temperature of the sheet. As the sheet continues to become hotter, it rapidly becomes fluid. The next condition to occur is the ideal forming temperature. Unfortunately, with most crystalline materials, this is only a few degrees below the melt temperature. Consequently, much of this type of material is *cold formed* at the *orienting* temperature or slightly above. This situation can set up an excessive amount of internal stresses, causing a lower heat distortion point, increased warpage, and less impact strength. This explains why some crystalline materials are difficult to thermoform. Polypropylene resin suppliers in particular have improved the behavior of this polymer to correct these problems.

Crystalline materials require a greater amount of heat than do amorphous plastics to reach the Tg. Once at this temperature, little additional heat is required to reach the forming temperature. Nylon, polypropylene, polyethylene, and acetal are common examples of crystalline materials.

Commonly used materials

Polypropylene

- *Characteristics:* Notch sensitive; edges must be smooth; surface easily marred when hot; may warp or distort if removed from the mold too rapidly (ideally leave overnight)
- *Common uses:* All orthoses where rigidity is required
- *Typical shrink*: 1.5% to 2%

Copolymer

- *Characteristics:* Will cold flow (creep); not as rigid or brittle as polypropylene; blanching or crazing develops at areas of high or cyclic stress; moderately notch sensitive (polish edges to avoid crazing)
- *Common uses:* All orthoses where some flexibility is required; prosthetic check sockets
- *Typical shrink*: 1.5% to 2%

Polyethylene

- *Characteristics:* Flexible and easy to vacuum form; cold flow under pressure with sustained use; thinner gauges can be cut by hand; not particularly notch sensitive (however, edges should be polished)
- *Common uses:* Spinal and upper limb orthoses; orthoses in which greater flexibility is required
- *Typical shrink*: low density, 1.5% to 3%; high density, 3% to 3.5%

Surlyn (Ionomer)

- *Characteristics:* Transparent (for optimum clarity, material should be worked over a bare, wet, warm cast); not as rigid or brittle as polypropylene; very tough; cold flows; may be solvent bonded; not affected by cold; notch sensitive (tears rather than cracks); can be worked at a wide range of temperatures
- *Common uses:* Check sockets; all orthoses

Copolyester (Durr-Plex)

- *Characteristics:* Very rigid and brittle; difficult to judge proper working temperature; for best results and to reduce brittleness work with a warm cast (140°F)
- *Common uses:* Check sockets

Polycarbonate

- *Characteristics:* Hydrophilic (must be hydrated 48 hours at 275°F for ⅜-inch-thick material; rigid at proper working temperature; sensitive to acetone and other solvents
- *Common uses:* Check sockets

Kydex

- *Characteristics:* Abrasion resistance; dimensionally stable; rigid; can be drape formed without vacuum
- *Common uses:* Thoracolumbosacral orthosis (TLSO) body jackets; cervical orthoses

Thermoforming processing temperature

Cast and set

The set temperature is the temperature at which the thermoplastic sheet hardens and can be safely taken from the cast (Table 3-12). This generally is defined as the heat distortion temperature at 66 psi (ASTM D 648). The closer the cast temperature is to the set temperature, without exceeding it, the less are the internal stress and warping.

Lower processing limit

This is the lowest possible temperature for the sheet before it is completely formed (Table 3-12). Material formed at or below this limit has severely increased internal stress that can cause warpage, lower impact strength, and other poor physical properties.

Normal forming

This is the temperature the sheet should reach for proper forming conditions under normal circumstances (Table 3-12). The core of the sheet should be at this temperature. The normal forming temperature is determined by heating the sheet to the highest temperature at which it still has enough hot strength or elasticity to be handled yet is below the degrading temperature.

Table 3-12 Theromoforming processing temperature (°F)

Material	Cast and Set	Lower Limit	Normal Forming	Upper Limit
Polypropylene	190	290	310–325	331
Copolymer	190	290	310–325	331
High-density polyethylene	180	260	275	331
Low-density polyethylene	180	260	275	331
Surlyn	130	200	250	450
Copolyester	170	250	300	330
Polycarbonate	280	335	375	400
Kydex	—	—	380–390	400

Upper limit

This is the temperature at which the thermoplastic sheet begins to degrade or decompose (Table 3-12). It is crucial to ensure that the sheet temperature stays less than this amount. When using radiant heat, the sheet surface temperature should be carefully monitored to avoid degradation while waiting for the "core" of the material to reach forming temperature. These limits can be exceeded for only a short time, with minimum impairment to the sheet properties.

The practitioner should know the thermal conductivity of the plastic, particularly how long the material must be at a particular temperature for a given thickness to ensure that the core has been elevated to the forming temperature.

The least amount of internal stress is obtained by a hot cast, hot sheet, and a rapid vacuum.

Sheet selection

When selecting a sheet of plastic for forming, several factors must be considered: (1) depth of draw, (2) desired finished thickness, (3) rigidity, and (4) shrink. The deeper the draw, the larger the sheet should be. By forcing a small sheet to stretch over a deep draw, shrink, additional stress, and uneven wall thickness can occur in the finished product.

A rule of thumb for forming sockets is the material sheet size should be twice as large as the depth of the draw to allow for the natural flow of material. An 8-inch draw requires a 16-inch piece of material. If the plastic is forced over a longer pull, the stress in the plastic and the probability of increased shrink are increased. This sizing must be adjusted by considering the size of vacuum systems, finished wall thickness desired, available sheet sizes, and temperature of the cast.

Sheet heating considerations

Once the type of material and the sheet size have been selected, the plastic is heated. The sheet of plastic should be supported in the center of the oven, allowing air to circulate on all sides. If the sheet is supported against the side of the oven, the air flow in that area is reduced and causes uneven heating.

To ensure even heating of the sheet, the oven must be calibrated. To calibrate the oven, support a frame or grid inside the oven at the same position the plastic will be heated. Using an accurate thermometer, take rapid readings every 4 to 6 inches, left to right and front to rear. Note any variations. If the variations are >5°F, baffle or shadow the hot areas so that the heat is as even as possible.

During heating of the plastic, minimize the number of times the oven doors are opened. Door openings affect the heat cycles and may produce hot and cold spots throughout the sheet. When the plastic is completely heated and removed from the oven, avoid drafts from the doors, windows, or air conditioning vents, which also can cause cold spots in the sheet. Cold spots can cause uneven wall thickness, difficulties in forming, warping, and irregular surface finishes.

As the sheet is heated, the heat is transferred to the sheet by the circulating hot air. Heat also is transferred to the sheet through the metal frame if it is clamped tightly to the sheet. The metal frame transfers heat to the sheet much faster than does the air around the plastic. This can be seen in increased thinning along the edges. To overcome this effect,

Table 3-13 *K* factor (K = btu/hr-ft^2-°F)

Material	K Factor	Heat Transfer Rate*
Air (ref.)	0.106	0.76
Wool felt	0.021	1.00
Spruce	0.052	2.50
Maple	0.094	4.50
Epoxy	0.131	6.20
Plaster of Paris	0.174	8.3
Alum-filled epoxy	0.50–0.99	24–47
Acrylic	1.4	67
Stainless steel	9.4	448
Bronze	20.5	976
Steel	26.0	1238
Kirksite	60.4	2876
Aluminum	115	5476

*Heat transfer rate factor—compared to wool felt.

insulate the plastic from the frame. For possible insulating materials, see *K* factor in Table 3-13.

The hot air comes in contact with the surface of the plastic, and heat transfer begins. The heat migrates toward the center of the sheet, increasing the total sheet temperature. In this process, uneven heating in the sheet occurs because the outer surface is hotter than the internal core temperature (Fig. 3-65).

To heat a sheet more quickly, practitioners commonly set the oven temperature higher than the upper limit temperature of the material. This should not be done because excessive heat can be absorbed by the plastic, and the surface of the material will begin to deteriorate.

If a sheet of polypropylene is heated with an oven set at 375°F to 400°F (190°C–200°C), the plastic surface temperature is close to the oven temperature. The upper limit for polypropylene is 331°F (166°C). At the point the material turns from milky to clear, the material has reached the lower processing limit or the Tg point. The sheet now has a temperature gradient of 375°F (190°C) at the surface to 290°F (143°C)

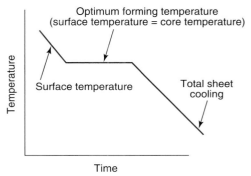

Fig. 3-65 Surface temperature.

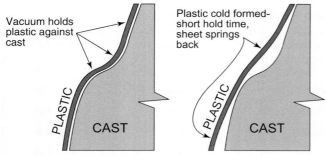

Vacuum holds plastic against cast

Plastic cold formed-short hold time, sheet springs back

PLASTIC

CAST

PLASTIC

CAST

Fig. 3-66 Effect of inadequate vacuum hold time.

at the core. The plastic formed at this point has stresses, uneven forming, and uneven surface finishes. The sheet must reach equilibrium before it is formed.

A blast of cool air on the surface helps reduce the surface temperature and solidify the surface for a better finish. This procedure is tricky because the sheet is so close to the lower processing temperature. If the sheet cools too rapidly, it tends to warp from internal stresses. Referring back to the *K* factors (Table 3-13), plaster of Paris has a significantly greater *K* factor than air. When forming over a plaster cast, the plaster removes the heat much faster than the outside air. The effects of this uneven cooling can be seen in body jackets. Body jacket plastic is formed directly on the plaster cast and has a tendency to curl inward after removal. Conversely, plastic that is formed against a foam liner has a tendency to curl outward after removal.

It is important to maintain the vacuum on the part until the entire plastic sheet reaches the set temperature of the plastic. With the low thermal conductivity of plastic, it takes several minutes for the core temperature to drop to the set temperature. Not uncommonly, vacuum is maintained on a thick part for >1 hour.

Figure 3-66 shows the effect of removing the vacuum too soon. The memory of the sheet causes the return to its original flat shape.

Another effect that occurs is thickening of material on the first surface contacted by the hot plastic (Fig. 3-67). The plaster cast chills the plastic and prevents it from forming with uniform thickness over the entire cast.

Heating thermoplastics

The three methods of heating are convection, conduction, and radiation.

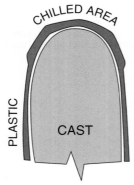

CHILLED AREA

PLASTIC

CAST

Fig. 3-67 Thickening effect.

Convection

This is the slowest heating process. Convection heat transfer takes place when a material is exposed to a moving fluid (e.g., recirculating hot air) that is at a higher temperature.

Convection heating in the thermoforming industry is done with the use of a hot-air recirculating oven. The oven temperature is carefully maintained at the thermoforming temperature of the particular material to be formed. Air is a greater insulator, and plastic materials absorb heat slowly, so this method of heating is relatively slow. The specific heat of the particular material governs the heating cycle. When comparing convection heating with radiant heating, convection heating is extremely slow. For example, a 0.125-inch-thick acrylic sheet has a specific heat of 0.35. In a well-baffled hot-air recirculating oven running at the forming temperature of 360°F (approximately 180°C) throughout, about 1 minute of heating is required for every 10 mm of sheet thickness. This timing should always be checked with the material supplier because the amount of time varies with the material. With use of radiant heat and the proper wave length, 0.125-inch acrylic sheet can be brought to a core temperature of approximately 350°F to 360°F (180°C) in just over two minutes.

The main advantage of convection heat is its uniformity of heating and the ability to keep the sheet surfaces from getting hotter than the oven temperature. This method is recommended when heating (1) heavy-gauge foam sheets, (2) very thick, solid sheets, (3) sheet stocks where the thickness is difficult to control accurately, and (4) sheets where surfaces have been planished (heat-press polished) and when (5) surfaces might degrade easily if overheated.

The most accurate hot-air recirculating ovens are electrically powered and for this reason are used whenever precise temperature control and heating are needed.

Conduction

This is a faster method than convection heating but slower than radiant heating. Heat transfer by conduction takes place when temperature gradients exist within a material.

Most conduction heater plates used in thermoforming are Teflon-coated aluminum plates that are electrically heated. Uniform heat can be maintained with electric heaters. The surface of the hot plate should have a uniform temperature and the same heat sink distribution throughout. As in convection heating, the contact plates usually are run at the same temperature as the forming temperature of the sheet. This prevents degradation of the surface and gives extremely uniform heat even when sheet thickness varies.

Radiation

Radiation is the energy transmitted between two separated bodies (for thermoformers that is the sheet and the radiant heater surface) at different temperatures by means of electromagnetic waves. It is the most energy-efficient way of heating sheet material. Infrared wavelength radiation elements are the usual source of heat; the specific wavelength is related to a given temperature of a specific radiant heater.

All types of radiation have an important property in common: they travel with the same velocity (the speed of light). This radiation can be considered a transporter of energy. As the radiant emitter is directly exposed to the material to be processed, a high percentage of the electromagnetic waves is absorbed within the plastic sheet only if the emitter operates at the proper wavelength, and the wavelength is determined strictly by the emitter-surface temperature. *Tuning* the radiant heater to the particular material's best absorbing range can be an advantage. Convection and conduction have to absorb and give up heat through contact with only the surface of the sheet and then transferred to the "core" by conduction; thus, they are much slower and more inefficient than radiant heat.

Description of the most popular heating elements

Small-diameter coiled Nichrome wire

Efficiency: New 16% to 18%; 6 months, 8% to 10%
Average life: 1500 hours

Although small-diameter coiled Nichrome wire is least expensive, it is inefficient and heats nonuniformly with use.

Tubular rods and metal panels

Efficiency: New, 42%; 6 months, 21%
Average life: 3000 hours

Tubular rods are inexpensive, heat nonuniformly with use, and are difficult to screen or mask for profile heat.

Ceramic panels and quartz panels

Efficiency: New, 55% to 62%; 6 months, 48% to 55%
Average life: 1200 to 1500 hours

Ceramic and quartz panels are the most cost efficient because they heat uniformly, are efficient, and are ideal for profile heating.

Gas fired, infrared-type

Efficiency: New, 40% to 45%; 6 months, 25%
Average life: 1000 to 6000 hours

Gas-fired, infrared-type heating elements are inexpensive initially and inexpensive to operate but do not heat uniformly.

Conclusion

Successful orthotic management requires a clear understanding of the condition being treated and a realistic plan to address the biomechanical deficits presented. A thorough knowledge of the principles summarized in this chapter is the final prerequisite to ensuring that the orthosis provided is durable, safe, and unobtrusive and performs the required function for as long as required. The engineering principles highlighted here are the fundamentals of modern orthotic design, quality device management, and patient safety practices. These principles form the basis of the manufacturers' property charts, instructional sheets, and directions.

Understanding these fundamentals provides the practitioner with the skills needed to perform the appropriate assessment of designs, materials, and failures and most importantly the ability to justify the decisions, practices, and techniques used to create the device.

Appendix

Thermal stress
Example 1

A straight aluminum wire 100 feet long is subject to a tensile stress of 10,000 psi. Determine the total elongation of the wire. What temperature change would produce this same elongation? Take $E = 10^7$ psi and $\alpha = 12.5 \times 10^{-6}$°F. The total elongation is given by Equation 3-7:

$$\Delta L = \frac{FL_0}{AE} = \frac{(10,000)(100 \times 12)}{10^7}$$

From Equation 3-6, it can be seen that a rise in temperature of ΔT would cause this same expansion if:

$$1.20 = (12.5 \times 10^{-6})(100 \times 12)\Delta T$$
$$\Delta T = 78.2°F$$

Centroids and center of gravity
Example 2

Calculate the centroid coordinates for a **P**-shaped object (Fig. 3-A1). This object can be divided into two rectangles (A_1 and A_2), one triangle (A_3), and a semicircle (A_4). Next draw a 'Cartesian coordinate' system with the origin at the bottom left. The centroid is calculated from Equation 3-9 as follows:

$$\frac{\bar{x}_1 A_1 + \bar{x}_2 A_2 + \bar{x}_3 A_3 + \bar{x}_4 A_4}{A_1 + A_2 + A_3 + A_4}$$

$$\frac{\bar{y}_1 A_1 + \bar{y}_2 A_2 + \bar{y}_3 A_3 + \bar{y}_4 A_4}{A_1 + A_2 + A_3 + A_4}$$

Moment of inertia and parallel axis theorem
Example 3

To increase mediolateral stability in a KAFO, a standard ⅝-inch × ³⁄₁₆-inch sidebar on a KAFO is reinforced by welding ⅝-inch × ³⁄₁₆-inch reinforcing ribs perpendicular to the sidebar proximal to the mechanical knee

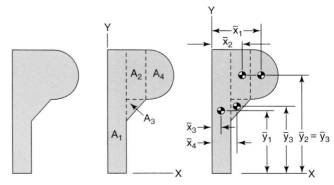

Fig. 3-A1 Centroid analysis.

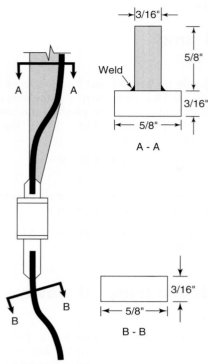

Fig. 3-A2 Knee joint reinforcement.

joint (Fig. 3-A2). Calculate the moment of inertia of the sidebar proximally (A–A) and distally (B–B) to the mechanical knee joint. The proximal sidebar cross section at A–A is more complicated and is determined first.

Proximal (Fig. 3-A3)

The moment of inertia for the proximal (A–A) section about the centroidal axis must be calculated from the parallel axis theorem:

$$I_{cc} = I_{xx} - Ad^2 = \text{parallel axis theorem}$$

However, the moment of inertia about the base I_{xx} and vertical centroid d must be determined first. If section (A–A) is divided into two rectangles (Fig. 3-A3), then total moment of inertia of the two rectangles about the base is:

$$I_{xx} = (I_1 + A_1 d_1^2) + (I_2 + A_2 d_2^2)$$

$$d = \bar{y} = \frac{A_1 \bar{y}_1 + A_2 \bar{y}_2}{A_1 + A_2}$$

The variable d in the parallel axis theorem is, in this case, the same as the y-centroid. Given that $A_1 = A_2 = \frac{5}{8}$ inch × $\frac{3}{16}$ inch = 0.117 in² and that $y_1 = \frac{3}{16} + \frac{1}{2}(\frac{5}{8}) = 0.5$

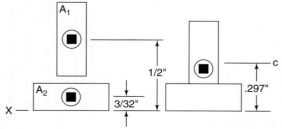

Fig. 3-A3 Section A–A centroid.

and $y_2 = \frac{1}{2}(\frac{3}{16}) = 0.09375$ inch, the y-centroid of section A–A is:

$$d = \bar{y} = \frac{(0.117)(0.5) + (0.117)(0.09375)}{0.234}$$

$$d = \bar{y} = 0.297 \text{ inch (for section } A-A)$$

In general, $I = bh^3/12$ for a rectangle:

$$I_1 = \frac{(\frac{3}{16})(\frac{5}{8})^3}{12} = 0.00381 \text{ in}^4$$

$$I_1 = \frac{(\frac{5}{8})(\frac{3}{16})^3}{12} = 0.00034 \text{ in}^4$$

$$A_1 d^2 = (\frac{5}{8})(\frac{3}{16})(\frac{1}{2})^2 = 0.0293 \text{ in}^4$$

$$A_2 d^2 = (\frac{5}{8})(\frac{3}{16})(0.297)^2 = 0.00103 \text{ in}^4$$

$$I_{xx} = (0.00381 + 0.0293 + 0.00034 + 0.00103) \text{ in}^4$$
$$= 0.0345 \text{ in}^4$$
$$= \text{moment of inertia about base of section } A-A$$

Solving for Ad^2:

$$A = (2)(\frac{5}{8})(\frac{3}{16}) = 0.234 \text{ in}^2 = d^2 = y^2 = (0.297)^2 = 0.08823 \text{ in}^4$$
$$Ad^2 = (0.234 \text{ in}^2)(0.0882 \text{ in}^2) = 0/0207 \text{ in}^4$$

Apply the parallel axis theorem:

$$I_{cc} = I_{xx} - Ad^2 = \text{parallel axis theorem}$$
$$I_{cc} = 0/0345 \text{ in}^4 - 0.0207 \text{ in}^4 = 0.0138 \text{ in}^4$$

Distal (Fig. 3-A4, *section B–B*):

$$I_{cc} = \frac{(\frac{5}{8})(\frac{3}{16})^3}{12} = I_{cc} = 0.00034 \text{ in}^4$$

Note that I_{cc} (proximal)$/I_{cc}$ (distal) = 40.6; that is, the proximal section of the sidebar is over 40 times as stiff as the distal section.

BEAM STRESS AND DEFLECTION
Example 4

The conventional AFO and KAFO contain sidebars that are subjected to bending stress in the mediolateral (coronal) and anteroposterior (sagittal) planes. The sidebars may be treated as a freely supported beam with a midspan load. For example, consider the valgum condition illustrated in Fig. 3-A5. The torque responsible for the valgum is given by:

$$T_{val} = F_{fr} \times L_{fr},$$

where F_{fr} = single limb stance floor reaction (pounds), and L_{fr} = floor reaction lever at knee joint (inches).

Assume that mediolateral flexibility in both the knee and the subtalar joints allows correction of the valgum deformity. A laterally directed force at the medial condyle F_{mc} restrains

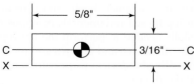

Fig. 3-A4 Section B–B centroid.

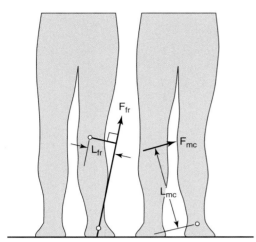

Fig. 3-A5 Valgum control.

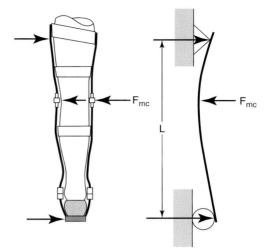

Fig. 3-A6 KAFO free body diagram.

(or corrects) the valgum deformity. This force and its lever to the subtalar joint L_{mc} must produce at least as much torque as the deforming force and lever, or:

$$F_{mc} \times L_{mc} \geq F_{fr} \times L_{fr}$$
$$F_{mc} \geq (F_{mc} \times L_{fr}) \div L_{mc}$$

Typical values for the variables in the above equation are F_{fr} = body weight (assume 150 lb), L_{fr} = 4 inches, and L_{mc} = 17 inches. Under these circumstances, the medially directed force would be F_{mc} = 35.3 lb. The free body diagram of a KAFO that experiences this force is shown in Fig. 3-A6.

The freely supported KAFO with medially directed valgum force (Fig. 3-A6) is replaced with two sidebars rigidly attached by way of the calf and distal thigh bands (Fig. 3-A6). This double-sidebar arrangement is replaced with a single beam composed of double-thickness sidebars (Fig. 3-A6). The medially directed valgum force is a distance $L/2$ from both the proximal and the distal ends. Recall from

Equation 3-17 that the stress in a freely supported beam is given by:

$$\sigma = \frac{3FL}{2bh^2} = 6025 \text{ psi}$$

where F = 35.3 lb, L = 10 inches (assumed distance from distal thigh band to calf band), b = ⅜ inch = anteroposterior thickness of sidebar, and h = ⅜ inch = 2 × 3/16 inch = mediolateral thickness of two sidebars.

Recall from Equation 3-21 that the maximum deflection of a freely supported beam is given by:

$$y_{max} = \frac{FL^3}{-48EI} = -0.267 \text{ inch}$$

where E = Young's modulus = 10^7 psi, and

$$I = \frac{bh^3}{12} = \frac{(⅝)(⅜)^3}{12} = 2.75 \times 10^{-3} \text{ in}^4$$

The stress in the sidebars is > 6000 psi, and the deflection is −0.267 inch (minus sign indicates inward).

Chapter

4

Principles of fabrication

Terry J. Supan

Key Points

- Although meticulous fabrication remains essential for creating an optimal orthosis, the methods and materials currently used create much stronger, thinner, lighter, and more biomechanically sophisticated orthoses than previously possible.

- Most custom orthoses are formed over accurate three-dimensional positive models derived from casting or electronic digitization of the affected body segments.

- Total contact orthoses made from thermoplastic or thermoset plastics predominate, but the historic metal bar and band orthoses still are used, particularly in the developing world.

- Computer-aided design and computer-aided manufacture methods are available to even the smallest orthotic facility and can be used to expedite fitting as well as to facilitate off-site manufacturing at a specialized fabrication center.

- Sound clinical judgment, combined with conscientious fitting and adjustment of well-designed orthoses, remains the hallmark of optimal orthotic treatment.

This chapter provides the neophyte orthotist, the prescribing physician, and other allied health personnel with a brief overview of the fabrication techniques necessary to produce the various types of orthoses used at the present time. It is interesting to note that more than one third of the original 1950 edition of this book, *Orthopaedic Appliance Atlas*, Volume 1, was devoted to fabrication methods and materials used by the "brace maker." Reflecting the evolution of the field since then, this edition emphasizes the changing role of orthoses and their clinical function rather than how each individual type of orthosis is made.

Data collection: measurements and impressions

The key to a properly designed and functioning orthosis is accurate collection of a patient's data. Accurate physical measurements and other data ensure that the device correctly fits the patient's body segment. Techniques have changed over the years, but the principles have remained essentially the same. Currently, instead of a two-dimensional tracing of the limb profile, a three-dimensional model is created. Plaster molds and computer-aided design (CAD) programs derived from measurements or optical scans now are available to orthotists.

Although the traditional metal and leather orthosis is not used often in the developed world, this style still may be necessary when there is a requirement for skeletal unloading or increased transverse plane resistance, or when the patient has become accustomed to wearing this type of orthosis. The patient with postpolio paralysis who has used an ischial weight-bearing knee–ankle–foot orthosis (KAFO) for decades is an example of a patient who may prefer this type of device. Metal and leather orthoses still are commonly used in the developing world.

Fabrication of a metal structure usually begins with anatomical measurements to obtain the required dimensions of the body segment to be supported. These measurements will give the orthotist the appropriate circumferences and diameters for the metal frame of the orthosis and the locations of the mechanical joints. Physical measurements are followed by a tracing of the profile of the torso or the limb. Tracings can be made with the patient supine (Fig. 4-1), but tracings also can be made with the patient standing against the wall, as when a profile of the torso is required for a spinal orthosis. Care must be taken to keep the tracing tool both

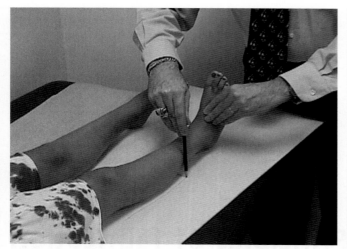

Fig. 4-1 Two-dimensional tracing process used to produce a metal ankle–foot orthosis.

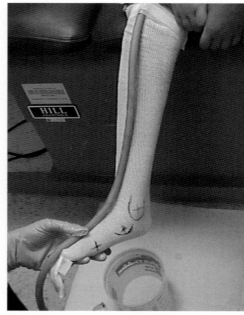

Fig. 4-2 Right limb being prepared for impression to produce the mold for a plastic ankle–foot orthosis. The flexible tube aids in mold removal. Indelible pencil markings indicate malleoli, navicular, and other key bony prominences.

perpendicular to the paper surface and parallel to the body, or the resulting diameter will be either too wide or too narrow, and the orthosis will not fit correctly. Typically, for fabrication the tracing must be reversed to provide a posterior view of the body because the bands of the orthosis usually are located behind the leg.

Physical assessment and measurements also are required when a total contact orthosis is being made. In general, a three-dimensional model of the limb or torso is required to create such an intimately fitting orthosis. Historically this is made by molding a plaster of Paris bandage around the body segment. A thin layer of stockinette is slipped over the body segment to protect the skin, then plaster rolls are applied to create a thin and accurate impression. Unlike fracture management, no web roll or other padding material is applied under the cast because such padding would distort the dimensions of the mold. Because a cast saw is often used to remove the mold after the plaster hardens, 0.5-inch tubing typically is incorporated to protect the patient's skin from the blade (Fig. 4-2). An indelible pencil is used to mark bony prominences and joint axes before the plaster is applied. This water-soluble pencil allows the marks to transfer to the interior of the plaster impression and later transfer a second time to the liquid plaster, which will fill the mold to produce a positive model. The orthotist will have not only a dimensionally stable model but also accurate delineations of the critical location for mechanical joints and areas requiring pressure relief (e.g., fibular head and peroneal nerve).

Low-density polyurethane foam can be used to make the impression when only a replica of the plantar surface of the feet is necessary. The foam is compressed under partial weight-bearing as the patient gently pushes into the material, which retains the foot's plantar contour (Fig. 4-3). The orthotist may need to guide the dorsum of the instep, metatarsal heads, and toes to ensure an accurate mold. The orthotist can modify the foam impression to create further relief in the negative before it is filled with liquid plaster. The foam is easily removed once the plaster has hardened, forming the positive model.

Use of synthetic casting tape for three-dimensional molds is increasingly common because the noise of the cast saw and the cleanup required with plaster bandage can be avoided

with use of water-activated resins. The body segment is prepared in the same manner as for a plaster cast with the stockinette and the indelible markings. The flexible tube is placed on the anterior surface of the body, and the casting material is wrapped and molded to the segment. After the resin has gelled but before it has completely hardened, the tube is pulled out from under the mold, forming a channel. A pair of heavy-duty bandage scissors or cast shears can be used to open the mold and remove it from around the body, thus avoiding the need for a cast saw (Fig. 4-4). The synthetic tape impression is sealed and filled with liquid plaster, and the pencil marks transfer to the positive plaster model.

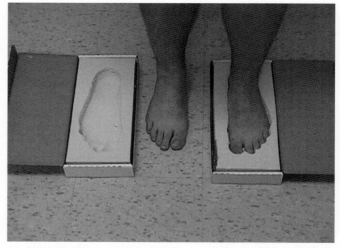

Fig. 4-3 Foam impressions of the plantar surface of the patient's feet. The orthotist must control the amount of weight bearing to prevent excessive compression of the foam casting material.

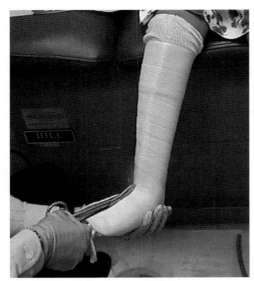

Fig. 4-4 Heavy-duty shears can be used to open the semihardened mold. The flexible tube has been removed from under the impression to create a channel for the tip of the shears.

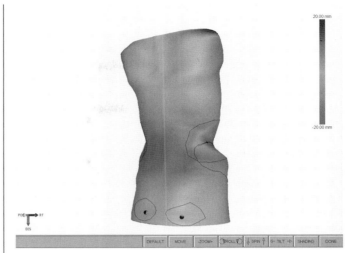

Fig. 4-5 Digitized image of torso used to produce a scoliosis thoraco-lumbosacral orthosis. This particular computer-aided design image is based on measurements and templates from prior successful orthoses. The computer-aided design image also can be produced by digitization of the patient's entire torso. (Courtesy Vorum Corporation.)

CAD allows the orthotist to create a positive model, with less inconvenience to the patient. Two techniques are used to collect the data: measurements and scanning. The data are handled by a computer program, which creates an image of the model. The orthotist then manipulates the data/image to rectify the positive model of the patient's torso, head, or limb. The information is exported to computer-aided manufacturing (CAM) equipment, which is used to carve the modified positive model that is used to fabricate the custom orthosis.

Spinal orthoses can be made from measurement data. The circumferences and diameters of the torso are processed by a software program to create a three-dimensional model that is viewed on the computer screen. The images then are modified to more closely match the clinical needs of the patient (Fig. 4-5). Derotation and scoliosis corrective forces can be specified on the computer model to create the desired orthotic design. Once the orthotist is satisfied with the image(s), the data are sent to the CAM equipment, which produces a positive model. The custom-made orthosis is vacuum formed over the model.

Noncontact scanning is another common method of data collection. The patient can be placed in the scanner equipment (e.g., for manufacture of plagiocephaly orthoses), or a hand-held optical or laser scanner can be passed over the body segment or inside a mold (Fig. 4-6). The collected data then are imported into the computer program. The orthotist can modify the digital image on the computer screen rather than physically modifying the plaster model, which remains the traditional method. The data from the rectified positive model are downloaded to a CAM lathe for positive model creation.

CAM is often done by a central fabrication company because the cost of the CAM equipment can be prohibitive for a smaller orthotic facility. The modified data can be transmitted to the fabrication laboratory via the Internet, and the completed orthosis is shipped to the orthotist for patient fitting.

Metal components

The process for incorporating metal components is similar whether a metal orthosis is being fabricated or metal joints

are being added to a plastic orthosis. When the two-dimensional tracing is used, the model must be "laid out" to ensure proper device fit (Fig. 4-7). The joints must be at the proper axis location, and they must be "square" or parallel in all planes. Clearance between the patient's bony anatomy and the mechanical joints must be optimal. The sidebar material is contoured to the profile of the tracing. For a KAFO or ankle–foot orthosis (AFO), the bands are contoured to match the shape and width of the leg. When the bands are attached to the sidebars, care is taken to match the profile of the leg in the sagittal plane as well. This step also applies when a stirrup is to be attached to the shoe.

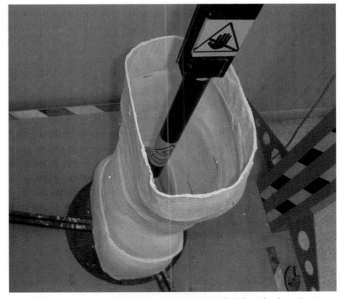

Fig. 4-6 Laser scanning wand can be used to digitize the interior contours of a custom mold of the patient's torso. Resulting data are imported into a computer-aided design software program for electronic rectification by the orthotist. (Courtesy Vorum Corporation.)

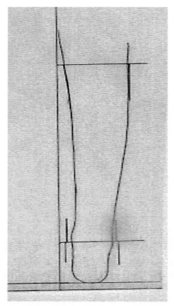

Fig. 4-7 Reversed tracing used to design and blueprint fabrication of a metal ankle–foot orthosis. In this example, the height and width of the ankle joints and the calf band have been established.

An alignment fixture is required to maintain joint congruity during fabrication (Fig. 4-8). The three-dimensional model is modified and the joint axis location determined. The metal sidebars are formed to the shape of the model in both the coronal and sagittal planes. Care must be taken not to work harden the metal and to sand and polish any scratches created during the contouring of the bars. Excessive bending of the metal or nicks create high-stress areas that could lead to failure of the metal in clinical use. Once the metal components are attached to the plastic cuffs or the alloy bands, the joints must be reexamined

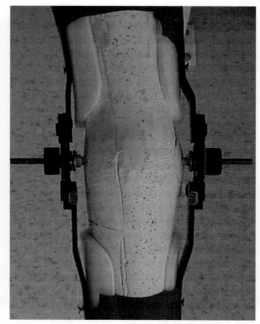

Fig. 4-8 Fixture used to align the knee joints on a custom-made knee orthosis. The fixture maintains the joints in proper location while the sidebars are being contoured.

for congruity and corrected as necessary. Meticulous fabrication is important because binding of the joints interferes with clinical function and results in premature wear of the parts.

When shaping the components, bending fixtures or irons are used to contour the metal. Bends should be "fluid" over as long a distance as possible and should not be abrupt. The radius of the bend is based on the distance between the heads of the bending irons or the contact points of the fixture. The bend will be located at the halfway point between those contact points. If possible, the majority of the contouring should be done before any attachment holes are drilled into the metal. Bends made afterward could create stress risers in the metal or damage threads tapped into the parts. The same care is necessary for any predrilled parts that are already threaded.

Thermoplastic Materials

Both sheet thermoplastics and thermoset resin plastics are used in orthoses. The fabrication processes are quite different, as are the functional characteristics of the plastic sections of the orthoses. Thermoplastics usually are vacuum formed, and the resulting orthosis is more flexible and can be readily modified postproduction. Thermoset plastics go through a polymerization process, usually are more rigid, and cannot be heat modified postproduction without destroying the molecular structure of the plastic. Preparation of the positive model is the same for both types of plastic orthoses.

Model preparations begin with sealing of the negative impression to create a mold. Liquid molding plaster is mixed and poured into the mold. A metal mandrel is placed into the plaster, and, once the plaster has hardened, the mandrel is used in a special vise to hold the positive model (Fig. 4-9). The indelible pencil marks will have transferred onto the model but may need to be reinforced for clarity. Any artifact in the plaster is smoothed, the desired buildups are made over bony areas, and joint fixture/dummies are applied to the exterior of the model (Fig. 4-10). Biomechanical changes are made to the model at this time.

For vacuum forming of thermoplastic material, stockinette material typically is used as a wick to rapidly evacuate the air during the forming process. Clarity, stiffness, durability, or resistance to torsion all can be affected by the choice of plastic and its thickness.

The vacuum forming process consists of heating the sheet plastic until it is flexible and autoadhesive, then draping the plastic over the positive model and applying vacuum to remove all of the air between the plastic and the model (Fig. 4-11). Once the thermal molding is completed, the plastic is allowed to gradually cool and solidify.

Equipment necessary to fabricate custom orthoses includes ovens to heat the thermoplastic, vises to hold the positive models during rectification, vacuum forming equipment and fixtures, and machine tools for sanding, grinding, polishing, cutting, and dust collection. Because the size of the positive model varies with the size of the patient, very large ovens are used to heat the plastic sheet material to the correct temperature, which can be up to 450°F. Infrared or convection ovens also may be used to process sheet thermoplastics.

Reinforcements can be added to the thermoplastic during the vacuum forming process when extra stiffness is necessary. Either base plastic or composite inserts can be used for this purpose. Changing the trim lines of the orthosis or creating

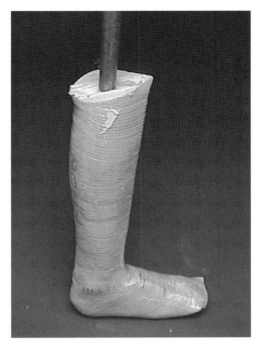

Fig. 4-9 The mold of the limb is filled with liquid plaster of Paris. A metal pipe, placed into the plaster before it hardens, creates a mandrel that is used to hold the model while the orthosis is being created. After the plaster hardens, the outer mold is removed, creating a precise positive model of the patient's limb.

corrugations also will affect the flexibility of the device. Composite inserts are heated at the same time as the base thermoplastic and applied to the model. The thermoplastic is immediately draped over the outside of the model, sandwiching the reinforcing insert between the plastic and the model (Fig. 4-12).

Additional thickness of the base plastic can be used to stiffen the final result (Fig. 4-13). All plastic pieces are heated at the same time so that they are the same temperature during the forming process and will thermobond to one another.

A change in geometric shape will change the stiffness of the plastic (Fig. 4-14). The ankle and knee are made more stable by having the plastic trim lines anterior to the malleoli; trim lines

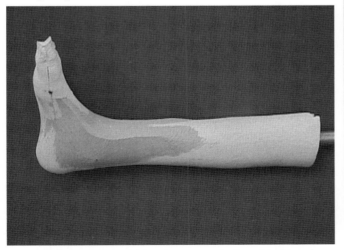

Fig. 4-10 The plaster model has been smoothed, and buildups have been added over the bony prominences to create appropriate reliefs. Further modifications will be made to create the proper biomechanical forces before the model is ready for thermoplastic vacuum forming.

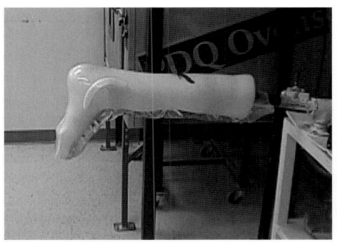

Fig. 4-11 Polypropylene plastic has been vacuum formed over the model. The hot plastic seals to itself and the evacuation fixture. As the air is removed, atmospheric pressure forces the inside of the softened plastic against the contours of the model. The foam corrugation at the ankle stiffens the ankle–foot orthosis in this region without increasing overall weight.

posterior to the malleoli will allow more dorsiflexion and plantar flexion. Placing a corrugation on the exterior of the model is another method for increasing localized stiffness.

Once the plastic has been removed from the positive model, the initial trim lines are established and the edges are polished smooth to prevent both rough spots that could scratch the skin and stress risers that could result in early failure of the plastic. Any edges that impinge on the patient's skin can be flared away from the body by either heat modification or beveling the inside edge of plastic.

Thermoset lamination techniques

When a more rigid orthosis is desired, thermoset lamination materials can be used instead of the vacuum-formed thermoplastics. Laminates, used primarily in prostheses and lower limb

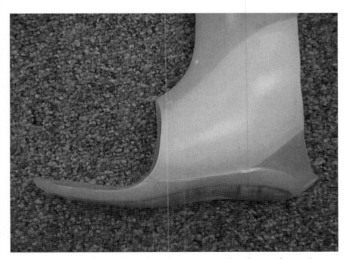

Fig. 4-12 During the vacuum forming process, the thermoformed composite insert is sandwiched between two layers of polypropylene to stiffen the sole plate of this orthosis. All three pieces of plastic are heated at the same time to ensure a strong thermal bond between the dissimilar materials.

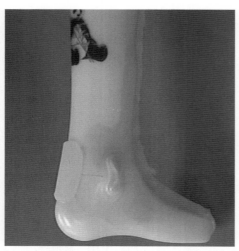

Fig. 4-13 This articulated ankle–foot orthosis will require a plantar flexion stop, so an extra layer of plastic has been added to the Achilles tendon area. The edges of the extra plastic will be blended into the base plastic later in the process.

orthoses, are made from different types of fabric matrix and monomer resins. A chemical catalyst is added that causes conversion of the monomer resin to a polymer that surrounds the reinforcing matrix. The most common resins used for orthoses are polyester, epoxy, and acrylic. The most commonly used fabrics are nylon, carbon fiber, and Kevlar. Many orthoses are reinforced with two or more of these materials in a specific manner determined by the biomechanical loads to be applied in clinical use. The functional goals and structural strength desired determine which resin and matrix are used in the orthosis (Fig. 4-15).

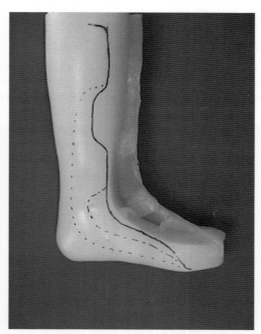

Fig. 4-14 Varying the trim lines from anterior to posterior will change the biomechanical function of the ankle–foot orthosis. Trim lines well anterior to the apex of the malleoli will prevent or limit ankle motion, encouraging knee extension during stance. Trim lines posterior to the ankle will provide dorsiflexion assistance during swing phase but will not significantly restrict sagittal plane ankle motion during stance phase. Varus or valgus control flanges proximal to the ankle can be used to enhance biomechanical control of the subtalar joints in the coronal plane.

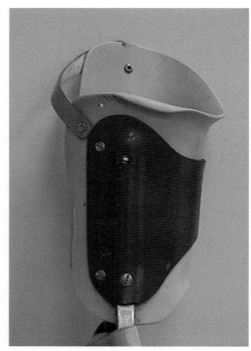

Fig. 4-15 Thermoset, carbon/graphite lamination is used to produce a very rigid but lightweight external band for the proximal section of this knee–ankle–foot orthosis. The internal plastic is flexible, improving comfort to the patient while providing good biomechanical control of the limb.

Vacuum-assisted lamination techniques are commonly used to create a custom orthosis. The model is prepared the same way as when a vacuum-formed thermoplastic orthosis is being fabricated. A polyvinyl alcohol (PVA) barrier, usually in the form of a bag, is placed over the modified model and evacuated. The layers of the appropriate reinforcing fabric then are stretched taut over the model. A second PVA layer/bag is placed over the fabric and attached to a vacuum source. A catalyst that changes the monomer resin into the polymer is added to the resin, the resin is poured into the PVA bag, and the negative pressure caused by the vacuum source pulls the resin into the mold, saturating the fabric. Once the chemical reaction has occurred, the vacuum is shut off, and the plastic component is removed from the model as in the thermoplastic technique.

Use of carbon fiber composite materials preimpregnated with epoxy resin is one of the strongest fabrication methods available. Curing the work piece requires simultaneous application of heat and pressure, so curing often is done in an autoclave. The cost of the equipment and the labor-intensive process make the fabrication of such "prepreg" orthoses expensive and more difficult for a smaller orthotic facility. Most prepreg orthoses are either premade or fabricated by a central fabricator (Figs. 4-16 and 4-17).

Computer-aided manufacture

CAM is the second half of the CAD/CAM process. Rectified positive models usually are carved from rigid foam blanks on a CAM lathe. The modified data from the CAD process are either downloaded to a carver in the local facility or sent to a central fabrication laboratory (Fig. 4-18). Once the model has been carved, the orthosis usually is fabricated in the normal manner using thermoplastic or thermoset materials. Because of their relatively simple overall geometric shape, models for

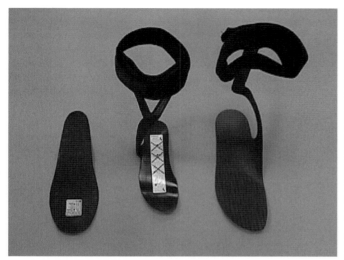

Fig. 4-16 Ankle–foot orthoses premade from carbon composite material preimpregnated with optimal liquid resin by the manufacturer. This fabrication technique produces a very lightweight orthosis with varying degrees of flexibility and rigidity, depending on the fiber orientation.

spinal orthoses, plagiocephaly cranial orthoses, and knee orthoses can be made easily using CAD. Models for KAFOs and AFOs are much more difficult to carve because of the complex shapes of the leg and the foot.

In addition to its use in creating custom-made orthoses, CAM is practical for large production runs of prefabricated orthoses. Computer control helps to ensure uniformity of injection molded parts, reproduce multiple models used for vacuum forming, and reduce the costs of production runs.

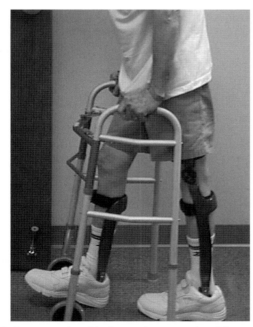

Fig. 4-17 Custom-made ankle–foot orthoses, produced from a mold of the patient's leg, incorporate carbon composite sidebars and bands with titanium joints. The biomechanical function is analogous to that of metal orthoses, but these devices are much lighter in weight than even aluminum alloy equivalents.

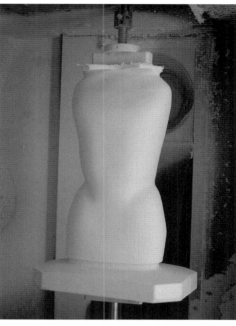

Fig. 4-18 Thoracolumbosacral orthosis model produced using a computed-aided design/computer-aided manufacturing program. The orthotist can electronically rectify the raw shape and then send the electronic carving instructions to the remote manufacturing facility. The computerized lathe carves the urethane foam block into the desired shape created by the orthotist. Once manufactured, the thoracolumbosacral orthosis is returned to the practitioner for fitting, trimming, finishing, and delivery to the patient. (Courtesy Vorum Corporation.)

Research is under way to develop innovative CAM methods that could permit direct fabrication of the final orthosis without the need for a positive model. This approach, if successful, may not only reduce the cost of fabrication but also may permit the orthotist to create novel structures that are not practical with present fabrication methods. Another potential advantage of CAD/CAM methods is the ability to store an electronic definition of the orthosis for future applications.

Conclusion

Although orthoses still are created using traditional materials and fabrication methods, the use of total contact plastic devices is increasingly prevalent. Vacuum-molded thermoplastics, thermoset laminations, and carbon composite prepreg fabrication methods are increasingly common because these modern techniques create an orthosis that is lighter, stronger, and more biomechanically effective than orthoses made with less sophisticated techniques.

Use of CAD offers even the small orthotic facility the ability to use noncontact imaging and software-based modifications to create a custom orthosis. Use of CAM permits fabrication of complex orthoses in laboratories far from the patient care facility and to the precise specifications of the orthotist.

Despite numerous advances in materials and fabrication techniques, the most critical element in the creation of a well-fitted, highly functional orthosis remains the clinical judgment and technical skill of the orthotist treating the patient.

Chapter

5

Normal and pathologic gait

Jacquelin Perry

Key Points

- Walking involves a complex interaction of hip, knee, ankle, and foot motions to advance the body in the desired line of progression.
- Forces with ever-changing alignment are imposed on the supporting limb by the weight of the body. Selective muscle action controls these motions and forces for two essential functions: weight-bearing stability and progression over the supporting foot.
- The physical strain of walking is reduced by two accessory functions: shock absorption and energy conservation.
- Effectiveness of these gait mechanics is summarized by the individual's stride characteristics (e.g., velocity) and energetics.

Normal gait

Each limb blends the patterns of motion, passive force, and muscular control into a sequence of activity (called a *gait cycle* or a *stride*), which is repeated endlessly until the desired destination is reached. The two limbs perform in a reciprocal manner, offset by 50% of the gait cycle. The head, neck, trunk, and pelvis are self-contained passengers riding on the limb's locomotor system.[15]

Basic functions

The normal interactions of joint motion and muscle activity of walking serve four basic functions. Although each is described as a separate event, they occur in an overlapping fashion during the stride.

Weight-bearing stability

In a serial fashion, the extensor muscles maintain the limb's ability to support body weight. This begins with the hamstrings and quadriceps preparing the swinging limb for stance. Responding to the rapid drop of body weight onto the foot, the hip extensors and quadriceps stabilize the flexed hip and knee, while the hip abductors support the pelvis. As body weight progresses over the foot, the ankle plantar flexors restrain the tibia and provide indirect extensor stability of the hip and knee.

This pattern of muscle control is dictated by the changing alignment of the body weight line (vector) with the individual joints. As the vector moves away from the joint center, a rotational moment develops that must be controlled by opposing muscles to preserve postural stability.

Progression

To advance the weight-bearing limb over the supporting foot (i.e., stance limb progression), three rocker actions are used. A fourth rocker initiates swing limb advancement. The sites of progression are the heel, ankle, forefoot, and toe.

1. *Heel rocker:* Following floor contact, the descent of body weight through the tibia plantar flexes the ankle while the pretibial muscles slow the rate of foot drop. This creates an unstable period of heel-only support, which rolls the limb forward on the rounded calcaneus.
2. *Ankle rocker:* As momentum advances the body vector, ankle dorsiflexion allows the stance limb to roll forward over the stationary foot. Stance stability depends on graded restraint by the ankle plantar flexor muscles.
3. *Forefoot rocker:* Heel rise moves body weight across the forefoot. Both the foot and the limb roll forward over the

unstable area of support provided by the rounded metatarsal heads.

4. *Toe rocker:* Advancement of the body weight vector to the metatarsophalangeal (MP) joint allows the foot to dorsiflex rapidly about the base of the toes. The knee is unlocked and swing limb advancement initiated. Dorsiflexion availability at the ankle and MP joints is the critical factor.

The two forces stimulating progression are forward fall of body weight and momentum created by the swinging limb. From a quiet stance, forward fall is initiated by flexion of the swing limb and calf muscle relaxation, which allows the weight-bearing tibia to advance.

Shock absorption

The impact of rapid body weight transfer onto the limb is dissipated by knee flexion redirecting the force to the quadriceps. This action is initiated by the heel rocker.

Energy conservation

Selective relaxation of muscle action by substitution of momentum or passive positioning can conserve energy. Cocontraction of antagonists is rare. The normal occurrences are use of hamstrings and quadriceps during limb loading and anterior and posterior tibialis during medial foot control.

Floor contact pattern

The simplest system for subdividing the continuum of activity that constitutes walking uses the timing of foot–floor contact as a frame of reference. The instant of initial floor contact has been designated as the start of the gait cycle. Within each cycle, the period of floor contact by any part of the foot is called *stance*. This is followed by an interval of midair limb advancement called *swing*. At the beginning and end of stance, there is an interval when both limbs are in contact with the floor for weight transfer. These intervals are called *initial* and *terminal double stance*. In between is a longer interval of *single-limb stance*, at which time the other foot is in the air. A more functional term is *single-limb support*. The limitation of this temporal classification system is that the divisions impart minimal indications of function.

Functional phases of gait

To understand the purpose of individual joint motions and their modes of control, it is necessary to consider the action of the whole limb as the posture of each segment is influenced by the others. During a gait cycle, the limb moves through eight functionally distinct postural sequences, which are called *phases of gait*. Each has one or more events that are critical to accomplishing its purpose. These phases are combined into three primary tasks by the synergistic patterns of the muscles controlling the limb. Transitional actions between stance and swing create an overlap in the phase sequence. The actions in the final phase of swing (*terminal swing*) also prepare the limb for stance. Similarly, the final phase of stance (*preswing*) prepares the limb for swing before the toe is lifted.

Task I: Weight acceptance

Phase 1—Initial contact: The way the foot contacts the floor is the first influence on the pattern of limb loading.

Phase 2—Loading response: Three major functions are shock absorption to blunt the floor impact force, limb stability to accept body weight, and preservation of progression.

Task II: Stance limb progression (single-limb support)

Phase 3—Midstance: The ankle serves as a rocker that allows the limb to advance over the stationary foot.

Phase 4—Terminal stance: The forefoot provides a rocker that allows both the foot and the limb to roll forward.

Task III: Swing limb advancement

Phase 5—Preswing: Actions at the ankle and hip of the unloaded limb initiate knee flexion in preparation for swing.

Phase 6—Initial swing: Muscle action at the hip, knee, and ankle lift the foot and advance the limb.

Phase 7—Midswing: The limb is advanced by continued hip flexion and early knee extension. With the tibia vertical, active foot support is required.

Phase 8—Terminal swing: Limb advancement is completed by knee extension, while further hip flexion is inhibited in preparation for stance.

Individual joint motion patterns

During stance, loading the heel initiates motion at each joint. Prompt response by the muscles provides an eccentric force that limits the arc of joint motion and also serves as a shock-absorbing mechanism. Recent investigations of eccentric muscle function, using portable ultrasound sensors (taped over the target muscle) have differentiated muscle fascicles from tendon during walking and jumping. These findings have redefined eccentric muscle action, which commonly is defined as a lengthening contraction. However, an ultrasound display of the muscle fascicles showed no increase in length.[9] The gain in length was stretch of the tendon while the muscle exerted an isometric contraction to stabilize the joint; muscles only shorten or maintain neutral length.[12]

Ankle and foot

During each stride, the ankle passes through four arcs of motion (Fig. 5-1). At the onset of stance, the ankle is in neutral dorsiflexion, and floor contact is by the heel. Rapid loading of the heel causes the ankle to quickly plantar flex and then return to neutral before forefoot contact. Ultrasound analysis of muscle function at this time identified that the motion was the result of tibialis anterior tendon stretch.[6] Release of the stretch force occurred as the heel lever shortened with the advancement of the vector across the heel. Following forefoot contact with the ground, ankle motion reverses to 10 degrees dorsiflexion as the tibia advances over the stationary foot for stance limb progression. Then the ankle plantar flexes 20 degrees during the final phase of stance (preswing). As toe-off starts swing, the foot again dorsiflexes under control of the pretibial muscles. Full elevation of the foot to neutral, however, is not completed until midswing.

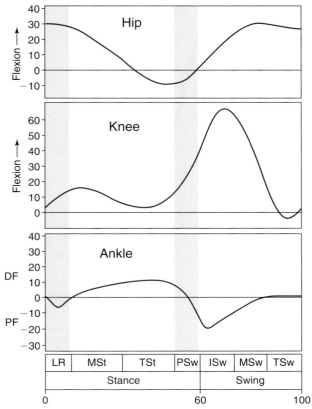

Fig. 5-1 Typical motion pattern of the limb during a gait cycle: Hip *(top)*, knee *(middle)*, and ankle *(bottom)*. *DF*, Dorsiflexion; *PF*, plantar flexion; *LR*, loading response; *MSt*, midstance; *TSt*, terminal stance; *PSw*, preswing; *ISw*, initial swing; *MSw*, midswing; *TSw*, terminal swing. *0*, Onset of gait cycle; *60*, end of stance; *100*, end of gait cycle.

The subtalar joint moves into eversion following initial floor contact by the heel. This unlocks the midtarsal joint, allowing it to dorsiflex slightly (arch flattens) following forefoot impact with the floor. Then the subtalar joint progressively inverts and locks the midtarsal joint through late midstance and terminal stance.

MP joint dorsiflexion is an essential component of heel rise. The foot rolls up over the base of the toes, particularly the great toe, as the trailing limb advances.[14]

Dorsiflexion control is provided by the pretibial muscles (tibialis anterior, extensor hallucis longus, and extensor digitorum) during the loading response in addition to swing. The soleus and gastrocnemius control the tibia during stance limb progression. During terminal stance the EMG intensity of the gastrocnemius and soleus muscle mass increases rapidly in response to the dorsiflexion moment generated by the advancement of the body mass over the forefoot rocker. This same moment also stretches the tendon and gains 5 degrees of dorsiflexion at the ankle.[9] In preswing, the tension of the Achilles tendon is abruptly released by the rapid transfer of body weight to the other limb. This creates a large power burst of plantar flexion by elastic recoil. The muscle mass is inactive (no EMG).[9] The "push off" power generated is sufficient to initiate swing.[12]

Subtalar inversion control is created by the anterior tibialis, posterior tibialis, and soleus. The peroneus brevis and

peroneus longus muscles restrain inversion as they produce an eversion force on the lateral side of the foot. Midtarsal restraint of the dorsiflexing forces created by body weight advancement is provided by the intrinsic flexor muscles as well as the subtalar muscles and the long toe flexors. The primary role of the flexor hallucis longus and flexor digitorum longus is to stabilize the MP joint during heel rise.

Knee

Within each gait cycle, the knee alternately flexes and extends both in stance and in swing (see Fig. 5-1). From a position of full extension at initial contact, the knee rapidly flexes 18 degrees during weight acceptance. Ultrasound analysis shows this motion is the result of patellar tendon stretch while the quadriceps muscle is undergoing an isometric contraction.[6] This is followed by progressive extension throughout the period of single stance, reaching a final position of 5 degrees flexion. The knee then rapidly flexes to 40 degrees during preswing and continues to 60 degrees in initial swing. From this position, the knee then extends to neutral.

The quadriceps restrains knee flexion in stance and assists extension. All the vasti respond simultaneously. The gluteus maximus through its iliotibial band insertion also contributes to knee extensor stability. Brief and occasional action of the rectus femoris (and less frequently the vastus intermedius) restrains excessive preswing flexion. Knee flexion in swing is aided by the short head of the biceps femoris. Terminal swing knee extension is limited by the hamstring muscle group.

Hip

The major hip motions occur in the plane of progression (see Fig. 5-1). This consists of an arc of extension through stance, reaching 10 degrees hyperextension in terminal stance. A similar arc of flexion occurs from preswing through midswing. The resulting 35-degree flexed posture is maintained in terminal swing and loading response. In the other planes, there are small (4 to 5 degree) arcs of postural accommodation, which are described as pelvic motions.

Hip extensor muscle action begins with the hamstrings in terminal swing and proceeds to the gluteus maximus and adductor magnus during the loading response. Lateral stability of the hip in stance is provided by the gluteus medius–gluteus minimus complex and the tensor fascia lata.

Hip flexion results from serial activation of several muscles: adductor longus (plus rectus femoris), iliacus, sartorius, and gracilis.

Pelvis

The pelvis moves through small (5 degree) arcs in each plane as it yields to body weight in stance and follows the advancing limb in swing. Stability is provided by the muscles of the weight-bearing hip.

Head and trunk

The basic function of the head and trunk is to maintain an upright posture. The small (5 degree) arcs of motion that

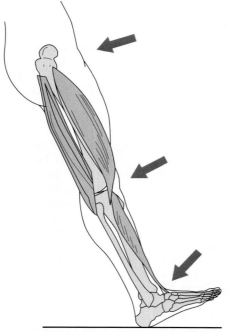

Fig. 5-2 Terminal swing pattern of muscle control. The limb is positioned for stance by synergistic action of the hamstrings (posterior thigh), quadriceps (anterior thigh), and tibialis anterior (anterior leg).

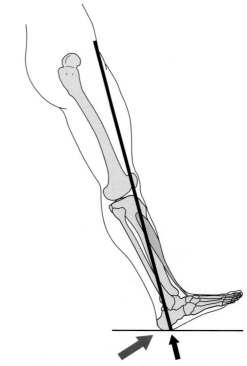

Fig. 5-3 Initial contact by the heel with pretibial muscle control (tibialis anterior shown) establishes the heel rocker. *Vertical line* represents the body weight vector. Both ground impact *(large arrow)* and base of the body weight vector *(small arrow)* are at the heel.

occur reflect the uneven support provided by the reciprocal actions of the two limbs. Motion is greatest in the lumbar area and decreases at each higher segment. The spinal muscles act to preserve balance, absorb shock, and minimize head displacement.

Integrated function of the limb

Task I: Weight acceptance

Weight acceptance is the first determinant of the ability to walk. Two objectives determine the events that occur during this task: establishment of a stable limb for weight bearing and minimization of the shock of floor impact. The last phase of swing and the first two stance phases are dedicated to optimum weight acceptance.

Phase 8—Terminal swing: To prepare the swinging limb for stance, hip flexion is interrupted, the knee extends, and the ankle remains dorsiflexed (Fig. 5-2).

Rapid, intense action by the hamstring muscles (semimembranosus, semitendinosus, biceps femoris long head) stops hip flexion and terminates swing. These muscles then reduce their intensity and allow the quadriceps to extend the knee. The continuation of mild hamstring action prevents knee hyperextension from the residual tibial momentum. Pretibial muscle action supports the dorsiflexed foot.

Phase 1—Initial contact: Floor contact by the heel is the critical event (Fig. 5-3). Its purpose is to initiate the heel rocker for progression and shock absorption. The significant postures are ankle dorsiflexion and full knee extension. Initial floor contact by the heel is a forceful

event, which begins with 1 cm of free fall between the foot and the ground. The impact registers 50% to 125% body weight during the first 10 to 20 ms of stance (1% to 2% of the gait cycle).[17,19] The heel responds to the impact by initiating small arcs of ankle plantar flexion and subtalar inversion. Anterior tibialis control of the foot determines heel rocker effectiveness.

Phase 2—Loading response (initial double stance): This is a highly demanding phase. At the ankle, the pretibial muscles (especially the anterior tibialis) preserve the heel rocker by intense isometric activity, while stretch of the anterior tibialis tendon allows a small arc of plantar flexion for shock absorption. This reverses the early plantar flexion arc to neutral (6° at 6% of the gait cycle) by the end of the loading response.[18] The limb is destabilized by the heel rocker and then supported by strong extensor muscular response. There are three critical events (Fig. 5-4).

For both shock absorption and progression, the heel rocker drives the foot toward the floor as the limb is loaded. Response of the pretibial muscles to decelerate the dropping foot pulls the tibia forward. This places the vector behind the knee, leading to rapid knee flexion for shock absorption. Prompt quadriceps response opposes the vector's flexor moment to preserve knee stability and absorb the shock of the initial floor impact. Knee extensor stability is aided by the femoral stability gained from the adductor magnus and gluteus maximus. Prompt relaxation of the hamstring muscles avoids an unnecessary flexor force.

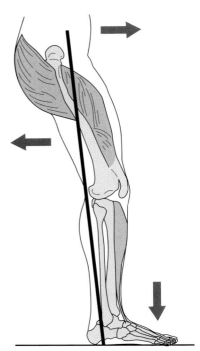

Fig. 5-4 Loading response vector *(vertical line)* is anterior to the hip (flexor moment is restrained by the gluteus maximus), posterior to the knee (quadriceps restraint of the flexor moment), and posterior to the ankle (plantar flexor moment is restrained by the tibialis anterior).

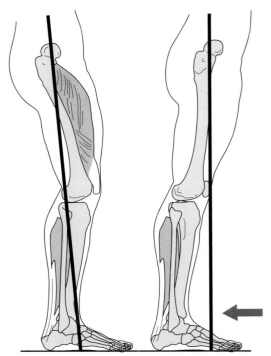

Fig. 5-5 Midstance progression of the limb over the stationary foot generates two patterns of muscle action. In early midstance *(left)*, the vector is behind the hip (no muscle action required), closer to the knee (less quadriceps) and anterior to the ankle (this dorsiflexor moment is retrained by the soleus). By late midstance *(right)*, the vector is anterior to the knee, and no quadriceps action is needed. Ankle dorsiflexor moment has increased.

At the hip, there is a rapid response by the abductor muscle group to stabilize the pelvis, which lost its contralateral support with the transfer of body weight to the forward limb.

Task II: Stance limb progression

The basic function is advancement of the limb (and body) over the supporting foot. This is the second determinant of the ability to walk. Two phases of single-limb support are involved as the means of progression differ.

Phase 3—Midstance: The critical event is ankle dorsiflexion for progression of the stance limb over a stationary, flat foot (Fig. 5-5). As momentum from the contralateral swing limb moves the vector along the foot, the soleus (quickly assisted by the gastrocnemius) modulates the tibial advancement so the lower leg proceeds less rapidly than the femur. This provides passive extension of the hip and knee for weight-bearing stability. As a result, the hip extensor and quadriceps muscles rapidly relax and stability of the hip and knee become dependent on the strength of the plantar flexor muscles.

At the hip, there also is a major adducting moment as lifting the other limb for swing removes the support for that side of the pelvis (Fig. 5-6). This creates a large medial vector, which is restrained by the gluteus medius.

Phase 4—Terminal stance (late single stance): Heel rise is the critical event that continues progression (Fig. 5-7). Free

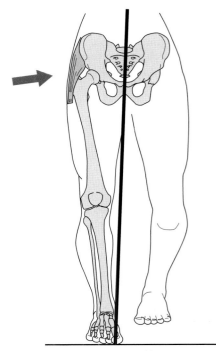

Fig. 5-6 Single-limb stance creates an adductor moment at the hip as the pelvis, with midline vector medial to hip, is unsupported. Gluteus medius action restrains adductor moment.

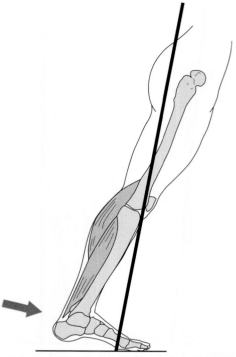

Fig. 5-7 Terminal stance progression advances the vector across the forefoot, and the heel rises. The vector remains behind the hip and knee joints (knee hyperextension moment is restrained by the gastrocnemius). Vector alignment at the ankle creates a maximal dorsiflexion moment, which is restrained by the soleus and gastrocnemius.

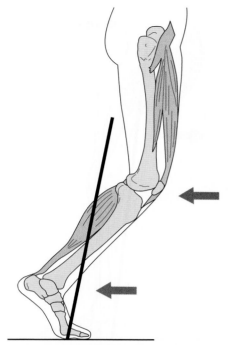

Fig. 5-8 Preswing transfer of body weight to the other limb reduces the vector. The base of the vector now is at the metatarsophalangeal joint. The unloaded foot falls forward with the tibia as it follows the dorsiflexion moment. Gastrosoleus tension induces ankle plantar flexion. The knee flexes in response to the posterior moment, with rectus femoris restraint if needed. Posterior hip moment is opposed by the flexor component of the adductor longus and rectus femoris.

dorsiflexion mobility of the MP joints also is essential. Both the foot and the limb roll forward over the forefoot rocker. The soleus and gastrocnemius muscles virtually lock the slightly dorsiflexed ankle, thus making the forefoot the site of limb rotation.

This creates a lever (ankle to metatarsal heads), which enlarges the arc of limb rotation. Heel height is preserved while greater advancement of the center of mass adds to step length. Heel rise is 3.5 cm at contralateral initial contact.[14]

Task III: Limb advancement

The ability to lift the foot is the third determinant of walking ability. Flexing the limb for floor clearance and swing advancement begins in the terminal double-support period of stance. Because the purpose is limb advancement rather than weight bearing, the phase has been titled *preswing*. The other actions occur throughout swing.

Phase 5—Preswing: Passive knee flexion to 40 degrees is the critical event because this is the primary contributor to foot clearance of the floor in swing (Fig. 5-8).

Following floor contact by the other foot, body weight is rapidly transferred to that limb to catch the forward fall. The equally abrupt unloading of the trailing limb initiates a series of actions commonly called *push-off*. A rapid arc of ankle plantar flexion to 20 degrees is accompanied by passive knee flexion to 40 degrees, increased toe dorsiflexion, and release of the extended hip. The initial force is a large burst of plantar

flexion power. Because there is no corresponding EMG, the source of the power is attributed to elastic energy generated by the abrupt release of the previously tense soleus and gastrocnemius muscles: push-off positions the limb for swing and initiates the action, allowing several small forces to be effective. As the limb's trailing posture reduces the foot's floor contact to the anterior margins of the metatarsal heads and the toes (fourth rocker), there is no stabilizing force, so the foot and the leg are free to roll forward. This is accelerated by the rapid ankle plantar flexion stimulated by the release of the tension stored in the eccentrically stretched soleus and gastrocnemius. Passive knee flexion is initiated. Unloading the limb also releases the tension in the hip flexors. This force combined with adductor longus action initiates early hip flexion and assists knee flexion.

Phase 6—Initial swing: The critical event is knee flexion sufficient for the toe to clear the floor as the thigh advances. This involves total limb flexion (Fig. 5-9). Hip flexion may be a passive continuation of the preswing events or result from direct action by the iliacus, sartorius, and gracilis. Attainment of full knee flexion largely depends on the imbalance between the forward momentum of the femur generated by hip flexion and inertia of the tibia. Active assistance also is provided by the biceps femoris, short head. Brisk activation of the pretibial muscles initiates ankle dorsiflexion, but the arc is incomplete in initial swing.

Phase 7—Midswing: Ankle dorsiflexion to neutral is the critical event for floor clearance at this time (Fig. 5-10). Additional hip flexion and partial knee extension

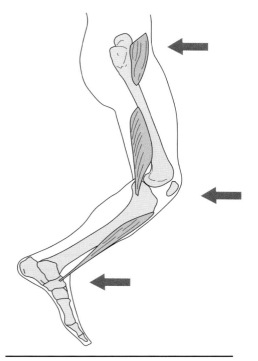

Fig. 5-9 Initial swing advancement of the limb by simultaneous active flexion at the hip (iliacus) and knee (biceps femoris, short head) and ankle dorsiflexion (tibialis anterior).

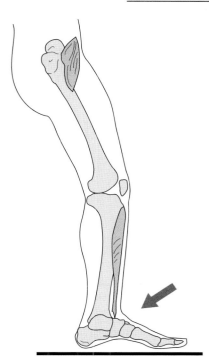

Fig. 5-10 Midswing limb advancement continues with residual active hip flexion, passive knee extension, and persistent ankle dorsiflexion to neutral by the pretibial muscles.

advance the limb. The relative vertical posture of the lower leg requires pretibial muscle support of the ankle.

Phase 8—Terminal swing: Forward swing of the limb for step length is accomplished by knee extension (see Fig. 5-2). The other actions relate to preparing the limb for stance as previously described.

Pathologic gait

Many types of disease and injury impair the patient's ability to walk. To the extent possible, patients accommodate their disability by altering the motion of adjacent joints or changing the timing and intensity of the controlling muscles. These substitutions increase the energy cost of walking. When the physiologic effort or pain exceeds the individual's tolerance, the disability becomes visible. To improve the patient's gait, the clinician must accurately identify the functional errors, differentiate the primary dysfunction from substitutive actions, correlate these events with the patient's pathology, and select the optimum corrective measures.

Pathologic patterns

Systematic gait analysis can identify the specific modes of dysfunction. Interpretation of these findings for clinical management depends on an understanding of the functional penalties the different pathologies impose and the patient's ability to substitute.

To facilitate interpretation, the wide spectrum of causes that challenge the ability to walk has been grouped into four functional categories according to their anatomic and pathologic qualities.

Structural impairment

Although some lesions lead to hypermobility, restricted passive motion and malalignment are the more common problems. The contributing pathologies are contractures, skeletal deformity, and musculoskeletal pain.

Contractures Freedom to move and attain optimal postures is readily impaired by fibrous connective tissue stiffness. Inactivity during the acute phase of illness, rigid immobilization for early healing, and stretch inhibition by spasticity are the major causes.

Fibrous tissue is present in every component of the musculoskeletal system (fascial sheaths, muscular aponeuroses, joint capsules, and ligaments). Stiffness is the inability of the strong, relatively inelastic collagen fibers to alter their alignment. Normally the collagen fibers move within the gel-like proteoglycan matrix that provides both support and lubrication.[1] With inactivity, the proteoglycan ground substance suffers chemical deterioration and loss of water. Measurable changes may occur within 2 weeks.[2]

Clinically, the two levels of contracture are elastic and rigid. Both resist manual testing. An *elastic contracture* yields under body weight to allow near-normal function. A *rigid contracture* obstructs motion in both stance and swing. Walking can be significantly impaired by contractures. The most significant contractures are ankle plantar flexion, knee flexion, and hip flexion.

Plantar flexion contractures of a "mere" 15 degrees can significantly impair stance limb progression. With the foot flat, body weight cannot be balanced over the foot without substitutive posturing (Fig. 5-11). The vigorous walker substitutes a premature heel rise to roll on the forefoot. Less able

67

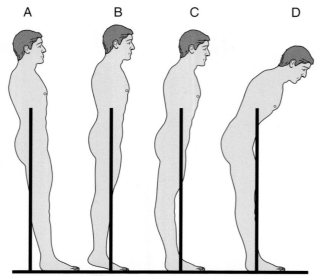

Fig. 5-11 A 15-degree plantar flexion contracture effects on standing balance and postural compensations. **A,** Flatfoot stance places the body vector behind the area of support, balance impossible. **B,** Heel rise shifts the vector over the forefoot, standing balance attained. Knee hyperextension (when available) **(C)** and forward trunk lean **(D)** move the vector over the flatfoot.

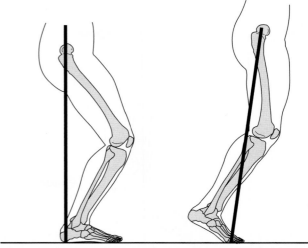

Fig. 5-13 Standing balance with knee flexion contracture. Either excessive ankle dorsiflexion and hip flexion *(left)* or a proportional heel rise is necessary.

persons use knee hyperextension or a forward trunk lean to advance their body vector over the stationary foot. These substitutions are only partially effective. Stride length is shortened.

Knee flexion contractures threaten stance stability. With the trunk erect, the body vector is behind the knee joint, leading to a greater demand on the quadriceps (Fig. 5-12). Based on a cadaver model, the inconspicuous 15-degree flexion angle requires a 20% quadriceps effort.[16] Increasing knee flexion to 30 degrees raises the required quadriceps force to 50% of maximum. Patients with limited strength lose their ability to walk. Also, the quadriceps action creates an equal compressive load on the joint, causing increased pain in arthritic patients.

Standing with a flexed knee requires increased ankle dorsiflexion. With limited ankle mobility, there is an early heel rise (Fig. 5-13). Inadequate knee alignment in terminal swing shortens stride length.

Hip flexion contractures threaten both stance stability and progression. The body vector becomes anterior to the supporting foot (Fig. 5-14). To stand erect, either the spine must provide excessive lordosis or the limb must be realigned by a flexed knee. Children commonly develop the needed spinal mobility, but few adults have sufficient flexibility. Crutch support then is needed.

Skeletal malalignment Deformed joint surfaces and supporting shafts can be further impaired by continued weight bearing. In 1892, Wolff observed that changes in a person's weight-bearing pattern could alter the internal architecture of bones.[4] Children are most susceptible because their growing tissue accommodates the abnormal stresses. Asymmetrical

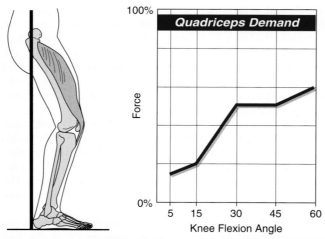

Fig. 5-12 Knee flexion contracture displacement of the vector behind the knee *(left)*. Quadriceps demand is increased *(heavy line)* as the flexed posture becomes greater. The difference between 15-degree and 30-degree knee flexion is severe *(right)*.

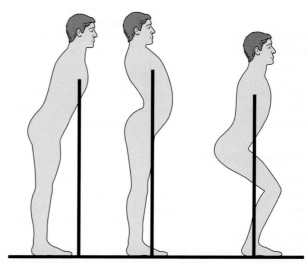

Fig. 5-14 Hip flexion contracture displacement of the vector anterior to the area of foot support *(left)*. Excessive trunk hyperextension *(center)* and knee flexion *(right)* are postures used to recover standing balance.

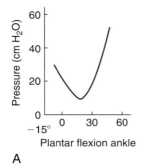 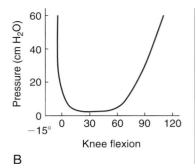

Fig. 5-15 Influence of joint position on intra-articular pressure created by joint swelling (experimental distention). **A,** Ankle joint pressure is minimal at 15 degrees plantar flexion. **B,** Knee joint pressure is least at 30 degrees flexion. *Vertical axis* is intra-articular pressure. *Horizontal axis* is joint position. (Modified from Eyring EJ, Murray WR: *J Bone Joint Surg* 46A:1235–1241, 1964.)

forces discourage new growth on the compressed side while inducing overgrowth contralaterally.[11] Adults, lacking the adaptability of growing tissues, react with degenerative changes that lead to pain and loss of function. During walking, the malalignments are seen as motion errors.

Musculoskeletal pain A common reaction to joint trauma or inflammation is swelling. The accumulated fluid makes the enveloping joint capsule tense and painful. In response, the swollen joints assume a resting position with minimal intra-articular pressure. For the ankle, it is 15 degrees plantar flexion (Fig. 5-15, *A*), whereas the knee and hip approximate 30 degrees flexion (Fig. 5-15, *B*).[8]

Swelling within the joint inhibits muscle action to avoid their compressive forces. Experimental testing of this response at the knee by progressive distention leads to quadriceps inhibition (Fig. 5-16).[7] Recovery of muscle action by intra-articular anesthesia confirmed the existence of a protective feedback mechanism. Secondary deformity and muscle weakness compromise the patient's ability to walk.

Motor unit insufficiency

Muscle weakness is the clinical penalty of having fewer motor units available to generate the forces needed for walking. Several different types of pathology (e.g., lower motor neuron diseases) can cause motor unit loss by selectively

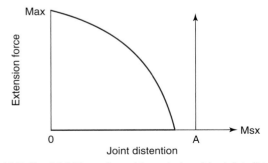

Fig. 5-16 Reflex inhibition of quadriceps induced by joint distention. Anesthesia of the distended joint restored quadriceps action *(A)*. *Vertical axis* (extension force) represents quadriceps action. *Horizontal axis* is intensity of the joint distention. (Modified from deAndrade MS, Grant C, Dixon A: *J Bone Joint Surg* 47A:313–322, 1965.)

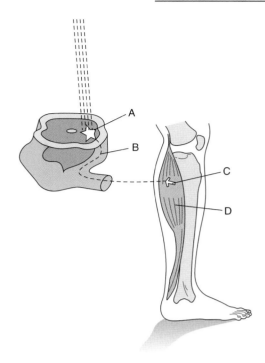

Fig. 5-17 Motor unit components. *A,* Anterior horn cell; *B,* root of the axon; *C,* myoneural junction; *D,* muscle fibers. (From Perry J, Hislop HJ: *Lower extremity bracing*, New York, 1967, American Physical Association.)

invading one component of the motor unit. Although each disease has its unique characteristics, the common characteristic is that patients have an excellent ability to substitute for the local weakness because normal sensation and control have been retained.

A motor unit has four major components: anterior horn cell, axon, myoneural junction, and muscle fibers (Fig. 5-17). From the cell body lying within the anterior horn of the spinal cord, an axon extends to the muscle and then divides into multiple branches. Each axonal branch connects to a muscle fiber through a myoneural junction (endplate) that chemically transmits the activating signals from nerve to muscle. The multiple muscle fibers under that cell's control generate the force used to create or restrain motion. In the lower limb, the muscles contain about 500 motor units, each containing 200 to 1000 muscle fibers.[10]

Poliomyelitis is an acute viral invasion of the anterior horn cells that causes a random pattern of paralysis. Anterior horn cell recovery averages 47% (range 12% to 91%).[5] Additional function is gained through axon sprouting to adopt orphaned muscle fibers,[18] enabling most patients to resume a normal lifestyle. *Postpolio syndrome* is a second problem. Overuse of the subnormal neuromuscular system for at least 30 years has led to a significant loss of function. Affected adults now experience new muscle weakness, fatigue, and pain. Because of patients' substitutive expertise, careful gait analysis is required to identify their disability. Often the postural substitutions are the only signs of disability.

Strength is judged by the manual muscle test, but the examiner's maximum manual force does not equal the ability of the larger muscles.[3] Grade 5 (normal) for the quadriceps averaged 50%. Grade 4 (good) was only 40% of true normal

Table 5-1 Manual muscle test grades and Beasley equivalents

True normal		100%
Manual Grades	**(MRC)**	**Beasley**
Normal	5	75%
(quadriceps)		(50%)
Good	4	40%
Fair	3	20%
Poor	2	5%

Source: Medical Research Council: Aids to investigators of peripheral nerve lesions, *Memorandum No. 7*, ed 2, London, 1943, Her Majesty's Stationery Office.
MRC, Medical Research Council.

(Table 5-1). Stationary dynamometry is indicated when clinical strength and symptoms disagree.

Guillain-Barré syndrome is a self-limiting inflammatory disease of unknown origin that strikes the roots of the axons as they exit the spinal cord. Patients are clinically similar to those with poliomyelitis except that the involvement is symmetrical and recovery is more rapid. Sensory involvement, if present, is minor (mild dysesthesia).

Myasthenia gravis is an autoimmune disease that involves the neuromuscular junction. It is managed medically rather than with use of orthoses. The disease is included here merely to complete the picture of motor unit pathology.

Muscular dystrophy is a bilaterally symmetrical, progressive degeneration of the muscle fibers. Among the differing patterns of involvement, Duchenne pseudohypertrophic form is most common. Within the lower limbs, progressive weakness begins in the pelvic girdle and extends distally. Fatty connective tissue replacement of the lost muscle fibers makes contracture formation a significant factor.

Peripheral sensory and motor impairment

The addition of a sensory loss to muscle paralysis reduces the patient's ability to substitute. One common cause is a cauda equina spinal cord injury. The cause may be congenital (spina bifida) or acute trauma. Impaired sensation occurs first on the soles of the feet. This delays awareness of floor contact. With complete foot and ankle paralysis, the patient must rely on the position sense within the flexed knee. Walking ability

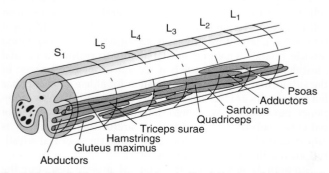

Fig. 5-18 Distribution of anterior horn cells within the spinal cord, indicating functional levels. Note the S1 cluster of triceps surae, hamstrings, and gluteals and the L2–3 cluster of quadriceps, hip flexors, and adductors. (Modified from Sharrard WJW: *J Bone Joint Surg* 37B:540, 1955.)

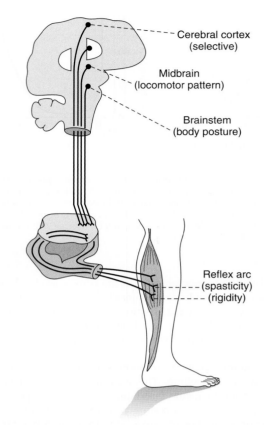

Fig. 5-19 Centers of upper neuron motor control. Levels below cortex (selective control) represent primitive control mechanism: midbrain (locomotion), brainstem (body position), and intramuscular spindle (stretch reflex arc, spasticity, rigidity).

decreases with each higher level of spinal cord impairment (Fig. 5-18). Adults have less potential to walk than do children.

Sacral (S1, S2) lesions primarily impair the posterior calf muscles (soleus and gastrocnemius). There also is early weakening of the hip extensor and abductor muscles.

Low lumbar (L5, L4) lesions increase the impairment, extending the paralysis to the hamstrings and most of the foot muscles. Excessive ankle dorsiflexion and knee flexion are the prominent postures in midstance. Heel contact persists through stance.

Upper lumbar (L3) lesions involve the quadriceps. The patient lacks the strength needed to independently support a flexed knee. Continued presence of L2 neural control preserves hip flexion for initiating a step.

The walking potential of each neurologic level is reduced by hip flexion contractures and bilateral involvement.

Central control dysfunction

Within the brain and spinal cord, several *upper motor neuron* pathways control the anterior horn cells (Fig. 5-19). These central control systems determine what muscles are activated. Brain lesions such as a stroke, acute head trauma, and cerebral palsy are the most common causes. Spinal cord injuries in the cervical and thoracic areas also create central control dysfunction. Spasticity is a universal characteristic. Beyond this, the nature of the resulting motion varies with the particular control pathways involved.

Selective control allows independent movement of one joint or muscle relative to the direction, intensity, and duration of action. This determines the patient's ability to respond accurately to manual muscle testing. Walking relies on selective control for simultaneous action by the knee extensors and ankle dorsiflexors during weight acceptance, for quadriceps relaxation while the soleus increases its activity in stance progression, and for other sources of gait smoothness. Impaired selective control by itself results in muscle weakness.

Primitive control activates the muscles through basic synergies and reflex responses. Normally these are background actions that simplify function, but they become dominant when their suppressive pathways are damaged. The three basic levels of primitive control are locomotor synergies, postural reflexes, and stretch reflexes.

Locomotor synergies provide two mass patterns of muscle action. An *extensor pattern* simultaneously activates the hip and knee extensors and the ankle plantar flexors. This meets the demand for early midstance but inhibits the ankle dorsiflexion needed for a heel rocker and obstructs the integration of knee flexion and ankle plantar flexion for preswing. The *flexion pattern* activates the ankle dorsiflexors in concert with the hip and knee flexor muscles. This is appropriate for initial swing but contradicts the needs of terminal swing. Although the limb synergies lie within the spinal cord, a locomotor center within the midbrain allows voluntary use of the patterns for walking.

Postural reflexes relate to both the body and the limb. A straight knee increases the tone in all of the extensor muscles, including the ankle plantar flexors. Conversely, limb flexion relaxes the extensors and augments the flexors. Being upright increases extensor tone compared to lying supine. Hence, limb and body posture modify the findings of a clinical examination.

Stretch reflexes vary with stimulus intensity. Clonus is the usual response to a quick stretch. Sustained muscle action follows a slow stretch. This latter finding means clinical examination cannot differentiate contracture from spasticity unless the neural pathway has been inactivated by anesthesia.

Gait of an upper motor neuron lesion is typified by the relative stiffness of the action and only midrange mobility. However, individual patients differ considerably because of the variability in the severity of selective control impairment and relative emergence of the more primitive controls.

Gait analysis process

The purpose of gait analysis is to identify the patient's walking disability. *Observation*, the basic clinical approach, is most effective when done systematically. In serial fashion, each joint is analyzed separately for its motion pattern throughout the gait cycle. Starting with the foot and ankle and advancing up the limb provides the easiest visualization of the activity. For each pertinent gait phase, deviations from normal are identified. Interpretations to differentiate primary deficits from substitutive posturing are made by correlating the actions of all segments according to the gait phases (Fig. 5-20). The causes of primary deviations are deduced from the clinical records of strength, range of motion, and, for spastic patients, upright spasticity and motor control. *Laboratory analysis* is indicated when problems remain. These data should be analyzed by the same format.

Gait motion errors represent either inadequate or excessive performance of the normal action. Their phasing has been emphasized because it facilitates visualization and interpretation. The functional significance of a gait error in one phase often becomes more evident when its development within the sequence of activity is noted. This relationship is displayed in many of the figures.

Gait deviations
Ankle

Because the ankle normally moves into selected arcs of dorsiflexion and plantar flexion, abnormal function could involve excessive or inadequate motion in either direction. To simplify the analysis, the term *excessive dorsiflexion* also relates to inadequate plantar flexion. Similarly, *excessive plantar flexion* includes inadequate dorsiflexion.

Excessive ankle dorsiflexion

Although occasionally present in swing, excessive ankle dorsiflexion is a functional problem only in stance. There are two distinct patterns of dysfunction.

Weight acceptance Loss of passive ankle plantar flexion range causes a prolonged heel rocker. Following heel contact, forefoot drop to the floor is delayed until the tibia rolls forward to a vertical position (Fig. 5-21). The result is excessive knee flexion and prolonged quadriceps activity. The cause may be a solid shell ankle–foot orthosis, prosthetic foot, or combined fusion of the ankle and subtalar joints in neutral.

Stance limb progression The tibia advances over the foot in midstance or terminal stance either at an excessive rate or to an excessive dorsiflexion arc. Terminal stance heel rise is either delayed or absent. Weakness of the soleus and gastrocnemius is the most common cause. The secondary effect is persistent or excessive knee flexion. A weak elastic contracture becomes the final restraining force (Fig. 5-22). Posturing to approach foot flat support in the presence of fixed knee flexion is a secondary cause (Fig. 5-23, *B*).

Excessive ankle plantar flexion

The two basic patterns of dysfunction are paralytic passive drop foot (anterior insufficiency) and posterior restraint from contracture, spasticity, primitive extensor synergy, or deliberate posturing.

Passive drop foot Two gait tasks are involved.

Swing limb advancement. The presence of a drop foot is most conspicuous in midswing. Also, this is the only phase in swing when the deviation is functionally significant. In initial swing, foot dorsiflexion is incomplete, and floor clearance is not dependent on the foot's position. With the tibia vertical in midswing, the passive drop at the ankle places the foot below horizontal (Fig. 5-24). The forefoot prematurely contacts the floor (foot drag) if there is no substitutive effort.

Weight acceptance. Initial contact generally is made with the forefoot, and the heel rocker is lost (Fig. 5-25, *B*). The loading

Reference Limb:		Weight acceptance		Single limb support		Swing limb advancement			
L ☐ R ☐		Stability Fwd progression Shock absorption		Stability Fwd progression		Foot clearance Limb advancement			
Diagnosis:									
		IC	LR	MSt	TSt	PSw	ISw	MSw	TSw
Trunk	Normal ROM	Upright	Upright	Upright	Upright	Upright	Upright	Upright	Upright
	Forward lean								
	Backward lean								
	Lateral lean								
Pelvis	Normal ROM	Level	Level	Level	Level	Level	Level	Level	Level
	Contralateral drop								
Hip	Normal ROM	25° flex	25° flex	0°	Apparent hyperext	0°	15° flex	25° flex	25° flex
	Limited flexion								
	Inadequate extension								
	Past retract								
Knee	Normal ROM	0°	15° flex	0°	0°	40° flex	60° flex	25° flex	0°
	Limited flexion								
	Excess flexion								
	Inadequate extension								
Ankle	Normal ROM	0°	10° PF	5° DF	10° DF	20° PF	10° PF	0°	0°
	Forefoot contact								
	Foot flat contact								
	Excess dorsiflexion								
	Excess plantar flexion								
	No heel off								
	Drag								

Fig. 5-20 Observational gait analysis form. *Left vertical column* lists the major deviations. *Right group of eight columns* identify the phases of gait. *Horizontal rows* designate the phases where each deviation has major significance *(white spaces)*, minor significance *(shaded)*, and no significance *(black area)*. IC, Initial contact; LR, loading response; MSt, midstance; TSt, terminal stance; PSw, preswing; ISw, initial swing; MSw, midswing; TSw, terminal swing. (Courtesy of Rancho Physical Therapy and Pathokinesiology Services: Observational Gait Analysis, 1993, LAREI.)

response that follows forefoot contact is a passive drop of the limb. Ankle plantar flexion is reduced and foot flat contact initiated (Fig. 5-25, *C*). The lack of a heel rocker effect results in persistent knee extension. The subsequent stance phases are normal if a passive drop foot is the patient's only problem. Inadequate function of the tibialis anterior and long toe extensor muscles is the cause of a passive drop foot gait.

Plantar flexor rigidity Excessive ankle plantar flexion caused by overly tense posterior structures (muscles or capsule) can begin in terminal swing (which positions the foot for initial contact) or any subsequent phase in stance, depending on the severity and timing of the plantar flexor force.

Weight acceptance. Three associated factors determine the functional significance of excessive posterior restraint: knee position at initial contact, vigor (speed) of the patient's gait, and elasticity of the plantar flexor force. These factors result in several weight acceptance patterns.

Initial contact with an extended knee and only 15 degrees plantar flexion allows minimal heel strike (Fig. 5-26, *A*). Loading response includes a rapid forefoot contact (Fig. 5-26, *B*) and a lack of knee flexion. More conspicuous evidence of plantar flexor restraint is the loss of ankle dorsiflexion in midstance (Fig. 5-26, *C*).

Initial contact with excessive ankle plantar flexion and a flexed knee is by the forefoot (Fig. 5-27). The subsequent loading response varies with the strength of the plantar flexor force and gait speed. With a slow gait and tissue elasticity, the heel drops to the floor and the knee extends (Fig. 5-28, *A*). Tibial advancement is delayed or obstructed relative to elasticity of the restraining tissues (Fig. 5-28, *B*). Fast walkers with sufficient plantar flexor strength to support body weight maintain a heel-off, forefoot support posture (Fig. 5-29, *B*). Both the heel rocker and shock-absorbing knee flexion are inhibited.

Stance limb progression. The ankle rocker either is curtailed or lost (Fig. 5-26, *C*). Tibial advancement is inhibited unless there is a premature heel rise (Fig. 5-28, *B*). An early forefoot rocker makes metatarsal loading prolonged and excessive (Fig. 5-29, *B* and *C*). It also challenges the integrity of the midfoot plantar support (Figs. 5-28, *C*, and 5-29, *B*). Limitations in stance progression result in a short step by the other limb.

The obstructive forces generally are gastrocnemius-soleus contracture or spasticity. Persons with normal control and weak quadriceps may voluntarily mimic the pattern of a mild, elastic contracture.

Swing limb advancement. Both midswing and terminal swing display excessive plantar flexion when the cause is a

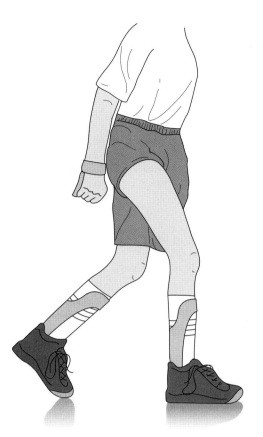

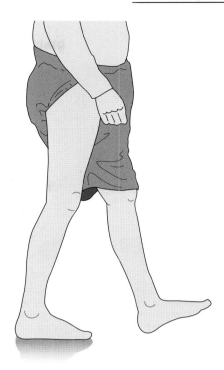

Fig. 5-22 Excessive ankle dorsiflexion from calf muscle weakness (right limb). Stance limb progression (terminal stance) with prolonged heel contact (foot flat), dorsiflexed ankle, and excessive knee flexion.

Fig. 5-21 Excessive dorsiflexion. Right limb in loading response with excessive ankle dorsiflexion, excessive knee flexion, and foot flat. Left limb in preswing with inadequate ankle plantar flexion. The patient's rigid ankle–foot orthosis prevents optimum function in both phases.

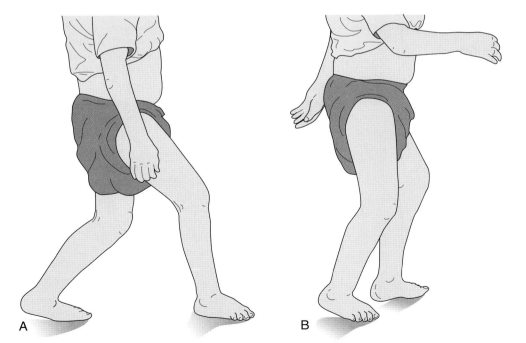

Fig. 5-23 Excessive ankle dorsiflexion to accommodate excessive knee flexion. A, Weight acceptance with the limb reaching forward. Excessive knee flexion does not challenge the ankle or the flat foot contact. B, Stance limb progression (midstance). Alignment of body weight over the supporting foot requires excessive ankle dorsiflexion and premature heel rise to accommodate the flexed knee.

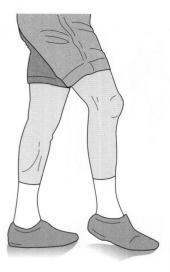

Fig. 5-24 Passive drop foot with drag (right limb). Swing limb advancement (midswing): Excessive ankle plantar flexion with normal flexion at the hip and knee causes premature forefoot floor contact. Further progression of limb is inhibited.

contracture. Elastic contractures that stretched under body weight in stance create a plantar flexed posture in swing because the dorsiflexor muscles are a much weaker force. When the cause of the excessive ankle plantar flexion is primitive pattern control, ankle position differs in midswing and terminal swing. Midswing is normal as the ankle is dorsiflexed as part of the flexor pattern. In terminal swing, the ankle actively plantar flexes in synergy with knee extension.

Foot

Loss of neutral foot alignment may occur in any gait phase. Functional significance, however, relates only to stance.

Excessive inversion (varus)

Subtalar joint inversion displaces floor contact to the lateral side of the foot (Fig. 5-30). Continued inversion following heel rise leads to persistent forefoot weight bearing on the fifth metatarsal head. First metatarsal floor contact is delayed or absent. Unstable weight bearing is the result. Common causes are soleus contracture; overactivity of the anterior tibialis, posterior tibialis, and soleus muscles; or primary bony malformation (clubfoot).

Excessive eversion (vagus)

Subtalar joint eversion leads to medial heel weight bearing, a flat arch, and premature first metatarsal loading (Fig. 5-31). Generally the cause is invertor muscle weakness. Occasionally, peroneal muscle overactivity is the cause.

Knee

Because the knee is in some degree of flexion throughout the gait cycle, function deviations relate to the magnitude of the motion in the individual phases. Significant deviations are excessive flexion, inadequate flexion, and excessive extension. Posturing at the knee may result from faulty ankle function as well as intrinsic knee dysfunction.

Excessive knee flexion

Excessive knee flexion is the most common knee dysfunction. Every phase of gait except initial swing can be impaired.

Weight acceptance. Weight-bearing stability is threatened by the added quadriceps demand of an overly flexed knee (see Fig. 5-23). Causes are flexion contracture, overly intense hamstring muscle activity in spastic patients, or lack of ankle plantar flexion.

Stance limb progression. Inability to extend the knee progressively from its initial flexed position prolongs quadriceps demand (see Fig. 5-23, *B*). In addition, the flexed knee may obligate forefoot support and excessive ankle dorsiflexion, creating weight-bearing instability. Progression of the body over the supporting foot is inhibited by lack of femoral advancement on the tibia.

Swing limb advancement. In midswing, increased knee flexion is a common voluntary effort to avoid a toe drag from a plantar flexed foot while the tibia is vertical (see Fig. 5-25, *A*). With premature and overly intense spastic hamstring action,

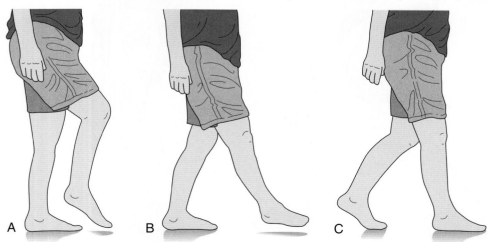

Fig. 5-25 Passive drop foot with floor clearance (right limb). **A,** Midswing with excessive ankle plantar flexion and excessive knee and hip flexion provides toe clearance. **B,** Terminal swing with excessive ankle plantar flexion, fully extended knee, and flexed hip for forward reach positioning the foot for forefoot contact. **C,** Loading response with foot flat and less ankle plantar flexion. Shock-absorbing knee flexion is absent.

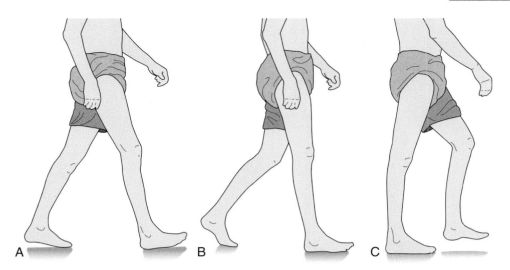

Fig. 5-26 Mild rigid excessive ankle plantar flexion. **A,** Low heel strike (nearly foot flat) posturing of right ankle in terminal swing. **B,** Weight acceptance with a rapid foot flat contact and extension of the knee. Knee flexion for shock absorption absent. **C,** Stance limb progression (midstance) with foot flat contact, inadequate ankle dorsiflexion, and knee hyperextension.

as occurs in cerebral palsy diplegia (Fig. 5-32), tibial advancement is restricted. The result is persistent knee flexion in terminal swing with inadequate knee posturing for stance (Fig. 5-33).

Inadequate knee flexion

Weight acceptance. Without knee flexion, the shock-absorbing mechanism is absent, leading to greater joint impact. The most common cause is excessive ankle plantar flexion

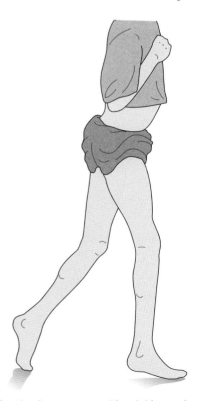

Fig. 5-27 Forefoot loading response with a rigid excessive ankle plantar flexion. Heel rocker is lost and replaced with premature heel rise and mild forward lean (right limb).

(passive or rigid; see Figs. 5-25 and 5-26). Persons also voluntarily avoid knee flexion to protect a weak quadriceps.

Swing limb advancement. In preswing, flexion less than 40 degrees inadequately prepares the limb for swing. Likely causes are continued action of the vasti as part of a spastic extensor pattern or inadequate terminal stance rocker because of persistent heel contact and absent dorsiflexion.

During initial swing, inadequate knee flexion causes toe drag unless the patient can substitute other motions (Fig. 5-34). The absence of a trailing foot posture reduces the need for knee flexion. Several factors contribute. Out-of-phase quadriceps action is the most common. When dynamic inhibition is limited to the rectus femoris, with or without vastus intermedius activity, surgical release can improve the patient's range (Fig. 5-35). Other situations that limit initial swing knee flexion are inadequate preswing flexion, hip flexor weakness, and premature hamstring action.

Excessive knee extension

Excessive knee extension may be frank hyperextension (Fig. 5-36) or an extensor thrust (see Fig. 5-26, *C*). The latter term is used when the limb is rapidly driven backward but the knee lacks a passive range of hyperextension. Causes are rigid ankle plantar flexion (contracture or spasticity), spastic overactivity of the vasti, and voluntary premature soleus action to stabilize a knee with insufficient quadriceps strength. The time of knee hyperextension varies with the cause. It may follow forefoot contact or be delayed into midstance (see Fig. 5-35) or terminal stance.

Knee varus (adduction) and vagus (abduction)

Knee varus (adduction) and vagus (abduction) are static knee postures related to the alignment of the joint surfaces or bony shafts.

Hip

Dysfunction at the hip relates to both thigh and pelvis postures. Inappropriate thigh posturing is reflected as inadequate

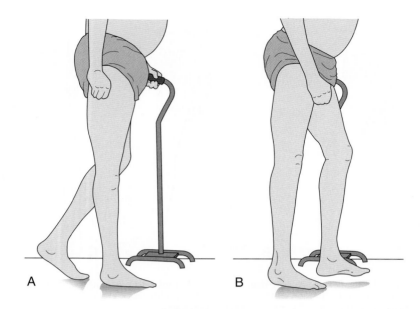

Fig. 5-28 Foot flat weight acceptance. **A,** Knee flexion absent. **B,** Stance limb progression with excessive ankle plantar flexion and premature heel rise.

flexion in swing and inadequate extension in stance. Excessive adduction and abduction are infrequent findings.

Inadequate hip flexion

Swing limb advancement. The critical time is initial swing. Primary hip flexor weakness is infrequent because grade 2+ is sufficient in flaccid paralysis. In spastic patients, inadequate hip flexion most often is caused by premature hamstring action or represents inhibition by a stiff knee gait (Fig. 5-37).

Weight acceptance. Inadequate hip flexion that continues into terminal swing limits the limb's forward reach for stance (Fig. 5-38).

Inadequate hip extension

Stance limb progression is the only task that is impaired. Without hip extension, the patient is denied a trailing limb position in late midstance and terminal stance (see Fig. 5-23, *B*). Stride length is shortened. Direct causes are avoidance of stretching a painful joint capsule, hip flexion contracture, or spasticity. Common indirect causes are postural adaptations for balance over a plantar flexed ankle or a flexed knee (see Fig. 5-37, *B*).

Hip past-retract. In terminal swing, a voluntary substitution is used to gain knee extension when the quadriceps muscle is paralyzed. Rapid, excessive hip flexion advances both the

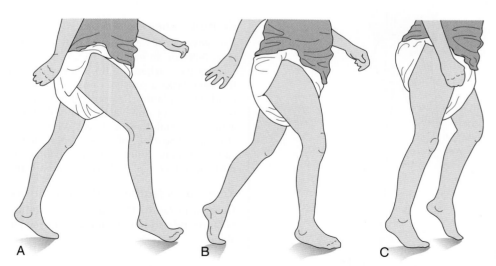

Fig. 5-29 Excessive ankle plantar flexion and excessive knee flexion (right limb). **A,** Initial contact by the forefoot. **B,** Loading response weight bearing partially reduces excessive plantar flexion, and posterior tibial thrust decreases excessive knee flexion. Midfoot dorsiflexes under the forefoot load. **C,** Midstance forward alignment of body on foot redirects the ankle plantar flexion force to increase ankle posture and height of heel rise. Excessive knee flexion is reduced.

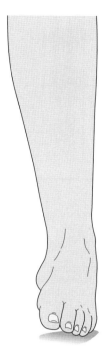

Fig. 5-30 Excessive inversion of the foot (varus). Floor contact has been shifted to the lateral side of the foot. The medial forefoot lacks floor contact. Overactivity of the anterior tibialis is apparent. Participation by the posterior tibialis cannot be assessed visually.

thigh and the tibia. Then, rapid hip extension retracts the thigh while inertia sustains the forward tibia.

Pelvis

Malalignments of the pelvis are secondary reactions to demands at the hip.

Contralateral pelvic drop

Weight acceptance. Transfer of body weight to the stance limb in preparation for swing removes the support of the opposite

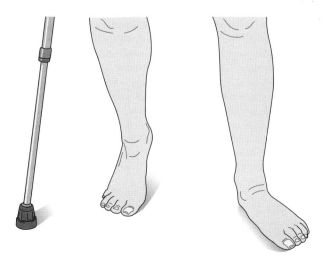

Fig. 5-31 Excessive eversion of the foot (valgus). Weight has been shifted toward the medial side of the foot, the arch is low, and the great toe is slightly rolled under.

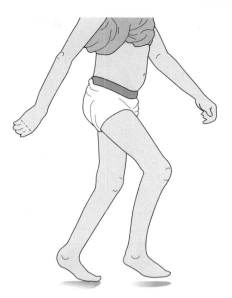

Fig. 5-32 Excessive knee flexion (bilateral). Swing limb advancement (right) knee flexion greater than hip flexion, which prevents tibia becoming vertical. Stance limb progression (left) knee does not attain full extension.

side. Hip abductor muscle weakness (gluteus medius, gluteus minimus, and upper gluteus maximus) allows the unsupported contralateral pelvis to drop (Fig. 5-39). Demand on the abductor muscle complex is aggravated by a long leg. Protection is provided by a tight iliotibial band or prepositioning into adduction by a short leg.

Pelvic hike

Swing limb advancement. Elevation of the ipsilateral side of the pelvis is used for foot clearance when hip and/or knee flexion is inadequate (Fig. 5-40).

Excessive rotation

Swing limb advancement. Anterior pelvic motion substitutes the trunk muscles for weak hip flexors to assist limb advancement.

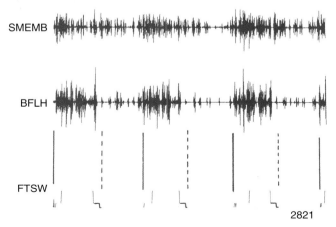

2821

Fig. 5-33 Dynamic electromyography of hamstring muscles showing nearly continuous activity of semimembranosus (SMEMB) and biceps femoris, long head (BFLH) with most intense action in stance. Footswitch (FTSW) "staircase" indicates stance. *Vertical solid line* is onset of stance. *Dotted line* is onset of swing.

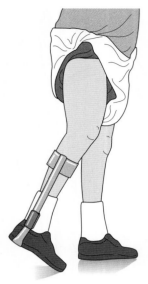

Fig. 5-34 Inadequate knee flexion (right limb). Swing limb advancement. Initial swing knee flexion is approximately 20 degrees rather than the normal 60 degrees. Ankle–foot orthosis support of the ankle shows toe drag results from the limited posture of the knee, not the foot.

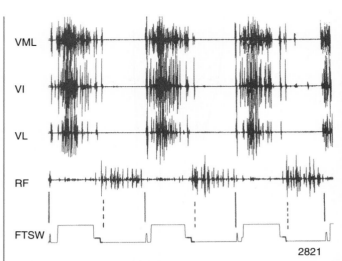

Fig. 5-35 Dynamic electromyogram of quadriceps. Vastus medialis longus (VML), vastus intermedius (VI), and vastus longus (VL) show intense and prolonged action in stance, which diminishes in preswing and is absent in swing. Rectus femoris (RF) overactivity (intensity and duration) is present throughout swing. *Solid vertical bar* is onset of stance. *Dashed vertical line* is onset of swing. FSW (footswitches) stair profile indicates sequence of floor contact: brief heel "scuff," return to baseline, support by heel and fifth metatarsal head, and contact only by fifth metatarsal and toes.

Stance limb progression. Posterior rotation and drop in terminal stance provide mild leg lengthening to accommodate persistent heel contact.

Trunk

Normal trunk motions are so small (5 degrees) that any visible deviation from the upright posture is abnormal. Patients with intrinsic spine deformity (scoliosis, lordosis, kyphosis) or paralysis have a constant posture abnormality that may increase the demand on the lower limbs to preserve standing balance.

Variable postural deviations of the trunk (*trunk leans*) are used to preserve standing balance by displacing the body vector or to assist limb advancement. Each deviation has a functional significance.

Forward trunk lean

Weight acceptance. Quadriceps demand is reduced by moving the vector anterior to the knee. Muscle weakness is an indication.

Stance progression. Anterior displacement of the body vector is used to restore standing balance over a plantar

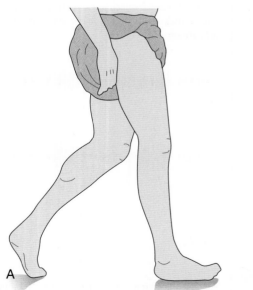
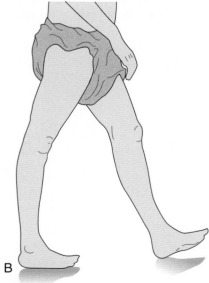

Fig. 5-36 Excessive knee extension (hyperextension) secondary to ankle plantar flexion contracture, right limb. **A,** Forward alignment of limb in weight acceptance allows a normal knee and ankle posture. **B,** Terminal stance advancement of thigh over the tibia restrained by plantar flexion contracture and lack of heel rise results in knee hyperextension.

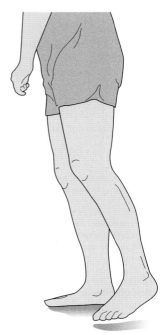

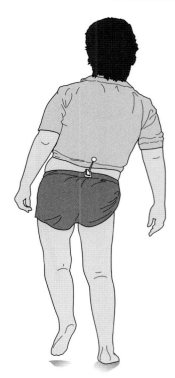

Fig. 5-37 Inadequate hip flexion (left). Swing limb advancement with inadequate flexion and hip, knee and ankle dorsiflexion. Right lateral lean for floor clearance.

Fig. 5-39 Contralateral pelvic drop and ipsilateral trunk lean indicate abductor muscle weakness.

flexed ankle or flexed knee (see Fig. 5-38). Excessive hip flexion that lacks compensatory lordosis also creates a forward trunk lean.

Backward trunk lean

Weight acceptance and stance progression. Posterior displacement of the body vector reduces the demand on weak hip extensor muscles (Fig. 5-41). The protective alignment begins with floor contact. Hip flexion contracture increases the amount of backward lean required to preserve standing balance. Bilateral posterior arm position adds further balance protection.

Swing limb advancement. In initial swing, a backward lean accompanied by anterior pelvic tilt assists limb advancement when the hip flexors are weak.

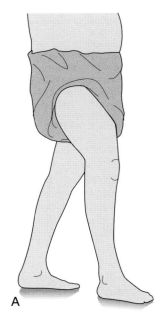

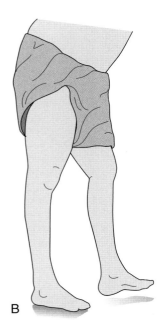

A   B

Fig. 5-38 Inadequate hip flexion (right). **A,** Weight acceptance with trunk erect, short forward reach, excessive ankle plantar flexion, and forefoot contact. **B,** Stance limb advancement with forward trunk for balance over plantar flexed ankle.

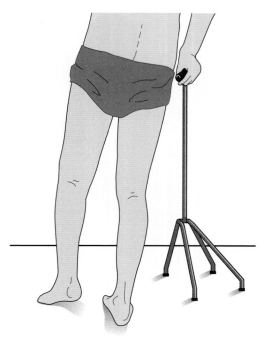

Fig. 5-40 Ipsilateral pelvic hike for floor clearance with inadequate hip and knee flexion.

Lateral trunk lean

Weight acceptance through stance progression. An ipsilateral lean is used to reduce the demand on the hip abductor muscles (see Fig. 5-39). The amount of lateral trunk lean is proportional to the severity of weakness.

Swing limb advancement. Combined contralateral lateral lean of the trunk and ipsilateral pelvic hike is another substitution to assist limb advancement (see Fig. 5-40).

References

1. Akeson WH, et al: The connective tissue response to immobility: biochemical changes in periarticular connective tissue of the immobilized rabbit knee, *Clin Orthop Rel Res* 93:356–362, 1973.
2. Akeson WH, et al: Biomedical and biochemical changes in the periarticular connective tissue during contracture development in the immobilized rabbit knee, *Connect Tissue Res* 2:315–323, 1974.
3. Beasley WC: Quantitative muscle testing: principles and applications to research and clinical services, *Arch Phys Med Rehabil* 42:398–425, 1961.
4. Bick EM: *Source book of orthopedics*, New York, 1968, Hofner Publishing.
5. Bodian D: Motoneuron disease and recovery in experimental poliomyelitis. In Halstead LS, Weichers DO, editors: *Late effects of poliomyelitis*, Miami, FL, 1985, Symposia Foundation.
6. Chelbourn GS, Busic AL, Graham KK, Stucky HA: Fascicle length change of the human tibialis anterior and vastus lateralis during walking, *J Ortho Sports Med* 37:372–379, 2007.
7. deAndrade MS, Grant C, Dixon A: Joint distension and reflex muscle inhibition in the knee, *J Bone Joint Surg* 47A:313–322, 1965.
8. Eyring EJ, Murray WR: The effect of joint position on the pressure of intra-articular effusion, *J Bone Joint Surg* 46A:1235–1241, 1964.
9. Fukunaga T, Kubo K, Kawakami Y, Fukashiro S, Kanehisa H, Maganaris CN: In vivo behavior of human muscle tendon during walking, *Proc Royal Society of London B*, 229–233, 268, 2001.
10. Feinstein B, et al: Morphological studies of motor units in normal human muscles, *Acta Anat* 23:127, 1955.
11. Haas SL: Retardation of bone growth by wire loop, *J Bone Joint Surg* 27A:25, 1945.
12. Lichtwark GA, Bougoulias K, Wilson AM: Muscle fascicle and series elastic element length changes along the length of the human gastrocnemius during walking and running, *J Biomech* 40:157–164, 2005.
13. Medical Research Council: *Aids to investigators of peripheral nerve lesions*, Memorandum No. 7, ed 2, London, 1943, Her Majesty's Stationery Office.
14. Murray MP, Clarkson BH: The vertical pathways of the foot during level walking: I. Range of variability in normal men, *Phys Ther* 46:585–589, 1966.
15. Perry J: *Gait analysis, normal and pathological function*, Thorofare, NJ, 1992, Charles B. Slack.
16. Perry J, Antonelli D, Ford W: Analysis of knee-joint forces during flexed-knee stance, *J Bone Joint Surg* 57A:961–967, 1975.
17. Simon SR, Paul IL, Mansour J, Munro M, Abernathy PJ, Radin EL: Peak dynamic force in human gait, *J Biomech* 14:817–822, 1981.
18. Weiss P, Edds MV: Spontaneous recovery of muscle following partial denervation, *Am J Physiol* 145:587–607, 1946.
19. Wittle MW: Generation and attenuation of transient impulsive forces beneath the foot, *Gait Posture* 10:264–275, 1999.

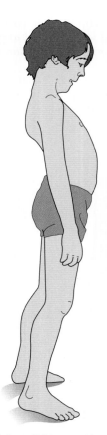

Fig. 5-41 Backward trunk lean. With poor hip extensor muscles and a hip flexion contracture, standing balance gained by trunk lordosis and both arms slightly posterior to substitute for weak hip extensors. Note the ankle dorsiflexion used to align the body mass center over the foot.

2

Spinal orthoses

In previous editions of the *Atlas*, topics such as biomechanics and components were brought together in separate sections under the headings of Basics and Principles, and Materials and Components. For this edition, the editors have combined all of the issues dealing with a given anatomical region into separate sections. The editors have asked the authors to give outcome evidence where possible and have encouraged all authors to base their chapters on clinical relevancy. As a result, it is hoped that each section and each chapter will speak to all readers, regardless of their discipline or background.

The principles of biomechanics underlie the effective function of all orthoses. Chapter 6, Biomechanics of the Spine, by Patwardhan et al., guides the reader from an understanding of basic anatomical and structural integrity to mechanical considerations in the disease process. The same authors contribute to later chapters, discussing biomechanics when relevant to treatment considerations.

In Chapter 7, Principles and Components of Spinal Orthoses, Romo et al. build upon earlier work by T. Gavin, Patwardhan, Bunch, D. Gavin, Levin, and Fenwick, revising their chapter by categorizing all of the different types of spinal orthoses. Although a complete discussion of componentry is given, the strict clinical application of these components is also presented in separate chapters dealing with specific indications. The reader will find Chapter 7 complementary to the other chapters.

The strength of Chapter 8, Orthoses for Spinal Pain, by Strenge and Fisk, is its evidence-based approach. The authors demonstrate well the paucity of outcomes data on the efficacy of spinal orthoses for treatment of spinal pain. That is not to say that spinal orthoses have no role in painful conditions. What it does say is that there is room for a great deal of additional clinical studies.

In Chapter 9, Orthoses for Spinal Deformities, Donald Katz demonstrates his understanding of the use of spinal orthoses for treatment of deformities. His work at Texas Scottish Rite Hospital for Children and his activity with the orthotic committee of the Scoliosis Research Society are apparent in this chapter. Once again the evidence in the literature must be carefully weighed before unsubstantiated claims can be made about the effectiveness of a given brace. With braces named for almost as many cities as there are treatment centers, an adequate base of outcome data is still lacking. The prospective randomized study using the need for surgery as an endpoint has not yet been performed. The exhaustive bibliography at the end of Katz's chapter is a good starting point for the reader interested in what investigators have accomplished.

In Chapter 10, Orthoses for Spinal Trauma and Postoperative Care, Malas et al. remind us of the principles behind the role of a well-made orthosis in this time of aggressive surgical management of spinal fractures. In areas underserved by surgeons, spinal orthoses for treatment of spinal fractures may be one solution for these injuries. This is not to say that spinal orthoses do not have an important role in the industrialized world. Malas et al. set out the indications and limitations for the use of spinal orthoses in the treatment of Spinal Trauma and Postoperative Care.

Chapter 11, Orthoses for Osteoporosis, by Meade et al., is a new addition to the fourth edition of the Atlas. Osteoporosis now is a common household word, with ever increasing awareness of the consequences of a sedentary livestyle and of increasing longevity. The authors report on a new orthotic design that is showing some promise for persons with insufficiency fractures of the spine. Long-term outcomes are lacking, but their thinking is clear.

In Section 2, the editors have attempted to pull together authors who actively use orthoses for treatment in their respective areas of expertise. Prospective outcome studies that can narrow the number of different orthoses used for treatment of spinal conditions are needed.

John R. Fisk

Chapter

6

Biomechanics of the spine

Avinash G. Patwardhan, Kevin P. Meade, and Thomas M. Gavin

Key Points

- The primary biomechanical function of the spinal column is to support the substantial loads induced during activities of daily living while allowing physiologic mobility.

- This chapter presents a framework for understanding these biomechanical functions of the spine by first discussing the stability of the osteoligamentous spinal column and the role played by the muscles. The chapter progresses to a discussion of the stability of a healthy spinal segment, followed by the effects of injuries, degeneration, and surgical procedures on load sharing between the components of a spinal segment.

- The chapter presents a brief discussion of the biomechanics of spinal fusion implants as well as orthoses used for stabilizing an unstable spine.

Physiologic loads

Mechanical loading of the spine is an important factor in the etiology of spinal disorders. It also affects the outcome of orthotic treatments for spinal disorders. Loads on the human spine are produced by (1) gravitational forces due to the mass of body segments, (2) external forces and moments induced by a physical activity, and (3) muscle tension. These loads are shared by the osseoligamentous tissues and muscles of the spine. Tensile forces in the paraspinal muscles, which exert a compressive load on the spine, balance the moments created by gravitational and external loads (Fig. 6-1). Because these muscles have a small moment arm from the spinal segment, they amplify the compressive load on the osseoligamentous spine.

The human spine is subjected to large compressive preloads during activities of daily living. The internal compressive forces on the ligamentous spine have been estimated for different physical tasks using kinematic and electromyographic data in conjunction with three-dimensional biomechanical models. The compressive force on the human lumbar spine is estimated to range from 200 to 300 N during supine and recumbent postures to 1400 N during relaxed standing with the trunk flexed 30 degrees. The compressive force may be substantially larger when an individual is holding a weight in the hands in the static standing posture and even more so during dynamic lifting. The human cervical spine also withstands substantial compressive preloads in vivo. Cervical preload approaches three times the weight of the head due to muscle coactivation forces in balancing the head in the neutral posture. The compressive preload on the cervical spine increases during flexion, extension, and other activities of daily living and is estimated to reach 1200 N in activities involving maximal isometric muscle efforts. In normal individuals, the spine sustains these loads without causing injuries to bony, soft tissue, or neurologic structures.

Stability of the spinal column
Load-bearing ability of the osteoligamentous spine

In the absence of muscle forces, the osteoligamentous spine cannot support vertical compressive loads of in vivo magnitude. Experiments in which a vertical load was applied at the cephalic end of cervical, thoracolumbar, or lumbar spine specimens caused buckling of the spines at load levels well below those seen in vivo. The stability of the spine, characterized by a critical load (maximum load carrying capacity, or

83

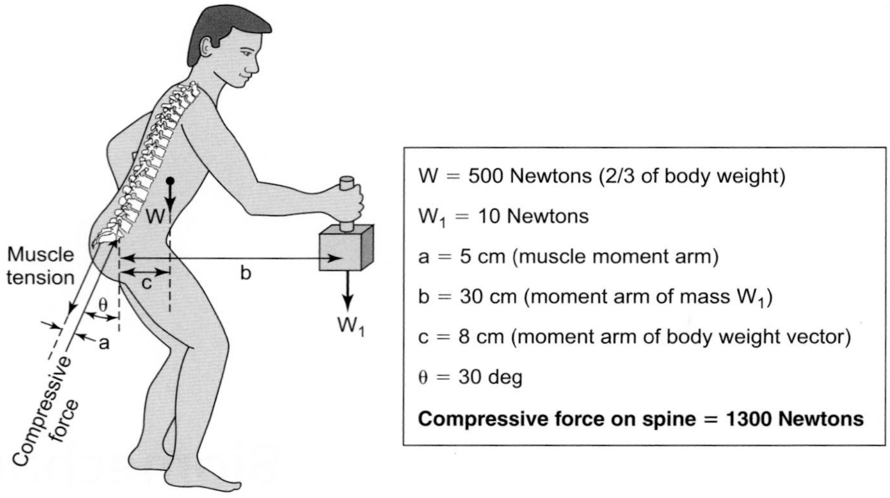

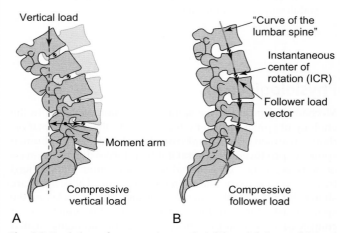

Fig. 6-1 Loads on the spine. The compressive force acting on the spine is magnified by the small moment arm of the muscles. (Adapted from Mow VC, Flatow EL, Ateshian GA: Biomechanics. In Buckwalter JA, Einhorn TA, Simon SR, editors: *Orthopaedic basic science,* Rosemont, Ill, 2000, American Academy of Orthopaedic Surgeons.)

W = 500 Newtons (2/3 of body weight)

W_1 = 10 Newtons

a = 5 cm (muscle moment arm)

b = 30 cm (moment arm of mass W_1)

c = 8 cm (moment arm of body weight vector)

θ = 30 deg

Compressive force on spine = 1300 Newtons

Euler buckling load of spinal column), was determined by these experiments. When the load exceeded the critical value, the spine, constrained to move only in the frontal plane in these experiments, became unstable and buckled. The cervical spine buckled at a vertical load of approximately 10 N, the thoracolumbar spine at 20 N, and the lumbar spine at 88 N, all well below the compressive loads expected in vivo during activities of daily living. When a compressive load is applied in a vertical direction to a multisegment spine specimen, segmental bending moments and shear forces are induced as a result of the inherent curvature of the spine. This load application causes large changes in the specimen's posture at relatively small loads. Further loading can cause damage to the soft tissue or bony structures.

Role of muscles

Some investigators have modeled the muscles as springs in order to explain their role in preventing a buckling instability of the spinal column. Simulation of active muscle forces in experiments on the ligamentous spine is difficult because of the large number of muscles and the uncertainty in load sharing among the various muscles during different activities. The simulated muscle actions must provide stability to the ligamentous spine to carry compressive loads while permitting the mobility needed to perform the activities of daily living.

Analysis using muscle models of the trunk support the argument that the individual spinal segments, often referred to as functional spinal units (FSUs), are subjected to nearly pure compressive loads in vivo. Attempts to determine joint loads based on the assumption of a vertical load on the spine have resulted in serious overprediction of shear forces on the FSU. Calculations of spine models, taking into consideration the activity of paraspinal and abdominal muscles, demonstrated that, in weight-holding tasks, the compressive force on the lumbosacral disc increased with increasing trunk inclination and the amount of weight lifted, whereas the maximum anteroposterior shear force remained small (approximately 20% to 25% of the compressive force). The obliquity of the short lumbar extensor muscles allows them to share anterior shear forces resulting from lifting a load.

When these muscles are activated to contribute a balancing extensor moment, they help to offset the anterior shear force on the lumbar FSU.

Stability of the spinal column under a follower load

It can be reasoned that coactivation of trunk muscles alters the direction of the internal compressive force vector such that its path follows the lordotic and kyphotic curves of the spine, passing through the instantaneous center of rotation of each segment (Fig. 6-2). This would minimize the segmental bending moments and shear forces induced by the compressive load, allowing the ligamentous spine to support loads that otherwise would cause buckling and providing a greater margin of safety against both instability and tissue injury. The load vector described is called a *follower load.*

Experiments on human cadaveric specimens of lumbar (L1–5), thoracolumbar (T2–sacrum), and cervical spines

Fig. 6-2 Depiction of compressive vertical **(A)** and follower **(B)** load vectors. The compressive follower load vector in the sagittal plane passes through the flexion–extension instantaneous center of rotation of each segment, minimizing the coupled flexion–extension angular changes.

(C2–7) as well as mathematical models have demonstrated that (1) the ligamentous spine with multiple motion segments can withstand physiologic compressive loads without tissue injury or instability if the compressive load vector is applied along a follower load path approximating the curve of the ligamentous spine, (2) the ligamentous spine subjected to compressive preloads of in vivo magnitude along the follower load path permits physiologic mobility under flexion–extension moments, and (3) the follower preload simulates the resultant vector of muscles that allow the spine to support physiologic compressive loads. Intradiscal pressures in human cadaveric lumbar spines under a follower preload are comparable to those measured in vivo, and spinal stability is increased without compromising its mobility in flexion–extension and lateral bending. A superimposed follower preload renders more physiologic the in vitro loading of the ligamentous spine with pure moments.

The follower load concept suggests a new hypothesis for the role of muscle coactivation in providing in vivo spine stability. Coactivation of trunk muscles (e.g., lumbar multifidus, longissimus lumborum, iliocostalis lumborum) could alter the direction of the resultant internal force such that its path follows the curve of the spine (follower load path), allowing the ligamentous spine to support compressive loads that otherwise would cause buckling of the column. Muscle dysfunction can induce abnormal shear forces at the lumbar FSU, leading to segmental instability in the presence of disc degeneration. On the other hand, a compressive follower preload produced by coordinated muscle action could stabilize shear instability in a degenerative FSU. This suggests a role for muscle conditioning and therapy in treating degenerative spine conditions.

Stability of the functional spinal unit
Three-joint complex

A spinal motion segment is the smallest functional unit of the osteoligamentous spine and exhibits the generic characteristics of the spine. The FSU consists of two vertebral bodies connected by an intervertebral disc, facet joints, and ligaments (except at the C1–2 segment, where no intervertebral disc is present). The FSU can be viewed as a three-joint complex consisting of the disc (a cartilaginous joint) and two facet joints (synovial joints). A dynamic relationship exists between the intervertebral disc and facet joints in sharing physiologic loads.

The intervertebral disc carries substantial loads as a result of gravitational and muscle forces. It is the major anterior load-bearing element in axial compression and flexion. In the young healthy spine, load transmission from vertebra to vertebra occurs primarily through the disc's nucleus pulposus. As load is applied to the healthy disc, forces are distributed equally in all directions from within the nucleus, placing the annulus fibers in tension. The collagen fibers of the annulus fibrosis are well suited to resisting tension along the fiber direction. The pressure in the nucleus pulposus stretches the fibers in the annulus, and the resistance of the fibers to tensile loading allows the annulus to contribute to load sharing. The annulus fibrosis is well suited to resisting torsion as a result of the characteristic orientation of fibers in the each layer.

The intervertebral disc provides most of the motion segment's stiffness in compression, whereas ligaments and facets contribute significantly to resisting bending moments and axial torsion.

Facet joints provide a posterior load path and have an important role in determining the limits of motion in the FSU. Biomechanical studies demonstrated that facets in the lumbar spine carry 10% to 20% of the compressive load when a person is in the standing upright position. The proportion of the total load shared by the disc increases with flexion. Load transmission through the articular facet surfaces as well as through the tips of the inferior facets in extension relieves some of the load on the intervertebral disc. Maintenance of cervical and lumbar lordosis helps to reduce the load on the disc, whereas flexion increases disc loading. The contribution of the facet joints to the stability of an FSU is also dependent on the capsular ligament and the level within the spine. For example, thoracic facets have limited capsular reinforcement, which facilitates axial rotation, in contrast to the lumbar spine, where the facet capsule is well developed and capable of stabilizing the spine against rotation and lateral bending.

Segmental instability

Injuries, degeneration, and surgical procedures can significantly alter normal load sharing between the components of an FSU and can cause abnormal motion response under physiologic loads. Instability is quantified in terms of loss of stiffness or increase in flexibility of an FSU. Stiffness of an FSU is a measure of how much load is required to produce a given motion. Flexibility is the inverse of stiffness; it is a measure of the motion produced by a given load. An FSU is unstable if the stiffness is too small or flexibility is too large. It is helpful to think about FSU instability in terms of macroinstability and microinstability.

Macroinstability

Macroinstability implies gross disruption of the spinal column, such as that caused by a fracture leading to disruption of load transmission from one vertebra to another. Macroinstability can lead to progression of the deformity at the injury site and neurologic deficit. Examples of macroinstability include instability caused by injuries of the thoracolumbar spine such as compression fracture, fracture–dislocation, traumatic spondylolisthesis, burst fracture, as well as tumors, infections, and iatrogenic causes. Thinking about the spine as a structure made of three load-bearing columns is helpful in appreciating the severity of clinical and biomechanical macroinstability. The *anterior* column is formed by the anterior longitudinal ligament, anterior annulus fibrosis, and anterior part of the vertebral body. The *middle* column is formed by the posterior longitudinal ligament, posterior annulus fibrosis, and posterior wall of the vertebral body. The *posterior* column is formed by the posterior arch, supraspinous and interspinous ligaments, facet joints, and ligamentum flavum. Compression fracture involves failure of the anterior column, with the middle column being totally intact. The burst fracture involves failure of both the anterior and middle columns. The seat-belt–type injury represents failure of the middle and posterior columns. Finally, the fracture–dislocation injury represents failure of all three load-bearing columns.

Loss of load-carrying capacity of the spine is influenced by the number of columns disrupted. Disruption of a single column, such as the anterior column, due to a compression fracture results in minimal loss of load-carrying capacity. The instability associated with a two-column disruption, such as that caused by a burst fracture or a flexion–distraction seatbelt injury, is more severe. Burst fractures cause significant instability (loss of stiffness relative to intact segment) in flexion, lateral bending, and axial rotation. That is, the injured segments undergo excessively large motion compared to the intact or uninjured segment for the same amount of load. If, in addition to the two-column burst fracture, the facets are disrupted, a significantly larger loss of stiffness may be seen in axial rotation. A fracture–dislocation is an example of a three-column disruption and is at the high end of the macroinstability spectrum.

Microinstability

The instability associated with degenerative disorders of the lumbar spine can be viewed as microinstability. Failure or degeneration of any one element of the three-joint complex can alter the normal load sharing between these elements, leading to symptoms of back and leg pain. It also may set into motion a chain reaction (degenerative cascade) leading to degeneration and pain at other elements of the FSU.

Disc degeneration is thought to precede all other changes within the aging FSU. Degenerative changes in a disc are associated with a loss of proteoglycans in the nucleus that, in turn, leads to a decrease in the ability of the nucleus to generate fluid pressure. With disc dehydration and narrowing of the disc space, the annular fibers of the disc are no longer subjected to the same tensile stresses as they would be in a healthy disc with the hydrated nucleus. Instead the annulus in a degenerated disc is more likely to bear the axial load under direct compression from the vertebra above. Early degenerative changes in the disc render the FSU more flexible. Facet degeneration is most commonly a result of segmental instability. As narrowing of the disc space occurs as a result of degeneration, the facets begin to undergo subluxation until the tips of the inferior facets impinge on the lamina below, causing the facets to increase their share of load transmission. Typically, in patients suffering from facet syndrome, symptoms are aggravated by an extension maneuver because facet loading increases in extension. Increased peak pressures within the facet joint may give rise to degeneration of the joint cartilage. Thinning of the cartilage may cause capsular ligament laxity and allow abnormal motion or hypermobility of the facets joints. Cartilage degeneration seems to further increase the segmental movements that already were increased with disc degeneration. The final stage of the degenerative cascade is associated with attempted stabilization. The abnormal pressure and focal degeneration give rise to formation of bony hypertrophy and osteophytes and a decrease in segmental mobility. Occasionally, an uneven collapse of the disc space causes acute angular deformities within the three-joint complex, and the patient may present with complaints of both neurogenic as well as low back pain.

During the process of three-joint complex degeneration, surgical intervention may be necessary to alleviate disabling symptoms. The combination of the surgical procedure (e.g., discectomy, facetectomy, foraminotomy, laminectomy) and

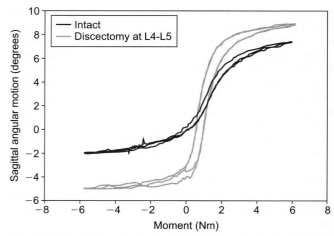

Fig. 6-3 Moment versus angular displacement curve for an L4–5 segment: intact, and after unilateral hemifacetectomy with partial discectomy.

the phase of degeneration affects the biomechanical stability of the FSU and the clinical outcome. Biomechanical studies on human cadaveric spines showed that disruption of the ligamentum flavum and posterolateral annular integrity and removal of the nucleus content, simulating partial discectomy for disc herniations, significantly increase primary motions in flexion, axial rotation, and lateral bending. Significant changes to FSU motion occur with nucleus pulposus removal as opposed to removal of the annulus. Hemilaminotomy–partial discectomy increases angular motion over that seen in the intact FSU. Unilateral hemifacetectomy has little effect on angular motion in flexion–extension and lateral bending but may cause a small increase in axial rotation. Subsequent discectomy significantly increases angular motion in flexion–extension without a preload (Fig. 6-3); however, a physiologic compressive preload of 400 N tends to reduce the instability produced after discectomy. Discectomy also significantly increases angular motion in axial rotation in the absence of a compressive preload. Hemilaminotomy with partial discectomy is the gold standard for surgical treatment of symptomatic radiculopathy caused by a herniated disc. Although discectomy is quite effective in relieving radicular symptoms, persistent mechanical low back pain is not uncommon. The back pain may relate to disc degeneration and the ensuing altered kinematics at the involved segment, which may be exacerbated by surgical treatment. Nonphysiologic motions may lead to altered stresses across the motion segment stabilizers, including the facet joints and the supporting musculoligamentous structures, which could contribute to postdiscectomy mechanical back pain. However, the true source of back pain remains unknown despite our many attempts to define it.

Procedures performed for pathologies in the late degenerative phase, such as decompressive laminectomy or facetectomy for degenerative spondylolisthesis, may lead to instability. Significant instability may result from bilateral hemifacetectomy. Unilateral or bilateral total facetectomy was shown to produce an increase in segmental motion of 65% in flexion, 78% in extension, 15% in lateral bending, and 126% in rotation. These procedures may require postdecompression stabilization.

Biomechanics of stabilization

Spinal fusion

Options for surgical stabilization range from uninstrumented fusion to fusion aided by the combination of anterior and posterior instrumentation. There is consensus in the literature concerning the ideal mechanical environment to promote spinal fusion; a greater degree of immobilization of adjacent vertebrae enhances the chances of obtaining a solid bony fusion. Spinal instrumentation increases the rigidity of segments at the fusion site, reducing the relative motion between the vertebrae during the biologic healing process. Posterior spinal implants typically act as tension band devices. When the load-bearing function of the anterior column is not compromised, posterior stabilization systems can enhance spinal stability. Posterior instrumentation typically consists of two longitudinal components (e.g., plates or rods) and segmental attachments to the vertebrae, forming a solid construct. The rigidity of the construct depends on the size and shape of the longitudinal components, the number of vertebrae spanned by the implant, the method of their attachment to the vertebrae, and the cross-links between the longitudinal components.

Implants that use wires or hooks to attach the longitudinal components to the vertebrae can resist tensile forces but cannot effectively resist angular deformity caused by loads experienced during activities of daily living in the presence of compromised load-bearing ability of the anterior column. On the other hand, a spinal instrumentation that uses transpedicular screws has the ability to resist both compressive and tensile forces, as well as bending moments. Transpedicular screws, which span all three columns, can transfer compressive loads and bending moment from the anterior column, through the pedicle to the longitudinal components of the instrumentation. Thus, fixation using transpedicular screws results in more rigid constructs than sublaminar wire or hooks. However, in the presence of failure of anterior elements as a load-sharing component, the possibility of screw failure (loosening or breakage) is high. This is common in highly comminuted fractures of the vertebral body, treated by hyperdistraction with posterior instrumentation.

Although transpedicular fixation allows three-column bony purchase, reports indicate the potential for continued micromotion in the intervertebral space, providing a possible explanation for persisting back pain despite solid fusion. Furthermore, in the presence of chronic instability, screw loosening or breakage is possible if the anterior column support is lacking. This may also be the case when stabilizing the macroinstability associated with substantial disruption of two of the three load-bearing columns. To enhance stability, it may be necessary to augment the load-bearing capacity of the anterior column (i.e., use an interbody spacer such as a cage); this provides the anterior support that allows posterior instrumentation to act as a tension band.

Whether an interbody fusion device should be used as a stand-alone device is a matter of debate. In the early postoperative period, the stability of a stand-alone interbody device depends primarily on the compressive forces on the interbody implant that are produced by tension in the remaining lateral and posterolateral annulus fibrosus and ligaments resulting from disc space distraction. A biomechanical study showed that the disc-space distraction force (and hence the compressive force on the interbody device) significantly increased in proportion to the degree of distraction. However, the distraction force reduced in magnitude by more than 20% in the first 15 minutes due to stress relaxation of the soft tissues, suggesting that the "tightness of fit" that the surgeon notes immediately after interbody cage insertion will degrade in the very early postoperative period. Furthermore, excessive disc-space distraction can result in changes in spinal alignment and stretching or tearing of the posterior ligaments and facet capsules. Distraction of the facet joints can cause pain and loss of segmental stiffness or hypermobility in extension. On the other hand, if disc-space distraction is inadequate, the compressive preload on the interbody implant may not be sufficient; resulting in motion at the implant–bone interface in the early postoperative period. This can lead to delayed fusion and/or pseudarthrosis and, in some instances, dislodgement or migration of the fusion cage itself. Supplemental stabilization using translaminar facet screws, pedicle screws, or external spinal orthoses can enhance the stability of the FSU treated with interbody cages.

Spinal orthoses

Orthoses have been used as nonoperative alternatives to spinal fusion in some cases of microinstability and macroinstability and as postoperative adjuncts to protect the surgical constructs used for stabilizing macroinstability in the thoracolumbar spine. The postoperative orthosis should limit the gross motion of the trunk during activities of normal daily living, thereby protecting the surgical construct from large loads created from torso motion until solid biologic fusion occurs. Another function of a postoperative orthosis is to protect the surgical construct from the planes of motion in which the construct may be vulnerable to failure. For most surgical constructs, these motions are flexion and/or torsion. The molded thoracolumbosacral orthosis (TLSO) provides the most overall restriction of trunk motion in flexion–extension, lateral bending, and axial rotation. The corset provides an intermediate degree of gross motion restriction, and the elastic corset is only minimally restrictive. A custom-molded TLSO reduces intervertebral motion in the lumbar spine; however, it is more effective in reducing motion at the upper lumbar levels than at lower levels. A thigh extension may be needed to further limit motion at the lower lumbar and lumbosacral levels. Thus, augmenting the surgical construct used for stabilizing macroinstabilities may be possible by appropriate selection of a postoperative orthosis.

Cervical orthoses are primarily used to limit flexion–extension, rotation, lateral bending, and translational motion in the cervical spine. For the upper cervical spine (occiput–C2), four-poster orthoses are best for reducing flexion–extension motion. The two-poster orthoses also are effective in reducing flexion; however, these orthoses have limited effectiveness in lateral bending and rotation. To immobilize odontoid injuries, the halo orthosis clearly is superior because it limits motions in all planes. The halo orthosis is not significantly better than the four-poster orthosis at immobilizing the midcervical spine (C3–5). Rigid collars provide a moderate amount of immobilization at the midcervical levels but tend to lose effectiveness at the upper (occiput–C2) and lower cervical segments (C6–7). In order to achieve immobilization in flexion–extension at the lower cervical segments, the four-poster is the most effective orthosis, whereas the two-poster is effective for flexion alone. The halo is the best orthosis for all planes in the upper and lower cervical spine, whereas rigid collars provide adequate stabilization for microinstabilities in the midcervical spine.

Bibliography

Physiologic loads

Han J S, Goel VK, Ahn JY, Winterbottom J, McGowan D, Weinstein J, Cook T: Loads in the spinal structures during lifting: development of a three-dimensional comprehensive biomechanical model, *Eur Spine J* 4:153–168, 1995.

Wilke HJ, Rohlmann A, Neller S, Graichen F, Claes L, Bergmann G: A novel approach to determine trunk muscle forces during flexion and extension: a comparison of data from an in vitro experiment and in vivo measurements, *Spine* 28:2585–2593, 2003.

Wilke HJ, Neef P, Caimi M, Hoogland T, Claes LE: New in vivo measurements of pressures in the intervertebral disc in daily life, *Spine* 24:755–762, 1999.

Stability of the spinal column

Arjmand N, Shirazi-Adl A: Model and in vivo studies on human trunk load partitioning and stability in isometric forward flexions, *J Biomech* 39:510–521, 2006.

Patwardhan AG, Havey R, Carandang G, Simonds J, et al: Effect of compressive follower preload on the flexion-extension response of the human lumbar spine, *J Orthop Res* 21:540–546, 2003.

Panjabi M, Cholewicki J, Nibu K, et al: Critical load of the human cervical spine: an in vitro experimental study, *Clin Biomech* 13:11, 1998.

Patwardhan A, Havey R, Ghanayem A, et al: Load carrying capacity of the human cervical spine in compression is increased under a follower load, *Spine* 25:1548–1554, 2000.

Patwardhan A, Havey R, Meade K, Lee B, Dunlap B: A follower load increases the load-carrying capacity of the lumbar spine in compression, *Spine* 24:1003–1009, 1999.

Stability of the functional spinal unit

Abumi K, Panjabi MM, Kramer KM, Duranceau J, Oxland T, Crisco JJ: Biomechanical evaluation of lumbar spinal stability after graded facetectomies, *Spine* 15:1142–1147, 1990.

Fujiwara A, Lim TH, An HS, et al: The effect of disc degeneration and facet joint osteoarthritis on the segmental flexibility of the lumbar spine, *Spine* 25:3036–3044, 2000.

Goel VK, Nishiyama K, Weinstein J, Liu YK: Mechanical properties of lumbar spinal motion segments as affected by partial disc removal, *Spine* 11:1008–1012, 1986.

Krismer M, Haid C, Behensky H, Kapfinger P, Landauer F, Rachbauer F: Motion in lumbar functional spine units during side bending and axial rotation moments depending on the degree of disc degeneration, *Spine* 25:2020–2027, 2000.

Frei H, Oxland TR, Nolte LP: Thoracolumbar spine mechanics contrasted under compression and shear loading, *J Orthop Res* 20:1333–1338, 2002.

Rohlmann A, Neller S, Claes L, Bergmann G, Wilke HJ: Influence of a follower load on intradiscal pressure and intersegmental rotation of the lumbar spine, *Spine* 26:E557–E561, 2001.

Rohlmann A, Zander T, Schmidt H, Wilke HJ, Bergmann G: Analysis of the influence of disc degeneration on the mechanical behavior of a lumbar motion segment using the finite element method, *J Biomech* 39:2484–2490, 2006.

Shirazi-Adl A: Analysis of large compression loads on lumbar spine in flexion and in torsion using a novel wrapping element, *J Biomech* 39:267–275, 2006.

Biomechanics of stabilization

Gavin TM, Carandang G, Havey RM, Flanagan P, Ghanayem AJ, Patwardhan AG: Biomechanical analysis of cervical orthoses in flexion and extension: a comparison of cervical collars and cervical thoracic orthoses, *J Rehab Res Dev* 40:527–538, 2003.

Patwardhan A, Carandang G, Ghanayem A, et al: Compressive preload improves the stability of the anterior lumbar interbody fusion (ALIF) cage construct, *J Bone Joint Surg Am* 85A:1749–1756, 2003.

Vander Kooi D, Abad G, Basford JR, Maus TP, Yaszemski MJ, Kaufman KR: Lumbar spine stabilization with a thoracolumbosacral orthosis: evaluation with video fluoroscopy, *Spine* 29:100–104, 2004.

Shono Y, Kaneda K, Abumi K, et al: Stability of posterior spinal instrumentation and its effects on adjacent motion segments in the lumbosacral spine, *Spine* 23:1550–1558, 1998.

Principles and components of spinal orthoses

H. Duane Romo, Thomas M. Gavin, Avinash G. Patwardhan, Wilton H. Bunch, Donna Q. Gavin, Phyllis D. Levine, and Laura Fenwick

Key Points

- Custom devices will always be required for patients with atypical dimensions or significant bony prominences. The intimacy of fit is best accommodated by custom-molded contours.

- Custom contours are especially indicated when high corrective forces are applied through the devices for treatment of spinal deformities, such as scoliosis. In cases of spinal injury, general immobilization across the involved spinal segment(s) is required.

- Several manufacturers now provide reasonably priced prefabricated devices that approximate the functionality of custom designs. These functionally similar devices differ in material selection and even durability.

- The choice of a custom or prefabricated orthosis will be determined by the level(s) of injury and the amount of stabilization required and must be determined on a case-by-case basis.

Spinal orthoses are recommended for three basic reasons: abdominal support, pain management, and motion/positional control. Trunk support is indicated when patients have weakened spinal or abdominal musculature. When spinal pain impedes functional capabilities, a spinal orthosis may be indicated to reduce the intensity of the pain.[17,36,43,44,46] Motion control is necessitated when motion would aggravate a fracture or other pathology. Spinal orthoses are used to reposition the spine into a more anatomically correct alignment, as in cases of scoliosis or kyphosis.

Spinal orthoses are generally categorized by the vertebral level that they are intended to treat. Specific examples include the sacral orthosis (SO), lumbosacral orthosis (LSO), and thoracolumbosacral orthosis (TLSO). Whenever possible, popular eponym adjectives are used. For a complete catalogue of eponymic orthoses, the reader is referred to the text *Orthotics Etcetera*.[30,31]

Semirigid spinal orthoses (corsets)

Commercially available corsets come in various sizes, shapes, and fabrics. Corset design is based on the area of the body requiring stabilization, the amount of control necessary, and the anatomical dimensions of the patient.

With an inelastic construction consisting of soft canvas or Dacron and fortification with both rigid and flexible stays, corsets can provide some degree of immobilization of the spine, although not to the same degree as rigid TLSOs. Spring steel posterior stays, if present, can be contoured to accommodate a deformity or to encourage postural correction. Many authors recommend reduced lordosis to manage lumbosacral muscle strain.[31,43,49] Corsets worn sufficiently tight result in increased intracavitary pressure, which contributes to abdominal support and reduced axial load on the vertebral bodies.[21,35,37,42]

Corsets can be effective in managing pain caused by muscle strain because they reduce the activity of the spinal and abdominal musculature. However, when corsets are used long term, musculature can atrophy and increase the chance of reinjury. Therefore, corsets should be used only as long as necessary.

Orthotic examples of corsets

Sacroiliac corsets are meant to provide assistance to the pelvis only. These garments encompass the pelvis with endpoints inferior to the waist and superior to the pubis (Fig. 7-1, *A*)

These corsets offer minimal support to the spine and typically are used to effect a slight increase in abdominal circumferential pressure for mild conditions.

Lumbosacral corsets encompass the pelvis and abdomen. In exerting circumferential pressure, they increase intracavitary pressure in the abdomen and transmit a semirigid three-point pressure system on the lumbar spine (Fig. 7-1, *B*). The trim lines of the lumbosacral corset are inferior to the xiphoid process and superior to the pubic symphysis anteriorly and extend between the inferior angle of the scapula and the sacrococcygeal junction posteriorly. On female corset styles, the posterior trim line may extend to the gluteal fold posteriorly to reduce migration in patients with significant hip development.

Thoracolumbosacral corsets increase the leverage of the corset system (Fig. 7-1, *C*). The trim lines of this style are the same as in lumbosacral garments except posteriorly, where the superior edge terminates inferior to the scapular spine. In addition, shoulder straps provide a posteriorly directed force meant to extend the thoracic spine. Thoracolumbosacral corsets serve mostly as a kinesthetic reminder to control motion in the thoracic spine; they do not provide sufficient rigidity to prevent such motion. For this reason, thoracolumbosacral corsets have been discussed as providing trunk support but not motion control.

Rigid spinal orthoses

A number of commercially available spinal orthoses offer greater rigidity than provided by corsets. These orthoses may control motion in specific planes. Some devices restrict motion in only one plane, whereas others restrict motion in all three planes. A number of manufacturers provide orthoses offering similar controls. Therefore, specific rigid orthosis selection can vary significantly based on the level of injury and the stability of the spine. Another important consideration in device selection is the patient's "gadget tolerance." Donning and doffing of the device may prove excessively challenging for a particular patient and thus should be considered when selecting an orthosis that aims to preserve the patient's independence. Once the planar motion(s) requiring control is identified, physician or orthotist preference often is the final determination of the final brand used.

In order to provide a frame of reference for orthosis selection based on planar control, components of traditional metal spinal orthoses are described. These components, in various combinations, provide differing controls for the spine.

Components of conventional (metal) spinal orthoses

The components used to construct most common metal spinal orthoses typically are aluminum alloys that are radiolucent and malleable yet of sufficient strength to hold their shape. Ideally, orthoses are custom fabricated to fit specific landmarks so that the devices provide adequate motion control through the best possible leverage. Figure 7-2 shows some common components.

The *thoracic band* is located so that the superior edge rests 24 mm inferior to the inferior angle of the scapulae. The band may be horizontal across the back or convex superiorly to provide the greatest height in the midline while allowing for relief of the scapulae. Lateral to the scapula, the component dips inferiorly to relieve for the axilla. The component ends just anterior to the lateral midline of the body or the midaxillary trochanteric line, a line defined by a bisection of the body at the axilla and trochanter.

At the midline, the inferior edge of the *pelvic band* rests at the sacrococcygeal junction. Lateral to the midline, the component usually dips inferiorly to contain the gluteal musculature. The rationale for this curve is to provide the greatest leverage for the orthosis. This component also ends just anterior to the midaxillary trochanteric line. Norton and Brown[39] described an alteration to this pelvic band design that increases motion control at the lumbosacral junction. They described a pelvic section having inferior projections from the lateral bars that terminate in disks resting over the trochanters. A strap that fastens anteriorly is connected to these disks, offering additional leverage in the sagittal plane. The disks increase the leverage for coronal plane motion control as well.

The *paraspinal bars* are contoured to follow the paraspinal musculature. On LSOs, the bars may appear vertical and pass from the pelvic band to the thoracic band. For thoracolumbar styles, the space between the paraspinal bars often narrows toward the superior end to follow the reduction in coronal diameter of the vertebrae. In TLSOs, the paraspinal bars terminate inferior to the spine of the scapula.

The *lateral bars* follow the midaxillary trochanteric line from the superior edge of the thoracic band to the inferior edge of the pelvic band.

The *interscapular band* is contained within the lateral borders of the scapulae, with its inferior edge superior to the inferior borders of the scapulae. All metal orthoses can be worn with either a corset or an anterior panel of corset material.

Orthotic examples of rigid orthoses: Conventional spinal orthoses and contemporary equivalents

LSO: Sagittal control

This orthosis (also known as *LSO: chairback style*) consists of a thoracic band, pelvic band, and two paraspinal bars (Fig. 7-2, *A*). Fitting parameters are the same as described for each of the components. This device is indicated for reduction of gross motion in the sagittal plane, including both flexion and extension. The mechanism consists of 2 three-point pressure systems. Flexion control is achieved via two posteriorly directed forces (at the xiphoid level and the pubic level on the corset panel) and one anteriorly directed force at the midpoint of the paraspinal bars. Extension control is achieved via two anteriorly directed forces (arising from the thoracic and pelvic bands) and one posteriorly directed force from the midpoint of the corset panel. An equivalent commercially available LSO that provides sagittal control is shown in Figure 7-3. This orthosis uses preformed anterior and posterior acrylonitrile-butadiene-styrene (ABS) plastic panels lined with soft breathable foam. Closures on each side allow for adjustment of support. The panels can be heated and reshaped to accommodate anatomical contours.

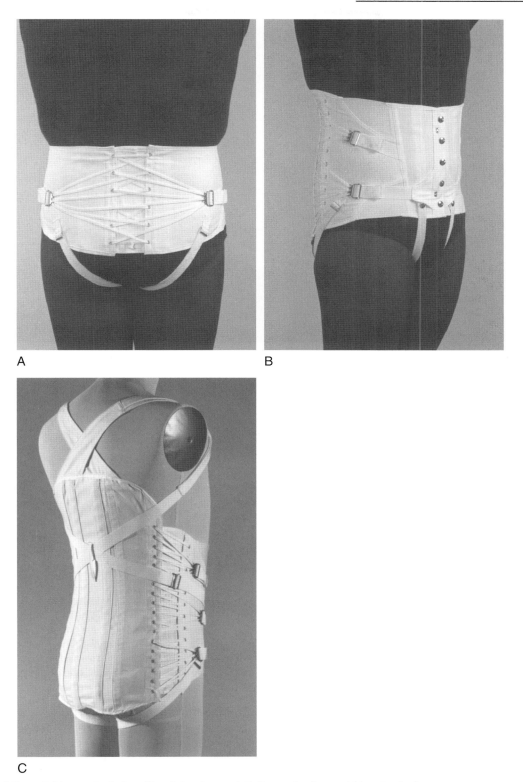

Fig. 7-1 Commercially available corsets. **A**, Sacroiliac. **B**, Lumbosacral. **C**, Thoracolumbosacral (dorsolumbar).

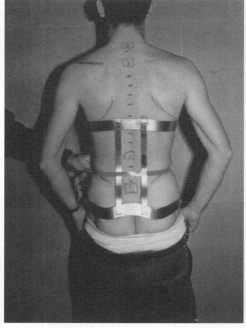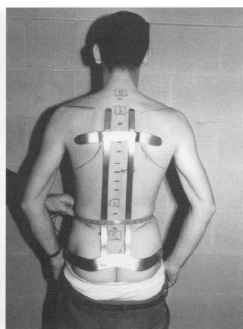

Fig. 7-2 Custom-fabricated orthoses show the appropriate location for some common spinal orthotic components, such as the thoracic band, pelvic band, paraspinal bars, lumbosacral length, thoracolumbosacral length, and interscapular band.

A   B

LSO: Sagittal–coronal control

This orthosis includes a component of coronal control by the addition of lateral bars. The eponym for this orthosis, *LSO: Knight style*, refers to Knight, who described a version of the orthosis in *Orthopaedia* in 1884.[2] The current form of this orthosis consists of a thoracic band, pelvic band, paraspinal bars, and lateral bars. In addition to the three-point pressure systems described for restriction of sagittal plane motion, this orthosis adds three-point pressure systems in the coronal plane to limit lateral flexion (Fig. 7-4). A functionally equivalent, commercially available thermoplastic LSO offering sagittal–coronal control is shown in Figure 7-4. This anterior-opening design integrates rigid sides that provide motion restriction in the coronal plane. The frame can be recontoured by heating and reshaping as necessary. The soft inner liner is made of breathable foam for increased patient comfort.

LSO: Extension–coronal control (Williams flexion)

This dynamic orthosis consists of a thoracic band, pelvic band, lateral bars, and oblique bars (Fig. 7-5). The oblique bars provide structural integrity. The attachments at the thoracic band and lateral bars are mobile. This orthosis articulates to allow motion in the sagittal plane. As the device is worn, an inelastic pelvic strap is tightened so that free flexion can occur, but extension is stopped. Williams originally described this orthosis in 1937 for treatment of spondylolisthesis,[51] and the device still may be prescribed for this pathology.[17,26,32]

TLSO: Flexion control (hyperextension orthosis)

This orthosis is commercially available in various styles and sizes from a number of manufacturers (Fig. 7-6). One style consists of an aluminum frame with pads at the pubis, sternum, and lateral midline of the trunk. This *TLSO: Jewett style* is named for Jewett, who described the device in 1937.[23] Other styles provide similar motion control. Control is achieved through a single three-point pressure system. The system applies two posteriorly directed forces, one at the sternal pad and one at the pubic pad, and an equal but opposite anteriorly directed force from the lumbar pad. When worn, the orthosis restricts flexion of the spine.[10,48]

TLSO: Sagittal control

The eponym *TLSO: Taylor style* is named for Taylor, the New York orthopedist who described it in 1863.[45] The orthosis consists of a pelvic band, paraspinal bars, an interscapular band, and axillary straps (Fig. 7-7). This orthosis provides 2 three-point pressure systems in flexion and extension for the thoracic and lumbar spine. The interscapular band provides one of the anteriorly directed forces to limit extension, and the axillary straps provide one of the posteriorly directed forces to reduce the range of flexion.

TLSO: Sagittal-coronal control

This combination orthosis has the apt eponym *TLSO: Knight-Taylor style*. It is fabricated with a thoracic band, pelvic band, paraspinal bars, lateral bars, interscapular band, and axillary straps. Through these components, the orthosis limits flexion, extension, and lateral flexion of the thoracic and lumbar spine. The three-point pressure systems in the sagittal plane for the TLSO: sagittal–coronal control are shown in Figure 7-8. The commercially available California Knight-Taylor Spinal System (Orthomerica) provides sagittal-coronal control (Fig. 7-9). Its padded frame, formed in shape and contour similar to a traditional Knight-Taylor orthosis, provides sagittal and coronal motion restriction for the spine.

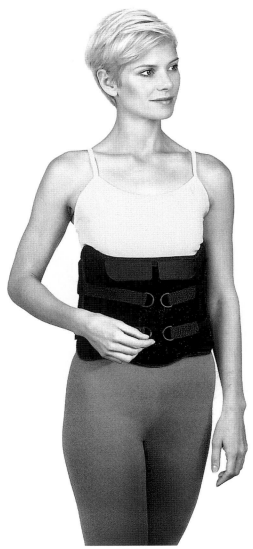

Fig. 7-3 California soft spinal system, lumbosacral orthosis. (Courtesy Orthomerica Products.)

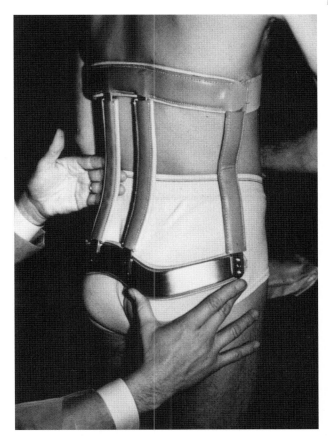

Fig. 7-4 Conventional lumbosacral orthosis: sagittal-coronal control. Note the location of the lateral bars. The lateral bars follow the midaxillary–trochanteric line, an imaginary line that connects the lateral midline at axilla level with the lateral midline at the trochanter level.

TLSO: Triplanar control

This variation of the Knight-Taylor orthosis consists of a thoracic band with subclavicular extensions, pelvic band, paraspinal bars, and lateral bars. The inclusion of subclavicular extensions, which are colloquially referred to as *cowhorn projections*, adds transverse plane control to this orthosis. As a person attempts right or left rotation of the thoracic spine, counterforces from the thoracic band and subclavicular extension limit motion (Fig. 7-10, *A*). One example of a commercially available triplanar control TLSO is shown in Figure 7-10, *B*. This orthosis has been shown to be similar in effectiveness to the above orthosis and to be quite comfortable for the patient.[9,27]

TLSO: Triplanar control, custom-fabricated body jacket

If maximal control is required, a custom-fabricated rigid thermoplastic TLSO is indicated. This orthosis also is referred to as a *TLSO body jacket*. It is fabricated over a model of the patient. The model either is created from a direct mold of the torso or is generated using numerous anatomical measurements. This orthotic design is capable of providing the most effective triplanar stabilization due to its intimate fit of the torso and pelvis. The orthosis, if worn sufficiently tight, provides increased intracavitary pressure. Rigidity can be varied somewhat by the composition and thickness of the thermoplastic. This design can be lined with soft, closed-cell foam and ventilated for increased patient comfort.

The body jacket can be of a bivalve design (Fig. 7-11, *A*), or it may have a single anterior opening for donning (Fig. 7-11, *B*). The bivalve design probably is best suited for patients with variable volume. The anterior and posterior shells of the orthosis can spread apart or compress together while maintaining their mediolateral dimensions. In this way, volume can be accommodated without sacrificing coronal plane stability. A TLSO using an anterior opening does not accommodate volume fluctuation well but may be simpler for patients to don, so this device may be more suitable for nonsurgical patients.

The height of the TLSO is determined by the spinal level requiring stabilization. For the xiphoid-level body jacket, trim lines typically are 1 inch superior to the xiphoid. When this orthosis is fit on a female patient, the orthosis should terminate under the breasts to prevent impingement of soft tissues. If more proximal stabilization is required, the orthosis can

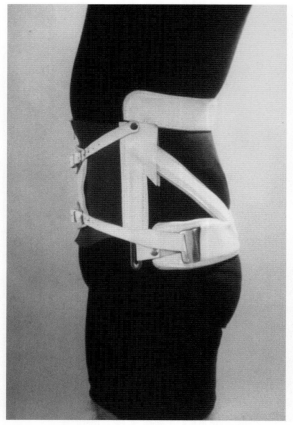

Fig. 7-5 Lumbosacral orthosis: extension-coronal control. The oblique bars follow the body contour. The oblique bars provide structural integrity for the orthosis but do not contribute to control of motion.

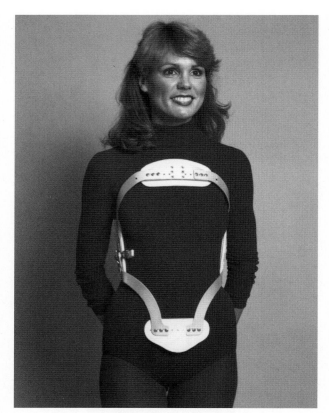

Fig. 7-6 Thoracolumbosacral orthosis: flexion control; Jewett style. (Courtesy Ben Moss, Florida Brace Corp.)

encase the breasts and terminate 1 inch distal to the sternal notch anteriorly. A variation of this design uses a xiphoid-level jacket and a padded metal sternal extension (Fig. 7-12). This variation provides similar proximal stabilization but remains cooler for patients of either gender; however, it is especially beneficial in providing relief of the breasts for female patients.

TLSO: Triplanar control, soft body jacket

A relatively recent introduction to the multitude of custom TLSO designs is the soft body jacket. This orthosis is composed of a rigid frame surrounded by soft closed-cell foam (Fig. 7-13). The frame can be external or sandwiched between two layers of foam. The foam extends to the customary trim lines. The frame terminates approximately 1 to 1.5 inches inside the foam edges. Soft body jacket designs typically use an anterior opening. Advantages of this design are that it is softer and much lighter than typical body jackets. These features are helpful when treating the elderly in whom subcutaneous padding is minimal. For this population, weight and comfort are important for increased patient compliance.

Cervical orthoses

Cervical orthoses are indicated for two primary reasons: pain management and motion control of the cervical spine. The vast majority of devices are prefabricated. Several designs offer different levels of stabilization for the cervical spine. Similar to spinal orthoses, the devices in this category also are identified by the level at which spinal stabilization is sought. In some cases, stabilization is required only over the cervical spine; this is considered a *cervical orthosis* (CO). If maximal stabilization is indicated, the orthotic design extends to the thorax, often using the shoulders and upper thoracic spine as a foundation for additional cervical spine immobilization.

Orthotic examples of cervical orthoses

CO: Cervical

Prefabricated cervical orthoses can be generally categorized as soft, semirigid, and hard. Examples of soft, semirigid, and hard collars are shown in Figures 7-14, 7-15, and 7-16, respectively. The soft cervical orthosis, also known as a *foam collar*, functions primarily as a kinesthetic reminder for the individual to reduce excessive motion. Semirigid and hard cervical collar styles are available in a great variety of prefabricated styles. As a group, these orthoses reduce cervical motion in the sagittal plane[18] more than foam collars do but still provide little control of lateral flexion and rotation. Additional control of the cervical spine can be provided by poster-style orthoses. Two-poster and four-poster designs of cervical orthoses are shown in Figures 7-17 and 7-18. These orthoses offer more rigid immobilization of the cervical spine because of the occipital pad, mandibular pad, and sternal and thoracic pads. Many of the aforementioned orthoses can be modified with a thoracic extension to provide more effective stabilization for motion control of the lower cervical spine.[11]

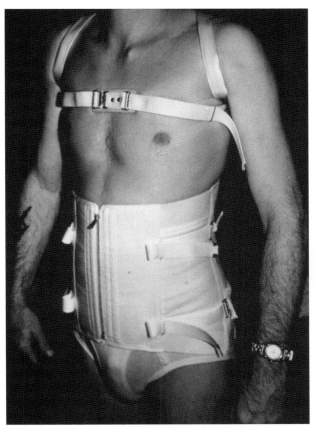

Fig. 7-7 Conventional thoracolumbosacral orthosis: sagittal control; Taylor style.

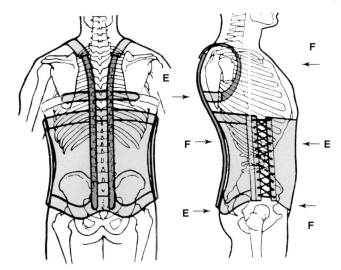

Fig. 7-8 Conventional thoracolumbosacral orthosis: sagittal-coronal control with three-point pressure systems delineated. *E*, Extension control; *F*, flexion control. (From *American Academy of Orthopaedic Surgeons: atlas of orthotics*, ed 2, St. Louis, 1985, CV Mosby.)

CTO: Cervicothoracic

A commercially available cervicothoracic orthosis that is frequently used for motion control is the sternal occipital mandibular immobilizer (Fig. 7-19). This orthosis consists of a sternal plate with shoulder components, mandibular pad and bar, and occipital pad and bars. It provides good motion control of flexion, especially in the lower cervical segments, but it actually allows some extension motion because of a swivel-type occipital pad.[25]

The halo cervicothoracic orthosis provides triplanar motion control in the cervical spine (Fig. 7-20). This orthosis consists of a halo ring fixed to the skull with pins, a chest jacket, and a superstructure that connects the ring and jacket. This orthosis provides the best endpoint control of the cervical spine; however, its lack of total contact allows the occurrence of a phenomenon called *intersegmental snaking*. A total contact cervicothoracic orthosis such as a Minerva or Miami JTO (Fig. 7-21) might provide better intersegmental immobilization of the cervical spine.[3,33] Despite the intersegmental motion, however, halo fixation usually is best for fracture healing.[22,25,47]

Orthoses for spinal deformity

The primary clinical goal of orthoses indicated for spinal deformity is preventing the progression of aberrant curvature. This is accomplished by stabilizing the spine over the pelvis through various means. The orthotic design is dependent on the level and magnitude of the curve(s) present. Several orthoses offer various amounts of correction, but the basic principles of stabilization are the same: endpoint control, transverse load, curve correction, and a combined effect.

Principles and components of orthoses for spinal deformity

Endpoint control denotes the mechanical constraints on the spine provided by an orthosis. The purpose of the pelvic interface of all orthoses is to fix the orthosis rigidly to the base of the spine. For example, the neck ring of the Milwaukee brace limits lateral sway by keeping the head and neck centered over the pelvis.

Endpoint control increases the critical load of a spinal curve. Stabilizing the superior end of the spine by means of a hinge (Fig. 7-22, *B*) results in a theoretical critical load value that is eight times that for the column shown in Figure 7-22, *A*. The mechanical analogy (Fig. 7-22, *B*) is an approximation of the constraints imposed by an orthosis on the endpoints of the scoliotic curve. For example, even though the neck ring of the Milwaukee brace limits lateral sway of the neck, the superior endpoint of the scoliotic curve (usually T5) is caudal to the neck ring and is not subjected to the same kinematic constraint as the Euler model (Fig. 7-22, *B*). Thus, the actual beneficial effect of the neck ring on the stability of a scoliotic curve may be much less than predicted by the mechanical analogy. However, this illustration of the concept does emphasize the importance of achieving endpoint control in orthotic stabilization of scoliosis.

All scoliosis orthoses provide some form of a transversely directed load to the curvature of the scoliotic spine. A non-translatory transverse load directed at the apex of the curve increases the critical load that the spine can carry. In Figure 7-23, *B*, the solid line represents the critical load of an unsupported spine of increasing degree of curvature; the

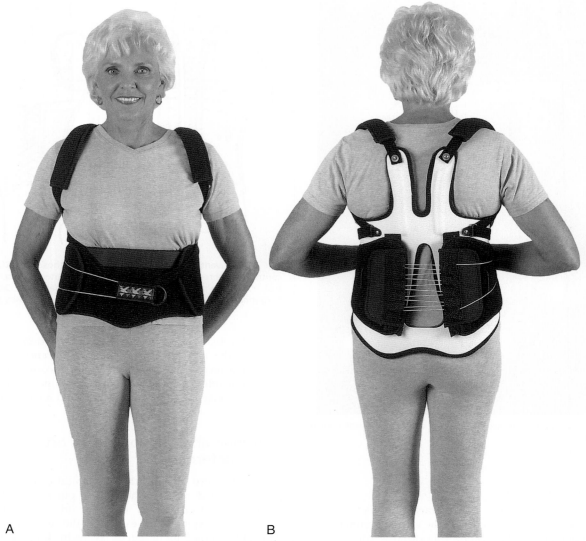

Fig. 7-9 Contemporary thoracolumbosacral orthosis: sagittal-coronal control; California Knight-Taylor spinal system. **A**, Anterior. **B**, Posterior. (Courtesy Orthomerica Products.)

dashed line indicates the critical load of the spine with a transverse support applied at the apex of the curve. For curves of 25 to 30 degrees, the transverse support raises the critical load from approximately 50% of normal to approximately 70% of normal. This increase is shown as the vertical bar labeled A. This increase may be enough to prevent the curve from progressing. For curves of this magnitude, long-term maintenance of this degree of curvature is a satisfactory result because progression after skeletal maturity is rare.

With increasing curvature, the effect of transverse support is reduced. In contrast to the smaller curves, the critical load of a 45-degree curve increases from approximately 20% of normal to approximately 30%. This is shown in Figure 7-23, *B*, as the vertical bar labeled B. The resultant stability may not be enough, and progression may occur even with the orthosis.

Curve correction in the orthosis has the greatest effect on the critical load. Reducing a curve of 30 degrees to 20 degrees in the orthosis increases the stability of the curve from

approximately 50% of normal to approximately 80% of normal. This result is shown in Figure 7-23, *C*, by the arrow and vertical bar labeled A.

This effect also is significant for larger curves. A curve of 45 degrees has a critical load of approximately 20% of normal. If the curve can be reduced to 30 degrees, the critical load increases to approximately 50% of normal. This is shown in Figure 7-23, *C*, as the arrow and vertical bar labeled B.

A comparison of results illustrates that, for any given curvature, reducing the curve magnitude improves the load-carrying capacity of the spine far more than does transverse support alone (Fig. 7-23, *B* and *C*). This is particularly true for larger curves. This analysis provides an explanation for the observation that satisfactory results in curves greater than 40 degrees require a reduction of curve magnitude to approximately 50% of the initial curve.[29]

The effects of curve correction and continued transverse support are additive (Fig. 7-23, *D*). Once a curve of 45 degrees is reduced in the orthosis to 30 degrees, the pads can be reset to provide continued lateral support to the curve, further

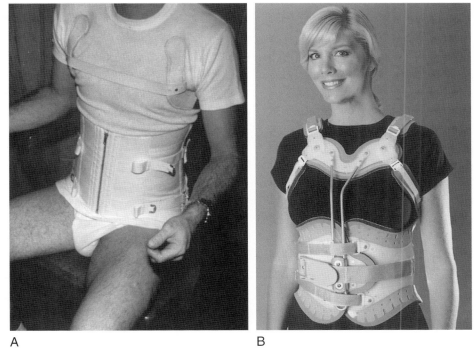

A   B

Fig. 7-10 A, Conventional thoracolumbosacral orthosis (TLSO): sagittal-coronal control. Note the subclavicular extensions of the TLSO. **B,** Contemporary TLSO: sagittal-coronal control. Aspen TLSO. (Courtesy Aspen Medical Products.)

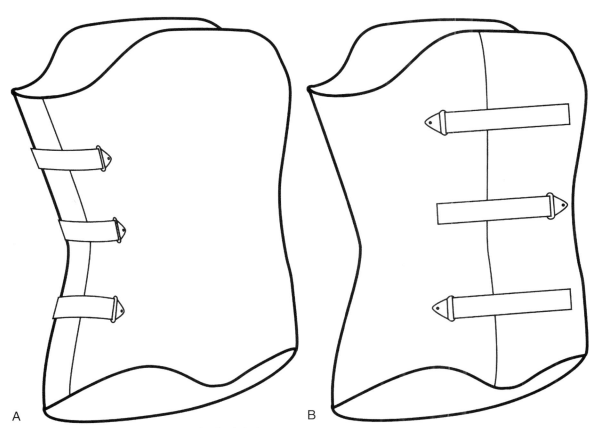

A   B

Fig. 7-11 A, Bivalved body jacket. **B,** Anterior-opening body jacket.

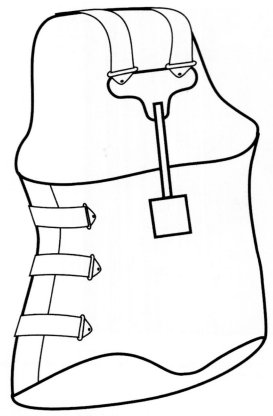

Fig. 7-12 Xiphoid-level bivalved body jacket with sternal extension. This design provides enhanced thoracic sagittal control with increased patient comfort.

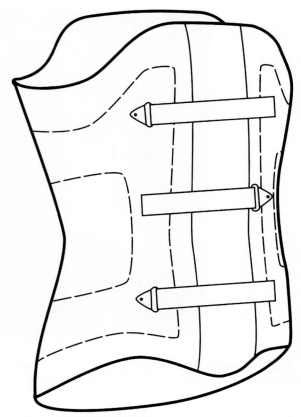

Fig. 7-13 Bivalved soft body jacket. The rigid frame is denoted by the dotted lines. Foam extends over the frame and terminates at the trim lines of the custom orthosis, creating a lightweight, supportive, comfortable design.

increasing the critical load. With this cumulative orthosis adjustment, the critical load can be increased from approximately 20% of normal to approximately 70% of normal. Thus, with significant curve correction in the orthosis and continued lateral support, curves of larger magnitude sometimes can be controlled.

Cervicothoracolumbosacral orthoses

Present-day criteria for nonoperative orthotic treatment of spinal deformities originated in the 1950s with Blount and Moe.[4] They began using the Milwaukee brace, a device that was fabricated from steel and leather and extended from the pelvis to the mandible and occiput. The device provided longitudinal distraction along with a lateral pad against the most displaced ribs on the convex side of the deformity. The purpose of the orthosis was to control scoliosis in an effort to prevent or delay surgery.[8,14,38]

With the older Milwaukee brace, distraction under the mandible caused orthodontic deformities.[6] The neck ring of the present-day Milwaukee brace is composed of stainless steel and no longer presses on the mandible; the device includes a throat mold and two occipital pads. Some active distraction is achieved when the patient extends the neck.[4] With the development of low-profile neck rings (Fig. 7-24) came complete abandonment of the concept of distraction. These rings function primarily to reduce sway of the vertebral column, keeping the upper thoracic spine constrained over the sacrum.[5,19,40,41] Euler's analogy shows a theoretical

eightfold increase in stability when a flexible linear column is fixed at the base and constrained near the top, although the residual motion still permitted in the Milwaukee brace suggests a much less actual increase in stability.[19]

Pad placement Thoracic and lumbar pads are used to achieve curve reduction via transverse loading of the deformed spine. They function as translatory variables in space, positioned directly between the constants of the neck ring and the superstructure.

The *thoracic pad* of the Milwaukee brace is fashioned in an L shape and often is fabricated from low-density polyethylene, with foam padding on the patient side. This pad is shaped in an arc from posterior to anterior, contouring to the torso. Size is patient specific, so a custom design is required. The pad is fitted on the convex side of the curve and is placed over the rib that articulates with the apical vertebra and the next rib inferior (Fig. 7-25, *A*).[16,19] The transverse span of the pad covers the medial aspect of the convex-side paraspinal musculature to the midcoronal line. This pad spans the entire posterolateral quadrant of the trunk. The posterior vertical aspect of the L pad is fitted under the convex-side paraspinal bar of the superstructure so that this bar can be contoured inward to assist in the anterior derotational force.[16]

Because the thoracic pad is mounted on a flexible Dacron strap, a transverse outrigger made of aluminum is used on the anterior bar to bridge the strap away from the patient in the area anterior to the midcoronal line. Anterior contact is in

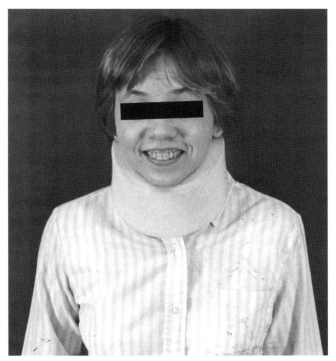

Fig. 7-14 Soft foam collar.

direct opposition to the force of the thoracic pad and diminishes load.

For the patient with hypokyphosis, the thoracic pad is placed directly lateral so that the anterior derotational force is eliminated.[16,19,28] This is achieved by moving the pad anteriorly on the strap to a direct lateral position and either shortening or eliminating the anterior outrigger. The neck ring should be centered more anteriorly to midline in an effort to induce a kyphotic force.

The *lumbar pad* is triangular so that it can be placed inferior to the costal ribs and superior to the iliac crest. This pad usually is fashioned from high-density foam and is contoured to the waist. Placement should be directly over the curve apex on the convex-side posterolateral quadrant. The transverse span is similar to that of the thoracic pad, on the convex-side posterolateral quadrant (Fig. 7-25, *B*).

Pad loading For patients with more than one curve, the curve of greatest mechanical stiffness or primary curve should be loaded and shifted first. This process allows the torso to shift toward the concavity of the primary curve and thus is the load effecting greatest trunk shift. Once that shift is accomplished, the more flexible compensatory curve can be loaded. This load on the compensatory curve is mostly transverse force and only minimally shifts the torso.[16,19]

For double primary curves, each curve should be loaded and shifted equally because the stiffnesses of these curves are considered equal. Thus, multiple curves with differential stiffnesses can be treated with differential loads, whereas curves with equal stiffness should be loaded relatively equally.

Thoracic and lumbar pad force Pad force is the primary mechanism for reducing spinal curvature. The loading vector for thoracic and lumbar pads should be anteromedial,

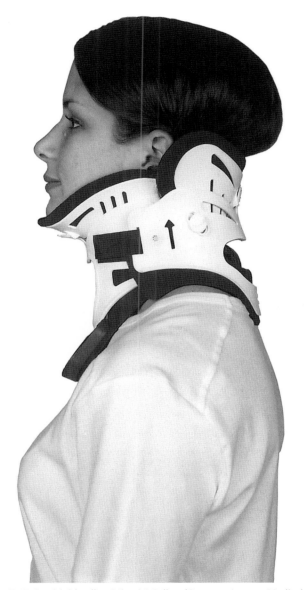

Fig. 7-15 Semirigid collar: Miami J Collar. (Courtesy Jerome Medical.)

except for a thoracic pad used for a hypokyphotic spine, which is medial only.[16,19,28] To optimize results, pads should be kept at maximum force during treatment. Because viscoelastic relaxation of the spine occurs in the soft tissues and the curvature reduces, the pads, which are adjustable, can be tightened periodically.

Force is evaluated clinically by the degree of skin redness under the pads and patient comfort in the orthosis. For lighter skin, redness should be apparent in the pad areas but should disappear within 35 minutes after the orthosis is removed. This finding ensures that force has not exceeded skin tolerance, thus avoiding skin breakdown. If redness dissipates within 15 minutes after the orthosis is removed, the pads should be tightened because they are not applying optimal force. The greatest increase in pad tightening is made after the patient has worn the orthosis for 1 month. Thereafter, the pads are checked every 3 months to ensure maximal force still is present and to reposition the height of the pads to compensate for patient growth.

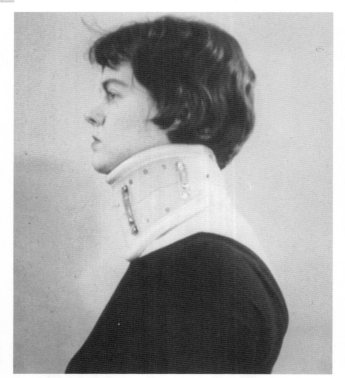

Fig. 7-16 Hard collar.

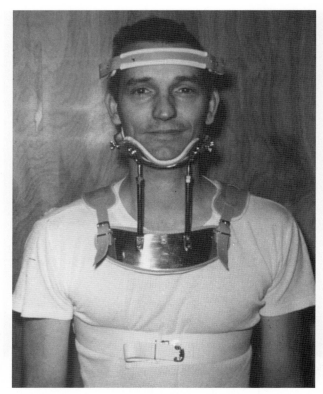

Fig. 7-18 Four-poster style cervical orthosis, anterior view.

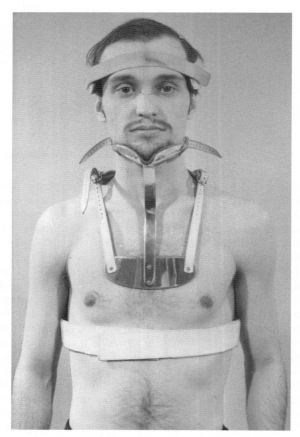

Fig. 7-17 Two-poster style cervical orthosis, anterior view.

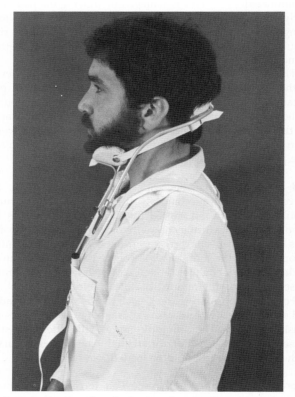

Fig. 7-19 Cervicothoracic orthosis, sternal occipital mandibular immobilizer style.

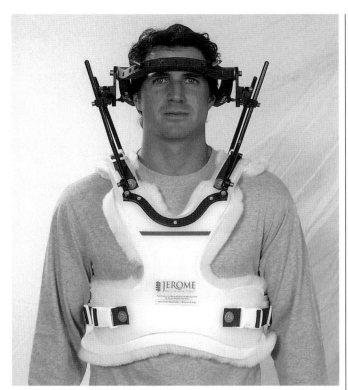

Fig. 7-20 Ambulatory halo orthosis: ReSolve halo. (Courtesy Jerome Medical.)

Triangulation of forces The lumbar pad force of the Milwaukee brace is countered from both the pelvic interface and the thoracic pad. This setup triangulates the force into a three-point system. The thoracic pad triangulates from either the contralateral pelvic interface or the lumbar pad as a caudad counterforce but requires the addition of an axillary sling (Fig. 7-26) as the concave-side cephalad counterforce. The counterforces play a primary role, not only in righting and stabilizing the orthosis in the coronal plane but also acting as a mechanical constraint at the concave-side cephalad endpoint. For double curves that require both thoracic and lumbar pads, four points of contact yield 2 three-point force triangulations (Fig. 7-27).

Axillary sling load is relative to the load of the thoracic pad. The pad is tightened to the point at which the orthosis is vertical and the patient's torso is centered or compensated.

High thoracic curves Orthotic treatment of scoliotic curves in the cervicothoracic spine is controversial. The literature is devoid of information on orthotic treatment outcome studies, biomechanics of treatment, and natural history studies for these curves. The task of reducing these cephalad curves using an orthosis is formidable at best. Blount and Moe[4] reported that the shoulder ring flange (Fig. 7-28, *A*) is the component used to load these high curves as well as depress the convex-side shoulder (which raises after transverse load is applied). Traditionally, these curves could be loaded only minimally because the contralateral side of the neck ring contacted the patient in reaction to the transverse axillary force, creating a neck ring reaction, a decompensated torso, and patient

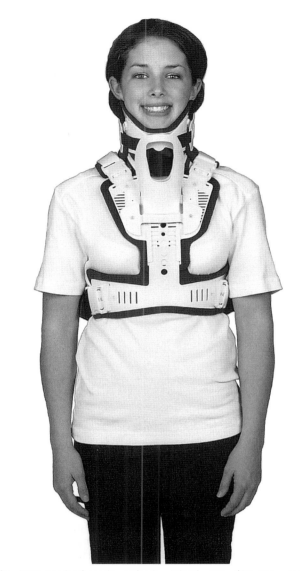

Fig. 7-21 Cervicothoracic orthosis: Miami JTO. (Courtesy Jerome Medical.)

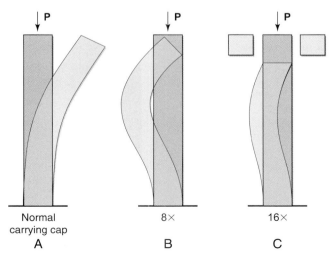

Fig. 7-22 Elastic buckling of a straight column with different boundary conditions. **A,** Column with one end fixed and the other free. **B,** Column with one end fixed and the other pinned. **C,** Column with both ends fixed.

101

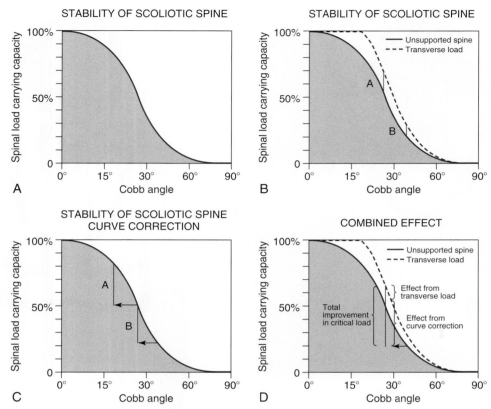

Fig. 7-23 **A**, Effect of curve magnitude on stability of the scoliotic spine. **B**, Effect of an apical transverse load on spinal stability. **C**, Effect of correcting (reducing) the scoliotic curve. **D**, Combined effect is optimal when an orthosis is used to treat scoliosis. (Redrawn from Bunch WH, Patwardhan AG: *Scoliosis: making clinical decisions*, St. Louis, 1989, CV Mosby.)

discomfort. Without maximal loading at the axillary (T5) level, these high curves do not reduce in magnitude, and the result is poor.

Gavin et al.[19] reported a method for reorienting the straps on the shoulder ring to depress the shoulder proportionate to the amount of transverse axillary load so that the patient's neck maintains a neutral position in the center of the neck ring without a neck ring reaction, thus allowing maximal transverse loading (Fig. 7-28, *B*). Figure 7-28, *C* and *D*, shows a patient with a double thoracic curve of 40 and 39 degrees that reduced to 25 and 25 degrees with use of a Milwaukee brace and a well-fitted shoulder ring. Because this force

Fig. 7-24 **A**, Metal low-profile neck ring. **B**, Friddle low-profile neck rings. (From Gavin TM, Shurr DG, Patwardhan AG: Orthotic treatment for spinal disorders. In Weinstein SL, editor: *The pediatric spine*, New York, 1993, Raven Press.)

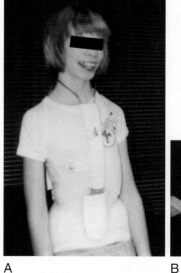

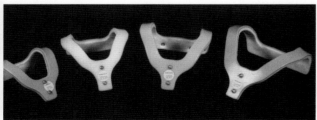

A   B

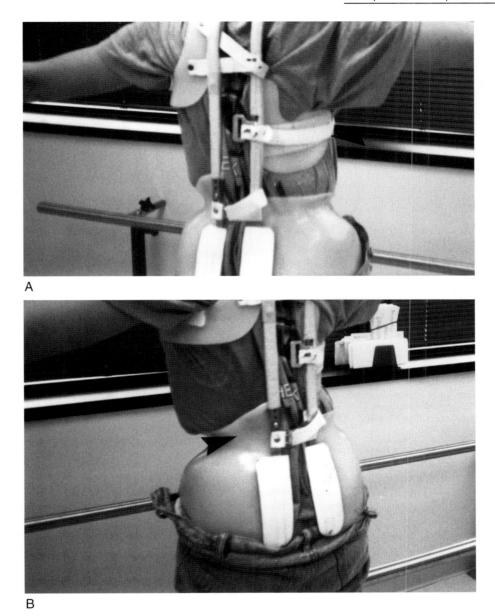

A

B

Fig. 7-25 A, Conventional thoracic pad for Milwaukee orthosis. **B,** Conventional lumbar pad for Milwaukee orthosis.

system nullifies the neck ring reaction, it is theoretically possible to accomplish this setup in a TLSO such as that pictured in Figure 7-29. In this figure, a patient with a double thoracic curve of 21 and 28 degrees was fitted in a TLSO having proper coupling of axillary and shoulder forces, and her curves reduced to 13 and 11 degrees.

Outcome studies of results of orthotic treatment of high thoracic scoliosis are difficult because of the small patient populations having high thoracic curves and the lack of data on the natural history of these curves.

Thoracolumbosacral orthoses

TLSOs are indicated for treatment of curves with apices at or below T8.[15,16,19,28] TLSO application for nonoperative treatment of scoliosis began with the Boston brace (Fig. 7-30). The concept started as a method for treating curves with apices at and caudad to T10 with the pelvic aspect of a

cervicothoracolumbosacral orthosis, thus eliminating the superstructure.[13,24] The Boston brace has evolved into a system of prefabricated TLSO modules custom fitted for specific patient needs. It currently is used to treat all curves with apices as cephalad as T8 and is the TLSO most widely used for scoliosis treatment. In contrast to the Milwaukee brace (which still is the only cervicothoracolumbosacral orthosis used for treatment of spinal deformity), a multitude of TLSOs have been developed. The Lyonnaise orthosis originally was developed in France, with modifications used in the United States (Fig. 7-31). The Lyonnaise orthosis was the first TLSO used for treatment of thoracic curves with apices as cephalad as T8 as well as treatment of more caudad lumbar and thoracolumbar curves. The Miami orthosis is a custom-molded orthosis similar to the Boston brace in many regards, with variations in trim line.[34] The Wilmington orthosis (Fig. 7-32) is a custom-molded TLSO fabricated from a Risser frame

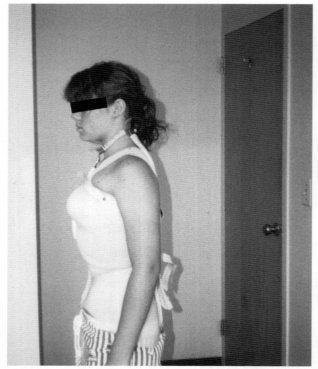

Fig. 7-26 Axillary sling. Note direct lateral placement. (From Gavin TM, Shurr DG, Patwardhan AG: Orthotic treatment for spinal disorders. In Weinstein SL, editor: *The pediatric spine*, New York, 1993, Raven Press.)

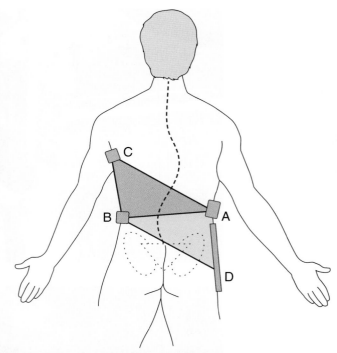

Fig. 7-27 Six-point double-force triangulation provided by four points of contact. (From Bunch WH, Patwardhan AG: *Scoliosis: making clinical decisions*, St. Louis, 1989, CV Mosby.)

plaster impression taken with maximal curve correction.[7] Usually an anteroposterior radiograph of the patient in the impression is obtained to predict curve correction in the orthosis. The Rosenberger orthosis (Fig. 7-33) is a custom-molded TLSO fabricated from a plaster impression taken with curvature correction that uses a Dacron thoracic sling to load thoracic curves.[15]

Pad placement Many different orthoses for nonoperative treatment of scoliosis are available. Each orthosis has distinct characteristics, but all orthoses have some basic similarities. All scoliosis orthoses begin with the same parameters of pad placement, pad loading, pad force, and outcome expectations. All TLSOs use the same pad placement as the Milwaukee brace. Because the TLSO does not have a neck ring to ensure compensated alignment of the cervicothoracic spine, improper placement of counterforce in the TLSO can cause spinal decompensation.

Pad loading The loading sequence for TLSO pads is the same as that suggested for the Milwaukee brace. Primary curves must be loaded and shifted first so that compensatory curve loading is performed with minimal translation of the trunk. For the Boston, Miami, and Lyonnaise orthoses (which load the curves via pads mounted on the wall of the orthosis), increases in loads and shifts must be done by thickening the pad. Transverse loading for the Wilmington orthosis is done in the Risser frame impression and is not adjustable in the orthosis. This process requires periodic refabrication if loading must be changed after the curve reduces. The Rosenberger orthosis uses an adjustable sling, so this orthosis can be adjusted with relative ease.

For the patient with idiopathic scoliosis, it is exceptionally important to monitor the fit of the orthosis periodically and to keep the pad force maximal and pads repositioned despite patient growth. Pad pressure is based on the criterion for the Milwaukee brace: maximum tolerable pressure.[1]

The advantages of the TLSO are use of a minimal orthosis for maximum result, good cosmesis, low weight, and lack of metal superstructure that can tear clothing. The disadvantages of the TLSO are lack of longitudinal adjustment possible from a superstructure and lack of a neck ring to prevent sway of the cervicothoracic spine.

Orthotic examples of TLSOs

Low-profile TLSO

Boston The Boston brace is a modular, one-piece, posterior-opening TLSO made from polypropylene. This orthosis extends anteriorly from the xyphoid process to the symphysis pubis, with posterior and lateral trim lines varied for each curve pattern. This orthosis is modular and does not require a plaster impression, but it must be custom fitted for individual size and curve pattern. On the convex side of the curve, the Boston is trimmed one level superior to the apex of the curve to provide a wall to function as a thoracic or lumbar pad mount. On the concave side of the curve, an opening is cut opposite the pad to allow an open area for the concave-side trunk shift on the level of the primary curve. Above the cutout, a band of plastic is left intact to provide concave-side superior endpoint counterforce to function in the same manner as the axillary sling of the Milwaukee brace (Fig. 7-34).

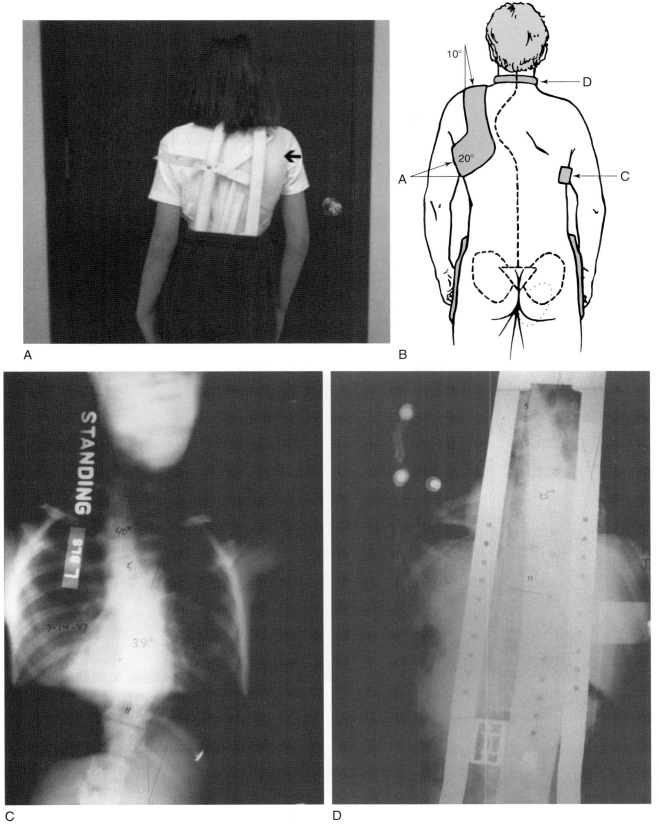

A

B

C

D

Fig. 7-28 A, Custom-molded shoulder ring for high thoracic curves. **B,** Clinical vectors for strap pull of shoulder ring. **C,** Preorthosis radiograph showing left high thoracic curve of 40 degrees and right midthoracic curve of 39 degrees. **D,** Milwaukee orthosis with shoulder ring and thoracic pad; both curves reduced to 25 degrees

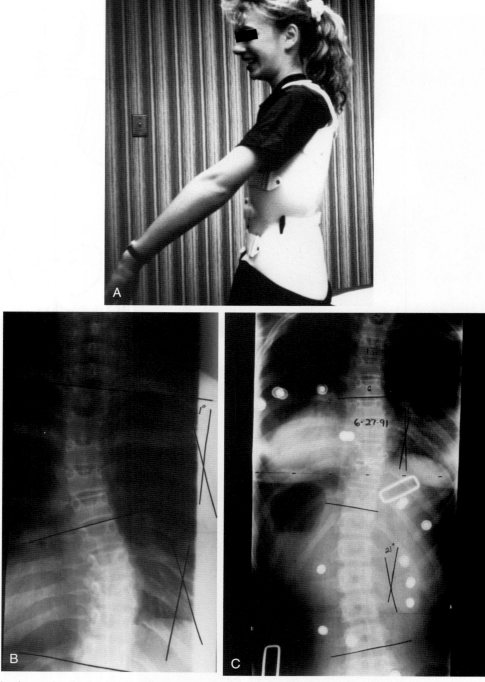

Fig. 7-29 A, Thoracolumbosacral orthosis with shoulder component for high thoracic curve. **B,** Preorthosis radiograph showing a left high thoracic curve of 21 degrees and a midthoracic curve of 28 degrees. **C,** In-brace radiograph showing the high thoracic curve reduced to 13 degrees and the right midthoracic curve reduced to 11 degrees.

Rosenberger The Rosenberger orthosis is a custom-molded, low-density, polyethylene, anterior-opening TLSO. This orthosis is fabricated from a bivalved plaster impression carried out on an examination table with corrective forces applied during casting. Although the impression is bivalved and does not require a Risser frame, the procedure is similar to that used for the Wilmington orthosis. This orthosis extends anteriorly from the pubis to the xiphoid process.

The convex-side trim line is one rib level superior to apical height, similar to the Boston or Miami orthosis, but the concave side is similar to the Wilmington orthosis in that there is no cutout for trunk shift (because the shift is built into the orthosis). The concave-side trim line terminates at the superior endpoint of the superior curve being treated. This orthosis is unique in that it uses adjustable floating slings for curve loading (Fig. 7-35) so that loading can

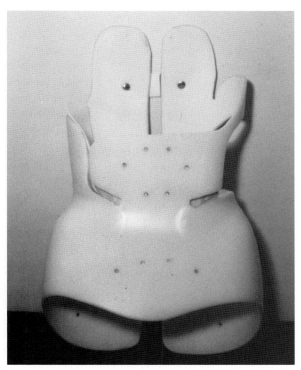

Fig. 7-30 Boston brace. (Courtesy Jeff Miller, CO, National Orthotics and Prosthetics Corp. Boston, Boston Children's Hospital Medical Center. From Gavin TM, Shurr DG, Patwardhan AG: Orthotic treatment for spinal disorders. In Weinstein SL, editor: *The pediatric spine*, New York, 1993, Raven Press.)

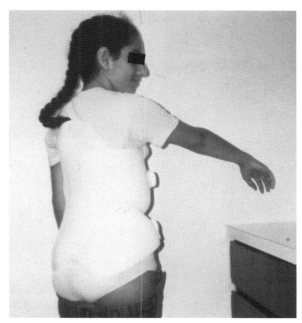

Fig. 7-32 Wilmington orthosis.

exceed that achieved by the corrected walls of the orthosis.[15,16,41]

Miami The Miami orthosis is a one-piece, posterior-opening polypropylene TLSO that is custom molded from a plaster impression. This orthosis offers many of the advantages of the Boston brace, but, in contrast to the Boston, it is custom molded and trimmed short enough to allow forward bending of the patient.[34] Lateral trimline heights and concave-side cutout areas for trunk shift are similar to those for the Boston and Lyonnaise orthoses and are varied according to curve pattern.

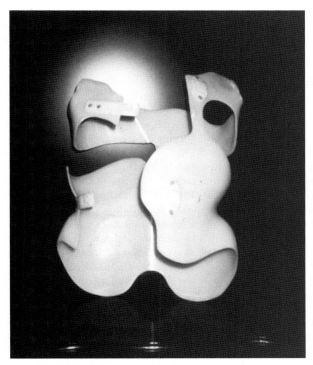

Fig. 7-31 Modified Lyonnaise orthosis. Note lack of aluminum structure and steel hinges. (Courtesy L. Dreher Jouett, CPO, Dreher-Jouett, Chicago.)

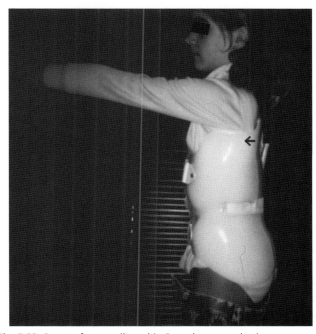

Fig. 7-33 Counterforce wall used in Rosenberger orthosis.

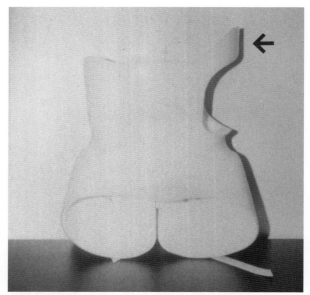

Fig. 7-34 Counterforce band used in the Boston brace. (From Bunch WH, Patwardhan AG: *Scoliosis: making clinical decisions*, St. Louis, 1989, CV Mosby.)

Lyonnaise The Lyonnaise orthosis is a one-piece, anterior-opening orthosis custom fabricated from a plaster impression and fashioned from polypropylene. This orthosis extends anteriorly from the sternal notch to the symphysis pubis. It has lateral trim lines, openings, and counterforce parameters with function similar to that of the Boston orthosis. The original fabrication used two lateral shells of custom-molded plastic joined posteriorly by a longitudinal aluminum bar and steel hinges allowing for function as an anterior-opening

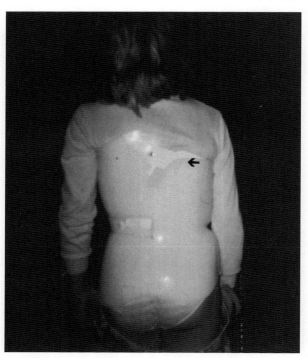

Fig. 7-35 Rosenberger orthosis. Note use of thoracic sling.

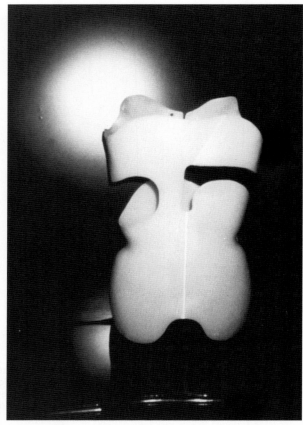

Fig. 7-36 Modified Lyonnaise orthosis lacks the superstructure of aluminum and the steel hinges used in the traditional Lyonnaise orthosis. (Courtesy L. Dreher Jouett, CPO, Dreher-Jouett, Chicago.)

orthosis. Modifications have changed the original fabrication to a one-piece molded structure with a posterior seam used for hinge function, which eliminates the metal structure and lightens the orthosis (Fig. 7-36).

Wilmington jacket The Wilmington orthosis is unique in that it is casted by molding the plaster impression while the patient is on the Risser frame. This impression is designed similar to the localizer cast because the curves are reduced and analyzed by radiography before proceeding with fabrication.[7] This orthosis originally was designed to be fashioned from low-temperature plastic (Orthoplast). Many clinicians prefer the high-temperature, vacuum-formed, low-density polyethylene material (Fig. 7-37) because it provides greater longevity without material degradation. This orthosis is a one-piece, anterior-opening orthosis with anterior trim line from symphysis pubis to sternal notch and bilateral heights to axilla. This orthosis does not have concave-side cutouts, varied trim lines, or wall-mounted pads because all loads, counterforces, and concave-side areas for trunk shift are fabricated into the orthosis.

Charleston bending brace Green[20] reported that part-time orthotic treatment can yield good results and that the protocol of full-time treatment is not necessary. Edmonsson and Morris[12] found that patients who were not cooperative with full-time wearing did not do as well as the full-time wearers. In the study by Edmonsson and Morris, the difference was

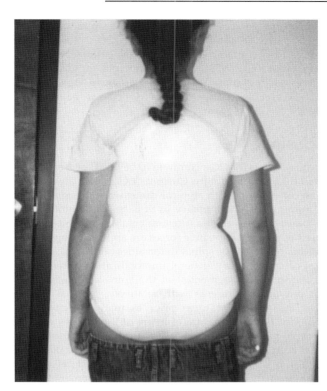

Fig. 7-37 Wilmington orthosis. Modification includes use of poly-ethylene in fabrication. Note contours of orthosis walls and trim-line heights. (From Gavin TM, Shurr DG, Patwardhan AG: Orthotic treatment for spinal disorders. In Weinstein SL, editor: *The pediatric spine*, New York, 1993, Raven Press.)

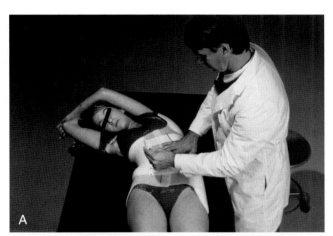

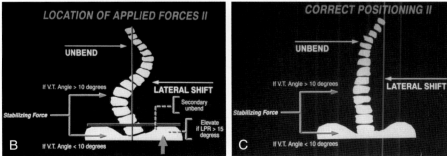

Fig. 7-38 A, Charleston bending brace. Note sidebending contour of orthosis. **B, C,** Curve unbending principles of the Charleston bending brace. (Courtesy Ralph Hooper, CPO, Charleston Bending Brace Research and Education Foundation, Winter Park, Fla.)

25% long-term correction for full-time wearers but only 14% for partially compliant patients. One present-day alternative to part-time orthotic treatment is the Charleston bending brace (Fig. 7-38, *A*). The principle of unbending the curves for nighttime use only is shown in Fig. 7-38, *B* and *C*. Acceptable results using this orthosis have been reported.[50]

Conclusion

Numerous orthotic devices continue to be used for treatment of spinal injury or instability. Custom devices will always be required for patients with atypical dimensions or significant bony prominences; the intimacy of fit is best accommodated by custom-molded contours. Custom contours are especially indicated when high corrective forces are applied through the devices for treatment of spinal deformities such as scoliosis. In cases of spinal injury, general immobilization is required across the involved segment(s) of the spine. Typically, this patient population presents with relatively "normal" contours of the spine and torso prior to injury. In cases of spinal injury, the acute nature of many of the injuries necessitates rapid treatment. Internal spinal fixation technique also has advanced significantly. In some cases, these enhanced techniques may preclude additional external stabilization with orthotic devices. In response to these developments, several manufacturers now provide reasonably priced prefabricated devices that are functionally equivalent to custom designs. These functionally similar devices differ in material selection and even durability. The choice of a prefabricated device often is mediated by physician preference. Regardless of the device selected for treatment of the spine, the choice of a custom or prefabricated orthosis will be determined by the level(s) of injury and the amount of stabilization required and must be determined on a case-by-case basis.

References

1. Andriacchi TP, et al: Milwaukee brace corrections of idiopathic scoliosis, *J Bone Joint Surg* 58A:806, 1976.
2. Andry N: *Orthopaedia*, Philadelphia, 1961, JB Lippincott (facsimile reproduction of the first edition in English, London, 1743).
3. Benzel E: A comparison of the Minerva and Halo jackets for stabilization of the cervical spine, *J Neurosurg* 70:411–414, 1989.
4. Blount WP, Moe JH: *The Milwaukee brace*, Baltimore, 1973, Williams & Wilkins.
5. Bunch W, Patwardhan A: Clinical experience in orthotic treatment. In: Bunch WH, Patwardhan AG, editors: *Scoliosis: making clinical decisions*, St. Louis, 1989, CV Mosby.
6. Bunch WH, Patwardhan AG, editors: *Scoliosis: making clinical decisions*, St. Louis, 1989, CV Mosby.
7. Bunnell WP, MacEwen GD, Jayakumar S: The use of plastic jackets in the non-operative treatment of idiopathic scoliosis, *J Bone Joint Surg* 62A:31–38, 1980.
8. Carr W, et al: Treatment of idiopathic scoliosis in the Milwaukee brace, *J Bone Joint Surg* 62A:599–612, 1980.
9. Cholewicki J, et al: Comparison of motion restriction and trunk stiffness provided by three thoracolumbosacral orthoses (TLSOs), *J Spinal Disord Tech* 16:461–468, 2003.
10. Chow GH, et al: Functional outcome of thoracolumbar burst fractures managed with hyperextension casting or bracing and early mobilization, *Spine* 21:2170–2175, 1996.
11. Colachis SC Jr, Strohm BR, Ganter EL: Cervical spine motion in normal women: radiographic study of effect of cervical collars, *Arch Phys Med Rehabil* 54:161, 1973.
12. Edmonsson A, Morris J: Follow-up study of Milwaukee brace treatment in patients with idiopathic scoliosis, *Clin Orthop* 126:58–61, 1977.
13. Emans J: The Boston bracing system for idiopathic scoliosis: follow-up results in 295 patients, *Spine* 11:792–801, 1986.
14. Galante J, et al: Forces acting in the Milwaukee brace on patients undergoing treatment for idiopathic scoliosis, *J Bone Joint Surg* 52A:498, 1970.
15. Gavin T, Bunch WH, Dvonch V: The Rosenberger scoliosis orthosis, *J Assoc Child Prosthet Orthot Clin* 21:35–38, 1986.
16. Gavin TM: Fabrication and fitting of orthoses. In: Bunch WH, Patwardhan AG, editors: *Scoliosis: making clinical decisions*, St. Louis, 1989, CV Mosby.
17. Gavin TM, et al: Preliminary results of orthotic treatment for chronic low back pain, *J Pros Orthos* 5:5/25–9/29, 1993.
18. Gavin TM, Carandang G, Havey R, et al: Biomechanical analysis of cervical collars and cervical thoracic orthoses, *J Rehabil Res Dev* 40:527–538, 2003.
19. Gavin TM, Shurr DG, Patwardhan AG: Orthotic treatment for spinal disorders. Weinstein SL, editor: *The pediatric spine*, New York, 1993, Raven Press.
20. Green NE: Part-time bracing of idiopathic scoliosis, *Orthop Trans* 5:22, 1981.
21. Harris EE: A new orthotics terminology—a guide to its use for prescription and fee schedules, *Orthot Prosthet* 27:6–19, 1973.
22. Harris JD: Cervical orthoses. In: *Orthotics etcetera*, ed 3, Baltimore, 1986, Williams & Wilkins.
23. Jewett EL: Hyperextension back brace, *J Bone Joint Surg* 19:1128, 1937.
24. Jodoin A, et al: Treatment of idiopathic scoliosis by the Boston brace system: early results, *Orthop Trans* 5:22, 1981.
25. Johnson RM, et al: Cervical orthoses—a study comparing their effectiveness in restricting cervical motion in normal subjects, *J Bone Joint Surg* 59A:332, 1977.
26. Kim SS, Denis F, Lonstein JE, et al: Factors affecting fusion rate in adult spondylolisthesis, *Spine* 15:979–984, 1990.
27. Krag MH, Fox J, Haugh LD: Comparison of three lumbar orthoses using motion assessment during task performance, *Spine* 28:2359–2367, 2003.
28. Lonstein JE: Orthotic treatment of spinal deformities. *American Academy of Orthopaedic Surgeons: atlas of orthotics*, St. Louis, 1985, CV Mosby.
29. Lonstein JE, Winter RB: The Milwaukee brace for the treatment of adolescent idiopathic scoliosis—a review of one thousand twenty patients, *J Bone Joint Surg* 76:1207–1221, 1994.
30. Lucas D: Spinal bracing. In: *Orthotics etcetera*, Baltimore, 1966, Williams & Wilkins.
31. Lucas D, et al: Spinal orthotics for pain and instability. In: *Orthotics etcetera*, ed 3, Baltimore, 1986, Williams & Wilkins.
32. Lusskin R: Pain patterns in spondylolisthesis, *Clin Orthop* 40:125–136, 1965.
33. Maiman D, et al: The effect of the thermoplastic Minerva body jacket on cervical spine motion, *Neurosurgery* 25:363–367, 1989.
34. McCollough NC III, et al: Miami TLSO in the management of scoliosis: preliminary results in 100 cases, *J Pediatr Orthop* 1:141–152, 1981.
35. McGill SM, et al: The effect of an abdominal belt on trunk muscle activity and intra-abdominal pressure during squat lifts, *Ergonomics* 33:147–160, 1990.
36. Micheli LJ, Hall JE, Miller ME: Use of the modified Boston brace for back injuries in athletes, *Am J Sports Med* 8:351–356, 1980.
37. Morris JM, Lucas D, Bresler B: Role of the trunk in stability of the spine, *J Bone Joint Surg* 43A:327–351, 1961.
38. Mulcahy T, et al: A follow-up study of forces acting in the Milwaukee brace on patients undergoing treatment for idiopathic scoliosis, *Clin Orthop* 93:53, 1973.
39. Norton PL, Brown T: The immobilizing efficiency of the back braces: their effect on the posture and motion of the lumbosacral spine, *J Bone Joint Surg* 39A:111–139, 1957.
40. Patwardhan AG, et al: Orthotic stabilization of idiopathic scoliotic curves: a biomechanical comparison of the Milwaukee brace and low profile orthoses. In: Erdman AG, editor: *Advances in bioengineering*, 1987, ASME.
41. Patwardhan AG, et al: Biomechanics of adolescent idiopathic scoliosis: natural history and treatment. In: Goel VK, Weinstein JN, editors: *Biomechanics of the spine: clinical and surgical perspective*, Boca Raton, FL, 1990, CRC Press.
42. Perry J: The use of external support in the treatment of low back pain, *J Bone Joint Surg* 52A:1440–1442, 1970.
43. Salter RB: *Textbook of disorders and injuries of the musculoskeletal system*, ed 2, Baltimore, 1983, Williams & Wilkins.
44. *Spinal orthotics*, New York, 1973, New York University Postgraduate Medical School.
45. Taylor CF: On the mechanical treatment of Pott's disease of the spine—the spinal assistant, treatise, *N Y S Med Soc* 6:67, 1863.

46. Thompson A: Appliances for the spine and trunk. In: *American Academy of Orthopedic Surgeons: orthopedic appliance atlas*, vol. I, Ann Arbor, Mich, 1952, Edwards Bros.
47. Triggs KJ: Length dependence of a halo orthosis on cervical immobilization, *J Spinal Disord* 6:34–37, 1993.
48. van Leeuwen PJ, et al: Assessment of spinal movement by thoraco-lumbar-sacral orthoses, *J Rehabil Res Dev* 37:395–403, 2000.

49. Waters RL, Morris JM: Effects of spinal supports on the electrical activity of muscles of the trunk, *J Bone Joint Surg* 52A:51–60, 1970.
50. Wilhemy JK, Farrow B, Zeller JL: Five year study evaluating the use of the Charleston night brace for the treatment of idiopathic scoliosis, *Proceedings of the 25th Annual Meeting of the Scoliosis Research Society, Honolulu,* 1990.
51. Williams PC: Lesions of the lumbosacral spine—lordosis brace, *J Bone Joint Surg* 19:702, 1937.

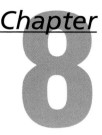

Chapter

8

Orthoses for spinal pain

K. Brandon Strenge and John R. Fisk

Key Points

- The available literature is inconclusive regarding the effectiveness of orthoses for treatment of spinal pain.
- The mechanisms of action of spinal orthoses remain controversial based on the available literature.
- Despite a lack of supporting evidence, orthoses are commonly prescribed for treatment of spinal pain from a variety of causes, with a number of patients achieving pain relief from device use.
- Practicing physicians should have knowledge of spinal orthoses as treatment alternatives within a comprehensive management plan for patients suffering from spinal pain.

Historical perspective

Orthoses have been used in the management of spinal pathology for hundreds of years, with the earliest reported use from ancient Egypt more than 2500 years ago.[91] Most of the early orthotic devices, which were specifically designed for treatment of spinal deformities, used wood and iron frames, leather straps, paper cellulose, and glue.[11] The development of new composite materials, polymer resins, and thermoplastics has led to a number of commercially available orthoses that are extremely lightweight and comfortable, almost completely replacing the heavy, cumbersome devices of the past. Use of polypropylene and other thermoplastics has allowed production of relatively inexpensive, rapidly fabricated custom-molded orthoses and a proliferation of orthotic use for a wide variety of orthopaedic conditions.

Spinal orthoses for back pain
Pathophysiology

Back pain is one of the most common disabling conditions experienced by individuals throughout the industrialized world, affecting more than half of Americans at some time during their lives. Epidemiologic studies have reported that the lifetime prevalence of experiencing low-back pain is as high as 80% in the general population.[34]

Often symptoms can be related to a specific injury or action, such as lifting a heavy object or twisting of the back; however, in many cases no traumatic cause can be ascertained. Alternatively, many cases of low-back pain are associated with demonstrable pathologic lesions such as disk herniations or spondylosis. Low-back pain that occurs in the absence of an identifiable cause, such as bony injury or disk pathology, is termed *nonspecific* low-back pain.

In 80% to 90% of patients presenting with disabling low-back pain, the precise diagnosis is unknown.[92] Dillane et al.[27] found that 79% of men and 89% of women who presented with a first episode of back pain to a general practice office were classified as having back pain of unknown origin. Some authors have estimated that only 15% of chronic low-back pain cases have an identifiable pathoanatomic explanation.[74]

Almost all structures of the spine, including the intervertebral disk, supporting spinal ligaments, facet joint capsules, and paraspinal musculature, are potential sources of pain. Innervation of the spinal column is complex and overlapping, which can partially explain the difficulty in localizing pain to specific anatomic elements.

The posterior longitudinal ligament, outer lamina of the posterior annulus fibrosus, and ventral dural sac and blood vessels of the vertebral body are innervated by branches

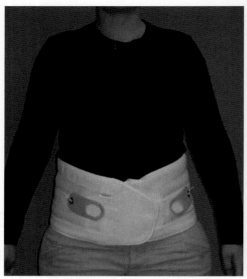
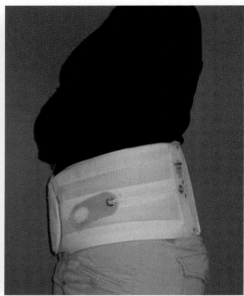

A   B

Fig. 8-1 Flexible lumbar corset. (Photos Courtesy of Dr. Daryl G Barth, CPO, of Orthotic and Prosthetic Associates of Central Illinois.)

of the sinuvertebral nerve, which is formed by ventral rami and autonomic roots from gray rami communicantes. Transverse and descending branches supply the posterior longitudinal ligament at the level of nerve entry, with an ascending branch to the next cranial level providing overlapping innervation at each spinal level. Segmental branches from ventral rami supply the ventral annulus fibrosus and anterior longitudinal ligament. The dorsal rami divide into multiple branches innervating the paraspinal musculature and facet joint capsules.

Treatment recommendations

The vast majority of nonspecific low-back pain is managed conservatively with rest, analgesics, antiinflammatory medications, physical therapy, manipulation, and, in many cases, orthoses. Lumbar supports continue to be one of the most common methods of handling the impairment and disability caused by low-back pain, despite the lack of knowledge regarding their true physiologic effect or their effectiveness in relieving symptoms.[2,53] One study found that 99% of orthopaedic surgeons had prescribed an orthosis at some time for their patients with low-back pain.[78] A survey of patients indicated that 27% of patients with back pain for at least 2 weeks had used braces to relieve their complaints; the percentage increased to 37% in patients who experienced pain for 6 months or longer.[25]

Lumbar orthotic management

Orthoses used for treatment of low-back pain are categorized by the body region incorporated, with sacroiliac (SIO), lumbosacral (LSO), and thoracolumbosacral (TLSO) orthoses the standardized terminology used. Each of these orthotic devices can be divided into flexible and rigid designs based upon material characteristics. Flexible lumbar orthoses include lumbar support bands and belts as well as some lightweight corsets. Rigid lumbar orthoses include mainly corsets and braces.

Contemporary corsets (Fig. 8-1) are composed of sturdy, lightweight canvas or elastic material. Vertical reinforcing stays usually are necessary to prevent the upper margin from curling away from the trunk. In the front, corsets extend from a point just below the xiphoid process to a point just above the pubic symphysis. Corsets cover the back from below the inferior border of the scapulae to the gluteal folds. Some corsets include posterior reinforcements made of rigid thermoplastic or metal that can be custom molded to the patient. Perineal straps usually are included, mainly for use by men, to prevent the garment from sliding upward with forward flexion; however, these straps can be uncomfortable and often are removed. Women's corsets usually include garters to aid with prevention of upward displacement. Abdominal belts cover the pelvis, extending from the iliac crests to the pubic symphysis anteriorly and gluteal folds posteriorly.

Rigid trunk orthoses or braces (Fig. 8-2) include stiff plastic or upholstered metal bands in both the vertical and horizontal planes, in contrast to corsets, which provide no horizontal reinforcement. When prescribed for pain relief, pelvic and thoracic bands are included that lie flat on the torso and terminate at the lateral midline. Frame-like constructs of some trunk orthoses make them cooler to wear than corsets. It is important that the rigid orthoses be fitted with the patient in both the standing and sitting positions to accommodate pelvic tilt and prevent pressure on the upper thighs or buttocks. Some rigid orthoses have inflatable pads that allow continued adjustment of fit. Custom-molded designs are available.

Mechanisms of action of lumbar orthoses

Several potential mechanisms of action for the pain-relieving ability of spinal orthoses have been proposed in the literature. The mechanical effectiveness of orthoses could result from intersegmental motion restriction, gross motion restriction, or decreased load on the spinal column. Other rationales include increased abdominal pressure, reduced muscle

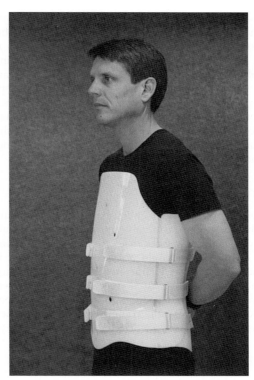

Fig. 8-2 Rigid lumbar brace, prefabricated thoracolumbosacral orthosis. (From Botte MJ, Garfin SR, Bergmann K, et al: Spinal orthoses for traumatic and degenerative disease. In Herkowitz HN, Garfin SR, Balderston RA, et al., editors: *The spine*, ed 4, Philadelphia, 1999, WB Saunders.)

fatigue, increased postural awareness or proprioception, as well as the miscellaneous effects of massage, heat, and placebo. Unfortunately, conflicting results in the literature have led to criticism of most hypotheses based on theoretical grounds, with the mechanisms of action remaining a matter of considerable debate.[14,83] Quite possibly, a combination of factors, varying from patient to patient, results in the pain relief experienced by patients using lumbar orthoses.

Motion restriction

The effect most often expected from a brace is restriction of motion; however, available literature investigating different orthoses and their ability to restrict motion has reported inconsistent results. Excessive trunk motion, especially axial rotation, often is assumed to be the cause of back injury. Orthoses are prescribed to prevent this excessive motion and thus reduce low-back pain.[5]

Norton and Brown[76] inserted pins into the spinous processes of lumbar vertebrae and found surprisingly small effects on intersegmental flexion and extension movements when several different braces were used. The orthoses were unable to eliminate intervertebral motion, and the more rigid braces actually increased motion at the lumbosacral junction. This finding was confirmed by Lumsden and Morris[58] using similar techniques but studying mainly rotation. Increased motion at L5–S1 with use of lumbar orthoses also was demonstrated by Miller et al.,[67] leading some authors to suggest that fixation of the pelvis is essential in restricting motion.[58,100] Another study using flexion and extension lateral radiography

found lumbar supports were able to restrict the sagittal movements of the lumbosacral spine, although considerable variation between individuals was noted.[30]

More recently, roentgen stereophotogrammetric analysis has failed to show a stabilizing effect on sagittal, vertical, or transverse intervertebral translations with use of either a molded rigid orthosis or a canvas corset with a molded plastic posterior support.[4] The authors concluded that an external lumbar support can decrease the overall load on the lumbar spine by restricting gross motions of the trunk but appears to have no stabilizing effect on the intervertebral mobility of the lower lumbar spine. This concept had been suggested previously,[55] with gross motion restrictions thought to be of greater importance than intersegmental motion restrictions in the effectiveness of orthoses in patients with low-back pain.[73]

An extensive literature review focusing on proposed mechanisms of action concluded that lumbar supports reduce trunk motion with respect to flexion, extension, and lateral bending but provide no significant effect on rotation.[99] In essence, no orthotic device has the ability to completely eliminate motion within the spinal column, and specific orthoses display a great deal of variability in motion restriction.

Unloading of the spinal column

Another common rationale for use of lumbosacral orthoses is based on the premise that the devices directly or indirectly provide some assistance to trunk extensor moment, reducing the activation of erector spinae muscles and consequently the magnitude of spinal compression forces. In *direct unloading*, the orthosis actually bears some of the load that would otherwise be transmitted through the lumbar trunk. In *indirect unloading*, the orthosis transmits little load but raises the intraabdominal pressure enough to unload the vertebral column.[73] By compressing the abdomen, lumbar corsets and braces convert the trunk into a semirigid cylinder, reducing the usual paraspinal musculature workload by shifting a portion of the load from the spine to the entire trunk. A larger percentage of the upper body weight then is supported by the abdomen, relieving the vertebral column to some degree and requiring less back muscle force to extend the trunk.

In an attempt to demonstrate the spine unloading function of braces, numerous studies have examined intraabdominal pressure, differences in trunk musculature electromyogram, and changes in vertebral compression forces. Bartelink[6] was the first to suggest that an increase in intraabdominal pressure could be used to unload the spine. Early work by Morris et al.[71] showed that braces and corsets increased the intraabdominal pressure of the wearer by 10 to 15 mm Hg at rest. Morris and Lucas[70] studied static lifting postures and found that myoelectric activity in the abdominal muscles decreased when braces were worn; however, intraabdominal and intrathoracic pressures were unchanged. Nachemson and Morris[72] tested an inflatable corset and found that intraabdominal pressures remained generally low and inconsistent.

Waters and Morris[103] measured the effect of chairback braces and lumbosacral corsets on the myoelectric activity of trunk muscles during level walking and found a great deal of variability in muscle activity. Nachemson et al.[74] found inconsistent trends in the effect of orthoses on the myoelectric activity of trunk muscle and encountered no significant changes in intragastric pressure. This finding was supported by Lantz and Schultz,[56] who reported that none of the orthoses they tested was consistently effective in reducing myoelectric activity, and that, in many cases, electromyographic signals increased when the orthoses were worn. They concluded that wearing a lumbar orthosis is mechanically effective only sometimes, often is not effective, and sometimes is counterproductive. They also indicated that the load restrictions were not dramatic even when wearing an lumbar orthosis was effective.[56]

On the other hand, Cholewicki[16] suggested that although the additional support supplied by a lumbosacral orthosis may produce only a modest overall reduction in trunk muscle activity as measured by electromyography, the device still may be of functional significance in patients suffering from low-back pain. These patients exhibit increased trunk muscle contraction during activities of daily living, presumably in an effort to enhance the stability of the lumbar spines, thus creating a significant physiologic burden.[98]

In healthy subjects, as little as 2% of maximal voluntary activation from all trunk muscles may be sufficient to stabilize the spine in a neutral, upright standing position.[17] Ergonomic studies have shown that static muscle contractions sustained above 5% maximal voluntary activation lead to muscle fatigue and pain, with contractions below 5% maintainable indefinitely.[8,51] A small reduction in trunk muscle activity may be sufficient to bring contractions to below the 5% threshold; therefore, lumbosacral orthoses may provide symptomatic relief to some patients with low-back pain by reducing their necessary static trunk muscle contraction, preventing muscle fatigue that may compound their existing pain.[17]

Spine compression forces during lifting tasks have been investigated to determine the unloading effect produced by orthoses. An often cited study by Nachemson and Morris[72] demonstrated a 25% decrease in intradiskal pressure with use of an inflatable corset in normal subjects standing upright. Lumbar belts have been suggested to modify trunk kinematics, resulting in lower spinal loads; however, reductions in spine compression force were not observed when task kinematics were controlled.[63,87,108] Postural shrinkage, proposed as an indicator of the cumulative mechanical stress placed on the spine during physical activity, has been compared in patients with and without orthoses, but results have been inconsistent.[60,84]

Although both positive and negative results have been reported,[56,57,60] collectively the scientific literature does not appear to support the hypothesis that orthoses reduce the activity of erector spinae muscles, increase intraabdominal pressure, or significantly impact compression forces.[99]

Proprioception

Some articles discussing lumbar supports have suggested various mechanisms of action that imply proprioceptive enhancement, such as improving posture, increasing awareness of pelvis and spine positioning, reminding patients to lift properly, and reminding patients not to overstress the back. This increase in proprioceptive input may be effective in relieving pain by reminding patients of their position in space and stopping patients from placing their trunk in harmful positions. McNair and Heine[66] described improved trunk proprioception through increasing afferent input via the mechanoreceptors in the skin with use of lumbar bracing. Newcomer et al.[75] demonstrated an improvement in repositioning error, a commonly used method of measuring proprioception with position sense, in subjects wearing a lumbar support. These studies support the concept that braces provide enhanced proprioception through increased cutaneous input, but some authors have suggested that bracing also may activate mechanoreceptors of the underlying musculature and joint capsules, providing another source of proprioceptive input.

Patient factors

Many of the investigations on lumbar bracing mechanisms of action have found considerable interindividual variation in mobility with and without use of supports, implying that patient characteristics could be as, or perhaps more, important than actual corset characteristics in spinal immobilization. In a study that focused on central obesity measured using waist-to-hip ratio, Todo[95] specifically investigated interindividual differences and commented that the efficacy of lumbosacral corsets may be affected by central obesity.

Miscellaneous

Local temperature elevation, an increased feeling of safety, and the placebo effect have been suggested as other potential mechanisms alleviating low-back pain with use of spinal orthoses.[2] Thick or padded material incorporated into lumbar supports has been shown to increase lumbar skin temperature by almost 2°C, perhaps supporting the concept that increased warmth improves low-back pain.[40] However, this finding has been criticized because the amount of padding necessary to potentiate this effect is more than usually found in standard orthoses or corsets.[11]

Authors have described the development of psychological dependence on orthoses as a result of the sense of security or safety provided by the devices. Ahlgren and Hansen[1] conducted a survey of randomly selected patients for whom a corset had been prescribed for back pain and found that 50% were still using their corset 4 years later, perhaps because patients had developed this type of dependence.

Given the inconsistent literature on the mechanisms of action of orthotic devices, many have attributed the pain-relieving properties of the devices to a placebo effect.[47] Proving or disproving these beliefs is a nearly impossible task because "blinding" of patients cannot be accomplished as easily as with other treatment modalities.

Side effects and other considerations

Because bracing attempts to control the position of the spine through the application of external forces, orthotic designs must account for regional variations of the surrounding anatomy, such as the vital soft-tissue structures of the anterior neck, the rigid thoracic rib cage, and the bony pelvis. The surrounding soft-tissue envelope has a substantial effect on the ability of an externally applied force to control spinal movement, but it also can be an area of potential complications. Adverse effects of wearing lumbar orthoses include local pain, skin breakdown, gastrointestinal disorders, decreased vital capacity, increased lower extremity venous pressure, higher blood pressure, and higher heart rates.[14,64]

Concern has been expressed over the possibility of disuse atrophy of the lumbar muscles with use of lumbar supports, leading some authors to deprecate the use of lumbar supports.[83] One study indicated that more than 40% of corset wearers reported subjective weakness of the trunk musculature.[2] Walsh and Schwartz[102] found no significant change in abdominal muscle strength after 6 months of lumbar brace use by a group of warehouse workers. Another study actually found an increase in isometric trunk flexor strength after 2 months of using a soft lumbar belt, with an insignificant decrease in trunk extensor strength.[44] Eisinger et al.[29] demonstrated statistically significant weakness of both concentric and eccentric trunk extension as well as concentric trunk flexion in patients who used lumbar orthotics for chronic low-back pain. Taking these findings into account, some believe orthoses should be used only intermittently and selectively recommend that any bracing technique should include a strong abdominal exercise program with postural reeducation to prevent muscular atrophy once the patient achieves symptomatic relief.[21,90]

In the experience of some authors, the usefulness of orthotic devices is limited because many of the devices are so uncomfortable that patients soon stop wearing them. Any motion restriction achieved likely can be attributed to the discomfort caused by the pressure of the orthosis on the skin and bony prominences of the patient.[96] Buchalter et al.[13] demonstrated an inverse relationship between a brace's ability to restrict motion and patient comfort. They found that the most comfortable brace, an elastic corset, was the least restrictive of the braces tested, whereas the Raney jacket provided maximal restriction but was the most uncomfortable to wear.

Outcome studies and effectiveness of lumbar orthoses for spinal pain

The natural history of low-back pain is extremely variable, thus compromising the ability to objectively evaluate treatment strategies for efficacy. Whether or not due to an identifiable injury, symptoms may resolve spontaneously within a few days or weeks, or they may persist for months or years. Approximately 40% of patients will have resolution of symptoms within 1 week, 60% within 3 weeks, and well over 90% after 2 months.[27] These often quoted percentages have fueled a recommendation for essentially "benign neglect" in the first several months of symptom occurrence.[62] However, contemporary literature supports the concept that although many patients experience improvement, up to 75% have one or more relapses, and 72% continue to have pain at 1 year.[97,101]

Another limitation inherent to all studies evaluating the pain-relieving efficacy of orthoses is the inability to achieve a blind methodology.[24] Spratt et al.[92] added that the undoubtedly heterogeneous pathology comprising patients grouped together as having nonspecific or idiopathic back pain makes difficult the evaluation of treatment strategies. In support of this concept, Willner[105] found that pain deriving from a spondylolisthesis appeared to respond to lumbar bracing more favorably than back pain with no specific identifiable cause.

The literature on the effectiveness of orthoses in the treatment of spinal pain has revealed inconsistent results.

Two early studies are conflicting. Million et al.[68] demonstrated superior pain relief with use of a lumbar corset incorporating a rigid plastic support; however, Coxhead et al.[22] found no treatment at all was as effective as use of a corset. Similarly, Hsieh et al.[46] and Pope et al.[82] did not find differences in pain relief with use of a corset, soft-tissue massage, manipulation, or transcutaneous muscular stimulation. In contrast, Valle-Jones et al.[96] demonstrated a significant difference with respect to pain, limitation of activity, ability to work, and use of analgesics in favor of lumbar support use for back pain after a 3-week period.

Koes and van den Hoogen[53] concluded in a systematic review that the effectiveness of lumbar supports in the treatment of low-back pain remains controversial, adding that the methodologic quality of available randomized trials varies widely. Similarly, in a systematic review of the available literature using the Cochrane database, Jellema et al.[48] found "limited" evidence that lumbar supports are more effective than no treatment at all for low-back pain. Unfortunately, whether lumbar supports are more effective than other treatments remains unclear.

Conclusion

Evidence on the effectiveness of orthoses in the treatment of low-back pain is conflicting. Some devices likely are more effective than others in reducing pain; however, a variety of factors, including interindividual differences, appear to influence the pain-relieving characteristics of the devices. With more aggressive rehabilitation focusing on range of motion and increased activity becoming the standard of care for many orthopaedic conditions, many surgeons appear to be strictly opposed to immobilization of patients with low-back pain in orthotic devices.[42] On the other hand, a great number of physicians will continue to prescribe orthoses for treatment of low-back pain based largely on empiric or anecdotal evidence, and with many patients will achieve some measure of pain relief, regardless of the actual mechanism of action.

Spinal orthoses for cervical pain
Pathophysiology

Neck pain is a common problem in the industrialized world, estimated to affect approximately 10% of the population at any given time.[12,61] Common conditions thought to cause neck pain are degenerative disk disease, with or without disk herniation, and degenerative arthritis of the facet joints. Other less understood conditions reported to cause neck pain are posttraumatic neck pain syndrome, commonly known as *whiplash*, and pain following repetitive activities in the occupational setting.

The relationship between neck pain and degenerative changes and disk herniations found on imaging studies is not always clear. Degenerative conditions are extremely common with increasing age and are often found incidentally in asymptomatic people. Osteophytes and other degenerative changes are almost universally found on cervical radiographs of middle-aged patients.[33,37,94] Long-term studies have shown that the degenerative process actually slows down and may again become asymptomatic with further increases in age.[37]

Numerous epidemiologic studies on low-back pain are available, but relatively few investigations of neck pain have been conducted. It is generally believed that neck pain is not as common as low-back pain, and that neck pain, if present, may not be as disabling and thus may not have as great an economic impact on society with respect to lost work and medical expenses.

Gore et al.[38] evaluated the natural history of neck pain in a retrospective review of 205 patients followed clinically and radiographically over a 10-year period. Although 79% of patients had diminished pain and 43% had near complete relief of symptoms, approximately one third of the study group reported persistent moderate-to-severe pain. This finding emphasizes that neck pain frequently is not a self-limiting problem and that many patients will have long-term symptoms that are potentially disabling.

Treatment recommendations

Because a large percentage of patients experience symptoms that diminish or completely resolve within a few weeks, most patients with neck pain, with or without radiculopathy, can be managed nonoperatively in the early stages. Initial treatment strategies include activity modification that avoids neck extension and heavy lifting, use of analgesics and antiinflammatory medications, and physical therapy with heat and ultrasound modalities, injections, and cervical traction.

Cervical orthoses have become an extremely important component of most contemporary trauma protocols, with cervical spine protection and immobilization one of the first requirements for safe extrication and transport of traumatized individuals. As these devices have evolved to become lightweight and relatively comfortable, they have been incorporated into the treatment algorithm for the management of neck pain resulting from a variety of causes other than trauma, including painful degenerative conditions and postoperative immobilization.

Cervical orthotic management

Orthotic devices used for treatment of the cervical spine can be divided into two broad categories, cervical orthoses (CO) and cervicothoracic orthoses (CTO), depending on whether or not the trunk is incorporated into the design. CTOs are most commonly used in the trauma setting for immobilization of lower cervical and upper thoracic spine fractures. Cervical orthoses are prescribed much more frequently and can be subdivided into soft collars, rigid collars, and cervical orthoses that incorporate the head (see Chapter 7).

Soft collars (Fig. 8-3) are the most comfortable cervical orthoses available. However, they provide only limited motion restriction, decreasing flexion and extension by 5% to 15%, lateral bending by 5% to 10%, and axial rotation by 10% to 17%. Hard cervical collars (Fig. 8-4) are more durable than soft collars when used for the longer term. Motion restriction is estimated at 20% to 25% flexion and extension, slightly better than that achieved using soft collars. Cervical orthoses may provide better head stabilization by incorporating a chin, occiput, or forehead strap.

As a group, cervical orthoses with a head control component restrict cervical flexion and extension, lateral bending, and axial rotation by approximately 60%, with some degree of

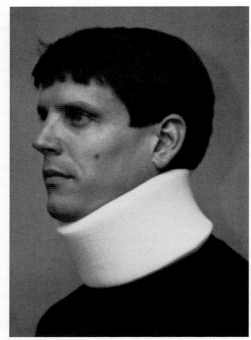

Fig. 8-3 Soft cervical collar. (From Botte MJ, Garfin SR, Bergmann K, et al: Spinal orthoses for traumatic and degenerative disease. In Herkowitz HN, Garfin SR, Balderston RA, et al., editors: *The spine*, ed 4, Philadelphia, 1999, WB Saunders.)

variability among commercially available brands. Nearly all designs have an anterior hole for tracheotomy access, if required. Many devices have available thoracic extensions that reportedly increase motion restriction from the lower cervical to upper thoracic segments.

One example of a premade cervical orthosis is shown in Figure 8-5. This two-piece semirigid cervical orthosis is made

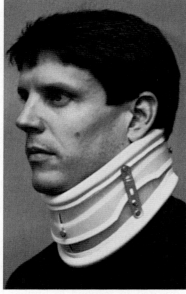

Fig. 8-4 Hard cervical collar. (From Botte MJ, Garfin SR, Bergmann K, et al: Spinal orthoses for traumatic and degenerative disease. In Herkowitz HN, Garfin SR, Balderston RA, et al., editors: *The spine*, ed 4, Philadelphia, 1999, WB Saunders.)

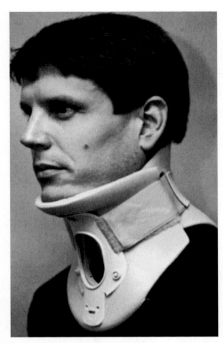

Fig. 8-5 Philadelphia cervical collar. (From Botte MJ, Garfin SR, Bergmann K, et al: Spinal orthoses for traumatic and degenerative disease. In Herkowitz HN, Garfin SR, Balderston RA, et al., editors: *The spine*, ed 4, Philadelphia, 1999, WB Saunders.)

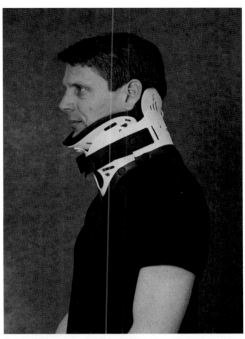

Fig. 8-6 Miami J-style cervical orthosis. (From Botte MJ, Garfin SR, Bergmann K, et al: Spinal orthoses for traumatic and degenerative disease. In Herkowitz HN, Garfin SR, Balderston RA, et al., editors: *The spine*, ed 4, Philadelphia, 1999, WB Saunders.)

of polyethylene foam and has plastic struts anteriorly and posteriorly for support. The upper portion of the orthosis supports the lower jaw and occiput; the lower portion covers the upper thoracic region. Hook-and-loop straps unite the anterior and posterior shells, which are available in approximately 20 different sizes. Liners of jersey-knit cotton are available for added comfort and moisture absorption. Other examples are shown in Figures 8-6, 8-7, and 8-8.

CTOs provide greater motion restriction in the middle to lower cervical spine by incorporating the trunk, with added pressure from anterior and posterior orthotic extensions connected with circumferential straps. Most designs feature two to four rigid uprights or posts that connect the chin and occiput supports to the trunk plates. CTOs improve cervical motion restriction in all planes, with flexion and extension decreased 70% to 80%, lateral bending decreased 60%, and axial rotation decreased 60% to 70%. Unfortunately, the increased immobilization afforded by CTOs is associated with considerably decreased patient comfort. Specific examples of CTOs are shown in Figures 8-9, 8-10, and 8-11. Although these devices can be used for relief of spinal pain, they are most often used for immobilization of vertebral fractures amenable to nonoperative management.

Mechanisms of action of cervical orthoses

The specific mechanisms of action of cervical orthoses have been studied in much less detail than orthotics of the lumbosacral spine; however, the pain-relieving effects of the two are thought to be similar. The most cited, and therefore researched, reason for prescribing cervical collars is motion restriction, which can be useful for limiting or preventing cervical pain, protecting spinal instability either preoperatively

or postoperatively, and protecting the cervical spine in emergency situations immediately following trauma. In addition to the mechanical restraint provided, wearing of cervical collars probably provides the benefits of improved proprioception and decreased loading to injured muscles or

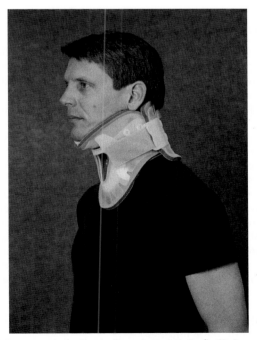

Fig. 8-7 Aspen cervical orthosis. (From Botte MJ, Garfin SR, Bergmann K, et al: Spinal orthoses for traumatic and degenerative disease. In Herkowitz HN, Garfin SR, Balderston RA, et al., editors: *The spine*, ed 4, Philadelphia, 1999, WB Saunders.)

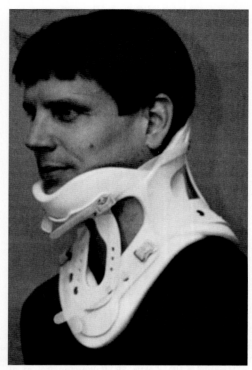

Fig. 8-8 Malibu cervical brace. (From Botte MJ, Garfin SR, Bergmann K, et al: Spinal orthoses for traumatic and degenerative disease. In Herkowitz HN, Garfin SR, Balderston RA, et al., editors: *The spine*, ed 4, Philadelphia, 1999, WB Saunders.)

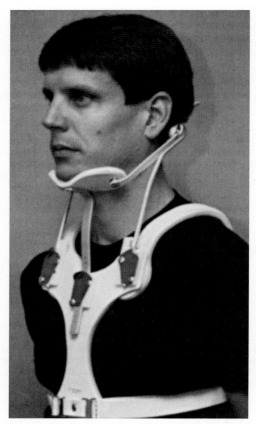

Fig. 8-9 Sterno-occipito-mandibular immobilizer (SOMI) brace. (From Botte MJ, Garfin SR, Bergmann K, et al: Spinal orthoses for traumatic and degenerative disease. In Herkowitz HN, Garfin SR, Balderston RA, et al., editors: *The spine*, ed 4, Philadelphia, 1999, WB Saunders.)

ligaments by increased support to the region.[88] Other potential benefits include increasing the local temperature of the soft tissues of the cervical region by reducing heat loss and providing a placebo effect.

Motion restriction

Much of the literature on the ability of cervical orthoses to restrict motion pertains to immobilization of the cervical spine with respect to trauma situations. Patients extricated from acute trauma environments require immediate cervical immobilization to minimize or hopefully prevent spinal cord injuries and their devastating consequences. Naturally the motion-restricting ability of specific orthoses is of great concern for these applications, where the least amount of motion possible is desired in the event potentially unstable fractures are present.

The mechanical aspects of the collar-immobilized cervical spine were first reported by Jones[50] in 1960 using cineradiography to analyze the motion restriction provided by various cervical collars. Hartman et al.[41] used similar techniques to compare motion restriction in soft and semirigid collars with both two-poster and four-poster cervical orthoses and found soft collars restricted less than 10% of total motion in all three planes. In support of this finding, subsequent work by other authors concluded that soft foam collars did little to limit cervical motion and that more rigid plastic collars were only slightly more effective.[20,49]

Using roentgenograms, Johnson et al.[49] evaluated the effectiveness of five cervical orthoses in restricting sagittal motion in normal subjects and found that cervicothoracic orthoses with rigid connections between the anterior and posterior chest components were superior. Interestingly, they also noted that motion between the occiput and C1 increased in all orthoses tested when compared to the unrestricted spine. Using roentgenographic data, Fisher et al.[32] found that four-poster and sterno-occipito-mandibular immobilizer (SOMI) orthoses were significantly more restrictive at the midcervical levels compared with soft collars and Philadelphia collars, but they also found that the Camp collar provided the best immobilization at the C1–2 level. In a similar study using radiography, Colachis et al.[20] compared the sagittal motion restriction of four different cervical orthoses in normal women and determined that adding chin and occiput supports substantially improved motion restriction.

McGuire et al.[65] found no significant differences in the immobilizing power of the NecLoc and Stifneck emergency collars compared with the more traditional Philadelphia collar in flexion–extension and translation on C4–5 destabilized cadaver specimens. Kaufman et al.[52] compared NecLoc, Philadelphia, and soft collars using goniometry in normal subjects and determined that the NecLoc collar was significantly better in immobilizing the cervical spine in all three planes of motion. Lunsford et al.[59] found that four contemporary collars (Philadelphia, Miami J, Malibu, and Newport Extended Wear) were not as effective as the poster-type or halo-vest orthoses but were effective in limiting cervical motion by approximately 40% to 60%. Sandler et al.[88]

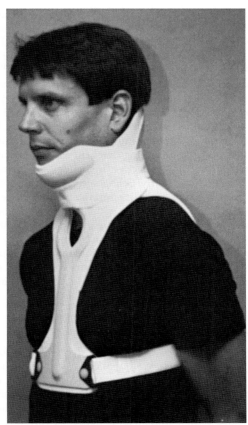

Fig. 8-10 Yale brace. (From Botte MJ, Garfin SR, Bergmann K, et al: Spinal orthoses for traumatic and degenerative disease. In Herkowitz HN, Garfin SR, Balderston RA, et al., editors: *The spine*, ed 4, Philadelphia, 1999, WB Saunders.)

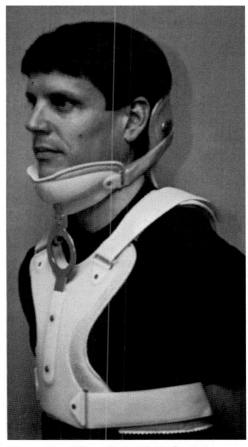

Fig. 8-11 Minerva brace. (From Botte MJ, Garfin SR, Bergmann K, et al: Spinal orthoses for traumatic and degenerative disease. In Herkowitz HN, Garfin SR, Balderston RA, et al., editors: *The spine*, ed 4, Philadelphia, 1999, WB Saunders.)

ranked the soft collar, Philadelphia collar, Philadelphia collar with thoracic extension, and SOMI brace from least restrictive to most restrictive, respectively. Askins and Eismont[3] found the NecLoc orthosis was statistically superior in restricting cervical flexion, extension, rotation, and lateral tilt, with the Miami J-collar the next most restrictive orthosis. To summarize, all cervical orthoses restrict motion to some extent, and a fair amount of variability exists among specific designs, but no orthosis provides a particularly high level of mechanical restriction of motion.[88]

The capacity of cervical orthoses to immobilize the neck in extrication situations has been studied. Cline et al.[19] found radiographically that their short board technique, consisting of a short board with Kerlix head and chin straps, was superior to three commonly used extrication collars (Philadelphia, Hare, and rigid plastic) for immobilization, adding that the collars did not seem to offer any additional support to the short board technique used alone. Using goniometry, Podolsky et al.[81] compared cervical immobilization in all three planes in normal supine subjects and determined that the Philadelphia collar in combination with forehead tape and sandbags was best, a conclusion supported by others.[26] Graziano et al.[39] radiographically measured sagittal and coronal plane motion restriction in normal subjects using common extrication and transport devices and found that the XP-One collar, which splints the head and torso, was superior.

Using both optoelectronic motion measurements and videofluoroscopy, Gavin et al.[35] found that the Miami J-collar and Aspen collar significantly reduced gross and intervertebral motion of the cervical spine in flexion and extension, but interestingly the Aspen collar was better in restricting motion at the C5–6 level. Using a similar three-dimensional motion analysis system, Zhang et al.[107] found that two newer collars, the C-Breeze and XTW, restricted cervical motion in a comparable fashion to both Miami J-collars and Aspen collars.

Side effects and other considerations

The ability of cervical orthotic devices to apply external forces to the spine is significantly compromised by the soft-tissue structures of the anterior neck region, including the esophagus, trachea, carotid arteries, and jugular veins. All contemporary orthoses account for this anatomy and therefore apply external pressure on nearby structures to obtain the desired motion restriction and support. Understandably, a complication frequently associated with cervical orthoses is skin breakdown and ulceration over the bony prominences of the head and neck region, including the chin, mandible, clavicles, sternum, and occiput. Studies have estimated that the incidence of pressure ulcer development related to use of cervical orthoses ranges from 38% to 55%.[15,18,23,43] Friction between facial hair, especially beards, and the orthotic liner or interface material can lead to ingrown hair. Although these problems are of most concern during neck immobilization for prolonged periods in nonambulatory obtunded or critically ill patients, the same anatomical regions can become sources of discomfort or irritation due to inappropriate orthotic fit or poor design in any patient.

Plaisier et al.[80] evaluated the pressure exerted by four different cervical orthoses on the occiput, chin, and body of the mandible by measuring the capillary closing pressure (CCP). They found that the Stifneck collar exceeded CCP in both the supine and upright positions, the Philadelphia collar exceeded CCP only in the supine position, and Miami J-collars and Aspen orthoses did not exceed the CCP in either position. Black et al.[9] concluded that both the Philadelphia and Aspen collars have the potential to exert enough pressure to lead to the development of skin ulceration. To date, no randomized clinical trials have compared the incidence of pressure ulcers with use of one orthosis versus another.[7]

Many other problems with long-term use of cervical orthotic devices in nonambulatory patients have been reported, including marginal mandibular nerve palsy,[86] increased intracranial pressure,[54,69,84] delayed extubation or difficulty weaning from the ventilator, decreased tidal volume,[28] dysphagia and potential aspiration,[45,93] and additional injuries caused to the spinal cord during patient transfers because of the false sense of security offered by the devices.[104]

As with orthotic devices used for other anatomic body regions, there appears to be an inverse relationship between comfort and restrictive effectiveness, with the most comfortable orthoses being the least effective in restricting cervical motion. One study has suggested that most cervical orthoses are loosened by patients because the devices have been fit too "tightly."[31] This orthotic discomfort has been ascribed not only to strap tightness but also to an overall "confining" effect. When an orthosis must be worn for an extended period, comfort can be the primary concern, and restrictive efficacy often is sacrificed.[52] With this in mind, soft and semirigid collars usually are the treatment of choice for management of cervical pain because these devices offer improved comfort. Cervicothoracic orthoses are rarely used in the absence of spinal instability.

Similar to the concerns associated with chronic use of lumbar orthoses and braces, concerns about muscle weakness and atrophy with cervical orthotic use have been raised. However, in contrast to the literature on lumbar devices, no studies regarding weakness of the cervical musculature as it relates to collar use have been reported. Also suggested but not specifically studied are the physical and psychological dependence issues surrounding the chronic use of cervical collars. Finally, some authors who have denounced lumbar braces for treatment of low-back pain also have dismissed cervical orthoses as primarily placebos in most patients.[47]

Outcome studies and effectiveness of orthoses for cervical pain

Relatively few studies have objectively evaluated the efficacy of the various cervical orthoses in use today; most of the literature has discussed the efficacy of orthoses in the treatment of whiplash injuries. Gennis et al.[36] determined that most patients with whiplash-type injuries have persistent pain for at least 6 weeks, and they stated that soft cervical collars did not appear to influence the duration or degree of persistent pain experienced by patients. Borchgrevink et al.[10] found better outcomes in patients who were encouraged to continue engaging in their normal, preinjury activities than in patients who took sick leave from work and were immobilized during the first 14 days after neck sprain or whiplash injuries. Peeters et al.[77] do not support neck immobilization, concluding that "rest makes rusty" and finding that active interventions have a tendency to be more effective in patients suffering from whiplash injuries. Similarly, Schnabel et al.[89] found exercise therapy was superior to collar immobilization in reducing pain intensity and disability in patients with whiplash injuries. One study evaluating the treatment of patients with long-lasting cervical radicular pain found cervical collars were equally effective as both physiotherapy and surgery.[79] Overall, caution is needed when drawing conclusions regarding the efficacy of orthotic treatment in patients with neck pain because of the lack of consistent literature.

Conclusion

Although cervical orthoses are commonly prescribed for treatment of neck pain from a variety of conditions, evidence supporting their specific mechanisms of action or clinical effectiveness is lacking. Most often, cervical collars are used to restrict neck motion, thus relieving pain. However, the available literature demonstrates a large degree of variation among specific orthoses with regard to their motion-restriction capabilities, with no device able to completely eliminate motion. Active rehabilitation programs with resumption of daily activities and physical therapy appear to be more effective than collar immobilization in the group of patients suffering from whiplash-type injuries, but no conclusive evidence supports or refutes orthotic use for treatment of other causes of neck pain.

Supporting Evidence

- Evidence reported in the literature regarding the effectiveness of orthoses for treatment of spinal pain is conflicting.
- Evidence supporting the pain relief mechanisms of spinal orthoses is inconclusive.

References

1. Ahlgren SA, Hansen T: The use of lumbosacral corsets prescribed for low back pain, *Prosthet Orthot Int* 6:139–146, 1978.
2. Alaranta H, Hurri H: Compliance and subjective relief by corset treatment in chronic low back pain, *Scand J Rehabil Med* 20:133–136, 1988.
3. Askins V, Eismont FJ: Efficacy of five cervical orthoses in restricting cervical motion, *Spine* 22:1193–1198, 1997.
4. Axelsson P, Johnsson R, Strömqvist B: Effect of lumbar orthosis on intervertebral mobility. A roentgen stereophotogrammetric analysis, *Spine* 17:678–681, 1992.
5. Barron BA, Feuerstein M: Industrial back belts and low back pain: mechanisms and outcomes, *J Occup Rehabil* 4:125–139, 1991.
6. Bartelink DL: Role of abdominal pressure in relieving pressure on lumbar intervertebral discs, *J Bone Joint Surg* 46A:517–524, 1957.
7. Belanger L, Cobb J, Bernardo A, et al: In search of the "superior" cervical orthosis: Philadelphia cervical orthosis versus Aspen cervical orthosis, *SCI Nurs* 21:158–160, 2004.

8. Björkstén M, Jonsson B: Endurance limit of force in long-term intermittent static contractions, *Scand J Work Environ Health* 3:23–27, 1977.

9. Black CA, Buderer NM, Blaylock B, et al: Comparative study of risk factors for breakdown with cervical orthotic devices: Philadelphia and Aspen, *J Trauma Nurs* 5:62–66, 1998.

10. Borchgrevink GE, Kaasa A, McDonagh D, et al: Acute treatment of whiplash neck sprain injuries. A randomized trial of treatment during the first 14 days after a car accident, *Spine* 23:25–31, 1998.

11. Botte MJ, Garfin SR, Bergmann K, et al: Spinal orthoses for traumatic and degenerative disease. In Herkowitz HN, Garfin SR, Balderston RA, et al., editor: *The spine*, ed 4, Philadelphia, 1999, WB Saunders.

12. Bovim G, Schrader H, Sand T: Neck pain in the general population, *Spine* 19:1307–1309, 1994.

13. Buchalter D, Kahanovitz N, Viola K, et al: Three-dimensional spinal motion measurements. Part 2: a noninvasive assessment of lumbar brace immobilization of the spine, *J Spinal Disord* 1:284–286, 1988.

14. Calmels P, Fayolle-Minon I: An update on orthotic devices for the lumbar spine based on a review of the literature, *Rev Rheum Engl Ed* 63:285–291, 1996.

15. Chendrasekhar A, Moorman DW, Timberlake GA: An evaluation of the effects of semi-rigid collars in patients with severe closed head injury, *Am Surg* 64:604–606, 1998.

16. Cholewicki J: The effects of lumbosacral orthoses on spine stability: what changes in EMG can be expected? *J Orthop Res* 22:1150–1155, 2004.

17. Cholewicki J, Panjabi MM, Khachatryan A: Stabilizing function of the trunk flexor-extensor muscles around a neutral spine posture, *Spine* 22:2207–2212, 1997.

18. Clancy MJ: Clearing the cervical spine of adult victims of trauma, *J Accid Emerg Med* 16:208–214, 1999.

19. Cline JR, Scheidel E, Bigsby EF: A comparison of methods of cervical immobilization used in patient extrication and transport, *J Trauma* 25:649–653, 1985.

20. Colachis SC, Strohm BR, Ganter EL: Cervical spine motion in normal women: radiographic study of the effect of cervical collars, *Arch Phys Med Rehabil* 54:161–169, 1973.

21. Coplans CW: The low-compression corset, *S Afr Med J* 66:456–457, 1984.

22. Coxhead CE, Inskip H, Meade TW, et al: Multicentre trial of physiotherapy in the management of sciatic symptoms, *Lancet* 1:1065–1068, 1981.

23. Davis JW, Parks SN, Detlefs CL, et al: Clearing the cervical spine in obtunded patients: the use of dynamic fluoroscopy, *J Trauma* 39:435–438, 1995.

24. Deyo RA: Conservative therapy for low back pain, *JAMA* 250:1057–1062, 1983.

25. Deyo RA, Tsui-Wu YJ: Descriptive epidemiology of low-back pain and its related medical care in the United States, *Spine* 12:264–268, 1987.

26. Dick T, Land R: Spinal immobilization devices, *J Emerg Serv* 14:26, 1982.

27. Dillane JB, Fry J, Kalton G: Acute back syndrome: a study from general practice, *BMJ* 2:82–84, 1966.

28. Dodd FM, Simon E, McKeown D, et al: The effect of a cervical collar on the tidal volume of anaesthetised adult patients, *Anaesthesia* 50:961–963, 1995.

29. Eisinger DB, Kumar R, Woodrow R: Effect of lumbar orthotics on trunk muscle strength, *Am J Phys Med Rehabil* 75:194–197, 1996.

30. Fidler MW, Plasmans MT: The effect of four types of support on the segmental mobility of the lumbosacral spine, *J Bone Joint Surg* 65A:943–947, 1983.

31. Fisher SV: Proper fitting of the cervical orthosis, *Arch Phys Med Rehabil* 59:505–507, 1978.

32. Fisher SV, Bowar JF, Awad EA, Gullikson G: Cervical orthoses effect on cervical spine motion: roentgenographic and goniometric method of study, *Arch Phys Med Rehabil* 58:109–115, 1977.

33. Friedenberg ZB, Miller WT: Degenerative disc disease of the cervical spine: a comparative study of asymptomatic and symptomatic patients, *J Bone Joint Surg Am* 45:1171–1178, 1963.

34. Frymoyer JW: Back pain and sciatica, *N Engl J Med* 318:291–300, 1988.

35. Gavin TM, Carandang G, Havey R, et al: Biomechanical analysis of cervical orthoses in flexion and extension: a comparison of cervical collars and cervical thoracic orthoses, *J Rehabil Res Dev* 40:527–537, 2003.

36. Gennis P, Miller L, Gallagher EJ, et al: The effect of soft cervical collars on persistent neck pain in patients with whiplash injury, *Acad Emerg Med* 3:568–573, 1996.

37. Gore DR, Sepic SB, Gardner GM: Roentgenographic findings of the cervical spine in asymptomatic people, *Spine* 11:521–524, 1986.

38. Gore DR, Sepic SB, Gardner GM, et al: Neck pain: a long-term follow-up of 205 patients, *Spine* 12:1–5, 1987.

39. Graziano AF, Scheidel EA, Cline JR, et al: A radiographic comparison of prehospital cervical immobilization methods, *Ann Emerg Med* 16:1127–1131, 1987.

40. Grew ND, Deane G: The physical effect of lumbar spinal supports, *Prosthet Orthot Int* 6:79–87, 1982.

41. Hartman JT, Palumbo F, Hill BJ: Cineradiography of the braced normal cervical spine, *Clin Orthop Related Res* 109:97–102, 1975.

42. Helliwell PS, Wright V: What are the indications for the use of a lumbar corset in low back pain? *Br J Rheumatol* 30:62, 1991.

43. Hewitt S: Skin necrosis caused by a semi-rigid cervical collar in a ventilated patient with multiple injuries, *Injury* 25:323–324, 1994.

44. Holmstrom E, Moritz U: Effect of lumbar belts on trunk muscle strength and endurance: a follow-up study of construction workers, *J Spinal Disord* 5:260–266, 1992.

45. Houghton DJ, Curley JW: Dysphagia caused by a hard cervical collar, *Br J Neurosurg* 10:501–502, 1996.

46. Hsieh CJ, Phillips RB, Adams AH, et al: Functional outcomes of low back pain: comparison of four treatment groups in a randomized controlled trial, *J Manipulative Physiol Ther* 15:4–9, 1992.

47. Huston GJ: Everyday aids and appliances. Collars and corsets, *BMJ* 296:276, 1988.

48. Jellema P, van Tulder MW, van Poppel MNM, et al: Lumbar supports for prevention and treatment of low back pain: a systematic review within the framework of the Cochrane Back Review Group, *Spine* 26:377–386, 2001.

49. Johnson RM, Hart DL, Simmons EF, et al: Cervical orthoses. A study comparing their effectiveness in restricting cervical motion in normal subjects, *J Bone Joint Surg Am* 59:332–339, 1977.

50. Jones MD: Cineradiographic studies of the collar-immobilized cervical spine, *J Neurosurg* 17:633, 1960.

51. Jonsson B: Quantitative electromyographic evaluation of muscular load during work, *Scand J Rehabil Med Suppl* 6:69–74, 1978.

52. Kaufman WA, Lunsford TR, Lunsford BR, et al: Comparison of three prefabricated cervical collars, *Orthot Prosthet* 39:21–28, 1986.

53. Koes BW, van den Hoogen HMM: Efficacy of bed rest and orthoses of low back pain, *Eur J Phys Med Rehabil* 4:86–93, 1994.

54. Kolb JC, Summers RL, Galli RL: Cervical collar-induced changes in intracranial pressure, *Am J Emerg Med* 17:135–137, 1999.

55. Lantz SA, Schultz AB: Lumbar spine orthosis wearing. I. Restriction of gross body motions, *Spine* 11:834–837, 1986.

56. Lantz SA, Schultz AB: Lumbar spine orthosis wearing. II. Effect on trunk muscle myoelectric activity, *Spine* 11:838–842, 1986.

57. Lavender SA, Shakeel K, Andersson GB, et al: Effects of a lifting belt on spine moments and muscle recruitments after an unexpected sudden loading, *Spine* 25:1569–1578, 2000.

58. Lumsden RM, Morris JM: An in vivo study of axial rotation and immobilization at the lumbosacral joint, *J Bone Joint Surg* 50A:1591–1602, 1968.

59. Lunsford TR, Davidson M, Lunsford BR: The effectiveness of four contemporary cervical orthoses in restricting cervical motion, *J Prosthet Orthot* 6:93–99, 1994.

60. Magnusson M, Pope MH, Hansson T: Does a back support have a positive biomechanical effect?, *Appl Ergonom* 27:201–205, 1996.

61. Makela M, Heliovaara M, Sievers K, et al: Prevalence, determinants, and consequences of chronic neck pain in Finland, *Am J Epidemiol* 134:1356–1357, 1991.

62. Malanga GA, Nadler SF: Nonoperative treatment of low back pain, *Mayo Clin Proc* 74:1135–1148, 1999.

63. Marras WS, Jorgensen MJ, Davis KG: Effect of foot movement and an elastic lumbar back support on spinal loading during free-dynamic symmetric and asymmetric lifting exertions, *Ergonomics* 43:653–668, 2000.

64. McGill SM: Abdominal belts in industry: a position paper on their assets, liabilities and use, *Am Ind Hygiene Assoc* 54:752–754, 1993.

65. McGuire RA, Degnan G, Amundson GM: Evaluation of current extrication orthoses in immobilization of the unstable cervical spine, *Spine* 15:1064–1067, 1990.

66. McNair PJ, Heine PJ: Trunk proprioception: enhancement through lumbar bracing, *Arch Phys Med Rehabil* 89:96–99, 1999.

67. Miller RA, Hardcastle P, Renwick SE: Lower spinal mobility and external immobilization in the normal and pathologic condition, *Orthop Rev* 21:753–757, 1992.

68. Million R, Nilsen KH, Jayson MIV, et al: Evaluation of low back pain and assessment of lumbar corsets with and without back supports, *Ann Rheum Dis* 40:449–454, 1981.

69. Mobbs RJ, Stoodley MA, Fuller J: Effect of cervical hard collar on intracranial pressure after head injury, *Aust N Z J Surg* 72:389–391, 2002.

70. Morris JM, Lucas DB: Physiological considerations in bracing of the spine, *Orthop Prosthet Appl* 1:37–44, 1963.

71. Morris JM, Lucas DB, Bresler B: Role of the trunk in stability of the spine, *J Bone Joint Surg* 43A:327–351, 1961.

72. Nachemson AL, Morris J: In vivo measurements of intradiscal pressure, *J Bone Joint Surg* 46A:1077–1092, 1964.

73. Nachemson AL, Schultz AB, Andersson G: Mechanical effectiveness of lumbar spine orthoses, *Scand J Rehab Med (Suppl)* 9:139–149, 1983.

74. Nachemson AL, Schultz AB, Berkson MH: Mechanical properties of human lumbar spine motion segments: influences of age, sex, disc level and degeneration, *Spine* 4:1–8, 1978.

75. Newcomer K, Laskowski ER, Yu B, et al: The effects of a lumbar support on repositioning error in subjects with low back pain, *Arch Phys Med Rehabil* 82:906–910, 2001.

76. Norton PL, Brown T: The immobilizing efficiency of back braces. Their effect on the posture and motion of the lumbosacral spine, *J Bone Joint Surg* 39A:111–138, 1957.

77. Peeters GG, Verhagen AP, de Bie RA, et al: The efficacy of conservative treatment in patients with whiplash injury: a systematic review of clinical trials, *Spine* 26:E64–E73, 2001.

78. Perry J: The use of external support in the treatment of low back pain. Report of the Subcommittee on Orthotics of the Committee on Prosthetic-Orthotic Education, National Academy of Sciences, National Research Council, *J Bone Joint Surg* 52A:1440–1442, 1970.

79. Persson LC, Carlsson CA, Carlsson JY: Long-lasting cervical radicular pain managed with surgery, physiotherapy, or a cervical collar. A prospective, randomized study, *Spine* 22:751–758, 1997.

80. Plaisier B, Gabram SGA, Schwartz RJ, et al: Prospective evaluation of craniofacial pressure in four different cervical orthoses, *J Trauma* 37:714–720, 1994.

81. Podolsky S, Baraff LJ, Simon RR, et al: Efficacy of cervical spine immobilization methods, *J Trauma* 23:461–465, 1983.

82. Pope MH, Phillips RB, Haugh LD, et al: A prospective randomized three week trial of spinal manipulation, transcutaneous muscle stimulation, massage and corset in the treatment of subacute low back pain, *Spine* 19:2571–2577, 1994.

83. Quinet RJ, Hadler NM: Diagnosis and treatment of backache, *Semin Arthritis Rheum* 8:261–287, 1979.

84. Rabinowitz D, Bridger RS, Lambert MI: Lifting technique and abdominal belt usage: a biomechanical, physiological and subjective investigation, *Safety Sci* 28:155–164, 1998.

85. Raphael JH, Chotai R: Effects of the cervical collar on cerebrospinal fluid pressure, *Anaesthesia* 49:437–439, 1994.

86. Rodgers JA, Rodgers WB: Marginal mandibular nerve palsy due to compression by a cervical hard collar, *J Orthop Trauma* 9:177–179, 1995.

87. Rohlmann A, Bergmann G, Graichen F, Neff G: Braces do not reduce loads on internal spinal fixation devices, *Clin Biomech* 14:97–102, 1999.

88. Sandler AJ, Dvorak J, Humke T, et al: The effectiveness of various cervical orthoses. An in vivo comparison of the mechanical stability provided by several widely used models, *Spine* 21:1624–1629, 1996.

89. Schnabel M, Ferrari R, Vassiliou T, et al: Randomised, controlled outcome study of active mobilisation compared with collar therapy for whiplash injury, *Emerg Med J* 21:306–310, 2004.

90. Selby DK: Conservative care of nonspecific low back pain, *Orthop Clin North Am* 13:427–437, 1982.

91. Smith GE: The most ancient splint, *BMJ* 1:732, 1908.

92. Spratt KF, Weinstein JN, Lehmann TR, et al: Efficacy of flexion and extension treatments incorporating braces for low-back pain patients with retrodisplacement, spondylolisthesis, or normal sagittal translation, *Spine* 18:1839–1849, 1993.

93. Stambolis V, Brady S, Klos D, et al: The effects of cervical bracing upon swallowing in young, normal, healthy volunteers, *Dysphagia* 18:39–45, 2003.

94. Teresi LM, Lufkin RB, Reicher MA, et al: Asymptomatic degenerative disk disease and spondylosis of the cervical spine: MR imaging, *Radiology* 164:83–88, 1987.

95. Toda Y: Impact of waist/hip ratio on the therapeutic efficacy of lumbosacral corsets for chronic muscular low back pain, *J Orthop Sci* 7:644–649, 2002.

96. Valle-Jones JC, Walsh H, O'Hara J, et al: Controlled trial of a back support in patients with non-specific low back pain, *Curr Med Res Opin* 12:604–613, 1992.

97. van der Hoogen HJ, Koes BW, van Eijk JT, et al: On the course of low back pain in general practice: a one year follow up study, *Ann Rheum Dis* 57:13–19, 1998.

98. van Dieen JH, Cholewicki J, Radebold A: Trunk muscle recruitment patterns in patients with low back pain enhance the stability of the lumbar spine, *Spine* 28:834–841, 2003.

99. van Poppel MNM, de Looze MP, Koes BW, et al: Mechanisms of action of lumbar supports, *Spine* 25:2103–2113, 2000.

100. Vogt L, Pfeifer K, Portscher M, et al: Lumbar corsets: their effect on three-dimensional kinematics of the pelvis, *J Rehabil Res Dev* 37:495–499, 2000.

101. Wahlgren DR, Atkinson JH, Epping-Jordan JE, et al: One-year follow-up of first onset low back pain, *Pain* 73:213–221, 1997.

102. Walsh NE, Schwartz RK: The influence of prophylactic orthoses on abdominal strength and back injury in the workplace, *Am J Phys Med Rehabil* 69:245–250, 1990.

103. Waters RL, Morris JM: Effects of spinal supports on the electrical activity of muscles of the trunk, *J Bone Joint Surg* 52A:51–60, 1970.

104. Webber-Jones JE, Thomas CA, Bordeaux RE: The management and prevention of rigid cervical collar complications, *Orthop Nurs* 21:19–25, 2002.

105. Willner S: Effect of a rigid brace on back pain, *Acta Orthop Scand* 56:40–42, 1985.

106. Woldstad JC, Sherman BR: The effects of a back belt on posture, strength, and spinal compressive force during static lift exertions, *Int J Ind Ergonom* 22:409–416, 1998.

107. Zhang S, Wortley M, Clowers K, et al: Evaluation of efficacy and 3D kinematic characteristics of cervical orthoses, *Clin Biomech* 20:264–269, 2005.

Orthoses for spinal deformities

Donald E. Katz

Key Points

- The use of orthoses for treatment of spinal deformities is controversial.
- The greatest challenge in evaluating the efficacy and usefulness of spinal orthoses emanates from the lack of a clear understanding of the natural history of various disorders for which orthoses are prescribed.
- Increasing evidence in the literature supports the value of orthotic treatment for various forms of spinal deformity.

The use of orthoses in the treatment of spinal deformity is controversial. Most often, they are used to prevent further progression or to effect mild correction of an existing deformity in a growing child or adolescent. The greatest challenge in evaluating the efficacy and usefulness of spinal orthoses emanates from a lack of a clear understanding of the natural history of various disorders for which these orthoses are prescribed. Because of the multifactorial aspects of a plethora of disease processes that can cause deformities of the spine, the inability to accurately predict the behavior of deformities that are left untreated makes it difficult to formulate reliable prescription criteria for a given population. Great strides in understanding these processes have been made over of the last several decades, but because of the complex nature of various pathologies, additional research is ongoing. Increasing evidence in the literature supports the value of orthotic treatment for various forms of spinal deformity. It is therefore incumbent upon those who prescribe and provide orthoses for spinal deformity to fully understand the complexities of this form of patient care.

This chapter focuses on scoliotic and kyphotic deformities of the spine. While a multitude of pathologies can cause these deformities, this chapter will focus primarily on the most common forms thought to benefit from spinal orthoses: idiopathic scoliosis and Scheuermann's kyphosis.

Scoliosis

Pathophysiology and natural history

Scoliosis can be defined as a lateral curvature of the spine, greater than 10 degrees as measured by the Cobb method.[36] Because lateral curvature of the spine is typically associated with vertebral rotation within the curve, a three-dimensional deformity occurs. There is coronal plane translation of a series of vertebrae away from midline; transverse plane deformity by way of vertebral rotation in relation to each other because of the nature of the intervertebral articulations of the posterior elements[132]; and, more commonly in idiopathic thoracic curves, an anterior translation in the sagittal plane, resulting in a hypokyphotic, or even lordotic relationship of the effected vertebrae.[45] A host of terms is used to describe the various types of scoliosis (Table 9-1)[78]

Idiopathic scoliosis

Idiopathic scoliosis (IS), termed as such because of the unknown cause or etiology of the deformity, is the most common form of scoliosis. A thorough physical examination by a qualified physician, including a radiographic analysis to rule out numerous potential differential diagnoses, is required to make the diagnosis. The type of IS is defined by the age of onset.[83] If a scoliosis is recognized in patients less than 3 years of age, it is considered *infantile idiopathic scoliosis*. A scoliosis detected between the ages of 3 and 10 years of age is considered *juvenile idiopathic scoliosis*. The most common form of idiopathic scoliosis is *adolescent idiopathic scoliosis*

Table 9-1 Glossary of terms describing different types of scoliotic curves

Term	Definition
Adult scoliosis:	Spinal curvature present after skeletal maturity. It may be due to any cause.
Cervicothoracic curve:	Any spinal curvature in which the apex is at C7 or T1.
Compensatory curve:	A secondary curve located above or below the structural component that develops in order to maintain normal body alignment.
Congenital scoliosis:	Scoliosis due to bony abnormalities of the spine that are present at birth. These anomalies are classified as failure of vertebral formation and/ or failure of segmentation.
Double curve:	Scoliosis in which there are two lateral curves in the same spine.
Double major curve:	Scoliosis in which there are two structural curves that usually are of similar size and rotation.
Double thoracic curve:	Scoliosis with a structural upper thoracic curve, a larger, more deforming lower thoracic curve, and a relatively nonstructural lumbar curve.
Hysterical scoliosis:	A nonstructural deformity of the spine that develops as a manifestation of a psychological disorder.
Idiopathic scoliosis:	A structural curve for which the cause has not been definitely established.
Kyphoscoliosis:	Noted as an increased round-back on the lateral radiograph, the condition may represent a true kyphotic deformity (as seen in some pathologic conditions) or it may represent such excessive rotation of the spine that the lateral radiograph is actually reflecting the scoliotic deformity. (In idiopathic scoliosis, true kyphotic deformity does not occur.)
Lordoscoliosis:	Structural scoliosis associated with increased swayback or loss of normal kyphosis within the measured curve; nearly always present in idiopathic scoliosis.
Lumbar curve:	A spinal curvature in which the apex is between L1 and L4.
Lumbosacral curve:	A spinal curvature in which the apex is at L5 or below.
Neuromuscular scoliosis:	Scoliosis due to a neurologic disorder of the central nervous system or muscle.
Nonstructural (functional) curve:	A curvature that does not have a fixed deformity and may be compensatory in nature. The curve may be a result of leg length discrepancy (and so disappears when the patient is supine), poor posture, muscle spasm, or other cause.
Primary curve:	The first or earliest curve present.
Structural curve:	Represents a segment of the spine that has a fixed lateral curvature.
Thoracic curve:	A spinal curvature in which the apex is between T2 and T11.
Thoracolumbar curve:	A spinal curvature in which the apex is at T12, L1, or the T12-L1 interspace.

(AIS) and is termed as such when the curve is detected after age 10 years but prior to skeletal maturity. A scoliosis that is detected after skeletal maturity is termed *adult scoliosis*. More recently, however, due to the relationship that exists between the rate of spinal growth and the progression of deformity, the terms *early-onset idiopathic scoliosis* (EIS) and *late-onset idiopathic scoliosis* (LIS) have come into favor. Even though scoliosis can develop at any age during growth, the two primary periods of rapid growth occur in the first few years of life and then again during the adolescent growth spurt. Mehta[113] pointed out that the fastest rate of growth in children is in the first year of life, with a growth rate of 20 to 25 cm in those twelve months. This is nearly twice the growth rate of the adolescent growth spurt, where growth of 12 to 14 cm per year can be seen. An increase in height at the rate of 9 cm per year is considered a reasonable threshold to identify this peak period during adolescence.[25] The increase in height during the second year of life (12 to 13 cm per year) is similar to the rate seen during the adolescent growth spurt. With regard to the specific growth velocity of the spine as measured between the T1 and L5 segments, it is greatest from birth to age 5 years, with marked deceleration between ages 5 and 10 years. Similarly, the onset of scoliosis between the ages of 5 of 10 is less common.[43,48] For this reason, the term *early-onset scoliosis* has been used to reflect the presence of scoliosis prior to 5 years of age, including all possible etiologies, whereas the term *late-onset scoliosis* applies to scoliosis detected after age 5,[44] and is most commonly associated with the onset of scoliosis that occurs just before puberty.

Some critical differences exist between the prognosis of patients with EIS and of those with LIS. EIS is diagnosed within the first 6 months of life in the majority of children,[78] is seen more often in boys than in girls (with most having left-sided thoracic curve patterns),[182] and has the capacity to spontaneously resolve in some patients.[47,83,98,111,112] The most reliable indicators for differentiating resolving from progressive scoliosis are the rib-vertebra angle difference (RVAD), which is the angular difference between the concave and convex side ribs in relation to the apical thoracic vertebra, and the amount of apical vertebral rotation, as defined by Phase I and Phase II rotation as first reported by Mehta[111] in 1972 (Fig. 9-1). A RVAD < 20 degrees indicates a high likelihood of curve resolution whereas curves with a RVAD of 20 degrees or greater are more likely to be progressive. A phase 2 relationship between the rib head and apical vertebra on the convex side implies that progression of the curve is almost certain (Fig. 9-2). In Mehta's initial study, 46 of 86 patients with phase 1 curves resolved, and of those, 83% had a RVAD < 20 degrees. The average RVAD of those that progressed was 25.5 degrees (compared to 11.7 degrees in those that resolved); 84% had a RVAD of 20 degrees or greater. The usefulness of the RVAD was strongly supported by Ferreira et al.,[57] who reported that 67 of 68 patients with resolving curves had a RVAD < 20 degrees, and all were classified as phase I. In 40 patients with progressive curves, 37 had a RVAD of 20 degrees or greater. Diedrich et al.[47] reported on the long-term observation of resolving infantile scoliosis. In their study of 42 patients, 34 of whom were followed more than 25 years, 85% of those having a RVAD of less than 20 degrees had a resolving curve, whereas 90% of those who had a progressive curve had a RVAD of 20 degrees or more.

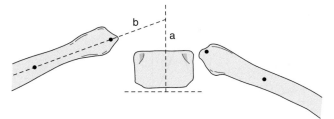

Fig. 9-1 How to measure the rib–vertebra angle difference (RVAD). A line is drawn perpendicular to the inferior endplate of the apical thoracic vertebra. Another line is drawn between two points that bisect the head and neck of the rib articulating with the apex. The angle between the perpendicular line (a) and the rib line (b) is measured. The same procedure is repeated for the rib on the opposite side. The concave-convex side angles = the RVAD. (Adapted from Gillingham BL, Fan RA, Akbarnia BA: *J Am Acad Orthop Surg* 14:101–112, 2006.)

Pulmonary compromise is a much more significant concern in those diagnosed with EIS compared to those with LIS. This is because of the presence of a potentially progressive chest wall deformity associated with the scoliosis during the time in which the lungs are rapidly developing. There is a 10-fold increase in the number of alveoli between birth and adulthood, with the majority of this increase occurring during the first 8 years of life.[53] There is also an increase in the number of respiratory branches, from 21 to 23, between the ages of 3 months and 8 years.[49] The incomplete maturation of the lung and pulmonary vasculature has been reported as the primary reason for ventilation defects seen in patients with early-onset scoliosis.[119] While the influence of compressive forces acting upon the lung tissue is still under investigation, there is an apparent correlation between the age of scoliosis onset and the diminished number of alveoli that develop. The most hypoplastic lungs are found in those with the earliest onset of EIS.[24] The result can be a restrictive pattern of lung disease that includes reductions

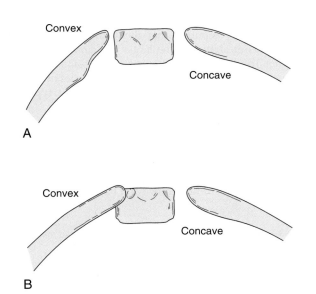

Fig. 9-2 Differentiating phase 1 (**A**) and phase 2 (**B**) rib-vertebra relationship for infantile curve types. Phase I shows no overlapping of the rib head and vertebral body. Phase II shows the rib head intersecting the vertebral body, which is indicative of greater rotation and an increased risk of further curve progression. (Adapted from Gillingham BL, Fan RA, Akbarnia BA: *J Am Acad Orthop Surg* 14:101–112, 2006.)

in vital capacity and total lung capacity. In children with EIS, the amount of vital capacity reduction is also influenced by the location and severity of the curve.[67] This is unique to these young patients, as those with LIS demonstrate little or no reduction of vital capacity in response to the presence of their curve.[119] Ultimately, patients with EIS who also demonstrate significant respiratory compromise due to the early age of onset and size of their curve are at greater risk for life-threatening respiratory failure at or before late middle age.[24,131]

Understanding the natural history of LIS is essential to clinical decision-making. This is true not only for determining when observation or treatment is indicated, but also for determining when treatment is effective. AIS is the most common form of idiopathic scoliosis, affecting 1.5% to 3.0% of children who are at least 10 years of age. Curves exceeding 20 degrees affect between 0.3% and 0.5%, and curves exceeding 30 degrees are found in 0.2% to 0.3% of adolescents.[78] Curve progression is typically defined as a measured difference of 5 degrees or greater,[100,167] however a 10-degree change has been reported as being required for 95% certainty that an observed change was not caused by measurement error alone, but is instead indicative of true progression.[31]

Less than 1% of children screened for scoliosis and less than 10% of those who are positively identified as having a curve of at least 10 degrees will require active treatment.[165] The goal of an evaluating physician is to make an accurate diagnosis and to identify which patients are most likely to progress and thus require treatment, either with an orthosis or with surgery. When prescribed, the goal of the orthosis is to prevent further progression of a curve that would otherwise worsen if left untreated. Factors that have the most influence on whether or not a curve secondary to AIS will progress are patient gender, remaining growth, curve magnitude, and curve pattern.[28,100,123]

With respect to gender, the prevalence of AIS is similar in boys and girls with smaller curves, but girls are more likely to experience curve progression (Table 9-2).[9,39,99,143] Boys with comparable curves have been estimated to have about one tenth the risk of curve progression as girls,[165] however one report suggests the difference is less.[86]

The amount of growth remaining is typically estimated by two maturity indices: the Risser sign and, in girls, the onset of menstruation; however the single most accurate indicator is to monitor growth. The Risser sign is a skeletal marker based on the ossification of the iliac apophysis.[140] It is interpreted by viewing a standing posterior-anterior radiograph of the spine and pelvis, where ossification of the pelvis begins laterally and progresses medially until maturation (Fig. 9-3).

Table 9-2 Prevalence of gender for idiopathic scoliosis as related to the severity of the curve in 1,222 subjects

Curve	Girls	Boys	Girls:Boys
6°–10°	316	322	1:1
11°–20°	299	208	1.4:1
21° or more	65	12	5.4:1
Under treatment	36	5	7.2:1

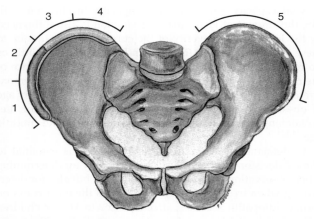

Fig. 9-3 In the skeletally immature patient, the Risser sign ranges from grade 0 (no ossification) to grade 5 (all four quadrants show ossification of the iliac apophysis). When the ossified apophysis has fused completely to the ilium (Risser grade 5), the patient is skeletally mature. (From Herring JA: *Tachdjian's pediatric orthopaedics*, ed 3, Philadelphia, 2002, WB Saunders.)

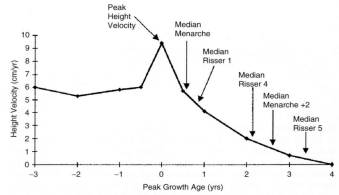

Fig. 9-4 Plot of height velocity curve with median occurrence of menarche, age at menarche plus 2 years, and Risser grades 1, 4, and 5 in 120 female patients treated for AIS. (From Little DG, Song KM, Katz D, et al: Relationship of peak height velocity to other maturity indicators in idiopathic scoliosis in girls. *J Bone Joint Surg Am* 82:685–693, 2000.)

The range of the Risser sign is from 0 to 5, with 0 indicating no ossification and 5 indicating a fully ossified ilium, which indicates skeletal maturity. A Risser sign of 0, 1, or, to a lesser extent, 2, is indicative of significant growth remaining, which can equate to a greater risk for curve progression in some patients with AIS. Some studies have questioned the usefulness of the Risser sign as a reliable measurement of skeletal maturity,[15,81,96,97,150,152,184] including reports of differing interpretations on how the excursion of the iliac apophysis is scored.[16,185] In girls, the onset of the menstrual cycle is a physiologic indicator that is helpful in estimating remaining growth. A premenarchal girl is most likely to be in a very active growth period, whereas after menarche, the girl enters the deceleration phase of growth where curve progression becomes less likely.

A third indicator of skeletal maturity, the peak height velocity, is more difficult to immediately assess than the Risser sign or menarchal status in girls, but it has gained greater recognition as a more accurate tool to assess the amount of growth remaining in the adolescent with idiopathic scoliosis. Peak height velocity (PHV) is calculated from changes in a patient's height measurements over time, typically recorded in intervals no less than 4 and not more than 6 months. The average PHV for girls has been reported as about 8.0 cm per year and 9.5 cm per year for boys in the groups studied.[25,54]

Little et al.[96] reported on the relationship of growth rates, as expressed in overall height velocities, to other maturity indicators in girls with AIS. The timing of peak height velocity, also known as peak growth age (PGA), was plotted against other maturity indicators, including chronological age, Risser sign, and menarchal status, to determine its usefulness as a prognostic tool for curve progression. PGA was found to have a stronger correlation with curve progression than any other maturity indicator (age, Risser sign, or menarchal status). The authors also cited the apparent relevance of the timing of PGA as related to curve size as a prognostic indicator of curve progression. Reporting on 88 of 120 girls who demonstrated progression of their primary curve despite being braced, 60 of these patients had a curve of more than 30 degrees at PGA, and in 50 (83%) of these 60 patients the curve

progressed to 45 degrees or more. The remaining 28 patients had a curve of 30 degrees or less at peak height velocity, with only one curve (4%) progressing to 45 degrees or more. The authors suggested a significant relationship that exists between the size of a primary curve size, with 30 degrees as an important threshold, and the timing of PGA. Lastly, and of particular clinical interest, the median time in which PGA was achieved in this population was earlier than that of the median time of menarche and Risser 1 (Fig. 9-4). The usefulness of PGA as a clinical tool in boys with AIS has also been reported.[152]

The size of a curve at the time of detection combined with estimating the degree of maturity is very helpful in predicting the risk for progression in AIS. Lonstein and Carlson[100] described the relationship between maturity and curve progression. In their review of 727 school-age children (575 girls, 152 boys), with initial curves of 5 to 29 degrees, they described three primary prognostic factors in predicting curve progression in a growing child: curve size, chronological age, and Risser sign. They reported that the younger the child, the lesser the Risser sign; and the larger the curve at discovery, the higher the likelihood for curve progression (Table 9-3). A scoliosis that reaches a magnitude of 25 degrees in an immature patient, even if detected during an initial visit, typically is considered a candidate for orthotic treatment.[101,123]

Natural history studies also have reported the usefulness of curve pattern in predicting curve progression. Opinion in the literature tends to agree that single lumbar and single thoracolumbar curves are the least likely to progress and are the most receptive to brace treatment. Compiling data from various natural history studies, Bunch and Patwardhan[26] reported

Table 9-3 Incidence of curve progression based on curve magnitude and Risser sign

Risser Sign	Percentage of Curves That Progressed	
	Curves 5–19 Degrees	Curves 20–29 Degrees
Grade 0 and 1	22%	68%
Grade 2, 3, or 4	1.6%	23%

Table 9-4 The relationship of curve progression with curve pattern in immature patients

	Percentage of Curves that Progressed			
	Thoracic	**Double**	**T/L**	**Lumbar**
Clarisse[35]	42%	67%	47%	12%
Fustier[61]	54%	75%	69%	25%
Bunnell[28]	44%	27%	27%	18%
Lonstein[100]	26%	27%	12%	9%

Reproduced from Bunch WH and Patwardhan AG: *Scoliosis: Making clinical decisions.* C.V. Mosby Co. Chapter 4, pg. 57, 1989.

single thoracic and double curve patterns are more likely to progress (by as much as a factor of two) than single lumbar or single thoracolumbar curve patterns (Table 9-4).[27,35,61,100]

The natural history of scoliosis after skeletal maturity is reached is an important consideration in the context of appropriate use of orthoses during growth. Orthoses should be used in patients whose curve size and pattern would be both cosmetically acceptable and stable throughout adulthood if successfully stabilized with orthotic management during growth. Weinstein and Ponseti[167] reported on a series of 102 untreated scoliosis patients representing 133 curves with available radiographs, with an average follow-up of 40.5 years. Sixty-eight percent of the curves progressed after skeletal maturity. Curves that were less than 30 degrees at skeletal maturity tended not to progress regardless of curve pattern. Progression of curves greater than 30 degrees appeared to be related to the amount of vertebral rotation. Curves that measured between 50 and 75 degrees at skeletal maturity, particularly thoracic curves, progressed the most; the latter at a rate of nearly 1 degree per year. Lumbar curves less then 50 degrees tended to progress when accompanied by a transitory shift between the lower vertebrae. In a follow up series, Weinstein et al.[166] studied outcomes related to health and general function in patients with untreated AIS. Citing previous long-term studies as having a more heterogeneous population of both true idiopathic and non-IS patients, Weinstein et al. argued that late-onset IS (LIS) was a distinct entity with a unique natural history compared to other forms of "idiopathic" scoliosis. Defining LIS as "a structural lateral curvature of the spine arising in otherwise normal children usually during puberty," the authors compared 117 prospectively evaluated, untreated patients with 62 age- and sex-matched volunteers. Reporting on 50 years of follow up, this review stated that those with LIS were significantly more likely to experience shortness of breath in the presence of a thoracic curve of more than 80 degrees compared to controls. LIS patients were also significantly more likely to report chronic back pain than controls. There was no significant difference, however, in the estimated probability of survival between the two groups. Others have cited no difference in mortality rate between patients with AIS and the general population.[131] Thus the authors concluded that untreated adults with LIS demonstrated little physical impairment other than back pain and cosmetic concerns compared to age- and sex-matched controls. Chronic low-back pain is more common

in adults with scoliosis, but it does not interfere with a patient's ability to work or perform activities.[122,166]

Historical perspective

The history of using external support for spinal deformity dates back centuries. Ambroise Paré (1510–1590) is credited as the first to write extensively on the use of metal braces, similar to armor, to treat patients with scoliosis. In the 18th century, recognizing what the S shape the spine could assume in the growing child, Nicolas Andry (1658–1712) wrote of straightening children by "repressing" the "protuberances" that result from the underlying spinal deformity with the use of external supports.[7] Throughout the 19th century the Europeans were credited with developing various orthotic designs to correct spinal deformities through the use of steel, leather, and plaster.[65] In 1946, Walter Blount first described the Milwaukee brace, which was developed as an alternative to various forms of hinge and turnbuckle plaster casts such as those described by Hibbs[79] and Risser[139] in the operative treatment of scoliosis.[19] Early designs of the Milwaukee brace were described by Richard Bidwell, a certified orthotist, in an effort to make it more reproducible.[18] Moe and Kettleson[116] first described use of the Milwaukee brace for nonoperative treatment of idiopathic scoliosis in 1970. They described additional refinements that decreased the overall bulk of the system, including removal of the chin pad distraction because it caused orthodontic and facial deformities.

In the 1960s and 1970s, many studies were published dealing with the effects of using orthoses in the nonoperative treatment of idiopathic scoliosis. One early report suggested that patients who were compliant with their prescriptions could expect about 25% correction of thoracic curves and 20% of lumbar curves.[90] More adequate follow-up analysis, however, revealed that the dramatic improvement of some curves was offset by the substantial degeneration of others.[114] One report stated that while a mean overall improvement of 2 to 4 degrees was seen when comparing curve sizes at the beginning of Milwaukee brace treatment to that of post-treatment follow up, 80% of patients demonstrated a measurable amount of curve progression after discontinuing use of the brace.[32] It was becoming clear that permanent, post-treatment curve correction from orthotic treatment was not a realistic expectation; however prevention of further curve progression in the growing child or adolescent seemed possible.

Around this same time, the Boston brace was introduced as a low-profile alternative to the Milwaukee brace in the treatment of thoracolumbar or lumbar curves, and eventually for curves with apices as high as the seventh thoracic vertebra.[52,84,94,164] Other low-profile, underarm thermoplastic designs, such as the Wilmington, Miami, and Rosenberger thoracolumbosacral orthoses (TLSOs), were also introduced.[29,64,109] Most reports suggested that approximately four out of five adolescents treated with an orthosis for idiopathic scoliosis would not experience any significant curve progression.[52,70,115] Patients were enrolled into many studies; however, the factors influencing the risk of further scoliotic curve progression had not yet been well defined. While the early brace studies had included patients at high risk for progression, those studies also included patients not sharing this risk. Despite the identification of some keen insights, such as the importance of in-brace correction to increase the likelihood of a positive outcome, the early research on a brace's ability to halt curve progression became suspect once practitioners developed a greater understanding of the natural history of the disease.

Studies have shown that the corrective forces of a brace are passive in nature and that the predominant corrective component is the transverse loading of the spine through the use of corrective pads.[6,34,63,120,129,181] Early theories suggested scoliosis braces worked partly by a kinesthetic reminder, meaning the patient would actively pull away from an irritating stimulus placed at the apex on the convex side of a curve.[17,38,74] However, Wynarsky and Schultz[181] reported no difference in trunk musculature electromyographic activity in patients with idiopathic thoracic curves while in and out of a Boston brace, and the electromyographic analysis while the brace was worn would not approach values that could have a significant biomechanical influence on the size of the curve.

Current issues

A number of questions for study remain regarding the use of orthoses in the treatment of idiopathic scoliosis. A consensus conference report from the American Academy of Orthotists and Prosthetists documented both the current understanding of how best to utilize orthoses in the treatment of idiopathic scoliosis and Scheuermann's kyphosis as well as a list of research priorities to help advance understanding of this practice.[1] The priorities include the need to better understand the effect an orthosis has in altering the natural history of curve progression, the best use of a variety of orthotic designs, and the most appropriate application of forces to act upon the spine in a way that is most tolerable for the patient. New designs for orthoses intended to treat spinal deformity are often introduced to the medical community and public, but often in the absence of clinical evidence verifying their usefulness compared either to designs that have been subject to significant study, or to what is understood to be the natural history of the disorder being treated.

Current research

In an effort to form a consensus from the literature on the effectiveness of bracing (including whether part-time bracing controls curve progression as effectively as full-time bracing), the Prevalence and Natural History Committee of the Scoliosis Research Society conducted a meta-analysis on more than 1,900 patients from 20 studies.[144] They concluded that bracing (with TLSOs or the Milwaukee orthosis) is indeed effective in controlling curve progression in idiopathic scoliosis and that full-time (23 hours per day) bracing is more effective than part-time (8 to 16 hours per day) bracing. The latter finding is further supported by more recent studies.[87,88,135,172]

Evaluation of compliance with brace wearing remains very subjective and differs depending on whether the child or the parents are giving the report. Better objective means of documenting compliance would be useful in determining the effectiveness of full-time bracing in comparison to part-time bracing. Newer technology now allows objective assessment of compliance. Temperature sensors or pressure switches combined with data loggers have been imbedded into orthoses.[75,76,103-105,124,125,135,156,162] In the future, when these data loggers can be economically fabricated into orthoses, then objective evidence of compliance will be routinely available. From the subjective information currently available, it appears that the highest success rate from a bracing program can be expected when a patient is instructed to wear the orthosis for 20 or more hours per day. However, it also appears that the use of orthoses specifically designed for nighttime-only use exerts a favorable influence on the natural history of adolescent idiopathic scoliosis for patients with single lumbar or thoracolumbar curve magnitudes of 35 degrees or less.[38,82,88,133,134,186]

Hypokyphosis in thoracic scoliosis secondary to AIS is well documented in the literature.[2,41,45,107,136,141,151] Early reports on bracing suggested orthoses should decrease lumbar lordosis to enhance the reduction of a scoliotic curve.[95,160,164,174] More recent research, however, has questioned the appropriateness of aiming to tuck the pelvis in an attempt to delordose the lumbar spine as a strategic orthotic maneuver in the treatment of idiopathic scoliosis, because of the positive correlation between lumbar lordosis and thoracic kyphosis. More specifically, if the goal of a scoliosis orthosis is to return the spine to a more normal alignment, further reduction of thoracic kyphosis in an already hypokyphotic spine is contrary to that goal. Some authors have suggested that forces within an orthosis need to be reequilibrated not only to decrease the amount of flattening of thoracic kyphosis that can occur with an anterior translation of the thorax,[10,72,93] but even to increase lumbar lordosis[72,169] in an effort to increase thoracic kyphosis, all while reducing the scoliosis in the coronal plane. The impact of altering the sagittal spinal alignment on outcome while aiming to reduce the Cobb angle in the coronal plane in the orthotic treatment of idiopathic scoliosis is not well understood. The need remains for further research on the most appropriate application of forces within an orthosis to most appropriately address the three-dimensional aspects of a scoliotic deformity.

The use of computer-assisted manufacturing (CAD/CAM) has been investigated for spinal orthoses.[38,51,178,179] Initial reports on the use of CAD/CAM have focused primarily on those requiring lower-extremity prostheses. Technologic improvements that impact the means by which a digital image of a patient's torso is captured and a greater ability to electronically manipulate the orthotic design are increasing the use of CAD/CAM for those requiring spinal orthoses for deformity. Two reports by Wong et al. suggested CAD/CAM manufacturing of spinal orthoses for AIS required less time[179] than the more conventional rectification of a plaster model without compromising the amount of in-brace correction achieved.[178] Use of this technology to design and manufacture custom orthoses for spinal deformity will likely increase in as it becomes more comprehensive and cost effective.

Treatment recommendations

The aim of orthotic treatment of idiopathic scoliosis may differ based on the age of onset and size of the curve. In infants with EIS in whom the curve is less than 25 degrees and the RVAD is less than 20 degrees at the time of initial evaluation, active treatment is not required and radiographic follow-up should take place every 4 to 6 months.[92] Having the infant sleep in the prone position rather than supine may be of benefit. Most infantile curves that resolve do so by age 1 to

2 years.[33,98,110,157] Occasionally, several years may pass before the curve has resolved.[163] Follow-up should continue even after resolution, because scoliosis may recur in adolescence.

Nonoperative treatment should be undertaken without delay in those having infantile scoliosis and a demonstrated progression of the curve. Left untreated, these curves can easily exceed 70 degrees by age 10 years. Further worsening can occur during the periods of rapid adolescent growth. The goal of brace treatment is to control curve progression until sufficient patient size and skeletal growth have been achieved, to allow a one-time spinal stabilization procedure to be performed. Parents should have a clear understanding early on that operative intervention is almost always necessary. A curve that resolves in a brace would probably have resolved without treatment. For the young child with a flexible curvature, the physician should consider using either a custom molded TLSO or a modified Milwaukee brace, preferably worn full-time. Successful management requires strong parental support, along with frequent adjustments by the orthotist.

In a recent prospective study of 136 children with progressive infantile scoliosis who were treated before age 4 years, Mehta demonstrated that scoliosis could actually be reversed by utilizing the patients' growth in combination with serial casts.[112] Ninety-four of the 136 children were treated in the early stages of progression (average age 1 year 7 months), and their scoliosis resolved by the average age of 3 years 6 months. In this group of patients who were successfully managed this way, the succession of corrective plaster casts were ceased when radiographs showed a balanced trunk, minimal apical rotation, and complete or almost-complete correction of the curve. The patients were then treated with custom-molded TLSOs to maintain the correction that had been achieved through casting. Citing the critical importance of compliant wear, if after 6 months the deformity remained corrected, the patient was weaned from the orthosis, with treatment discontinued soon thereafter. No further treatment was needed in these individuals over the course of 10 years of follow-up. In those referred with larger curves (average 52 degrees), or referred for treatment at an older age (average age 2 years and 6 months), treatment could reduce but not reverse the deformity. Many of these patients eventually underwent spinal fusion, with more of them expected to need fusion in the future.

Juvenile idiopathic scoliosis is diagnosed in children ages 3 to 10 years. The female-male ratio ranges from 1.6:1 to 4.4:1, with the difference increasing with age.[58,142] Convex-right thoracic curve patterns are most common in juvenile scoliosis. Relatively few patients have thoracolumbar or lumbar curves. Patients with juvenile-onset scoliosis are more likely to have curves that progress and are less likely to respond to bracing. They are more likely to require surgical treatment than those with AIS.[108,176] Use of the RVAD has not been found to predict progression of curves in juvenile scoliosis,[158] but may be an indication of treatment effectiveness. Patients with progressive curves have a steady increase in the RVAD, while those whose curves resolve usually show a decrease in the RVAD. If the RVAD does not improve following bracing, then it is likely that spinal fusion will be required. The level of the most rotated vertebra at the apex of the primary curve appears to be the most useful factor in determining the prognosis of patients with juvenile idiopathic

scoliosis. Those with the apex of the curve at T8, T9, or T10 have an 80% chance of requiring spinal arthrodesis by age 15 years.[142] The predictive value of two other factors once thought to be associated with a poor prognosis—thoracic kyphosis of less than 20 degrees, and left-sided curves in boys—has recently been questioned.

Most adolescents with idiopathic scoliosis will not require treatment because of the low probability that their curves will progress.[3,100] Therefore treatment is warranted only for those patients whose scoliotic curves are at substantial risk of worsening over time or for patients with severe curves at presentation. Actively growing adolescents (Risser ≤ 2) with curves between 30 and 45 degrees should have an orthosis prescribed at the time of their initial visit.[144] In the very immature patient (Risser 0 and premenarchal if female) with a curve exceeding 25 degrees, bracing should also be started immediately.[101,144] While most adolescents are treated with an orthosis for curves less than 40 degrees, successful treatment of larger curves has also been reported.[87,172] In most cases, growing adolescents with curves exceeding 45 to 50 degrees cannot be stabilized with an orthosis. Skeletally mature individuals with curves exceeding 50 to 55 degrees also are at risk for continued curve progression and therefore should be considered for surgical treatment.[167] Possible exceptions include patients with well-balanced double curves of less than 60 degrees whose clinical appearance is acceptable to them. Continued observation is recommended to establish if further progression of their scoliosis occurs, which would necessitate surgery.

Orthotic management and best practice

To be considered effective, orthotic treatment must prevent curve progression in those who are most at risk (curves of 25 to 45 degrees in Risser 0 or 1 patients), result in an acceptable cosmetic appearance at the end of treatment, and reduce the need for surgery. In other words, use of an orthosis must improve the patient's outcome when compared with the expected natural history. Given the likelihood that an orthosis generally will not improve the amount of deformity to a significant degree after treatment is complete, patients being considered for orthotic management should have deformities that are considered cosmetically acceptable, and they should be willing to wear the brace as prescribed. Low-profile TLSOs are the most commonly used orthoses at present, but their use is generally restricted to patients whose curve apex is at T7 or below. Fortunately, this is the case in most curve patterns in adolescents with idiopathic scoliosis.

Numerous reports in the literature attest to the effectiveness of orthotic treatment of adolescent idiopathic scoliosis.[4,6,11,12,34,37,38,50,52,56,59,62,66,70,87–89,93,101,117,123,125,128,133,134,144,159,161,168,170,172,173,175,177,180] In most of these studies, bracing was considered effective if the primary curve being treated either improved or remained within 5 to 6 degrees of its original magnitude on completion of treatment. Some of these studies included low-risk patients (Risser 3 to 5, curves less than 20 degrees), patients still undergoing treatment, patients who had had previous treatment, and children younger than 10 years. In some studies, patients may have been eliminated from the patient population because of noncompliance. All of these factors make comparisons between studies difficult, particularly when one is trying to assess the effectiveness of bracing in patients most at risk. Recently, the Bracing committee of the Scoliosis Research Society made recommendations concerning inclusion criteria for future AIS brace studies.[137] Optimal inclusion criteria were thought to consist of patients age 10 years and older when the orthosis is prescribed, Risser 0 to 2, primary curve magnitude 25 to 40 degrees, no prior treatment, and, if female, either premenarchal or less than one year post-menarchal. Some of the more recent literature has been more consistent in focusing on this population at greatest risk.[4,38,87,88,101,123,127,134,159,172] These studies, along with a 1997 meta-analysis of the bracing literature,[144] strongly reinforce the idea that bracing is effective in controlling curve progression. This perception is not universal, however, as there are some studies that question whether orthotic management provides any benefit in scoliosis.[46,68,69,154]

Numerous orthoses are available today, many of which are named after their place of origin. Examples include the Milwaukee brace,[101] the Boston brace,[52,74] the Wilmington brace,[4,13] the Miami TLSO,[109] the Rosenberger orthosis,[64,154] the Charleston brace,[133] the Providence brace,[38] the SpineCor orthosis (from Canada),[37] and the Cheneau orthosis (from Europe).[80] It is important for prescribing physicians and orthotists to understand the most appropriate use of these various orthoses due to their distinct differences in both design and prescribed use.

The Milwaukee brace, introduced by Blount, Schmidt, and Bidwell in 1946, was the first design in the 20th century to be fully described in the medical literature. While the designs used today may differ in varying degrees to that which was originally described, the basic principles of how corrective forces are applied to the spine remain essentially the same. The Milwaukee brace exemplifies the principle of creating a foundation for control by firmly grasping the pelvis with a thermoplastic pelvic girdle, attaching a metal suprastructure over the torso to create a rigid framework from which a series of corrective pads and straps can be strategically attached to maximize the corrective force being applied to a given spinal deformity. The primary advantage of this open orthotic design is the ability to apply corrective forces at the convexity of a deformity in a way that's unencumbered by a concave side force that could prevent the torso and spine from sufficiently shifting in a corrective manner.

With the Milwaukee brace's open design, the location, magnitude and direction of the forces being applied can be easily adjusted. For instance, in the presence of significant hypokyphosis of a thoracic curve, the corrective pad can be easily lateralized to apply a more medially directed force. This would be preferable to a more posteriorly located pad that would apply more of an anteriorly directed force, as this could worsen the amount of existing hypokyphosis. Reports on the biomechanical effectiveness of this orthotic design have yielded insights relating to the most appropriate placement of corrective forces.[6,26,63,120] For both thoracic and lumbar curves, maximal stability of a scoliotic curve is achieved when a corrective force is placed at the curve apex on the convex side.[6,129,149] The effectiveness of this corrective force diminishes with each vertebral level a corrective pad is moved either caudad or cephalad away from the apex of the curve. Corrective forces may also be complementary to each other in providing maximal spine stability. For instance, in

a thoracic curve maximum stability is achieved with a force placed at the apex of the curve in combination with a concave-side counterforce at the level of the superior endpoint of the curve. The presence of a concave-side lumbar counterforce serves to maintain a positive contact between the force applied at the apex and at a lumbar curve. This will render the spine more stable.[26] Further, biomechanical studies have suggested that a Milwaukee brace is capable of providing greater stability to a primary thoracic curve, whereas a low-profile thermoplastic TLSO can offer greater stability to a primary lumbar curve pattern.[130]

The Milwaukee brace has been shown to be effective in controlling curve progression in idiopathic scoliosis, with the largest recent series reported by Lonstein and Winter.[101] The authors found that patients with curves between 20 and 39 degrees who used the Milwaukee brace were less likely to have curve progression exceeding 5 degrees when compared with a similar patient population that received no treatment. However, as with all braces, the success achieved with the Milwaukee brace has not been universal.[125] Today, when there is a strong emphasis on self-image, use of the Milwaukee brace has decreased greatly and has largely been replaced by the use of equally effective lower-profile braces. Low-profile TLSOs such as the Boston brace, Wilmington brace, and Miami TLSO can often be hidden under looser-fitting clothing, providing the adolescent with a more acceptable alternative.

The Boston brace was introduced in 1971 by Hall and Miller.[74] Its design consists of a prefabricated, symmetric thoracolumbar-pelvic module that is customized to the patient based on shape and the radiographic parameters needing to be addressed. It is based on the principle of applying corrective forces at the convexity of the curve while providing relief opposite these areas of pressure through windows cut in the plastic and other methods. Each orthosis is individually designed and fit by the orthotist based on a blueprint created from the patient's full-length radiograph. The Boston brace has been shown to be as effective in controlling curve progression as the Milwaukee brace and is one of the most common orthoses used today.[52,87,88,117,128,172,173] The brace is effective in treating either single- or double-curve patterns in which the apex of the most cephalad curve is located at T7 or below. To control a thoracic curve whose apex is higher requires a suprastructure as a component of the brace. Rarely is this actually done.

The Wilmington brace was described in 1980.[29] It is custom-made from a positive mold of the patient's torso in which the scoliosis is maximally corrected in a Risser- or Cotrel-type cast. The indications for the Wilmington brace are the same as those for the Boston brace. It also has the same limitations (i.e., it is not effective in curves with an apex above T7–8). This brace has not enjoyed the popularity of the Boston brace, although it continues to be used by several institutions.[4,62]

The number of hours per day that an orthosis must be worn remains uncertain. Originally, 20 to 22 hours per day was advocated for the Milwaukee brace in immature adolescents with progressive curves. This same recommendation was made for the lower-profile TLSOs. Faced with this situation, adolescents understandably experienced some emotional distress, and poor compliance with brace wear was not uncommon.[42] As a result, the idea of part-time use of braces evolved, setting the goal of 16 hours of daily use. Although there have been several studies reporting that part-time use of these orthoses appears to be as effective as full-time wear in controlling curve progression,[4,52,70] other reports emphasize that the outcome is better when a greater number of hours per day are spent in-brace.[87,172]

The Charleston brace was developed based on the concept that part-time use may be effective.[55,133,134] Worn at night for only 8 to 10 hours, this orthosis is designed to take advantage of the recumbent position to shift the convexity of the curve as much as possible toward the midline, and unbending the curve above the apex in the opposite direction for maximum side-bending correction. Due to the aggressive side-bending force that the orthosis applies, it cannot be worn in the upright position, thus making wear feasible only when the patient is recumbent. The main appeal of this brace is the limited number of hours of daily use, all of which are accomplished during sleep.

Despite several studies that have reported that the Charleston brace is as effective as the Milwaukee and Boston braces,[55,66,133,134,159] some skeptics doubt that such a limited amount of time spent in a brace can successfully control curve progression. In a comparison of the Boston brace with the Charleston brace in 319 patients, Katz et al.[88] found that in patients with curves between 36 and 45 degrees, 83% treated with a Charleston brace experienced curve progression of more than 5 degrees, compared with 43% of patients treated with a Boston brace.[88] When choosing between the two braces, the authors concluded that the Charleston brace should be reserved for single lumbar or thoracolumbar curves with magnitudes of 35 degrees or less. Subsequent investigations from other centers have come to the similar conclusions with regard to the use of nighttime orthoses for these select patients.[82,186]

The Providence brace is another orthosis used at night only. Made using CAD/CAM technology, it has been reported effective in females with AIS.[38,186] The Providence brace is similar to the Charleston brace in design with regard to shifting the convexity of the curve to midline. The Providence brace differs from the Charleston primarily by being designed not to unbend the curve in the opposite direction superior to the apex.

Scheuermann's kyphosis

Pathophysiology

Scheuermann described a spinal pathology consisting of vertebral endplate irregularities and wedging. Sorensen set the radiographic criteria: (a) more then 5 degrees of anterior wedging of three consecutive adjacent vertebral bodies at the apex of the kyphosis; (b) irregular vertebral apophyseal lines, combined with flattening and wedging; (c) narrowing of the intervertebral disk spaces; and (d) a variable presence of Schmorl nodes[148] (the penetration of disk material and subsequent alteration of the endochondral ossification process of the anterior vertebral body). Clinically, it is characterized by a rigid deformity that cannot be reasonably corrected by passive manipulation or by the patient's active extension. There is also a distinct dorsal kyphosis as seen laterally with the Adams forward bending test. These patients will often have a more athletic body habitus and may present with tightness in their pectoral muscles and hamstrings. The deformity may be hidden in others by obesity.

Scheuermann's kyphosis is a form of kyphotic deformity that is unique in its severity and rigidity across the involved vertebral segments. It is characterized by wedging of the anterior vertebral bodies caused by growth disturbances of the vertebral endplates. From a treatment perspective, it is important to distinguish Scheuermann's kyphosis from adolescent postural roundback.

The normal range of thoracic kyphosis is considered to be 20 to 45 degrees[60] using the Cobb method of measurement on a standing lateral radiograph of the spine. This degree of kyphosis is exceeded in both Scheuermann's kyphosis and postural kyphosis. Those with a postural deformity can more easily reduce their kyphosis by active contraction of the erector spinae muscles and they lack the vertebral wedging described with Scheuermann's disease.[147,153] However, in some cases it can be quite structural. The reported incidence of Scheuermann's kyphosis ranges from 0.4% to as high as 10% of adolescents between 10 and 14 years of age.[8,23,121] Scheuermann reported a male predominance (male/female ratio of 7.3:1), as did Murray et al., albeit a lower ratio of 2.2:1. Others however have reported an equal male/female ratios,[118,153] and Bradford et al. reported a greater female incidence.[22] Inconsistent diagnostic and inclusion criteria between the study populations cited contribute to the variability of gender bias.

Historical perspective

References to increased kyphosis in adolescence, or a roundback deformity, can be found in the medical literature beginning in the 19th century. Prior to the availability of radiographs, this deformity was believed to be secondary to muscular deficiencies or congenital anomalies.[77] In 1920, Holger Scheuermann identified the radiographic characteristics in a typically juvenile kyphotic disorder that could be distinguished by a more fixed angular deformity with wedging of the vertebral bodies and irregularities of the vertebral apophyses.[147]

While initially described as a deformity of the thoracic spine, Scheuermann's disease can also occur in the thoracolumbar and lumbar spine. Thoracic Scheuermann's kyphosis is defined as having an apex between T7 and T9, and thoracolumbar between T10 and T12. Lumbar Scheuermann's disease will typically lack the clinical deformity seen in thoracic or thoracolumbar types because of its location, and it is more commonly associated with male patients presenting with complaints of backache.[20,71] Further, lumbar Scheuermann's disease is seen more typically in athletic patients and in those who perform hard labor or some form of overuse activity and have Schmorl nodes over several segments of the lumbar spine.

Several investigations have sought to better understand the natural history of Scheuermann's kyphosis. Back pain and fatigue are common complaints in those diagnosed but typically are mild and diminish with maturation. Pain, when present, can be relieved effectively with orthotic management. Patients so affected are more likely to be compliant with brace-wear. Long-term studies have found that most patient complaints disappear with skeletal maturity, and while some may have functional limitations, such limitations are not associated with pain nor do they cause a significant interference with activities of daily living.[121,153] However, one report on adults with more severe deformities (> 75 degrees) and untreated Scheuermann's disease can have severe thoracic pain secondary to degenerative disk disease and spondylolysis in the lumbar spine caudal to the kyphotic deformity. That said, progression of the kyphosis, which might be expected to have a high correlation with increasing symptoms, is poorly related to pain. Murray et al.[121] found those with average angles ranging from 65 to 85 degrees were more symptomatic than those with lesser or greater angles.

Neurologic complications in Scheuermann's disease are rare,[14,21,91,126,145,155,183] and are more likely to occur in male patients.[5,85,126] Bradford reported on three types of neural compression: (1) extradural spinal cyst, (2) compression of the cord at the apex of the kyphos, and (3) disk hernia at the apex of the kyphos.[21] Most reports suggest no obvious correlation with the magnitude of deformity present, but complications appeared more likely when the deformity was more sharply angulated rather than being present over a larger number of vertebral segments. In the rare cases where disk ruptures occur, they typically are at the apex of a thoracic deformity.[85,102]

Treatment recommendations

Because of the relatively benign natural history of the disease, treatment, both nonsurgical and surgical, is often contraindicated in adolescents.[77] Most patients have few symptoms and a deformity that is considered cosmetically acceptable. For patients who are approaching skeletal maturity with mild symptoms, exercise programs to strengthen spinal extensors (to correct thoracic or thoracolumbar kyphosis) and abdominal muscles (to reduce lumbar hyperlordosis) are commonly recommended.[121] In the skeletally immature patient with significant symptoms or progressive deformity, more vigorous forms of treatment are indicated.

The use of orthoses has been shown to have a positive influence on the expected natural history of Scheuermann's disease.[22,40,118,146] The goal in using an orthosis is to diminish any pain present, to control the deformity, and to reconstitute the anterior vertebral height through the application of spinal extension forces. Ideally, an orthosis is used in the early stages of the disease, where satisfactory extension flexibility affords a reasonable reduction of the deformity while the orthosis is being worn. When used in the treatment of thoracic curves ranging from 50 to 75 degrees, the Milwaukee brace has been shown to be an effective design in applying both a passive force at the midthoracic level of the spine and an extension inducement as the patient reacts actively in response to the neck ring. It is equally important to reduce lumbar lordosis in an effort to improve the overall sagittal spinal alignment. Flexibility across the kyphotic segment is needed to treat a patient successfully with an orthosis. Those with more rigid curves may benefit from a passive antigravity cast prior to use of an orthosis.[22] For a thoracolumbar deformity, a thermoplastic TLSO with appropriate anterior sternal extensions is preferred because it can apply a posteriorly directed force sufficiently cephalad to the apex of the curve, but in a design that offers a lower profile for improved appearance.[73,171]

The initial use of an orthosis should be full-time, with the patient allowed to remove the brace 1 to 2 hours each day for exercise. Radiographs should be obtained at 3- to 4-month intervals to assess for improvement. With each visit, the orthotist should adjust the posterior kyphosis pads to provide further correction. Bracing should be continued until skeletal maturity. Realistically, this is difficult to achieve as the adolescent tends to become less compliant with brace wear over time. Males may require additional encouragement to use the orthosis longer since they achieve skeletal maturity later in adolescence. Full-time wear is typically indicated for 12 to 18 months. With documented reduction of deformity and evidence of progression toward bone maturity, part-time wear for maintenance purposes is advised until complete skeletal maturity has been achieved.[40] Sachs et al. reported no statistical difference between the results of patients who wore their Milwaukee brace full-time for 11 months compared to those who wore it for 8 to 10 months.[146]

Orthotic management

In general, the use of orthoses in the treatment of Scheuermann's disease is less common but more challenging compared to orthotic management of idiopathic scoliosis. Because most cases involve the more cephalad segments of the thoracic spine, it can be difficult to apply forces adequate to reduce the size of the deformity while the brace is being worn. In turn, it can be equally difficult for the patient to tolerate an orthosis extending high into the thorax, especially when a suprastructure and some form of a neck-ring is required. That said, when orthotic treatment is indicated and agreed upon, the prescribing orthopedist and the orthotist must understand basic orthotic options and how best to utilize varying strategies to increase the likelihood of an acceptable outcome. Both the Milwaukee brace and the lower-profile TLSO apply 3-point corrective forces at and around the apex of the kyphotic segment. However, the actual mechanisms of the Milwaukee and TLSO designs differ.

The Milwaukee brace, with either a circumferential neck ring or lower-profile suprastructure design, relies on both passive and active forces to provide reduction of thoracic Scheuermann's kyphosis. The most inferior point of pressure comes from the thermoplastic pelvic portion of the orthosis, also referred to as the "girdle." The importance of an accurately fitted pelvic girdle cannot be overemphasized. It provides the inferior base of support upon which all other components of the brace design depend. The pelvic girdle should fulfill three primary criteria: (1) It should decrease lumbar lordosis; (2) it should be shaped to lock onto the pelvis without impinging on the iliac crests, and (3) it should have a snug-fitting and appropriately contoured waist groove to prevent superior or inferior migration of the orthosis.[30]

The second location for force application, which is the primary application for correction of the kyphotic deformity, comes from pads exerting an anteriorly directed pressure at and just inferior to the apical vertebrae of the curve. These pads are mounted on the posterior, paraspinal uprights of the orthoses' suprastructure.

The cephalad and third point of force application (directed posteriorly) depends on an active response by the patient rather than on passive pressure. The neck ring, whether of a high- or low-profile design, invokes a noxious, posteriorly directed stimulus superior to the apex of the thoracic kyphosis. Also known as a "kinesthetic reminder," this superior third point of force application relies on the patient to actively pull away, thus further reducing the degree of the kyphosis while wearing the orthosis. In theory, the more traditional, circumferential neck ring is used for higher thoracic curves (e.g., apex T6 and above), while the lower-profile neck ring designs are more suited to midthoracic curves (e.g., apices of T7 or T8). Little science exists, however, to substantiate the concept of a the patient providing the active correction elicited either by the standard neck ring design or by a superior sternal pad. The success that the Milwaukee brace design actually achieves in the treatment of Scheuermann's kyphosis does suggest, however anecdotally, that some level of active correction takes place. Without it, brace reduction of thoracic kyphosis would be negligible, because no posteriorly directed force can be exerted at the cervical (throat) level, and very little can be applied at the level of the sternal notch.

The thermoplastic TLSO is more typically used in the treatment of low thoracic or thoracolumbar kyphosis. Relying more on passive correction of the kyphotic deformity rather than the active correction of a patient's posture by kinesthetic reminder, the deformity must be low enough in the spine to allow the exertion of a posteriorly directed corrective force that is adequately superior to the apex of the curve. A TLSO is typically custom molded to the patient, utilizing a casting technique which passively decreases the kyphotic deformity. A mold is often taken with the patient lying in the supine position with the hips flexed to reduce lumbar lordosis. The patient is placed over a bolster located at the apex of the kyphosis. Fabrication of the inferior portion of the orthosis is similar to that described in the making of a pelvic girdle for a Milwaukee brace. Because a metal superstructure is not used in the brace design, pads are mounted on the interior wall of the posterior aspect of the orthosis at and below the apex of the kyphosis. Superior to the curve's apex, a posteriorly directed, corrective force is applied by a pad at the level of the manubrium, extending laterally to the deltopectoral grooves. Care must be taken to provide adequate relief to the lower anterior chest wall to enable maximal in-brace correction. This is usually achieved by fashioning a large window between the abdominal apron and the sternal extension of the orthosis.

Because progressive correction of a kyphotic deformity with an orthosis is advised, the orthotist needs to consider various methods to achieve this goal. Increasing the amount of corrective force on a kyphotic spine in the Milwaukee brace can be achieved in multiple ways. The orthotist can use any one or a combination of the following adjustments:

1. Thicken the pads mounted to the paraspinal bars;
2. Contour the paraspinal bars into more of an antikyphotic posture;
3. Raise the anterior superstructure, increasing the amount of effort required to dynamically decrease the kyphotic posture. Great care must be taken in order to not exceed the amount of corrective posture a patient is capable of maintaining, especially while seated.
4. The neck ring can be translated more posteriorly, typically by lowering the posterior and raising the anterior superstructure in relation to the pelvic girdle. This action necessitates a dynamic postural correction by the patient;

5. The amount of lumbar lordosis can be decreased by contouring the relationship between the inferior portion of the paraspinal uprights and the anterior superstructure.

A TLSO can be adjusted to apply greater corrective forces by increasing the thickness of the pads utilized in the passive correction of the deformity. For this simple change to be effective, it is important for the orthotist to confirm the existence of an adequate void to allow the anterior expansion of the thorax.

Best practice

As with other spinal deformities that may be progressive during growth, Scheuermann's kyphosis can be treated successfully with an orthosis as long as treatment begins in the earlier stages of the disease. In general, orthotic treatment should begin while the patient is skeletally immature (Risser 2 or less) having a deformity that is cosmetically or functionally unacceptable This scenario is seen more typically in those with a curve at or near 60 degrees. Orthotic management can be effective in relieving pain from the inflammatory process in Scheuermann's disease. In anticipation that a more rigid thoracic curve will be encountered in Scheuermann's kyphosis than in juvenile roundback or postural kyphosis, a curve must have at least some flexibility for an orthosis to be considered. With a treatment goal of progressively reducing the amount of existing kyphotic deformity, success will be possible only with a deformity that is flexible enough to allow a reduction of the curve, thus allowing reconstitution of the anterior vertebral height with sufficient time for active growth before maturity. If flexibility across the kyphotic segment is inadequate, an antigravity corrective cast should precede use of an orthosis.

Several studies have demonstrated the efficacy of bracing in the treatment of Scheuermann's kyphosis.[22,73,106,118,138,146] All of these studies, however, are retrospective, have varying inclusion criteria, and lack control groups. Bradford et al.[22] published the first report on the efficacy of orthotic treatment in this population. Of 223 patients reviewed, 75 had completed treatment with a Milwaukee brace. The average kyphosis at the beginning of treatment for these patients was 58.9 degrees (range, 45 to 92 degrees) and 34.9 degrees at the completion of treatment. The authors reported an overall 40% decrease in mean thoracic kyphosis; a decrease in vertebral wedging averaging of 41%, and a mean decrease in lumbar lordosis of 36%. With an average treatment duration of 34 months, the best average correction was to 30 degrees in-brace, which was achieved an average of 8.9 months into treatment. Eighteen patients (24%) were reported to have what were described as unsatisfactory results: one having an increase in kyphosis from 43 to 55 degrees and one showing no improvement; the remaining 16 subjects showed improvement, but with a failure to correct their kyphosis to less than 45 degrees. Forty-six of the 75 patients were seen at an average postbrace discontinuation follow-up of 16.8 months with an average kyphosis of 35.9 degrees. The authors suggested kyphosis greater than 65 degrees, skeletal maturity at the time of discovery, and vertebral wedging averaging more than 10 degrees were factors that limited the amount of correction obtained with a Milwaukee brace. The same center later reported on 120 of 274 subjects with Scheuermann's kyphosis having at least 5 years follow up after the completion of treatment with a Milwaukee brace.[146] Initial correction of approximately 50% was followed by a loss of correction in follow-up. The average time of brace wear was 14 months full-time and 18 months part-time.

Montgomery and Erwin reported similar findings of loss of correction after a minimum of 18 months follow-up in 21 of 62 patients treated with a Milwaukee brace.[118] All subjects had open iliac apophyses at the onset of treatment, and duration of brace wear averaged 18 months (10 to 36 month range) followed by an average of 6 months of part-time wear after maximum correction was obtained. Pretreatment kyphosis averaged 62 degrees compared to a posttreatment average of 41 degrees. Maximum correction was typically obtained within 6 to 12 months, but the authors cautioned that shorter treatment duration could compromise the amount of sustained correction. The healing of the vertebral wedging was emphasized as the primary factor that should determine a treatment end point, with 18 months of full-time brace wear thought to be the minimum required to achieve 5 degrees or less of wedging. Loss of correction averaged 15 degrees in long-term follow-up. The authors also reported problems with brace acceptance, with 17% of the patients rejecting the brace, most being male subjects. Ultimately, the reports showing a loss of correction in follow-up illustrate the importance of significantly reducing the deformity to a degree that would exceed the threshold of cosmetic acceptability at the time of brace discontinuation.

As in the treatment of idiopathic scoliosis, the use of a TLSO in those with Scheuermann's kyphosis was undertaken largely in hopes of increasing patient acceptance. Gutowski and Renshaw[73] reported on 75 patients treated with either a Boston lumbar or a Milwaukee brace in the treatment of Scheuermann's disease or abnormal juvenile roundback. Twenty-three (31%) of the patients completely rejected their orthosis within the first 4 months of treatment. The remaining 52 patients were reported as a group, citing virtually identical treatment results in the 41 with Scheuermann's disease compared with the 11 with juvenile roundback. The Boston brace was prescribed for younger patients with smaller, more flexible curves. The authors hypothesized that if the amount of lumbar lordosis is effectively reduced with the lower profile Boston brace, a dynamic straightening of the concomitant excessive thoracic kyphosis would occur. The average pretreatment kyphosis in 36 patients treated with the Boston brace measured 60 degrees, and the average curve size at the time of brace discontinuation was 44 degrees (a 27% improvement). Of the 16 patients treated with a Milwaukee brace, the average curve size at the start of treatment measured 71 degrees, which was reduced to an average kyphosis of 46 degrees at the end of treatment (a 35% improvement). Based on patient and family self-reports in this retrospective review, the authors reported satisfactory compliance in 27 of 44 patients (61%) who were prescribed to wear the Boston brace, compared to 9 of 31 (29%) patients who were prescribed to wear the Milwaukee brace. The authors concluded the Boston brace was a satisfactory alternative to the Milwaukee brace in those with flexible kyphotic curves less than 70 degrees in size.

Citing a desire to increase patient compliance in the treatment of Scheuermann's thoracic kyphosis, one report on the use of a custom-molded TLSO fabricated from a corrective negative mold from a casting table demonstrated a treatment effectiveness in 73% of subjects reviewed.[138] In this retrospective review of 34, roughly one third (12 subjects) were determined to be noncompliant and thus excluded from study's results. Of the 22 subjects who completed treatment (14 boys and 8 girls), 9 showed improvement, 7 remained unchanged, and 6 demonstrated progression of at least 5 degrees. Of the 16 patients considered a treatment success, the mean improvement was 9 degrees (the average pre-brace kyphosis measuring 64 degrees, compared to an average curve of 55 degrees at the time of brace discontinuation due to maturity). The average increase in curve size for the 6 patients who worsened was 9 degrees (59 degrees to 68 degrees). Curve flexibility was a positive predictor of treatment success; however, lack of flexibility was not found to be a contraindication for treatment. With an average treatment duration for all subjects reviewed of 23 months, the authors recommended a minimum of/16 months of wear to increase the likelihood of a either improving or halting progression of the kyphotic deformity.

References

1. The American Academy of Orthotists and Prosthetists: *Orthotic treatment of idiopathic scoliosis and Scheuermann's kyphosis*, Campbell JH, editor: Dallas, 2003, Lippincott Williams & Wilkins.
2. Adams W: *Lectures on the pathology and treatment of lateral and other forms of curvature of the spine*, London, 1865, J Churchill and Sons.
3. Albanese S: Idiopathic scoliosis: etiology and evaluation; natural history and nonsurgical management. In Richards B, editor: *Orthopaedic Knowledge Update: Pediatrics*, Rosemont, Il, 1996, American Academy of Orthopaedic Surgeons, pp. 97–98.
4. Allington NJ, Bowen JR: Adolescent idiopathic scoliosis: treatment with the Wilmington brace. A comparison of full-time and part-time use. *J Bone Joint Surg Am* 78:1056–1062, 1996.
5. Anderson M, Hwang SC, Green WT: Growth of the normal trunk in boys and girls during the second decade of life; related to age, maturity, and ossification of the iliac epiphyses. *J Bone Joint Surg Am* 47:1554–1564, 1965.
6. Andriacchi T, Schultz AB, Belytschko TB, et al: Milwaukee brace correction of idiopathic scoliosis. *J Bone Joint Surg Am* 58:806–815, 1976.
7. Andry N: *Orthopaedia*, Philadelphia, 1743, JB Lippincott.
8. Ascani E, Salsano V, Giglio G: The incidence and early detection of spinal deformities. A study based on the screening of 16,104 schoolchildren. *Ital J Orthop Traumatol* 3:111–117, 1977.
9. Asher M, Green P, Orrick J: A six-year report: spinal deformity screening in Kansas school children. *J Kans Med Soc* 81:568–571, 1980.
10. Aubin CE, Dansereau J, de Guise JA, et al: Rib cage-spine coupling patterns involved in brace treatment of adolescent idiopathic scoliosis. *Spine* 22:629–635, 1997.
11. Bassett GS, Bunnell WP: Effect of a thoracolumbosacral orthosis on lateral trunk shift in idiopathic scoliosis. *J Pediatr Orthop* 6:182–185, 1986.
12. Bassett GS, Bunnell WP: Influence of the Wilmington brace on spinal decompensation in adolescent idiopathic scoliosis. *Clin Orthop* 223:164-169, 1987.
13. Bassett GS, Bunnell WP, MacEwen GD: Treatment of idiopathic scoliosis with the Wilmington brace. Results in patients with a twenty to thirty-nine-degree curve. *J Bone Joint Surg Am* 68:602–605, 1986.
14. Bhojraj SY, Dandawate AV: Progressive cord compression secondary to thoracic disc lesions in Scheuermann's kyphosis managed by posterolateral decompression, interbody fusion and pedicular fixation. A new approach to management of a rare clinical entity. *Eur Spine J* 3:66–69, 1994.
15. Biondi J, Weiner DS, Bethem D, et al: Correlation of Risser sign and bone age determination in adolescent idiopathic scoliosis. *J Pediatr Orthop* 5:697–701, 1985.
16. Bitan FD, Veliskakis KP, Campbell BC: Differences in the Risser grading systems in the United States and France. *Clin Orthop Relat Res* 190–195, 2005.

17. Blount WP, Moe JH: *The Milwaukee Brace*, Baltimore, 1973, Williams and Wilkins.

18. Blount WP, Schmidt AC, Bidwell RG: Making the Milwaukee brace. *J Bone Joint Surg Am* 40-A:526–528 passim, 1958.

19. Blount WP, Schmidt AC, Keever ED, et al: The Milwaukee brace in the operative treatment of scoliosis. *J Bone Joint Surg Am* 40-A:511–525, 1958.

20. Blumenthal SL, Roach J, Herring JA: Lumbar Scheuermann's. A clinical series and classification. *Spine* 12:929–932, 1987.

21. Bradford DS, Garica A: Neurological complications in Scheuermann's disease. A case report and review of the literature. *J Bone Joint Surg Am* 51:567–572, 1969.

22. Bradford DS, Moe JH, Montalvo FJ, et al: Scheuermann's kyphosis and roundback deformity. Results of Milwaukee brace treatment. *J Bone Joint Surg Am* 56:740–758, 1974.

23. Bradford DS, Moe JH, Winter RB: Kyphosis and postural roundback deformity in children and adolescents. *Minn Med* 56:114–120, 1973.

24. Branthwaite MA: Cardiorespiratory consequences of unfused idiopathic scoliosis. *British Br J Dis Chest* 80:360–369, 1986.

25. Buckler JMH: *A longitudinal study of adolescent growth*, London, 1990, Springer.

26. Bunch WH, Patwardhan AG: *Scoliosis: making clinical decisions*, St. Louis, 1989, Mosby.

27. Bunnell WP: A Study of the natural history of idiopathic scoliosis. *Orthop Trans* 6, 1983.

28. Bunnell WP: The natural history of idiopathic scoliosis before skeletal maturity. *Spine* 11:773–776, 1986.

29. Bunnell WP, MacEwen GD, Jayakumar S: The use of plastic jackets in the non-operative treatment of idiopathic scoliosis. Preliminary report. *J Bone Joint Surg Am* 62:31–38, 1980.

30. Carlson J: A Thoraco-Lumbo-Sacral-Orthosis for Idiopathic Scoliosis—Part II. *Gillette Children's Hospital Instructional Manual* 1981.

31. Carman DL, Browne RH, Birch JG: Measurement of scoliosis and kyphosis radiographs. Intraobserver and interobserver variation. *J Bone Joint Surg Am* 72:328–333, 1990.

32. Carr WA, Moe JH, Winter RB, et al: Treatment of idiopathic scoliosis in the Milwaukee brace. *J Bone Joint Surg Am* 62:599–612, 1980.

33. Ceballos T, Ferrer-Torrelles M, Castillo F, et al: Prognosis in infantile idiopathic scoliosis. *J Bone Joint Surg Am* 62:863–875, 1980.

34. Chase A, Bader DL, Houghton GR: The biomechanical effectiveness of the Boston brace in the management of adolescent idiopathic scoliosis. *Spine* 14:636–642, 1989.

35. Clarisse P: *Pronostic evolutif des scoliosis idiopathiques mineures de 10 degrees a 29 degrees, en periode de croissance*, Lyon, Universite Claude-Bernard, 1974.

36. Cobb J: Outline for the study of scoliosis. *AAOS Instr Course Lect* 5:261, 1948.

37. Coillard C, Leroux MA, Zabjek KF, et al: SpineCor—a non-rigid brace for the treatment of idiopathic scoliosis: post-treatment results. *Eur Spine J* 12:141–148, 2003.

38. D'Amato CR, Griggs S, McCoy B: Nighttime bracing with the Providence brace in adolescent girls with idiopathic scoliosis. *Spine* 26:2006–2012, 2001.

39. Daruwalla JS, Balasubramaniam P, Chay SO, et al: Idiopathic scoliosis. Prevalence and ethnic distribution in Singapore schoolchildren. *J Bone Joint Surg Br* 67:182–184, 1985.

40. De Smedt A, Fabry G, Mulier JC: Milwaukee brace treatment of Scheuermann's kyphosis. *Acta Orthop Belg* 41:597–605, 1975.

41. Deane G, Duthie RB: A new projectional look at articulated scoliotic spines. *Acta Orthop Scand* 44:351–365, 1973.

42. Di Raimondo CV, Green NE: Brace-wear compliance in patients with adolescent idiopathic scoliosis. *J Pediatr Orthop* 8:143–146, 1988.

43. Dickson RA: Early onset idiopathic scoliosis. In Weinstein SL, editor: *The Pediatric Spine: Principles and Practice*, New York, 1994, Raven Press, pp. 709–714.

44. Dickson RA, Archer IA: Surgical treatment of late-onset idiopathic thoracic scoliosis. The Leeds procedure. *J Bone Joint Surg Br* 69:709–714, 1987.

45. Dickson RA, Lawton JO, Archer IA, et al: The pathogenesis of idiopathic scoliosis. Biplanar spinal asymmetry. *J Bone Joint Surg Br* 66:8–15, 1984.

46. Dickson RA, Weinstein SL: Bracing (and screening)—yes or no? *J Bone Joint Surg Br* 81:193–198, 1999.

47. Diedrich O, von Strempel A, Schloz M, et al: Long-term observation and management of resolving infantile idiopathic scoliosis—a 25-year follow-up. *J Bone Joint Surg Br* 84:1030–1035, 2002.

48. Dimeglio A: Growth of the spine before age 5 years. *J Pediatr Orthop B* 102-107, 1993.

49. Dunnill MS: Postnatal growth of the lung. *Thorax* 17:329–333, 1962.

50. Edelmann P: Brace treatment in idiopathic scoliosis. *Acta Orthop Belg* 58 (Suppl 1):85–90, 1992.

51. Eldeeb H, Boubekri N, Asfour S, et al: Design of thoracolumbosacral orthosis (TLSO) braces using CT/MR. *J Comput Assist Tomogr* 25:963–970, 2001.

52. Emans JB, Kaelin A, Bancel P, et al: The Boston bracing system for idiopathic scoliosis. Follow-up results in 295 paients. *Spine* 11:792–801, 1986.

53. Emery JL, Mithal A: The number of alveoli in the terminal respiratory unit of man during late intrauterine life and childhood. *Arch Dis Child* 35:544–547, 1960.

54. Faust M: Somatic development of adolescent girls. *Monogr Soc Res Child Dev* 42:1–90, 1977.

55. Federico DJ RT: Results of treatment of idiopathic scoliosis with the Charleston Bending Brace. *Spine* 15:886–887, 1990.

56. Fernandez-Feliberti R, Flynn J, Ramirez N, et al: Effectiveness of TLSO bracing in the conservative treatment of idiopathic scoliosis. *J Pediatr Orthop* 15:176–181, 1995.

57. Ferreira JH, de Janeiro R, James JI: Progressive and resolving infantile idiopathic scoliosis. The differential diagnosis. *J Bone Joint Surg Br* 54:648–655, 1972.

58. Figueiredo UM, James JI: Juvenile idiopathic scoliosis. *J Bone Joint Surg Br* 63-B:61–66, 1981.

59. Fiore N, Onimus M, Ferre B, et al: Treatment of lumbar and dorso-lumbar scoliosis using the Boston orthosis and the 3-valve orthosis. Comparative study of the results in the frontal and horizontal planes. *Rev Chir Orthop* 74:569–575, 1988.

60. Fon GT, Pitt MJ, Thies AC Jr.: Thoracic kyphosis: range in normal subjects. *Am J Roentgenol* 134:979–983, 1980.

61. Fustier T: *Evolution radiologique sponeanee des scoliosis idiopathiques de moins de 45 degrees en periode de croissance* Lyon, Universite Claude-Bernard, 1980.

62. Gabos PG, Bojescul JA, Bowen JR, et al: Long-term follow-up of female patients with idiopathic scoliosis treated with the Wilmington orthosis. *J Bone Joint Surg Am* 86-A:1891–1899, 2004.

63. Galante J, Schultz A, Dewald RL, et al: Forces acting in the Milwaukee brace on patients undergoing treatment for idiopathic scoliosis. *J Bone Joint Surg Am* 52:498–506, 1970.

64. Gavin TM, Bunch WH, Dvonch VM: The Rosenberger scoliosis orthosis. *J Assoc Child Prosthet Orthot Clin* 3:35–38, 1986.

65. Gavin TM, Shurr DG, Patwardhan AG: Orthotic Treatment for Spinal Disorders: *The Pediatric Spine: Principles and Practice*, New York, 1994, Raven Press, 1994.

66. Gepstein R, Leitner Y, Zohar E, et al: Effectiveness of the Charleston bending brace in the treatment of single-curve idiopathic scoliosis. *J Pediatr Orthop* 22:84–87, 2002.

67. Gillingham BL, Fan RA, Akbarnia BA: Early onset idiopathic scoliosis. *J Am Acad Orthop Surg* 14:101–112, 2006.

68. Goldberg CJ, Dowling FE, Fogarty EE: Adolescent idiopathic scoliosis—early menarche, normal growth. *Spine* 18:529–535, 1993.

69. Goldberg CJ, Moore DP, Fogarty EE, et al: Adolescent idiopathic scoliosis: the effect of brace treatment on the incidence of surgery. *Spine* 26:42–47, 2001.

70. Green NE: Part-time bracing of adolescent idiopathic scoliosis. *J Bone Joint Surg Am* 68:738–742, 1986.

71. Greene TL, Hensinger RN, Hunter LY: Back pain and vertebral changes simulating Scheuermann's disease. *J Pediatr Orthop* 5:1–7, 1985.

72. Griffet J, Thevenot L, Barral F: Presentation of GTB orthoses for hyperlordotic treatment of idiopathic scoliosis. *Eur J Pediatr Surg* 8:163–167, 1998.

73. Gutowski WT, Renshaw TS: Orthotic results in adolescent kyphosis. *Spine* 13:485–489, 1988.

74. Hall JE, Miller ME, Schumann W, et al: A refined concept in the orthotic management of idiopathic scoliosis. *Prosthet Orthot Int* 29:7–13, 1975.

75. Havey R, Gavin T, Patwardhan A, et al: A reliable and accurate method for measuring orthosis wearing time. *Spine* 27:211–214, 2002.

76. Helfenstein A, Lankes M, Ohlert K, et al: The objective determination of compliance in treatment of adolescent idiopathic scoliosis with spinal orthoses. *Spine* 31:339–344, 2006.

77. Herring: Kyphosis. In Herring JA, editor: *Tachdjian's Pediatric Orthopaedics*, edition. W.B. Saunders Company, 2002, pp. 323–350.

78. Herring JA: Scoliosis. In Herring JA, editor: *Tachdjian's Pediatric Orthopaedics*, edition. W.B. Saunders Company, 2002, pp. 213–321.

79. Hibbs RA, Risser JC, Ferguson AB: Scoliosis treated by the fusion operation. An end-result study of three hundred and sixty cases. *J Bone Joint Surg* 13:91–104, 1931.

80. Hopf C, Heine J: [Long-term results of the conservative treatment of scoliosis using the Cheneau brace]. *Z Orthop Ihre Grenzgeb* 123:312–322, 1985.

81. Hoppenfeld S, Lonner B, Murthy V, et al: The rib epiphysis and other growth centers as indicators of the end of spinal growth. *Spine* 29:47–50, 2004.

82. Howard A, Wright JG, Hedden D: A comparative study of TLSO, Charleston, and Milwaukee braces for idiopathic scoliosis. *Spine* 23:2404–2411, 1998.

83. James J: Idiopathic scoliosis: the prognosis, diagnosis, and operative indications related to curve patterns and the age of onset. *J Bone Joint Surg* 36-B:36–49, 1954.

84. Jonasson-Rajala E, Josefsson E, Lundberg B, etal: Boston thoracic brace in the treatment of idiopathic scoliosis. Initial correction. *Clin Orthop Relat Res* 37–41, 1984.

85. Kapetanos GA, Hantzidis PT, Anagnostidis KS, et al: Thoracic cord compression caused by disk herniation in Scheuermann's disease: A case report and review of the literature. *Eur Spine J* 15 (Suppl 17): 553–558, 2006.

86. Karol LA, Johnston CE, 2nd, Browne RH, et al: Progression of the curve in boys who have idiopathic scoliosis. *J Bone Joint Surg Am* 75:1804–1810, 1993.

87. Katz DE, Durrani AA: Factors that influence outcome in bracing large curves in patients with adolescent idiopathic scoliosis. *Spine* 26:2354–2361, 2001.

88. Katz DE, Richards BS, Browne RH, et al: A comparison between the Boston brace and the Charleston bending brace in adolescent idiopathic scoliosis. *Spine* 22:1302–1312, 1997.

89. Kehl DK, Morrissy RT: Brace treatment in adolescent idiopathic scoliosis. An update on concepts and technique. *Clin Orthop Relat Res* 34–43, 1988.

90. Keiser RP, Shufflebarger HL: The Milwaukee brace in idiopathic scoliosis: evaluation of 123 completed cases. *Clin Orthop Relat Res* 19–24, 1976.

91. Klein DM, Weiss RL, Allen JE: Scheuermann's dorsal kyphosis and spinal cord compression: case report. *Neurosurg* 18:628–631, 1986.

92. Koop SE: Infantile and juvenile idiopathic scoliosis. *Orthop Clin North Am* 19:331–337, 1988.

93. Labelle H, Dansereau J, Bellefleur C, et al: Three-dimensional effect of the Boston brace on the thoracic spine and rib cage. *Spine* 21:59–64, 1996.

94. Laurnen EL, Tupper JW, Mullen MP: The Boston brace in thoracic scoliosis. A preliminary report. *Spine* 8:388–395, 1983.

95. Lindh M: The effect of sagittal curve changes on brace correction of idiopathic scoliosis. *Spine* 5:26–36, 1980.

96. Little DG, Song KM, Katz D, et al: Relationship of peak height velocity to other maturity indicators in idiopathic scoliosis in girls. *J Bone Joint Surg Am* 82:685–693, 2000.

97. Little DG, Sussman MD: The Risser sign: a critical analysis. *J Pediatr Orthop* 14:569–575, 1994.

98. Lloyd-Roberts GC, Pilcher MF: Structural idiopathic scoliosis in infancy: a study of the natural history of 100 patients. *J Bone Joint Surg Br* 47:520–523, 1965.

99. Lonstein JE, Bjorklund S, Wanninger MH, et al: Voluntary school screening for scoliosis in Minnesota. *J Bone Joint Surg Am* 64:481–488, 1982.

100. Lonstein JE, Carlson JM: The prediction of curve progression in untreated idiopathic scoliosis during growth. *J Bone Joint Surg Am* 66:1061–1071, 1984.

101. Lonstein JE, Winter RB: The Milwaukee brace for the treatment of adolescent idiopathic scoliosis. A review of one thousand and twenty patients. *J Bone Joint Surg Am* 76:1207–1221, 1994.

102. Lonstein JE, Winter RB, Moe JH, et al: Neurologic deficits secondary to spinal deformity. A review of the literature and report of 43 cases. *Spine* 5:331–355, 1980.

103. Lou E, Hill DL, Raso JV, et al: Smart orthosis for the treatment of adolescent idiopathic scoliosis. *Med Biol Eng Comput* 43:746–750, 2005.

104. Lou E, Raso JV, Hill DL, et al: The daily force pattern of spinal orthoses in subjects with adolescent idiopathic scoliosis. *Prosthet Orthot Int* 26:58–63, 2002.

105. Lou E, Raso JV, Hill DL, et al: Correlation between quantity and quality of orthosis wear and treatment outcomes in adolescent idiopathic scoliosis. *Prosthet Orthot Int* 28:49–54, 2004.

106. Lowe TG: Scheuermann disease. *J Bone Joint Surg Am* 72:940–945, 1990.

107. Mac-Thiong JM, Labelle H, Charlebois M, et al: Sagittal plane analysis of the spine and pelvis in adolescent idiopathic scoliosis according to the coronal curve type. *Spine* 28:1404–1409, 2003.

108. Masso PD, Meeropol E, Lennon E: Juvenile-onset scoliosis followed up to adulthood: orthopaedic and functional outcomes. *J Pediatr Orthop* 22:279–284, 2002.

109. McCollough NC 3rd, Schultz M, Javech N, et al: Miami TLSO in the management of scoliosis: preliminary results in 100 cases. *J Pediatr Orthop* 1:141–152, 1981.

110. McMaster MJ: Infantile idiopathic scoliosis: can it be prevented? *J Bone Joint Surg Br* 65:612–617, 1983.

111. Mehta MH: The rib-vertebra angle in the early diagnosis between resolving and progressive infantile scoliosis. *J Bone Joint Surg Br* 54:230–243, 1972.

112. Mehta MH: Growth as a corrective force in the early treatment of progressive infantile scoliosis. *J Bone Joint Surg Br* 87:1237–1247, 2005.

113. Mehta MH, Morel G: The non-operative treatment of infantile idiopathic scoliosis. In Zorab PA, Siegler D, editors: *Scoliosis*, London, 1980, London Academic Press pp. 71–84.

114. Mellencamp DD, Blount WP, Anderson AJ: Milwaukee brace treatment of idiopathic scoliosis: late results. *Clin Orthop Relat Res* 126:47–57, 1977.

115. Miller JA, Nachemson AL, Schultz AB: Effectiveness of braces in mild idiopathic scoliosis. *Spine* 9:632–635, 1984.

116. Moe JH, Kettleson DN: Idiopathic scoliosis. Analysis of curve patterns and the preliminary results of Milwaukee-brace treatment in one hundred sixty-nine patients. *J Bone Joint Surg Am* 52:1509–1533, 1970.

117. Montgomery F, Willner S: Prognosis of brace-treated scoliosis. Comparison of the Boston and Milwaukee methods in 244 girls. *Acta Orthop Scand* 60:383–385, 1989.

118. Montgomery SP, Erwin WE: Scheuermann's kyphosis—long-term results of Milwaukee braces treatment. *Spine* 6:5–8, 1981.

119. Muirhead A, Conner AN: The assessment of lung function in children with scoliosis. *J Bone Joint Surg Br* 67:699–702, 1985.

120. Mulcahy T, Galante J, DeWald R, et al: A follow-up study of forces acting on the Milwaukee brace on patients undergoing treatment for idiopathic scoliosis. *Clin Orthop Relat Res* 93:53–68, 1973.

121. Murray PM, Weinstein SL, Spratt KF: The natural history and long-term follow-up of Scheuermann kyphosis. *J Bone Joint Surg Am* 75:236–248, 1993.

122. Nachemson A: A long-term follow-up study of non-treated scoliosis. *Acta Orthop Scand* 39:466–476, 1968.

123. Nachemson AL, Peterson LE: Effectiveness of treatment with a brace in girls who have adolescent idiopathic scoliosis. A prospective, controlled study based on data from the Brace Study of the Scoliosis Research Society [see comments]. *J Bone Joint Surg Am* 77:815–822, 1995.

124. Nicholson GP, Ferguson-Pell MW, Smith K, et al: The objective measurement of spinal orthosis use for the treatment of adolescent idiopathic scoliosis. *Spine* 28:2243–2250; discussion 2250–2241, 2003.

125. Noonan KJ, Weinstein SL, Jacobson WC, et al: Use of the Milwaukee brace for progressive idiopathic scoliosis. *J Bone Joint Surg Am* 78:557–567, 1996.

126. Normelli HC, Svensson O, Aaro SI: Cord compression in Scheuermann's kyphosis. A case report. *Acta Orthop Scand* 62:70–72, 1991.

127. O'Neill PJ, Karol LA, Shindle MK, et al: Decreased orthotic effectiveness in overweight patients with adolescent idiopathic scoliosis. *J Bone Joint Surg Am* 87:1069–1074, 2005.

128. Olafsson Y, Saraste H, Soderlund V, et al: Boston brace in the treatment of idiopathic scoliosis. *J Pediatr Orthop* 15:524–527, 1995.

129. Patwardhan AG, Bunch WH, Meade KP, et al: A biomechanical analog of curve progression and orthotic stabilization in idiopathic scoliosis. *J Biomech* 19:103–117, 1986.

130. Patwardhan AG, Gavin TM, Bunch WH, et al: Biomechanical comparison of the Milwaukee brace (CTLSO) and the TLSO for treatment of idiopathic scoliosis. *J Prosthet Orthot* 8:115–122, 1996.

131. Pehrsson K, Larsson S, Oden A, et al: Long-term follow-up of patients with untreated scoliosis. A study of mortality, causes of death, and symptoms. *Spine* 17:1091–1096, 1992.

132. Perdriolle R, Vidal J: Thoracic idiopathic scoliosis curve evolution and prognosis. *Spine* 10:785–791, 1985.

133. Price CT, Scott DS, Reed FE Jr., et al: Nighttime bracing for adolescent idiopathic scoliosis with the Charleston bending brace. Preliminary report. *Spine* 15:1294–1299, 1990.

134. Price CT SD, Reed FR: Nightitime bracing for adolescent idiopathic scoliosis with the Charleston bending brace: Long-term follow-up. *J Ped Orthop* 17:703–707, 1997.

135. Rahman T, Bowen JR, Takemitsu M, et al: The association between brace compliance and outcome for patients with idiopathic scoliosis. *J Pediatr Orthop* 25:420–422, 2005.

136. Raso VJ, Russell GG, Hill DL, et al: Thoracic lordosis in idiopathic scoliosis. *J Pediatr Orthop* 11:599–602, 1991.

137. Richards BS, Bernstein RM, D'Amato CR, et al: Standardization of criteria for adolescent idiopathic scoliosis brace studies: SRS Committee on Bracing and Nonoperative Management. *Spine* 30:2068–2077, 2005.

138. Riddle EC, Bowen JR, Shah SA, et al: The duPont kyphosis brace for the treatment of adolescent Scheuermann kyphosis. *J South Orthop Assoc* 12:135–140, 2003.

139. Risser JC: The application of body casts for the correction of scoliosis. *Instruct Course Lect* 12:255–259, 1955.

140. Risser JC: The iliac apophysis; an invaluable sign in the management of scoliosis. *Clin Orthop* 11:111–119, 1958.

141. Roaf R: The basic anatomy of scoliosis. *J Bone Joint Surg Br* 48:786–792, 1966.

142. Robinson CM, McMaster MJ: Juvenile idiopathic scoliosis. Curve patterns and prognosis in one hundred and nine patients. *J Bone Joint Surg Am* 78:1140–1148, 1996.

143. Rogala EJ, Drummond DS, Gurr J: Scoliosis: incidence and natural history. A prospective epidemiological study. *J Bone Joint Surg Am* 60:173–176, 1978.

144. Rowe DE, Bernstein SM, Riddick MF, et al: A meta-analysis of the efficacy of non-operative treatments for idiopathic scoliosis. *J Bone Joint Surg Am* 79:664–674, 1997.

145. Ryan MD, Taylor TK: Acute spinal cord compression in Scheuermann's disease. *J Bone Joint Surg Br* 64:409–412, 1982.

146. Sachs B, Bradford D, Winter R, et al: Scheuermann kyphosis. Follow-up of Milwaukee-brace treatment. *J Bone Joint Surg Am* 69:50–57, 1987.

147. Scheuermann H: Kyfosis dorsalis juvenilis. *Ugeskr Laeger* 82:385–393, 1920.

148. Schmorl G, Junghans H: *Die gesunde und kranke Wirbelsaeule in Roentgenbild*, Leipzig, 1932, Theime Verlag.

149. Schultz AB: The use of mathematical models for studies of scoliosis biomechanics. *Spine* 16:1211–1216, 1991.

150. Shuren N, Kasser JR, Emans JB, et al: Reevaluation of the use of the Risser sign in idiopathic scoliosis. *Spine* 17:359–361, 1992.

151. Somerville EW: Rotational lordosis; the development of single curve. *J Bone Joint Surg Br* 34-B:421–427, 1952.

152. Song KM, Little DG: Peak height velocity as a maturity indicator for males with idiopathic scoliosis. *J Pediatr Orthop* 20:286–288, 2000.

153. Sorensen K: *Scheuermann's juvenile kyphosis*. Copenhagen, Mundsgaard, 1964.

154. Spoonamore MJ, Dolan LA, Weinstein SL: Use of the Rosenberger brace in the treatment of progressive adolescent idiopathic scoliosis. *Spine* 29:1458–1464, 2004.

155. Stambough JL, VanLoveren HR, Cheeks ML: Spinal cord compression in Scheuermann's kyphosis: case report. *Neurosurg* 30:127–130, 1992.

156. Takemitsu M, Bowen JR, Rahman T, et al: Compliance monitoring of brace treatment for patients with idiopathic scoliosis. *Spine* 29:2070–2074, 2004.

157. Thompson SK, Bentley G: Prognosis in infantile idiopathic scoliosis. *J Bone Joint Surg Br* 62-B:151–154, 1980.

158. Tolo VT, Gillespie R: The characteristics of juvenile idiopathic scoliosis and results of its treatment. *J Bone Joint Surg Br* 60-B:181–188, 1978.

159. Trivedi JM, Thomson JD: Results of Charleston bracing in skeletally immature patients with idiopathic scoliosis. *J Pediatr Orthop* 21:277–280, 2001.

160. Uden A, Willner S: The effect of lumbar flexion and Boston Thoracic Brace on the curves in idiopathic scoliosis. *Spine* 8:846–850, 1983.

161. Upadhyay SS, Nelson IW, Ho EK, et al: New prognostic factors to predict the final outcome of brace treatment in adolescent idiopathic scoliosis. *Spine* 20:537–545, 1995.

162. Vandal S, Rivard CH, Bradet R: Measuring the compliance behavior of adolescents wearing orthopedic braces. *Issues Compr Pediatr Nurs* 22:59–73, 1999.

163. Ventura N, Huguet R, Ey A, et al: Infantile idiopathic scoliosis in the newborn. *Int Orthop* 22:82–86, 1998.

164. Watts HG, Hall JE, Stanish W: The Boston brace system for the treatment of low thoracic and lumbar scoliosis by the use of a girdle without superstructure. *Clin Orthop Relat Res* 126:87–92, 1977.

165. Weinstein SL: Adolescent idiopathic scoliosis: prevalence and natural history. In Weinstein SL, editor: *The pediatric spine: principles and practice*. New York, Raven Press, 1994, pp. 463–478.

166. Weinstein SL, Dolan LA, Spratt KF, et al: Health and function of patients with untreated idiopathic scoliosis: a 50-year natural history study. *JAMA* 289:567, 2003.

167. Weinstein SL, Ponseti IV: Curve progression in idiopathic scoliosis. *J Bone Joint Surg Am* 65:447–455, 1983.

168. Weiss HR: Adolescent idiopathic scoliosis: the effect of brace treatment on the incidence of surgery. *Spine* 26:2058–2059, 2001.

169. Weiss HR, Dallmayer R, Gallo D: Sagittal counter forces (SCF) in the treatment of idiopathic scoliosis: a preliminary report. *Pediatr Rehabil* 9:24–30, 2006.

170. Weiss HR, Weiss GM: Brace treatment during pubertal growth spurt in girls with idiopathic scoliosis (IS): a prospective trial comparing two different concepts. *Pediatr Rehabil* 8:199–206, 2005.

171. Wenger D, Rang M: *The art and practice of children's orthopaedics*, New York, 1993, Raven Press.

172. Wiley JW, Thomson JD, Mitchell TM, et al: Effectiveness of the Boston brace in treatment of large curves in adolescent idiopathic scoliosis. *Spine* 25:2326–2332, 2000.

173. Willers U, Normelli H, Aaro S, et al: Long-term results of Boston brace treatment on vertebral rotation in idiopathic scoliosis. *Spine* 18:432–435, 1993.

174. Willner S: Effect of the Boston thoracic brace on the frontal and sagittal curves of the spine. *Acta Orthop Scand* 55:457–460, 1984.

175. Winter RB: The pendulum has swung too far. Bracing for adolescent idiopathic scoliosis in the 1990s. *Orthop Clin North Am* 25:195–204, 1994.

176. Winter RB: A tale of two brothers: ultra-long-term follow-up of juvenile idiopathic scoliosis. *J Spinal Disord Tech* 17:446–450, 2004.

177. Winter RB, Lonstein JE, Drogt J, et al: The effectiveness of bracing in the nonoperative treatment of idiopathic scoliosis. *Spine* 11:790–791, 1986.

178. Wong MS, Cheng JC, Lo KH: A comparison of treatment effectiveness between the CAD/CAM method and the manual method for managing adolescent idiopathic scoliosis. *Prosthet Orthop Int* 29:105–111, 2005.

179. Wong MS, Cheng JC, Wong MW, et al: A work study of the CAD/CAM method and conventional manual method in the fabrication of spinal orthoses for patients with adolescent idiopathic scoliosis. *Prosthet Orthop Int* 29:93–104, 2005.

180. Wong MS, Mak AF, Luk KD, et al: Effectiveness and biomechanics of spinal orthoses in the treatment of adolescent idiopathic scoliosis (AIS). *Prosthet Orthot Int* 24:148–162, 2000.

181. Wynarsky G, Schultz AB: Trunk muscle activities in braced scoliosis patients. *Spine* 14:1283–1286, 1989.

182. Wynne-Davies R, Littlejohn A, Gormley J: Aetiology and interrelationship of some common skeletal deformities. (Talipes equinovarus and calcaneovalgus, metatarsus varus, congenital dislocation of the hip, and infantile idiopathic scoliosis). *J Med Genet* 19:321–328, 1982.

183. Yablon JS, Kasdon DL, Levine H: Thoracic cord compression in Scheuermann's disease. *Spine* 13:896–898, 1988.

184. Yasuhiro I: The accuracy of Risser staging. *Spine* 20:1868–1871, 1995.

185. Yoshikuni N: [Bone maturation in scoliosis patients, comparison of the degrees of ossification of the iliac crest and carpal bone age]. *Nippon Seikeigeka Gakkai Zasshi* 62:313–320, 1988.

186. Yrjonen T, Ylikoski M, Schlenzka D, et al: Effectiveness of the Providence nighttime bracing in adolescent idiopathic scoliosis: a comparative study of 36 female patients. *Eur Spine J* 15:1139–1143, 2006.

Orthoses for spinal trauma and postoperative care

Bryan S. Malas, Kevin P. Meade, Avinash G. Patwardhan, and Thomas M. Gavin

Key Points

- The treatment team must agree upon vocabulary used for terms characterizing the "stability" and "instability" of fractures.

- Only stable spine fractures can be treated orthotically; the exception is unstable fractures of the upper cervical spine.

- The primary orthotic goal is to increase spinal stability in all three anatomical planes by immobilization.

- An understanding of the mechanism for injury of traumatic spine fractures and associated sequelae is necessary before orthotic management is pursued as a treatment pathway.

- Orthotic goals and biomechanical principles of orthotic treatment should be clearly defined and understood when managing fractures nonoperatively or postoperatively.

- When orthotic management is selected as an alternative to surgery, standards for orthotic outcomes should be similar to the standards for surgical outcomes.

- Evidence suggests that certain types of compression, seat belt, and burst fractures respond well to orthotic management as the primary course of treatment.

- Scientific evidence supporting or refuting the efficacy of postoperative orthotic management is limited.

- Utilization of viscoelastic creep during measurement, impression, and fitting may be an important consideration for spinal alignment and/or fracture reduction.

- For the majority of spinal injuries at the macro level, the primary orthotic goal is protecting the spinal column from loads and stresses that would likely cause progression of the spinal deformity and not allow for adequate healing of the injury.[29,37]

Pathophysiology

With the exception of some fractures of the upper cervical spine and bilateral facet fractures, orthotic treatment of spinal trauma may be indicated only for clinically stable spinal fractures. Thus, the treatment team must have a common understanding of the definitions of the terms clinical "stability" and "instability" of the spine.

Before proceeding with orthotic treatment procedures, it is incumbent on the orthotist to independently verify the stability of the injury to the spine. The mechanism of injury, results of clinical examination, and radiologic evidence should be considered. In general, if the integrity of the anterior and/or posterior ligamentous complex is compromised, the injury should be considered unstable (Table 10-1).

Cervical spine fractures

An axial load applied to the top of the head and transferred through the condyles of the occiput can fracture the ring of the first cervical vertebra. This is known as a *Jefferson fracture*. Typically, C1 is split into multiple fragments, and the injury is unstable in all three anatomical planes. In the absence of external support, the patient is at high risk for neurologic damage because motion of the head is not constrained.

A *hangman fracture* is a fracture through the pedicles of C2 that separates the posterior neural arch from the vertebral body. The mechanism of injury, which consists of hyperextension followed by distraction, is called *traumatic spondylolisthesis*. The spinal cord may be compressed, with possible transient neurologic findings. This injury

Table 10-1 Criteria for stability of spine

History of Mechanism of Injury	Physical and Neurologic Examinations	X-ray Examination Specific Criteria
Flexion-rotation Excessive flexion	Palpable spine defect Motor/reflex/sensation alteration Abrasions on the back	Spinous process separation Articular process dislocation and/or fracture
Disruption of posterior ligamentous complex	Disruption of posterior ligamentous complex	Disruption of posterior ligamentous complex

Hoppenfeld S: Orthopedic neurology: a diagnostic guide to neurologic levels, Philadephia, Lippincott Williams & Wilkins, 1977

also is unstable in all three anatomical planes, and the risk of neurologic damage is high in the absence of external support.

Fractures of the odontoid are caused by a combination of shear and compression loading and may result from a blow to the back of the head. In the rare case where the fracture is through the tip of the odontoid (*type I* fracture), the injury is stable. A *type II* odontoid fracture is through the base of the odontoid body. With a type III fracture, the fracture line is into the body of the vertebra. Types II and III are considered unstable; however, the clinical outcome is better for type III fractures because of the higher rate of bony union.

Compression fractures in the region C3–7 are hyperflexion injuries where the endplates of the vertebra may be damaged and the vertebral body fractured. The most common level of injury is C5, and the brachial plexus may be involved.[14] Hyperextension injuries (e.g., from whiplash) are mostly soft-tissue injuries, and the anterior longitudinal ligament may be ruptured. A full clinical assessment must be performed to determine whether the injury is stable.[25]

Facet joint dislocations

Facet joint dislocations involve disruption of the joint capsule and possibly the posterior ligament. Unilateral facet fractures are caused by lateral flexion and rotation and result in narrowing of the spinal canal and neural foramen. For example, a T3–4 unilateral facet fracture may be a shoulder belt injury from a motor vehicle accident. The vertebral body usually is dislocated less than 50% anteriorly, and approximately 75% of patients have no neurologic involvement. Unilateral facet joint dislocations are considered stable fractures but may result in isolated paralysis, such as Brown-Séquard syndrome (one-sided paralysis).

In bilateral facet dislocations, the facet capsules, posterior ligament, and intervertebral disc are disrupted. The mechanism of injury is severe flexion with some rotation, with the vertebral body displaced by more than half of its anterior-posterior dimension. Approximately 85% of patients have neurologic lesions because of the greater narrowing of the spinal canal. The most common level of injury is C5–6 where the range of motion is greatest (except for C1–2). Risk factors include spondylosis, degenerative disc disease,

decreased range of motion, and age over 50 years. These fractures are considered unstable.

Thoracic and thoracolumbar spine fractures

Normal thoracic kyphosis ranges from 20 to 50 degrees.[2] Because of the kyphotic posture, the thoracic spine is especially vulnerable to flexion injuries. On the other hand, the ribs and their articulations provide considerable additional stability by restricting the mobility of the vertebrae. The lower thoracic vertebrae from T9–12 are considered transitional vertebrae and have more mobility.

Compression fractures are characterized by impaction of the anterior aspect of the vertebral body. The mechanisms of injury involve flexion and compression of the affected segments. These fractures are stable so long as the anterior and posterior longitudinal ligaments as well as the posterior ligamentous complex are intact. Moreover, the spinous processes must not be separated.

Spinal trauma can be categorized with the Denis classification[7] of acute thoracolumbar spinal injuries using a three-column theory (Fig. 10-1). If the anterior column of the spine alone is injured (Denis type I), the mechanism of injury is flexion followed by compression. If the anterior and middle columns are injured, causing a burst fracture (Denis type II), the mechanism of injury is compression followed by flexion. The posterior and middle columns can be injured through the mechanism of flexion followed by distraction (Denis type III). They can be through bone (Chance fracture), soft tissue (slice fracture), or a combination of the two. Fractures through soft tissue usually are treated surgically.

The Chance fracture often results from a motor vehicle accident. They are referred to as *lap belt injuries* because they occur when the occupant is wearing a lap belt with no shoulder harness. Other causes include the abdomen hitting a solid object such as a tree or pole. The most common Chance fracture involves the posterior elements of the involved vertebra and possibly the posterior aspect of the vertebra. The second type of Chance fracture involves the posterior elements as before; in addition there is a significant transverse fracture of the vertebral body. The third type of Chance fracture involves the interspinous ligaments, facets, and disc. In all types, the pedicles and the transverse and spinous processes are intact. Clearly, as the amount of damage increases, the likelihood of having a stable fracture decreases.

According to Denis,[7] approximately 50% of all fractures occur between T11–12 and L1–L2 levels, and almost half of thoracolumbar fractures that occur are compression fractures.

Lumbar spine fractures

Compression fractures typically occur in the upper part of the lumbar spine. Regardless of the location, it is essential to check for the integrity of the anterior longitudinal ligament, which is well developed in the lumbar region and is largely responsible for stability in this region of the spine.

Spondylolysis is the fracture of the pars interarticularis and is a stable condition. Spondylolisthesis is the anterior migration of one vertebral body over another and may or may not be stable.

COMPRESSION FRACTURES (DENIS TYPE 1)
Mechanism of injury: spinal flexion with compression
Subtype   I-A   Anterior fracture only
           I-B   Anterior fracture with lateral
                  components

BURST FRACTURES (DENIS TYPE II)
Mechanism of injury: spinal compression with flexion
Subtype   II-A   Fracture of both end plates or
                  retropulsion, or both, of the
                  posterior wall as a free fragment
           II-B   Fracture of the superior end plate;
                  occasional retropulsion of inferior
                  wall as a free fragment
           II-C   Fracture of the inferior end plate
           II-D   Burst fracture with rotational injury
           II-E   Burst fracture with lateral flexion
                  injury

SEAT BELT INJURIES (DENIS TYPE III)
Mechanism of injury: spinal flexion with distraction
Subtype   III-A (Chance fracture) single segments,
                  posterior or middle column
                  opening
           III-B (Slice fracture) single segments,
                  posterior and middle column
                  opening through soft and bony
                  Tissue
           III-C Two segments, posterior and
                  middle column opening through
                  soft and bony tissue
           III-D Two segments, posterior and
                  middle column opening through
                  soft tissue only

FRACTURE DISLOCATIONS (DENIS TYPE IV)
Mechanism of injury: translation, flexion, rotation,
With shear
Subtype   IV-A   Flexion and rotation injury with
                  disruption through bone or
                  intervertebral disk, or both
           IV-B   Due to shear (anterior-posterior
                  or posterior-anterior) with fracture
                  and dislocation of facet joints
           IV-C   Ligamentous and injury to posterior
                  and middle column, with failure
                  (marked instability) of the
                  anterior column
           IV-D   Oblique shear forces resulting in
                  significant instability of involved
                  segment (bone or disk)

Fig. 10-1 Classification system for traumatic fractures of the thoraco-lumbar spine. (From Lusardi MM, Nielsen CC: *Orthotics and prosthetics in rehabilitation.* Philadelphia, WB Saunders, 2007.)

Postoperative care

Early ambulation postoperatively is often in the patient's best interest. However, additional loads that may be placed on the spine during gait must not damage the surgical construct of a spinal fusion. Besides upright posture and ambulation, even greater loads may be present in the seated posture, and caution must be exercised. Thus, the splinting effect of the orthosis may be helpful in protecting the surgical construct, bone–construct interface, and, if appropriate, biologic fusion. The excessive tissue between the spine and the orthosis may

make the orthosis less effective in stabilizing the construct and preventing unwanted movements that may damage it and slow the healing process. Knowledge of common surgical procedures and surgical construct characteristics are important. Specifically, a good understanding of planes of motion where the construct is susceptible to failure can help with appropriate orthotic treatment.

Complicating factors

Obesity occurs in near epidemic proportions in the United States.[34] The presence of substantial excess adipose tissue may deteriorate the performance of an orthosis by compromising its stabilizing effects.[1] Because the orthotic practitioner likely will treat patients with the comorbidity of obesity, strategies should be in place to cope with this complication.[14]

Historical perspective
Spinal trauma

Orthotic treatments of spinal trauma have evolved over centuries. They all are based on the ideas of immobilization of the fracture to reduce pain and reduction of the deformities associated with particular injuries. Early devices were made of materials such as whalebone and wood. Plaster body casts became popular in more modern times. Orthoses for spinal trauma formerly constructed with metal components in the early to middle twentieth century have been replaced by orthoses constructed from thermoplastics. In 2006, ever increasing numbers of prefabricated orthoses were being used to treat spinal trauma.

Understanding the historical traditional approaches to spinal trauma and treatment provides a foundation for learning from previous successes and decreasing the probability of future mistakes. These approaches are related specifically to the mechanism of injury (of the trauma) and the mechanism of action (orthotic treatment) addressing the injury. The mechanism of injury in the past (and frequently in the present) was routinely categorized by terms such as lateral flexion, compression, rotation, and extension injuries. Although this approach can have meaningful clinical application, it also runs the risk of oversimplifying complex injury mechanisms that then are managed orthotically in an inappropriate manner (Fig. 10-2).[37]

For example, a patient may present with an anterior compression fracture that resulted from a small compressive load but also associated with a major forward bending moment that has simultaneously disrupted the posterior ligamentous structures. The result is a motion segment more susceptible to instability secondary to shear. This also has been liberally reported as the main factor for destabilization of a compression fracture.[21,37,38] If the focus remains only on the compression fracture, then the logical orthotic treatment may result in use of a Jewett three-point hyperextension orthosis. Although the lumbar pad is an important element of this three-point hyperextension addressing the compression fracture, it also introduces the element of shear with its anteriorly directed transverse force. Ultimately the patient is at greater risk for further instability and increased discomfort. In this example, a better knowledge of the mechanism of injury may have resulted in a more logical and predictable treatment strategy and outcome.

	Level		Type	Mechanism of Injury	Remarks	Orthoses
Upper cervical	C1		Jefferson	Axial load	Tri-planar instability	Halo-vest
	C2		Hangman	Hyperextension plus distraction	Traumatic spondylolisthesis, tri-planar instability	Halo-vest
			Odontoid	Shear plus compression	Type I - stable, Types II & III - unstable	Halo-vest
Lower cervical	C3-C7		Anterior compression	Hyperflexion	C5 most common level, possible brachial plexus involvement	Rigid collar
			Whiplash	Hyperextension	Soft tissue injury to anterior longitudinal ligament likely, long-term risk for chronic forward head posture.	Soft collar
Cervicothoracic junction–injuries spanning this level require a CTO or CTLSO						
Upper thoracic	T1-T8	Denis Classification applies to all thoracic and lumbar levels.	Denis I - Anterior Compression	Flexion plus compression	Three-fourths of thoracolumbar fractures are of this type, two-thirds of those occur at T12-L1-L2. Anterior column damage only in most cases. Posterior ligamentous injury may indicate instability.	Hyperextension is the mechanism of action. Common choices: corsets, Jewett (milder injuries), and TLSOs (custom or pre-fab).
			Denis II - Burst	Compression plus flexion	Anterior and middle columns are damaged. Fracture of superior endplate is more common. There may be retropulsion of one or more fragments from the posterior wall.	
Lower thoracic	T9-T12		Denis III - Chance and Slice	Flexion plus distraction ("seat belt injury")	Chance: Posterior and middle column damage to vertebral body. Slice: Posterior and middle column damage to intervertebral disc. Surgery is indicated.	
Thoracolumbar junction–T12-L1-L2 are very common fracture sites and require a TLSO						
Upper lumbar	L1-L2		Denis IV - Fracture dislocation	Translation, Flexion, Rotation, Shear	Complete disruption of anterior, middle, and posterior columns. Surgery is indicated.	N/A
Lower lumbar	L3-L5	Other	Spondylolysis and spondylolisthesis	May be a sports-related injury from gymnastics. In adults, may cause chronic LBP.	Common in the lower lumbar spine especially L4-L5 and L5-S1. Spondylolisthesis usually requires posterior pelvic tilt in the orthosis.	Custom LSO or TLSO

Fig. 10-2 Summary of main fracture types. *CTO*, Cervicothoracic orthosis; *LBP*, lower back pain; *LSO*, lumbosacral orthosis; *TLSO*, thoracolumbosacral orthosis.

Using the previous case as an example, the mechanism of action must be investigated thoroughly before a decision regarding orthotic treatment. In this case, the issue requiring greatest attention is not the hyperextension itself but how the hyperextension was achieved. A three-point hyperextension orthosis introduces the appropriate mechanism of hyperextension, but at the expense of introducing shear to the fracture site. A total-contact polymer thoracolumbosacral orthosis (TLSO) is a reasonable alternative because the patient can be hyperextended using a sagittal bending moment while not introducing shear. In addition to addressing the compression fracture, this orthosis likely will be more comfortable for the patient. It is important to note that the degree of ligamentous injury could eliminate completely the option for orthotic treatment and warrant future surgery. However, this case serves a purpose and underscores the need for greater consideration for the mechanism of injury and mechanism of action. Although previous thinking should not be abandoned, it should be the foundation for greater attention to detail and for a clear decision about the specific mechanism of action of orthotic treatment.

Postoperative care

In the early days of spinal fusion, body jackets commonly were used postoperatively. Of course, the goal was to provide additional stability to the surgical construct to allow it to heal properly. Today, the role of postoperative orthoses remains controversial. Some argue that modern surgical techniques and devices provide all the stability necessary to allow for proper healing without an orthosis. On the other hand, surgical failures still occur, especially when postoperative bracing is omitted from the treatment plan. One of the problems with settling the controversy is that insufficient research demonstrates the efficacy of postoperative spinal orthoses in specific surgical procedures.

Current issues and research

Choices of spinal orthoses for trauma and postoperative care include prefabricated and custom devices. However, definitive answers to the basic questions of when to use spinal orthoses and whether they are effective remain incomplete, and further research is needed. It is useful to divide the discussion between (a) nonsurgical treatments of spinal trauma and (b) postoperative care. In each case, orthotic management may or may not be part of the treatment plan.

When an orthosis is part of the treatment plan, the prescribing physician must decide from among prefabricated, made to measure, and custom-fit devices. The efficacy of the different choices often is not well understood, and further research is needed.

Nonsurgical treatments of spinal trauma

Cervical fractures

The primary orthotic goal is to immobilize a fracture of the cervical spine. The orthotist may be faced with the questions of which orthosis to recommend, and, in particular, whether the recommended device should be a cervical orthosis or a cervicothoracic orthosis. These devices are used for both nonoperative and postoperative care. To shed light on the issue, Gavin et al.[11] analyzed two cervical orthoses (Aspen and Miami J) and two cervicothoracic orthoses (Aspen two-post and Aspen four-post) using video fluoroscopy. They concluded that cervicothoracic orthoses provided significantly more reduction of cervical intervertebral and gross range of motion in 20 normal subjects compared to cervical orthoses. The two collars performed the same.

In the elderly, half of cervical spine fractures occur at the C1-C2 level. Fractures of the odontoid are the most common cervical fractures in patients older than 70 years and account for 10% to 15% of all fractures of the cervical spine.[30,33] Tashjian et al.[33] studied 78 patients older than 65 years with type II or type III fractures of the odontoid, which were considered unstable. They found that the patients managed with a halo vest had a mortality rate of 21% as well as higher rates of complications such as pneumonia and cardiac arrest compared with patients managed surgically or with a rigid cervical orthosis. The study also suggested that when managing an elderly patient having an odontoid fracture with a halo vest, extreme caution and daily supervision are required.

Injuries to the cervical spine resulting from motor vehicle accidents are common. Reduction or reversal of cervical lordosis that can lead to abnormal forward head posture is associated with whiplash injuries. With the head forward of its normal position, loads on the posterior musculature and vertebral bodies can increase significantly. Cervical kyphosis is a known primary risk factor for chronic pain in whiplash-associated disorders.[15] Some evidence indicates that correcting the posture can relieve the symptoms to a great extent.[9] An orthosis for this purpose should use the mechanism of retraction of the head rather than extension.[25]

Thoracolumbar fractures

Nonsurgical treatment of anterior compression fractures remains controversial. There is a broad spectrum of opinions on whether orthotic management should be part of the treatment plan. Some studies, such as that by Ohana et al.,[27] suggest that up to 30% of single-column anterior compression fractures may be treated with early ambulation and hyperextension exercises and that an orthosis is not required. A retrospective study by Dai[5] of 54 patients with lower lumbar fractures stated that conservative management is indicated for stable compression fractures and surgery for other fractures.

Nonsurgical management of traumatic thoracolumbar burst fractures also is controversial. Advocates of surgical treatment cite spinal realignment, reduction of deformity, neurologic stability, and pain reduction as indications for surgical intervention. Proponents of nonsurgical treatment (bed rest, body cast, orthotic management) argue that results are comparable to long-term surgical outcomes without the risks of surgery. Although some evidence supports nonsurgical treatment, the difficulty lies in determining the amount of stability necessary for nonsurgical treatment to be as effective as surgical treatment. It is important to note that success of orthotic management should not be measured only by the fit of the orthosis.

Weinstein et al.[36] assessed the long-term effects of nonsurgical management of traumatic burst fractures. The average time from injury to follow-up was 20.2 years. Results indicated that patients with no neurologic deficit who were treated conservatively had good long-term effects. Work ability was not affected in 88% of individuals. Only three of 42 patients required surgery, and none of the 42 patients showed neurologic deterioration.[1] In another study, Krompinger et al.[18] found that nonsurgical treatment was effective when canal compromise was less than 50% and kyphotic angle less than 30 degrees. A study by Knight et al.[16] comparing surgical to nonsurgical treatment of thoracolumbar burst fractures indicates no significant difference in treatment outcomes between the two options. Although the surgical group revealed more significant deformity, the mild deformity responded effectively to nonsurgical treatment, and individuals were able to decrease, on average, their hospital stay and were able to return to work sooner than the surgical group. In a study by Chow et al.,[4] hyperextension casting and orthotic management were used to treat 24 patients with thoracolumbar burst fractures and determine functional outcome. At final follow-up (mean 34.3 months), 79% of patients complained of little to no pain; 75% returned to work; 75% stated that they had little to no restriction at work; and only 4% stated that they were dissatisfied with the nonsurgical treatment.

Although evidence appears to support nonsurgical management as an alternative to surgical treatment for thoracolumbar burst fractures, remaining questions about the different types of nonsurgical treatments and the most effective type of treatment warrant further research. Additional research is needed to determine the level of burst fracture deformity that will respond best to nonsurgical management.

Postoperative care

Implants used for surgical treatment of spinal trauma are designed to support the construct until fusion is established. The fused bone then supports the loads that previously were taken up by the implant. Some studies support the contention that no additional external support is needed to help the fusion heal and that no orthosis is required. However, other studies support the use of postoperative orthoses because they are thought to protect the construct from unwanted external loads that may compromise the healing process. In a retrospective study of 109 patients who had undergone a spinal fusion for thoracic and/or lumbar spinal trauma, Benzel and Larson[1] argue in favor of postoperative splinting for early ambulation.

For individuals presenting with fractures or instrumentation at or superior to T3, it is important to consider using over-the-shoulder straps to extend the lever of the existing TLSO. This will discourage further vertebral sway and increase stability. The line of pull of the over-the-shoulder straps should be based on the mechanism of injury and the motion being reduced. For fractures at T2 or above, the combined TLSO and over-the-shoulder straps appear to lose some of their effectiveness, requiring the use of a cervicothoracic orthosis.

---

[1]In this study, 17% (7/42) of patients exhibited neurologic improvement using the Frankel scale for neurologic status.

Orthotic management and treatment

Nonoperative management

Nonoperative management of spinal trauma consists of bed rest, moderate activity, and/or orthotic management. For certain fracture types, nonoperative treatment is a reasonable alternative to surgery and offers comparable long-term results. For other fracture types, the choice between operative and nonoperative treatment remains controversial. However, other types of fractures appear to respond only to operative management. In all cases, agreement regarding spinal stability/instability and what defines successful management should be the foundation for making treatment decisions. Consideration of orthotic management is based on stability, fracture type, comorbidity, and intended outcome. Many studies have compared nonoperative to operative treatment, but few have compared the various types of orthotic treatments with one another.

To appreciate the efficacy of orthotic management, it is necessary to review management based on individual fracture types. Fracture types can be divided into cervical and thoracolumbar injuries. For thoracolumbar injuries, the Denis classification[7] describes four major types of spinal fractures: (a) compression fractures, (b) burst fractures, (c) seatbelt fractures, and (d) fracture dislocation.

The practitioner managing patients with a traumatic spinal fracture must have a clear knowledge of the goal of orthotic management and what outcome is deemed successful. In many instances, the orthosis could meet all fitting expectations and yet fail to achieve acceptable geometric alignment of the injury and long-term functional outcome. As a result, orthotic management may be abandoned in favor of surgical intervention rather than a design change to improve the effectiveness of the orthosis.

If orthotic management is a reasonable alternative to surgery, then it should be held to the same rigorous standards that define success for similar spinal injuries managed surgically. This includes the geometric changes (kyphotic angle and restoration of vertebral height) of the fracture site based on treatment and long-term outcomes such as capacity to work, pain reduction, and restoration of activities of daily living.

For the majority of spinal injuries at the macro level, the primary orthotic goal is protecting the spinal column from loads and stresses that would likely cause progression of the spinal deformity and not allow for adequate healing of the injury.[29,37] To achieve this goal, the orthotic design should have the ability to (a) limit gross vertebral sway (motion) of the spinal column, (b) limit intersegmental motion at the injured site, and (c) provide proper spinal alignment/realignment as it relates to the injured site. Limitation of both gross and localized motion minimizes bending moments that could prevent healing and cause further deformity. Spinal alignment/realignment attempts to restore the anatomical geometry of the injured site and has the ability to shift the axial load path away from the injured site. When orthotic management is indicated for Denis classification types I, II, and III, the mechanism of action for this orthosis should include sagittal hyperextension. Information for nonoperative management of traumatic spinal injuries is given in Box 10-1.

> **BOX 10-1**
> **Important Considerations for the Nonoperative Management of Traumatic Spinal Injuries**
>
> - Cause of injury
> - Type of injury
> - Extent of soft tissue injury
> - Level/location of pain
> - Neurologic status
> - Additional injuries
> - Position that increases/decreases pain

Thoracolumbar compression fractures

Single-column compression fractures with a loss of one third or less of the original anterior height of the vertebra can be managed effectively with initial bed rest to allow elastic recoil of the injury. This can be followed with a regimen of specific exercises and activities.[37]

For more involved compression fractures, TLSO anterior control may be sufficient to resist further deformity but is dependent upon the percent loss of segmental stiffness. According to Patwardhan et al.,[29] single-level injuries with up to 50% loss of segmental stiffness can be managed with Jewett-style TLSO anterior control to effectively restore normal resistance to the deformity. With loss of segmental stiffness between 50% and 85%, the orthosis can effectively restore resistance to deformity when associated with restricted patient activity level in the orthosis. In cases where segmental stiffness loss exceeds 85%, the orthosis does not appear to effectively prevent progression of the deformity. Under circumstances where the compression fracture does not respond favorably to TLSO anterior control, orthotic management need not necessarily be abandoned; rather, alternative consideration may warrant use of a total-contact polymer TLSO.

Thoracolumbar burst fractures

Orthotic management for burst fractures remains controversial, yet evidence suggests that it is a reasonable alternative to surgery.[6,22,39] The mechanism of injury for a burst fracture and the resulting instability dictate to a large degree the appropriate orthotic treatment plan. For burst fractures, the typical mechanism of injury is axial compression plus sagittal flexion (Figs. 10-3 and 10-4). Although the resulting deformity could persist into further flexion and loss of vertebral height, studies indicate significant instability in the transverse plane as well.[24]

This transverse instability should alert the orthotic practitioner to the need for more aggressive orthotic treatment. For this reason, the most effective orthotic treatment is the total-contact polymer TLSO. This design can maintain sagittal hyperextension with concomitant management of the rotation deficit. Although evidence suggests that TLSO anterior control can be effective for some burst fractures, the underlying transverse instability is best managed by the total-contact polymer TLSO.[20] Because the total-contact TLSO has been shown to limit gross trunk motion more effectively than other orthotic designs, it should be the preferred method of treatment for burst.[8,19] For fractures in the more inferior lumbar region, consideration should be given to a thigh

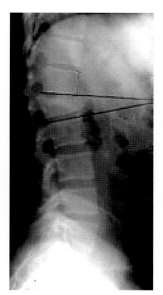

Fig. 10-3 Preorthosis radiograph depicts a burst fracture with disruption of the anterior and middle columns.

extension as the effectiveness of segmental motion control diminishes.[10,23,26]

The effectiveness of orthotic management for burst fractures can be measured against geometric and functional outcomes that include the following:

- Reduced kyphotic angle (neutral)
- Decreased percentage of sagittal vertebral compression
- Decreased percentage of canal compromise
- No change in neurologic status
- Decreased level of pain
- Improvement or return to previous activities of daily living
- Ability to return to work

Similar outcome measures are routinely used to determine not only success but also the type of surgical procedure. Ligamentous and neurologic status are factors that influence the physician's decision to decompress anteriorly or posteriorly. Reconstruction and stabilization of the spine may include use of a strut graft or cage and a side-mounted plate or rod system.[35]

Seat belt fractures

Seat belt injuries are the result of mechanisms related to flexion and distraction. In this type of presentation, the injury propagates from posterior to anterior. For a bony Chance fracture, the posterior and middle columns are compromised, but the soft tissue remains intact. For a ligamentous Chance or slice fracture, the injury propagates from posterior to anterior and through the soft tissue instead. In this scenario, the intervertebral disc likely has sustained injury. Although distinct bony or soft-tissue seat belt injuries do occur, a combination of osseous and soft-tissue damage across a motion segment is not uncommon (Figs. 10-5 through 10-8).

Successful orthotic management for this type of injury usually is predicated on the ability to maintain appropriate sagittal hyperextension. When the posterior and middle columns are osseous injuries, orthotic treatment has been cited to be very effective when the mechanism of action for the orthosis is hyperextension.[3,12] However, as a greater percentage of soft-tissue damage is included in this category of injury, the success of orthotic management becomes less predictable.

The most common types of orthotic management for this injury are TLSO anterior control and the total-contact polymer TLSO. Although evidence indicates that TLSO anterior control can be successful, it does have limitations and may not have the design capability to hyperextend the patient enough to reduce the injury. Second, the TLSO anterior control design includes a posterior lumbar pad, which induces an anteriorly directed force when the device is worn by the patient. This anteriorly directed shear force increases the possibility of translation across the injured site. In our experience,

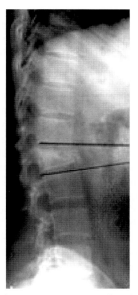

Fig. 10-4 In-orthosis (custom polymer TLSO) radiograph of the same patient shown in Fig. 10-3 reveals proper segmental hyperextension and reduction of the kyphotic angle for this burst fracture.

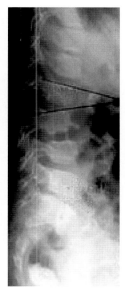

Fig. 10-5 Preorthosis (custom polymer TLSO) radiograph shows disruption of the posterior and middle columns resulting in a Chance fracture.

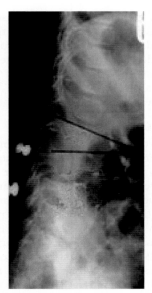

Fig. 10-6 In-orthosis radiograph reveals only minimal extension at the injured segment. As a result, a second custom polymer TLSO with greater sagittal hyperextension was fabricated.

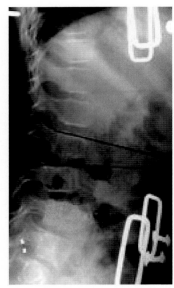

Fig. 10-8 After nearly 5 months in the second TLSO, the in-orthosis film reveals that proper sagittal extension continues to be maintained for the Chance fracture.

patients who wear this type of orthosis experience greater discomfort in the region just inferior to the shear force exerted by the lumbar pad. These factors should be carefully considered when determining appropriate orthotic treatment. In this case, use of a total-contact polymer TLSO has the advantage of creating hyperextension by introducing a sagittal bending moment without the component of shear. This may increase patient compliance and improve the possibility of reducing the fracture.

For fractures with a significant amount of compromised soft tissue and kyphotic angulation, surgery can be pursued as an alternative to orthotic management. Options include short segmental compression with open reduction, posterior

instrumentation, and combined posterior fusion. Clinical outcome is based on back pain and function, kyphotic angulation, solid union of fusion, and neurologic status.[32]

Impression process for hyperextension

When using a custom-molded polymer TLSO to manage Chance or burst fractures, the practitioner should be prepared to spend up to 2 hours during the initial measurement and impression phase of treatment. After initial assessment, application of the stockinette, and measurement/landmark identification, the patient should be placed recumbent and in the supine position. A small bolster (e.g., a towel) should be placed under the patient and located under the fracture site to facilitate spinal hyperextension. It is important to progressively increase the bolster over time (10 to 30 minutes) and in small increments to foster proper viscoelastic change in order to achieve maximum hyperextension.[28] If the process occurs too quickly, the patient likely will experience more discomfort and be unwilling to continue with the process (Figs. 10-9 and 10-10).

After maximum hyperextension is achieved and the patient still in a supine position, the sternal angle and pubic angle should be measured and recorded for later reconciliation during positive cast modification (Fig. 10-11). After the anterior impression has set, the patient is placed into a prone position, and measurements and landmarks are identified and recorded, including the degree of lordosis as measured with a surface gauge goniometer along the spinous processes. The patient is asked to elevate onto his or her elbows to create hyperextension while in a prone position. This angle is measured and recorded. If the patient is unable to sustain independently the position, pillows can be used effectively to maintain the desired hyperextension. Posterior plaster splints are applied and remain in place until set. Once the impression is removed and the cast modification process begins, it is important to pay particular attention to achieving the desired sagittal angles obtained during the impression process.

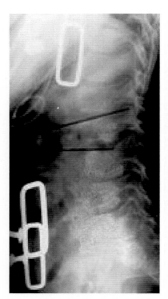

Fig. 10-7 In-orthosis radiograph for the second custom polymer TLSO depicts much better results.

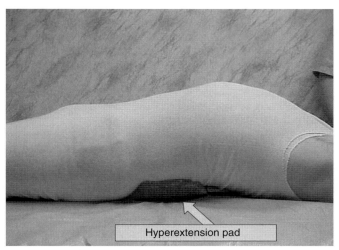

Fig. 10-9 Placement of the bolster in relationship to the fracture site is important for proper spinal geometry and is most effective when the practitioner allows for proper viscoelastic changes to occur over a period of 20 to 30 minutes. An unwillingness to wait for this process may increase the patient's discomfort and decrease the chances of adequately reducing the fracture.

Cervical injuries

Hangman fractures (traumatic spondylolisthesis of C2) The hangman fracture typically is characterized by a bilateral fracture through the pedicles and is secondary to hyperextension. A hangman fracture with concomitant facet dislocation is considered unstable. It has a high incidence of neurologic compromise and must be managed initially with cervical traction. For fractures without facet dislocation, conservative treatment with a cervical orthosis is considered appropriate. Effective orthotic designs should include a longer lever arm posteriorly and short anteriorly in order to encourage cervical flexion through kinesthetic reminder and the patient's intact righting reflex. In some cases, the halo vest may be indicated as a better form of nonsurgical treatment and increased stability.

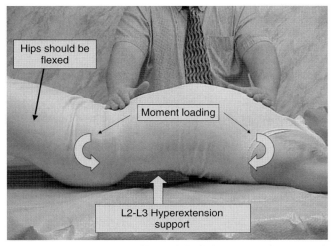

Fig. 10-10 To facilitate the effects of the bolster, a gentle posteriorly directed force at the pubis and superior sternum should be a consideration after the anterior splints have been applied. The patient is likely to tolerate this maneuver better if it is preceded by incremental increases in the height of the bolster using the principles of viscoelastic change.

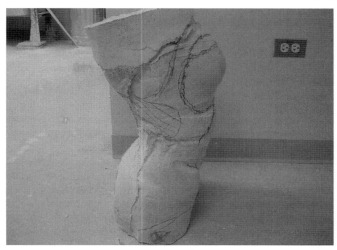

Fig. 10-11 View of the positive cast in the sagittal plane reveals the sagittal hyperextension that must be captured in the impression and subsequent positive cast. This alignment can improve geometry and limit or reduce the deforming force on the fracture site as it heals.

Odontoid fractures Odontoid fractures are classified as type I, II, and III. *Type I* is a fracture of the tip of the dens and is considered a stable fracture. A *type II* odontoid fracture occurs at the base of the dens and has the highest incidence of nonunion compared to type I and III fractures. Several theories account for the high incidence of nonunion, but the lack of blood supply to this area and the relatively small amount of cancellous bone appear to be the chief reasons for nonunion. The lack of blood supply and subsequent nonunion appear to result from envelopment of the dens in a synovial capsule that prevents it from receiving periosteal blood supply. Conservative treatment of type II fracture has involved either a cervical orthosis or halo vest. For the elderly population, a cervical orthosis is recommended as the initial treatment option because higher incidences of morbidity and mortality have been reported with use of the halo vest in this population.[13] A *type III* fracture occurs into the body, tends be more stable, and has a better blood supply. Type III appears to respond well to conservative treatment with a cervical orthosis, primarily due to its inherent stability.

Jefferson fractures The Jefferson fracture is a fracture of the C1 atlas that results from axial compression. The downward force of the occipital condyles causes the lateral masses of C1 to fracture and be displaced laterally. The degree of lateral displacement determines the level of stability. Associated with the lateral displacement are fractures of the anterior and posterior arches of C1. Conservative treatment is indicated when lateral displacement is less than 7 mm and can be managed using a halo vest.

Postoperative orthotic management

The need for postoperative orthotic management as an adjunct to previous surgical management is controversial. The lack of evidence and limited research supporting or refuting the efficacy of postoperative management is an important question that needs to be answered. In most cases, evidence is empirical at best. The purpose of postoperative management is to protect the surgical construct and construct–bone interface from failure secondary to planar motion that usually includes a combination of rotation and a second motion.

Early mobilization and decreased pain are described as benefits to postoperative management. The total-contact polymer TLSO remains the ideal orthosis because it has the best opportunity to address combined motions detrimental to the surgical site. Bivalve TLSOs remain the most practical option for donning and doffing because the patient is likely to be fit in a recumbent position. For patients in whom the surgery site extends down to and includes the sacrum, the addition of a thigh extension to the TLSO that provides a longer lever arm for greater stability and protection of the surgical sight is recommended. According to Schimandle et al.,[31] patients who wore a thigh extension in addition to the TLSO had a 20% decrease in failure at the site of the fusion. Equally important is the decision of what limb to place the thigh extension. In a separate study using videofluoroscopy, both rotation and intervertebral motion were decreased when a TLSO was used compared to no TLSO.[17] These motions were further decreased with use of a thigh extension. It is recommended that the thigh extension be placed on the limb with one or more of the following presentations: (a) autograph harvested from the iliac crest; (b) lower limb weakness that is greater than the contralateral limb; and (c) the limb nearest the inside of the car door for ease of getting in and out of a vehicle.

Patients typically remain in the orthosis for 4 to 6 months or until biologic fusion has occurred. This time frame may be less for younger patients and longer for older patients, but it also is dependent upon the underlying pathology and the health of the bone. Early weaning or decreasing the original height of the TLSO may have the adverse effect of adding a stress riser and making the fusion more susceptible to failure. Information for orthotic postoperative management is given in Box 10-2.

Best practices

Application of the principles discussed in this chapter is illustrated through a case study. The intention is to draw attention to several common clinical issues that arise in orthotic management of spinal trauma and how best to address them.

Case study

Anterior compression fractures of the thoracolumbar junction constitute approximately 50% of all thoracolumbar fractures.

BOX 10-2
Important Considerations for Orthotic Postoperative Management

- Reason for surgery
- Type of surgery
- Surgical complications that alter or affect orthotic treatment
- Level of surgery
- Surgical construct (if any) that was used
- Origin/location of bone graft
- Co-morbidity

Orthotic management of these fractures is common and is considered routine by many orthotic practitioners. In many cases this is true. However, the following "typical" example demonstrates the need to critically evaluate the orthotic recommendation in all cases, whether or not considered routine.

Clinical information

A male patient, approximately 35 years of age, presented with a stable anterior compression fracture of L1 from a motor vehicle accident. His main complaint was pain. As shown on the sagittal plane x-ray film (Fig. 10-12), there is approximately 20% to 25% reduction in the height of the anterior column, supporting the clinical characterization of a stable fracture. Note the fragment coming off the anterior superior region of the vertebra. A transverse plane magnetic resonance image shows evidence of an asymmetric insult to the vertebral body, with more damage on the left side. A coronal plane x-ray film reveals a small left lateral curvature of the lumbar spine. As may be expected, a three-point hyperextension orthosis (Jewett orthosis) was prescribed and fitted to the patient. Figures 10-13 and 10-14 show several views of the patient in the orthosis. Unfortunately, the patient's symptoms did not resolve, and the pain increased.

Troubleshooting

The outcome of this case emphasizes the importance not only of careful attention to fitting parameters but also of the appropriateness of the orthotic recommendation. Once a particular orthosis is prescribed, undetected errors in fitting may mislead the treatment team to an incorrect conclusion regarding the appropriateness of the orthosis. On the other hand, if the initial orthotic recommendation is inappropriate, no amount of correction to the fitting parameters will yield the desired outcome. Thus, a detailed critical clinical evaluation of the patient, that is, searching for the precise nature of the damage to the spine and how to treat it, is no substitute for more routine and perhaps more superficial approaches.

In assessing the fitting parameters of the Jewett orthosis, the orthosis appears to be shifted in the transverse and coronal plane. For an orthosis with a primary function of limiting sagittal flexion and encouraging hyperextension, this type of shift is problematic because the direction of the force application is no longer specific to just the sagittal plane.

In retrospect, the asymmetry of the damage to the L1 vertebra appears to indicate greater mobility in the coronal plane to the left. Therefore, pushing more in that direction with the posterior pad force increases the deformity and may contribute to the patient's increased pain. Moreover, the damage to the left is more consistent with a two-column burst fracture. Considering this finding, a more likely recommendation might have been a TLSO to provide transverse plane stability, which is not one of the mechanisms of action of a three-point hyperextension orthosis such as the Jewett orthosis.

The initial recommendation of a three-point hyperextension orthosis apparently was inappropriate, given the damage to the L1 vertebra. Even correcting the fitting errors did not improve the outcome. Therefore, in evaluating the orthotic management for spinal trauma, the answer to the fundamental question of the desired mechanism of action of the orthosis

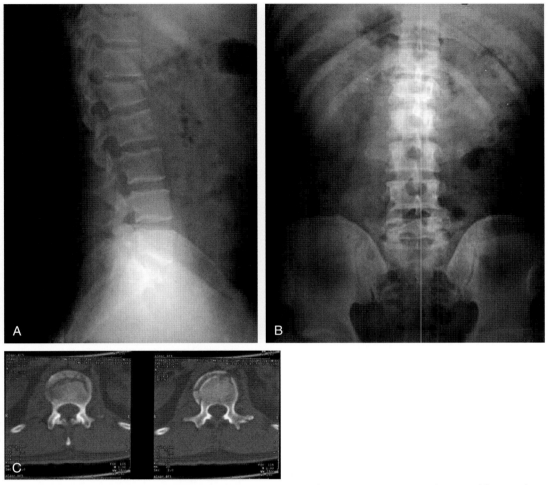

Fig. 10-12 A, Sagittal plane x-ray film. **B,** Coronal plane x-ray film. **C,** Transverse plane magnetic resonance images of fractured vertebra.

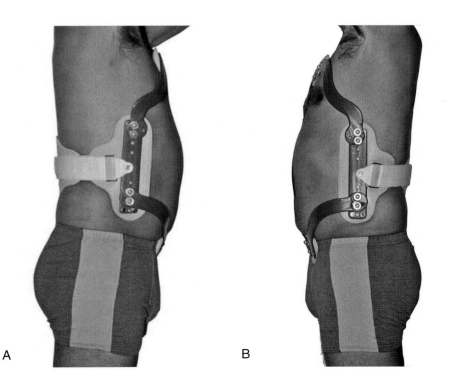

Fig. 10-13 A, Sagittal plane, in orthosis, right side. **B,** Sagittal plane, in orthosis, left side.

Fig. 10-14 A, Coronal plane, in orthosis, anterior view. **B**, Coronal plane, in orthosis, posterior view.

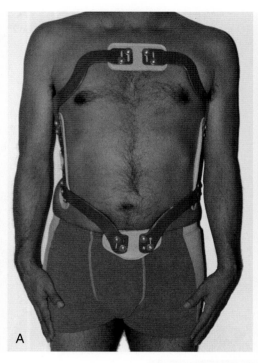

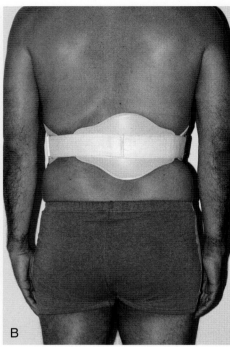

A

B

must be reevaluated if the treatment outcome is not the desired one.

Supporting evidence

Cervical spine

Gavin TM, Carandang G, Havey R, et al Biomechanical analysis of cervical orthoses in flexion and extension: a comparison of cervical collars and cervical orthoses, *J Rehab Res Dev* 40:527-538, 2003.

Tashjian RZ, Majercik S, et al Halo-vest immobilization increases early morbidity and mortality in elderly odontoid fractures, *J Trauma* 60:199-203, 2006.

Thoracolumbar spine

Shen W-J, Liu T-J, Shen Y-S: Nonoperative treatment versus posterior fixation for thoracolumbar junction burst fractures without neurological deficit, *Spine* 26:1038-1045, 2001.

Thomas KC, Bailey CS, Dvorak MF, et al: Comparison of operative and nonoperative treatment for thoracolumbar burst fractures in patients without neurological deficit: a systematic review, *J Neurosurg Spine* 4:351-358, 2006.

Postoperative care

Benzel EC, Larson SJ: Postoperative stabilization of the posttraumatic thoracic and lumbar spine: a review of concepts and orthotic techniques, *J Spinal Disord* 2:47-51, 1989.

References

1. Benzel EC, Larson SJ: Postoperative stabilization of the posttraumatic thoracic and lumbar spine: a review of concepts and orthotic techniques, *J Spinal Disord* 2:47–51, 1989.
2. Bernhardt M, Bridwell KH: Segmental analysis of the sagittal plane alignment of the normal thoracic and lumbar spines and the thoracolumbar junction, *Spine* 14:17, 1989.
3. Chance GQ: Note on a type of flexion fracture of the spine, *Br J Radiol* 21:452, 1948.
4. Chow GH, Nelson BJ, Gebhard JS, et al: Functional outcome of thoracolumbar burst fractures managed with hyperextension casting or bracing and early mobilization, *Spine* 21:2170–2175, 1996.
5. Dai L-Y: Lower lumbar spine fractures: management options, *Int J Care Injured* 33:579–582, 2002.
6. Davies WE, Morris JH, Hill V: An analysis of conservative (nonsurgical) management of thoracolumbar fractures and fracture dislocations with neural damage, *J Bone Joint Surg* 62A:324, 1980.
7. Denis F: The three-column spine and its significance in the classification of acute thoracolumbar spinal injuries, *Spine* 8:817–831, 1983.
8. Dorsky S, Buchalter D, Kahanovitz N, Nordin M: A three dimensional analysis of lumbar brace immobilization utilizing a noninvasive technique, *Proceedings of the 33rd Annual Meeting, Orthopaedic Research Society*, San Francisco, California, 1987.
9. Ferrantelli JR, Harrison DE, Harrison DD, Stewart D: Conservative treatment of a patient with previously unresponsive whiplash-associated disorders using clinical biomechanics of posture rehabilitation methods, *J Manipulative Physiol Ther* 28:205:e1–e8.
10. Fidler MW, Plasmans CMT: The effect of four types of support on the segmental mobility of the lumbosacral spine, *J Bone Joint Surg* 65A:943–947, 1983.
11. Gavin TM, Carandang G, Havey R, et al: Biomechanical analysis of cervical orthoses in flexion and extension: a comparison of cervical collars and cervical orthoses, *J Rehabil Res Dev* 40:527–538, 2003.
12. Gertzbein SD, Court-Brown CM: The rationale for management of flexion/distraction injuries of the thoracolumbar spine based on a new classification, *Proceedings of the 22nd Annual Meeting of the Scoliosis Research Society*, Vancouver, B.C., Canada, September 1987.
13. Glaser JA, Whitehall R, Stamp WG, Jane JA: Complications associated with the halo-vest—a review of 245 cases, *J Neurosurg* 65:762–769, 1986.
14. Hoppenfeld S: Orthopedic neurology: a diagnostic guide to neurologic levels, Philadelphia, Lippincott Williams & Wilkins, 1977.
15. Kai Y, Oyama M, Kurose S: Traumatic thoracic outlet syndrome, *Orthop Traumatol* 47:1169–1171, 1998.
16. Knight RQ, Stornelli DP, Chan DP, Devanny JR: Comparison of operative versus nonoperative treatment of lumbar burst fractures, *Clin Orthop Relat Res* 293:112–121, 1993.
17. Kooi DV, Abad G, Basford JR, Maus TP: Lumbar spine stabilization with a thoracolumbar orthosis, *Spine* 29:100–104, 2004.
18. Krompinger WJ, Fredrickson BE, Mino DE, Yuan HA: Conservative treatment of fractures of the thoracic and lumbar spine, *Orthop Clin North Am* 17:161, 1986.

19. Lantz SA, Schultz AB: Lumbar spine orthosis wearing—I. Restriction of gross body motions, *Spine* 11:834–837, 1986a.

20. Lantz SA, Schultz AB: Lumbar spine orthosis wearing—II. Effect on trunk muscle myoelectric activity, *Spine* 11:838–842, 1986b.

21. Lindahl R, Willen J, Irstam L: Computed tomography of bone fragments in the spinal canal: an experimental study, *Spine* 8:181–186, 1983.

22. McEvoy RD, Bradford DS: The management of burst fractures of the thoracic and lumbar spine: experience in 53 patients, *Spine* 10:631–637, 1985.

23. Morris JM, Lucas DB: Physiological considerations in bracing of the spine, *Orthop Prosth Appl 37* 44, 1963.

24. Nagel DA, Koogle TA, Piziali RL, Perkash I: Stability of the upper lumbar spine following progressive disruptions and the application of individual internal and external fixation devices, *J Bone Joint Surg* 63A:62–70, 1981.

25. Neuman D: *Kinesiology of the musculoskeletal system: foundation for physical rehabilitation*, St. Louis, Elsevier Health Sciences, 2002.

26. Norton PL, Brown T: The immobilizing efficiency of the back braces; their effect on the posture and motion of the lumbosacral spine, *J Bone Joint Surg* 39A:111–139, 1957.

27. Ohana N, Sheinis D, Rath E, et al: Is there a need for lumbar orthosis in mild compression fractures of the lumbar spine?: a retrospective study comparing the radiographic results, *J Spinal Disord* 13:305–308, 2000.

28. Oliver MJ, Twomey LT: Extension creep in the lumbar spine, *Clin Biomech* 10:363–368, 1995.

29. Patwardhan AG, Li S, Gavin TM, et al: Orthotic stabilization of thoracolumbar injuries: a biomechanical analysis of the Jewett hyperextension orthosis, *Spine* 15:654–661, 1990.

30. Ryan MD, Henderson JJ: The epidemiology of fractures and fracture-dislocations of the cervical spine, *Injury* 23:38–40, 1992.

31. Schimandle JH, Weigel M, Edwards CC: Indications for thigh cuff bracing following instrumented lumbosacral fusions, Presented at the eight annual meeting of the North American Spine Society, San Diego, California, October 1993.

32. Shih SL, Wang ST, Ma HL, et al: Surgical treatment of seat belt type injury of the thoracolumbar spine, *Chin Med J* 60:74–80, 1997.

33. Tashjian RZ, Majercik S, et al: Halo-vest immobilization increases early morbidity and mortality in elderly odontoid fractures, *J Trauma* 60:199–203, 2006.

34. U.S. Department of Health and Human Services: *Weight-control information network statistics related to overweight and obesity.* Available at: http://win.niddk.nih.gov/statistics/index.htm, accessed September 9, 2006.

35. Vaccaro AR, Lim MR, Hurlbert RJ, et al: Surgical decision making for unstable thoracolumbar spine injuries: results of a consensus panel review by the spine trauma study group, *J Spinal Disord Tech* 19:1–10, 2006.

36. Weinstein JN, Collalto P, Lehmann TR: Thoracolumbar "burst" fractures treated conservatively: a long-term follow-up, *Spine* 13:33–38, 1988.

37. White A, Panjabi M: *Clinical biomechanics of the spine*, ed 2, Philadelphia: JB Lippincott, 1990.

38. Whitesides TE: Traumatic kyphosis of the thoracolumbar spine, *Clin Orthop* 128:79–92, 1977.

39. Willen J, Lindahl S, Nordwall A: Unstable thoracolumbar fractures: a comparative clinical study of conservative treatment and Harrington instrumentation, *Spine* 10:111–122, 1985.

Chapter

11

Orthoses for osteoporosis

Kevin P. Meade, Bryan S. Malas, Avinash G. Patwardhan, and Thomas M. Gavin

Key Points

- According to the Centers for Disease Control and Prevention, osteoporosis is a disease characterized by low bone mass and deterioration of bone tissue, which can lead to an increased risk for fractures.
- Prevention of vertebral compression fractures (VCFs) from osteoporosis as part of the treatment plan is an important consideration.
- The consequences of VCFs due to osteoporosis include acute and/or chronic back pain, functional limitations, and mood impairment.
- Three categories of treatment options for VCFs are pharmacologic, nonpharmacologic, and surgical.
- A limited number of orthoses have scientific support for their efficacy in treating VCFs.
- A multidisciplinary team approach is necessary to treat patients with VCFs due to osteoporosis.

Pathophysiology of osteoporosis

An understanding of the potential role of orthotic management of vertebral compression fractures (VCFs) begins with an understanding of osteoporosis itself. Osteoporosis is a disorder in which mineralized bone density is below normal, resulting in a bone structure that is vulnerable to fractures. The compromised bone structure is characterized by a reduction in bone mass that is related to an imbalance in bone formation and resorption. Osteoporosis is the most common of the metabolic bone diseases described as osteopenia, meaning "too little bone."[11] A decrease in bone mass normally begins in a person's early thirties and continues throughout life. Osteoporosis is defined as a bone mineral density greater than 2.5 standard deviations below the young adult mean for normal bone mineral density. It results from an imbalance in bone turnover such that the amount of new bone production cannot keep up with the amount of bone resorption, that is, bone resorption is greater than bone deposition.

The majority of primary osteoporosis can be described as type I or type II. Type I affects women and is associated with estrogen deficiency occurring 5 to 10 years after menopause (Table 11-1). Trabecular osteogenesis is primarily affected and results in a diminished capacity to support compressive loads. As a result, vertebral bodies, the distal radius, and the hip are common sites at greater risk for fractures. Type II osteoporosis affects both males and females. It is due to calcium deficiency and is associated with aging. In type II osteoporosis, both trabecular and cortical bone are affected. Because cortical bone provides support, especially for bending and torsional loads, the femoral neck, proximal tibia, humerus, pelvis, and vertebral bodies are at higher risk for fractures.

Osteoporosis is a significant public health problem, with 100 million people at risk worldwide and 28 million people at risk in the United States alone.[21] An estimated 1.5 million fragility fractures occur annually, including 700,000 spine, 300,000 hip, 250,000 wrist, and 250,000 other fractures related to osteoporosis. Even more compelling is the economic cost associated with osteoporotic fractures. In 1995 the United States spent over $13.8 billion on hospital and nursing home direct costs ($38 million daily). Projected expenditures for 2030 are more than $60 billion, or $164 million per day.[36] More than 260,000 patients with a first-time symptomatic VCF are diagnosed each year. There are more than 150,000 hospitalizations per year, with an 8-day average stay and $12,300 average charge.[37] Typically, there are 14 hospital bed days per VCF, which is comparable to the 18 hospital

Table 11-1 Classification of osteoporosis

Classification	Clinical course	Remarks
Primary		
Involutional		
Type I (postmenopausal)	Affects women only within menopause, lasts 15–20 yr	Predominantly trabecular bone loss in axial skeleton
Type II (age-associated)	Men or women > 70 yr	Proportional loss of trabecular and cortical bone
Idiopathic juvenile	Age 8–14 yr, self-limited (2–4 yr)	Normal growth; consider secondary forms
Idiopathic young adult	Mild to severe, self-limited (5–10 yr)	
Secondary (type III)		
Endocrine Gastrointestinal Bone marrow disorders Connective tissue disorders Malnutrition Lymphoproliferative diseases Medications Calcium poisoning Others	Dependent on underlying cause	Usually reversible to some extent after treatment of primary disease
Regional		
Reflex sympathetic dystrophy	Three overlapping clinical stages: typical course lasts 6–9 mo, followed by spontaneous or assisted resolution	Radiographic changes may be seen in the first 3–4 wk as patchy demineralization of affected area; triple-phase bone scan shows increased uptake in involved extremity before radiographic changes; brief tapering dose of corticosteroids often warranted
Transient regional osteoporosis	Localized, migratory, predominantly involves hip, usually self-limited (6–9 mo)	Rare; diagnosis by clinical suspicion, radiograph, and bone scan; treatment similar to that for reflex sympathetic dystrophy

From O'Young BJ, Young MA, Stiens SA, editors: *Physical medicine and rehabilitation secrets*, ed 2, Philadelphia, 2002, Hanley & Belfus.

bed days for hip fractures. Moreover, there is increased long-term morbidity and mortality in patients with VCF.[13]

VCFs can present with acute pain, or they can be silent and have no associated pain. Nearly one third of the latter patients will experience chronic pain.[5] A large percentage of cases go undiagnosed. VCFs typically are caused by falls, but they may result from something as innocuous as a cough or sneeze. The risk for VCFs is amplified as these events occur in the presence of compromised bone integrity. Eighty-four percent of patients with radiographic evidence of VCF report associated back pain. VCFs lead to progressive sagittal deformity (hyperkyphosis), and the changes in spinal biomechanics increase the risk of further fractures in the vertebrae above or below the fracture site.[24]

Hyperkyphosis is a common postural deformity secondary to VCF. The degree of kyphosis correlates with physical function and mobility (independent of pain), pulmonary function, mental well-being, and risk of new fractures.[14,27,35] Lung function in patients with thoracic and lumbar VCFs is affected and leads to increased mortality.[39] Hyperkyphosis can lead to ligamentous stretching, diminished functional vital capacity, inferior costal margin and pelvic rim contact and discomfort, chronic low back pain, abdominal crowding, depression, muscle imbalance, and painful, chronic intravertebral pseudarthrosis. In the case of muscle imbalance, the kyphotic deformity progressively elongates the paraspinal muscle extensors

and leads to overall muscle weakness. Involutional muscle loss, called *sarcopenia*, is common in the elderly and can be an important factor contributing to muscle weakness.[9,38,47] The severity of the VCF and associated pain can lead to diminished function, decreased mobility, physical deconditioning, and consequently accelerated bone loss.

Clinical signs of VCF include sudden onset of back pain with little or no trauma,[23] loss of height, spinal deformity (dowager's hump), protuberant abdomen, and diminished vital capacity. In patients with thoracic or lumbar VCF, lung function (forced vital capacity, forced expiratory volume in 1 second) is significantly reduced. One thoracic VCF causes 9% loss of vital capacity.[26] A prospective study of 9575 women followed for more than 8 years demonstrated that patients with VCF have a 23% to 34% increased mortality rate compared to patients without VCF. The most common cause of death is pulmonary disease, including chronic obstructive pulmonary disease (COPD) and pneumonia (hazard ratio 2.1).[21]

VCFs and their secondary effects remain a constant challenge for the medical team and should be addressed as quickly as possible. In particular, strategies addressing postural deformity reduction should be a major orthotic consideration because a person's ability to function on a daily basis can be dramatically improved and pain medication reduced.

Historical perspective

Treatment of osteoporosis is divided into pharmacologic, nonpharmacologic, and surgical options that address either the acute pain from a recent VCF or the chronic pain that may follow.[45] The distinction is essential because the treatment goals, methods, and timeline are different for each category. Historically, for orthotic treatment, it appears that devices originally intended for acute pain have been used often for chronic pain. This situation has contributed to disappointing failures of orthotic treatment of VCFs from osteoporosis and should be avoided.

Much interest has focused on developing effective pharmacologic treatments to reduce bone loss, which is the hallmark of osteoporosis and the primary underlying cause of fractures. Options include drug therapies such as bisphosphonates to decrease bone resorption, estrogen/hormone replacement to counteract the postmenopausal increased rate of bone loss, and calcitonin to reduce osteoclastic bone resorption.[21] However, the efficacy of pharmacologic treatments in reducing the risk of falls, fractures, and skeletal deformities is unclear and "should not be overrated."[45]

The primary types of nonpharmacologic treatments of osteoporosis include exercise, physical management of pain, orthotic treatment, and gait training.[45] The goals are to reduce the rate of bone resorption, improve the strength of bone, and enhance the overall quality of life. Improving muscle strength, especially in the lower extremities, can reduce the risk of falls.[28] There is general agreement that preventing fractures is preferable to treating the complications that may arise from them. Thus, prevention programs, including screening for osteoporosis, are now being emphasized.[6]

As a consequence of diminished bone strength, many patients with acute VCFs from osteoporosis are not candidates for spinal fusion, and less invasive procedures such as vertebroplasty and kyphoplasty have been developed.[20] These procedures can relieve pain and stabilize the fracture, but the long-term benefits in preventing additional fractures are not well understood.[10]

Orthotic management of VCFs from osteoporosis is used as part of nonpharmacologic treatment. Few studies have investigated the efficacy of specific orthotic interventions in spinal osteoporosis.[16,17,32] Thus, there is a substantial need for research addressing this issue. Traditional orthotic approaches (e.g., three-point bending orthoses) have concentrated on preventing excessive spinal flexion to reduce pain from VCFs. These orthoses do not substantially correct the anteroposterior standing imbalance that often is present, nor do they provide stability in the transverse plane. However, correcting standing posture has been found to be a more fruitful approach.[12]

Concerns have been expressed about the effects of long-term use of spinal orthoses in treating osteoporosis, such as the possibility of muscle atrophy. Indeed, the condition known as sarcopenia (i.e., involutional loss of functional muscle motor units) has been identified as a potentially important condition that may worsen osteoporosis. Therefore, it is essential to include, as part of orthotic treatment, a carefully designed physical therapy routine and to intentionally manage the effects of sarcopenia, if present. A successful nonpharmacologic treatment can be achieved through a team approach, with the physicians, physical therapist, and orthotist working toward the goals of treatment.

Current issues

Prevention of osteoporotic vertebral compression fractures

Osteoporosis often goes undiagnosed until after the first painful fracture occurs. At that point, attention is focused on resolving the acute pain and returning the patient to the activities of daily living, which can be an expensive undertaking. Given that preventing a fracture is preferable to treating one, screening for osteoporosis is an important consideration for the patient. Although opinions vary on the value of screening for osteoporosis based on bone mineral density measurements alone,[2,8] there is general agreement that taking steps such as exercising more, increasing calcium intake through dietary and/or pharmacologic means, smoking cessation, and lowering alcohol consumption help to prevent bone degradation.[6]

Efficacy of treatment options

Sinaki et al.[45] reported several studies on nonpharmacologic treatment of vertebral fractures. Nonpharmacologic treatment is intended to relieve pain and return function to the patient. It may include exercise, orthotic management, and gait training. Orthotic management options are limited, and few studies on the effectiveness of specific orthoses have been reported.

Pharmacologic treatment of osteoporosis is intended to treat pain and to slow or reverse the progression of disease.[21] Calcitonin and bisphosphonates inhibit osteoclasts and slow bone resorption. Several substances have been shown to increase bone mass, including sodium fluoride, anabolic steroids, testosterone, and parathyroid hormone. However, they may have serious side effects if not used correctly. For pain control, the choices are nonsteroidal antiinflammatory drugs and opioids. Possible side effects of opioids that may compromise orthotic management include drowsiness and dizziness.

Augmentation of VCF with bone cement has emerged as a *minimally invasive* surgical treatment for patients who have not responded to other therapies. There are two distinct procedures: *vertebroplasty*, in which bone cement is percutaneously injected into the fractured vertebral body to stabilize it but does not correct the deformity, and *kyphoplasty*, in which bone cement is injected after percutaneous reduction of the vertebral body deformity using inflatable bone tamps (balloons). The goals of these treatments are to reduce pain and to restore the normal weight-bearing function of the spine so that the risk of future fractures is reduced.[10,33]

Vertebroplasty can result in pain reduction, but it does not correct spinal alignment, and complications are associated with cement leakage. Increased risk for new VCFs has been reported after vertebroplasty.[24] The excessive kyphosis leads to increased forward bending moments, which can lead to paraspinal muscle fatigue and increased strain at the facet capsules, contributing to chronic pain. Some patients attempt to improve standing posture by flexing their knees to counterbalance the increased forward bending moments.

However, this can lead to muscle contractions, impaired gait velocity and balance, and increased risk of falls. The presence of two or more VCFs can increase the risk of hip fractures, independent of bone mass. In contrast, kyphoplasty can reduce the vertebral deformity and restore normal spinal alignment, but it requires more surgical expertise and is much more expensive.

Current research

Pharmacologic treatment studies

Improving pharmacologic treatments of osteoporosis is a topic of ongoing research. Variability in the response to pharmacotherapy makes difficult the prediction of success or failure in an individual patient. Moreover, the outcome of pharmacologic treatment may not be known for years. The emerging field of *pharmacogenomics of osteoporosis* aims to use genetic information to predict the outcomes of pharmacologic treatments and could lead to new drug therapies for osteoporosis.[31]

Nonpharmacologic treatment studies

Broadly speaking, spinal orthoses are used for both short-term management of acute pain from VCFs as well as long-term management of chronic pain. However, in each case they are used differently and have different orthotic goals. A possible problem in orthotic management is the use of an orthosis intended for acute pain for treatment of chronic pain and vice versa. Unfortunately, few research studies have evaluated the efficacy of specific devices for orthotic management of spinal problems due to osteoporosis. Thus, this aspect of nonpharmacologic treatment requires further study.

Surgical treatment of vertebral compression fractures from osteoporosis

Several studies have reported on the risk of adjacent fractures after vertebroplasty and kyphoplasty. This risk is significantly increased in patients with severe secondary osteoporosis and is greater in the first 30 to 60 days after both vertebroplasty and kyphoplasty.[24] However, the available studies do not allow definite conclusions because of the lack of good-quality prospective randomized trials. As a result, the potential therapeutic benefits of vertebroplasty and kyphoplasty procedures in altering the fracture risk in adjacent, nonaugmented vertebral bodies are not well known.

A well-recognized risk factor for adjacent fracture is the kyphotic deformity[24] consisting of vertebral deformity of the fractured vertebra caused by a loss of anterior height and regional kyphotic deformity that contributes to increased forward bending moments. The reported percentage of vertebral kyphosis reduction ranges from 39% to 65%,[22,34] whereas the restoration of vertebral body height ranges from 35% to 68%.[7,11] Spinal extension inducing "postural reduction" of VCFs also has been reported. In a prospective study of 41 consecutive patients with 65 VCFs who underwent vertebroplasty, McKiernan et al.[29] achieved improvement of kyphotic deformity in 23 fractures using spinal extension. In a prospective clinical study, Kim et al.[18] described the

ability of postural reduction to achieve significant correction of anterior vertebral body height and vertebral kyphotic deformity in 90% of patients with acute VCFs of onset less than 8 weeks.

A cadaveric study showed that spinal extension was effective in recovering the anterior height loss.[10] However, the middle height of the fractured vertebra was better restored by balloon inflation. The combination of balloon inflation and extension resulted in improved correction of both the vertebral and segmental kyphotic deformities, better than achieved with individual modalities alone. Therefore, based upon knowledge gained by studying vertebroplasty and kyphoplasty, spinal orthoses may have a role in postural reduction of VCF deformity. They also may prove useful as an adjunct to vertebroplasty and kyphoplasty. This finding supports further clinical studies assessing the efficacy of spinal orthotic devices in the treatment of osteoporotic VCFs.

Treatment recommendations

Treatment recommendations for VCFs from osteoporosis are classified as pharmacologic, nonpharmacologic, or surgical. An important consideration is whether the patient is being treated for acute pain from a new VCF or for chronic back pain. The possible interactions between different treatment modalities must be considered to avoid increasing risks for falls and other trauma.

Few orthotic recommendations for spinal problems resulting from osteoporosis are available. Moreover, even fewer studies support the efficacy of available orthoses. Some conventional orthoses, such as the total-contact polymer thoracolumbosacral orthosis (TLSO), often can be ruled out because of large spinal deformities that may be present, uncomfortable fit over bony prominences, or restriction of pulmonary capacity.

Posture training support

The posture training support (PTS) is one of two spinal orthoses for osteoporosis that have any scientific study supporting or refuting their efficacy.[17,45] The PTS, called a "weighted kypho-orthosis," provides a weight suspended just inferior to the scapulae (Fig. 11-1). The weight can be increased to as much as 2.5 lb in several increments. Patients are encouraged to try different levels of weight to determine which is most effective. Too much weight will not benefit the patient, and compliance will suffer.

The PTS is indicated in cases of excess dorsal kyphosis possibly involving iliocostal contact or iliocostal friction syndrome. Two mechanisms of action are hypothesized. First, anterior compression forces on the spine are reduced by the countermoment produced by the posterior weight. Second, the device encourages active back extension through proprioceptive input and helps increase back extensor strength. The PTS is designed to aid physical therapy and, as the study showed, help increase the strength of the paraspinal muscles.[17]

The PTS appears to be the least invasive orthotic recommendation and is cosmetically acceptable, with a high level of patient compliance. Because of its unobtrusive nature, the PTS does not appear to have any serious disadvantages.

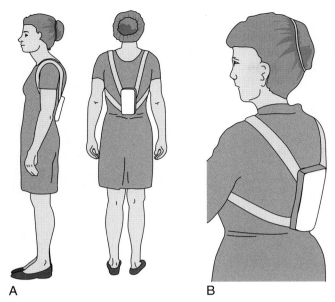

Fig. 11-1 Posture training support (PTS). The weight below the scapulae acts to improve standing posture and tends to retract the shoulders and strengthen the paraspinal muscles.

However, the challenge is determining which candidates are suitable for this orthotic recommendation. Also, a patient's desire for a less invasive orthotic intervention should not result in substituting this orthosis for one that is more appropriate given the patient's clinical presentation.

Lumbosacral corset and dorsolumbosacral corset

Both the lumbosacral corset and dorsolumbosacral corsets are total-contact orthoses. They increase the intracavity pressure and provide resistance to axial loading. They also serve as a kinesthetic reminder in all three anatomical planes. Possible orthotic goals of these devices include reduction of pain by axial unloading, reduction of muscle strain, and/or improvement of standing balance by moving the position of the center of gravity posteriorly. Orthotic management may be contraindicated in all three instances if a severe respiratory condition is present. For select patients with COPD, orthotic management may help increase vital capacity and should be considered as a treatment option.

The dorsolumbosacral corset differs from the lumbosacral corset because of the addition of a dorsal thoracic piece extending to the midthoracic spine, with straps over the shoulders. Its mechanism of action is distinct from the lumbosacral corset in that it provides forces to help retract the shoulders and limit thoracic spine motion.

Three-point hyperextension orthoses

Three-point hyperextension orthoses are indicated for stable compression fractures in the lower thoracic/upper lumbar spine. They are sometimes prescribed to treat acute pain secondary to VCFs resulting from osteoporosis. However, many current designs are not tolerated well by the patient,

especially for long-term use, and appear to offer little benefit in correcting standing posture. Patients may complain of excessive pressure on the pubis and sternum as well as the weight of the orthosis, which tends to increase the anteroposterior (AP) imbalance in posture. Although some of these problems could be eased by adjusting the orthosis, the fact that little correction of standing posture is achieved is a clear disadvantage independent of fit. Moreover, traditional three-point hyperextension orthoses do not provide stabilization in the transverse plane. Possible orthotic goals of this device include unloading of the fracture site to decrease pain and preventing excessive flexion.

Spinomed (TLSO–sagittal plane control)

The Spinomed is the second of two orthoses for osteoporosis that has scientific study regarding its efficacy.[33] It resembles the traditional Knight-Taylor orthosis (TLSO–sagittal plane control) in its mechanism of action. Unlike the Knight-Taylor orthosis, the Spinomed has very high compliance rates. This TLSO, which weighs approximately 450 g, consists of a metallic "back pad" that can be molded by hand without heating and a system of hook-and-loop straps (Fig. 11-2). It is worn similar to how a backpack is worn. It is indicated more for management of chronic pain resulting from VCFs.

The study by Pfeifer et al.[33] was a prospective, randomized, controlled crossover study of 62 ambulatory females over age 60 years with at least one VCF and a kyphosis angle greater than 60 degrees. Results showed that 6 months of wearing the orthosis for 2 hours per day significantly increased body height, strength of the back extensors and abdominal flexors, relaxed vital capacity, 1-second forced expiratory volume, and overall well-being. Significant decreases in kyphosis angle, postural sway magnitude and velocity, and pain also were observed.

The posteriorly directed forces provided by the shoulder straps may help achieve orthotic goals such as correcting the unbalanced anterior posture in the sagittal plane, retracting the shoulders, and increasing back extensor strength. The back pad is in total contact and can provide hyperextension of selected segments by adjustments to its shape. Because of the corset front, intracavity pressure increases. The study also demonstrated the potential for the orthotic goal of strengthening the paraspinal muscles.

Advantages include a high rate of patient compliance, strengthening of the paraspinal muscles, the device's light weight and highly noninvasive nature, ease of donning and doffing the device, and hand-moldable shape of the device's posterior piece. There do not appear to be any significant disadvantages. As with the PTS, the most important consideration is the appropriateness of the orthosis in meeting the needs of the patient.

Posterior shell TLSO

The posterior shell TLSO consists of a plastic posterior shell, a soft corset front, and a system of straps (Fig. 11-3). Similar to the Spinomed, the shoulder straps provide posteriorly directed forces that help correct the unbalanced anterior posture in the sagittal plane (Fig. 11-4). However, unlike the Spinomed, the plastic posterior shell is not designed to be in total contact

Fig. 11-2 Spinomed orthosis, anterior **(A)** and posterior **(B)** views. Note the corset front and hand-moldable metallic back piece. The shoulder straps help retract the shoulders. (Retrieved from www.mediusa.com/ortho pedics/mediortho/spinomed.shtml)

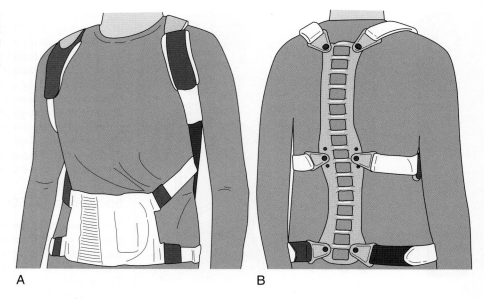

A

B

at the superior portion in the initial phase of orthotic treatment, but it may achieve contact in the later phase of orthotic treatment. This orthosis has not been scientifically studied to validate or refute its efficacy. However, Gavin et al.[12] fit more than 75 of these orthoses over a 10-year period (1988–1998) and reported good success in correcting posture and reducing pain.

Possible orthotic goals of the posterior shell TLSO include restoration of sagittal plane standing posture alignment, reduction of internal rotation of the shoulders, improvement of vital capacity, restoration of heel-to-toe gait pattern, and improvement of seated posture. Advantages include its use as a viable nonsurgical alternative to vertebroplasty or kyphoplasty, soft corset front for comfort, improved cosmesis of the patient, improved mobility and endurance, act as a seating orthosis, and ability to accommodate changes in the patient's weight.

Disadvantages include difficulty in donning the orthosis and excessive weight. These disadvantages surface especially for patients who have conditions such as rheumatoid arthritis, who are of small stature, and/or who may not have a caretaker to help donning and doffing.

The posterior shell TLSO is an excellent device to gradually "right" these patients in the sagittal plane (see Fig. 11-4). When the device is properly fabricated and fitted, caregivers are instructed to increase the shoulder strap tightness daily over 1 month to achieve this goal. Usually, once the patient is realigned, he or she can ambulate without a walker and for a significantly longer period of time. Although clinical studies are forthcoming, it is our experience that most of this geriatric population will continue to wear the posterior shell once they have accomplished the repositioning during the first month.

Conclusion

Although currently a limited number of spinal orthoses for osteoporosis are available, new devices appear from time to time. Therefore, it would be unwise to limit the choices only to the devices discussed in this chapter. The orthotic practitioner should be vigilant in seeking out new options for treatment while keeping in mind the desired mechanisms of actions of the orthosis.

Orthotic management of osteoporosis
Overview

Individuals with osteoporosis and secondary spinal deformity present a unique and complex set of problems that, if not fully evaluated, can lead to unsuccessful treatment. This can quickly become a reality if the rigors of comprehensive orthotic care are not viewed as ongoing for the patient. The patient with osteoporosis likely will present with a multitude of ever changing challenges and will require constant review. Individuals with a diagnosis of osteoporosis with at least one VCF and who range in age from 55 to 80 years show a significant impairment of quality of life compared to healthy individuals of the same age and gender.[25] It is not uncommon for these individuals to have diminished function both physically and socially. It is important that these factors receive as much attention as the more obvious musculoskeletal deficits and associated pain if orthotic treatment is to be successful.

Traditionally, orthoses for persons with VCFs secondary to osteoporosis are thought to be a burden and not well received by the patient and the healthcare worker alike. Unfortunately, in many instances the orthotist is likely to read and fill the prescription rather than acknowledge these issues and pursue a comprehensive patient history and physical assessment. Moreover, the orthotist is unlikely to initiate dialogue with the physician and/or medical team members and remains isolated in providing orthotic care. The orthotist may simply fill the prescription in an attempt to address the VCF and associated pain. The patient often is prescribed a dorsolumbar corset or a three-point hyperextension orthosis.[4] Upon failure of the orthosis, which was intended to reduce pain and improve the quality of life, the device usually is discarded and orthotic management abandoned completely.

To avoid rejection of orthotic management of osteoporosis, additional consideration should involve the concept of

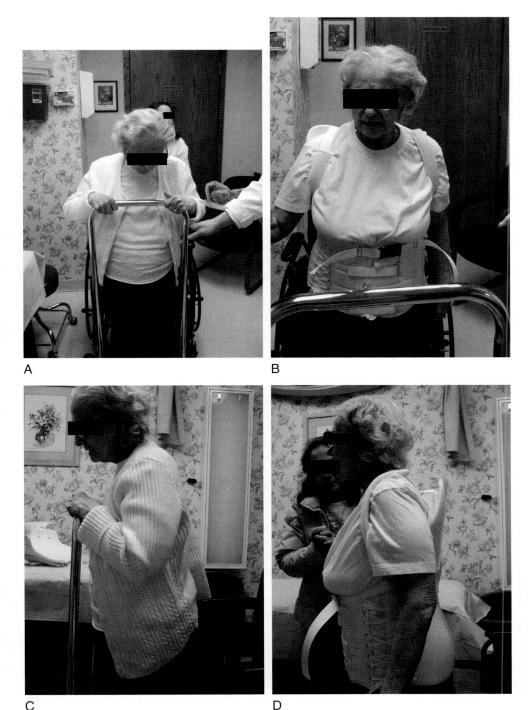

A

B

C

D

Fig. 11-3 Posterior shell thoracolumbosacral orthosis (TLSO). Anterior view without orthosis **(A)** and with orthosis **(B)**. Observe the gap between the shoulders and superior edge of the orthosis that will close over time. Lateral view without orthosis **(C)** and with orthosis **(D)**. Note the corset front and straps that retract the shoulders.

a well-coordinated multidisciplinary team approach to properly manage the individual with osteoporosis. In particular, a multifaceted approach is suggested to optimize recovery from a VCF secondary to osteoporosis.[48] Interdisciplinary strategies for management of patients with osteoporosis may include proprioceptive dynamic posture training, pharmacotherapy. muscle strengthening and coordination, orthotic management, and/or surgical management.[33] These strategies should be in response to well-defined goals determined through discussion with the patient and medical team. Goals common to this population can include reduction of

acute and or chronic pain, risk reduction for falling, and management of VCFs. Collectively the impact of these goals should be to improve the patient's quality of life, defined as the summation of physical, social, and mental function.[15]

At the time orthotic strategies are introduced as part of the overall treatment plan, the patient will present with a likely clinical scenario and chief complaint of back pain.[19,43] In many cases the patient will describe a list of current or previous treatment strategies that can include nutrition, drug therapy, and physical therapy. Often the patient will present

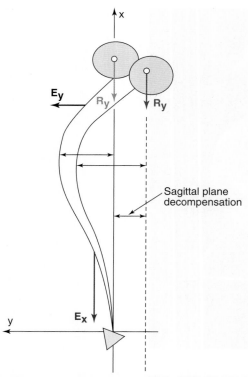

Fig. 11-4 Mechanism of action of the posterior shell thoracolumbosacral orthosis (TLSO): sagittal plane view. For a patient with significant sagittal plane decompensation, the weight line is displaced forward (Ry) and causes an increased forward bending moment, which is resisted by the paraspinal muscles (Ex) with a small moment arm. The posterior shell TLSO overcomes this by applying forces at the shoulders (Ex) over a much larger moment arm, which can correct standing posture and shift the weight line posteriorly.

with VCFs of the midthoracic and upper lumbar regions of the spine. Many of these patients exhibit a progressive loss of lumbar lordosis as a consequence of VCFs. This results in a sagittal plane malalignment where the head and shoulders are abnormally anterior to the sacrum. There may be loss of vertical height and the presence of kyphotic deformity resulting in negative psychological self-image.[46]

Muscle fatigue and weakness, which can be caused by a combination of hyperkyphosis, muscle disuse, and/or sarcopenia, may be present and may increase as the patient becomes less active. Closer examination may reveal paraspinal musculature that is in a state of abnormal elongation, where the muscle is in a compromised length–tension state and is unable to overcome the deforming force. In many cases, physical therapy alone may not be sufficient, and orthotic treatment is required to restore a close to normal length–tension state for certain paraspinal muscles.

Acute pain management

If the first VCF causes acute pain, then there are three types of treatments: nonpharmacologic, pharmacologic, and surgical. Ideally, nonpharmacologic and pharmacologic treatments go hand in hand in an attempt to prevent a second fracture. Orthotic management may be introduced at this point to stabilize and unload the fracture, encouraging early ambulation. Some patients are candidates for vertebroplasty or

kyphoplasty and may exercise that option. In that instance, a postoperative orthosis might be prescribed to help restore anterior vertebral height.

An example of an inappropriate device for acute pain from VCF is the PTS. The PTS is not designed to immobilize the fracture site or to provide the stability needed for relief of pain and healing of the fracture. It is intended for the rehabilitation process for chronic pain. To provide adequate fracture stabilization and vertebral body unloading, certain design characteristics should be incorporated into an orthosis. For proper fracture stabilization, the length of the orthosis should be long enough to limit further sagittal flexion and kyphotic deformity localized to the fracture site. In this case, appropriate length should extend posteriorly from the sacrococcygeal junction inferiorly to the level of the spine of the scapula superiorly. Over-the-shoulder straps or axillary straps can further augment fracture stabilization. The ability to unload the deforming force on the VCF is best addressed when the orthosis is able to maintain proper sagittal alignment, which may or may not entail increasing lordosis for the lumbar spine. This postural change, if properly achieved, likely will shift the axial load path from the VCF to the more posterior elements and allow for proper healing of the fracture.

Chronic pain management

Following resolution of acute pain, chronic pain may result. Moreover, if the first VCF did not produce acute pain, it may produce chronic pain. Once again, the three types of treatments may play a role. In cases where surgery is not performed, the goals of orthotic treatment for chronic pain differ from acute pain; that is, more emphasis is placed on correcting the patient's posture as an aid for strengthening the paraspinal muscles.

An example of an inappropriate device for chronic pain management is the three-point hyperextension orthosis. A three-point hyperextension orthosis does not have the design features that would encourage sufficient lumbar lordosis to improve the patient's standing posture. Additionally, little evidence indicates that this orthosis can achieve proper sagittal alignment to facilitate strengthening of the paraspinal muscles. The three-point hyperextension orthosis does have design features that specifically treat anterior compression fractures of the lower thoracic and upper lumbar regions of the spine by providing resistance to spinal flexion. The orthotic practitioner should be keenly aware of the differences between this chronic pain and acute traumatic fractures. Each warrants a different regimen of orthotic treatment and consideration if management is to be successful.

Clinical assessment and orthotic recommendation (Box 11-1)

Clinical signs and symptoms are central to assessing the patient and making a sound orthotic recommendation. Acute or chronic pain greatly influences the orthotic recommendation and should be distinguished from the outset. For each possible orthotic recommendation, it must be determined if the patient has the functional capacity to properly don, doff, and comply with the recommended use of the orthosis. This can be determined by considering complicating medical conditions (e.g., rheumatoid arthritis or COPD), psychological conditions (e.g., dementia or depression), and the patient's living environment. Clearly, input from the other members of the treatment team is essential.

Patient assessment should include medical history, knowledge of the patient's living environment, and patient's ability to perform activities of daily living. Medical history should include previous/current fractures, previous/current treatment (e.g., physical therapy, pharmacologic, surgery), other medical conditions (e.g., diabetes), and occurrence of falls.[23] From a functional standpoint, the orthotic practitioner should assess the patient's ability to go from sitting to standing and the patient's ambulatory capability. Manual muscle testing and range of motion should be assessed, particularly for the upper extremities, to determine the patient's ability to don and doff an orthosis. Quality-of-life determination is equally essential and can be used as an outcome measure for successful orthotic treatment. Visual and/or cognitive impairment may require alternative strategies for proper orthotic management and should be reviewed. All elements of pain and pain relief should be thoroughly assessed, as this will become a strong outcome measure of orthotic success. Pain should be assessed in the following areas: chronic versus acute, duration, location, type of pain, degree of pain, and postural alignment that relieves pain. Finally, the orthotist should assess the patient's current level of independence to determine the likelihood that the patient will be able to effectively utilize an orthosis. Unquestionably, the orthotic recommendation also depends on the goals of the patient.

Measurements for patient assessment and sizing the orthosis (Box 11-2)

Measurements are essential not only for proper sizing of the orthosis but also for patient assessment. Although some measurements may not be needed in order to choose the size of a particular orthosis, it is highly desirable to accurately and consistently record the measurements at follow-up to help in early detection of progressive deterioration of the patient's condition. Making use of standard orthometry forms aids in communication across the treatment team and quantifies perceptions of changes in the patient.

A simple quantitative measurement of AP balance is to use a plumb line at the acromion and measure the distance of this line to the greater trochanter in the sagittal plane.

Frequently, patients will have an anterior displacement of the plumb line of several centimeters anterior to the greater trochanter. As such, restoration of standing balance often is one of the primary orthotic goals.

With the exception of the posterior shell TLSO, the sizing of orthoses discussed in the treatment recommendations is based mainly upon measurements. However, it is important to also record these measurements for the posterior shell TLSO because of potential inaccuracies in the plaster impression. Regardless, to assure accuracy and consistency, an agreed upon consistent set of measurement units should be used.

Plaster impression technique for the posterior shell TLSO (Box 11-3)

Devices requiring plaster impressions are the polymer TLSO and the posterior shell TLSO. If a polymer TLSO is prescribed, standard procedures apply. However, there are some special considerations for the plaster impression for the posterior shell TLSO.

The impression is taken with the patient in a prone position, with the ultimate goal of improving sagittal alignment of the head over the pelvis and reducing sagittal plane decompensation. This can be achieved by either shifting of the patient's postural alignment posterior (see Fig. 11-4) or hyperextension of the lumbar spine. In both cases, the principle of viscoelastic creep should be applied. After stockinette, landmarks, and measurements are applied and recorded, the patient lies on the examination table in a prone position for a period of 15 to 20 minutes.[3] The orthotic practitioner should place a pillow or pad under the superior and anterior aspect of the torso and in the region of the chest. If able, the patient can use his or her elbows for additional support to maintain this position. If additional lordosis is required, more pillows or padding should be introduced gradually to facilitate proper viscoelastic change. Vertical plaster splints are placed on the posterior aspect of the patient and should extend laterally past the midaxillary trochanteric line, superiorly to the level of the spine of the scapula, and inferiorly to the level of the sacrococcygeal junction or gluteus fold for females.

Fitting the orthosis and follow-up (Box 11-4)

For all orthotic recommendations, the orthotic practitioner, in addition to establishing and verifying fitting parameters, may need to help define strategies such that the patient can effectively don and doff the orthosis. These strategies are dependent on whether the person lives independently, with family, or in an assisted living environment.

For the posterior shell, some special considerations include fitting the orthosis supine (reverse of the impression) and allowing the patient's back to "relax" into the orthosis. The straps are tightened in that position. The donning process takes 20 to 30 minutes in order to take advantage of the viscoelastic creep of the tissues. Some patients are unable to position themselves supine on the examination table, even with help. In that case, the patient may be possible to don the orthosis while seated in a recliner. Such a strategy also may be helpful when the patient dons the orthosis at home. Equally important is the ability of the patient or caretaker to doff the orthosis. The orthotic practitioner should visually observe this action before the patient visit is concluded. All donning and doffing performed by the patient or caretaker should be documented because this status can change with each scheduled visit.

Conclusion

It is essential that an orthosis intended primarily for acute pain resulting from a VCF not be used for chronic pain and vice versa. An instructive clinical example is a patient who presents using a three-point hyperextension spinal orthosis for management of chronic pain. The orthosis may have been prescribed only for the acute pain phase but, because of lack of proper follow-up and reassessment, was never changed. Often, these patients complain of excessive pressure on the sternum and pubis and may abandon use of the orthosis altogether. This noncompliance may be perceived as failure of orthotic management. Because of the high incidence of osteoporosis and the aging of the adult population, demand for orthotic management of VCFs is likely to increase sharply in the future. Orthotists must be prepared to provide the best possible orthotic management options available.

Best practices

Ideally, orthotic management of VCFs from osteoporosis should be part of a broader treatment plan that may include pharmacologic and nonpharmacologic approaches. Because osteoporosis usually is a progressive degenerative process, the needs of the patient change over time, so timely periodic reassessment is required. The orthotic practitioner must take steps to avoid managing the osteoporotic patient in isolation—a sure way to undermine the chances for successful treatment outcomes. Following is a summary of several best practices for treating a patient with VCFs from osteoporosis.

Direct the treatment plan toward relieving symptoms and improving function

The independence of patients who already may have significant restrictions is seriously threatened by the consequences of VCFs, such as pain and loss of function.

Design the treatment plan with a multidisciplinary team approach

Osteoporosis is rarely the only pathology present in the patient. It often is accompanied by conditions such as COPD, leg-length discrepancy, diminished mood, and pain, which emphasize the need for a multidisciplinary team approach to designing the treatment plan.

Agree on clear goals of orthotic treatment

To use an orthosis properly, the osteoporotic patient may need to make significant changes in his or her environment and possibly accept outside help for donning and doffing the orthosis. This will be easier if the goals as well as the potential benefits are clear. It is best to recommend the least invasive device that accomplishes the orthotic goals.

Educate the patient and caregivers on the proper fit and functioning of the orthosis

Compliance with the recommendations of the treatment plan is crucial for patients with osteoporosis because they are at high risk for further deterioration of their physical condition even over short periods of time.

Agree upon the timing of follow-up visits and take steps to ensure the patients follow it

When treating osteoporosis, time is of the essence. Major setbacks can occur over short time periods in this population. Missing even a few days of orthosis-wearing time can greatly reduce gains made over longer periods.

Emphasize the importance of strengthening the paraspinal muscles

Many studies suggest that muscle strengthening is a key factor in improving function in these patients. Rather than viewing a spinal orthosis as an immobilization device, it should be seen as an aid to improving function by restoring posture and relieving pain.

Do not use an orthosis intended to treat acute pain to treat chronic pain and vice versa

A common error to avoid is recommending an orthosis intended for acute pain management to manage chronic pain. In acute pain management, the orthosis is more immobilizing so the fracture can be stabilized. However, the same orthosis used in the same way to manage chronic pain may do more harm than good because immobilization over a long time period is known to lead to further bone and muscle loss.

Supporting evidence

General information

Pfeifer M, Sinaki M, Geusens P, et al: Musculoskeletal rehabilitation in osteoporosis: a review, *J Bone Miner Res* 19:1208-1214, 2004.

Nonpharmacologic treatment

Sinaki M: Nonpharmacologic interventions—exercise, fall prevention, and the role of physical medicine, *Clin Geriatr Med* 19:337-359, 2003.

Efficacy of specific orthotic devices

Kaplan RS, Sinaki M, Hameister MD: Effect of back supports on back strength in patients with osteoporosis: a pilot study, *Mayo Clin Proc* 71:235-241, 1996.

Pfeifer M, Begerow B, Minne HW: Effects of a new spinal orthosis on posture, trunk strength an quality of life in women with postmenopausal osteoporosis: a randomized trial, *Am J Phys Med Rehabil* 83:177-186, 2004.

Vertebroplasty and kyphoplasty

Gaitanis IN, Carandang G, Phillips FM, et al: Restoring geometric and loading alignment of the thoracic spine with a VCF: effects of balloon (bone tamp) inflation and spinal extension, *Spine* 5:45-54, 2005.

Multidisciplinary team approach to treatment

Nguyen DMT: The role of physical medicine and rehabilitation in pain management, *Clin Geriatr Med* 12:517-529, 1996.

References

1. Andersson GBJ, Bostrom MPG, Eyre DR, et al: Consensus summary on the diagnosis and treatment of osteoporosis, *Spine* 22(24S):63S–65S, 1997.
2. Berg AO: Screening for osteoporosis in postmenopausal women: recommendations and rationale, *Am J Nurs* 103:73–80, 2003.
3. Bunch WH: Posterior fusion for idiopathic scoliosis. In: *AAOS instructional course lectures*, St. Louis, 1985, CV Mosby Co.
4. Cohen LD: Fractures of the osteoporotic spine, *Orthop Clin North Am* 2:143–150, 1990.
5. Cyteval C, Sarrabere MP, Roux JO, et al: Acute osteoporotic vertebral collapse: open study on percutaneous injection of acrylic surgical cement in 20 patients, *AJR Am J Roentgenol* 173:1685–1690, 1999.
6. Department of Health and Human Services–Centers for Disease Control and Prevention: Bone health campaign. Available from: http://www.cdc.gov/nccdphp/dnpa/bonehealth/.
7. Dudeney S, Lieberman I, Phillips F: Kyphoplasty for osteoporotic vertebral compression fractures, *Osteoporos Int* 11:S178, 2000; (abstract).
8. Felson DT, Zhang Y, Hannan MT, et al: The effect of postmenopausal estrogen therapy on bone density in elderly women, *N Engl J Med* 329:1141–1146, 1993.
9. Foster-Burns SB: Sarcopenia and decreased muscle strength in the elderly woman: resistance training as a safe and effective intervention, *J Women Aging* 11:75–85, 1999.
10. Gaitanis IN, Carandang G, Phillips FM, et al: Restoring geometric and loading alignment of the thoracic spine with a VCF: effects of balloon (bone tamp) inflation and spinal extension, *Spine J* 5:45–54, 2005.
11. Garfin SR, Yuan HA, Reiley MA: New technologies in spine: kyphoplasty and vertebroplasty for the treatment of painful osteoporotic compression fractures, *Spine* 26(14), 1511–2001.
12. Gavin TM, Patwardhan AV, Meade KP, et al: Class II posterior shell TLSO improves treatment of thoracolumbar fractures. *Am Prosthet Orthos News* 5:1-4, 1999, Available from: http://www.oandp.com/facilities/ia/ampro/spring994.htm.
13. Jalava T, Sarna S, Pylkkanen L, et al: Association between vertebral fracture and increased mortality in osteoporotic patients, *J Bone Miner Res* 18:1254–1260, 2003.
14. Kado DM, Browner WS, Palermo L, et al: Vertebral fractures and mortality in older women: a prospective study. Study of Osteoporotic Fractures Research Group, *Arch Intern Med* 159:1215–1220, 1999.
15. Kanis JA, McCloskey EV: Epidemiology of vertebral osteoporosis, *Bone* 13:S1–S10, 1992.
16. Kaplan RS, Sinaki M: Posture training support: preliminary report on a series of patients with diminished symptomatic complications of osteoporosis, *Mayo Clin Proc* 68:1171–1176, 1993.
17. Kaplan RS, Sinaki M, Hameister MD: Effect of back supports on back strength in patients with osteoporosis: a pilot study, *Mayo Clin Proc* 71:235–241, 1996.
18. Kim YS, Chin DK, Cho YE, et al: Percutaneous vertebroplasty: new technique using a postural reduction for acute osteoporotic vertebral compression fracture, Paper presented at the World Spine II Meeting, August 10–13, 2003, Chicago, Illinois.
19. Leidig-Bruckner G, Minne HW, Schlaich C, et al: Clinical grading of osteoporosis: quality of life components and spinal deformity in women with chronic low back pain and women with vertebral osteoporosis, *J Bone Miner Res* 12:663–674, 1997.
20. Levine SA, Perin LA, Hayes D, Wayes WS: An evidence-based evaluation of percutaneous vertebroplasty, *Managed Care* 9:56–61, 2000.
21. Levy CE, Rosenbuth J, Lanyi VF, et al: Metabolic bone disease. In O'Young BJ, Young MA, Stiens SA, editors: *Physical medicine and rehabilitation secrets*, ed 2, Philadelphia, 2002, Hanley & Belfus.
22. Lieberman IH, Dudeney S, Reinhardt MK, et al: Initial outcome and efficacy of "kyphoplasty" in the treatment of painful osteoporotic vertebral compression fractures, *Spine* 26:1631–1638, 2001.
23. Lin JT, Lane JM: Rehabilitation of the older adult with an osteoporosis-related fracture, *Clin Geriatr Med* 22:435–447, 2006.
24. Linville DA: Vertebroplasty and kyphoplasty, *South Med J* 95:583–587, 2002.
25. Lips P, Cooper C, Agnusdei D, et al: Quality of life in patients with vertebral fractures: validation of the quality of life questionnaire of the European Foundation for Osteoporosis (QUALEFFO), *Osteoporos Int* 10:150–160, 1999.
26. Lombardi I, Oliveira LM, Mayer AF, et al: Evaluation of pulmonary function and quality of life in women with osteoporosis, *Osteoporos Int* 16:1247–1253, 2005.
27. Lyles KW, Gold DT, Shipp KM, et al: Association of osteoporotic compression fractures with impaired functional status, *Am J Med* 94:595–601, 1993.

28. Lynn SG, Sinaki M, Westerlind KC: Balance characteristics of persons with osteoporosis, *Arch Phys Med Rehabil* 78:273–277, 1997.

29. McKiernan F, Jensen R, Faciszewski T: The dynamic mobility of vertebral compression fractures, *J Bone Miner Res* 18:24–29, 2003.

30. Nguyen DMT: The role of physical medicine and rehabilitation in pain management, *Clin Geriatr Med* 12:517–529, 1996.

31. Nguyen TV, Eisman JA: Pharmacogenomics of osteoporosis: opportunities and challenges, *J Musculoskel Neuronal Interact* 6:62–72, 2006.

32. Pfeifer M, Begerow B, Minne HW: Effects of a new spinal orthosis on posture, trunk strength and quality of life in women with postmenopausal osteoporosis: a randomized trial, *Am J Phys Med Rehabil* 83:177–186, 2004.

33. Pfeifer M, Sinaki M, Geusens P, et al: Musculoskeletal rehabilitation in osteoporosis: a review, *J Bone Miner Res* 19:1208–1214, 2004.

34. Phillips FM, Todd Wetzel F, Lieberman I, et al: An in vivo comparison of the potential for extravertebral cement leak after vertebroplasty and kyphoplasty, *Spine* 27:2173–2179, 2002.

35. Pluijm SM, Tromp AM, Smit JH, et al: Consequences of vertebral deformities in older men and women, *J Bone Miner Res* 15:1564–1572, 2000.

36. Ray NF, Chan JK, Thamer M, et al: Medical expenditures for the treatment of osteoporotic fractures in the United States in 1995: report from the National Osteoporosis Foundation, *J Bone Miner Res* 12:24–35, 1997.

37. Riggs BL, Melton LJ III: The worldwide problem of osteoporosis: insights afforded by epidemiology, *Bone* 17:505S–511S, 1995.

38. Roubenoff R, Hughes VA: Sarcopenia: current concepts, *J Gerontol A Biol Sci Med Sci* 55:M716–M724, 2000.

39. Schlaich C, Minnie HW, Bruckner T, et al: Reduced pulmonary function in patients with spinal osteoporotic fractures, *Osteoporos Int* 8:261–267, 1998.

40. Schneider EL, Guralnik JM: The aging of America. Impact on health care costs, *JAMA* 263:2335–2350, 1990.

41. Sinaki M, Brey RH, Hughes CA, et al: Balance disorder and increased risk of falls in osteoporosis and kyphosis: significance of kyphotic posture and muscle strength, *Osteoporos Int* 16:1004–1010, 2005.

42. Sinaki M, Itoi E, Rojers JW, et al: Correlation of back extensor strength with thoracic kyphosis and lumbar lordosis in estrogen-deficient women, *Am J Phys Med Rehabil* 75:370–374, 1996.

43. Sinaki M: Postmenopausal spinal osteoporosis: flexion versus extension exercises, *Arch Phys Med Rehabil* 65:593–596, 1984.

44. Sinaki M, Offord KP: Physical activity in postmenopausal women: effect on back muscle strength and bone mineral density of the spine, *Arch Phys Med Rehabil* 69:277–280, 1988.

45. Sinaki M: Exercise and physical therapy: osteoporosis. In Riggs BL, Milton J, editors: *Etiology, diagnosis and management.* New York, 1988, Raven Press.

46. Sinaki M: Nonpharmacologic interventions—exercise, fall prevention, and the role of physical medicine, *Clin Geriatr Med* 19:337–359, 2003.

47. Walsh MC, Hunter GR, Livingstone MB: Sarcopenia in premenopausal and postmenopausal women with osteopenia, osteoporosis and normal bone mineral density, *Osteoporos Int* 17:61–67, 2006.

48. Wu SS, Lachmann EL, Nagler W: Current medical, rehabilitation, and surgical management of VCFs, *J Womens Health* 12:17–26, 2003.

Upper limb orthoses

Section 3 brings together the material dealing with the upper limb. It begins with a very strong chapter on biomechanics. Chapter 12 is an up-to-date report of not only orthotic biomechanics but more importantly the physiologic biomechanics of the entire upper limb. The authors present a detailed discussion of the current thinking that provides a strong foundation for appreciating the biomechanics and function of upper limb orthotics.

Chapter 13 provides a conceptual foundation for the classification of upper limb orthoses and offers an overview of key principles in their design. Exemplars are depicted in black and white drawings, from very simple to more complex designs, illustrating specific approaches that have proven to be clinically useful.

Chapter 14 deals with cerebrospastic disorders, which are increasing numerically. Orthoses have a limited but important role in the prevention of upper extremity deformities. After much testing for safety and effectiveness, botulism toxin now is readily available to assist in the management of the increased muscle tone following brain tissue insult. Its use augments diagnostic nerve blocks and assists orthoses post chemodenervation.

Chapter 15 introduces the reader to new material in this edition of the *Atlas*, functional electrical stimulation as a method for enhancing upper limb function. It goes beyond conventional wrist-driven orthoses into a new arena for improved mobility. Wrist-driven wrist–hand orthoses may give way to implanted stimulators that can affect more physiologic function.

Chapter 16 presents a clear discussion on the process of deformation of the hand after burns. This leads naturally to a better understanding of how splinting and orthotic management can help prevent these deformities.

Chapter 17 discusses the importance of an integrated team approach to successful management of upper extremity arthritic deformities. The authors emphasize the need to monitor the many problems that arise from the basic disorder. Rheumatoid arthritis—a progressive, chronic, systemic disease—continues to present unique challenges.

Chapter 18 brings out the importance of orthotic use in the treatment of brachial plexus injuries. The chapter includes recently developed surgical techniques utilizing primary nerve repair, the interposition of nerve cable grafts, tendon/muscle transfers, and free-functioning muscle transfers performed at various periods following injury

The authors discuss management of glenohumeral subluxation and the role of dynamic and static wrist orthoses. They point out that as surgical alternatives improve, the need for orthoses is becoming more limited. The biomechanical principles of orthoses give insight to the problems that must be addressed by a surgical approach.

The authors of Chapter 19, key contributors in the development of functional fracture bracing, review the physiologic principles and scientific evidence underlying this form of treatment. Specific applications for selected upper limb diaphyseal fractures are presented, focusing on the practical considerations that are necessary for a successful outcome. Contraindications and risk factors are reviewed.

Chapter 20 represents a well-illustrated discussion showing currently available protective equipment to the upper extremity in sports. The authors emphasize the need for properly fitted, well-maintained, durable, and lightweight protective equipment.

In Chapter 21, the authors begin with a list of six common overuse disorders of the upper limb. They present an overview of the management of these disorders and end with a discussion of the role of orthoses. As with many chapters in this edition of the Atlas, the reader is left with a better understanding of all the issues involved with management of a specific disorder, not just orthotic management.

John D. Hsu

Upper limb orthoses

Chapter

12

Biomechanics of the upper limb

Marjorie Johnson Hilliard, Kai-Nan An, Steven L. Moran, and Richard A. Berger

Key Points

- Achieving a functional range of motion, rather than a normal range of motion, can be an acceptable goal. This functional range of motion, however, can be represented as an overall average or task specific.
- At its most fundamental level, a functional hand requires a stable platform of the wrist and forearm and at least two sensate digits with opposable power.
- Synergistic motion between the wrist and fingers is efficient and should be incorporated when possible into orthotic and prosthetic designs.
- The motion and functionality of the thumb should be top priorities due to its critical role in hand function.
- Joint stability is equally important to joint motion as a functional consideration for orthotics and prosthetics.

Upper extremity function allows for complex task accomplishment in reaching, prehension, and manipulation. The upper extremity can be examined as a linkage system. The main effector of the upper extremity is the hand; the wrist, elbow, and shoulder act to place the hand in space. The description and analysis of function can be assisted by studies using biomechanical principles. Application of this information is especially relevant for orthotic design and prescription. This chapter discusses upper extremity biomechanics according to the main joint functions of motion, stability, and strength. The final section addresses specific needs created by trauma or congenital deformity.

Motion

Description of motion

Biomechanically anatomical joints are described according to joint axes and degrees of freedom. For example, the interphalangeal (IP) joint is considered to be a uniaxial joint with one degree of freedom, allowing motion in the one plane. The type and range of movement of a joint are dependent upon passive constraint provided by the shape and contour of the joint surfaces, ligaments, and soft tissue, as well as active facilitation by the neuromuscular system.

The description of motion becomes detailed when multiaxial joints, such as the glenohumeral joint, are studied. The eulerian angle system is a method that has utility in describing three-dimensional rotation.[4,5] This method takes into consideration the fact that three-dimensional rotation is sequence dependent. This description can be applied clinically to describe the range of joint motion as well as specify joint position in orthotic prescription.

Normal range of motion arcs versus functional motion requirements

When studying upper extremity motion, it is important to delineate between the normal arc of movement standards for specific joints and the functional arc of motion required for most daily activities. For example, although the elbow has a normal arc of flexion–extension of 0 to 150 degrees and pronation and supination of 75 to 85 degrees, respectively,[15] the full arc of motion is not generally used for most activities of daily living. A study of the functional elbow arc of motion conducted by Morrey et al.[66] revealed that 15 activities of

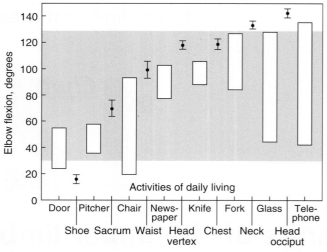

Fig. 12-1 Functional arc of elbow motion for activities of daily living is approximately 100 degrees, between 30 and 130 degrees. (From An KN, Morrey BF: Biomechanics. In Morrey BF editor: *Joint replacement arthroplasty*, New York, 1991, Churchill Livingstone.)

daily living can be carried out with an arc of motion of 30 to 130 degrees of flexion–extension (Fig. 12-1). Furthermore, these same activities required an equal amount of 50 degrees of pronation and 50 degrees of supination. Those activities that use an arc of motion require it be about equally centered between pronation and supination. Note that the activities studied were related to activities of daily living. Special requirements for other activities, including occupational tasks, have not been clearly elucidated. Figure 12-2 illustrates the importance of forearm supination and pronation in positioning the upper extremity for feeding and dressing tasks.

Similarly, the wrist has a normal arc of flexion of 80 to 85 degrees, approximately 70 degrees of extension, 20 degrees of radial deviation, and 30 degrees of ulnar deviation.[2]

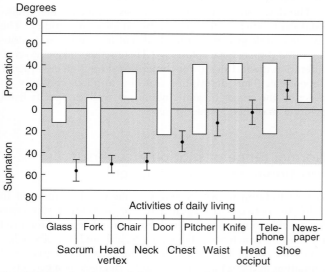

Fig. 12-2 Functional arc of forearm rotation is approximately 50 degrees of pronation and 50 degrees of supination for most activities of daily living. (From An KN, Morrey BF: Biomechanics. In Morrey BF editor: *Joint replacement arthroplasty*, New York, 1991, Churchill Livingstone.)

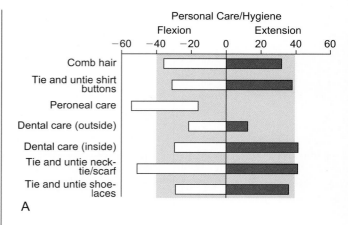

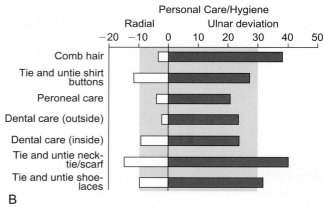

Fig. 12-3 Range of wrist motion required during personal care and hygiene activities. **A,** Extension–flexion. **B,** Ulnar–radial deviation. The gray striped area represents 70% of the maximum motion (40 degrees extension, 40 degrees flexion, 10 degrees radial deviation, 30 degrees ulnar deviation). (From Ryu J, Cooney WP III, Askew LJ, et al: *J Hand Surg* 16A:409-419, 1991.)

Ryu et al.[84] examined 40 normal subjects (20 men and 20 women) to determine the range of motion required to perform activities of daily living. The amount of wrist flexion and extension, as well as radial and ulnar deviation, were measured simultaneously using a biaxial wrist electrogoniometer. The entire battery of evaluated tasks could be accomplished with 60 degrees of extension, 54 degrees of flexion, 40 degrees of ulnar deviation, and 17 degrees of radial deviation. The majority of the hand placement and range of motion tasks studied in this project could be accomplished with 70% of the maximal range of wrist motion (Fig. 12-3). This converts to 40 degrees each of wrist flexion and extension and 40 degrees of combined radial–ulnar deviation (30 degrees of ulnar deviation, 10 degrees of radial deviation). The knowledge of functional range of motion requirements for activities of daily living can act as a guide when developing orthotic assistive devices. It should be an objective to provide devices that will allow motion in order to perform functional tasks and, ideally, occupational tasks.

Compensatory motion in the upper extremity

Contrary to accepted thought, the primary functions of the shoulder complex and elbow are mutually exclusive. It has been observed clinically that patients can tolerate elbow flexion contractures of about 30 degrees without much functional impairment. On the other hand, it also is well recognized that with motion loss greater than 30 degrees, patients readily complain of functional impairment. To better understand the implications of this loss of motion, it should be recognized that the shoulder functions as a ball and socket joint, allowing the hand to move in a spherical boundary in space.[65] As the elbow moves into a more extended position, a new sphere surface may be described. Thus, the effective sphere of influence of the hand extends from the patient as far into space as the link at the elbow allows. It has been calculated that a loss of elbow motion of 30 degrees, 45 degrees, and 60 degrees leads to loss of functional volume of the hand by 28%, 39%, and 60% respectively.

A study by O'Neill et al.[79] analyzed compensatory motion in the upper extremity after simulated elbow arthrodesis. The 3Space Tracker System (Polhemus, Inc., Colchester, VT) was used to measure shoulder motion, a biaxial wrist goniometer was used to measure wrist compensation, and all subjects were videotaped to qualitatively observe other compensatory motion. Ten healthy male subjects were asked to complete a series of tasks that represented use of the elbow in functional tasks. They were fitted with a custom adjustable brace that simulated elbow arthrodesis at 50, 70, 90, and 100 degrees of flexion and asked to repeat the tasks. Unlike other joints, elbow arthrodesis at any angle resulted in a significant impairment because the adjacent shoulder and wrist joints could not compensate to allow completion of activities. In upper extremity orthotic design, it is important to apply this information to understand the role and limits of compensatory motion of adjacent joints in providing function after injury or disease.

Synergistic motion of wrist and hand

Awareness of the relationship between wrist joint position and tendon excursion is essential for understanding motor control of the fingers and hand. Positioning the wrist in the direction opposite that of the fingers alters the functional length of the digital tendons so that synergistic finger movement can be attained. Wrist extension is synergistic to finger flexion and increases the length of the finger flexor muscles, allowing increased flexion with stretch.[100] In contrast, wrist flexion is synergistic to finger extension, with wrist flexion placing tension on the long extensors, facilitating finger extension. This relationship has application in tendon-splinting techniques with respect to affecting tendon excursion through positioning and the potential benefits of synergistic wrist motion and metacarpophalangeal (MP) joint motion in promoting flexor tendon gliding after repair. Also, synergistic wrist motion principles are the basis for many orthotic designs that provide assistive function of the hand with quadriplegia.

In a study by Horii et al.,[46] the efficacy of a new technique that used synergistic wrist motion (S-splint) was compared with traditional dorsal splinting methods used for mobilization of the flexor tendon after repair: the Kleinert splint (K-splint) and the Brooke Army Hospital/Walter Reed modified Kleinert splint with a palmar bar (P-splint). The results of this study question the anticipated tendon excursion associated with postoperative splinting. They demonstrated that the measured tendon excursion under a condition of low tendon tension was almost half that of theoretically predicted values. In zone II, the magnitude of excursion introduced by the three mobilization methods were in descending order: S-splint, P-splint, K-splint ($P <.05$). The differential tendon excursion between the flexor digitorum profundus and the flexor digitorum superficialis had a mean value of 3 mm and was not significantly different among the three methods. Passive proximal interphalangeal (PIP) joint motion was the most effective means of providing increased amplitude of tendon gliding in zone II. Passive distal interphalangeal (DIP) joint motion did not increase excursion in zone II as much as had been predicted. Further study is needed to test new designs of splints in vivo.

Stability

It is believed that any joint constraint, in part, consists of static and dynamic elements. The static factors can be divided into articular, capsular, ligamentous, and intraarticular pressure components. Dynamic stability originates from muscle activity.

Shoulder

In the normal shoulder, the articulating surfaces of the humerus and glenoid provide minimal stability to the shoulder.[9] The contact area between the two articulating surfaces is relatively small, with only 25% to 30% of the humeral head in contact with the glenoid surface in any anatomical location. Because the glenohumeral joint does not possess inherent bony stability, it relies to a greater extent on capsular, ligamentous, and dynamic muscular activity for constraint.

The capsule and ligamentous structures of the shoulder function in a coordinated manner to resist joint translation. This occurs primarily by resisting displacement but secondarily by soft tissue constraints imparting increased joint contact pressure opposite the direction of the displacement. Dempster[30] studied the relationship between increased joint contact pressure and resistance to translation. The influence of atmospheric pressure or intraarticular pressure on the stability of the shoulder has been assessed in experimental and analytic investigations.[9] The shoulder was seen to subluxate inferiorly by as much as 2 cm after capsular puncture, with marked alteration in joint constraint while performing passive motion. Venting of the capsule in cadaveric specimens was found to have a significant effect on the position of the humeral head. The mean intraarticular pressure was -76 cm H_2O without load, and values decreased in a linear fashion with increased load.

Dynamic shoulder stability during activity is achieved by the shoulder musculature.[85] The role of the rotator cuff in shoulder joint stability is well recognized. Howell et al.[48] demonstrated in a cadaveric study that the humeral head is positioned in the center of the glenoid in the horizontal plane by a centering mechanism provided by the active rotator cuff. Even in an unbalanced situation, without equal simulated muscle contraction from the anterior or the posterior cuff components, the activity of the remaining cuff centers the humerus on the glenoid surface. Thus, compression of the articular surfaces and the centering effect are believed to be accomplished by secondary tightening of the ligaments. The central role of the deltoid muscle in elevating the arm is countered by depressive action of the anterior and posterior rotator cuff musculature. Thus, the shoulder rotators stabilize the joint by increasing the compressive force between the glenohumeral articular surfaces.

Joint stability can be enhanced by the barrier effect of the contracted muscle. The subscapularis is an important dynamic stabilizer, acting as an anterior barrier to resist anteroinferior humeral head displacement with abduction and external rotation. Because the cross-sectional areas of the rotator cuff musculature anteriorly and posteriorly are essentially equal, the torque generated by these groups is balanced with respect to a force couple that resists both anterior and posterior humeral head translation.

Itoi et al.[50] investigated the stabilizing effect of the long (LHB) and short head of the biceps (SHB) muscle. Anterior stability was analyzed in 13 cadaver shoulders. The LHB and SHB were replaced by spring devices, and translation tests of the arm at 90 degrees of abduction were performed by applying a 1.5-kg anterior force. The position of the humeral head was monitored by an electromagnetic tracking device with or without an anterior translational force; with loads of 0, 1.5, or 3 kg applied on either LHB or SHB tendons in 60, 90, or 120 degrees of external rotation; and with the capsule intact, vented, or damaged by a simulated Bankart lesion.

The authors concluded that the LHB and SHB have similar functions as anterior stabilizers of the glenohumeral joint with the arm in abduction and external rotation, and that their role increases as shoulder stability decreases. Both heads of the biceps, if contracted, have a stabilizing function in resisting anterior head displacement.

Elbow

The anterior bundle of the medial collateral ligament (MCL) has been implicated as the primary valgus stabilizer of the elbow, with the radial head serving as a secondary joint stabilizer.[8,54] Hotchkiss and Weiland[47] reported that all elbows became unstable after this structure was sectioned. In an unconstrained kinematic study using an electromagnetic tracking device, Morrey et al.[67] demonstrated moderate joint laxity after sectioning of the anterior bundle of the MCL, even with an intact radial head. Sojbjerg et al.[93] confirmed the importance of the anterior bundle of the MCL in a cadaveric model. Clinically, both Schwab et al.[90] and Conway et al.[24] emphasized the functional importance of the ligament reconstructions for patients with a deficiency of this structure.

Studies by O'Driscoll et al.[77] suggested that the lateral ulnar collateral ligament is a major stabilizing structure for both rotational and varus instability. Injury to this ligament results in posterolateral rotatory subluxation of the elbow, as demonstrated by feelings of instability and a positive pivot shift test. Reconstruction of this ligament has been shown to restore stability to the elbow both clinically and experimentally.[74,76]

An et al.[10] addressed in a cadaveric study the importance of the proximal ulna articular surface in providing joint stability. In this study, progressive excision of the proximal ulna resulted in a progressive decrease in the stability of the elbow. Valgus stress was in large measure (80%) resisted by the proximal portion of the greater sigmoid notch, whereas varus stress was primarily resisted by the distal portion of the joint surface (65%).

The coronoid process of the ulna is another important stabilizer of the elbow. A failure to reconstitute this structure after fractures occur has been correlated with elbow instability and a poor functional outcome.[83] The coronoid process appears to be an essential osseous block to prevent posterior subluxation of the elbow joint, especially with the elbow in extension.

Forearm joint

The forearm joint is a complex joint composed of the radius and ulna. In essence it is a bicondylar joint, with the proximal radioulnar joint (PRUJ) and distal radioulnar joint (DRUJ) serving as a condyle. The activity at either joint cannot be separated from the other joint due to the rigid body nature of the radius and ulna. The PRUJ is constrained by the mutual articulating surfaces of the cylindrical radial head and the lateral notch of the ulna, as well as the annular ligament and the joint capsule. The DRUJ is constrained by the articulating surfaces of the head of the ulnar and the sigmoid notch of the radius, as well as the distal radioulnar ligaments (forming the deep part of the triangular fibrocartilage complex) and the DRUJ joint capsule. In the center of the forearm, the interosseous membrane thickens to form the central band or ligament, which also contributes to forearm stability.[53,69,107]

The motion prescribed by the forearm can best be described as a pivoting behavior, with mobile hand–wrist–radius unit rotation around the fixed ulna.[103] There is nearly total rotation at the PRUJ, with a nearly fixed axis of rotation passing through the geometric center of the head of the radius. There is a combination of rotation and translation through the DRUJ, with the forearm axis of rotation passing through the fovea region at the base of the ulnar styloid process (Fig. 12-4). The intersection of the forearm axis of rotation

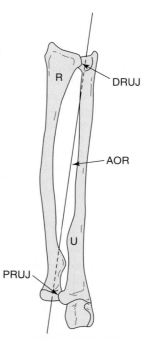

Fig. 12-4 The "forearm joint" is composed of the radius (R) and ulna (U), which articulate through the proximal radioulnar joint (PRUJ) and distal radioulnar joint (DRUJ). The axis of rotation (AOR) passes obliquely through the radial and ulnar heads.

and the cortex of the head of the ulna reciprocally translates posteriorly in supination and anteriorly in pronation.

The factors leading to instability of the DRUJ have been studied extensively, including the contribution of the interosseous membrane to DRUJ stability as well as the contributions of components of the triangular fibrocartilage complex.[1,42,89,97,106,107] Overall, the palmar radioulnar ligament and the dorsal DRUJ capsule can be considered the principal constraints against anterior translation of the radius relative to the ulna. The dorsal radioulnar ligament and the anterior DRUJ capsule are the principal constraints against posterior translation of the radius relative to the ulna. Clinically, the most common pattern of instability results from disruption of the common ligament attachment at the base of the ulnar styloid process, rendering both the dorsal and palmar radioulnar ligaments incompetent.[42]

The presence or absence of the ulnar head has become an important consideration in forearm stability. One of the most common procedures performed for painful arthritis of the DRUJ is the so-called Darrach resection, where the head of the ulna is simply excised.[28] This has led to the appreciation of residual instability and pain, largely from convergence of the radius onto the ulna.[63] A number of reconstructive procedures to restabilize the forearm joint following excision of the ulnar head have been proposed,[18,86–88] but the most efficacious procedure to date has been implantation of an ulnar head endoprosthesis to reestablish direct contact between the radius and ulna.[14,88,104]

Wrist

In the wrist, a complex system of ligamentous constraints and the articulations of the joint surfaces contribute to stability. This complex ligament system can be divided into extrinsic and intrinsic components. The palmar intrinsic ligaments of the distal row appear to be strongly connected to the carpal bones, as demonstrated by Garcia-Elias et al.[38,39]

The scapholunate and lunotriquetral ligaments are thought to be the most critical ligaments of the wrist, and they accept the greatest load and strain prior to failure.[73] Biplanar x-ray studies of normal and abnormal kinematics after sectioning of these ligaments have elucidated their importance in providing stability to the scaphoid and lunate.[45] The ultimate strength behavior, stress–strain curves, and joint kinematic pattern descriptions may be of value in developing repair or reconstruction techniques for the scapholunate and lunotriquetral ligaments.

Hand

Primary joint instability is related to muscle and tendon response to sustained pinch and grasp forces.[6,12] In contrast, the ligaments and capsules appear to play the role of initial stabilizer against instantaneous joint load and provide a second line of defense in maintaining joint stability.

The collateral ligament stabilizers of all joints in the hand are important soft tissues. Depending on the orientation of the fibers, various portions of the collateral ligament play different roles in joint stability. Understanding the anatomical characteristics and function of the capsuloligamentous structure is important for orthotic design when ligamentous structure is impaired.

Strength
Muscle mechanics

Three parameters have commonly been used to describe the size and morphology of the muscle.[7,17] Muscle fiber length is related to the potential for tendon excursion. The physiological cross-sectional area of a muscle is proportional to the maximum tension of the muscle. Because work equals force times distance, the muscle mass or volume is proportional to total work capacity.

The arrangement of the muscle fiber architecture further influences the characteristics of muscle contraction. Parallel muscle fibers produce a length–tension curve with maintained force throughout a greater distance than the sharply peaked length–tension curve of shorter fiber pennate muscles.[52,112] The muscle architecture has been defined based on the pennation angle. More recently, the concept of muscle index of architecture, i_a, has been adopted to describe the muscle architecture and the length–tension relationship. In general, the muscle fibers lie at an angle to the direction of induced motion. Two measurements can be taken at muscle optimum length: muscle fiber length and muscle belly length. The ratio of the mean fiber length to the muscle belly length is defined as the index of architecture.[112] Typically, the length–tension relationship of muscles is a function of different architecture indices.

Muscle moment arms around the joint determine the efficiency of the muscle in generating motion and torque; the larger the moment arm, the higher the torque and rotation angle generated for the same amount of muscle force and excursion. Determination of the potential moment arm contributions of muscles can provide insight into the balance of forces at a joint for planning tendon transfers or for designing orthotics to assist in providing mobility or stability with loss of function. A good example is examination of the tendon excursion and moment arms of the wrist muscles. Numerous investigators have examined tendon excursion and moment arm relationships at the wrist.[11,16,44,78] In a study by Horii et al., tendon excursion and joint rotation angles were measured using an electric potentiometer and an electromagnetic tracking device.[44] Instantaneous moment arms of each tendon then could be calculated based on the slope of the curve between tendon excursion and joint angular displacement. Five prime wrist motor tendons on freshly frozen cadavers were studied. Calculated tendon moment arms were found to be consistent throughout a full range of flexion–extension wrist motion and radioulnar deviation and corresponded closely to the anatomical location and orientation of the tendons. The flexor carpi ulnaris (FCU) tendon provided the largest moment contribution to the wrist joint. Forearm rotation did not affect the function of the wrist tendon except for the extensor carpi ulnaris. During flexion–extension motion, the excursion of the extensor carpi ulnaris decreased significantly from 10 to 4 mm, with the forearm in neutral and pronated positions. During radioulnar deviation, the excursion of the extensor carpi ulnaris increased from 14 to 17 mm, with the forearm in supinated and pronated positions. When a tendon transfer is planned, the entire tendon balance must be considered case by case. For example, the FCU tendon is recommended for reconstruction with radial nerve palsy.[40] However, the moment contribution of this muscle is large,[105] and one might predict that an imbalance of the wrist may result from the FCU transfer.

The maximum muscle tension that can be developed is directly related to the length of the muscle at contraction, which is dependent on the position of the joint. This concept is well illustrated by O'Driscoll et al.[75] in a study that analyzed the relationship between wrist position and grip strength. In their study, the position assumed by a normal wrist during unconstrained maximal grip and the relationship between wrist position and grip strength were investigated in 20 healthy subjects using a biaxial electrogoniometer and grip dynamometer. Grip strength and wrist position were recorded in the self-selected position and again while the subjects voluntarily deviated the wrist randomly into flexion, extension, or radial or ulnar deviation of 10 to 15 degrees. The self-selected position was 35 degrees of extension and 7 degrees of ulnar deviation. Grip strength was significantly less in any position of deviation from this self-selected position, even after accounting for fatigue. With the wrist in only 15 degrees of extension or in neutral radial–ulnar deviation, grip strength was reduced to two thirds to three fourths of normal. Gender did not affect wrist position. The dominant wrists were within 5 degrees of the nondominant wrists but were relatively less extended and in more ulnar deviation. Grip strength is significantly reduced when wrist position deviates from this self-selected optimal position. It has been hypothesized that as the wrist moves into ulnar deviation, the length–tension relationship affords a more effective functional length of the finger flexors, resulting in an increased level of force.

Orthotic and prosthetic considerations following hand injury

Traumatic injury often results in a loss of many of the relationships described. Mutilated hands, hands stricken with arthritis, and hands that are congenitally misshapen often require prosthetic or orthotic aids to regain or facilitate hand function. In addition to understanding the principles of normal hand mechanics, consideration of the essential components of hand function is important because it will aid therapists in their construction and fabrication of hand prosthesis and hand splints.

Functional hand essentials

In its most elemental form, the hand is composed of a stable wrist and at least two digits that can oppose with some power. One digit should be capable of motion so that it can grasp objects. The other digit need only act as a stable post against which the movable digit can pinch. To allow for prehensile movements, the digits require some form of cleft to divide them, which will allow for the accommodation of objects. The digits need to be sensate and pain-free. Insensate or chronically painful digits may offer little benefit over prosthetic replacement.[22,34,43] Requirements for functional sensation have been defined as two-point discrimination of less than 10 to 12 mm.[64]

The hand allows for prehension, which is the ability to grasp and manipulate objects. As defined by Tubiana et al.,[101] prehension "may be defined as all the functions that are put into play when an object is grasped by the hands-intent, permanent sensory control, and a mechanism of grip." Prehension requires that the hand be able to approach, grasp, and release an object.[82,101] Thus, if only two sensate digits remain to oppose each other, some prehension is possible.

In terms of biomechanical motion, the hand performs approximately seven basic maneuvers that compose the majority of hand function:

1. *Precision pinch* (*terminal pinch*). This involves flexion at the DIP joint of the index and at the IP joint of the thumb. The ends of the fingernails are brought together, as in lifting a paperclip from a tabletop.
2. *Oppositional pinch* (*subterminal pinch*). The pulp of the index and thumb are brought together with the DIP joints extended. This allows for generation of force through thumb opposition, first dorsal interosseous contraction and index profundus flexion. This often is measured with a dynamometer.
3. *Key pinch*. The thumb is adducted to the radial side of the middle phalanx of the index finger. Key pinch requires a stable post (usually the index finger) that has adequate length and an MP joint, which can resist the thumb adduction force.
4. *Directional grip* (*chuck grip*). The thumb and the index and long fingers come together to surround a cylindrical object. When using this grip, a rotational and axial force usually is applied to the held object (e.g., using a screwdriver).
5. *Hook grip*. This requires finger flexion at the IP joints and extension at the MP joints. It is the only type of functional grasp that does not require thumb function. This grip is used when lifting a suitcase.
6. *Power grasp*. The fingers are fully flexed while the thumb is flexed and opposed over the other digits, as in holding a baseball bat. Force if applied through the fingers into the palm.
7. *Span grasp*. The DIP and PIP joints flex to approximately 30 degrees and the thumb is abducted. Force is generated between the thumb and fingers as opposed to power grasp, where force is generated between the fingers and the palm. Stability is required at the thumb MP and IP. This grip is used to lift cylindrical objects.[32,92,101]

Postoperatively, the hand's ability to adopt these positions and exert force through them will impact how well the patient rehabilitates. These maneuvers are predicated on good sensation in the fingers and thumb. When assessing hand deficits (traumatic or congenital), it is easiest to think of the hand as containing four functional units: (1) opposable thumb, (2) index and long fingers, whose stable basal joints serve as fixed posts for pinch and power functions, (3) ring and small fingers, which represent the mobile unit of the hand, and (4) wrist. It also may help to think of only two major forms of hand motion as opposed to seven: thumb–finger pinch and digitopalmar grip. Pinch requires preservation of the thumb unit and a stable post. Patients who are able to add a third digit to pinch can achieve more precision. Pinch function tends to be preserved when the median nerve is intact and the thumb and index–long units of the hand are salvageable. Without median nerve function, thumb sensation and thenar function are lost, making fine motor movements negligible. In comparison, ulnar nerve function and the ring–small finger unit are more important for digitopalmar grip, where flexion and sensation in the ulnar digits are essential. Thumb preservation is important in power grasp to provide stability and control of directional forces. With these principles in mind, let us now examine how digital loss affects hand function.

Biomechanical impact following digital loss

Thumb

The functional importance of each digit has been debated. If the digits were to be prioritized, the thumb, with its importance in prehension and in all forms of grasp, takes top priority. It provides 40% of overall hand function in the uninjured setting.[94–96] Following mutilating trauma, when digits are missing or stiff, the thumb can account for greater than 50% of hand function.[110] Its uniqueness and versatility in humans are due to the position of the thumb axis. The thumb axis is based at the trapeziometacarpal (TMC) joint and is pronated and flexed approximately 80 degrees with respect to the other metacarpals in the hand.[70] This positioning allows for circumduction, which permits opposition.[25,26,49,70]

Opposition of the thumb is necessary for all useful prehension, and its preservation provides the basis for successful salvage procedures. Opposition of the thumb is the result of angulatory motion, which is produced through abduction at the TMC joint, flexion, and rotation of the TMC and MP joints.[27] Multiple muscles are required for functional opposition. These include the abductor pollicis brevis, opponens pollicis, and superficial head of the flexor pollicis brevis. These muscles act simultaneously on the TMC joint and the MP joint. The abductor pollicis brevis provides the major component of opposition, with the opponens pollicis and flexor pollicis brevis providing secondary motors for opposition.[17,27,49,51,70,71] The extensor pollicis longus (EPL) and adductor pollicis (ADP) are antagonists to thumb opposition, providing a supinating extension and adduction force.

Injuries distal to the IP joint (zone I injuries) may produce little functional deficit because oppositional length tends to be maintained.[29,102] Injuries, through the level of the MP, are the most common and represent significant loss of function. Unreconstructed injuries will result in a decrease in pinch dexterity and grip strength.[91] The MP joint of the thumb has no other mechanical equivalent in the hand. It has three degrees of freedom. It represents a ball-and-socket joint in extension; however, when the joint is flexed, tightening of the collateral ligaments causes the MP joint to function more like a hinge. The intrinsic muscles provide motion but also provide dynamic stability to the joint.

Injuries proximal to the MP joint result in damage to the thenar muscles, with resultant instability to the TMC joint. This produces a major stumbling block in thumb reconstruction because TMC stability is required for successful thumb reconstruction. Injuries at this level often will require special procedures to restore opposition and pinch.[57,91] In its most primitive form pinch can be recreated, as in the tetraplegic patient, with fusion of the IP and MP and reconstruction of the adductor musculature. However, for reconstruction of oppositional pinch, tendon transfers may be necessary.

Digital loss

For the most part, single digit amputation (with the exception of the thumb) will not result in the loss of essential hand function. Brown studied 183 surgeons who suffered partial or total digital amputations.[20] Only four surgeons were unable to continue operating after their injuries. Most surprising was the finding that 15 surgeons who had experienced thumb amputations through the metacarpal or MP joint level were able to continue operating with only minimal adaptation in their surgical practice. Brown[20] concluded that the motivation of the patient is more important than the actual number of retained digits when attempting to predict functional outcome for digital amputation. Of note, none of the surgeons had to perform repetitive strenuous activity with the hand, and grip strength presumably was not a major issue.[20]

Unlike single digit amputation, amputation of several digits remains a challenging problem. In the mutilated hand, multiple digital loss is the norm, as severely crushed and avulsed digits preclude replantation. Preservation of the thumb and a single digit will allow for some prehensile grasp, but for optimal function the reconstruction of an additional digit is recommended.[99,108–110] Preservation or reconstruction of the thumb and two digits allows for the possibility of chuck pinch, which is stronger than subterminal pinch. Use of a third digit confers lateral stability in power pinch. A third digit also allows patients to perform hook grip and power grasp. Span grasp now is possible as functional palmar space is increased, allowing for grasp of larger objects.[99,108–110] In injuries with loss of all fingers but sparing of the thumb, reconstructive goals should attempt to maintain useful thumb web space and an opposable ulnar post of adequate length[94,110]

Biomechanical impact of fusion

In several situations, the severity of trauma precludes any anatomical restoration of the joint surface. These situations may require fusion. Unfortunately, change in a single joint will have implications on the balance of the entire digit as well as the biomechanics of the hand. Of all fusions, DIP fusions are well tolerated and probably impart the least detriment to hand function. The DIP joint produces 15% of intrinsic digital flexion but contributes only 3% to the overall flexion arc of the finger.[61] Mechanical testing has shown that after simulated DIP fusion of the index and middle finger, grip strength decreases 20% to 25% compared to prefusion values. The decrease in grip strength may be secondary to the limited excursion of the profundus tendon following fusion; this can create a quadriga effect.

The PIP joint produces 85% of intrinsic digital flexion and contributes 20% to the overall arc of finger motion. PIP joint impairment can adversely affect the entire hand; however, a full range of PIP joint motion is not essential for hand function. An arc extending from 45 to 90 degrees can provide relatively normal function.[37] In addition, hyperextension of the MP joint can compensate for mild flexor contractures at the PIP level. This will allow the finger to move out of the plane of the palm when attempting to lay the hand flat or when placing objects into the palm.

PIP fusion in the index finger often is well tolerated, as the index's relatively independent profundus function does not impose a significant quadriga effect on the other fingers during power grasp. However, PIP fusion of the long finger has been shown to decrease the excursion of all profundus tendons, reducing grip strength. PIP fusion restricts profundus excursion to a greater extent than does DIP or MP fusion.[60,68,72] If both MP and PIP joints are injured, salvage of the MP joint through arthroplasty or other measures is preferred over PIP joint arthroplasty. Grip strength will be decreased due to a quadriga effect, but prehension can be maintained as long as the thumb or border digit is capable of opposition.

The MP joints probably represent the most important joint for hand function. They contribute 77% of the total arc of finger flexion.[33,37,61,62,98] Unlike the ginglymoid IP joint, which functions like a sloppy hinge joint, the condyloid MCP joint is diathroidal, allowing for flexion–extension, abduction–adduction, and some rotation.[13,33,36,55] Most prehension grips require that the digits extend and abduct at the MP joint.[36,114] Precision pinch requires flexion, rotation, and ulnar deviation at the MP joint.[13,36] During pinch the radial intrinsics as well as the collateral ligament to the index must resist the stress applied by the thumb. According to the American Medical Association's Guide to the Evaluation of Permanent Impairment, fusion of the MP joint results in 45% impairment of the involved finger.[3] Some have suggested that a single stiff MP joint can impair the entire hand's function.[41] A full range of motion, however, is not required for hand function. Most activities of daily living require only 50% of normal joint motion.[13,31,58] Studies have shown that obtaining 35 degrees of motion at the MP is satisfactory if the arc of motion is within the functional range and the joint is stable.[13] Many rheumatoid patients, who have undergone PIP and DIP fusions, maintain a useful hand through preservation of MP motion. Previously, MCP arthrodesis was recommended for border digits in heavy laborers; however, this indication may be reconsidered given the availability of new surface replacement arthroplasty.[58,59]

Wrist fusion

Although less common than finger fusion, immediate limited wrist fusion or total wrist fusion may be necessary following penetrating ballistic trauma, punch press-type injuries, or in cases of gross carpal instability. A stable wrist is necessary for power grasp. In addition, a stable wrist will prevent dissipation of finger flexion and extension forces as tendons pass over the carpus. The requirements for functional wrist motion have been debated. Palmer et al.[80] found that the normal wrist had an average flexion–extension arc of 133 degrees, but only 5 degrees of flexion and 30 degrees of extension were needed for the majority of activity. Brumfield and Champoux[21] found that 10 degrees of flexion and 35 degrees of extension allowed patients to complete the activities of daily living. However, Ryu et al.[84] found in 40 normal patients that the majority of activities of daily living could be accomplished with 40 degrees of flexion, 40 degrees of extension, 10 degrees of radial deviation, and 30 degrees of ulnar deviation.

Patients undergoing wrist fusion can lose the beneficial effect of tenodesis for any subsequent tendon transfer. In addition, wrist dorsiflexion is important for pushing off, rising from a chair, and performing a power grasp. However, fusion may be the only option for patients with substantial carpal loss.

Wrist fusion can have a negative impact on MP motion and thumb motion, presumably due to extensor adhesion.[35] A 25% decrease in grip strength may occur.[35,56] Strength with key pinch, subterminal pinch, and directional grip are better maintained at approximately 85% of the normal side. Maximum preservation of power grip has been found to occur in 15 degrees of extension and 15% of ulnar deviation.[81] Weiss et al.[111] found that patients felt they were able to accomplish 85% of the activities of daily living following total wrist fusion. Patients were least able to use a screwdriver and perform perineal care. Overall, skills that presented the most difficulty were those that required significant wrist flexion in small spaces, where compensatory movements by the shoulder and elbow are eliminated.

In severely mutilating trauma, preservation of wrist mobility imparts some function to a forearm stump with the addition of a prosthesis. Modern prosthetic techniques allow incorporation of the prosthesis to the wrist so that proximal straps and attachment to the elbow are unnecessary. Preservation of wrist motion also eliminates the need to incorporate a wrist articulation into the prosthetic unit.[19,22,23] Preservation of the DRUJ will further improve function, as 50% of forearm rotation can be transferred into the prosthesis.[113]

Conclusion

Orthotic design and prescription can be aided by an understanding of upper extremity biomechanical principles. Knowledge of the range of motion arcs required to perform functional tasks and the degree to which compensatory motion at adjacent joints can provide task accomplishment is especially relevant. For example, the wrist and shoulder cannot effectively compensate for loss of elbow motion.

Another important consideration is joint stability requirements for rehabilitation goals with orthotic use, as illustrated by the shoulder. Shoulder motion is highly complex, allowing movement in a sphere of motion placing the humerus at a fixed angle. Because of the multiaxial nature of this joint, effective orthotic management given the lack of dynamic stability of the rotator cuff muscles and long head of the biceps is difficult.

Strength parameters based on muscle mechanics can guide orthotic development based on considerations of tendon excursion, physiological cross-sectional area, moment arm determination, and the muscle–length tension relationship. The use of synergistic wrist motion in orthotic design and the application of the muscle–length tension relationship in optimally positioning the wrist for force production are two illustrations of the importance of understanding biomechanical principles. Further collaborative studies between clinicians and biomechanicians are needed for continued advancement of orthotic assistive devices.

References

1. af Ekenstam F, Hagert CG: Anatomical studies on the geometry and stability of the distal radio ulnar joint. *Scand J Plast Reconstr Surg*, 19:17-25, 1985.
2. American Academy of Orthopaedic Surgeons: *Joint motion: methods of measuring and recording*, Chicago, 1965, American Academy of Orthopaedic Surgeons.
3. American Medical Association: *Guides to the evaluation of permanent impairment*, Chicago, 1984, American Medical Association.

4. An KN, Browne AO, Korinek S, et al: Three-dimensional kinematics of glenohumeral elevation. *J Orthop Res*, 9:143-149, 1991.

5. An KN, Chao EY: Kinematic analysis of human movement. *Ann Biomed Eng*, 12:585-597, 1984.

6. An KN, Cooney WPI: Biomechanics, section II: the hand and the wrist. *Joint replacement arthroplasty*, New York, 1991, Churchill Livingstone.

7. An KN, Hui FC, Morrey BF, et al: Muscles across the elbow joint: a biomechanical analysis. *J Biomech*, 14:659-669, 1981.

8. An KN, Morrey BF: Biomechanics, section III: the elbow. *Joint replacement arthroplasty*, New York, 1991, Churchill Livingstone.

9. An KN, Morrey BF: Biomechanics, section IV: the shoulder. *Joint replacement arthroplasty*, New York, 1991, Churchill Livingstone.

10. An KN, Morrey BF, Chao EY: The effect of partial removal of proximal ulna on elbow constraint. *Clin Orthop Rel Res*, 209:270-279, 1986.

11. Armstrong TJ, Chaffin DB: An investigation of the relationship between displacements of the finger and wrist joint and the extrinsic finger flexor tendons. *J Biomech*, 11:119-128, 1978.

12. Basmajian JV: *Muscles alive*, Baltimore, 1962, Williams & Wilkins.

13. Beckenbaugh RD, Dobyns JH, Linscheid RL, et al: Review and analysis of silicone-rubber metacarpal phalangeal implants. *J Bone Joint Surg*, 58A:483-487, 1976.

14. Berger RA, Cooney WPI: Use of an ulnar head endoprosthesis for treatment of an unstable distal ulnar resection: review of mechanics, indications, and surgical technique. *Hand Clin*, 21:603-620, 2005.

15. Boone DC, Azen SP: Normal range of motion of joints in male subjects. *J Bone Joint Surg*, 61A:756-759, 1979.

16. Brand PW: *Clinical mechanics of the hand*, St. Louis, 1985, CV Mosby.

17. Brand PW, Beach RB, Thompson DE: Relative tension and potential excursion of muscles in the forearm and hand. *J Hand Surg*, 6A:209-219, 1981.

18. Breen TF, Jupiter JB: Extensor carpi ulnaris and flexor carpi ulnaris tenodesis for the unstable distal ulna. *J Hand Surg*, 14A:612-617, 1989.

19. Brown P: Sacrifice of the unsatisfactory hand. *J Hand Surg*, 4:417-423, 1979.

20. Brown PW: Less than–surgeons with amputated fingers. *J Hand Surg*, 7:31-37, 1982.

21. Brumfield RH, Champoux JA: A biomechanical study of normal functional wrist motion. *Clin Orthop Rel Res*, 187:23-25, 1984.

22. Burkhalter W: Mutilating injuries of the hand. *Hand Clin*, 2:45-68, 1986.

23. Childress DS, Hampton FL, Lambert CN, et al: Myoelectric immediate postsurgical procedure: a concept for the fitting the upper extremity amputee. *Artif Limbs*, 13:55-60, 1969.

24. Conway JE, Jobe FW, Glousman RE, et al: Medial instability of the elbow in throwing athletes. Treatment by repair or reconstruction of the ulnar collateral ligament. *J Bone Joint Surg*, 74A:67-83, 1992.

25. Cooney WP, Chao EYS: Biomechanical analysis of static forces in the thumb during hand function. *J Bone Joint Surg*, 59A:27-36, 1977.

26. Cooney WP, Linscheid RL, An KN: Opposition of the thumb: an anatomic and biomechanical study of tendon transfers. *J Hand Surg*, 9A:777-786, 1984.

27. Cooney WP, Lucca MJ, Chao EYS, et al: The kinesiology of the thumb trapeziometacarpal joint. *J Bone Joint Surg*, 63A:1371-1381, 1981.

28. Darrach W: Partial excision of lower shaft of ulna for deformity following Colle's fracture, 1913. *Clin Orthop Relat Res*, 275:3-4, 1992.

29. Dell'oca RL, Hentz VR: Thumb reconstruction. In Goldwyn RM, Cohen MN, editors: *The unfavorable result in plastic surgery*, Philadelphia, 2001, Lippincott.

30. Dempster WT: Mechanisms of shoulder movement. *Arch Phys Med Rehabil*, 46A:49-70, 1965.

31. Doi K, Kuwata N, Kawai S: Alumina ceramic finger implants: a preliminary biomaterial and clinical evaluation. *J Hand Surg*, 9A:740-749, 1984.

32. Duparc J, Alnot J-Y, May P: Single digit amputations. *Mutilating injuries of the hand*, Edinburgh, 1979, Churchill Livingstone.

33. Ellis PR, Tsai T: Management of the traumatized joint of the finger. *Clin Plast Surg*, 16:457-473, 1989.

34. Entin MA: Salvaging the basic hand. *Surg Clin North Am*, 48:1062-1081, 1968.

35. Field J, Herbert TJ, Prosser R: Total wrist fusion. *J Hand Surg*, 21B:429-433, 1996.

36. Flatt AE: *Care of the rheumatoid hand*, St. Louis, 1983, Mosby.

37. Foucher G, Hoang P, Citron N, et al: Joint reconstruction following trauma: comparison of microsurgical transfer and conventional methods: a report of 61 cases. *J Hand Surg*, 11B:388-393, 1986.

38. Garcia-Elias M, An KN, Cooney WP 3rd, et al: Stability of the transverse carpal arch: an experimental study. *J Hand Surg*, 14A:277-282, 1989.

39. Garcia-Elias M, An KN, Cooney WP, et al: Transverse stability of the carpus. An analytical study. *J Orthop Res*, 7:738-743, 1989.

40. Green DP: Radial nerve palsy. *Operative hand surgery*, New York, 1988, Churchill Livingstone.

41. Hagert CG, Branemark PI, Albrektsson T, et al: Metacarpalphalangeal joint replacement with osseointegrated endoprostheses. *Scand J Plast Reconstr Surg*, 20:207-218, 1986.

42. Haugstvedt JR, Berger RA, Berglund LJ, et al: An analysis of the constraint properties of the distal radioulnar ligament attachments to the ulna. *J Hand Surg*, 27A:61-67, 2002.

43. Hentz VR, Chase RA: The philosophy of salvage and repair for acute hand injuries. *Acute hand injuries: a multispecialty approach*, St. Louis, 1979, Mosby.

44. Horii E, An KN, Linscheid RL: Excursion of prime wrist tendons. *J Hand Surg*, 18A:83-90, 1993.

45. Horii E, Garcia-Elias M, An KN, et al: A kinematic study of luno-triquetral dissociations. *J Hand Surg*, 16A:355-362, 1991.

46. Horii E, Lin GT, Cooney WP, et al: Comparative flexor tendon excursion after passive mobilization: an in vitro study. *J Hand Surg*, 17A:559-566, 1992.

47. Hotchkiss RN, Weiland AJ: Valgus stability of the elbow. *J Orthop Res*, 5:372-377, 1987.

48. Howell SM, Galinat BJ, Renzi AJ, et al: Normal and abnormal mechanics of the glenohumeral joint in the horizontal plane. *J Bone Joint Surg*, 70A:227-232, 1988.

49. Imaeda T, An KN, Cooney WP: Functional anatomy and biomechanics of the thumb. *Hand Clin*, 8:9-15, 1992.

50. Itoi E, Kuechle DK, Newman SR, et al: Stabilising function of the biceps in stable and unstable shoulders [published erratum appears in J Bone Joint Surg Br 76:170, 1994]. *J Bone Joint Surg*, 75B:546-550, 1993.

51. Kaplan EB: *Function and surgical anatomy of the hand*, ed 2, Philadelphia, 1965, JB Lippincott.

52. Kaufman KR, An KN, Chao EY: Incorporation of muscle architecture into the muscle length-tension relationship. *J Biomech*, 22:943-948, 1989.

53. Kaufmann RA, Kozin SH, Barnes A, et al: Changes in strain distribution along the radius and ulna with loading and interosseous membrane section. *J Hand Surg*, 27A:93-97, 2002.

54. King GJW, Morrey BF, An KN: Stabilizers of the elbow. Review article. *J Shoulder Elbow Surg*, 2:165-174, 1993.

55. Krishnan J, Chipchase L: Passive and axial rotation of the metacarpophalangeal joint. *J Hand Surg*, 22B:270-273, 1997.

56. Labosky DA, Waggy CA: Apparent weakness of the median and ulnar motors in radial nerve palsy. *J Hand Surg*, 11:528-533, 1986.

57. Leung PC: Thumb reconstruction using second-toe transfer. *Hand*, 15:15-21, 1983.

58. Linscheid RL, Beckenbaugh RD: Arthroplasty of the metacarpal phalangeal joint. In Morrey BF, An KN, editors: *Reconstructive surgery of the joints*, ed 2, New York 1996, Churchill Livingstone.

59. Linscheid RL, Murray PM, Vidal MA, et al: Development of a surface replacement arthroplasty for proximal interphalangeal joints. *J Hand Surg*, 22A:286-298, 1997.

60. Lista FR, Neu BR, Murray JF, et al: Profundus tendon blockage (the quadriga syndrome) in the hand with a stiff finger. In: 43rd *Annual Meeting of the American Society for Surgery of the Hand*, Baltimore, 1988.

61. Littler JW, Herndon JH, Thompson JS: Examination of the hand. *Reconstructive plastic surgery*, Philadelphia, 1977, WB Saunders.

62. Littler JW: Surgical and functional anatomy. In Bowers WH, editor: *The interphalangeal joints*, New York, 1987, Churchill Livingstone.

63. McKee MD, Richards RR: Dynamic radio-ulnar convergence after the Darrach procedure. *J Bone Joint Surg*, 780B:413-418, 1996.

64. Moberg E: Reconstructive hand surgery in tetraplegia, stroke, and cerebral palsy: basic concepts in physiology and neurology. *J Hand Surg*, 1A:29-34, 1976.

65. Morrey BF: *Applied anatomy and biomechanics of the elbow joint*, St. Louis, 1986, Mosby.

66. Morrey BF, Askew LJ, Chao EY: A biomechanical study of normal functional elbow motion. *J Bone Joint Surg*, 63A:872-877, 1981.

67. Morrey BF, Tanaka S, An KN: Valgus stability of the elbow. A definition of primary and secondary constraints. *Clin Orthop Relat Res*, 265:187-195, 1991.

68. Murray JF, Carman W, MacKenzie JK: Transmetacarpal amputation of the index finger. Actual assessment of hand strength and complications. *J Hand Surg*, 2:471-481, 1977.

69. Murray PM: Diagnosis and treatment of longitudinal instability of the forearm. *Tech Hand Up Extrem Surg*, 9:29-34, 2005.

70. Napier JR: The attachments and function of the abductor pollicis brevis. *J Anat*, 86:335-341, 1952.

71. Napier JR: The form and function of the carpometacarpal joint of the thumb. *J Anat*, 89:362, 1955.

72. Neu BR, Murray JF, MacKenzie JK: Profundus tendon blockage: quadriga in finger amputations. *J Hand Surg*, 10A:878-883, 1985.

73. Nowak MD, Logan SE: Ultimate strength patterns of 10 clinically significant human wrist ligaments. In: *IEEE Engineering in Medicine and Biology Society 10th Annual International Conference*, 1988.

74. O'Driscoll SW, Bell DF, Morrey BF: Posterolateral rotatory instability of the elbow. *J Bone Joint Surg*, 73A:440-446, 1991.

75. O'Driscoll SW, Horii E, Ness R, et al: The relationship between wrist position, grasp size, and grip strength. *J Hand Surg*, 17A:169-177, 1992.

76. O'Driscoll SW, Morrey BF, Bell DF: Posterolateral rotatory instability of the elbow: clinical, pathoanatomic, and radiographic features. *J Bone Joint Surg*, 72B:543, 1990.

77. O'Driscoll SW, Morrey BF, Korinek S: The pathoanatomy and kinematics of posterolateral rotatory instability (pivot-shift) of the elbow. *Transactions of the Orthopaedic Research Society*, 1990.

78. Ohnishi N, Ryu J, Colbaugh R, et al: Tendon excursion and moment arm of wrist motors and extrinsic finger motors at the wrist. *Annual Meeting of the American Society for Surgery of the Hand, Ontario, Canada*, 1990.

79. O'Neill OR, Morrey BF, Tanaka S, et al: Compensatory motion in the upper extremity after elbow arthrodesis. *Clin Orthop Relat Res*, 281:89-96, 1992.

80. Palmer AK, Werner FW, Murphy D, et al: Functional wrist motion: a biomechanical study. *J Hand Surg*, 10A:39-46, 1985.

81. Pryce JC: The wrist position between neutral and ulnar deviation that facilitates the maximum power grip strength. *J Biomech*, 13:505-511, 1980.

82. Radischong P: Les problemes fondamentaux du retablissement de la prehension. *Ann Chir*, 25:927, 1971.

83. Regan WD, Morrey BF: Fractures of the coronoid process of the ulna. *J Bone Joint Surg*, 71A:1348-1354, 1989.

84. Ryu J, Cooney WPI, Askew LJ, et al: Functional ranges of motion of the wrist joint. *J Hand Surg*, 16A:409-419, 1991.

85. Saha AK: Dynamic stability of the glenohumeral joint. *Acta Orthop Scand*, 42:491-505, 1971.

86. Sauerbier M, Berger RA, Fujita M, et al: Radioulnar convergence after distal ulnar resection: mechanical performance of two commonly used soft tissue stabilizing procedures. *Acta Orthop Scand*, 74:420-428, 2003.

87. Sauerbier M, Fujita M, Hahn ME, et al: The dynamic radioulnar convergence of the Darrach procedure and the ulnar head hemiresection interposition arthroplasty: a biomechanical study. *J Hand Surg*, 27B:307-316, 2002.

88. Sauerbier M, Hahn ME, Fujita M, et al: Analysis of dynamic distal radioulnar convergence after ulnar head resection and endoprosthesis implantation. *J Hand Surg*, 27A:425-434, 2002.

89. Schuind F, An KN, Berglund LJ, et al: The distal radioulnar ligaments: a biomechanical study. *J Hand Surg*, 16A:1106-1114, 1991.

90. Schwab GH, Bennet JB, Woods GW, et al: Biomechanics of elbow instability: the role of the medial collateral ligament. *Clin Orthop Relat Res*, 146:42-52, 1980.

91. Shin AY, Bishop AT, Berger RA: Microvascular reconstruction of the traumatized thumb. *Hand Clin*, 15:347-371, 1999.

92. Smith P: *Lister's the hand*, London, 2002, Churchill Livingstone.

93. Sojbjerg JO, Ovesen J, Nielsen S: Experimental elbow instability after transection of the medial collateral ligament. *Clin Orthop Relat Res*, 218:186-190, 1987.

94. Soucacos PN: Indications and selection for digital amputation and replantation. *J Hand Surg*, 26B:572-581, 2001.

95. Soucacos PN, Beris AE, Malizos KN, et al: Transposition microsurgery in multiple digital amputations. *Microsurgery*, 15:469-473, 1994.

96. Strickland JW: Thumb reconstruction *Operative hand surgery*, ed 2, New York, 1998, Churchill Livingstone.

97. Stuart PR, Berger RA, Linscheid RL, et al: The dorsopalmar stability of the distal radioulnar joint. *J Hand Surg*, 25A:689-699, 2000.

98. Swanson AB: Flexible implant arthroplasty for arthritic finger joints. *J Bone Joint Surg*, 54A:435-455, 1972.

99. Tsai TM, Jupiter JB, Wolff TW, et al: Reconstruction of severe transmetacarpal mutilating hand injuries by combined second and third toe transfer. *J Hand Surg*, 6:319-328, 1981.

100. Tubania R: Architecture and functions of the hand. In Tubiana R, Thomine J-M, Mackin E, editors: *Examination of the hand and upper limb*, Philadelphia, 1984, WB Saunders.

101. Tubania R, Thomine J, Mackin E: Movements of the hand and wrist. *Examination of the hand and wrist*, St. Louis, 1996, Mosby-Year Book.

102. Urbaniak JR: Thumb reconstruction by microsurgery. *Instr Course Lect*, 33:425-446, 1984.

103. Van Roy P, Baeyens JP, Fauvart D, et al: Arthro-kinematics of the elbow: study of the carrying angle. *Ergonomics*, 48:1645-1656, 2005.

104. van Schoonhoven J, Fernandez DL, Bowers WH, et al: Salvage of failed resection arthroplasties of the distal radioulnar joint using a new ulnar head prosthesis. *J Hand Surg*, 25A:438-446, 2000.

105. Volz RG, Lieb M, Benjamin J: Biomechanics of the wrist. *Clin Orthop Relat Res*, 149:112-117, 1980.

106. Watanabe H, Berger RA, An KN, et al: Stability of the distal radioulnar joint contributed by the joint capsule. *J Hand Surg*, 29A:1114-1120, 2004.

107. Watanabe H, Berger RA, Berglund LJ, et al: Contribution of the interosseous membrane to distal radioulnar joint constraint. *J Hand Surg*, 30A:1164-1174, 2005.

108. Wei FC, Chen HC, Chuang CC, et al: Reconstruction of a hand amputated at the metacarpophalangeal level by means of combined second and third toes from each foot. A case report. *J Hand Surg*, 11A:340-344, 1986.

109. Wei FC, Chen HC, Chuang CC, et al: Simultaneous multiple toe transfers in hand reconstruction. *Plast Reconstr Surg*, 81:366-377, 1988.

110. Wei FC, Colony LH: Microsurgical reconstruction of opposable digits in mutilating hand injuries. *Clin Plast Surg*, 16:491-504, 1989.

111. Weiss AP, Wiedeman G, Quenzer D, et al: Upper extremity function after wrist arthrodesis. *J Hand Surg*, 20A:813-817, 1995.

112. Woittiez RD, Huijing PA, Boom HB, et al: A three-dimensional muscle model: a quantified relation between form and function of skeletal muscles. *J Morphol*, 182:95-113, 1984.

113. Wright TW, Hagen AD, Wood MB: Prosthetic usage in major upper extremity amputations. *J Hand Surg*, 20A:619-622, 1995.

114. Zancolli E*Structural and dynamic bases of hand surgery*, ed 2, Philadelphia, 1983, Lippincott.

Chapter

13

Principles and components of upper limb orthoses

Thomas R. Lunsford and Thomas V. DiBello

Key Points

- Upper limb orthoses are more often accepted by patients when a well-defined therapeutic program is in place and the orthoses provide a desired function that cannot be accomplished in any other fashion.
- Upper limb orthoses can be categorized according to whether the design elements are static or dynamic and further subdivided according to whether their primary purpose is therapeutic or functional.
- Low-temperature thermoplastic orthoses are often fabricated by the occupational therapist, whose role includes evaluating the need for orthoses, recommending devices, and training the patient in their use.
- The role of the certified orthotist usually is to recommend, design, fabricate, fit, and follow up on definitive upper limb orthoses that are constructed from durable metal and plastic alloys.

Upper limb orthoses are distinct from other orthoses because of the complexity of the human hand. Many simultaneous joint motions must be considered for either mobilization or immobilization (e.g., nine interphalangeal [IP], five metacarpophalangeal [MCP], wrist, forearm, elbow, three shoulder), short digital levers (which translates to high forces, high pressures, and skin intolerance), and little soft tissue padding for bands and other components. Orthotic design for the upper limb must give equal focus to mechanical efficiency and precision of fit because comfort is critical for acceptance. Therefore, the small segments, limitations in soft tissue padding, and multiplicity of joint motion create high demands, which require a clinician with both a keen problem-solving

sense and finely tuned fabrication skills.[4] Frequently, and by design, the useful period is limited; when the treatment goals are met, the orthosis is discontinued. The orthosis can be discarded if the patient finds another, more acceptable means of function or if the benefit of the orthosis is outweighed by the patient's lack of "gadget tolerance."

A client is more likely to accept an upper limb orthosis if its therapeutic purpose is well defined or if the orthosis provides a desired function that cannot be accomplished by any other means, such as substitution. Because even the best upper limb orthosis lacks mechanical versatility to grasp with equal ease objects that vary widely in size, shape, and weight, upper limb orthotic design tends to be optimized for a specific purpose. Combine this mechanical shortcoming with impaired sensation, reduced skin friction, and poor subcutaneous contouring, and individuals have to produce greater prehension force than the normal hand just to accomplish routine activities. In addition, an upper limb orthosis is conspicuous and advertises the disability. Despite these limitations, upper limb orthoses can offer appealing advantages for the limb left impaired by paralysis, deformity, or pain.

Frequently, upper limb orthoses are applied to insensate limbs, and a well-defined skin inspection regimen must be followed to avoid excessive pressure. In common practice, the patient initially wears the orthosis for a relatively short period (5 to 30 minutes), then removes the orthosis and inspects the skin for persistent red marks. Red marks should disappear within 20 minutes. If they do not, the orthosis should be adjusted to alleviate the excessive pressure on the skin. If the red marks disappear within the 20-minute period, wearing time can be gradually increased (e.g., by 15 minutes) until the patient can tolerate wearing the device for several hours.

To the novice, upper limb orthoses seem widely diversified and hopelessly unorganized. This probably is the result of the enormous versatility of the upper limb. With lower limb orthotic management, the general goals are to reduce walking or running deviations. Although the task of walking or running is defined by specific repeatable phases, no such simple definition can describe upper limb function. The upper limb is involved with so many activities that even identifying a specific goal or function can be difficult.

Upper limb orthoses can be categorized in several ways, for example, by pathology (e.g., spinal injury, arthritis, trauma, head injury), arthrosegmentally according to the joint encompassed (e.g., shoulder, elbow, wrist, hand, fingers), or treatment objective (e.g., promote healing, direct growth, prevent deformity, correct deformity, enhance function). The main categories selected for this chapter are *static* and *dynamic*. Under each of these primary categories, it is convenient to group upper limb orthoses further as either *therapeutic* or *functional*. To illustrate, one example of a static functional upper limb orthosis is a short opponens (static hand orthosis) with attachments for eating, reading, page turning, shaving, and grooming.

Temporary upper limb orthoses made from low-temperature thermoplastics are discussed separately. These devices typically are fitted immediately after surgery or trauma. Designs are developed using paper patterns, the plastic is heated in hot water, and the orthoses are formed directly on the patient's limb.

Static orthoses

Therapeutic

Orthoses in this category include the static wrist–hand orthosis (WHO), static hand orthosis (HdO), elbow orthosis (EO), shoulder–elbow orthosis (SEO), and shoulder–elbow–wrist orthosis (SEWO). Several specific therapeutic attachments to these basic devices are described. Although many other static orthoses are used occasionally for therapeutic purposes, space limitations preclude a listing or description of all custom-designed and custom-fabricated orthoses.

Static WHO

Clinical application: The static WHO (Fig. 13-1) supports the wrist joint, maintains the functional architecture of the hand, and prevents wrist–hand deformities. Occasionally the static WHO is used as a platform for other therapeutic attachments (e.g., MCP extension stop, IP extension assist, thumb extension assist). The static WHO illustrated in Fig. 13-1 is of the Rancho type. Several functionally equivalent metal and plastic designs are available, including those used at the Rehabilitation Institute in Chicago, The Institute for Rehabilitation and Research in Houston, and the Institute of Rehabilitation Medicine at New York University. The reader is referred to previous editions of this text for examples of alternative designs.

Patient population: Patients with severe weakness or paralysis of the wrist and hand musculature are appropriate candidates for the static WHO. Without support, these individuals are at risk for developing the "clawhand" deformity and/or overstretching weak muscles (Fig. 13-2). For example, quadriplegics usually exhibit the aforementioned weakness

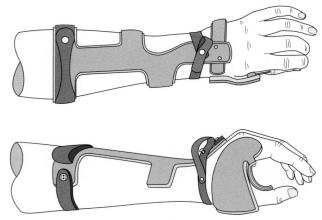

Fig. 13-1 Static wrist–hand orthosis (WHO).

and can benefit from a static WHO to preserve the functional posture of the hand and wrist (Figs. 13-1 and 13-2). It is important to prevent encumbering contractures or deformities in patients because they may later become candidates for a functional WHO. The static WHO is often indicated as a positional orthosis for C1–5 quadriplegics with zero wrist extensors and an *intrinsic minus* hand.

Attachments

Two of the most common attachments used with the static WHO are the MCP extension stop and the IP extension assist (Fig. 13-3). If there is loss of flexion range at the MCP joints and loss of extension range at the proximal IP joints, these two attachments can help prevent a clawhand deformity by preventing hyperextension of the MCP joints while encouraging extension of the IP joints of index through little fingers. Both of these attachments can be mounted on the same outrigger bar. This outrigger bar has two keyholes that facilitate installation and removal of the assembly.

The thumb can be maintained in opposition while allowing a limited range of motion with the addition of a swivel thumb (Fig. 13-4). The swivel thumb acts as a carpometacarpal flexion assist for the thumb and consists of a custom-contoured metal band over the proximal phalanx of the thumb, which is secured to the radial extension of the palmar piece with a simple cantilevered wire spring (Fig. 13-4).

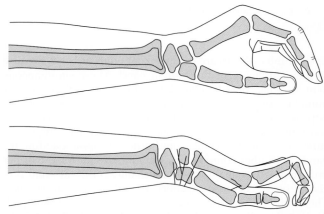

Fig. 13-2 Clawhand deformity (wrist flexed, MCPs hyperextended, thumb extended and abducted).

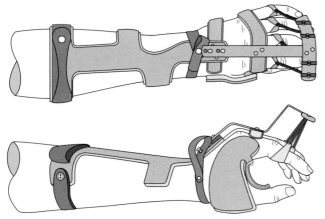

Fig. 13-3 Static WHO with MCP extension stop and IP extension assist.

Static hand orthosis

Clinical application: The static HdO (Fig. 13-5) maintains the functional position of the hand and prevents development of deformities. Occasionally the static HdO is used as a platform for other therapeutic attachments. All the attachments described for the static WHO can also be used with the static HdO. Again, the Rancho design is depicted here, and the reader is referred to previous editions of this text for examples of other functionally equivalent upper limb orthoses designs.

Patient population: Patients with weakness or paralysis of the hand intrinsic musculature and strong wrist extensors are appropriate candidates for the static HdO. Without this orthosis, these patients are at risk for developing a flat hand with the thumb carpometacarpal joint in extension. The C7 neurosegmental level quadriplegic exhibits this weakness and can benefit from a static HdO.

Elbow orthosis

Clinical application: EOs designed for reducing soft tissue contractures must be custom designed and custom fabricated with structural plastic (polypropylene) bands and total-contact flexible plastic (polyethylene) cuffs and straps. They must incorporate at least one of a variety of mechanisms for increasing range of motion. Application of low-magnitude, long-duration forces is preferable when attempting to reduce an elbow flexion or extension contracture (Fig. 13-6). This is necessary to avoid the antagonist response, which accompanies quick, intense stretching. With quick and/or intense orthotic forces, the outcome may be tightening of the muscles in series and parallel with the tight collagen fibers. In addition, the skin is at greater risk for breakdown

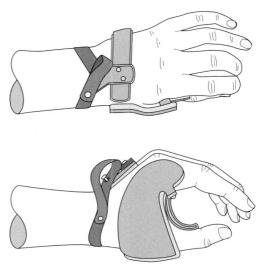

Fig. 13-5 Static hand orthosis (HdO).

with higher forces. Particular attention must be given to mechanical/anatomical joint alignment, and the arm and forearm must be restricted to pure rotation with minimum translation to avoid joint subluxation or dislocation. The contracture reduction force must be gradually increased therapeutically (Fig. 13-6; slowly expand or contract the turnbuckle) so that the soft tissue collagen adhesions responsible for contracture can undergo microtears without causing trauma to the joint. The bands and cuffs should be placed near the elbow joint so that the levers of the three-point contracture reduction force system are maximized, correction forces are minimized, and skin pressure is tolerable. The edges of the bands and cuffs should be flared to avoid excessive edge pressure and shear. The therapeutic strategy should be to tease the tissues into lengthening without provoking an antagonistic response, causing permanent red marks on the skin, or creating internal bruising.

Patient population: EOs are used for reduction of soft tissue contractures of the elbow that result in functional limitations. The need to reduce elbow flexion or extension contractures can result from trauma or disease. The largest population affected consists of individuals with spinal cord injury who depend on full range of motion of the elbow for alleviating ischial sitting pressure, propelling a manual wheelchair, or bringing the hand to the face.

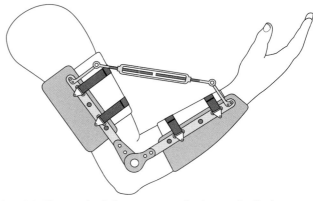

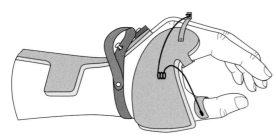

Fig. 13-4 Swivel thumb attached to static WHO.

Fig. 13-6 Elbow orthosis (contracture reduction application).

181

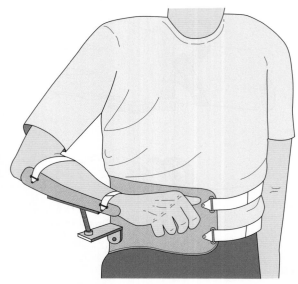

Fig. 13-7 Gunslinger shoulder–elbow orthosis (SEO).

Another common cause of restricted elbow motion is immobilization after trauma or surgery.

Shoulder–elbow orthosis

Clinical application: Support of a painful shoulder or traumatized brachial plexus–injured limb with an orthosis may be necessary. In many cases, a conventional arm sling suffices, provided there is no excessive force on the base of the neck and the use is short term. For long-term use, however, a sling offers very little function. The abduction orthosis, properly anchored on the hip, can be a successful alternative. Rancho Los Amigos Medical Center has developed a dynamic arm and shoulder support called the *gunslinger* (Fig. 13-7). The client's arm is strapped to a forearm trough, which is mechanically coupled to a plastic hemigirdle anchored on the patient's pelvis (iliac crest). The coupling between the forearm trough and iliac cap can be customized to permit a variety of motions, including glenohumeral joint internal/external rotation, flexion extension, and horizontal flexion/extension as well as flexion/extension of the elbow joint. The arm and hand are held in a cosmetically pleasing pose, and the hand is available for use, enabling early functional recovery. The gunslinger SEO is easy to put on and take off, and full deweighting of the arm is feasible.

Patient population: The brachial plexus–injured patient can benefit from application of the gunslinger SEO for both prevention of further stretch injury during the healing process and positioning of the hand in useful locations for functional activities. The iliac cap and arm trough can be concealed with a long-sleeve shirt, making the orthosis more cosmetically acceptable.

Some individuals with a brachial plexus injury have a normal hand and wrist (intrinsic plus hand and wrist, C7–8 spared) with proximal musculature weakness. In these cases, the gunslinger orthosis with a simple forearm trough is sufficient to support the arm, position it in space, and allow the hand to be functional. A painful, subluxing glenohumeral joint can be deweighted and can benefit from the gunslinger SEO with a simple forearm trough. However, if the wrist or hand also is weak or painful, either an extension to the

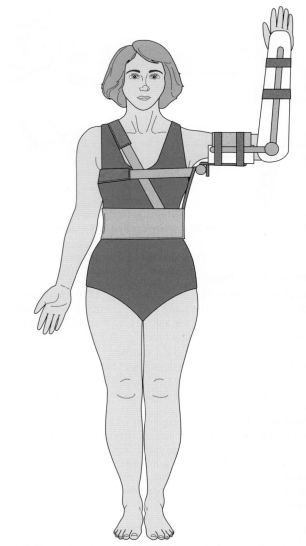

Fig. 13-8 Shoulder–elbow–wrist orthosis (SEWO).

forearm trough (cock-up palmar piece) or an attachable WHO is indicated.

Shoulder–elbow–wrist orthosis

Clinical application: SEWOs are frequently used to protect soft tissues or to prevent contractures of soft tissues. Occasionally, these orthoses are used to correct an existing deformity.

The specific design depends on the therapeutic goal prescribed. Interim SEWOs, used to relieve pain or promote healing, frequently are custom fitted to the patient from prefabricated kits or assemblies. The hardware usually is adjustable so that a few sizes fit all. SEWOs used for the long term are custom designed and custom fabricated, with carefully selected structural and biomechanical components. The bands and joints are not adjustable, and only the straps can accommodate physical changes in the patient.

The SEWO depicted in Fig. 13-8 transmits the weight of the upper limb to the ipsilateral pelvis, and the system is stabilized with trunk straps. When this type of SEWO is used by clients with an axillary burn, the objective is to provide as much contact as possible while keeping the glenohumeral joint in maximum abduction. The anatomical elbow joint may be immobilized or free motion allowed. Generally the wrist is supported in extension to protect the associated soft tissues against the forces of gravity.

The disadvantage of prefabricated and custom-fitted versus custom-designed and custom-fabricated SEWOs is that prefabricated orthoses require more follow-up to guard against excessive pressure or shear. This is especially true if the patient has sensory impairment. Also, prefabricated orthoses must be adjusted if the patient has episodes of edema, whereas a custom-fabricated device can be designed to reduce edema using total-contact bands and cuffs.

The orthosis shown in Fig. 13-8 is also known as the *airplane orthosis* because of the obvious resemblance when the device is used bilaterally. An alternate name for this orthosis is the *shoulder stabilizer*. By externally rotating the glenohumeral joint with the SEWO (Fig. 13-8), the internal rotators are stretched, and the tension on the deltoid and rotator cuff is relieved, which often are desirable after shoulder surgery.

It is possible to design the SEWO with maximum mobility for therapeutic purposes. Full range of abduction/adduction, flexion/extension, internal/external, and horizontal flexion/extension motions of the glenohumeral joint can be incorporated into the orthosis by careful selection of the subaxillary mechanical joints used. This permits postoperative rehabilitation without removing the orthosis.

Patient population: The airplane SEWO is an excellent orthosis to prescribe after rotator cuff repairs, anteroposterior capsular repairs, and postmanipulation. This orthosis is frequently prescribed for axillary burns to prevent contracture and alternatively to help reduce soft tissue contractures from a variety of reasons (e.g., long-term immobility). The wearing time for the airplane SEWO can be gradually increased while avoiding skin problems by routine inspection and modification of the orthosis when indicated.

Functional

Clinical application: The static WHO and HdO can be modified to provide functional activities by attaching clips and pockets that hold utensils, writing devices, page turners, and so forth. The static HdO shown in Fig. 13-9 has a butterfly-type clamp attached to the radial extension that clasps the shaft of a writing device. An alternative to the clamp is the truss stud configuration on the palmar extension of the palmar side (Fig. 13-10). Utensils and other attachments are adapted with a slotted plate that engages the truss studs on the palmar side to secure the attachments. A simple HdO can be modified with an aluminum rod to create an ulnar page turner (Fig. 13-11). The rubber end of an eyedropper is used on the end of the aluminum rod for friction to facilitate page turning. Numerous devices can be attached to an HdO or WHO, including toothbrushes, razors, combs, brushes, hygiene aids, eating utensils, arts and crafts implements, and devices unique to the injured individual's work environment.

Patient population: The static HdO or WHO usually is adapted in this fashion when rigid deformities exist in the hand and finger joints and supple prehension is not feasible, precluding use of more functional dynamic WHOs. Some individuals with spinal cord injury and residual quadriplegia lose the flexibility of their fingers and hand over time and

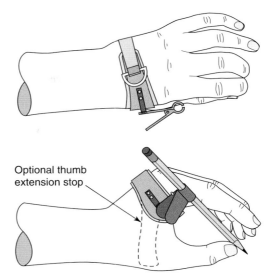

Fig. 13-9 Static HdO with butterfly writing clip.

become candidates for the HdO or WHO with a variety of attachments. In general, the HdO version is used when the patient's wrist extension musculature is strong enough to stabilize hand position during use.

Dynamic orthoses

Therapeutic

Wrist-action wrist–hand orthosis

Clinical application: The wrist-action wrist–hand orthosis (WAWHO) functions as a positional and therapeutic orthosis.[5] As with the static WHO, it maintains the functional position of the hand and prevents wrist and hand deformities (Fig. 13-12). Its therapeutic function is to protect and assist weak wrist extensors with mechanical wrist motion stops. Sometimes the WAWHO is used with a rubber band and pulley

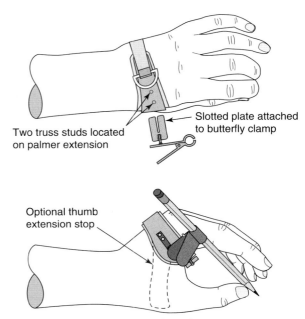

Fig. 13-10 Static HdO with truss stud attachment.

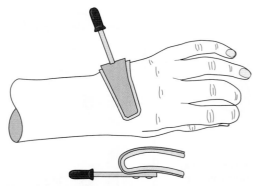

Fig. 13-11 Static HdO with ulnar page turner.

arrangement to assist wrist extension (Fig. 13-13). Also, if necessary, the previously described MCP extension stop and IP extension assist are added. Protection and strengthening of weak muscles are achieved by limiting wrist motion, while the functional position of the hand is maintained by the orthosis.

Patient population: Clients with weak [2 (poor) to 3 (fair)] wrist extensors and paralyzed hand muscles and clients who have potential for wrist extensor musculature return are appropriate candidates for a WAWHO. A WAWHO with extension assist is indicated for individuals with poor-to-fair wrist extensors or those with 3+ (fair+) wrist extensors with limited endurance (Fig. 13-13). The WAWHO has a hinge at the wrist that allows active extension and gravity-assisted flexion. A flexion stop (Figs. 13-12 and 13-13) is used to prevent prolonged stretching to the extensors, which may cause increased weakness. A rubber band can be used to assist weak extensors (Fig. 13-13). Progression usually consists of locking the wrist joint when muscles are less than fair (3) and loosening the wrist joint for periods of specific therapy. When wrist extensors are grade 3+ (fair+) or better with good endurance, static positioning is discontinued during the day, allowing more advanced functional training. Positioning at night is continued until functional hand position is maintained and no loss of range of motion or stretching occurs.

Elbow orthosis

Clinical application: EOs are frequently used immediately after trauma or surgery (Fig. 13-14). Usually a three-point force system in conjunction with a hydraulic lock of the semiliquid tissues surrounding the fragments is used to maintain

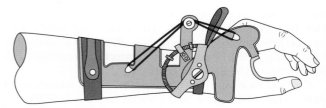

Fig. 13-13 WAWHO with wrist extension assist.

the fracture fragments as a single unit during the healing process. In the past, this was generally accomplished with a cast. However, a cast does not allow normal joint motion and eventually loosens, and the bone fragments may angulate. Compared to a cast, a well-fitting custom-fabricated EO is much lighter, is more comfortable, allows self-hygiene, and provides optimum control at the fracture site. As the patient gains or loses weight, the cuffs and straps opposing the bands can be tightened to maintain control. Many mechanical elbow joints are available. Most permit limited and adjustable range of motion at the elbow joint, to control mobility without sacrificing vital bone fixation.

Patient population: EOs are indicated after cast removal for stable fractures; postoperatively as an adjunct to internal fixation; for elbow dislocation management; and for strains, sprains, and muscle trauma. The design of an EO depends on the specific application. Postsurgical or posttrauma devices often are an "off the shelf" variety because they are used for a relatively short time. They tend to have soft cuffs with multiple straps and an adjustable mechanical elbow joint (Fig. 13-14).

In the case of a fracture, the therapeutic aim is to promote callus formation and simultaneously permit a safe, painless range of motion to stimulate healing and avoid the nuisance of an iatrogenic joint contracture.

Functional

Ratchet wrist–hand orthosis

Clinical application: The ratchet WHO is a functional prehension orthosis (Fig. 13-15) that enables the patient to grasp and release objects by using external power.[1] The ratchet WHO is manually controlled and substitutes for finger flexor and

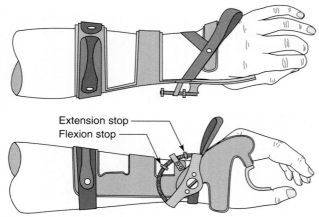

Extension stop
Flexion stop

Fig. 13-12 Wrist-action wrist–hand orthosis (WAWHO).

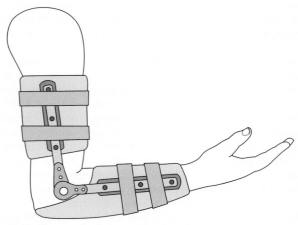

Fig. 13-14 Elbow orthosis (postsurgical application).

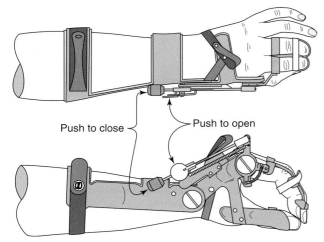

Fig. 13-15 Ratchet WHO.

extensor muscles that are less than grade 3 (fair). The wrist is stabilized for function, but the position can be changed for different activities. A thumb post is used to maintain abduction and to position the thumb in alignment with the finger pads. A finger piece assembly is provided to maintain the index and long fingers in position for pinch. A ratchet system is used so that the hand can be closed in discrete increments. Pinch is achieved by applying force on the proximal end of the ratchet bar (black knob) or by using the patient's own chin, other arm, or any stationary object to flex the index and long fingers toward the thumb to form a three-jaw chuck. When the ratchet disk is tapped, the ratchet lock is released and spring-assisted opening of the hand occurs.

The ratchet WHO allows the individual increased independence in a variety of functional activities without the need for multiple pieces of adaptive equipment (Fig. 13-16). Following a carefully organized and sequenced training program, a patient with C5 quadriplegia may attain independence in feeding, light hygiene (application of makeup, shaving, and hair grooming), desk top activities (e.g., writing and typing), and donning and doffing the orthosis. More complex desk tasks (more difficult writing, typing) are feasible using a well-organized desk arrangement. By using gross motion to close the hand, a functional three-point pinch is achievable.

An alternative to the Rancho type of ratchet WHO that also provides dynamic prehension with a locked wrist is the electric-powered prehension unit (EPPU), which was developed at The Institute for Rehabilitation and Research (TIRR) in Houston.

The EPPU is an externally powered prehension orthosis that derives energy from a rechargeable battery pack.

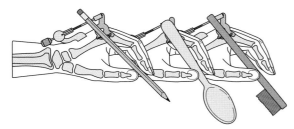

Fig. 13-16 Pen spring applications.

The battery pack supplies current to a geared-down DC motor that closes the hand with one polarity and opens it with the opposite polarity. Gross motion (e.g., forearm supination/pronation) operates a rocker-type electrical switch assembly that provides current from the battery pack to the motor. Typically, pronation produces prehension and supination hand opening.

Patient population: The ratchet WHO and EPPU are appropriate for patients with paralysis or severe weakness of the hand and wrist musculature. Some functional proximal strength is required to use the ratchet WHO. For optimal use, the individual should have at least 3+ (fair+) strength in shoulder flexion, abduction, external rotation, and internal rotation. Individuals with weaker proximal muscles may be able to use the ratchet WHO along with a mobile arm support (described in the section on mobile arm support). Other considerations that should be evaluated are endurance, range of motion limitations, spasticity, sensation, and the patient's motivation and social support. Originally, these orthoses were designed for upper limb paresis secondary to poliomyelitis. Today, these orthoses are used primarily for spinal-injured patients with no hand or wrist extension strength but at least grade 2 (poor) shoulder and elbow control (e.g., patients with functional C5 quadriplegia are appropriate candidates for the ratchet WHO and EPPU).

Wrist-driven wrist–hand orthosis

Clinical application: The wrist-driven WHO (WDWHO, or flexor hinge WHO) is a dynamic prehension orthosis for transferring power from the wrist extensors to the fingers (Fig. 13-17). Active wrist extension provides grasp, and gravity-assisted wrist flexion enables the patient to open the hand.

The proximal and distal IP joints of fingers 2 and 3 are immobilized along with the carpometacarpal and MCP joints of the thumb. Active wrist extension results in the fingers approximating the posted thumb. Conversely, passive (gravity-assisted) wrist flexion causes the hand to open. An adjustable actuating lever system at the wrist joint allows the user to fine-tune the wrist joint angle at which prehension occurs. This is necessary for achievement of maximum prehensile force. As with the ratchet WHO, the WDWHO replaces the need for multiple assistive devices.

Patient population: The WDWHO is an appropriate orthosis for the individual with paralysis or severe weakness of the hand. Wrist extensor strength must be at least grade

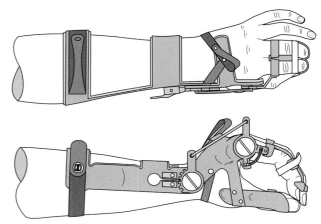

Fig. 13-17 Wrist-driven wrist–hand orthosis (WDWHO).

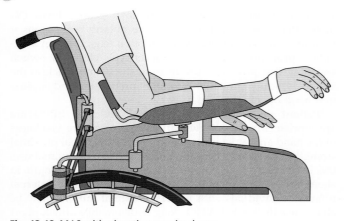

Fig. 13-18 MAS with elevating proximal arm.

3+ (fair+), and proximal strength must be functional. For individuals with wrist extensor grades of less than 3+ who are improving or are 3+ (fair+) with poor endurance, a rubber band wrist extension assist is indicated. Candidates for the WDWHO have a functional level of C5 with some C6 return (wrist extensors), C6, and C7 quadriplegia. By using active wrist extension, a functional three-point pinch is achieved.

If and when a patient begins to have return of function in the extrinsic muscles, the patient becomes a candidate for a WDWHO. In general, a patient who uses his or her orthosis for function throughout the day will gain wrist strength and consequently improved prehension.

Although rare, bilateral application of the WDWHO can be successful. Usually the patient's vocation or hobby is the determining factor. If the patient desires bilateral prehension and it cannot be achieved any other way, then bilateral application is feasible. The key is the motivation of the patient, not that of the clinician.

Mobile arm support

Clinical application: Mobile arm support (MAS) is an SEO that supports the weight of the arm and provides assistance to the shoulder and elbow motions through a linkage of bearings joints (Fig. 13-18). A properly installed and adjusted MAS enables patients to perform self-care and vocational and recreational activities and can decrease the patient's dependency on family or hospital personnel.

An MAS is therapeutic in that it can be adjusted to complement weak muscles so that they can function while being protected and strengthened. Joint range of motion can be maintained with use of an MAS. The MAS can provide considerable psychological value by enabling patients to perform meaningful activities despite severe disability.

The MAS can provide assistance for shoulder and elbow motions by

Using gravitational forces and occasionally tension from rubber bands or springs to substitute for or supplement loss of strength in shoulder and elbow musculature. For example, the inclined plane of an MAS may assist weak elbow extension, and the elastic mechanism assists shoulder elevation.
Supporting the weight of the arm so that weak muscles can move the arm over a useful range of motion.

The basic components of the MAS are the wheelchair mounting bracket, the proximal arm, the distal arm, and the forearm trough (Fig. 13-19). The standard proximal elevating arm is available with an optional feature to deweight the patient's arm (Fig. 13-19). The standard wheelchair mounting bracket is available with an optional pivot type of adjustment for tilting the axis of the proximal arm (Fig. 13-19).

Patient population: The MAS can increase upper limb function for patients who have severe arm paralysis because of disabilities such as muscular dystrophy, poliomyelitis, cervical spinal cord lesion, Guillain-Barré syndrome, and amyotrophic lateral sclerosis.

Patients should have sufficient muscle weakness or endurance limitation to warrant use of the support. Evaluation of the deltoid, elbow flexors, and external rotators is the most significant because of their importance in arm function. Criteria for MAS use are as follows:

Absent or weak elbow flexion (poor to fair)
Absent or weak shoulder flexion and abduction (poor to fair)
Absent or weak external rotation (poor to fair)
Limited endurance for sustained upper limb activity

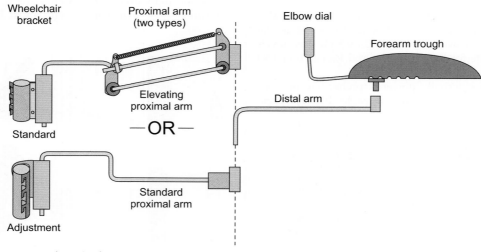

Fig. 13-19 MAS components and proximal arm options.

The patient must have adequate muscular strength to move the MAS. Neck, trunk, shoulder girdle, shoulder, and elbow may serve alone or in combination as power sources.

An exact minimum strength requirement to power an MAS is difficult to formulate, and a clinical trial often is necessary. The patient's basic coordination may be as important as the amount of muscle strength present. To have control over the lapboard range in the planes of horizontal motion at the elbow and at the shoulder, the patient must have some controlling muscles in both elbow and shoulder in order to position the arm in the MAS in the horizontal plane.

The individual with at least poor muscle strength, especially in the shoulder girdle, shoulder, elbow, or trunk, can operate the MAS more effectively and do more with it, and the MAS is much easier to adjust and to stabilize for function. Some hand function widens the scope of available activities but is not always a necessity. Lack of grasp may be substituted with the WDWHO or ratchet WHO.

Elbow orthosis

Clinical application: EOs designed to assist normal motion in functional activities are definitive in nature and should be custom designed and custom fabricated with the highest-quality components and materials and carefully fitted to provide durable function for many years. Functional EOs usually incorporate an elastic device with a locking mechanism to assist elbow flexion with multiple angular lock points (Fig. 13-20). The user initiates elbow flexion with residual musculature or using body mechanics. The elastic device (e.g., spiral spring) assists the flexion until one of the flexion stops is reached. A release on the stop permits the elbow either to advance to a new greater angle or to fall back into extension.

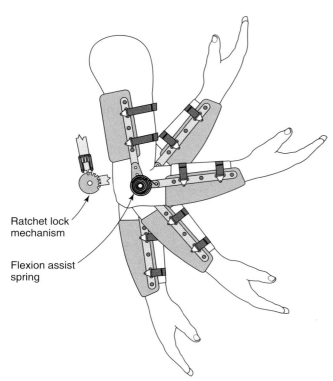

Ratchet lock mechanism

Flexion assist spring

Fig. 13-20 Elbow orthosis.

Patient population: Individuals with selective loss of elbow flexion secondary to a brachial plexus injury or congenital deficit are appropriate candidates for the EO with elbow flexion assist. Bilateral applications may be more successful than unilateral applications. This is because the normal side becomes dominant in the unilateral case, and the additional function provided by the orthosis in the presence of a normal contralateral limb often is insufficient to offset the stigma of wearing an orthosis. In the case of bilateral involvement, however, the orthosis is more likely to be accepted because no function is available without it. Unilateral applications tend to be acceptable when the wrist and hand are functional and only the elbow requires stabilization to complement the other normal side. Also, a successful outcome is more likely if the activity desired by the individual requires use of both the normal and the impaired sides.

Low-temperature thermoplastic orthoses

Because of their ease of fabrication, this group of upper limb orthoses meet the need for quickly available devices in the clinical setting. Because of a combination of the hand-forming technique used to produce them and the poor mechanical properties of the material, however, such orthoses are not well suited for long-term use or when intimacy of fit is required for function.

Such interim upper limb orthoses are generally fabricated from low-temperature thermoplastics, which can be formed in water heated to 140°F to 170°F. Higher-temperature thermoplastics can be used, but a plaster mold of the patient's forearm, wrist, or hand should be made to avoid burning the patient. In addition, the higher-temperature materials cannot be cut with scissors, so a power source must be used.

A large variety of both static and dynamic upper limb orthoses have been designed from low-temperature materials. The static orthoses may be protective, supportive, or corrective. Protective designs are intended to protect weak muscles from being stretched and therefore prevent contractures. Supportive orthoses are intended to support a joint or an arch in substitution for weak muscles. Supportive can mean *immobilize*, as in the case of a painful arthritic joint. Corrective designs may force the involved joint into a correct or near-correct alignment. Use of static orthoses must include concern for swelling and long-term immobility. Therapy should include a regimen of activities where the patient is encouraged to use the limb as often as possible.

The main advantages of low-temperature thermoplastic orthoses are that they can be fitted early after trauma or injury and that they are lightweight. For example, to prevent a deformity and position a limb in a functional position, it may be necessary to fit the patient within hours of the injury or admission. The disadvantages with using these materials is that they do not have sufficient stiffness to hold their form and prevent high-pressure spots and they have a less precise fit as a result of hand forming.

Dynamic upper limb orthoses using low-temperature plastics must be designed to provide specific forces in the correct direction, often using outriggers that are attached to the body of the main orthosis. Use of mechanical joints in parallel with

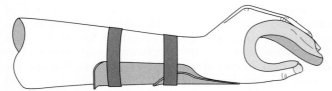

Fig. 13-21 Resting WHO.

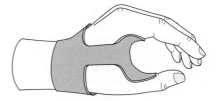

Fig. 13-22 HdO with thumb adduction stop (C-bar).

anatomical joints can decrease joint adhesions, maintain joint function, and prevent ankylosis of the joint. A large percentage of individuals requiring low-temperature dynamic orthoses are seen in acute-care hospitals following surgery or trauma to the forearm and hand and subsequently are seen as outpatients and in rehabilitation centers.

Resting wrist–hand orthosis

Clinical application: The resting WHO (Fig. 13-21) is designed to maintain the arches of the hand, keep the thumb abducted and flexed, and maintain the wrist in a functional position (30 degrees). The orthosis is made by placing the patient's limb on a piece of paper and drawing a pattern that encompasses the tips of the fingers, is expanded at the forearm for wraparound, and is slotted so that the thumb can be separated from the other fingers. If the affected side cannot be straightened for drawing the pattern, the unaffected side can be used and then reversed. When drawing the pattern, extra width must be allowed for padding. The pertinent joints and landmarks are noted. Many popular published patterns can be used as a guide to fabrication. Scissors or tin snips can be used to cut the chosen material (e.g., orthoplast). Heating the cut line with a heat gun facilitates the cutting. Orthoplast is heated in a long, shallow pan of hot water until the material is "rubbery," wiped dry, and then molded over the client's limb and secured with Ace wrap. After the orthosis cools, the straps can be added by using rivets or contact cement or by sandwiching between pieces of orthoplast with a solvent.

Patient population: Although the resting WHO is most often used to preserve the architecture of the hand and wrist on a patient with paralyzed musculature, it also can be used to reduce hypertonicity by abducting the fingers. This modification requires angular ridges between the digits and extra straps. This resting WHO is also used to alleviate wrist or hand pain by immobilizing these tissues. Because this orthosis can be readily formed and fitted in the clinic, it is suitable for preventing loss of motion after acute trauma (e.g., burns). Moreover, the large contacting area of the resting WHO can be beneficial in combating scar formation in the burn patient. Frequent skin inspection is particularly important in these cases.

Hand orthosis with thumb adduction stop

Clinical application: This upper limb orthosis is used to position the thumb in opposition and maintain the thumb web space, leaving the hand in a functional position for use (Fig. 13-22). If the dorsal and palmar extensions are formed snugly, the orthosis can sometimes be worn without straps.

Patterns for this orthosis should be custom designed by placing a flexible piece of paper around the appropriate portion of the patient's hand and sketching the pattern in place.

The hand part is formed first before the thumb web component can be formed. The thumb web component must allow IP flexion of the thumb and flexion of the second MCP joint.

Patient population: This HdO is particularly useful for acute intervention in a painful hand or in cases where a thumb contracture is threatening. The burn victim with palmar hand trauma or the arthritic patient with tender joints may benefit from use of this orthosis.

Hand orthosis with MCP extension stop

Clinical application: Intrinsic weakness of the hand can leave the hand in a resting posture that encourages MCP hyperextension. If the source of weakness is expected to resolve and the potential for function is good, an HdO with MCP extension stop is desired (Fig. 13-23). An oval-shaped piece of low-temperature thermoplastic is heated and wrapped around the dorsum of the patient's hand distal to the wrist and proximal to the proximal IP joints. A cutout in the pattern is made to avoid pressure on the MCP joints. A rectangular piece of orthoplast is formed into a "Tootsie Roll" shape, wrapped under the palmar aspect of the hand, and secured to the ulnar and radial sides of the oval. The design requires no straps if snugly fabricated.

Patient population: This orthosis is used when a condition results in an intrinsic minus hand that, if left untreated, would flatten and the MCP joints would hyperextend. This orthosis is also used when a median and radial nerve injury causes weakening of the transverse arch. If curvature is formed into the palmar roll, the normal palmar arch is preserved.

Dynamic dorsal wrist–hand orthosis

Clinical application: This orthosis provides a quick clinical means for positioning the hand and assisting wrist and MCP extension. The orthosis consists of three main components that accomplish these objectives (Fig. 13-24): the dorsal forearm piece, the palmar piece, and the MCP extension assist. The forearm and palmar pieces are connected with a rubber band, which assists wrist extension. For this feature to be effective, a large forearm strap is required to prevent distal migration of the forearm piece. The dorsum of the forearm piece provides a base of support for the wire outrigger to

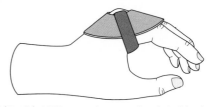

Fig. 13-23 HdO with MCP extension stop (lumbrical bar).

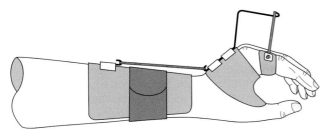

Fig. 13-24 Dorsal WHO with wrist extension assist and MCP extension assist.

which the rubber band for MCP extension is attached. One rubber band attached to the ends of the palmar phalangeal bar usually is sufficient to extend the MCP joint of the index through little fingers. The wire outrigger can be shaped to fine-tune the extension torque.

The patterns should be custom designed, heated to the appropriate temperature, and formed directly on the client. The small pads holding the hooks for the rubber bands are secured with a solvent (Carbona) or contact cement.

Patient population: Patients with a radial nerve injury resulting in weakness of wrist and MCP extension are typical candidates for this orthosis. For patients showing signs of muscle function return, rubber bands are used to assist clinically targeted motions. The rubber bands can be fine-tuned commensurate with the therapeutic changes.

General considerations

The edges of upper limb orthoses made from low-temperature thermoplastic, such as orthoplast, can be folded over to create a rounded, smooth finish. Reinforcing strips can be made the same way and attached with solvent or contact cement to certain weak areas (e.g., wrist area) of the orthosis. Instead of rolls of plastic, it may be desirable to create small corrugations by forming a small rectangular piece of plastic around a cylindrical object and then attaching to the main body of the orthosis where reinforcement is desired.

Hundreds of designs of low-temperature plastic upper limb orthoses are available. Only a few are presented here to give the reader a general idea of their potential. The designer is limited by his or her imagination and, to a certain degree, by the poor mechanical properties and bulk of low-temperature thermoplastic materials.

Team approach to orthoses management

With a well-organized team approach to orthotic management, patient acceptance of an orthosis can be high.[1] Both the certified orthotist and the occupational therapist have a vital role in ensuring a successful outcome. The occupational therapist evaluates the need for orthoses, recommends the devices, and trains clients in their use. In some cases, the occupational therapist fabricates low-temperature orthoses that can be readily applied during a short clinical encounter. The orthotist's role usually is to design, fabricate, and fit definitive upper limb orthoses fabricated from metal and high-temperature plastics.

To best meet the patient's orthotic needs, a team clinic is suggested. During this clinic, the orthotist, occupational therapist, and physician meet with the patient. The goals of the team clinic are as follows:

Ensure proper fitting and reevaluate fit over time as the patient's hand contours and functional needs may change

Facilitate patient compliance by incorporating the patient's feedback to the team discussion and teaching the patient about the fit and function of the orthosis

Provide ongoing "hands-on" training for both orthotic and occupational therapy students and staff

Provide a setting for ongoing dialogue among the orthotist, therapist, and patient

Facilitate brainstorming solutions to specific problems and consensus outcomes

The benefits of the team clinic can best be illustrated by an example. A patient presented after 1 month of using his WDWHO. The patient was able to use the WDWHO for hygiene and grooming and for tabletop activities. A problem occurred when the client was ready to begin self-catheterization. He was unable to hold the plastic tube tightly enough to insert it into the urethra. The nurse presented the problem in the team clinic. After discussion, the team decided to compromise finger opening for a tighter pinch by having the orthotist shorten the tenodesis bar and having the therapist provide additional training.

Training

To gain maximum use of the orthosis, the patient must be thoroughly trained. The occupational therapy training process involves the following steps.[1]

Education

The patient is instructed on the purpose and function of the orthosis. This learning can be facilitated by a peer who is successfully using the same orthosis.

Exploration and experimentation

Before starting with functional tasks, the therapist puts the orthosis on the patient, and the patient gets to "feel it out," open it, move it, and examine it. Step-by-step instructions are given. At this time, the patient observes but is not expected to attempt donning the orthosis. The patient is encouraged to experiment with the orthosis and become familiar with the mechanical principles before introducing objects or activities.

Prefunctional training

This step involves practicing grasp, hold, placement, and release of objects of various sizes, shapes, textures, and weights.

Functional activities

The sequence usually begins with passive maintenance of pinch while the patient performs some activity. Typing, prewriting, and fingerfood feeding (e.g., carrot sticks) are often used as initial activities. Feeding training is graded initially by providing a setup for cutting meat, opening containers, and placement of utensils.

Applying and removing

One school of thought is that this task should be taught only after the patient has achieved some proficiency using the orthosis because it is a more advanced skill and can be initially frustrating to the client. The patient is trained in removing the orthosis first because removing the device is easier than donning it. The other school of thought, however, is that the sooner the patient can don and doff the orthosis, the sooner he or she becomes less dependent on someone else's assistance. Which philosophy to follow depends on the amount of therapy time available and the wishes of the patient.

Advanced functional training

This area includes fine motor skills, such as activities using bilateral WDWHOs or ratchet WHOs. This training is done selectively only with patients who are skilled in using one orthosis and who have a specific functional need.

Follow-up

After the patient leaves the rehabilitation facility, his or her orthotic needs must be reevaluated periodically for maintenance of proper fit and optimal function.

Summary

The complexity of the human hand requires that orthotic design give equal emphasis to mechanical efficiency and accuracy of fit because comfort is critical for acceptance. Specific training and skill are required to meet the high design and fabrication demands that result from small segments (levers), limited soft tissue padding, and multiplicity of joints.

Upper limb orthoses are more often accepted by patients when a well-defined therapeutic program is in place and the orthoses provide a desired function that cannot be accomplished in any other fashion.[4] Perhaps the most important factor in patient acceptance is the orthotic team's open recognition that some level of compromise is necessary. Patients are quick to see through biased clouds of unrealistic enthusiasm.[4]

Specific orthoses are selected according to the patient's physical need. It is helpful to organize upper limb orthoses into groups that reflect need. Therefore, the orthoses reviewed for orthotic management of the patient with upper limb paresis or trauma were grouped primarily into *therapeutic* and *functional* categories. Each of these groups was further divided into *static* and *dynamic* subgroups. Examples of *static therapeutic* orthoses include the static WHO, which positions the wrist and hand for patients with absent or weak wrist and hand musculature, the static HdO, the wrist-action WHO, the EO, the SEO, and the SEWO. The *functional static* orthoses reviewed include the HdOs and WHOs with a variety of attachments. *Therapeutic dynamic* orthoses include the wrist-action wrist–hand orthosis (WAWHO) and the EO with adjustable joint range of motion for use after surgery or trauma. The *functional dynamic* orthoses described are the ratchet WHO, WDWHO, mobile arm support (MAS), and EO with flexion assist and multiple joint angle stops.

The ratchet WHO is a manually manipulated prehension orthosis for patients with C4 quadriplegia with some C5 return or C5 quadriplegia or similar loss of function and can be used in conjunction with an MAS. The WDWHO is a prehension orthosis powered by the wrist extensors and usually is prescribed for quadriplegics with 3+ (fair+) or greater wrist extensor strength and absent hand function.

The programs discussed include patient instruction on the orthotic purpose and mechanical principles, patient experimentation with the orthosis, and graded therapeutic and functional activity. With a carefully planned and implemented interdisciplinary training program, patient acceptance of an upper limb orthosis can be high. Upper limb orthoses can make major contributions to the management of dysfunction when properly selected, designed, fabricated, and fitted.

References

1. Baumgarten JM: Upper extremity adaptations for the person with quadriplegia. In Adkins H, editor: *Spinal cord injury*, New York, 1985, Churchill Livingstone.
2. Malick MH: *Manual on dynamic hand splinting with thermoplastic materials*, Pittsburgh, Penn, 1974, Harmarville Rehabilitation Center.
3. Malick MH: *Manual on static hand splinting*, ed 5, Pittsburgh, Penn, 1976, Harmarville Rehabilitation Center.
4. Perry J: Prescription principles. In: *AAOS: atlas of orthotics*, St. Louis, 1975, CV Mosby.
5. Wilson DJ, et al: *Spinal cord injury: a treatment guide for occupational therapists*, revised ed, Thorofare, NJ, 1984, Slack Inc.

Upper limb orthoses for the stroke and brain-injured patient

Chiara Mariani and Mary Ann E. Keenan

Key Points

- Stroke and brain injury are often complicated by the development of upper motor neuron syndrome.

- The majority of spontaneous motor recovery occurs within 6 months of stroke and traumatic brain injury. Definitive surgical procedures to reduce spasticity, such as neurectomies, tendon releases, and transfers, are delayed until the patient shows minimal further improvement in motor control.

- The prolonged period of spontaneous neurologic recovery is further complicated by spasticity (resistance to quick stretch), rigidity (resistance to slow stretch), impairment of motor control, synergistic patterns of movement, synkinesis (involuntary movement in one limb or limb segment when another part is moved [associated distant movement]), and immobility.

- Nerve blocks, chemodenervation, and casting techniques are used commonly and aggressively.

General principles

Stroke and brain injury are often complicated by the development of upper motor neuron syndrome.[23,22,39,52] Upper motor neuron syndrome is characterized by impairment of motor control, spasticity, muscle weakness, stereotypical patterns of movement (synergy), and stimulation of distant movement by noxious stimuli (synkinesis). Often the spasticity is severe and prevents adequate range of motion therapy

of joints or maintenance of acceptable limb position. Contractures can occur despite the most conscientious and aggressive treatments.

Even when joint motion can be maintained by knowledgeable therapists, it commonly requires much force that is painful for the patient, potentially harmful to limbs, and time consuming for caregivers to provide. Lesser degrees of spasticity can impede a patient's function or require the use of positioning devices that interfere with the use of an extremity.

Prevention of deformity and myostatic contractures in the presence of severe spasticity is challenging. Splints applied to only one side of an extremity are not sufficient to control excessive spasticity and may result in skin breakdown from motion of the extremity against the splint.[5] If used inappropriately, an orthosis may conceal the severity of a deformity or may cause additional deformity. It is important to treat the underlying spasticity in order to utilize orthoses effectively.

Treatment options for temporary control of spasticity

The majority of spontaneous motor recovery occurs within 6 months of stroke and traumatic brain injury. Definitive surgical procedures to reduce spasticity, such as neurectomies, tendon releases, and transfers, are delayed until the patient shows minimal further improvement in motor control.[10,36,48]

The prolonged period of spontaneous neurologic recovery is further complicated by spasticity (resistance to quick stretch), rigidity (resistance to slow stretch), impairment of motor control, synergistic patterns of movement, synkinesis (involuntary movement in one limb or limb segment when another part is moved [associated distant movement]), and immobility. These phenomena make temporary control of spasticity difficult but essential. Nerve blocks, chemodenervation, and casting techniques are used commonly and aggressively.[6,7,9,13,15,17,22,23,26,51]

Anesthetic nerve blocks

Anesthetic nerve blocks can be used to temporarily eliminate muscle tone. They can be used diagnostically to evaluate what portion of a deformity is dynamic (occurring because of muscle spasticity) and what portion is secondary to myostatic contracture. Repeated blocks of local anesthetics give a carryover effect to decrease muscle tone.

Phenol nerve blocks

When muscle spasticity requires control for an extended period but the patient still has potential for spontaneous improvement, a phenol nerve block may be indicated.[6,7,13,19,27,28,35,37,41,44,45,53,54,69] Phenol exerts two actions on the nerves. The first is a *short-term effect*. The short-term effect is similar to that produced by a local anesthetic and is directly proportional to the thickness of the nerve fibers. The second is a *long-term effect* that results from protein denaturation.

Phenol, a derivative of benzene, denatures the protein membrane of peripheral nerves when used in aqueous concentrations of 5% or more. When phenol is injected in or near a nerve, it reduces neural traffic along the nerve; hence, it is useful for temporary treatment of spasticity. Onset of the destructive process may begin to show effects several days after injection, but phenol also has a local anesthetic feature that allows a clinician and the patient to see "partial results" shortly after the phenol block is performed. The denaturing process induced by phenol continues for several weeks, but regeneration eventually occurs within 3 to 5 months.

Histologic studies have shown that phenol destroys axons of all sizes in a patchy distribution. The effect is more pronounced on the outer aspect of the nerve bundle, onto which phenol is dripped. When phenol is percutaneously injected, the nerve block likely will be incomplete. This effect is particularly beneficial in situations where a spastic muscle has retained volitional capacity, because under these circumstances it is desirable to reduce spasticity while preserving volitional capacity of a given muscle or muscle group.

The technique of phenol injection is based on electrical stimulation. Nerve branches are injected as close as possible to the motor points of the involved muscle. A surface stimulator is briefly used to approximate the percutaneous stimulation site in advance. A 25-gauge Teflon-coated hypodermic is advanced toward the motor nerve. Electrical stimulation is adjusted by noting whether muscle contraction of the index muscle occurs. As one gets closer to the motor nerve, less current intensity is required to produce a contractile response. The motor nerve is injected when minimal current produces a visible or palpable contraction of the muscle. Generally 4 to 7 mL of 5% to 7% aqueous phenol is injected at each site. As with any injection, care must be taken to avoid injection into a blood vessel; this is accomplished by aspirating prior to the injection.

Chemodenervation

Use of botulinum toxin also exemplifies a temporary, localized approach to controlling spasticity.[15,17,20,22,23,26,29,30,59,61,62,63,66,68] Ordinarily, an action potential propagating down a motor nerve to the neuromuscular junction triggers the release of acetylcholine (ACh) from presynaptic storage sites in the nerve terminal into the synaptic space. The released quanta of ACh, after traversing the synapse and attaching onto receptors located on the postsynaptic muscle membrane, cause its depolarization. This activates a biochemical sequence that ultimately leads to forceful muscle contraction. Botulinum toxin type A is a protein produced by *Clostridium botulinum* that inhibits the calcium-mediated release of ACh at the neuromuscular junction. Botulinum toxin A attaches to the presynaptic nerve terminal, and a component of the toxin crosses the nerve cell membrane. This component interferes with "fusion proteins" affiliated with vesicles of ACh and thereby prevents release of ACh from their storage vesicles.

Clinical benefit lasts 3 to 5 months but may be more variable. Botulinum toxin is injected directly into an offending muscle. Depending on the size of the muscle being injected, dosing has ranged between 10 and 200 units (U), depending on the size of the muscle. Current practice is to wait at least 12 weeks before reinjection and not to administer a total of more than 400 U in a single treatment session. Because this upper limit of 400 U can be reached rather quickly when injecting a few large proximal muscles or many smaller-sized distal muscles, a different strategy is needed for the limb requiring many proximal and distal injections. In this circumstance, botulinum toxin A and phenol can be combined, with the former injected into smaller distal muscles and the latter aimed at larger proximal ones. A 3- to 7-day delay between injections of botulinum toxin A and the onset of its clinical effect is typical.

The technique of injection varies. Some physicians prefer to inject through a syringe attached to a hypodermic needle that doubles as a monopolar electromyographic (EMG) recording electrode. Patients may be asked to make an effort to contract the targeted muscle, or the muscle may be contracting involuntarily. After the needle electrode is inserted, injection is made when EMG activity is recorded. For deep or small spastic muscles (e.g., tibialis posterior, long toe flexors, or finger flexors), electrical stimulation is preferred as a means of localizing the muscle prior to injection.

Because botulinum toxin is the most potent biologic toxin known and the cost is relatively high, the smallest possible dose should be used to achieve results. Most studies have reported side effects in 20% to 30% of patients per treatment cycle. The incidence of adverse effects varies based on the dosage used (i.e., the higher the dose, the more frequent the adverse effects); however, it has been reported that incidence of complications is not related to the total dose of botulinum toxin used. Local pain at the injection site is the most commonly reported side effect. Other adverse effects (e.g., local hematoma, generalized fatigue, lethargy, dizziness, flu-like syndrome, pain in neighboring muscles) also have been reported.

Causes of limited joint motion

The brain-injured patient is likely to have quadriplegic involvement, concomitant peripheral nerve injuries, residual deformities from fractures, and limitation of joint motion from heterotopic ossification.[11,47,49] Distinguishing from among several possible causes of decreased range of motion often is difficult in a brain-injured patient. The causes of decreased motion to be considered are increased muscle tone, myostatic contracture, heterotopic ossification, undetected fracture or dislocation, pain, or lack of patient cooperation secondary to decreased cognition.[8,10,31] The stroke patient tends to be older. Limited joint motion can be associated with degenerative arthritis. Congenital deformities can be present.

Arthritis, fractures, or dislocations may not exhibit a clinical deformity but can be detected easily by plain radiographs. Early heterotopic ossification is accompanied by an inflammatory reaction, with redness, warmth, severe pain, and steadily decreasing range of motion. Generally a radiograph shows evidence of the heterotopic bone as a hazy area of calcification forming in a periarticular location when it is suspected clinically.

Differentiating between the relative contributions of pain, increased muscle tone, and contracture can be more difficult. Diagnostic blocks using short-acting local anesthetic agents are extremely useful in assessing a spastic limb. The blocks can be performed at bedside or in the clinic setting without the use of special devices. By temporarily eliminating pain and muscle tone, patient cooperation is gained and the amount of fixed contracture can be measured. The strength and control of antagonistic muscle groups can be determined.

When focal intervention (chemodenervation, neurolysis, or surgery) is being considered, differentiating between the resistance to stretch offered by muscle contraction on a reflex basis versus resistance to stretch generated by inherent physical stiffness properties of muscle tissue is extremely important. EMG examination is another tool that can help make this distinction.[21,23,43,48]

General classification of orthoses

Orthoses can be constructed of different materials, such as plaster, metal, cloth, plastic, and thermoplastic. Thermoplastic materials usually are classified into high- and low-temperature types, based on the temperature at which they become pliable. Many upper limb orthoses are constructed of low-temperature thermoplastics. This material becomes pliable below 180°F, and it can be molded directly against the body. The materials used in orthotic devices include low-temperature thermoplastics that can be custom made for fit and other appropriations. Other materials include casting, metal, strapping, and hook-and-loop closure. Orthotic devices can be divided in two groups:

- *Static Orthoses:* These devices do not allow motion. They serve as rigid supports in cases of fractures and nerve injuries and in the postsurgical phase. Static orthoses may include an attachment for pens or eating utensils.
- *Dynamic/Functional Orthoses:* These devices permit motion. They are used to assist movement of weak muscles and to give some movement to the joint controlling (at the same time) the direction of the movement. Because of these features, they can be used after surgery to replace a static orthosis if the patient has some active motor control. Some dynamic splints have a dual or bilateral tension-providing mechanism that safely accommodates for spasms and limits or avoids soft tissue injuries. Dynamic splinting has a very limited role in treating spastic contractures and may trigger increased muscle tone if not used carefully.
- *Progressive Orthoses:* These devices are used to increase the range of motion of the affected joint, gradually increasing the amount of stretch created in the joint. They can be used to prevent or correct contractures. They also can be used if spasticity is present after a botulinum toxin injections.
- *Serial Orthoses:* These devices accomplish goals similar to those of progressive devices, but they are used in a series to gradually increase the range of motion of a joint.

Exact fit is a key element for many upper limb orthoses. In order to work properly, the orthosis must hold the body part in an exact position. If the orthosis does not fit exactly, it may not work and may actually cause harm.

The patient's motivation and attitude toward the orthosis are important components of the treatment plan. Most upper limb orthoses are removable, and patients can choose whether or not to use them. Health care professionals must work closely with the patient to ensure that the patient will accept the orthosis and use it properly.

Uses of orthotic devices
Contracture prevention

A combination of peripheral nerve blocks and casting or splinting techniques are commonly used to give temporary relief of spasticity.[10,56–58] Positioning a limb in the desired position for later function is important. Because the clinical situation may change quickly after a traumatic brain injury, a short-term orthosis such as a cast often is a practical choice.[5] Casting maintains muscle fiber length and diminishes muscle tone by decreasing sensory input. Lidocaine blocks are helpful when done prior to cast application, because relieving the spasticity allows for easier limb positioning. Casts are used prophylactically to prevent contracture formation in a nonfunctional position. A well-applied circular cast will protect the skin in unconscious patients. Casts are commonly used to treat pressure sores in these patients. Close neurovascular observation is necessary in head injury patients after circular plaster application because many cannot complain of pain secondary to a tight cast.

Orthoses as reinforcement after chemodenervation

When a decision to perform a botulinum toxin injection is made, an orthotic device can be used to maintain the injected muscles in a stretched position and to enhance the effect of the botulinum toxin. In this case, it is better to use progressive or serial orthoses that can be adjusted to increase the amount of stretch.

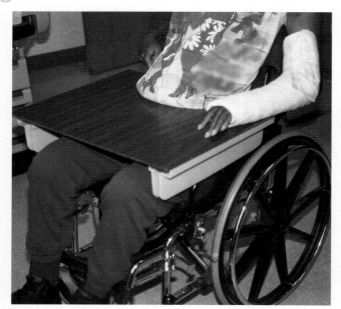

Fig. 14-1 Lap board.

The use of injections and orthoses can be an intermediate and transitory phase before surgery. The purpose is to give the patient a definitive idea of the surgical result. Orthoses also have an important role during the postsurgical phase.

Contracture correction

Correction of contractual deformities can be obtained by serial cast application done at weekly intervals or use of dropout casts.[5] Serial casting is most successful when a contracture has been present for less than 6 months. The patient is sedated, and an anesthetic nerve block is given if necessary to decrease the spasticity. The limb is manipulated for 10 minutes prior to cast application to gain increased joint motion. A well-padded cast is applied, holding the arm in the improved position. Care must be taken not to exert excessive force while applying the cast. The major correction in joint position should have been obtained by the manipulation.

Dropout casts utilize the force of gravity to passively assist in correction of an early contracture. These casts have be modified to allow motion in one direction while preventing motion in the opposite direction. Because gravity is needed for correction, these casts are used in patients who can be seated in an upright position or who are ambulatory.

Maintaining limb position

When the desired limb position has been achieved by serial or dropout casts, bivalved casts are frequently used. Bivalved casts or splints will maintain the limb in the desired position but can be removed several times daily to perform joint range of motion and skin care. Bivalved casts or splints should not be used if severe spasticity persists. They will not adequately immobilize the arm to prevent shearing of the skin against the cast, which quickly leads to decubitus formation.

Functional aids

Orthotics can be used to improve or assist function by positioning the limb adequately for use. Lap boards, arm slings, and other positioning devices should be considered as well as more conventional orthoses.

Shoulder orthoses

Spasticity can develop slowly following the onset of a brain injury. The extremity often begins in a flaccid state. Even as spasticity develops, the muscles supporting the shoulder are weak. The weight of the hanging arm can cause the shoulder to sublux inferiorly.[1,14,25,34,50,70]

A prospective study revealed that 34% of brain-injured patients admitted for rehabilitation had peripheral neuropathies that had not been previously diagnosed.[65] The most common were ulnar nerve compression at the elbow, median nerve impingement, and brachial plexus injuries. Many neuropathies are potentially preventable by careful positioning, padding, and treatment of spasticity.

Lap board

A lap board placed over the arms of a wheelchair can serve as a support for the upper extremity (Fig. 14-1). The thickness of the board is adjusted to support the arm. This device also assists the patient in maintaining an upright posture while seated.

Arm supports

A weak upper extremity can be supported using a sling suspended with springs from an overhead bar attached to a wheelchair (Fig. 14-2). This simple device is comfortable, inexpensive, and easy for the patient and caretakers to use.

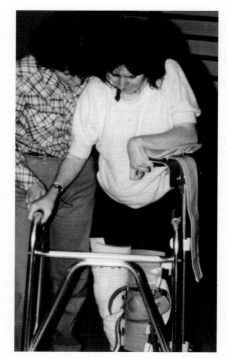

Fig. 14-2 Arm support.

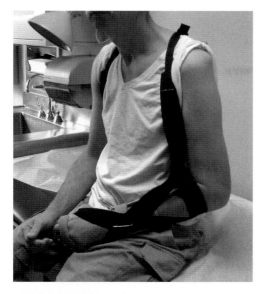

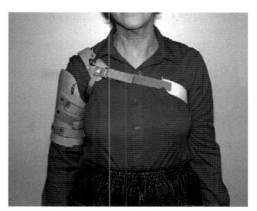

Fig. 14-4 Humeral cuff.

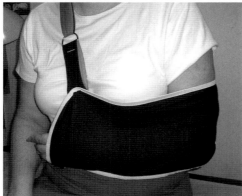

Fig. 14-3 Slings.

It provides support to prevent inferior subluxation of the glenohumeral joint and can be positioned to hold the arm in slight abduction and neutral rotation. This position is desirable to prevent adduction and formation of internal rotation contractures of the shoulder. Such contractures are painful and will interfere with hygiene and upper body dressing.

A forearm trough device can be used to support and position the arm. The device can be attached directly to the arm of a wheelchair. The trough is used to statically position a nonfunctional arm. The patient's forearm can be secured in position with padded straps. This is useful when there is a mild-to-moderate degree of spasticity in the adductor and internal rotator muscles of the shoulder.

A forearm trough can be attached to a hinged mobile support on the arm of the chair. This allows the arm to be placed in a variety of positions for functional use or training of the hand. By decreasing the amount of friction in the hinges, a relatively weak motion of the shoulder can be enhanced to position the hand and arm in a desired position. Alternately, the friction can be increased to provide greater stability.

Forearm and wrist orthoses are volar or dorsal and either gutter-based or circumferential. Ideally, the wrist should be positioned in 15 to 30 degrees of extension, except in carpal tunnel syndrome, when the wrist should be maintained at neutral to minimize median nerve compression.

Sling

A sling is the simplest and most common orthotic device used to position the arm (Fig. 14-3). Its advantages are low cost, ease of use, light weight, and portability. The sling remains the apparatus of choice in ambulatory patients with hemiplegic involvement.[1,3,14,25,64,70] The sling should be removed periodically to allow range of motion exercises of the shoulder and elbow.

Humeral cuff

A cuff applied circumferentially around the proximal humerus can be attached to a shoulder harness and used to maintain the humeral head reduced (Fig. 14-4). The cuff has the advantage of leaving the elbow and hand free. It also allows motion of the glenohumeral joint while maintaining reduction.

Abduction pillow

A bed-bound patient with paralysis or spasticity of the shoulder musculature is prone to develop an adduction and internal rotation contracture of the shoulder from prolonged immobility. A foam pillow is a useful device for positioning the shoulder in slight abduction and neutral rotation. This position facilitates care and prevents contractures and hygiene difficulties in the axilla.

Electrical stimulation

Electrical stimulation units can be considered dynamic orthotic devices. If the muscle weakness is believed to be transient, electrical stimulation of the deltoid and supraspinatus muscles can be used to prevent shoulder subluxation.[2,3,16,24,46,50,67] The expectation is that with further muscle recovery, the shoulder will remain in a reduced position. Treatment of chronic shoulder subluxation also can include electrical stimulation. Although usually successful in the short run, electrical stimulation as a permanent solution frequently is unacceptable to the patient.

Elbow orthoses

Flexor spasticity is common and frequently severe in stroke and brain-injured patients.[38] Flexion contractures are common.[31]

They are painful and lead to maceration of the antecubital skin. The flexed posture of the elbow places traction on the ulnar nerve in the cubital tunnel and positions the relatively immobile patient to place excess pressure directly on the nerve. Compression neuropathy of the ulnar nerve is seen in 10% of patients with brain injury.[18,40]

Elbow flexor spasticity must be diminished to allow correction of a contracture or permit static positioning of the elbow. During the initial 6 to 9 months after injury, spasticity is customarily treated by chemodenervation of the biceps, brachioradialis, and brachialis muscles.[22,23]

When neurologic recovery has stabilized, residual elbow flexor spasticity is treated surgically.[31,38,42,43] In an extremity that exhibits some volitional movement, the elbow flexor tendons are lengthened. When a contracture is present in an elbow that lacks volitional movement, the flexor tendons are transected. Residual flexion deformity even after surgical release is common.

Long arm cast

A long arm cast is an excellent static orthosis for positioning the elbow (Fig. 14-5). It is the most frequently used orthotic device for correcting a flexion contracture. After the spasticity has been diminished by blocks or surgery, the elbow is casted in maximum extension. The cast also can be used in a serial manner to gain further range of motion. In this situation, the cast is changed every 5 to 7 days. With each cast change, the elbow is gently manipulated into further extension. When full extension has been achieved, the cast is bivalved and a clamshell splint is fabricated. The elbow is immobilized in full extension for an additional 3 to 4 weeks to prevent recurrent deformity. The splints are removed several times daily for range of motion exercises.

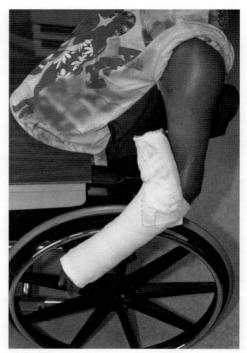

Fig. 14-6 Elbow dropout cast.

Dropout cast

A dropout cast can be used as a dynamic orthosis. The dropout cast is a modification of a long arm cast in which the posterior portion of the cast above the elbow joint has been removed (Fig. 14-6). This cast allows the elbow to extend further but prevents flexion. The cast is purposefully made heavy, or weights are added to the wrist to provide an extension force on the elbow. A dropout cast is effective only in patients who are in an upright position for much of the day because the arm must be hanging freely for the device to work. As the elbow extends further, the arm "drops out" of the cast. The cast is changed periodically as further elbow extension is gained.

Bivalved long arm cast

A bivalved cast or clamshell cast is another modification of the long arm cast (Fig. 14-7). The cast is lined with stockinette to provide a smooth inner surface. Straps are added to secure the anterior and posterior halves of the cast together. The cast can be removed several times daily to allow active or passive joint motion of the elbow to prevent stiffness. A bivalved cast cannot be used in the presence of severe spasticity because it will not sufficiently immobilize the arm to protect the skin from friction and breakdown. A bivalved cast must be reapplied carefully to assure proper alignment and prevent pressure on bony prominences. It requires a cooperative patient and a knowledgeable caretaker.

Dynamic elbow orthoses

A dynamic orthosis provides a force across the elbow joint to increase joint motion (Fig. 14-8).[33,64] Most commonly an extension force is needed in stroke and brain-injured patients.

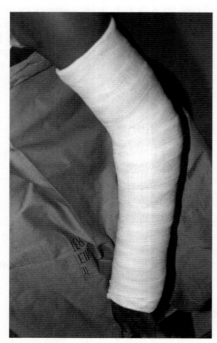

Fig. 14-5 Long arm cast.

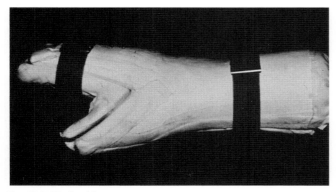

Fig. 14-7 Bivalved long arm cast.

Because a force is being applied, the skin must be monitored for signs of excessive pressure. Dynamic orthoses must be used with caution in patients with diminished awareness or limited communication abilities. Dynamic orthoses often permit motion within a prescribed range. They can be used to assist movement of weak muscles in the face while controlling the direction of the movement. Some dynamic splints have dual or bilateral tension-providing mechanisms. Such mechanisms provide safety by accommodating muscle spasms and limiting or avoiding soft tissue injuries. Because of these features, they can be used after chemodenervation or surgery to replace the static orthosis if the patient has some active motor control.

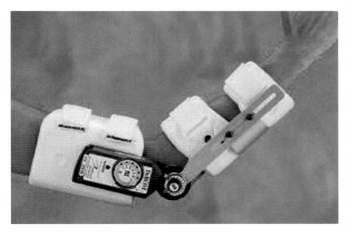

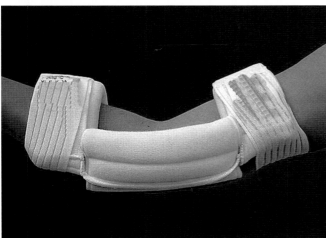

Fig. 14-8 Dynamic elbow orthoses.

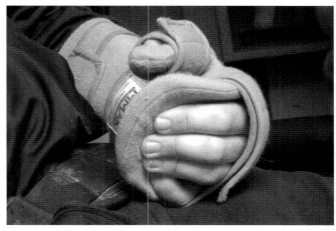

Fig. 14-9 Boutonnière deformities.

Wrist and hand orthoses

Spastic forearm flexor muscles causing wrist and finger flexion deformities are common. Decreasing muscle spasticity is important. A splint applied to a hand with uncontrolled muscle tone can cause a secondary abnormality, such as a boutonnière deformity of the proximal interphalangeal joints (Fig. 14-9). Casts and orthotic devices are used in an adjunctive manner to correct residual contractures or to position the wrist and hand.

During the first 6 to 9 months after onset of injury, flexor spasticity is treated by chemodenervation and nerve blocks. When neurologic recovery has ceased, the spastic extrinsic flexors are surgically lengthened. Specific types of forearm wrist–hand orthoses include casts, static wrist and hand splints, dynamic wrist orthoses, and finger orthoses.

Short arm cast

A short arm cast is an excellent orthotic device for positioning the wrist (Fig. 14-10). It is the most frequently used orthotic device for correcting a flexion contracture. After the spasticity has been diminished by blocks or surgery, the wrist is casted in maximum extension. As with the elbow, the cast is changed every 5 to 7 days. With each cast change, the wrist is gently

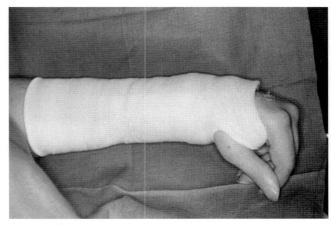

Fig. 14-10 Short arm cast.

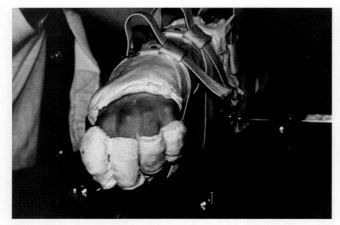

Fig. 14-11 Bivalved short arm cast.

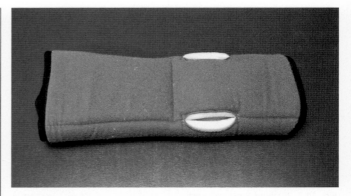

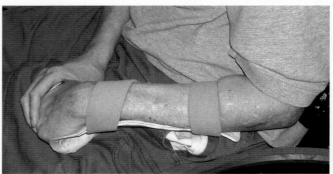

Fig. 14-12 Volar wrist splint.

manipulated into further extension. The cast is bivalved, and a clamshell splint is fabricated after full extension has been achieved (Fig. 14-11). The wrist is immobilized in full extension for an additional 3 to 4 weeks to prevent recurrent deformity. The splints are removed several times daily for range of motion exercises.

Bivalved short arm cast

A bivalved cast or clamshell cast is another modification of the short arm cast (Fig. 14-11). The cast is lined with stockinette to provide a smooth inner surface. Straps are added to secure the anterior and posterior halves of the cast together. The cast can be removed several times daily to allow active or passive joint motion of the wrist to prevent stiffness. A bivalved cast cannot be used in the presence of severe spasticity because it will not sufficiently immobilize the arm to protect the skin from friction and breakdown. A bivalved cast must be reapplied carefully to assure proper alignment and prevent pressure on bony prominences. It requires a cooperative patient and a knowledgeable caretaker.

Volar wrist splint

A light weight volar splint can be useful for maintaining the wrist in an extended position for hand function (Fig. 14-12). This most commonly is indicated following surgical lengthening of spastic extrinsic finger flexor muscles in a hand with modest volitional movement. By holding the wrist in slight extension, the patient can proceed with occupational therapy and functional training of finger motion.

A nonfunctional hand with severe flexion deformities is best treated by surgery. Patients with this condition tolerate orthotic devices poorly and tend to develop skin maceration. Because these patients commonly reside in skilled nursing facilities, the orthotic devices are easily lost or improperly applied. A superficialis to profundus tendon transfer combined with wrist arthrodesis is the treatment of choice.

Resting wrist–hand orthoses

A variety of resting wrist–hand orthoses are available, including both custom-made devices and premade splints

(Fig. 14-13). Many types of materials can be used. The orthosis can immobilize the wrist alone, or it can include the thumb and fingers. As with all hand orthoses, controlling the underlying muscle tone before using splints is important. Median nerve compression occurs with wrist flexion deformities. Forcing a wrist into an extended position can cause or increase pressure on the median nerve in the carpal canal.[55] This action not only is painful but can result in permanent nerve damage.

Spastic or contracted extrinsic finger flexors contribute to wrist flexion deformities. The superficial finger flexor muscles often display more severe spasticity than do the flexor profundus muscles. A wrist–hand orthosis can exacerbate boutonnière deformities if the extrinsic finger flexor tone is not diminished with chemodenervation or surgical lengthening (Fig. 14-9).

Dynamic wrist orthoses

Patients with a relatively flexible wrist flexion deformity can benefit from the use of a dynamic wrist extension orthosis (Fig. 14-14). The range of motion of the wrist can be adjusted as the deformity improves. As with all dynamic splints, the skin must be monitored closely for signs of excessive pressure.

Some patients develop a hyperextended wrist, which places increased stretch on the finger flexors and may exacerbate finger flexion deformities. Overactive wrist extensor muscles can be temporarily treated with chemodenervation or permanently relaxed by surgical lengthening. A dynamic wrist flexion device then is helpful for further correction of the wrist extension deformity (Fig. 14-15).

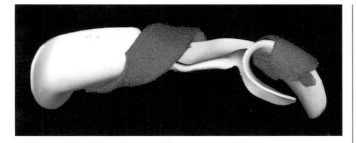

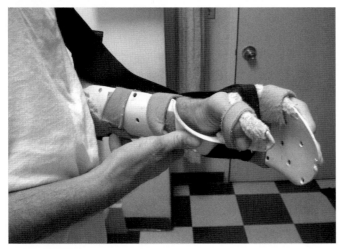

Fig. 14-13 Resting wrist–hand orthoses.

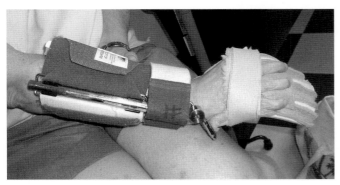

Fig. 14-14 Dynamic wrist extension orthosis.

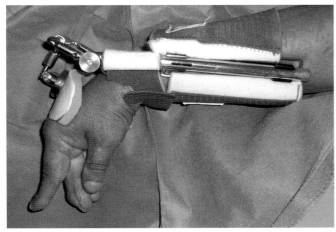

Fig. 14-15 Dynamic wrist flexion orthosis.

Finger and thumb orthoses

Finger positioning devices can be static or dynamic and can be used for maintaining a position or enhancing functional use of the hand. Electrical stimulation devices are available[3,4,12,32,60] and are used mainly as training aids. The longer-term carryover effects are not yet established.

Static hand splints

Static hand splints can be used to maintain the position of the fingers. They are not useful for improving the arc of motion. Surgery and hand therapy remain the best treatment options for improving finger position and mobility. Careful monitoring of skin and joint position is needed to prevent complications (Fig. 14-16). Soft hand rolls or splints are useful for preventing a worsening contracture and nail bed infections and for absorbing perspiration (Fig. 14-17). Excessive perspiration predisposes to skin maceration, malodor, and skin breakdown.

Dynamic hand splints

Many stroke and brain-injured patients regain active finger flexion and are capable of grasping objects. The problem is that only half of patients with active grasp have any active finger extension for hand opening. Chemodenervation or

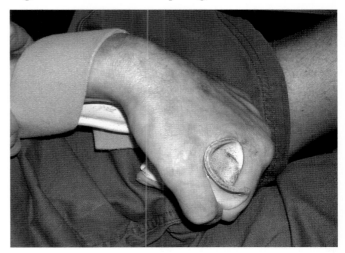

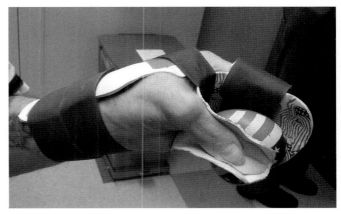

Fig. 14-16 Thumb flexion deformity in splint. In the top photo, positioning is incorrect; in the bottom photo, the thumb is in a better posture.

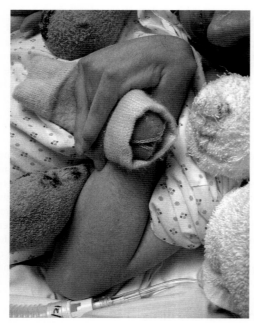

Fig. 14-17 Hand rolls.

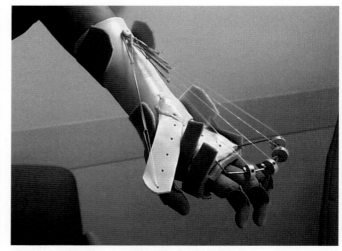

Fig. 14-19 Outrigger dynamic finger extension orthosis.

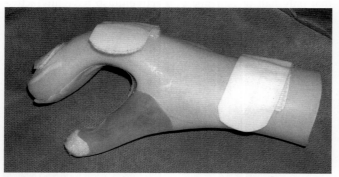

Fig. 14-18 Silicone mitt.

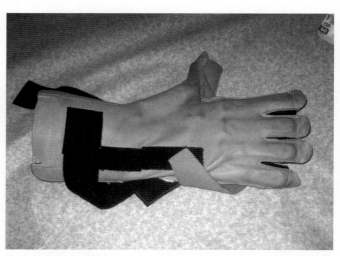

Fig. 14-20 Leaf spring glove.

surgical lengthening can provide relaxation of excessive finger flexor tone. Good hand function depends on the patient being able to open the hand. Finger extension can be supplied by dynamic orthoses.

Three types of orthoses are available. One design is a flexible silicone mitt (Fig. 14-18). The mitt places the fingers in an open position and the thumb abducted. This allows positioning of the hand around an object. The flexible nature of the silicone material allows the patient to close the hand and grasp the object. These orthoses are difficult to don, impede sensation, and cause uncomfortable perspiration of the hand. They are not well accepted by patients.

A second design is an outrigger splint, which uses rubber bands on slings placed beneath the proximal phalanx of the thumb and fingers (Fig. 14-19). The fingers are held in an open position and the thumb abducted. The patient can more easily position the hand to grasp an object. These orthoses are high in profile and not well accepted by patients.

The third design is a leaf spring glove (Fig. 14-20). Flexible strips are incorporated into the glove overlying the extensor surface of each finger. These strips provide active finger extension while allowing the patient to actively grasp. The finger tips of the glove are removed to improve sensation. Although lower in profile than the outrigger splints, the gloves are difficult to don, feel hot, and are not well tolerated.

Split ring orthoses

A simple split ring orthosis can be very useful for positioning the proximal interphalangeal joint for functional use of the hand (Fig. 14-21). The splint can be made of metal or plastic materials. It is low profile, lightweight, easy to don, and well tolerated by patients.

Thumb spica cast

The thumb-in-palm deformity is a frequent deformity in the spastic hand. This deformity is generally secondary to spasticity in the flexor pollicis longus muscle as well as the median and ulnar innervated thenar muscles.

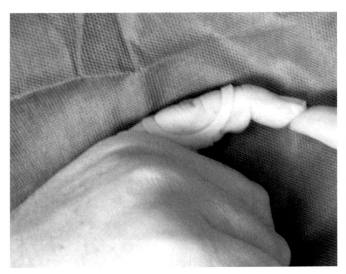

Fig. 14-21 Split ring orthosis for finger.

A thumb spica cast/splint is an excellent orthotic device for positioning the thumb. It is a commonly used orthotic device for correcting a thumb-in-palm contracture. As with all deformities in the spastic upper extremity, a thumb spica cast is used in conjunction with chemodenervation or surgery. The cast initially is applied as a circular device and later can be modified to a bivalved splint if needed.

Thumb abduction splint

A thumb abduction splint can be used to prevent or reposition a thumb that wants to rest in the palm. A lightweight splint that holds the thumb metacarpal in an abducted and slightly opposed position can be used to improve thumb function and pinch (Fig. 14-22). This type of orthosis cast is also used in conjunction with chemodenervation or surgery.

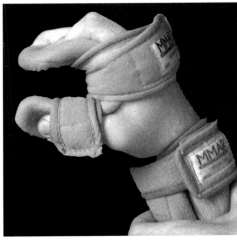

Fig. 14-22 Thumb abduction orthosis.

References

1. Ada L, Foongchomcheay A, Canning C: Supportive devices for preventing and treating subluxation of the shoulder after stroke, *Cochrane Database Syst Rev* CD003863, 2005.
2. Ada L, Foongchomcheay A: Efficacy of electrical stimulation in preventing or reducing subluxation of the shoulder after stroke: a meta-analysis, *Aust J Physiother* 48:257–267, 2002.
3. Aoyagi Y, Tsubahara A: Therapeutic orthosis and electrical stimulation for upper extremity hemiplegia after stroke: a review of effectiveness based on evidence, *Top Stroke Rehabil* 11:9–15, 2004.
4. Baker LL, et al: Electrical stimulation of wrist and fingers for hemiplegic patients, *Phys Ther* 59:1495–1499, 1979.
5. Booth BJ, Doyle M, Montgomery J: Serial casting for the management of spasticity in the head injured adult, *Phys Ther* 63:1960–1966, 1983.
6. Botte MJ, Abrams RA, Bodine-Fowler SC: Treatment of acquired muscle spasticity using phenol peripheral nerve blocks, *Orthopaedics* 18:151–159, 1995.
7. Botte MJ, Keenan MA: Percutaneous phenol blocks of the pectoralis major muscle to treat spastic deformities, *J Hand Surg Am* 13:147–149, 1988.
8. Botte MJ, Nickel VL, Akeson WH: Spasticity and contracture, *Clin Orthop Rel Res* 233:7–18, 1988.
9. Botte MJ, et al: Approaches to senior care #2. Orthopaedic management of the stroke patient. Part I. Pathophysiology, limb deformity, and patient evaluation, *Orthop Rev* 17:637–647, 1988.
10. Botte MJ, et al: Approaches to senior care #3. Orthopaedic management of the stroke patient. Part II: Treating deformities of the upper and lower extremities, *Orthop Rev* 17:891–910, 1988.
11. Botte MJ, et al: Heterotopic ossification in neuromuscular disorders, *Orthopedics* 20:335–341, 1997.
12. Bowman BR, Baker LL, Waters RL: Positional feedback and electrical stimulation: an automated treatment for the hemiplegic wrist, *Arch Phys Med Rehabil* 60:497–502, 1979.
13. Braun RM, et al: Phenol nerve block in the treatment of acquired spastic hemiplegia in the upper limb, *J Bone Joint Surg Am* 55:580–585, 1973.
14. Brooke MM, et al: Shoulder subluxation in hemiplegia: effects of three different supports, *Arch Phys Med Rehabil* 72:582–586, 1991.
15. Cardoso E, et al: Botulinum toxin type A for the treatment of the upper limb spasticity after stroke: a meta-analysis, *Arq Neuropsiquiatr* 63:30–33, 2005.
16. Chae J, Yu D, Walker M: Percutaneous, intramuscular neuromuscular electrical stimulation for the treatment of shoulder subluxation and pain in chronic hemiplegia: a case report, *Am J Phys Med Rehabil* 80:296–301, 2001.
17. Childers MK, et al: Comparison of two injection techniques using botulinum toxin in spastic hemiplegia, *Am J Phys Med Rehabil* 75:462–469, 1996.
18. Chua HC, Tan CB, Tjia H: A case of bilateral ulnar nerve palsy in a patient with traumatic brain injury and heterotopic ossification, *Singapore Med J* 38:447–448, 1997.
19. Copp EP, Keenan J: phenol nerve and motor point block in spasticity, *Rheumatol Phys Med* 11:287–292, 1972.
20. Dengler R, et al: Local botulinum toxin in the treatment of spastic drop foot, *J Neurol* 239:375–378, 1992.
21. Dickstein R, Heffes Y, Abulaffio N: Electromyographic and positional changes in the elbows of spastic hemiparetic patients during walking, *Electroencephalogr Clin Neurophysiol* 101:491–496, 1996.
22. Esquenazi A, Mayer N: Botulinum toxin for the management of muscle overactivity and spasticity after stroke, *Curr Atheroscler Rep* 3:295–298, 2001.
23. Esquenazi A, Mayer NH, Keenan MA: Dynamic polyelectromyography, neurolysis, and chemodenervation with botulinum toxin A for assessment and treatment of gait dysfunction, *Adv Neurol* 87:321–331, 2001.
24. Faghri PD, et al: The effects of functional electrical stimulation on shoulder subluxation, arm function recovery, and shoulder pain in hemiplegic stroke patients, *Arch Phys Med Rehabil* 75:73–79, 1994.
25. Foongchomcheay A, Ada L, Canning CG: Use of devices to prevent subluxation of the shoulder after stroke, *Physiother Res Int* 10:134–145, 2005.
26. Francisco GE: Botulinum toxin for post-stroke spastic hypertonia: a review of its efficacy and application in clinical practice, *Ann Acad Med Singapore* 36:22–29, 2007.
27. Garland DE, Lilling M, Keenan MA: Percutaneous phenol blocks to motor points of spastic forearm muscles in head-injured adults, *Arch Phys Med Rehabil* 65:243–245, 1984.
28. Garland DE, Lucie RS, Waters RL: Current uses of open phenol nerve block for adult acquired spasticity, *Clin Orthop Rel Res* 165:217–222, 1982.
29. Gordon MF, et al: Repeated dosing of botulinum toxin type A for upper limb spasticity following stroke, *Neurology* 63:1971–1973, 2004.

30. Hankey GJ: Botulinum toxin A injections improved wrist and finger spasticity after stroke, *ACP J Club* 138:22, 2003.
31. Hebela N, Keenan MA: Neuro-orthopedic management of the dysfunctional extremity in upper motor neuron syndromes, *Eura Medicophys* 40:145–156, 2004.
32. Hendricks HT, et al: Functional electrical stimulation by means of the "Ness Handmaster Orthosis" in chronic stroke patients: an exploratory study, *Clin Rehabil* 15:217–220, 2001.
33. Hicks JE, et al: Prosthetics, orthotics, and assistive devices. 4. Orthotic management of selected disorders, *Arch Phys Med Rehabil* 70(5-S):S210–S217, 1989.
34. Ikai T, et al: Evaluation and treatment of shoulder subluxation in hemiplegia: relationship between subluxation and pain, *Am J Phys Med Rehabil* 77:421–426, 1998.
35. Katz J, Knott LW, Feldman DJ: Peripheral nerve injections with phenol in management of spastic patients, *Arch Phys Med Rehabil* 48:97–99, 1967.
36. Keenan MA: Management of the spastic upper extremity in the neurologically impaired adult, *Clin Orthop Rel Res* 233:116–125, 1988.
37. Keenan MA, Botte MJ: Technique of percutaneous phenol block of the recurrent motor branch of the median nerve, *J Hand Surg Am* 12(5 Pt 1):806–807, 1987.
38. Keenan MA, Haider TT, Stone LR: Dynamic electromyography to assess elbow spasticity, *J Hand Surg Am* 15:607–614, 1990.
39. Keenan MA, Mehta S: Neuro-orthopedic management of shoulder deformity and dysfunction in brain-injured patients: a novel approach, *J Head Trauma Rehabil* 19:143–154, 2004.
40. Keenan MA, et al: Late ulnar neuropathy in the brain-injured adult, *J Hand Surg Am* 13:120–124, 1988.
41. Keenan MA, et al: Percutaneous phenol block of the musculocutaneous nerve to control elbow flexor spasticity, *J Hand Surg Am* 15:340–346, 1990.
42. Keenan MA, et al: Selective release of spastic elbow flexors in the patient with brain injury, *J Head Trauma Rehabil* 11:57–68, 1996.
43. Keenan MA, et al: The influence of dynamic polyelectromyography in formulating a surgical plan in treatment of spastic elbow flexion deformity, *Arch Phys Med Rehabil* 84:291–296, 2003.
44. Khalili AA, Betts HB: Peripheral nerve block with phenol in the management of spasticity, *JAMA* 200:1155–1157, 1967.
45. Khalili AA, et al: Management of spasticity by selective peripheral nerve block with dilute phenol solutions in clinical rehabilitation, *Arch Phys Med Rehabil* 45:513–519, 1964.
46. Kobayashi H, et al: Reduction in subluxation and improved muscle function of the hemiplegic shoulder joint after therapeutic electrical stimulation, *J Electromyogr Kinesiol* 9:327–336, 1999.
47. Kolessar DJ, Katz SD, Keenan ME: Functional outcome following surgical resection of heterotopic ossification in patients with brain injury, *J Head Trauma Rehabil* 11(4):78–87, 1996.
48. Kozin SH, Keenan MA: Using dynamic electromyography to guide surgical treatment of the spastic upper extremity in the brain-injured patient, *Clin Orthop Rel Res* 288:109–117, 1993.
49. Lazarus MD, et al: Heterotopic ossification resection about the elbow, *J Neurol Rehabil* 12:145–153, 1999.
50. Linn SL, Granat MH, Lees KR: Prevention of shoulder subluxation after stroke with electrical stimulation, *Stroke* 30:963–968, 1999.
51. Mayer NH, Esquenazi A, Keenan MA: Analysis and management of spasticity, contracture, and impaired motor control. In Horn ND, Zasler LJ, editors: *Medical rehabilitation of traumatic brain injury*, Philadelphia, 1996, Hanley & Belfus.
52. Mayer NH, et al: Approach to management of motor dysfunction after acquired brain injury, *Arab Medico* 18:65–70, 2000.
53. Mooney V, Frykman G, McLamb J: Current status of intraneural phenol injections, *Clin Orthop Rel Res* 63:122–131, 1969.
54. Moritz U: Phenol block of peripheral nerves, *Scand J Rehabil Med* 5:160–163, 1973.
55. Orcutt SA, et al: Carpal tunnel syndrome secondary to wrist and finger flexor spasticity, *J Hand Surg Am* 15:940–944, 1990.
56. Ough JL, et al: Treatment of spastic joint contractures in mentally disabled adults, *Orthop Clin North Am* 12:143–151, 1981.
57. Perry J: Contractures. A historical perspective, *Clin Orthop* 219:8–14, 1987.
58. Pomerance JF, Keenan MA: Correction of severe spastic flexion contractures in the nonfunctional hand, *J Hand Surg Am* 21:828–833, 1996.
59. Reiter F, et al: Low-dose botulinum toxin with ankle taping for the treatment of spastic equinovarus foot after stroke, *Arch Phys Med Rehabil* 79:532–535, 1998.
60. Ring H, Rosenthal N: Controlled study of neuroprosthetic functional electrical stimulation in sub-acute post-stroke rehabilitation, *J Rehabil Med* 37:32–36, 2005.
61. Sheean G: Botulinum toxin treatment of adult spasticity: a benefit-risk assessment, *Drug Saf* 29:31–48, 2006.
62. Simpson DM, et al: Botulinum toxin type A in the treatment of upper extremity spasticity: a randomized, double-blind, placebo-controlled trial, *Neurology* 46:1306–1310, 1996.
63. Slawek J, Bogucki A, Reclawowicz D: Botulinum toxin type A for upper limb spasticity following stroke: an open-label study with individualised, flexible injection regimens, *Neurol Sci* 26:32–39, 2005.
64. Sodring KM: Upper extremity orthoses for stroke patients, *Int J Rehabil Res* 3:33–38, 1980.
65. Stone L, Keenan MA: Peripheral nerve injuries in the adult with traumatic brain injury, *Clin Orthop Rel Res* 233:136–144, 1988.
66. Sun SF, et al: Application of combined botulinum toxin type A and modified constraint-induced movement therapy for an individual with chronic upper-extremity spasticity after stroke, *Phys Ther* 86:1387–1397, 2006.
67. Wang RY, Chan RC, Tsai MW: Functional electrical stimulation on chronic and acute hemiplegic shoulder subluxation, *Am J Phys Med Rehabil* 79:385–390, 2000.
68. Wilson DJ: Kinematic changes following botulinum toxin injection after traumatic brain injury, *Brain Injury* 11:157–167, 1997.
69. Wood KM: The use of phenol as a neurolytic agent, *Pain* 5:205–209, 1978.
70. Zorowitz RD, et al: Shoulder subluxation after stroke: a comparison of four supports, *Arch Phys Med Rehabil* 76:763–771, 1995.

Chapter

15

Upper limb orthoses for the person with spinal cord injury

M.J. Mulcahey

Key Points

- The goals of upper limb intervention for persons with spinal cord injury (SCI) are independence, ease of activity, spontaneity, and temporal aspects of activity performance.

- Resumption of meaningful roles is of primary importance in SCI rehabilitation.

- Anticipatory rehabilitation refers to rehabilitation that anticipates future treatments and technologies, preventing secondary deformities and avoiding irreversible treatments that will interfere with future interventions.

- Surgical reconstruction in the form of tendon transfers and other soft tissue reconstruction restores active arm and hand movement.

- Reconstructive surgery based on the International Classification of Surgery of the Hand in Tetraplegia should be offered to persons with tetraplegia.

- Neuroprostheses provide stimulated arm and hand function and will emerge as an effective method for restoring function.

- Orthoses remain a mainstay of SCI rehabilitation.

- Hybrid systems, which combine tendon transfers, neuro-prostheses, and orthoses, may result in superior outcomes over isolated treatment modalities.

- Low-cost, low-technology assistive devices remain pivotal in the rehabilitation of persons with SCI.

- Level I and II evidence supporting upper limb interventions for SCI is lacking.

Pathophysiology

The spinal cord is the major conduit through which motor, sensory, automatic, and conscious information travels between the brain and the body. Nerve roots that exit and enter the spinal cord excite groups of muscle cells, or myotomes, and receive sensory information from skin areas, or dermatomes. Nerve roots are numbered according to the vertebral level they exit and enter. For example, nerve roots that exit the spinal cord at the fifth cervical (C) vertebra excite C5 innervated muscles; likewise, sensory information from C5 dermatomes enter the vertebral canal at the fifth cervical vertebra. Spinal cord injury (SCI) interrupts the conduction of both sensory and motor signals and, based on the level of the injury, results in varying degrees of motor and sensory loss.

The cervical spinal cord is encased within seven cervical vertebrae. At the first and second levels, the diameter of the spinal cord is small in relation to the size of the spinal canal. The cord occupies only one third of the canal at C1–2 but occupies half of the canal at C7.[45] Because range of motion (ROM) is greatest at the C5, C6, and C7 vertebrae and as a result of the relationship between canal size and cord size in the lower cervical region, the majority of injuries occur at those levels.

Traumatic SCI generally results in disruption of the spinal cord architecture, followed by a complex pattern of pathophysiologic processes that exacerbate the injury.[65] Although they may be classified as functionally complete, the majority of traumatic injuries do not result in complete disruption of

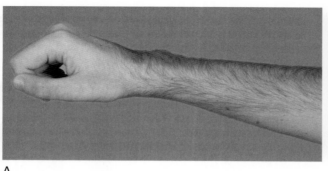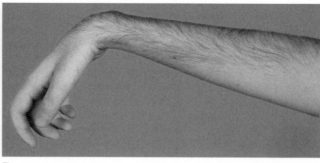

A   B

Fig. 15-1 Tenodesis hand. The hallmark of hand function in tetraplegia. **A,** After purposeful tightening of the flexor tendons, voluntary wrist extension results in passive grasp and pinch. **B,** With gravity-assisted wrist flexion, the fingers and thumb open passively.

the cord. Residual injury often is characterized by a peripheral rim of intact tissue with a central cystic cavity.[16,55,65] In a so-called "clinically complete" injury, peripherally preserved pathways can result in nonfunctioning residual axons secondary to loss of myelin locally, or they may be involved in the degree of spasticity exhibited. In incomplete SCI, in the condition called *central cord syndrome*, the rim of damage initially expands outward, but as the degree of injury resorbs back more centrally, the function effected by the periphery becomes preserved. Central cord syndrome typically is characterized by preserved bowel, bladder, and lower extremity function but dramatic loss of upper extremity function. The anatomical reason for this finding is the layering of the fibers in the lateral cortical spinal tract (primary motor tract). These fibers are layered such that the more distal functioning tracts are more peripheral, whereas the fibers for the upper extremity are more central in the tract and therefore more susceptible to damage that occurs from central to peripheral.

In the cervical spine, a unique set of injuries to the white matter and the gray matter results in a combination of central and peripheral injuries. Damage to the white matter affects motor control and sensory input from the periphery to the brain below the level of injury. Almost always at and surrounding the level of injury, evidence is seen of lower motor neuron (LMN) injury resulting in flaccid paralysis at the level of injury.[90,118] Muscles with LMN injury are at greater risk for contractures[22] as a result of shortening and scarring. In addition, muscles with LMN injury are not amenable to functional electrical stimulation (FES). Coulet et al.[22] have detailed the implications of SCI pathophysiology on upper extremity rehabilitation.

SCI most frequently occurs in young adults between the ages of 16 and 30 years,[37] with a recent increasing trend in injuries sustained by older persons.[100] In the United States, motor vehicle crashes and violence are the primary causes of SCI.[26] Approximately 3% to 5% of SCIs that occur each year in North America are sustained by individuals younger than 15 years and about 20% in those younger than 20 years.[39,41,59,100] Although boys more commonly sustain SCI than girls during childhood or adolescence, the frequency of SCI in boys and girls younger than 5 years is comparable.[39,41,112,132,133] The level and category of neurological injury vary as a function of age, with younger children more likely having paraplegia or complete injuries.[132,133]

The management, complications, and outcomes of adult and pediatric SCI have been extensively addressed in four notable comprehensive publications.[9,50,61,127]

Historical perspectives

Although high mortality rates after cervical SCI once were commonplace, today survival and discharge to the community are typical.[27] Although complications as a result of SCI still occur,[19] they are becoming less associated with medical and physical comorbidities and increasingly are related to challenges associated with resuming meaningful roles and productive work. This is particularly true for individuals with adult-onset tetraplegia who develop physical and select medical problems more frequently than their peers with paraplegia[121,122] but also realize greater challenges in dating, marriage, and productive employment.[135] Similarly, individuals with childhood-onset tetraplegia are underemployed, date less frequently than typically developing youth and young adults,[4] and, once they become adults, are more likely to be overeducated and underemployed.

Despite the dramatic progress in medicine, rehabilitation, and societal modifications, the upper limb remains obliged to assume new and demanding roles after SCI. After the introduction of antibiotics, high mortality rates among persons with tetraplegia declined, and early rehabilitation techniques focused on purposeful tightening of the finger flexor muscles to develop force between the thumb and index/middle fingers (Fig. 15-1).[45,139,141] Typically referred to as "natural tenodesis," "tenodesis action," "passive tenodesis," and "tenodesis hand,"[52,83,113] this pinch, which provides sufficient force to acquire light objects,[52] formed the basis for the wrist-driven flexor hinge splint[11] and the early techniques for surgical augmentation of the C6 hand.[17] Although the tenodesis hand remains a mainstay of rehabilitation in many SCI centers,[45,52,122,127] today's requirements for the upper limb of persons with SCI typically exceed what can be provided by the tenodesis hand. As such, new treatment paradigms have emerged over the last few decades. The evolution of surgical reconstruction and technology has resulted in upper extremity interventions that offer people with tetraplegia not only the long-standing goal of independence but also more contemporary goals associated with spontaneity, ease of activity, performance, and improved cosmesis.[31,34,45,58,69,73,93,95,101–103]

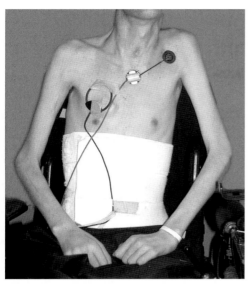

Fig. 15-2 External Freehand System. Electrodes are placed on the paralyzed muscles of the hand and forearm and channeled under the skin to an implanted receiver in the chest. A position sensor, placed on the shoulder, communicates with the internal receiver through radio frequency via an "antenna" that is placed on the skin over the implant.

Surgical reconstruction of the upper limb in tetraplegia: Historical perspective

Early reports of surgical reconstruction of the hand in tetraplegia describe using techniques similar to those used in polio,[17,123] with varying degrees of success and little acceptance among rehabilitation physisicans.[45] Erik Moberg is recognized as the father of upper extremity tendon transfers in SCI and, like other experts, pioneered the early reconstructive work. Despite positive outcomes, hand surgery continued to have little if any role in the general rehabilitation of persons with tetraplegia. However, in the last two decades of the 20th century, an international effort to build consensus on treatment techniques and share outcomes emerged.[44,73,81,82] As a direct result of this effort, surgical reconstruction of the upper extremity in select SCI centers worldwide has restored elbow extension,[91,94-96] wrist extension,[33,43] forearm rotation,[38] and hand grasp and release.[32,33,35,47,66]

Elbow extension has commonly been restored by transferring the posterior and part or all of the middle deltoid to the triceps.[44,82,91,94,95] However, evidence now suggests that the biceps-to-triceps transfer may provide superior outcomes.[91] Although the traditional goal of a tendon transfer for elbow extension has been to restore *control* of the arm and hand,[94] current tendon transfer planning considers restoration of power because of the promise of neurological recovery through regeneration and restorative therapies. For this reason, biceps transfer is being investigated as a preferred alternative to the traditional approach using the deltoid muscle.

Wrist extension provides tenodesis grasp in the absence of voluntary muscles. When combined with soft tissue reconstruction, transfer of the brachioradialis (BR) to the extensor carpi radialis brevis restores passive prehension to persons with a C5 SCI level of injury and has led to their ability to complete activities of daily living (ADLs).[33,44,46,82,94,95] Tendon transfers also have been performed to restore active finger and thumb flexion for pinch,[47,66,88] grasp,[32,35,88] and hand opening.[32,43] In combination, these tendon transfers enable persons with C6 and C7 SCI to acquire and hold objects that vary in size and weight using either palmar (gross) grasp or lateral (key) pinch. Tendon transfers for thumb and finger extension make release of objects possible without reliance on gravity-assisted wrist flexion. Restoration of active grasp and release eliminates the need for adaptive equipment for eating, brushing teeth, catheterizing, and other ADLs. When provided bilaterally, it restores bilateral abilities and improves the patient's ability to negotiate ramps, curbs, and uneven terrain while in the wheelchair by providing stronger grip of the tire rims. Tendon transfers also play an important role for ambulatory persons with incomplete tetraplegia who require restored function to maintain grasp of a walker or a crutch.

Neuroprosthesis for the upper limb in tetraplegia: Historical perspective

In addition to the contributions by Erik Moberg, the pioneering work in the area of FES by Hunter Peckham and Michael Keith represents one of the most influential efforts in the area of upper limb rehabilitation in tetraplegia. In cases of SCI, FES is the coordinated stimulation of two or more muscles to achieve a functional outcome.[85] The distinguishing feature between FES and therapeutic electrical stimulation (TES) is twofold. First, the primary purpose of FES is to enable an individual to perform an activity. In contrast, the primary purpose of TES is to provide a pattern of stimulation for therapeutic purposes such as muscle strengthening and ROM. The second primary distinction between FES and TES is the control source. The FES user has voluntary control of the stimulation parameters and variables via a switch or joint sensor and/or programming.[53] TES is preprogrammed and not under the user's volitional control.

Neuroprosthesis is a term coined to describe bracing of the limb by means of FES. The early work of Peckham and Keith using percutaneous electrical stimulation systems restored palmar and lateral grasp and release to persons with midcervical impairments[106,107] and demonstrated restored capabilities in ADL.[25,93,101,117,118,139] Successful outcomes of percutaneous work led to the development of an implantable neuroprosthesis[104,105,116] marketed under the name Freehand System.

The NeuroControl Freehand System, an eight-channel neuroprosthesis consisting of implanted and external components (Fig. 15-2) with capability to restore grasp and release function (Fig. 15-3), gained market approval by the United States Food and Drug Administration (FDA) after an international clinical trial demonstrated significance increases with FES in pinch and grasp forces, improved independence of every subject while using FES, and high satisfaction and preference for FES among users.[104] Subanalyses of the clinical trials data showed positive outcomes of the Freehand System on pediatric, adolescent, and adult performance of and satisfaction with ADLs[24,60,87,124,126] Because of the strong evidence supporting FES as an efficacious treatment and as a direct response to consumers' requests for the device early in recovery, the Freehand System also has been used successfully for restoring function during initial SCI rehabilitation.[86]

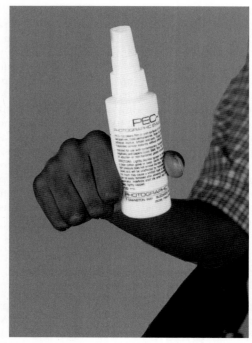

Fig. 15-3 Freehand System function. Stimulated grasp provides function for maintaining hold of objects such as a bottle.

stimulated grasp. Preliminary results with the bionic glove were positive, as evidenced by 24% and 49% improvement in the Functional Independence Measure and Quadriplegic Index of Function, respectively.[109] Plans for clinical deployment of the bionic glove are unclear.

The NESS H200 (Bioness Inc., Santa Clara, CA), formerly known as the Handmaster, consists of an arm–hand orthosis and a control box. Five surface electrodes contained within the orthosis deliver stimulation to the long extensor and flexor tendons of the fingers and thumb and to intrinsic thenar muscles.[120] Preliminary reports of 10 consecutive patients showed that six reestablished grasp patterns that enabled manipulation of objects that was not achievable without the device.[120] Although no prospective studies with large number of persons using the system have been performed, Alon and McBride[2] demonstrated positive outcomes of the NESS H200 in a series of patients with midcervical SCI.

Clinical directions of FES for the 21st century are well described by Peckham and Gorman[101] and include systems that will address multisystem functions, spontaneous and natural control mechanisms, and modularity, allowing for upgrades as technology advances. Hybrid systems likely will emerge as clinically relevant treatment paradigms emerge for upper limb neuroprostheses that combine FES, orthoses, and reconstructive surgery.

Orthotic intervention: Historical perspective

Until the introduction of neuroprostheses, the principles of upper extremity functional orthotic intervention for persons with tetraplegia remained relatively unchanged. Early work with patients with poliomyelitis[49] paved the way for orthotic treatment guidelines in tetraplegia,[28,48,64,95,97,99,140] many of which remain pertinent today.

Whether powered by external sources[3,6,75,128] or voluntary wrist extension,[5,54,62,75,80] the wrist-flexor hinged orthosis (Fig. 15-4) has been and continues to be a mainstay of orthotic prescription in tetraplegia rehabilitation. The first report on the wrist-driven flexor hinged orthosis described a static position of the stabilized thumb and partially flexed index and middle fingers that allowed for pinch with active wrist extension and opening with gravity-assisted wrist flexion.[97] If finger motion was preserved, a finger-driven orthosis

Yet, despite the evidence outcomes and other[23] support of neuroprostheses, marketing of the device was stopped in 2001.[57] Next-generation implantable neuroprostheses systems are under development[57,101] and are anticipated to reemerge in the 21st century as an intervention and treatment of choice for restoring upper extremity in persons with tetraplegia.

Some FES systems have used surface electrodes. The bionic glove, which was developed in 1989 by researchers at the University of Alberta, underwent multiple design modifications for improvement in functionality[109] for persons with midcervical tetraplegia. The glove requires the application of surface electrodes and donning of the glove that, when secure, holds the electrodes in place. Among nine users, only one reported difficulty in donning. Voluntary wrist extension provides the control source for

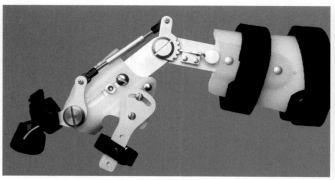

A

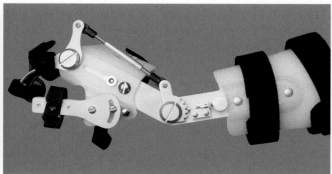

B

Fig. 15-4 Wrist-driven flexor hinge orthosis. A mainstay in SCI orthotic management, this dynamic orthosis augments the natural tenodesis hand such that with gravity-assisted wrist flexion, the orthosis augments passive hand opening **(A)**, and with wrist extension, the orthosis augments passive tenodesis pinch **(B)**.

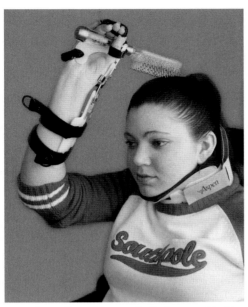

Fig. 15-5 Wrist-driven flexor hinge orthosis. Person with C6 tetraplegia holding a brush using a wrist-driven flexor hinge orthosis.

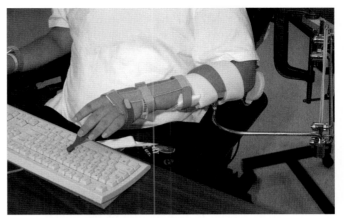

Fig. 15-6 Mobile arm support. Person with C4–5 tetraplegia using an MAS to facilitate use of proximal function for hand function. Note the dorsal wrist splint with universal cuff for maintaining the pencil for use during writing/typing.

was prescribed.[45] This variation has not remained a popular intervention most likely because of the splint's interference with sensory input to a sensate hand and poor cosmesis.

Nickle's wrist-drive flexor hinged orthosis, which was based on biomechanical principles of the hand[13] and commonly referred to as the "Rancho Splint" or "wrist-driven flexor hinge splint," was prescribed during stages of rehabilitation when training in multiple activities was being conducted.[56,98] For persons without wrist extension, cable-driven and gas-powered sources were used to activate the pinch.[6,29] Both sources of power were minimally accepted by the users because of the effort required, donning issues, and poor comfort; as a result, both have been phased out.[45] However, despite rejection of the externally powered flexor hinge splint by persons with higher cervical injuries, a variety of wrist-driven orthoses remain on the market for those with midcervical injuries. These wrist-driven orthoses are considered the standard of care for persons with midcervical tetraplegia for restoring simple ADL function (Fig. 15-5).[5,21,28,48,54,74,84]

Mobile arm supports (MAS) and suspension slings are designed to aid persons with high tetraplegia (C4 and above) with hand-to-mouth and tabletop activities. Although the terms are used interchangeably, as shown in Figure 15-6, MAS are mechanical devices that support the arm and forearm and assist with shoulder and elbow movement through a linkage of ball-bearing joints,[69,70,75,84,115,128] whereas suspension slings are kinetic devices that support the upper extremity.[84,127] The suspension feeder was first introduced for persons with polio[49] to assist with hand-to-mouth activities. Forearms rested in a trough and the arms were suspended by cables or springs from an overhead frame attached to the wheelchair. Although effective for some persons with weak residual proximal control, the suspension feeder eventually was rejected by the population with SCI because the bulkiness of the device made wheelchair

dimensions exceed accessible values, and portability from one environment to another was cumbersome.

Development of next-generation feeders focused on smaller devices positioned beneath the user's arm or mounted to the table. For example, the StandFeeder was a table-mounted unit with the pivot point located under the forearm,[69] and the C-Clamp Feeder was mounted to the tabletop and incorporated a forearm trough and the flexor hinged orthosis.[8]

Early work on the overhead suspension system and feeders paved the way for development of the ball-bearing feeder,[118] linkage feeder, and balanced forearm orthosis,[69] all of which are collectively referred to as MAS. Two of the first MAS introduced to persons with tetraplegia were developed by engineers at Rancho Los Amigos and Texas Institute for Rehabilitation and Research (TIRR).[69] The Rancho MAS, also called the Golden Arm, was successfully used by persons with polio who, despite no muscle activity, had full sensation in their limbs; the Golden Arm was rejected by those with SCI because of lack of sensory feedback while using the device.[69]

Engen's early work at TIRR provided important contributions to the philosophy of upper limb orthotic management that remain pertinent for SCI care today. In addition to engineering and design elements of the orthoses,[29] Engen believed that users must have easy control of the device and, as a result, custom made each MAS to meet the unique needs of individual patients. This custom approach to MAS restored three major arm and hand functions[69] and provided ease of function to the recipients. However, despite sound concepts and excellence in design, Engen's custom-made MAS was ill suited for commercial production and therefore eventually failed in successful clinical deployment.

The A.I. DuPont Hospital for Children has contributed to the evolution of MAS for persons with SCI.[42] Most recently they have focused on development of a power-assisted arm orthosis, the Wilmington Robotic Exoskeleton (WREX).[110,111] The WREX, which is mounted to the wheelchair, uses linear elastic elements to counter gravity and power assistance to shift the arm in response to the user. Preliminary trials of the WREX with persons having muscular dystrophy showed more than 50% reduction in the time to complete items on the Jebsen Test of Hand Function.[111] Development of free-standing arm units, such as the Action Arm (Flaghouse, Hasbrouck Heights, NJ) and the Zoncoarm (Technology for Education, Inner Grove Heights, MN), are being developed and illustrate the continued need for effective orthoses for high tetraplegia.

Current issues

Despite the evolution of upper extremity treatment for persons with tetraplegia, significant clinical challenges in SCI rehabilitation for persons with tetraplegia remain. No method effectively restores functional use of the upper limb in patients with high tetraplegia. Rehabilitation engineers in research laboratories continue to develop techniques, but pathways for clinical deployment are ill defined.[69] Tabletop feeding assists remain in use because of the limitations in restoring effortless and efficient upper extremity function to patients, particularly those with the most severe injuries.

Strong evidence supports use of neuroprostheses in patients with midcervical injuries, but knowledge of device availability and perceived complexity remain barriers to widespread use. Also, the only FDA-approved implantable FES system for upper limb function failed in the market because of the high cost and relatively small population with tetraplegia, and FES systems using surface electrodes have not gained acceptance by the rehabilitation community. Yet, despite these challenges, evidence in support of neuroprostheses is building, and promising clinical work continues. This work likely will impact standard of care within a few years.[101]

Evidence from clinical series and retrospective reviews in support of tendon transfers is strong, yet few centers offer a comprehensive program presumably because of the disconnect between the hand surgeon and rehabilitation physician.[66] Although the functional gains are enormous, the postoperative course associated with tendon transfers requires a temporary setback in independence, and, for some individuals who have been living with SCI, this sacrifice cannot be made because of financial, family, and work obligations. In recognition of this challenge, contemporary clinicians suggest that tendon transfers be considered during the immediate rehabilitation period when neurological stability is reached.

Orthotic intervention continues to be a mainstay in tetraplegia rehabilitation. Despite proposed recommendations,[21] acceptance and implementation of clinical practice guidelines are lacking, and most therapists have inadequate education on how to train people with SCI on the use of orthoses and neuroprostheses for activities.[69,101]

Other relevant issues should be considered. In the era of accountability and evidence-based practice, no level I studies support upper limb interventions in SCI. Although a plethora of literature on orthotic, reconstructive, and FES procedures is available, few prospective studies have used rigorous research methodology. A major barrier to outcomes research is the lack of a universally accepted outcome measure for upper limb function in SCI[69] and the relatively few number of persons with tetraplegia who are able or willing to participate in clinical outcomes trials.

There are broader issues as well. The 21st century brings an increase in the frequency of incomplete injuries and promising regeneration clinical trials that hold promise for some

degree of motor and sensory recovery. Persons with incomplete tetraplegia who have more atypical pain and spasticity may be less desirable candidates for hand surgery, FES, or orthoses. Conversely, some persons with incomplete tetraplegia may be fully ambulatory using assistive devices, thus placing much more demand on upper limb function, whether it be preserved or restored. Persons with complete and incomplete SCI are living longer, and new complications associated with aging, such as pain and degenerative changes of the upper limb, are becoming more prevalent.[20]

Treatment recommendations
Clinical practice guidelines

The Consortium for Spinal Cord Medicine has published clinical practice guidelines for upper limb function following SCI[20] and on outcomes following traumatic SCI[21]; both provide important upper extremity treatment guidelines for tetraplegic rehabilitation. Clinicians working with persons having SCI should know and understand these practice guidelines and integrate them into existing clinical pathways in the clinical setting.

Recommendations for evaluation of the upper limb in SCI

As described by Bryden et al.[15] and Landi et al.,[68] thorough evaluation of the upper limb is the foundation to successful treatment. The International Standards for Neurological Classification in Spinal Cord Injury (The Standards) remain the most widely used assessment of motor and sensory impairment after SCI. The muscle strength of 20 muscles (five upper and five lower limb on each side) is graded on an ordinal scale ranging from 0 (absent strength) to 5 (normal strength). Sensory testing to pinprick and light touch also is conducted, yielding a possible score of 56 for each sensation for each leg (112 total points for pinprick and 112 total points for light touch). From the motor and sensory examination, the neurological level and severity of the injury are determined. The Standards define neurological level as the most caudal segment where normal muscle and sensory function exist on both sides of the body. Centers specializing in SCI should be trained in the administration of The Standards and demonstrate competency in the examination and classification components. Teaching tools are available from the American Spinal Injury Association (ASIA), Atlanta, GA.

Although The Standards' motor and sensory examinations are internationally applied, they provide insufficient information for design of upper extremity treatment paradigms. As an adjunct, the International Classification for Surgery of the Hand in Tetraplegia (ICSHT) is recommended when planning for upper limb surgery.[82] As shown in Table 15-1, the ICSHT is a simple assessment of every muscle in the upper limb below the shoulder. Despite several shortcomings,[68] the ICSHT provides a foundation for decision-making about upper limb interventions[51,63] and augments the motor and sensory information gained from The Standards.

In addition to the motor and sensory systems, examination of joint ROM and pliability of the hand is essential because limitations in these areas will greatly impede application of

Table 15-1 Surgical treatment recommendations for persons with tetraplegia based on ICSHT and ASIA classification

ICSHT	ASIA	Key Muscle	Tendon Transfers and Augmentative Procedures to Optimize Hand Function
O(CU):0	C5	No grade 4 muscle below elbow	Possible elbow extension transfer
O(CU):1	C5	BR	Elbow extension transfer; BR > ECRL/B; FPL tenodesis; New Zealand FPL split
O(CU):2	C6	BR + ECRL	Elbow extension; BR to ECRL/B + FPL tenodesis; BR > FPL + ECRL > FDP; New Zealand FPL split
O(CU):3	C6	Above + ECRB	Elbow extension; BR > FPL + ECRL > FDP; New Zealand FPL split
O(CU):4	C6	Above + PT	Elbow extension; BR > FPL + PT > ABPL + EDC tenodesis; or PT > FPL + BR > EDC/EPL; New Zealand FPL split; intrinsic tenodesis
O(CU):5	C6	Above + FCR	As above
O(CU):6	C7	Above + EDC	As above without elbow extension; finger extension transfer also not indicated; intrinsic transfer or tenodesis
O(CU):7	C7	Above + EPL	As above without thumb extension transfer
O(CU):8	C8	Above + finger flexion	Transfer for thumb flexion
O(CU):9	C8–T1	Lacks intrinsics	Intrinsic transfer

ABPL, Abductor pollicis longus, *BR,* brachioradialis; *EDC,* extensor digitorum communis, *ECRB,* extensor carpi radialis brevis; *ECRL,* extensor carpi radialis longus; *EDC,* extensor digitalis communis; *EPL,* extensor pollicis longus; *FCR,* flexor carpi radialis; *FPL,* flexor pollicis longus; *PT,* pronator teres.

orthoses, neuroprostheses, and tendon transfers. Spasticity, muscle atrophy, and scarring due to LMN injury contribute to poor posturing and potentially fixed deformities. Electrodiagnostic testing in SCI has been popularized by the clinical deployment of neuroprostheses because of the need for intact LMN for viable electrostimulation. As a precursor to formal electrodiagnostics, clinicians can test LMN integrity by applying surface electrical stimulation to the forearm and hand muscles using a simple commercially available transepidermal nerve stimulation (TENs) unit. For patients with motor levels appropriate for neuroprosthesis, formal testing of the muscles' responses is recommended.[99]

The Capabilities of the Upper Extremity (CUE)[76,77] and the Grasp and Release Test (GRT)[125] are recommended for evaluation of hand function. The CUE is a 17-item questionnaire that asks patients to rate their ability to perform functional tasks with their arms on a seven-point ordinal scale. The questionnaire separates proximal arm function from hand function and has been shown to be effective in measuring outcomes after surgery to improve upper extremity function. The GRT, designed specifically for tetraplegia assessment, measures three variables: pinch strength, grasp strength, and hand function. Stroh-Wuolle et al.[125] first reported on the psychometrics of the GRT, which were further established by Mulcahey et al.[92] Clinically, the GRT has been an effective outcome measure for intervention studies of FES and tendon transfers.[88,97,98,117,127]

The Functional Independence Measure[40] continues to be widely used in SCI rehabilitation centers and is recommended as part of the assessment despite notable limitations.[15,16,89] Activity and participation have become important components in the overall assessment of upper extremity interventions in SCI and can be evaluated with the Craig Handicap and Reporting Technique (CHART),[136] Canadian Occupational Performance Measure (COPM),[72]

and Craig Hospital Inventory of Environmental Factors (CHIEF).[137,138] Current development and research on computer adaptive testing will make a significant contribution and likely change the culture of measurement. Comprehensive discussion on issues of outcomes instruments related to the upper extremity of persons with tetraplegia have been published.[15,68,88]

Recommendations for reconstructive procedures for the upper limb in tetraplegia

Recommendation for tendon transfers are given in Table 15-1. As summarized in Table 15-1, the greater the number of muscles an individual has under voluntary control, the greater the number of movements can be restored. There is a consensus on the clinical ladder for upper limb reconstruction in tetraplegia based on the number of residual muscles an individual has under volitional control.[63] Without exception, wrist extension should never be jeopardized, and restoration of pinch then grasp is a priority. Assuming sufficient preserved motors, restoration of hand opening is secondary.

What is less clear is the timing for surgery. Some believe that surgery for tendon transfers should be delayed until the patient is able to integrate the SCI into his or her self-image and until optimal performance in ADL is achieved.[45,51] Others suggest that sufficient natural history data are available to determine recovery patterns and to identify those who should undergo tendon transfers early in the rehabilitation process. Regardless of timing, tendon transfer surgery requires a temporary period of dependency on others and use of adaptive equipment and powered mobility. For more discussion on tendon transfer evaluation and technique, readers are referred to Hentz and LeClercq,[45] Kozin,[63] James,[51] and Mulcahey.[83]

Recommendations for serial casting for the upper limb in tetraplegia

Serial casting is the application of low-load prolonged stretch to shortened tissue with the objective of biologic remodeling or regrowth of tissue in the lengthened positions.[7,30] It has been shown to be one of the most effective interventions for enhancing passive ROM in patients having SCI with secondary joint tightness or recent contracture.[61] When considering serial casting, a thorough assessment of passive ROM, joint end feel, flexibility, sensation, volitional movement, muscle tone, skin integrity, and function should be performed.[30,143] In addition, an understanding of the mechanical principles of biological tissue,[13] alternative treatments,[12,30,79] candidate selection,[71,79] contraindications,[12,144] risk factors,[144] materials available for casting,[1] procedure for casting,[7,12,71] and preventive strategies[30] is important.

Because spontaneous fracture is a common secondary complication of SCI, a patient history of pathological fracture should be obtained prior to casting.[71] An injection of a localized muscle-blocking agent can be performed to reduce the soft tissue stresses to bone during the serial casting process. If the risk of pathological fracture is too high, an alternative approach such as chemodenervation[131] or surgical lengthening[45] should be considered. An understanding of the functional implications of potentially elongating a tight joint in a patient with SCI is important to assess. Some patients may rely on that passive limitation for enhancing functional performance. Conversely, some patients may not appreciate activities that would be available to them if they had a more supple hand. It is important to weigh the functional benefits against potential losses when considering serial casting in these cases.

Contraindications for serial casting include bony blocks or intraarticular restrictions,[144] unstable or unhealed fracture,[12] fluctuating edema, acute inflammatory conditions,[79] and acute thrombosis. Risk factors associated with serial casting include myositis ossifications,[144] skin redness, and fracture. These complications have been associated with an aggressive approach[144] and inadequate screening used to identify patients at greater risk. The types of cast materials used for serial casting include plaster of Paris and fiberglass or fiberglass-free, latex-free casting tape.[1]

Cast changes typically are scheduled anywhere from 3 to 5 days after initial application.[144] Cast cutting is performed using a sinusoidal motion along bisected lines. Once the cast is successfully cut, separators are used and the cast is removed. The clinician can use scissors or manually separate the web roll. Following stockinette removal, skin checks and skin care are performed while the arm is maintained in the extended position. The clinician reassess for changes in passive ROM, maintaining the limb in the lengthening position. Another session of warming and stretching ensues, followed by repeat casting. The procedure discussed is used for all joints except when casting the interphalangeal joints. For the latter case, a review of the work by Bell-Krotoski[7] is recommended.

Orthotic management

Orthotic and neuroprosthetic management in SCI involves static protective splinting, static functional orthoses, dynamic

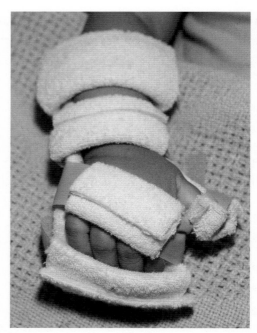

Fig. 15-7 Resting hand splint. The typical position of a static splint for SCI.

functional orthoses, and FES. The selection of orthotic intervention is dependent upon neurological level, time after injury, and desired goals and usually involves a combination of different types of splints and orthoses. The critical factor in deciding the type of orthosis is the strength of wrist extension. In general, for persons with poor or absent wrist extension, orthoses that cross the wrist and extend to the proximal forearm are needed. Conversely, for patients with against-gravity wrist extension strength, shorter, hand-based orthoses are sufficient.

Acute tetraplegia

Early protective splinting prevents overstretching of the ligaments, maintains a functional hand position, prevents deformity, and protects and stabilizes flaccid joints. Regular skin checks are necessary, and frequent adjustments to the splint should be anticipated. ROM exercises and proper bed positioning techniques are other critical components of upper extremity management in acute tetraplegia.[20,45,61]

A resting hand splint applied early after injury may help prevent edema by positioning the wrist in full extension and the metacarpophalangeal joints in flexion (Fig. 15-7). Tolerance for full-time wearing develops over a period of 1 week, starting with 2 hours on the first night and adding another hour each night until 8 hours of wearing is tolerated. Frequent adjustments to the splint are necessary because of changing edema, fluctuating tone, and volitional movement typically seen in acute stages of SCI.

Static splinting also prevents deformity and promotes a functional hand.[64] Although practice guidelines for splinting regimens are generally agreed upon,[21,45,64,84] there long has been controversy over the concept of tenodesis splinting. Tenodesis splinting, a form of static splinting to promote

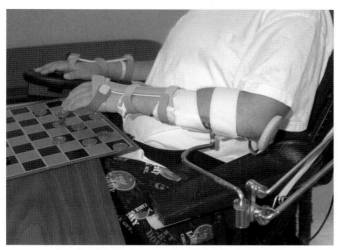

Fig. 15-8 Mobile arm support. Person with C5 tetraplegia demonstrating use of an MAS for leisure.

purposeful tightening of the flexor tendons to create a tenodesis hand, is implemented in some SCI centers early after injury. For tenodesis splinting, the wrist is held in extension and the fingers are taped or wrapped in flexion. Tenodesis splinting has been controversial because if incorrectly applied or worn too long, fixed flexion contractures may develop and compromise future treatment options.[45] Also, because persons with SCI desire a supple hand for socialization and interpersonal relations and because of advancements in neuroprostheses and surgical techniques that provide superior grasp strength over a tenodesis hand, tenodesis splinting should be used with prudence. I discourage tenodesis splinting because superior treatment is available and because tenodesis splinting may result in irreversible deformity that interferes with future options.

High-level tetraplegia (C1–4)

The goals of upper limb intervention for persons with high-level tetraplegia (C1–4) are to prevent and control development of paralytic deformities, protect insensate areas from injury, prevent and/or reduce edema, maintain a supple hand for human contact, and protect the limb from irreversible changes and preserve it for future treatment paradigms.

During waking hours, a long opponens wrist–hand orthosis should be used to support the proximal and distal transverse arch and the longitudinal arch. The wrist should be positioned in 30 degrees of extension and the thumb placed in full abduction (carpometacarpal joint) and extension (metacarpophalangeal joint). Night-time splinting supports the arches and holds the thumb in full abduction–extension but places the hand in an intrinsic plus posture.

Automatic, mechanical, and powered feeders should be prescribed for persons with high tetraplegia. Although daily use of feeders is unlikely due to prolonged time requirements, spillage, and poor ease of use, they provide some persons with C4 SCI the ability to eat (after setup), free of a personal care provider. Likewise, the MAS may provide some function to those with C4 tetraplegia (Fig. 15-8).

Although no neuroprostheses for high tetraplegia are available on the market, in the future FES will play an important role in the rehabilitation of persons with high tetraplegia. Preliminary reports have been promising,[10,14] and continued effort is underway to develop techniques to restore stimulatable arm and hand function for the patients most in need.

Midcervical SCI (ASIA C5–6; ICSHT Motor Groups 0–4)

Persons with midcervical injuries can be separated into two distinct functional groups: those with gravity-eliminated wrist extension strength and those with against-gravity wrist extension strength. Persons with C5 tetraplegia typically have adequate or good elbow flexion but poor or no wrist extension. Prescription of a neuroprosthesis for stimulatable pinch, grasp, and release provides optimal function as evidenced by the outcomes studies on the NeuroControl Freehand System[87,104,118] and the NESS H200.[2] Market availability of the next-generation implantable neuroprosthesis is anticipated after completion of clinical trials. Until then, the NESS H200 is commercially available from Bioness Inc.

The flexor hinge orthosis (Fig. 15-9) is the functional orthosis of choice for patients with C6 tetraplegia and remains within standard of care and despite findings of underuse after discharge.[3,62,78,114,142,143] It should be offered to the patient as an option for independent performance of activities even if a neuroprosthesis or tendon transfer has been provided.

Custom-made splints are needed for the youngest age group with tetraplegia because these devices are not commercially available for pediatric hands. Light material and frequent modifications are needed to accommodate constant growth, but with adequate design even children younger than 1 year can perform developmental ADL.

Without exception, low-technology, simple devices remain the most important equipment prescribed to persons with midcervical tetraplegia.[36] Independence in donning, light weight, low profile, and pleasing appearance are essential considerations in the provision of assistive devices. The universal cuff, with or without provision for wrist stabilization, is the single most important assistive device for patients with tetraplegia. It offers versatility and accommodates all types of objects, such as a toothbrush, pen, utensil, or razor (Fig. 15-10). Other equipment, such as writing splints, cup holder, and button hook, is essential in pursuit of independence. Readers are encouraged to review the practice guidelines for a complete list of recommendations for equipment.[22]

Low-level SCI

The goal of orthotic intervention for low cervical SCI is maintenance of the natural architecture of the hand and prevention of deformities due to muscle imbalance between the extrinsic and intrinsic hand muscles. Functional splinting may assist in promoting hand opening by preventing an intrinsic minus posture and wrist flexion (Fig. 15-11). For patients without grasping abilities, the universal cuff is most beneficial.

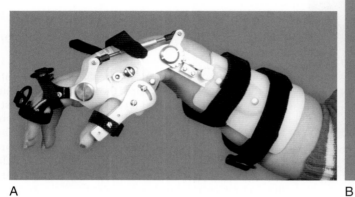

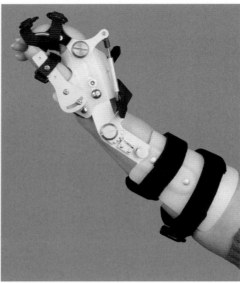

A   B

Fig. 15-9 Wrist-driven flexor hinge splint. Note how the orthosis augments the natural tenodesis by facilitating hand opening **(A)** and aligning the fingers and thumb for grasp and pinch **(B)**.

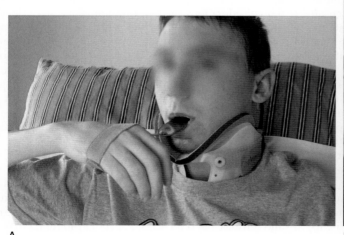

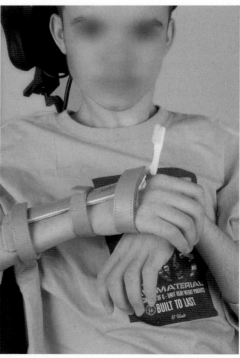

A   B

Fig. 15-10 Universal cuff. **A,** Most versatile splint for people with C6 tetraplegia. **B,** Dorsal-based wrist stabilizer is available for patients with C5 tetraplegia.

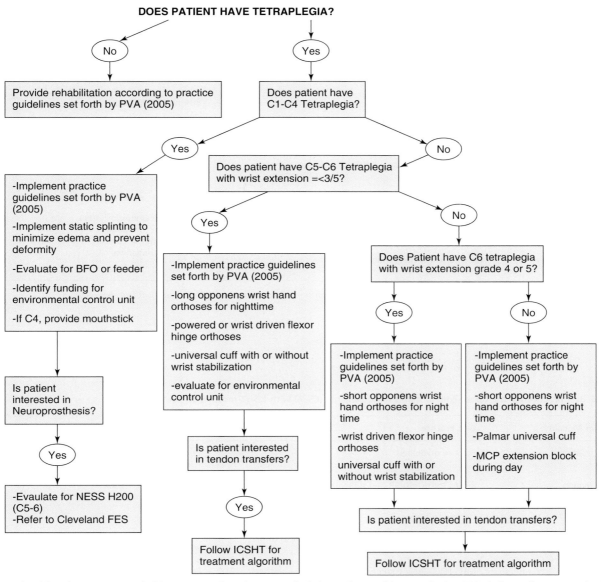

DOES PATIENT HAVE TETRAPLEGIA?

Fig. 15-11 Algorithm for treatment decisions concerning the upper limb in patients with tetraplegia. *BFO,* balance forearm orthosis; *MCP,* metacarpophalangeal.

Best practice

Although the concepts of "independence" and "function" remain central to rehabilitation of persons with tetraplegia, spontaneity, ease of activity, cosmesis, and temporal requirements of activity have emerged as core concepts. Twenty-first–century rehabilitation requires respect not only for independence but also for the quality of activity performance and social and cultural dimension of activity performance. Therefore, interventions for the upper limb of persons with tetraplegia must be cosmetically pleasing and enable ease of activity and spontaneity throughout the day. Because of advancements in regeneration and restorative SCI research, the concept of anticipatory rehabilitation must be understood. It is a term used to describe an approach to

rehabilitation that anticipates new interventions, thereby being proactive in protecting the limb from secondary paralytic deformities and avoiding irreversible treatments that may interfere with future interventions. Also, because persons with SCI are living longer, strategies to minimize overuse and pain are essential, and preventative measures, as outlined in the clinical guidelines,[20] should be administered.

Keeping these basic elements of "best practice" in mind, Tables 15-2 through 15-4 summarize best-practice recommendations for upper limb management of persons with high- and mid-level tetraplegia. Importantly, provision of one intervention (e.g., wrist-driven flexor hinge orthosis) does not necessarily preclude provision of another treatment (e.g., tendon transfers). Moreover, a combination of two or

Table 15-2 Best practice for the upper limb in high-level (C1–4) tetraplegia[a]

Treatment Modality	Best Practice	Best Evidence
General treatment	Clinical practice guidelines	Consortium for Spinal Cord Medicine Clinical Practice Guidelines[20,21] Bushnick[18] 2005
Neuroprostheses	Research-grade devices in select research centers	Betz et al.[10] 1992 Bryden et al.[14] 2005
Orthoses	Long opponens wrist–hand orthosis during nighttime and daytime	Hentz and LeClercq[45] 2002
	Mobile arm support (C4)	Landsberger et al.[69] 2005
Assistive devices	Environmental control	Garber and Gregorio[36] 1990 Consortium for Spinal Cord Medicine Clinical Practice Guidelines[21]
	Mouthstick	
	Automatic and mechanical feeders	

[a]*Tendon transfers are not a treatment option for this group because no volitional muscles are available for surgical transfer.*

Table 15-3 Best practice for the upper limb in mid-level tetraplegia (C5–6) with ICSHT motor classification 0–2

Treatment Modality	Best Practice	Best Evidence
General treatment	Practice guidelines	Consortium for Spinal Cord Medicine Clinical Practice Guidelines[20,21]
Surgical tendon transfers	Biceps to triceps (BR and supinator must be ≥ 4/5 strength) Deltoid to triceps BR to radial wrist extensor and FPL tenodesis **or** BR to FPL if wrist extension 3/5	Mulcahey et al.[91] 2004
Neuroprostheses	NESS-H200 (only commercially available neuroprosthesis for upper extremity)	Peckham et al.[104] 2001
Orthoses	Long opponens wrist–hand orthosis during nighttime Powered-driven (wrist extension strength ≤ 2) or wrist-driven (muscle strength 3/5) flexor hinge orthosis	Krajnik and Bridle[64] 1992
Assistive devices	Environmental control units Universal cuff via dorsal wrist splint Various adaptive equipment specific to activities of daily living (writing splint, etc.)	Consortium for Spinal Cord Medicine Clinical Practice Guidelines[21]
Hybrid intervention	Surgical transfer of BR to radial wrist extensors **and** wrist-driven (via tendon transfer) flexor hinge orthosis Surgical transfer of BR to radial wrist extensors **and** palmar-based universal cuff using wrist strength from tendon transfer	

BR, Brachioradialis; *FPL*, flexor pollicis longus.

Table 15-4 Best practice for the upper limb in mid-level tetraplegia (C6) with ICSHT motor classification 3–5

Treatment Modality	Best Practice	Best Evidence
General treatment	Practice guidelines	Consortium for Spinal Cord Medicine Clinical Practice Guidelines[20,21]
Surgical tendon transfers	Biceps to triceps	Mulcahey et al.[91] 2004
	Deltoid to triceps	
	Brachioradialis to FPL **and** one radial wrist extensor to FDP	
Orthoses	Wrist-driven flexor hinge orthosis during daytime	Krajnik and Bridle[64] 1992
	Short opponens splint during nighttime	
Assistive devices	Palmar universal cuff	Consortium for Spinal Cord Medicine Clinical Practice Guidelines[21]
	Various adaptive equipment specific to activities of daily living (writing splint, etc.)	

FDP, Flexor digitorum profundis; *FPL*, flexor pollicis longus.

more interventions (hybrid paradigms) are everyday practice and may result in superior outcomes. Figure 15-11 provides an algorithm to assist with clinical decision making related to management of the arm and hand of persons with tetraplegia.

References

1. Adkins LM: Cast changes: synthetic versus plaster, *Pediatr Nurs* 23:425–427, 1997.
2. Alon G, McBride K: Persons with C5 or C6 tetraplegia achieve selected functional gains using a neuroprosthesis, *Arch Phys Med Rehabil* 84:119–124, 2003.
3. Allen VR: Follow-up study of the wrist-drive flexor hinge splint use, *Am J Occup Ther* 25:398–401, 1971.
4. Anderson CJ, Vogel LC, Betz RR, Willis KM: Overview of adult outcomes in pediatric-onset spinal cord injuries: complications for transition to adulthood, *J Spinal Cord Med* 27:S98–S106, 2004.
5. Bacon G, Olszewski E: Sequential advancing flexion retention attachment: a locking device for the wrist driven flexor hinge splint, *Am J Occup Ther* 32:577–579, 1978.
6. Barber LM, Nickel VL: Carbon dioxide-powered arm and hand devices, *Am J Occup Ther* 20:217–220, 1966.
7. Bell-Krotoski JA: Plaster cylinder casting for contractures of the interphalangeal joints. In Hunter JM, Mackin EJ, Callahan AD, editors: *Rehabilitation of the hand*, ed 5, St. Louis, 2002, Mosby.
8. Bennett RL. The evolution of the Georgia Warm Springs Foundation Feeder, *Artif Limb* 10:5–9, 1966.
9. Betz RR, Mulcahey MJ: *The child with spinal cord injury*, Rosemont, Ill, 1996, American Academy of Orthopaedic Surgeons.
10. Betz RR, Mulcahey MJ, Smith BT, et al: Bipolar latissimus dorsi transposition and functional neuromuscular stimulation to restore elbow flexion in an individual with C4 quadriplegia and C5 denervation, *J Am Paraplegia Soc* 15:220–228, 1992.
11. Bisgrove J, Shrosbree R, Krey A: A new functional dynamic wrist extension-finger flexion hand splint-preliminary report, *J Assoc Phys Med Rehabil* 8:162–163, 1954.
12. Bonutti PM, Windau JE, Ables BA, Miller BG: Static progressive stretch to reestablish elbow range of motion, *Clin Orthop Relat Res* 303:128–134, 1994.
13. Brand PW, Hollister A: *Clinical mechanics of the hand*, ed 2, St. Louis, 1993, Mosby.
14. Bryden A, Kilgore K, Kirsch RF, Memberg WD, Peckham HP, Keith MW: An implanted neuroprosthesis for high tetraplegia, *Topics Spinal Cord Rehabil* 10:38–52, 2005.
15. Bryden A, Sinnott KA. Mulcahey MJ: Innovative strategies for improving upper extremity function in tetraplegia and considerations in measuring functional outcomes, *Topics Spinal Cord Injury Rehabil* 10:75–93, 2005.
16. Bunge RP, Puckett WR, Beccerra JL, et al: Observations on the pathology of human spinal cord injury. A review and classification of 22 new cases with details from a case of chronic cord compression with extensive focal demyelination, *Adv Neurol* 59:75–89, 1993.
17. Bunnell S: Tendon transfer in the hand and forearm. In: *American Academy of Orthopedic Surgery Instructional Course Lectures*, St. Louis, 1949, CV Mosby.
18. Buscnick T, issue editor: High tetraplegia: current practices and outcomes, *Topics Spinal Cord Rehabil* 10, 2005.
19. Cardenas DD, Hoffman JM, Kirshblum S, McKinley W: Etiology and incidence of rehospitalization after traumatic spinal cord injury: a multicenter analysis, *Arch Phys Med Rehabil* 85:1757–1763, 2004.
20. Consortium for Spinal Cord Medicine: Preservation of upper limb function following spinal cord injury: a clinical practice guideline for health care professionals, *J Spinal Cord Med* 5:433–470, 2005.
21. Consortium for Spinal Cord Medicine: Outcomes following traumatic SCI: clinical practice guidelines for health care professionals, *J Spinal Cord Med* 1999, Paralyzed Veterans of America.
22. Coulet B, Allieu Y, Chammes M: Injured metamere and functional surgery of the tetraplegic upper limb, *Hand Clin* 18:399–412, 2002.
23. Creasy GH, Kilgore KL, Brown-Triolo D, et al: Reduction of costs of disability using neuroprostheses, *Asst Technol* 12:67–75, 2000.
24. Davis SE, Mulcahey MJ, Betz RR: Freehand their hand: the role of occupational therapy in implementing FES in tetraplegia, *Technol Disabil* 11:29–34, 1999.
25. Davis SE, Mulcahey MJ, Smith BT, Betz RR: Outcome of functional electrical stimulation in the rehabilitation of a child with C5 tetraplegia, *J Spinal Cord Med* 22:107–113, 1999.
26. DeVivo MJ: Discharge disposition from model spinal cord injury care system rehabilitation programs, *Arch Phys Med Rehabil* 80:785–790, 1999.
27. Dijkers M, Abela MB, Gans BM, Gordon WA: The aftermath of spinal cord injury. In Stover S, DeLisa JA, Whiteneck G, editors: *Spinal cord injury. Clinical outcomes from the model systems*, Gaithersburg, Md, 1995, Aspen Publications.
28. DiPasquale-Lehnertz P: Orthotic intervention for development of hand function in C6 quadriplegia, *Am J Occup Ther* 48:138–144, 1994.
29. Engen TJ: Development of an externally powered upper extremity orthotic systems, *J Bone Joint Surg Br* 47:465–468, 1965.
30. Flowers KR, LaStayo P: Effect of total end range time on improving passive range of motion, *J Hand Ther* 7:150–157, 1994.
31. Freehafer AA: Tendon transfers in patients with cervical spinal cord injury, *J Hand Surg* 16A:804–809, 1991.

32. Freehafer AA, Kelly CM, Peckham PH: Tendon transfer for restoration of upper limb function after cervical spinal cord injury, *J Hand Surg* 9A:887–893, 1984.

33. Freehafer AA, Mast W: Transfer of the brachioradialis to improve wrist extension in high spinal cord injury, *J Bone Joint Surg* 49A:648, 1967.

34. Freehafer AA, Peckham PH, Keith MW: New concepts on treatment of the upper limb in the tetraplegic: surgical restoration and functional neuromuscular stimulation, *Hand Clin* 4:563–574, 1988.

35. Freehafer AA, Vonhaam A: Tendon transfer to improve grasp after injuries of the cervical spinal cord, *J Bone Joint Surg* 56A:951–959, 1974.

36. Garber SL, Gregorio TL: Upper extremity assistive devices: Assessment of use by spinal cord patients with quadriplegia, *Am J Occup Ther* 44:126–131, 1990.

37. Go BK, DeVivo MJ, Richards S: The epidemiology of spinal cord injury. In Stover S, DeLisa J, Whiteneck G, editors: *Spinal cord injury. Clinical outcomes from the model systems*, Gaithersburg, Md, 1995, Aspen Publications.

38. Gellman H, Kan D, Waters R, Nicosa A: Rerouting of the biceps brachii for paralytic supination contracture of the forearm in tetraplegia due to trauma, *J Bone Joint Surg* 76A:398–402, 1994.

39. Hadley MN, Zabramski JM, Browner CM, Rekate H, Sonntag VKH: Pediatric spinal trauma. Review of 122 cases of spinal cord and vertebral column injuries, *J Neurosurg* 68:18–24, 1988.

40. Hamilton BB, Ganger CV, Sherwin FS, Zielezny M, Tashman JS: A uniform national data system for medical rehabilitation. In Fuhrer MJ, editor: *Rehabilitation outcomes: analysis and measurement*. Baltimore, Md, 1987, Paul Brookes Publishing.

41. Hamilton MG, Myles ST: Pediatric spinal injury: review of 174 hospital admissions, *J Neurosurg* 77:700–704, 1992.

42. Harwin W, Strong S, Ramanathan R, et al: Design and preliminary evaluation of functional upper extremity orthoses, *Proceedings RESNA Conference 1999*, June 25–29, 633–663.

43. Hentz VR, Braun M, Keoshian LA: Upper limb reconstruction in quadriplegia: functional assessment and proposed treatment modifications, *J Hand Surg* 8A:119–131, 1983.

44. Hentz VR, House J, McDowell CL, Moberg EA: Rehabilitation and surgical reconstruction of the upper limb in tetraplegia: an update, *J Hand Surg* 17A:946–967, 1992.

45. Hentz VR, Leclercq C: *Surgical rehabilitation of the upper limb in tetraplegia*, Philadelphia, 2002, WB Saunders.

46. House JG, Gwathmey FW, Lundsgaard DK: Restoration of strong grasp and lateral pinch in tetraplegia due to cervical spinal cord injury, *J Hand Surg* 1A:152–159, 1976.

47. House JH, Shannon MA: Restoration of strong grasp and lateral pinch in tetraplegia: a comparison of two methods of thumb control in each patient, *J Hand Surg* 10A:22–29, 1985.

48. Hoy DJ, Guilford AW: The functional rachet orthotic system, *Orthot Prosthet* 32:21–24, 1978.

49. Irwin CE: Appliances for poliomyelitis patients. In Edwards JW, editor: *Orthopaedic appliances atlas*, Ann Arbor, Mich, 1952, American Academy of Orthopaedic Surgeons.

50. Jaffe K, editor: Special issue. Spinal cord injury. Current research outcomes from the model systems. *Arch Phys Med Rehabil* 85, 2004.

51. James M: Surgical treatment of the upper extremity: indications, patient assessment and procedures. In Betz RR, Mulcahey MJ, editors: *The child with spinal cord injury*, Rosemont, Ill, 1996, American Academy of Orthopaedic Surgeons.

52. Johansen ME, Murray WM: The unoperated hand: the role of passive forces in hand function after tetraplegia, *Hand Clin* 18:391–398, 2002.

53. Johnson MW, Peckham PH: Evaluation of shoulder movement as command control source, *IEEE Trans Biomed Eng* 37:876–885, 1990.

54. Jones RF, James R: A simple functional hand splint for C5-C6 quadriplegia, *Med J Aust* 1:998–1000, 1970.

55. Kakulas BA: The applied neuropathology of human spinal cord injury, *Spinal Cord* 37:79–88, 1999.

56. Kay HW: Clinical evaluation of the Engen plastic hand orthosis, *Artif Limbs* 13:13–26, 1969.

57. Keith MW, Hoyden H: Indications and future direction for the upper limb neuroprostheses in tetraplegic patients: a review, *Hand Clin* 18:519–528, 2002.

58. Keith MW, Peckham PH, Thrope GB, et al: Implantable functional neuromuscular stimulation in the tetraplegic hand, *J Hand Surg* 14A:524–530, 1989.

59. Kewalramani LS, Kraus JF, Sterling HM: Acute spinal-cord lesions in a pediatric population: epidemiological and clinical features, *Paraplegia* 18:206–219, 1980.

60. Kilgore KL, Peckham HP, Keith MW, et al: An implanted neuroprosthesis: a five patient review, *J Bone Joint Surg Am* 79:533–541, 1997.

61. Kirshblum S, Campagnolo DI, DeLias JA: *Spinal cord medicine*, Philadelphia, 2002, Lippincott Williams & Wilkins.

62. Knox CC, Engel WH, Siebens AA: Results of a survey on the use of a wrist-driven splint for prehension, *Am J Occup Ther* 25:109–111, 1971.

63. Kozin SH: Tetraplegia, *J Am Soc Surg Hand* 2:141–152, 2002.

64. Krajnik S, Bridle M: Hand splinting in quadriplegia: current practice, *Am J Occup Ther* 46:149–156, 1992.

65. Kwon BK, Tetzlaff W, Grauer JN, et al: Pathophysiology and pharmacologic treatment of acute spinal cord injury, *Spine J* 4:451–464, 2004.

66. Lamb DW, Chan KM: Surgical reconstruction of the upper limb in traumatic tetraplegia. A review of 41 patients, *J Bone Joint Surg* 65B:291–298, 1983.

67. Lamb DW, Landry R. The hand in quadriplegia, *Hand* 3:31–37, 1971.

68. Landi A, Mulcahey MJ, Caserta G, Della Rosa N: Tetraplegia: update on assessment, *Hand Clin* 18:377–389, 2002.

69. Landsberger S, Leung P, Vargas V, et al: Mobile arm supports: history, application and work in progress, *Topics Spinal Cord Injury Rehabil* 11:74–94, 2005.

70. Lathem PA, Gregorio TL, Garber SL: High level quadriplegia: an occupational therapy challenge, *Am J Occup Ther* 39:705–714, 1985.

71. Leahy P: Precasting work sheet: an assessment tool. A clinical report, *Phys Ther* 68:72–74, 1988.

72. Law M, Baptiste S, McColl M, Opzoomer A, Polatajko H, Pollock N: The Canadian occupational performance measure: an outcome measure for occupational therapy, *Can J Occup Ther* 57:82–87, 1990.

73. LeClercq C, editor: The tetraplegic upper limb, *Hand Clin* 18, 2002.

74. Lee AC: Survey of rancho flexor hinge splint users, *Br J Occup Ther* 51:197–198, 1988.

75. Malick MH, Meyer CM. *Manual on management of the quadriplegic upper extremity*, Pittsburgh, Penn, 1978, Harmerville Rehabilitation Center.

76. Marino RJ: Upper extremity capabilities in SCI, *Arch Phys Med Rehabil* 79:1512–1521, 1998.

77. Marino RJ, Shea JA, Stineman MG: The capabilities of upper extremity instrument: reliability and validity of a measure of functional limitation in tetraplegia, *Arch Phys Med Rehabil* 79:1512–1521, 1998.

78. Martin C: Functional hand orthosis for quadriplegia: long term use, *American Spinal Injury Association Abstract Digest* 372, 1987.

79. McClure PW, Blackburn LG, Dusold C: The use of splints in the treatment of joint stiffness: biologic rationale and algorithm for making clinical decisions, *Phys Ther* 74:1101–1107, 1994.

80. McCluer S., Conry JE: Modifications of the wrist driven flexor hinge splint, *Arch Phys Med Rehabil* 52:233–235, 1971.

81. McDowell CL, Moberg EA, Graham S: International conference on surgical rehabilitation of the upper limb in tetraplegia, *J Hand Surg* 4:387–390, 1979.

82. McDowell CL, Moberg EA, House JA: The second international conference or surgical rehabilitation at the upper limb in tetraplegia, *J Hand Surg* 11A:604–608, 1986.

83. Mulcahey MJ: Rehabilitation and outcomes of upper extremity tendon transfer surgery. In Betz RR, Mulcahey MJ, editors: *The child with spinal cord injury*. Rosemont Ill, 1996, American Academy Orthopedic Surgeons.

84. Mulcahey MJ: Upper extremity orthoses and splints. In Betz RR, Mulcahey MJ, editors: *The child with spinal cord injury*, Rosemont Ill, 1996, American Academy Orthopedic Surgeons.

85. Mulcahey MJ, Betz RR: Upper and lower extremity applications of functional electrical stimulation: a decade of research with children and adolescents with spinal injuries, *Pediatr Phys Ther* 9:113–122, 1997.

86. Mulcahey MJ, Betz RR, Kozin SH, et al: Implantation of the Freehand System during initial rehabilitation using minimally invasive techniques, *Spinal Cord* 42:146–155, 2004.

87. Mulcahey MJ, Betz RR, Smith BT, et al: Implanted functional electrical stimulation hand system in adolescents with spinal injuries: an evaluation, *Arch Phys Med Rehabil* 78:597–607, 1997.

88. Mulcahey MJ, Betz RR, Smith BT, Weiss AA: A prospective study of the outcomes of tendon transfers with children with tetraplegia, *J Pediatr Orthop* 19:319–328, 1999.

89. Mulcahey MJ, Hutchinson D, Kozin S: Assessment of the upper limb in tetraplegia: considerations in evaluation and outcomes research, *J Rehabil Res Dev* (In press).

90. Mulcahey MJ, Smith BT, Betz RR: Evaluation of the lower motor neuron integrity of upper extremity muscles in high level spinal cord injury, *Spinal Cord* 37:585–591, 1999.

91. Mulcahey MJ, Lutz C, Kozin S, Betz RR: Prospective evaluation of biceps to triceps and deltoid to triceps for elbow extension in tetraplegia, *J Hand Surg* 28A:964–971, 2003.

92. Mulcahey MJ, Smith BT, Betz RR: Psychometric rigor of the grasp and release test for measuring functional limitation of persons with tetraplegia: a preliminary analysis, *J Spinal Cord Med* 27:41–46, 2004.

93. Mulcahey MJ, Smith BT, Betz RR, Triolo RJ, Peckham PH: Functional neuromuscular stimulation: Outcomes in young people with tetraplegia, *J Am Paraplegia Soc* 17:20–35, 1994.

94. Moberg E: Surgical rehabilitation of the upper limb in tetraplegia, *Paraplegia* 28:462–469, 1990.

95. Moberg EA, Lamb DW: Surgical rehabilitation of the upper limb in tetraplegia, *Hand* 12:209–213, 1980.

96. Mohammand K, Rothwell A, Sinclair S, et al: Upper limb surgery for tetraplegia, *J Bone Joint Surg* 74B:873–879, 1992.

97. Newsom MJ, Keenan G, Maddry, Aguilar S: An occupational therapy training program for the C5-C6 quadriplegic, *Am J Occup Ther* 22:126–129, 1969.

98. Nickel V, Perry J: The flexor hinged hand, *J Bone Joint Surg* 40A:971, 1958.

99. Nickel V, Perry J, Garrett A: Development of useful function in the severely paralyzed hand, *J Bone Joint Surg* 45A:933–952, 1963.

100. Nobunaga AI, Go BK, Karunas RB: Recent demographic and injury trends in people served by the model spinal cord injury care systems, *Arch Phys Med Rehabil* 80:1372–1382, 1999.

101. Peckham PH, Gorman P: Functional electrical stimulation in the 21st century, *Topics Spinal Cord Rehabil* 10:126–150, 2004.

102. Peckham PH, Keith MW: Motor prostheses for restoration of upper extremity function. In Stein RB, Peckham PH, Popovic DB, editors: *Neural prostheses: replacing motor function after disease and disability*, New York, 1992, Oxford University Press.

103. Peckham PH, Keith MW, Kilgore KL: Restoration of upper extremity function in tetraplegia, *Topics Spinal Cord Injury Rehabil* 5:33–43, 1999.

104. Peckham PH, Keith MW, Kilgore KL, et al: Efficacy of an implanted neuroprosthesis for restoring hand grasp in tetraplegia: a multicenter study, *Arch Phys Med Rehabil* 82:1380–1388, 2001.

105. Peckham PH, Kilgore K, Keith MW, et al: An advanced neuroprosthesis system for restoration of hand and upper arm control employing an implantable controller, *J Hand Surg* 27A:265–276, 2002.

106. Peckham PH, Marsolais EB, Mortimer JT: Restoration of key grip and release in C6 tetraplegic through functional electrical stimulation, *J Hand Surg* 5:462–469, 1980.

107. Peckham PH, Mortimer JT, Marsolais EB: Controlled prehension and release in the C5 quadriplegic elicited by functional electrical stimulation of the paralyzed forearm musculature, *Ann Biomed Eng* 8:369–388, 1980.

108. Peckham PH, Mortimer JT, Marsolais EB: Upper and lower motor neuron lesions in the upper extremity muscles of tetraplegics, *Paraplegia* 14:115–121, 1976.

109. Prochazka A, Gauthier M, Wieler M, Kenwell Z: The bionic glove: an electrical stimulator garment that provides controlled grasp and hand opening in quadriplegia, *Arch Phys Med Rehabil* 78:608–614, 1997.

110. Rahman T, Alexander M, Scavina M: Powered orthosis for children with muscular dystrophy, Available at: http://www.nemours.org/internet?url=no/rsch/proj2713.html, Last accessed November 28, 2005.

111. Rahman T, Nam J, Sample W, Seliktar R: Development of WREX: A power-assisted arm orthosis, *Proceedings from the 2005 ACPOC Association Meeting*, Orlando, Florida, May 2005, 119–121.

112. Ruge JR, Sinson GP, McLone DG, Cerullo LJ: Pediatric spinal injury: the very young, *J Neurosurg* 68:25–30, 1988.

113. Sargent C, Braun MA: Occupational therapy management of the acute spinal cord injured patient, *Am J Occup Ther* 40:333–337, 1986.

114. Shepherd CC, Ruzicka SH: Tenodesis brace use by persons with spinal cord injuries, *Am J Occup Ther* 45:81–83, 1990.

115. Siebens A, Engel W, Peyrot A, et al: An assistive device for forearm lift, *Arch Phys Med Rehabil* 52:567–571, 1971.

116. Smith B, Buckett JR, Peckham HP, Keith MW, Roscoe DD: An externally powered, multichannel, implantable stimulator for versatile control of paralyzed muscle, *IEEE Trans Biomed Eng* 34:499–508, 1987.

117. Smith BT, Mulcahey MJ, Betz RR: Quantitative comparison of grasp and release abilities with and without functional neuromuscular stimulation in adolescents with tetraplegia, *Paraplegia* 34:16–23, 1996.

118. Smith BT, Mulcahey MJ, Triolo RJ, Betz RR: The application of a modified neuroprosthetic hand system in a child with C7 spinal cord injury. Case report, *Paraplegia* 30:598–606, 1992.

119. Smithson HH: Adaptation to ball bearing feeder, *Am J Occup Ther* 21:170, 1967.

120. Snoek GJ, Ijzerman MJ, Groen T, et al: Use of the NESS handmaster to restore hand function in tetraplegia: clinical experiences in ten patients, *Spinal Cord* 38:244–249, 2000.

121. Soderstrom G, Ducker T: Increased susceptibility of patients with cervical cord lesions to peptic gastrointestinal complications, *J Trauma* 25:1030–1038, 1990.

122. Staas WE, Formal CS, Freedman MK, Fried GW, Schmidt Read M: Spinal cord injury and spinal cord injury medicine. In Gans BM, editor: *Rehabilitation medicine*, ed 3, Philadelphia, 1998, Lippincott-Raven.

123. Street D, Stambaugh H: Finger flexor tenodesis, *Clin Orthop* 13:155–163, 1959.

124. Stroh-Wuolle K, Bryden A, Peckham HP, et al: Satisfaction with upper extremity surgery in individuals with tetraplegia, *Arch Phys Med Rehabil* 84:1145–1149, 2003.

125. Stroh-Wuolle K, Thrope G, Keith M, et al: Development of a quantitative hand grasp and release test for patients with tetraplegia using a hand neuroprosthesis, *J Hand Surg* 19A:209–218, 1994.

126. Stroh-Wuolle K, Van Doren C, Bryden A, et al: Satisfaction with and usage of a hand neuroprosthesis, *Arch Phys Med Rehabil* 80:206–213, 1999.

127. Stover S, DeLisa J, Whiteneck G: *Spinal cord injury: clinical outcomes from the model systems*, Gaithersburg, Md, 1995, Aspen Publications.

128. Sutton S: An overview of the management of the C6 quadriplegic patient's hand: an occupational therapy perspective, *Br J Occup Ther* 56:376–380, 1993.

129. Thenn JE, editor: *Mobile arm support: installation and use. A guide for occupational therapists*, Brookfield, Ill, 1975, Fred Sammons.

130. Trombly CA: Principles of operant conditioning: related to orthotic training in of quadriplegic patients, *Am J Occup Ther* 20:217–220, 1966.

131. Tynan M: Joint contractures in children with spinal cord injuries. In Betz RR, Mulcahey MJ, editors: *The child with a spinal cord injury*, Rosemont, Ill, 1996, American Academy of Orthopaedic Surgeons.

132. van Tuijl JH, Janssen-Potten YJM, Seelen HAM: Evaluation of upper extremity motor function tests in tetraplegics, *Spinal Cord* 40:51–64, 2002.

133. Vogel LC, DeVivo MJ: Etiology and demographics. In Betz RR, Mulcahey MJ, editors: *The child with a spinal cord injury*, Rosemont, Ill, 1996, American Academy of Orthopaedic Surgeons.

134. Vogel LC, DeVivo MJ: Pediatric spinal cord injury issues: etiology, demographics, and pathophysiology, *Topics Spinal Cord Injury Rehabil* 3:1–8, 1997.

135. Weiss AA. Tendon transfers in tetraplegia. In Betz R, Mulcahey MJ, editors: *The child with a spinal cord injury*, Rosemont, Ill, 1996, American Academy Orthopaedic Surgeons.

136. Whiteneck G, Charlifue S, Gerhart K, Overholser JD, Richardson G: Quantifying handicap: a new measure of long term rehabilitation outcomes, *Arch Phys Med Rehabil* 73:519–526, 1992.

137. Whiteneck G, Gerhart K, Cusick C: Identifying environmental factors that influence outcomes of people with traumatic brain injury, *J Head Trauma Rehabil* 19:191–204, 2004.

138. Whiteneck G, Meade MA, Dijkers M, Tate DG, Bushnik T, Forchheimer MB: Environmental factors and their role in participation and life satisfaction after spinal cord injury, *Arch Phys Med Rehabil* 85:1793–1803, 2004.

139. Wijman CA, Stroh KC, Van Doren CL, Thrope GB, Peckham PH, Keith MW: Functional evaluation of quadriplegic patients using a hand neuroprosthesis, *Arch Phys Med Rehabil* 71:1053–1057, 1990.

140. Wilson JN: Providing automatic grasp by flexor tenodesis, *J Bone Joint Surg* 38:1019, 1956.

141. Wilson DJ, McKenzie MW, Barber LM: *Spinal cord injury*, Thorofare, NJ, 1974, Charles B. Slack.

142. Wise M, Wharton G: Continues use of functional hand splints, *American Spinal Injury Association Abstract Digest* 45, 1980.

143. Wise M, Wharton G, Robinson T: Long term use of functional hand orthoses by quadriplegics. *American Spinal Injury Association Abstract Digest* 111–113, 1986.

144. Zander CL, Healy NL: Elbow flexion contractures treated with serial casts and conservative therapy, *J Hand Surg* 17:694–697, 1992.

Chapter

16

Orthoses for the burned hand

Bradon J. Wilhelmi, Mary C. Burns, and Damon Cooney

Key Points

- Typical deformities seen in the burned hand are hyperextension deformity of the metacarpophalangeal joints, flexion deformity of the interphalangeal (IP) joints, loss of transverse metacarpal arch, adduction contracture of the thumb, volar flexion contracture of the wrist, and shrinkage of the dorsal skin.

- A splint should position the hand in the position of antideformity, positioning the hand with the wrist in 15 to 30 degrees of extension, the metacarpophalangeal (MP) joints in 70 to 80 degrees of flexion, IP joints straight, and the thumb abducted. This position will place the MP collateral ligaments on maximal stretch, preserve the anatomical arches of the hand, and stretch the healing burn wounds, thus opposing the development of a "clawhand" deformity. Often this is called the "safe" or "intrinsic plus" position.

- Palmer hand burns will require an antideformity position of the palmer burn, consisting of wrist extension, MP joint extension, IP joint extension, digital abduction, and thumb abduction and extension: the "open palm" or "pancake" position. A palmar burn during the early initial inflammatory phase can be treated in a "safe position" splint to prevent fibrosis and shortening of the collateral ligaments.

- If the hand burn is circumferential and includes both dorsal and palmar surfaces, consideration should be given to alternating a safe position splint with the palmar stretch maximum extension splint during the course of each day.

- When patients are unable to participate in active motion regimens to the optimal degree or plateau with active motion protocols, dynamic splints can be considered once the wound has epithelialized.

Deep burns can result in more than just an unacceptable appearance but also profound functional consequences for the burned hand, such as loss of fingertips, mutilated nails, joint limitation, and painful scars. The patient must be well motivated in order to cope with and rehabilitate these problems. Restoration of function and appearance is the ultimate goal of treatment, and prevention of late deformities depends on successful early treatment.

Historical perspectives

With the increasing use of gunpowder in warfare, surgeons treating battlefield casualties encountered large numbers of patients suffering from burns to the extremities and hands.[5] Early pioneers in the treatment of these wounds, such as Ambrose Pare, William Clowes, Fabricius Hildanus, and Richard Wiseman, developed approaches to the treatment of burned hands.[5] This early work demonstrated the importance of the use of splints to prevent contractures. Contemporary approaches to splinting the burned hand have evolved from these concepts to emphasis on correct positioning of the hand and wrist and establishing the use of not only static but also dynamic splints to optimize early and late rehabilitation of these injuries.

Pathophysiology

The typical deformities seen in the burned hand are hyperextension deformity of the metacarpophalangeal joints, flexion deformity of the interphalangeal (IP) joints, loss of the transverse metacarpal arch, adduction contracture of the thumb, volar flexion contracture of the wrist, and shrinkage of the dorsal skin. The metacarpophalangeal joint assumes the hyperextended position because of with joint edema.

The metacarpophalangeal joint collateral ligaments are relaxed when this joint is extended because of the cam effect of the metacarpal head, which is longer in the dorsal–volar plane. This allows increased volume within the joint to accommodate edema. In contrast, edema in the IP joints results in a flexed posture and tightening of the volar plate. Persistent edema, infection, poor compliance with hand therapy, ineffective splinting, long immobilization, and loss of skin coverage all contribute to the development of the burned hand deformity. Success is best assessed by restoration of function, which often correlates with an improvement in appearance.

Current issues

Ideally, rehabilitation of the burned hand should be instituted immediately after the thermal injury.[7] A hand therapist should be involved in the care of the patient at presentation. The treatment plan is directly influenced by the depth of the burn and the requirement for surgery. Superficial burns do not require skin grafting and are treated with wound care and early active range of motion exercises. These patients usually do not develop contractures and do not require splints. Currently, deep partial thickness and full thickness burn wounds are treated with early excision and grafting. This goal of early excision of damaged tissue and skin grafting is to minimize the secondary problems of scar formation and contracture. Early excision is important for reducing the inflammatory phase, expediting wound coverage and healing to allow for earlier active motion rehabilitation.[7] At the time of excision and skin grafting, the patient is placed in a dorsal or volar splint made of plaster. The splint immobilizes the hand and wrist, to decrease shearing of the skin graft from the wound bed and increase graft survival. This requires immobilization for 5 days to optimize revascularization of the skin graft. This intraoperatively placed splint maintains the IP joints at 0 degrees of extension, the metacarpophalangeal joints in 70 degrees of flexion, the thumb in maximal abduction, and the wrist in neutral.

Treatment considerations and recommendations

Treatment of burns that involve the hand are complicated by the potential for exposure or injury to numerous important structures, including tendons, bones, and joints. Therefore, splinting and therapy protocols can be distinctly different for burns of the dorsal and palmar surfaces. The skin over the dorsum of the hand is thin, supple, and highly mobile, which allows for gliding of the underlying extensor tendons. When the dorsal surface is involved in burn injuries, significant functional disturbances may result. The close proximity of the underlying extensor tendons, especially on the dorsal surfaces of the fingers, makes these areas prone to tendon injuries and may result in deformities such as mallet fingers, boutonnière, and swan neck deformities. In performing excisions of dorsal burns, it is critical to preserve the extensor tendon apparatus, including the terminal extension, lateral bands, and central slip when possible. Palmar hand burns also result in significant deformities that can be very difficult to correct. Serious burns to the palmar surface of the hand

frequently cause devastating and sometimes uncorrectable flexion contractures. These burns can result in loss of the first web space, thus compromising use of the thumb. Fortunately, palmar burns frequently are only partial thickness and do not require excision and grafting owing to thickness of the glabellar skin. Sensory nerves of the hand are frequently injured both by the burn and possibly by required excision and debridement. Sensory involvement of both the dorsal and palmar surfaces poses an even more complex challenge. Circumferential third-degree burns and electrical burns of the hand can result in compartment syndrome and subsequent muscle loss. Loss of function and fibrosis of the intrinsic muscles are the most complex challenges to rehabilitation. It is critical to perform early escharotomies and compartment releases when indicated to prevent this muscle loss. Therefore, many factors must be considered as part of the evaluation of the acutely burned hand.

Edema is a major deterrent to successful outcome and should be addressed immediately following injury. Edema that is not controlled will be detrimental to the overall function of the hand because it compromises circulation and limits joint mobility. Protein-laden edema fluid accumulates in the joint capsules, collateral ligaments, and other soft tissues of the hand. Eventually this fluid becomes gelatinous and ultimately is replaced by dense fibrous tissue. The soft tissue structures of the hand thicken and shorten, resulting in a stiff hand and fixed contractures. If edema is controlled early, scar formation and stiffness can be lessened.

Generally, significant edema formation occurs within the first 48 to 72 hours after burn injury. Compression should not be used during this time because venous return may be impaired. Initially, emphasis should be placed on active range of motion (AROM) and elevation to control edema and keep the joints mobile. Elevation promotes venous return and prevents gravitational pooling of fluid in the dependent extremity. AROM provides a pumping action by means of active muscle contraction. This in turn assists with venous and lymphatic return to the central circulation. In patients with deep circumferential burns or burns accompanied by severe edema, overly aggressive range of motion should be avoided because it may aggravate swelling. These patients may benefit more from brief and frequent periods of AROM throughout the day. Active assisted range of motion (AAROM) may be initiated if necessary. Passive range of motion (PROM) is not recommended in the acute phase because forceful joint manipulations may disrupt the healing wounds. This in turn can cause additional inflammation and swelling, which will result in pain and loss of motion and increase scar formation and stiffness.

Wound healing is a complex process of collagen synthesis, with an end result of scar formation. If not managed properly, scar formation can result in deformities such as scar hypertrophy and soft tissue contractures. Wound contraction is a normal component of the healing process and is characterized by a shortening of collagen fibers. Unchecked, it may result in scar contractures. Hypertrophic scars are thick raised scars caused by deposition of disorganized layers of collagen fibers. Early application of pressure and sustained stretch to healing burn wounds may minimize the incidence of soft tissue contractures and scar hypertrophy, respectively.[2] Skin and soft tissue will adjust to the tension that is placed on it. Tissues can lose length (as in contracture) by losing cells, or they can increase in length by adding new cells. Remodeling occurs as a result of low-grade, gentle, sustained tension. By increasing tissue force over normal resting levels, cell proliferation is stimulated. Therefore, stretch over the scarred hand can initiate remodeling of collagen as well as increase the extensibility of collagen. Collagen fibers will tend to align along the lines of stress. Constant pressure on the healing wound will induce close approximation of collagen bundles by stimulating collagen cross-linking and reorganization of collagen into parallel fibers.[2] Remodeling of collagen fibers not only will inhibit scar contracture and hypertrophy but also will diminish vascular and lymphatic pooling and help reduce hypersensitivity of the skin.[2] Pressure therapy can be applied as early as 72 hours postinjury or after maximal edema has subsided. These early methods of pressure treatment may include compressive dressings or a figure-of-eight ace wrap over the burn dressing to provide light pressure. Fine mesh gauze can be draped between the web spaces of the digits to prevent scar syndactyly. Patients can be measured for custom-fit garments, such as Jobst garments, if they have no open areas larger than the size of a quarter. Temporary pressure garments may be used until custom garments are ready and a proper fit is assured. Temporary pressure may be provided with Isotoner gloves, elasticized stockings such as Tubigrip, coban ace wraps, and digital compression sleeves. Patients whose wounds heal within a 2-week period may not require customized pressure therapy because scarring may be minimal. Due to the expense of custom garments, theses patients can be managed with elastic stockinettes and Isotoner gloves. If development of heavy scarring later is determined, custom garments should be provided. Although a patient is fitted with a pressure glove, continuation of ROM exercises is necessary. Intermetacarpal glides and palmar stretches may help to counteract the transverse force of the glove and assist in maintaining the transverse palmar arch of the hand. Also, because the dorsum of the hand is convex and the palm is concave, the pressure will be greatest on the dorsum of the hand. The glove may bridge across the palm, providing little or no pressure to palmar scars. Custom insets on the palmar surface may be necessary to achieve even distribution of pressure. This can be accomplished with elastomer, Otoform, silicon gel sheeting, or foam inserts to the palm.

The burned hand must be carefully evaluated before motion exercises are initiated. Exposed tendons or deep dorsal burns over the fingers may result in tendon rupture and increased morbidity and deformity if not managed properly. If no tendons are exposed and the depth of the burn does not place underlying tendons at risk, AROM can be initiated immediately postinjury. In general, it is best to begin exercises with isolated joint motion and blocking to achieve differential tendon gliding. After each joint is exercised individually, composite joint motion or composite fist making can be instituted to provide stretching of all joint motion, or composite fist making can be instituted to provide stretching of all joint surfaces. Other necessary exercises include isolated extensor mechanism blocking to encourage IP extension (only if the central slip is intact), isolated MP joint motion, intrinsic stretches, web space stretches, thumb abduction and opposition, wrist flexion and extension, radial deviation, and ulnar deviation.[9] All are important components of a complete burned hand exercise regimen.

Ideally, the burn patient should be able to cooperate with an active assisted exercise program. The amount of exercise required frequently is greater than the amount of time the therapist can spend with the patient. For this reason, provision of clear instructions to the patient, the patients' family, and the nursing staff are of great importance. Such communication will allow the patient to perform an effective exercise program even when the therapist is unable to supervise. The patient should be instructed to exercise six to eight times daily. Exercising in warm water is beneficial and should be encouraged whenever possible. The warm water may help reduce pain and provide a soothing relaxing effect that may increase patient cooperation. The buoyancy may increase the ease of exercise. Exercising in water also allows the therapist to observe and monitor the wound. If the patient is unable to actively participate in an exercise program, then passive range of motion (PROM) exercises may be required. Such an approach may be dictated by patient disorientation or unconsciousness, or it may be used because of patient fear. In certain cases, use of a continuous passive motion device may be beneficial. PROM may be necessary as wound healing progresses and the antagonistic scar forces begin to exceed the patient's active abilities.

Orthotic management

Although splinting plays an integral part in early burn treatment, it should be used when the patient cannot exercise in a purposeful and supervised fashion or when correcting specific deformities but in a way that allows the patient motion of all other structures of the hand. When possible, the patient should be given directed tasks to perform with his or her burned hands, including self-care and activities of daily living. Proper positioning and splinting can help reduce edema and minimize contractures by providing a slow constant stretch, thus maintaining proper length of connective tissue and skin. The initial goal of splinting is preventing contracture rather than attempting to correct a contracture once it has occurred. Splinting may be necessary when the patient cannot voluntarily maintain adequate stretch of skin and soft tissue structures, such as when he or she is sedated. Splinting should be initiated at the first signs of decreased motion. This is often seen in the immediate post burn period but may present itself in later stages of wound healing. Splint position depends on the location of the burn and the amount of edema present. In general, a splint should position the hand in the position of antideformity. The most common deformity following a dorsal burn injury of the hand is the "clawhand" deformity, which positions the hand with the wrist in 15 to 30 degrees of extension, MP joints in 70 to 80 degrees of flexion, IP joints straight, and thumb abducted (Figs. 16-1 and 16-2). This position places the MP collateral ligaments on maximal stretch, preserves the anatomical arches of the hand, and stretches the healing burn wounds, thus opposing the development of a "clawhand" deformity. This often is called the "safe" or "intrinsic plus" position.

Palmer hand burns require a thorough evaluation to determine the type of splinting required. In general, the palmar skin will require maximum stretching to prevent the contracting forces of the healing burn. The antideformity position of the palmar burn consists of wrist extension, MP joint extension, IP joint extension, digital abduction, and thumb abduction and extension: the "open palm" or "pancake"

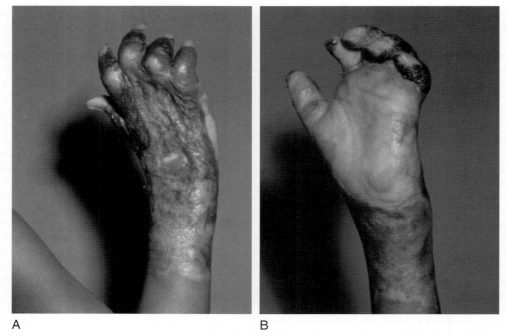

A   B

Fig. 16-1 The most common deformity after a dorsal burn injury of the hand is the "clawhand" deformity, which positions the hand with the wrist in 15 to 30 degrees of extension, the MP joints in 70 to 80 degrees of flexion, IP joints straight, and the thumb abducted.

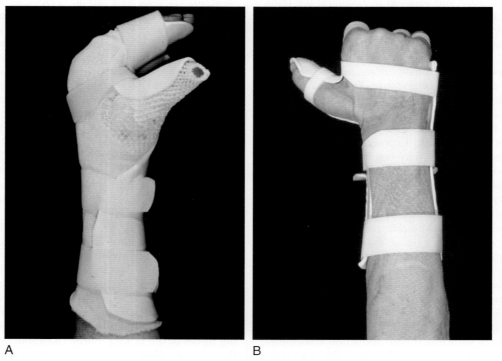

A   B

Fig. 16-2 This position places the MP collateral ligaments on maximal stretch, preserves the anatomical arches of the hand, and stretches the healing burn wounds, thus opposing the development of "clawhand" deformity. This often is called the "safe" or "intrinsic plus" position.

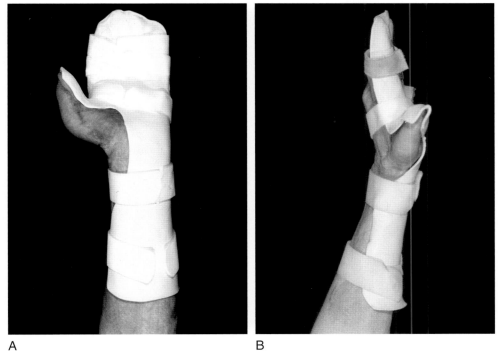

A   B

Fig. 16-3 Palmer hand burns require thorough evaluation to determine the type of splinting required. In general, the palmar skin will require maximum stretching to prevent the contracting forces of the healing burn. The antideformity position of the palmar burn consists of wrist extension, MP joint extension, IP joint extension, digital abduction, and thumb abduction and extension: the "open palm" or "pancake" position.

position (Fig. 16-3). With palmar burns, edema cannot be ignored. Both volar and dorsal edema may pull the hand into a "clawhand" position. Therefore, even with a palmar burn, during the initial inflammatory phase a "safe position" splint may prove to be beneficial in preventing fibrosis and shortening of the collateral ligaments. As edema subsides and wound healing and contraction begin, the palmar stretch, finger extension splint should be applied.

If the hand burn is circumferential and includes both dorsal and palmar surfaces, consideration should be given to alternating a safe position splint with the palmar stretch maximum extension splint during the course of each day.

The splint schedule depends on several factors and is individualized. The amount of edema formation is an important factor. Overuse of the hand may increase edema, but lack of motion may be equally injurious. The ability of the patient to maintain AROM and maintenance of proper positioning must be considered and brought into reasonable balance. Associated injuries, such as exposed tendons, peripheral neuropathies, and fractures, may require continuous immobilization. If the patient is unable to participate in an active exercise program, has significant pain, or demonstrates reluctance to move the injured hand, continuous splinting may be required between exercises. If the patient actively participates with exercises and daily living skills, then the splints may only be required at night. Initially, the patient may require adaptive equipment to perform daily tasks. This should be provided only when absolutely necessary and should be eliminated as soon as the patient is able to function reasonably well.

When patients are unable to participate in active motion regimens to the optimal degree or plateau with active motion protocols, dynamic splints can be considered once the wound has epithelialized. When patients are unable to actively close the fingers into the palm, a dynamic splint can be fashioned that utilizes rubber bands to passively encourage the digits to flex into the palm (Fig. 16-4). Alternatively, when patients are unable to optimally passively extend the digits, a dynamic outrigger can be used during periods throughout the day (Fig. 16-5).

When the patient has difficulty performing extension and flexion exercises, a dynamic splint can be fashioned that will assist with both passive flexion and extension (Fig. 16-6). When patients have suffered burns that involve the terminal extension of the extensor apparatus, a standard volar distal interphalangeal (DIP) splint indicated for treatment of mallet deformities can be used. The prefabricated Bunnell dynamic splint, which acts as a reverse knuckle bender, can be beneficial in patients who have lost the central slip and are developing a proximal interphalangeal (PIP) flexion contracture and boutonnière deformity. A dynamic splint can be fashioned to treat the wrist flexion deformity that can develop in burn patients (Fig. 16-7). Finally, a dynamic splint can be fabricated to help correct adduction contractures that occur in patients with web space burns (Fig. 16-8).

In the treatment of children with burn injuries, immediate splinting generally is required. Because most children will be unable to actively participate in a formal exercise program, continuous splint may be necessary. Children should wear

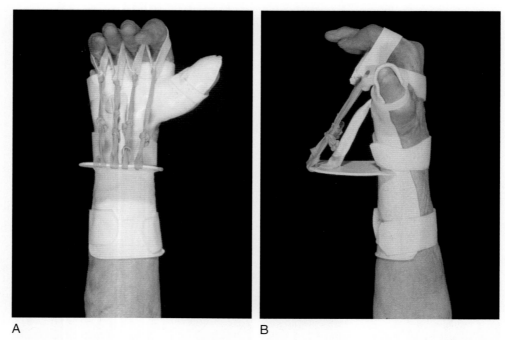

A   B

Fig. 16-4 When a patient is unable to actively close the fingers into the palm, a dynamic splint can be fashioned that utilizes rubber bands to passively encourage the digits to flex into the palm.

splints at night and during all naps. During normal play periods, the splints should be removed to permit active use of the hands, if possible.

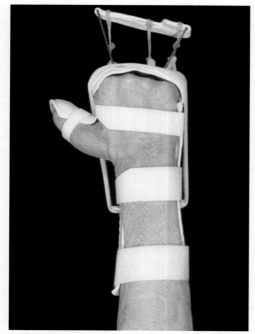

Fig. 16-5 When a patient is unable to optimally passively extend the digits, a dynamic outrigger can be used during periods throughout the day.

Best practice in the treatment of specific complications in the burned hand

Boutonnière deformity

Extensor tendons are frequently injured in burns of the hand because the dorsal skin of the hand is thin, and the tendons are more superficial.[3] Dorsal burns are more common than palmar burns. Therefore, it is important to consider potential extensor tendon involvement, especially over the PIP joint. Deep burns over the PIP joint can result in damage to the central slip.[4] Disruption of the central slip will result in volar subluxation of the lateral bands.[4] With the lateral bands volar to the axis of the PIP joint, they become flexors of the PIP join, pulling the DIP joint into hyperextension and causing a boutonnière deformity. If the burn is deep enough to threaten the central slip or cause exposure of the extensor tendons, then continual splinting is necessary. Exposed tendons will become dry, and imposition of stress upon these tendons likely will cause the tendons to rupture. The exposed tendons must be kept moist with wet-to-wet dressings, biologic dressings, or topical antibacterial ointment. The PIP joist should be continuously splinted in full extension for 6 to 8 weeks.[4] This will provide relaxation of the extensor tendons. If the central slip is damaged or ruptured, maintenance of finger extension will allow scar tissue to form across the damaged area, thereby restoring continuity of the extensor mechanism. Adjacent joints can be exercised cautiously, but the therapist must be aware of potential injury to the exposed or damaged structure. If the central slip is not totally destroyed, gently protected AROM may be possible. Composite flexion is generally not allowed. MP flexion may

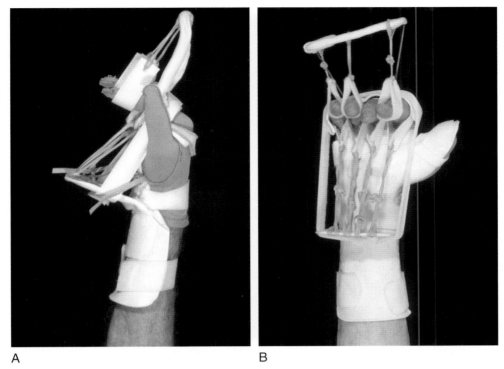

A   B

Fig. 16-6 When a patient has difficulty performing extension and flexion exercises, a dynamic splint can be fashioned that will assist with both passive flexion and extension.

be performed only with IP joints straight. Gentle PIP flexion, no greater than 30 degrees with MP joint and DIP joints extended, may be performed. Likewise, DIP flexion with the MP and PIP extended may be permitted.

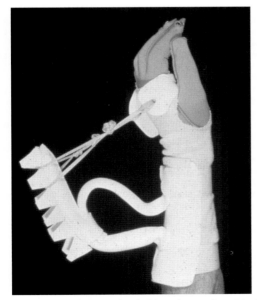

Fig. 16-7 A dynamic splint can be fashioned to assist with the wrist flexion deformity that can develop in burn patients.

Burn clawhand deformity

The burn clawhand deformity is a common occurrence after hand burns.[3] The burn clawhand deformity consists of MP joint hyperextension and PIP joint flexion. The fifth finger also may be involved, with a rotation of the distal phalanx and an abduction contracture caused by burns to the ulnar border of the hand. The most common cause of the clawhand is scar contracture of the dorsum of the hand involving the MP joints and pulling the MP joints into hyperextension. Hyperextension at the MP joint results in a relaxation of the extensor mechanism.[6] The flexor tendons then are unopposed, resulting in flexion of the IP joints. Volar burns over the IP joints of the digits also will pull the IP joints into flexion as the scar contracts. Other factors that may contribute to the clawhand deformity are damage to the extensor mechanism, skin shortening, and contraction of collateral ligaments. The clawhand deformity is preventable. Correct splinting and joint positioning and properly timed surgical interventions are essential elements in preventing this deformity.

Web space contractures

Burn scars of the web spaces produce narrowing of the web space, burn syndactyly, and decreased motion.[3] When the thumb web space is involved, prehension may be compromised and overall thumb mobility limited. In children, thumb web space contractures may restrict growth of the thumb.[1] Web space contractures can be difficult to correct.[1] Therefore, it is essential that they be treated early. For the thumb, a C-bar web spacer will be needed to prevent an

225

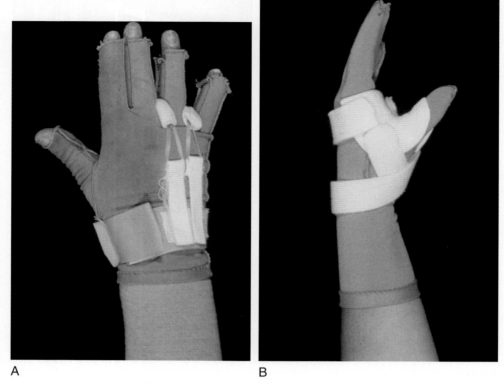

A   B

Fig. 16-8 A dynamic splint can be fabricated to help correct adduction contractures that occur in patients with web space burns.

adduction contracture.[1] During healing, this can be used continuously. Following healing, the C-bar web spacer can be used at night during the period of scar maturation. Pressure gloves are essential during scar maturation. However, it often is difficult to achieve good pressure to the web spaces with the gloves alone. Otoform web spacers can be fitted to the web spaces under the gloves to maintain constant pressure.[8] A dynamic digital web spacer can be devised for wear over the gloves to prevent scar syndactyly (Fig. 16-8).[8] In general, scar contractures are the primary cause of deformities in the burned hand. Failure to address them early will lead to permanent joint and ligament contractures. Treatment of these deformities are much more difficult than preventing them.

Conclusion

Rehabilitation of the burned hand is challenging, and successful rehabilitation begins shortly after the acute injury. Proper splinting and edema control are the mainstays of early rehabilitative efforts. Initiation of ROM exercises is based upon the severity of injury and an appreciation of the relative risks of tendon rupture and benefits derived by exercise. After the acute period, treatment consists of continued compliance

with therapy and use of compression garments to prevent contraction and hypertrophic scars. Prevention of deformity and maintenance or restoration of optimal hand function must be the principal goals of rehabilitative efforts.

References

1. Davlin LB, Aulicino PT: Post traumatic thumb index web space contractures: causes and treatment, *Atlas Hand Clin* 6:159–164, 2001.
2. Evans EB, Alvarado MI, Ott S, et al: Prevention and treatment of deformity in burned patients. In Herndon DN, editor: *Total burn care*, London, 1996, WB Saunders.
3. Hammond JS, War CG: Complications of the burn patient, *Crit Care Clin* 3:175, 1985.
4. Hobson L: Splinting for the proximal interphalangeal joint flexion contractures, *Atlas Hand Clin* 6:135–158, 2001.
5. Levine NS, Buchanan RT: The care of burned upper extremities, *Clin Plast Surg* 13:107–118, 1996.
6. Moscony A: Splinting for extension contractures of the digit, *Atlas Hand Clin* 6:117–134, 2001.
7. Nedelec B, Ghahary A, Scott PG, Tredget EE: Control of wound contraction: basic and clinical features, *Hand Clin* 16:289–302, 2000.
8. Schindeler-Grasse P, Paynter P: Splinting for the thumb contractures, *Atlas Hand Clin* 6:165–188, 2001.
9. Tilley W, McMahon S, Shukalak B: Rehabilitation of the burned upper extremity, *Hand Clin* 16:303–318, 2000.

Orthoses for the arthritic hand and wrist

Honor Duderstadt-Galloway, Monica R. Godinez, Alfred B. Swanson,
Troy D. Pierce, Judy Leonard, and Geneviève de Groot Swanson

Key Points

- Many health care professionals commonly see patients with some form of arthritis, especially rheumatoid arthritis (RA) and osteoarthritis (OA). RA and OA can be highly disabling conditions that can affect a person's life in many aspects (i.e., physically, psychologically, socially, economically, etc.). The severity of RA and OA can range from mild to severely disabling.

- Rheumatoid arthritis is a progressive, chronic, systemic disease marked by inflammatory changes of the joints, tendons, and their sheaths resulting in pain, weakness, and dysfunction. Inflammation caused by proliferative synovium results in erosions of articular cartilage, articular bone and soft tissue. This can cause rupture of tendons and the weakening of ligaments around the involved joints. In the hand, this eventually leads to muscle and tendon imbalance, ligamentous laxity, instability, and subluxation or complete dislocation of the joints.

- As explained by Yasuda, "[o]steoarthritis is a heterogeneous condition in which biomaterial properties of articular cartilage or bone are abnormal or there is excessive biomechanical loading, such as may occur after trauma to a joint or to normal cartilage or bone, or both."[46]

- Orthoses that are made for persons with arthritis are primarily used to reduce inflammation, reduce pain by helping to support and stabilize joints during function, protect joints from increased stress/demand, to prevent joint contractures, immobilize unstable joints, increase ROM, increase function, and "position joints for occupational performance"[11,46] (Yasuda; Deshaies).

The fabrication and application of an upper limb orthosis (splint or brace) for a person with arthritis requires a thorough knowledge of the disease process, knowledge of normal hand anatomy, and familiarity with the pathomechanics of the arthritic hand. Knowledge of the person's lifestyle, goals and expectations, attitudes, and preferences will help determine the most appropriate orthosis for the individual. Also necessary is an understanding of the person's living and working environments, social support, safety issues, ability to understand and follow through, and financial status. Examination of a person's upper limb clinical picture (including range of motion [ROM], muscle strength, sensory picture, dexterity, grasp and pinch, identification of any hand deformities, and analysis of overall hand function) is needed in order to effectively treat the patient with arthritis. Ongoing communication among the physician, orthotist, therapist, and patient is essential when addressing the upper limb orthotic needs of a person with arthritis.

Once the need for orthotic treatment is established, the appropriate type of splint must be chosen. Orthoses used in the rheumatoid hand are classified according to their function. *Resting orthoses* provide passive immobilization during the acute stage of inflammation, alleviating pain by resting involved joints and facilitating the use of uninvolved joints. *Static orthoses* have no moving parts. They are used primarily to provide support, stabilization, protection, or immobilization. *Static progressive splints* use nondynamic components, such as hook and loop closure, hinges, screws, or turnbuckles, to create a mobilizing force to regain joint motion. This differs from dynamic splinting in that it can be used without remolding and eases adjustments as motion improves. *Dynamic splints* use moving parts to permit, control, or restore movements, as stated and referenced by Deshaies: "They are primarily used to apply an intermittent gentle force with the goal of lengthening tissues to restore motion. Forces may be generated by springs, spring wires, rubber bands, or elastic cords. In addition, dynamic splints can be used to assist a weak or paralyzed muscle. Overall, in dynamic splinting, forces must be gentle and applied over a long period of time, and the line of pull must be at a 90 degree angle to the segment being mobilized."[11] Dynamic orthoses counteract the deforming forces of rheumatoid arthritis by providing a constant gentle traction, which is used to stretch scar tissue without excessive reaction. Controversy exists among physicians and therapists as to whether an orthosis can prevent or retard the deforming process of rheumatoid arthritis.

Dynamic orthoses are essential for postoperative rehabilitation of the rheumatic hand after implant resection arthroplasty and reconstruction. Orthoses used after hand reconstruction help maintain surgically achieved mobility and alignment, assist in postoperative strengthening, and decrease post-surgical adhesions. The greatest challenge in postoperative rehabilitation of finger joint arthroplasty is maintaining a proper balance between good healing of the surrounding scar tissue while applying proper amounts of tension across the scar to obtain a desired range of motion.

Treatment Recommendations: As stated by Deshaies,[11] as with any orthosis, the therapist must carefully monitor and teach the patient and caregiver to report any of the following problems related to orthotic use: impaired skin integrity (pressure areas, blisters, maceration, dermatologic reactions), pain, swelling, stiffness, sensory changes/problems, increased stress on unsplinted joints, and functional limitations.

Osteoarthritis of the hand most commonly affects the finger distal interphalangeal (DIP) and proximal interphalangeal (PIP) joints and the thumb carpometacarpal (CMC) joint. Common symptoms are joint tenderness sometimes accompanied by crepitus pain after use that is relieved by rest and progression of pain at rest and at night.[46] Preoperatively, static splints can be used particularly in resting the thumb CMC joint to decrease pain. Splints can also be used to immobilize the PIPs and DIPs. Postoperatively, dynamic splints may be used in the treatment of PIP implant resection arthroplasty.

Once the need for an orthosis is established, the therapist should consider whether the orthosis should be custom fabricated or prefabricated. **Treatment Recommendations:** When making a splint selection, key factors that must be considered are type, design, purpose, fit, comfort, cosmetic appearance, cost of fabrication, weight, ease of care, durability, ease of donning and doffing, effect on unsplinted joints, and effect on function, as well as those patient specific factors discussed earlier. As stated by Deshaies,[11] some studies show that the following factors can affect splint wear: flexibility of the splinting regimen combined with vigorous teaching to enable patients to understand the purpose and wearing schedule, individualized prescriptions focusing on the patient's comfort and preferences, strong family support, positive attitudes of the health care providers, and benefits that are immediately apparent to the patient.

Overall, the application of an orthosis, especially in the treatment of arthritis, is highly individualized. In all of these orthoses, the wearing time is individualized to meet the needs of each patient. Orthoses need to be evaluated for proper fit and usage after a trial application period. Adjustments are made as needed in conjunction with close follow-up with an orthotist or therapist. As with most medical intervention, patient education is of utmost importance to ensure compliance. Orthotics are of no value and may even be harmful if worn incorrectly. To avoid the problems that occur secondary to incorrect orthosis use or disuse, effective instruction is essential. **Treatment Recommendations:** Melvin[27] has outlined what she feels is vital information that should be taught to the patient: (1) the purpose of the splint, including the advantages and disadvantages; (2) when and for how long the splint should be worn; (3) what exercises to do in conjunction with the splint; (4) how to put the splint on and take it off; (5) how to determine if the splint is positioned correctly; (6) how to care for and clean the splint; and (7) how to check the skin for pressure areas.

Surface anatomy and arches of the hand

It is necessary to have knowledge of surface anatomy and of the structures that are represented by it when fabricating an orthosis. The surface anatomy of the hand often sets the boundaries of the orthosis. Crossing these boundaries often prevents motion at a joint, whereas clearing these boundaries allows motion and prevents stiffness of the adjacent joints (Fig. 17-1) For example, Moberg[28] has referred to a line proximal to the transverse fold of the palm, or distal palmar crease, as a life line of the hand. If the orthosis is extended distally, it limits range of motion of the metacarpophalangeal (MP) joints and impairs circulation by decreasing the pumping system. In cases where immobilization is needed, the

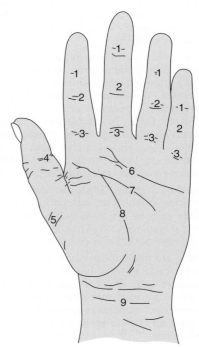

Fig. 17-1 The surface anatomy or creases of the hand often set the boundaries of a splint. Crossing a segmental crease often prevents motion at a joint, whereas clearing the crease allows motion. *1,* Distal creases; *2,* distal middle creases; *3,* distal proximal creases; *4,* distal thumb creases; *5,* proximal thumb creases; *6,* distal palmar crease; *7,* proximal palmar crease; *8,* thenar crease; *9,* wrist crease.

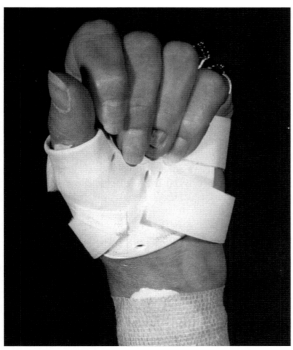

Fig. 17-2 On the thumb, the splint is extended as far as possible to the distal thumb crease to immobilize the MP joint yet clear the crease to allow thumb interphalangeal joint motion.

splint should be extended as far as possible to the next segmental crease to provide adequate support (Fig. 17-2). It is important that the structures to be protected are adequately supported and those that are to be left free for motion are allowed to move completely.

Proper orthotic fabrication and application depend on the understanding of the skeletal arches of the hand. The palm of the hand is concave and is formed by three skeletal arches. The distal transverse arch is deepened by the mobility of the first, fourth, and fifth metacarpals around the stability of the second and third metacarpals (Fig. 17-.3). This mobility is necessary for coordinated grasp and opposition. The longitudinal arch extends from the wrist to the tip of the third digit and is deepened by the composite flexion of the digits. This mobility is necessary for grasping. The third arch is the proximal transverse arch, which is located at the wrist. It is formed by the carpal bones and the ligaments. Flexor tendons, nerves, and

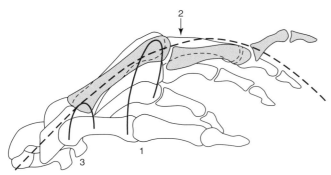

Fig. 17-3 Arches of the hand. *1,* Distal transverse arch; *2,* longitudinal arch; *3,* proximal transverse arch.

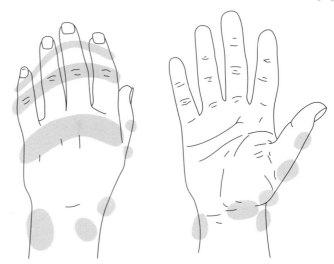

Fig. 17-4 Bony prominences of the hand. Splints must be contoured to prevent pressure over bony prominences, which can result in skin breakdown.

vascular structures fill this cavity. The longitudinal and distal transverse arches must be maintained in orthotic application to prevent flattening of the hand into a nonfunctional position. Orthotic application must be contoured to prevent pressure over bony prominences. Pressure points and skin breakdown can result from an improperly fitted orthosis (Fig. 17-4).

Wrist orthosis

The wrist is a key joint in proper hand function. The wrist joints and surrounding soft tissues are frequently affected by rheumatoid arthritis. It is estimated that 95% of persons with persistent RA develop bilateral wrist joint involvement.[46] Three pathological processes alter the carpus directly and produce deformity. These are cartilage degradation, synovial expansion with erosion, and ligamentous laxity. Cartilage degradation is often seen early in RA. Synovial expansion may cause bony erosion and may lead to ruptured tendons, especially the extensor tendons of the ulnar fingers or the flexor pollicis longus.[33b] Even without erosion, synovial expansion can lead to volar subluxation of the proximal carpal row that has been noted in 80% of RA wrists. The new positioning of all of the carpals can elicit pain. If pressure among the carpal links increases during gripping motions, pain increases as intercarpal pressure increases, which leads to a desire to reduce grip strength to reduce pain (Shapiro). Both cartilage loss and synovial expansion can lead to lax ligaments and thence to wrist instability and further carpal derangement, which in turn can lead to a radial shift of the carpus on the radius.[42a,46]

The distal radial ulnar joint is often involved in the arthritic process as well. The ability to supinate and pronate the forearm is affected by its arthritic involvement. Forearm rotation is an important function in positioning of the hand for maximum use. Destructive synovitis produces distal radial ulnar joint instability with dorsal subluxation of the ulna on the radius and palmar subluxation of the extensor carpi ulnaris tendon resulting in pain, weakness, and decreased range of motion. Position of the wrist influences the relative power of the extrinsic muscles of the hand. Extension of the wrist relaxes the

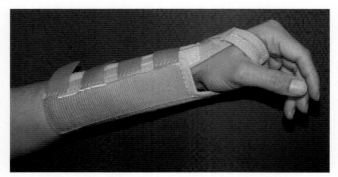

A

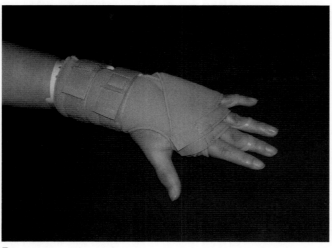

B

Fig. 17-5 A, Simple wrist cockup splint should allow full motion of the digits by clearing the thenar eminence and the distal palmar crease of the hand. **B,** Wrist orthosis that provides pain relief by immobilizing the wrist and supports the MP joints, preventing ulnar deviation. Patient also is wearing thermoplastic figure-of-eight (Oval-Eight) splints for swan neck deformities of the 3–5 digits.

extensors and increases the mechanical advantages of the flexor muscles. The opposite is true for wrist flexion. This concept must be understood when preparing orthoses for specific arthritic conditions of the wrist.

Wrist orthoses (WOs) may be used in acute stages of rheumatoid arthritis to decrease pain, assist in proper wrist positioning to increase maximum function, and provide stability of the wrist. The most commonly used WO is the wrist cockup splint. It is a simple, static orthosis that immobilizes the wrist and allows full MP flexion and thumb opposition. This simple WO positions the wrist in approximately 10 to 30 degrees of extension to allow maximum function. It stabilizes the wrist by preventing flexion and extension of the carpus but does not immobilize the distal radio ulnar joint, allowing the patient pronation and supination (Fig. 17-5, *A*). If supination and pronation prevention is desirable, as in distal radioulnar joint disease, the orthoses can be made to extend across the elbow a short distance. This allows some flexion and extension of the elbow, while blocking forearm and wrist rotation. The wrist cockup splint is applied volarly extending from the proximal third of the forearm ending just proximal to the palmar crease to allow full MP flexion and thumb opposition. The function of the splint is to immobilize the radio carpal joint, providing rest

and stability and allowing reduction of inflammation and pain. It also protects the extensor tendons, which may be at risk for rupture in the [patient with rheumatoid arthritis]. The simple volar splint may also be used to stabilize the wrist in a proper position after flexor synovectomy and carpal tunnel release preventing medial nerve and flexor tendon bowstringing while allowing full finger flexion.

Another orthosis used for acute stages of RA to decrease pain and offer support is the Freedom Arthritis Support Splint by Sammons Preston Rolyan, which immobilizes the wrist and keeps the fingers from ulnarly deviating (Fig. 17-5, *B*).

The orthosis may be appropriate for use preoperatively in a patient with severe wrist instability and a patient who is a candidate for wrist arthrodesis. It provides stability and simulates the fusion. It is important for the WO's to be avoided during active MP synovitis. Wrist immobilization may increase the deforming stresses to the MP joints. In these cases, a resting hand splint may be more appropriate.

The authors use the WOs routinely postoperatively after wrist implant resection arthroplasty or in limited radiocarpal fusion, after cast removal for an additional 6 to 12 weeks. The patient is then encouraged to use the wrist immobilizer when performing strenuous activities such as lifting. Wrist implant arthroplasty is indicated in case of arthritic or traumatic disability resulting in instability of the wrist from subluxation or dislocation of the radiocarpal joint. Wrist reconstruction usually should be performed before finger joint surgery in the person with rheumatoid arthritis. Some believe that wrist implant resection arthroplasty is contraindicated in workers performing heavy manual labor. It has been suggested that a wrist fusion might be a better alternative.

Postoperatively the limb is elevated for 3 to 5 days in a voluminous conforming hand dressing. A short arm cast, keeping the wrist in a neutral position, is applied and worn for 4 to 6 weeks thereafter. If MP joint arthroplasties are performed simultaneously, the outrigger from a high-profile dynamic extension splint may be incorporated in to the cast. During the period of plaster immobilization [of the wrist], the patient is encouraged to carry out active exercises for the MP and the interphalangeal (IP) joints. Isometric gripping exercises of the forearm muscles are started 2 to 3 weeks after surgery. The senior author has developed an isometric grip device (Grip-X) used for this purpose (Fig. 17-6). It is shaped to maintain proper anatomic position of digits and arches of the hand. Following cast removal, wrist exercises are progressively instituted. Flexion and extension exercises are carried out while the forearm is supported on a firm surface. Pronation/supination exercises for the forearm are begun as well. A good ratio of stability to mobility is sought because a joint that is too loose may be unstable. About 50% to 60% of normal flexion and extension movements is ideal after wrist implant resection arthroplasty. Three months after surgery, the active range of motion should approximate 30 degrees of flexion to 30 degrees of extension and 10 degrees of radial and ulnar deviation. The patient is cautioned against any activity such as heavy labor or certain sports that could produce repetitive stresses at the levels of the wrist joint, and the patient is encouraged to wear a WO if unable to avoid these activities.

The senior author has developed titanium carpal bone implants that can be used as spacers following resection of the thumb CMC joint, scaphoid or lunate. These implants can

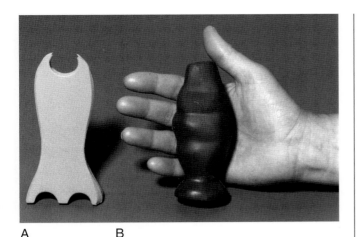

Fig. 17-6 A, Finger crutch (developed by Alfred B. Swanson) to help support the proximal phalanx in extension during PIP flexion exercises. **B,** Grip-S used for postoperative grip strengthening. Variations of these devices are available from rehabilitation and therapy supply catalogues.

satisfactorily maintain joint space and alignment after bone resection. Adequate capsuloligamentous support around carpal implants is essential for early and late stability. Adequate ligamentous repair must be obtained intraoperatively. The implant and the wrist capsule must be kept in an anatomic position during the healing period so that encapsulation becomes secure. Once the operative procedure is completed, the hand is elevated in a voluminous dressing 3 to 5 days post operatively. In scaphoid implant arthroplasty, a long arm thumb spica is applied postoperatively, after 3 to 5 days, with the wrist in 20 to 30 degrees of extension and

slight radial deviation. In lunate implant arthroplasty, a short arm cast with the wrist in slight extension is applied. The cast is worn for 6 to 8 weeks. The cast is removed after 8 weeks, and a cockup wrist splint is applied for the next 4 to 6 weeks, allowing the patient to remove it for range-of-motion exercises.

The resting hand orthosis (Fig. 17-7) provides static positioning to the wrist and digits. It is used in acute rheumatoid arthritis to decrease pain and to align the joints in a normal anatomic position to avoid the zigzag position. It immobilizes the wrist, fingers, and thumb of the patient with arthritis.

The resting hand orthoses are used to support the wrist, fingers and thumb. The normal resting position of the hand is determined anatomically by the bony architecture, capsular length, and resting tone of the wrist and hand muscles. This is typically 10 to 20 degrees of wrist extension, 20 to 30 degrees of metacarpophalangeal joint (MP) flexion, 0 to 20 degrees of proximal interphalangeal joint (PIP) flexion, the distal interphalangeal joints (DIPs) in slight flexion, the thumb CMC in slight extension and abduction, and the thumb MP and IP in slight flexion.[11,45a]

A volar or dorsal resting hand splint is commonly prescribed for patients with rheumatoid arthritis. Resting splints can reduces stress on joint capsules, synovial lining, and periarticular structures, thereby decreasing pain.[26] With this population, splinting should be in a position of comfort regardless of whether this is the ideal anatomical position.[13] During an acute exacerbation of the disease, splints are generally worn at night and during most of the day, removed at least once for hygiene and gentle range-of-motion exercises. It is recommended that splint use continue for several weeks after the pain and swelling have subsided.[11,13]

The resting [hand] orthosis is also used in a postoperative program after MP implant resection arthroplasties.

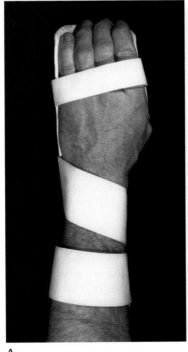
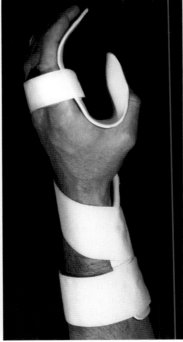

Fig. 17-7 Resting hand splint. **A,** Dorsal view. **B,** Side view.

Full-time wear of a dynamic MP splint is usually discontinued 6 weeks postoperatively, [and may be replaced by a resting hand orthosis. This may be used as a night splint to assist in maintaining proper digital alignment. It is recommended that the splint be worn at night, preoperatively as well as postoperatively. It may be used during the day, however, for additional rest during periods of acute inflammation. It should be noted that ongoing use of the resting hand orthosis can exacerbate joint stiffness. Night wear is often preferred in cases of acute rheumatoid arthritis, but when] worn during the day, it should be removed for pain-free range-of-motion exercises. It is important to achieve a balance between rest and activity in the rheumatoid hand.

When correcting MP ulnar deviation in the [hand] splint, the therapist must be concerned with the wrist position. If the digits align without correcting for the usual radial deviation found in the rheumatoid wrist, the wrist may be pulled into further radial deviation in the resting [hand] splint. The goal of splinting the zigzag deformity in the resting splint must also include correction of the wrist deformity. Straps can be applied to the resting [hand] splint to pull the wrist into ulnar deviation while keeping the fingers aligned in radial deviation, thus correcting the zigzag deformity.

Ulnar deviation orthoses in rheumatoid arthritis

Deformities of the MP joint are usually manifested by increased ulnar drift and palmar subluxation (Fig. 17-8). The MP joint becomes unstable when normal muscle balance is lost and the collateral ligaments are disrupted from the inflammatory process. The MP joint differs from the IP joints in that its movements are not simply flexion and extension but also involve some degree of rotation, abduction, and adduction. Because of this, the MP joint is subject to greater stresses.

Ulnar drift of the MP joints is uncommon in the early stages of RA. However, Wilson[44a] reports 45% of patients whose disease has persisted longer than 5 years demonstrate this deformity. Ulnar drift is a combination of deviation of the phalanx from the metacarpal head and lateral shift of the phalanx upon the metacarpal.[44a] The following are contributors to this deformity:

1. Synovitis within the MP joint alters the supporting structures. The radial collateral ligaments, which are weaker than their ulnar counterparts, stretch.
2. With resolution of the synovitis, the extensor tendons migrate toward the ulnar side, eventually ending up in the valleys between the metacarpal heads.
3. As the fingers flex, the flexors pull the digit ulnarly unopposed by the weakened radial collateral ligament.
4. Contractures of the intrinsic muscles caused by a reflex protective muscle spasm secondary to the synovitis contribute an MP volar displacing force. This disrupts the balance of the volar plate, sagittal bands, transverse metacarpal ligament, and collateral ligament.
5. When wrist synovitis causes radial deviation of the wrist, the dynamics of the finger flexor tendons change as they cross the MP, providing an ulnar force.

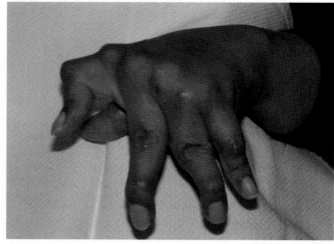

A

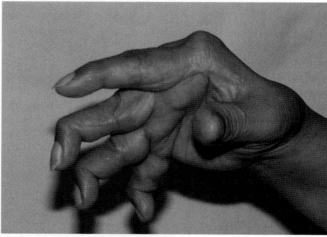

B

Fig. 17-8 A, Ulnar deviation (ulnar drift) and palmar subluxation, evident in the long, ring, and small fingers, are the most common deformities occurring in rheumatoid arthritis. The pronation deformity of the index also occurs frequently as a result of the rotational force applied by the thumb to the distal aspect of the index during lateral pinch. **B,** Deformities of the MP joint are usually manifested by increased ulnar drift and palmar subluxation.

6. MP joint cartilage loss and bony erosion lead to volar subluxation, again allowing the finger flexors to pull ulnarly during flexion.
7. Flexor tenosynovitis can also lead to volar subluxation at the MP joint.[11]

The ulnar deviation orthosis provides support to the MP joints, which restricts flexion and may assist in proper alignment by pulling the fingers radially out of ulnar deviation. The IP joints are left free to encourage proximal IP flexion during activities. This flexion may be beneficial if the patient develops swan-neck deformities. It also prevents further intrinsic tightening. This orthosis can include the wrist when it is involved. This orthosis is indicated in the acute stages of rheumatoid arthritis to decrease pain at the MP level and help prevent further deformities. It can also be used postoperatively after MP joint synovectomy to maintain

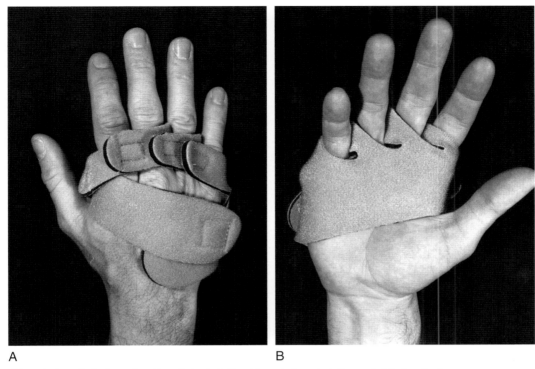

A   B

Fig. 17-9 A, Hand-based ulnar deviation splint (dorsal view). **B,** Hand-based ulnar deviation splint (volar view).

flexor and extensor tendon alignment. The ulnar deviation orthosis may be used as a night splint starting 6 weeks after MP implant resection arthroplasty to assist in maintaining joint alignment (Fig. 17-9).

The ulnar deviation orthoses may be fabricated in a variety of ways. All of the MP joints may be supported by a single platform or may be supported by individual finger separators. The splint may be applied to the palm and fingers only, if the wrist is not involved. This splint can also be used to treat swan-neck deformities that occur in conjunction with MP joint deformity. The splint supports the MP joints in near neutral position while allowing the flexion of the PIP and DIP joints, providing repetitive stretch to the tightened intrinsic muscles.

Thumb spica orthosis

The thumb spica orthosis may be hand or forearm based (Fig. 17-10). It provides support to the thumb CMC and MP joints. Indications may include acute rheumatoid arthritis or osteoarthritis of these joints to decrease pain and provide stability. During fabrication, the thumb should be positioned in abduction to be used as an oppositional post for the fingers. The patient should be instructed to wear the orthoses during daily activities to reduce pain and enhance function. It may be used at night to rest inflamed CMC and MP joints and provide better positioning. The orthosis may also be used postoperatively in patients who require additional stability after cast removal after trapezium or scaphoid implant resection arthroplasty. Following cast removal usually at 6 weeks, the splint is worn full-time except for bathing and gentle range of motion for 4 to 6 additional weeks.

The two most common thumb deformities are the boutonnière deformity (Fig. 17-11), which is characterized by MCP joint flexion and IP joint hyperextension, and the swan neck deformity (Fig. 17-12, *A*), which is characterized by MCP joint hyperextension and adduction and IP joint flexion. The origin of this deformity is synovitis at the CMC joint. Severe boutonniere deformities are usually treated with an MP joint fusion in the patient with rheumatoid arthritis; however, deformities can be stabilized with a thumb spica orthosis when they are mild.

The swan-neck deformity of the thumb is usually initiated by synovitis of the CMC joint followed by stretching of the joint capsule and radialward subluxation of the base of the metacarpal. Thumb abduction becomes painful, and a degree of adductor muscle spasm occurs. This imbalance of forces results in an adduction deformity of the metacarpal with contracture of the adductor pollicis muscle. As abduction of the thumb becomes more difficult, the distal joints are used to compensate for lack of motion. This results in hyperextension of the MP joints and IP joint flexion with resulting increased adduction of the first metacarpal. A self-perpetuating cycle of deformity ensues.

The swan-neck deformity can be treated in its mild cases or preoperatively by a long thumb spica orthosis (Fig. 17-12, *B*). The orthosis provides a stable post for opposition of the other fingers to the thumb, increasing function. Boutonniere deformities in which the MP joint is primarily involved can be treated with a short thumb spica splint, which does not immobilize the CMC joint and is thumb based (Fig. 17-10, *B*). Immobilization of the MP joint of the thumb often improves function by providing a more stable base to pinch.

233

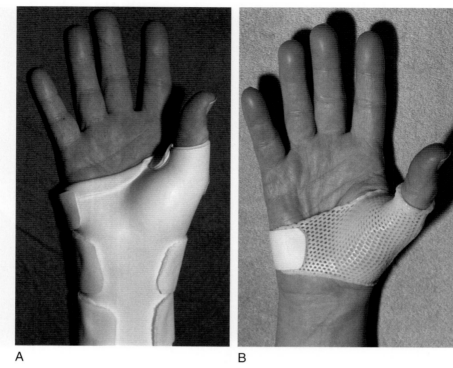

Fig. 17-10 A, Forearm-based thumb spica splint. **B**, Hand-based thumb spica splint.

Thumb interphalangeal joint orthosis

Instability and pain of the thumb IP joint [which results from OA or RA may present] in isolated deformities or in association with collapsed deformities such as swan-neck or boutonniere deformity. Immobilizing the IP joint with the use of aluminum and foam splint or small fabricated thermal plastic orthosis (Fig. 17-13) provides both stability and protection to the joint, allowing continued pinching activities without stretching of the supporting soft tissue and instability of the joint, which would make pinch difficult. The thumb IP orthosis may also be used in cases of pain and instability or when patients are considering an IP joint fusion to simulate the postoperative condition. At 6 to 8 weeks postoperatively, the splint may be used with IP joint fusions for protection following K-wire removal for an additional 2 to 6 weeks of immobilization.

Proximal interphalangeal joint orthoses

Swan-neck and boutonniere deformities are the most common finger deformities.[33a] Synovitis of the PIP joint produces a painful, swollen joint. If synovitis continues it spreads proximally under the central extensor slip, which becomes attenuated, and between the extensor and intrinsic tendons. When the central slip and lateral bands stretch, they migrate volarly and a boutonniere deformity is produced.[33a,44a] Nalebuff has described three stages of the boutonniere deformity.[28a] Stage I exhibits only a slight extensor lag, and a slight loss of DIP flexion occurs. A 40 degree PIP flexion deformity is considered stage II. In stage III, the PIP joint has a fixed flexion deformity.

If the initiating PIP synovitis is anterolateral, it can stretch the transverse retinacular ligament, allowing the lateral band to migrate dorsally, resulting in a PIP joint hyperextension, or swan-neck deformity. Lateral bands in this position prevent the normal volar and lateral shift that allows PIP flexion. With progression of the synovitis, joint erosion and finally destruction occur with fibrous articular adhesions or bony ankylosis.[45] The swan-neck deformity can also be caused by the destructive effect of the synovitis beginning at any one of the three digital joints (Rizio & Belsky).[46]

Preoperatively a static orthosis may be fabricated to prevent swan-neck or boutonniere deformities from becoming fixed and to improve hand function. A commonly used orthosis for this situation is a figure-of-eight ring orthosis (Fig. 17-14, *A*) or tripoint finger splint (Fig. 17-14, *B*, and Fig. 17-5, *B*). The orthosis applies pressure at three points on the finger, providing a correcting force opposite to that of the deformity. For example, in splinting the swan-neck deformity, the pressure is applied dorsally, proximally, and distally, to the PIP joint and volarly over the center of the joint. This results in a flexion force at the PIP joint, which consequently presents with PIP hyperextension and allows active PIP flexion. This splint may be used preoperatively and postoperatively. However, it is not recommended in the immediate postoperative period because of swelling. A dorsal PIP splint is better immediately postoperatively because it is less constricting. Prevention of hyperextension by splinting in flexion allows structures volar to the PIP joint to shorten and help prevent return of the deformity. For the boutonniere deformity, the orthosis is applied opposite that of the swan-neck deformity. There is

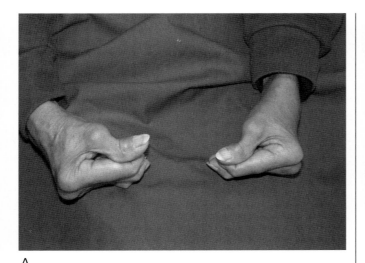

A

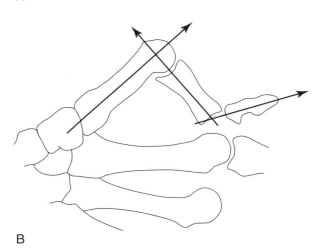

B

Fig. 17-11 Boutonnière deformity of thumb. **A,** This deformity is a common occurrence in rheumatoid arthritis and starts as synovitis of the MP joint. **B,** Pinch movements of functional adaptations accentuate the deformity, and a cycle of deformity is established.

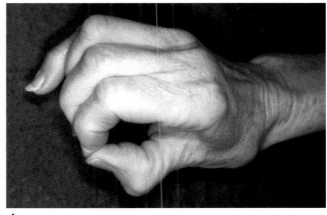

A

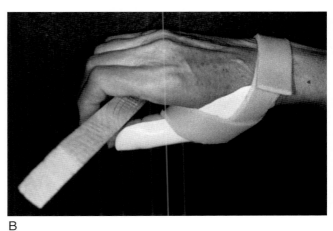

B

Fig. 17-12 A, Typical thumb swan neck deformity with first metacarpal adduction, CMC subluxation, hyperextension of the MP joint, and hyperflexion of the IP joint. **B,** Long dorsal thumb splint applied to correct MP and CMC deformities can provide the patient a stable base for pinch.

pressure over the central aspect of the PIP joint dorsally and proximal and distal to the PIP joint volarly resulting in an extension force preventing PIP flexion contractures.

Postoperatively, after PIP joint implant resection arthroplasty or surgical correction of PIP joint deformities, a dorsal orthosis may be used for protection and proper positioning between exercise periods. The orthosis may be fabricated from low-temperature plastics or padded aluminum. For surgical treatment of swan-neck deformity, a flexed orthosis is used for postoperative protection of the flexed PIP position after dermodesis, PIP fusion, sublimus tenodesis, or PIP manipulation (Fig. 17-15). A dorsal straight orthosis (Fig. 17-16) maintaining PIP extension is used for postoperative protection of boutonniere repair.

Implant resection arthroplasty has been used extensively over the last 45 years for the treatment of MP and PIP joint deformities. Implant resection arthroplasty can be indicated for isolated involvement of the PIP joint not associated with MP joint involvement in the presence of the following: (1) stiff arthritic PIP joint, (2) joint destruction with PIP lateral deviation, (3) boutonniere deformity with joint destruction, and (4) swan-neck deformity with joint destruction. The splinting programs for each of the aforementioned categories are addressed individually.

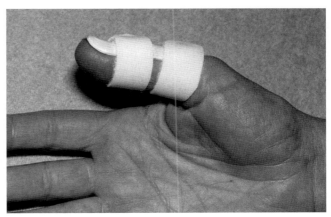

Fig. 17-13 Dorsal thumb IP splint.

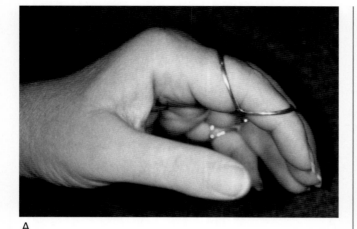

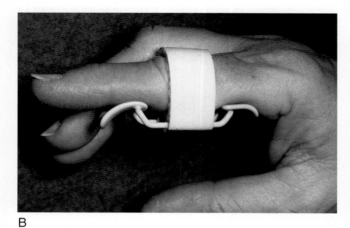

Fig. 17-14 A, Figure-of-eight ring splint prevents PIP joint hyperextension in a swan neck deformity. **B,** Tripoint finger splint is positioned for correction of a boutonnière deformity.

Joint implant arthroplasty
General considerations

Prior to surgical intervention of the wrist or hand, the patient should be seen by an occupational therapist to assess functional and clinical impairments. Assessment typically includes passive and active range of motion (PROM, AROM, including forearm pronation and supination) and maximum finger flexion for composite grasp. With digits in full flexion, measure the distance (in centimeters) from the distal tip of digit to the distal palmar crease. Strength should be tested within the limits of pain. Grasp and pinch are measured and recorded along with a description of mechanical compensation and pain or deformity where observed. The assessment should include the presence of any localized pain, swelling, triggering, joint deformity, or instability. The integrity of the skin and tendons should be documented. A sensory evaluation should be performed if there are indications of polyneuropathies or nerve compression as stated by Yasuda.[14,46] The patient may complain of burning, numbness, and tingling or of dropping objects. Hand function should be assessed, and the level of activities of daily living should be specified in the documentation.

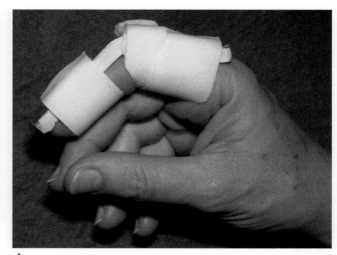

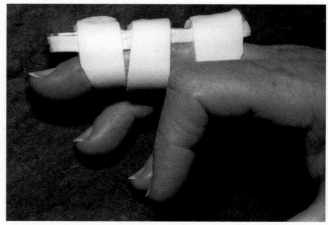

Fig. 17-15 A, Swan neck deformity is splinted postoperatively with a flexed padded aluminum orthosis. **B,** Distal hook and loop strap can be removed to allow for range of motion.

Fig. 17-16 Splinting the boutonnière deformity in extension postoperatively using an aluminum and foam splint, with hook and loop straps for easy adjustments.

In addition to these assessments, the Occupational Therapy Department at Rancho Los Amigos National Rehabilitation Center (OT, RLANRC) utilizes the following tools, which provide valuable information used to formulate the best possible rehabilitation program for the patient. The Pain Numerical Rating Scale [23] is one of several simple pain scales commonly used in current medical practice (some are based on a scale from 0 to 10; others on a scale from 1 to 10). A familiar tool to many patients, it provides a quick picture of the patient's perception of pain at that moment, and it enables the therapist to obtain a baseline pain level and to compare pain during various times or activities. For example, preoperative and postoperative pain, or pain at rest and during exercises can be compared. Another tool, the Arthritis Functional Hand Assessment,[2] requires approximately 1 hour to administer; however, it provides a very clear picture of functional deficits and the compensatory methods used for a functional grasp and pinch. Compensatory grasp and pinch should be considered preoperatively, as correction of a deformity may translate into functional loss if the patient relies on compensation in the presence of additional deformities. Two additional tools are the Typical Day Questionnaire and the Canadian Occupational Performance Measure (COPM).[18] The Typical Day Questionnaire looks at the functional activities performed over the course of a day and the context in which they are performed. It also provides an idea of the type of functional tasks the patient may expect to perform or resume postoperatively. The COPM is a tool that identifies the patient's functional goals and his or her perception of the importance, performance, and satisfaction with each goal that is identified. This provides an opportunity to initiate patient education and planning for restrictions during the postoperative period. "Because rehabilitation after MP joint replacement requires prolonged therapy and dynamic splinting for 3 to 6 months, pertinent social data (i.e., support at home for meal preparation and self-care postoperatively) and insurance considerations are all important to consider during the preoperative evaluation."[20]

Proximal interphalangeal joint implant arthroplasty

Pathophysiology
Once there is cartilage loss, instability, and deformity, joint restoration is no longer possible [and] it...becomes necessary to choose between two salvage procedures—**arthroplasty** (joint reconstruction) and **arthrodesis** (joint fusion). Both surgeries relieve pain, provide stability, correct or reduce deformity, and improve function. The arthroplasty provides the additional benefit of motion."[26] "Pain is diminished by the complete removal of the articular surfaces and diseased synovium. Function is improved by realignment of the joints, increased motion and stability, and decreased pain.... When possible the mobility provided by an arthroplasty is preferred for the ring and little fingers, where flexion improves grip strength. In the index and middle fingers, lateral stability is needed for strong pinch. If the surrounding joint structures are strong enough to ensure lateral stability, an arthroplasty is recommended. If the structures are weak or the bones are small, a fusion is often done in the index and middle fingers. Post surgical expectations for implant arthroplasty in a stiff PIP joint are relief of pain, increased stability or increased mobility (depending on initial status), improved functional use, and

improved cosmetic appearance.[26] (See later discussion under "Treatment Recommendations" for postoperative program for stiff PIP joint. Modifications will be indicated if reconstruction of the collateral ligaments or central tendon was performed.) When implant arthroplasty of a stiff PIP joint does *not* require reconstruction of the collateral ligaments or central tendon, active movements of flexion and extension should be started within 3-5 days after surgery.

Treatment Recommendations (the following protocol is taken from Melvin[26]):

1. First to fifth day:

    a. The hand is in a voluminous compression bandage and is elevated to reduce edema.
    b. ROM of the non-involved joints of the postoperative upper limb should be performed daily.

2. Second to fifth day:

    a. The compression bandage is removed.
    b. Active ROM at the PIP is started several times per day.
    Note: ...Early motion is contraindicated when tendon surgery is done in conjunction with arthroplasty.
    c. PIP joint is positioned in extension with a small dorsal aluminum splint (Fig. 17-16), except during exercise periods. If there has been prior swan-neck deformity or stiffness, the joint might be positioned into slight flexion (Fig. 17-15). In severe swan-neck deformities, the joint can also be taped into flexion at night.
    d. Flexion can be encouraged by stabilizing the MP joint in extension during active finger flexion, using either an orthosis or a device, which will allow PIP flexion while stabilizing the proximal phalanx and blocking MP flexion.

3. After discharge:
    Patients with bilateral arthritis will need instruction in joint-protection techniques and assistive devices for the nonsurgical hand. If patient does not have support at home, this should be done prior to discharge to identify potential problems.

    a. Third to fourth week: Orthosis can be discontinued during the day if the joint is stable; it is usually retained for protective night positioning. Communicate with the surgeon prior to discontinuing the splint.
    b. About sixth to eighth week: Orthosis can be discontinued." [26]

It is important that the orthosis be worn continuously, except for exercise sessions, for 4-6 weeks. The orthosis protects the joint while it is healing. The greatest challenge in postoperative rehabilitation of finger joint arthroplasty is maintaining a proper balance between good healing of the surrounding scar tissue while applying proper movements of tension across the scar to obtain the desired range of motion. The ideal ranges of motion after this surgery are from full extension to 45 degrees of flexion in the index finger, 60 degrees in the long finger, and 70 degrees in the ring and little fingers. An orthosis to hold the digit in extension is worn mainly at night but may also be worn

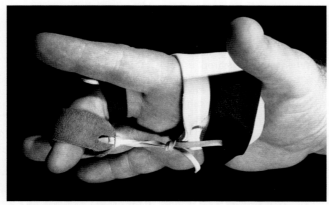

Fig. 17-17 Dynamic flexion splint can be applied three to five times daily for 10 to 20 minutes to increase range of motion if needed after PIP joint implant resection arthroplasty for a stiff joint.

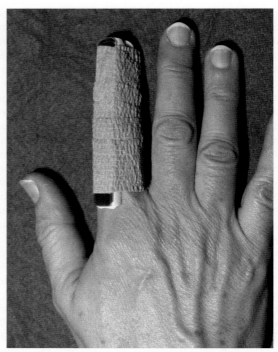

Fig. 17-18 Dorsal splint can be applied slightly laterally to correct any residual deformity. Can be fabricated of padded aluminum orthosis; however, low-temperature thermoplastic may provide improved conformity to finger contours.

continuously for several weeks postoperatively depending on the degree of extensor lag present. A dynamic flexion orthosis may be applied three to five times daily, for 10 to 20 minutes, if flexion is limited (Fig. 17-17). Nighttime extension splinting usually continues for a total of 3 months postoperatively.

Several orthoses have been developed for the postoperative rehabilitation of the PIP joint. Passive and active exercises of the PIP joint should be done, always taking care to support the MP joint in extension. This can be done with the use of a reverse lumbrical bar that supports the proximal phalanges and eliminates motion of the MP joints during flexion exercises. Various devices are available that support the proximal phalanx during flexion exercises and assist in maintaining finger alignment during gripping exercises (Fig. 17-6). Another device that works well is a modified volar wrist orthosis, fabricated from low-temperature thermoplastic with an appendage extending from the distal border to the volar aspect of the proximal phalanx of the postoperative joint, stopping just short of the joint in order to allow full available PIP flexion. Choose a strong low-temperature plastic with minimal stretching (e.g., Ezeform and Kay-Splint III). Straps are applied dorsally over the proximal and distal forearm, the palm, and the proximal phalanx. This orthosis has worked well, especially in the presence of wrist discomfort when the patient performs the exercises. It supports the wrist and the MP joint in extension, allowing movement to be localized at the PIP joint. Additionally, it is easily revised into a wrist support should it be needed after the therapeutic program is complete by removing the appendage and reshaping the distal border to accommodate the palmar arch and clear the distal palmar crease.

Proximal interphalangeal joint with lateral deviation

In addition to implant resection arthroplasty, these joints require soft tissue reconstruction of the collateral ligaments and central slip. The orthosis and postoperative program need to incorporate stability and proper alignment techniques; therefore the dorsal splint is placed laterally (Fig. 17-18) to correct any associated radial or ulnar deviation tendency postoperatively. Active range-of-motion exercises are usually *delayed* 7 to 14 days or longer at the index digit, which requires greater stability for pinch activities. The buddy taping system is used when active range-of-motion exercises are initiated to maintain alignment during motion (Fig. 17-19). The buddy system is applied only during exercise sessions, five to eight times a day, with the lateral extension orthosis in place the rest of the time. Day wear of the orthosis is usually discontinued after 6 weeks. Nighttime wear continues for 3 months postoperatively.

Swan neck deformity

After reconstruction of the PIP joint for a swan-neck deformity, it is important to achieve a 20- to 30-degree flexion contracture of the PIP joint. The orthosis is fabricated to keep the PIP joint in 30 to 40 degrees of flexion and the DIP in extension. The joint is immobilized for 3 weeks postoperatively. After 3 weeks, active range of motion is initiated, and the splint is used to block extension. The distal strap of the splint is removed 4 to 6 times a day for active range-of-motion exercises for 10 to 20 repetitions each (Fig. 17-15). The orthosis is worn day and night for the first 6 weeks. Nighttime splinting continues for 3 months postoperatively.

Boutonnière deformity

After PIP joint reconstruction for boutonniere deformity, it is important to maintain maximum PIP joint extension, while allowing DIP flexion. Therefore, an orthosis, taped in place

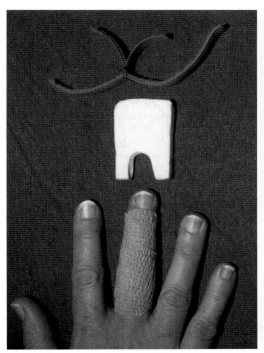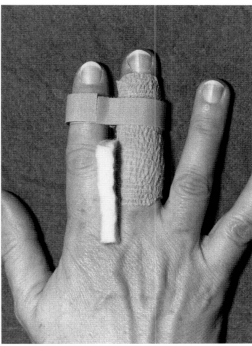

Fig. 17-19 The buddy system is used when active range of motion is initiated, usually after 2 weeks, after implant resection arthroplasty in patients with preoperative PIP joint deviation. Here the middle finger has received the implant and is aligned to the index digit. This allows protection of the collateral ligaments while allowing motion.

2 to 5 days after surgery, keeps the PIP joint extended and ends proximal to the DIP joint. The patient is instructed in hourly DIP active range-of-motion exercises. Active range of motion of the PIP joint is initiated usually at 2 to 3 weeks postoperatively. The orthosis is replaced after each exercise session (Fig. 17-16)....Daytime PIP joint splinting is usually discontinued after 6 to 8 weeks, but nighttime extension splinting may continue for 3 to 6 months postoperatively to maintain maximum PIP joint extension.

Dynamic metacarpophalangeal joint orthoses

General considerations

The metacarpophalangeal (MP) joint is perhaps the most important joint in the digit for function of the fingers.[1] It is subjected to significant mechanical stress as one goes about the daily business of living, such as reaching, grasping, lifting, holding, pinching, and pulling and manipulating objects.[9] Movement of this condylar joint occurs not only in the AP plane of flexion and extension, but also in the lateral plane of abduction and adduction and involves some passive axial rotation. The index finger normally tends to supinate to 45 degrees during pinch. Because of the anatomic configuration of the MP joint, the inherent stability is less than that of the IP joint and more vulnerable to the deforming forces present in RA.[12] Rheumatoid destruction typically results in both deformity and loss of function and commonly affects the MP joint.

Osteoarthritis and traumatic arthritis rarely affect the MP joints of the fingers. Therefore arthroplasty at this level is most often performed in patients with rheumatoid arthritis.

Soft tissue deformities in the MP joint are often severe, which greatly increases the difficulty of obtaining an ideal result from arthroplasty. Whereas arthrodesis is commonly indicated in the PIP and DIP joints, it is rarely performed at the MP joints because it significantly limits function. Fusion of all MP joints eliminates finger spread and is poorly accepted by patients. Fusion of the index finger only can provide for increased stability of pinch and protection against ulnar deviation of the remaining digits.[4]

Deformities of the MP joint in rheumatoid arthritis are usually manifested by increased ulnar drift and palmar subluxation (Fig. 17-8). The deformity often begins with the flexor tendons, which enter the fibrous sheath at an angle and exert an ulnad and palmad pull that is resisted in the normal hand (Fig. 17-20, *A*). When the rheumatoid process progresses, normal muscle balance is lost, and if the restraining structures of the ligament system are destroyed by the rheumatoid disease, resistance to the gradual deforming pull of the long flexors is lost, and the tendons are displaced distally, ulnar, and palmar (Fig. 17-20, *B*). The intrinsic muscles, which form a bridge between the extensor and flexor systems and provide direct flexor power across the MP joint, also become deforming elements once the disease has lengthened the restraining structures of the MP joint and extensor tendon hood. The extensor tendons are then weakened by their ulnad displacement, resulting in loss of balance between intrinsic and extrinsic muscles. The normal mechanical advantage of the ulnar intrinsic muscle is greatly increased once the deformity is established. This creates a cycle resulting in a continued ulnad and palmad dislocation, which results in the classic ulnar drift and volar dislocation of the MP joint seen in the hands of patients with rheumatoid arthritis.[1,17]

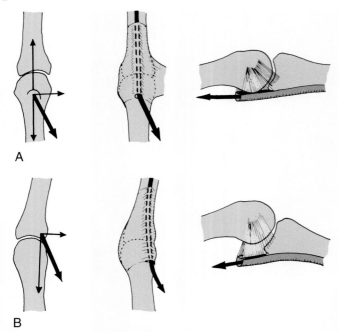

A

B

Fig. 17-20 A, Common flexor tendons enter the fibrous sheath at an angle, and the forces produced by their action have ulnar and palmar components (*left*). In a normal stable MP joint, the ulnar component has little or no displacement effect (*middle*), and resistance of capsule and ligaments prevents displacement of sheath inlet (*right*). **B,** When capsule and ligaments of the MP joint are distended and weakened by the rheumatoid process, resistance to these deforming forces is lost. The point of reflection of the sheath is displaced distally, ulnar and palmar (*left*). The ulnar component of the force produces ulnar deviation (*middle*) and palmar subluxation (*right*) of the proximal phalanx. This mechanism is especially deforming at the level of index and middle fingers.

Pathophysiology

The following factors affect the rheumatoid MP joint and ultimately result in volar subluxation or dislocation and ulnar deviation: MP synovitis, wrist deformity, intrinsic muscle imbalance, and flexor and extensor tendon forces.[45]

Pronation deformity [at the MP joint] of the index finger is a common disability of the rheumatoid hand (Fig. 17-8, *A*). In the normal hand, the pinch mechanism between the thumb and the index finger requires slight supination of the index finger so that the palmar surfaces can meet. In a pronation deformity, the less useful lateral surfaces are opposed. During pinch, the pronation deformity results in an ulnar-directed stress applied to the radial collateral ligaments of the MP joints. This further aggravates ulnar drift and MP subluxation.

Best Practice

MP joint deformities may significantly impair finger function. Deformities of this joint caused by inflammatory arthritis are best treated in their severest form by flexible implant resection arthroplasty. Flexible implant resection arthroplasty of the MP joints is indicated in rheumatoid or post-traumatic disabilities when:

1. The joints are fixed or stiff,
2. Radiographic evidence of joint destruction or subluxation is present,
3. Ulnar drift is not correctable by soft tissue surgery alone,

4. The intrinsic and extrinsic musculature and ligament systems are contracted, and
5. Associated stiffness is found in the IP joints

In addition, Melvin[26] adds:

6. Pain and
7. Functional limitations

The goals of this surgery are pain free functional arc of motion; 70 degrees of flexion for fourth and fifth fingers, and 60 to 65 degrees for the index and middle fingers. According to Feldon, Millender, and Nalebuff,[12] contraindications for this surgery are for those patients who, even in the presence of the above mentioned indications, are usually pain free and have good hand function.

"Too much motion leads to instability and possible recurrence of deformity, especially in the index finger, which is especially vulnerable to ulnar pressure. [In addition,] there is always a risk of less than ideal outcome (e.g., an extension lag and less than 70 degrees of flexion)...as well as fracture (failure) and infection. Therefore current practice is to recommend this surgery only if the ideal or even less than ideal results will improve function."[26] Melvin further states that cosmesis alone, in the absence of pain or significant functional deficits, is not an appropriate indication for this surgery even in the presence of significant deformity. Feldon, Millender, and Nalebuff [12] agree, stating that there is a group of people for whom surgery should not be suggested, although these patients have definite subluxation, ulnar drift, advanced radiographic changes, and a weakened grip, they are usually pain free and have good hand function. Surgery will not increase their function and would probably weaken their grip. An optimal treatment program for these patients would be to provide appropriate night splints and observe every 3 to 4 months for as long as they maintain satisfactory function. If they show progressive deformity and dysfunction, they will become candidates for operative treatment. "Many patients find they are not able to do more or different hand tasks postoperatively, but are able to do the same tasks, especially tasks requiring improved dexterity, with greater ease and without pain."[26]

Newer studies are needed, but a long-term study of 144 Swanson implant metacarpophalangeal arthroplasties has been conducted. It was concluded that excellent correction of ulnar drift, increased motion of the metacarpophalangeal joints, a more functional arc of motion of the metacarpophalangeal joints, and enhanced function of the hand can be expected after a successful procedure. The study further stated that with proper indications, good operative technique, an organized program of therapy, and a cooperative patient, this procedure can eliminate pain and can result in improvement in the function of the hand that is maintained over time.[17]

Key Point: Surgical prerequisites for MP arthroplasties are:

1. Intact neurovascular supply
2. Intact flexor and extensor tendons
3. Patient capable and motivated to follow precise postoperative splinting and exercise routine
4. Absence of infection and
5. adequate bone density to accept implant.[26,35]

Flexible implant arthroplasty of the MP joint, developed by Swanson has become the gold standard for MP arthroplasty. It has stood the test of time and meets the goals of providing a pain-free, mobile, stable, and durable joint. The basic concept of flexible implant resection arthroplasty can be summarized as follows:

$$\text{Bone resection} + \text{Implant} + \text{Encapsulation}$$

$$= \text{Functional joint}$$

The term *implant* is used to describe these devices because they are spacers rather than artificial joints. They function as a hinge and do not do all of the intricate gliding and rotational motions of a normal joint.[26] One of the most important functions of a flexible implant is to maintain internal alignment and spacing of the reconstructed joint; ...early motion is started with the implant acting as a dynamic spacer. The joint is thus rebuilt in a healing phenomenon called the encapsulation process, which is a major component of the flexible implant arthroplasty and essential to postoperative management.[26] The basic concept that collagen formation is dynamic and its development can be influenced in a controlled postoperative rehabilitation program must be understood by surgeons and therapists who treat rheumatoid patients. Madden et al.[21] state that in addition to a skilled surgeon, an organized postoperative management program is necessary for successful flexible implant resection arthroplasty. If motion is restricted during the healing phase, there is poor mobility of the joint; therefore, the host tissue or collagen reaction must be used advantageously by training it postoperatively. Prostheses that use cement fixation do not rely on the capsule or ligamentous structures for stability and the surgical and postoperative protocols are different than those for flexible implants. Since flexible implants are widely used and require the most postoperative therapy, the protocols presented here will be specific to this type of implant.[26]

Pathophysiology

The encapsulation process around the MP joint begins during the first week. During this time, the emphasis is on edema reduction with AROM, and gentle PROM performed within [the postoperative] splint. During the second week after surgery, collagen formation increases around the capsule and the implant. The reconstructed joints become more stable during this second postoperative week and continue to become stronger by the third postoperative week. This may be perceived by the patient and therapist as increased stiffness of the reconstructed joints. It is important to monitor the ROM of the MP joints during this time to ensure that the desired degree of motion is maintained during this phase of scar production and early maturation.[20]

Postoperative care

Key Point: The positioning and control of movement through dynamic orthotics and therapy during the first 6-8 weeks after reconstruction are as important as surgery.[26]

Use of a dynamic extension orthosis following MP implant resection arthroplasty involves a good understanding of the splint, splinting techniques, and postoperative rehabilitation principles. The dynamic extension orthosis has three major functions: to provide complete, adjustable correction of residual deformity; to control motion in the desired plane and range; and to assist flexion and extension power ensuring an adequate alternation of complete extension and flexion

ranges of motion in the joint. Although general postoperative protocols are similar, it is important to initiate communication with the surgeon performing the procedure regarding the specifics of the particular implant being used. Clear communication with regard to parameters for ROM, time lines for initiating active and passive motion, as well as any soft tissue reconstruction that may have been performed all are important components of the postoperative program. In addition to the goals for postoperative outcomes and a thorough understanding of the healing process, a clear understanding of the patients' postoperative expectations also are important.

After MP resection arthroplasty, the surgeon removes the dressings 2 days postoperatively, and fabrication of the custom-fit dynamic extension orthosis can be initiated per protocol agreed upon by the therapist and the surgeon performing the procedure. The goal of the dynamic orthosis used postoperatively for the MP resection arthroplasty is to support the digits in slight radial deviation and to encourage extension without hyperextension. The tension of the rubber band should be tight enough to guide the digits in a desired plane of motion while allowing 70 degrees of active flexion at the ring and little fingers. The response to dynamic splinting is rapid during the first few days. Initially the therapist may need to adjust the dynamic splint two or three times a week to prevent overcorrection or to gradually increase tension of the slings to facilitate MP joint extension. Placement and adjustment of the slings vary with the situation presented by each finger. The index finger often has a tendency toward pronation deformity preoperatively (Fig. 17-8). The patient then tends to use lateral pinch, which further exaggerates the ulnar deviation of the digits. The index finger must be supported in supination after surgery using the concept of the *force couple*. A force couple is defined as two equal and opposite forces that act along parallel lines and is obtained by applying a second outrigger to provide a supinatory torque. The index finger needs greater stability and less mobility at the MP joint to perform prehensile activities. In most cases, a string is used instead of a rubber band at the index finger to place the digit in the proper position and limit flexion for at least 2 to 3 weeks to achieve the goal of 0 extension and 45 degrees of flexion (Fig. 17-21).

In most cases, the long finger requires only a sling on the proximal phalanx to maintain a slight radial alignment. An additional lateral sling may be applied to the middle phalanx, if additional radial pull is needed or if correction of pronation tendency is required. The requirements of the ring finger are similar to those of the long finger with the exception that the rubber band tension may need to be reduced to allow 70 degrees of active flexion. The little finger may have weak flexor power, and rubber band tension may need to be reduced accordingly. In some cases, a buddy sling is applied to allow active assisted motion with the ring finger. This buddy sling needs to take into account the transverse arch to allow proper digital flexion. If the little finger has a supination tendency or tucks under the ring finger, the proximal phalanx sling can be placed radially to facilitate pronation. If further rotation is required, an additional outrigger is used to support a sling pulling ulnarly on the middle phalanx according to the force couple principle.

The importance of good patient education cannot be overstressed. The exercises are carried out for a short duration,

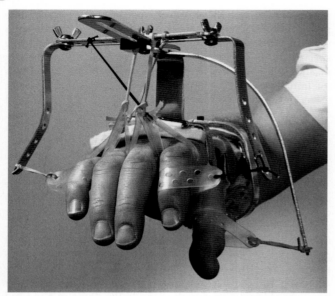

Fig. 17-21 High-profile hand splint preferred by Swanson clearly demonstrates all outriggers in place to supinate and stabilize the index finger using a string instead of a rubber band; pronate the little finger and allow motion through use of rubber bands; and abduct the thumb to avoid lateral pressure on the digits during active flexion. Note: This may also be achieved with a low-profile dynamic extension splint using an outrigger kit such as the Rolyan adjustable outrigger kit.

but are performed frequently during the day to train the new joint capsule in proper alignment. It is important that the exercises are carried out with the limb elevated to reduce edema. Active flexion exercises of all MP joints are performed for 5 to 10 repetitions; then are repeated five times for each MP joint individually. Patients who have good motion at the PIP joints may have difficulty isolating MP flexion. In these cases, a dorsal splint of padded aluminum or molded low-temperature thermoplastic is taped or strapped to the digit to immobilize the PIP joints, thus allowing localization of the flexion force at the MP joints. The range-of-motion goals at the MP joints after implant resection arthroplasty are: index finger, 0-45 degrees; long, 0-60 degrees; ring, 0-70 degrees; small, 0-70 degrees. If these goals are not reached with active exercises, passive range

of motion is initiated. A force no greater than 2 lb of pressure is applied to the proximal phalanx at each MP joint individually for five repetitions (Fig. 17-22). The surgeon may also wish to limit MP flexion in cases where greater stability is desired in the presence of good PIP motion. In this case, the rubber band is replaced with a dacron strap to provide a static sling arrangement. The lumbrical bar, available with the high-profile orthoses, can be used also to immobilize the MP joints.

The reconstructed joints start tightening up during the second postoperative week and are quite tight by the end of 3 weeks. If the desired range of motion has not been obtained by 4 weeks, it is difficult to gain further improvement in motion. If at 3 weeks the patient has good MP joint extension with poor flexion, dynamic flexion techniques are used. The therapist should be cautious with dynamic flexion devices because extension is usually more difficult to achieve. Passive flexion is achieved with finger slings on the proximal phalanges attached volarly to the flexion outrigger, which is secured to the base of the orthosis (Fig. 17-23). The slings should be placed so that the line of pull is directed toward the scaphoid bone. A figure-of-eight elbow strap may be needed to prevent distal migration of the splint during dynamic flexion. Dynamic flexion should be applied for only 20 minutes at a time, three to six times a day or more frequently if flexion limitations persist. At the sixth postoperative week, the extension portion of the splint is usually worn at night only for another 3 weeks. If there is persistent extensor lag or tendency for flexion contracture or deviation of the digits, part-time support by this orthosis must be continued for several more weeks or even months.

The patient should follow a prescribed rehabilitation program including active and passive exercises for at least 3 months after surgery to maintain desired range of motion. The range of motion is regularly measured to assess progress. Because collagen maturity, scar contraction, and tendon deficiencies vary from patient to patient, careful attention by the hand surgeon and therapist is required throughout the postoperative period. The patient's response to the rehabilitation program varies with the severity of preoperative deformities; the surgical procedure; the patient's physical and emotional state, ability to understand, and ability to cooperate; and individual collagen and scar tissue production. The program must be carried out with these variables in mind, realizing

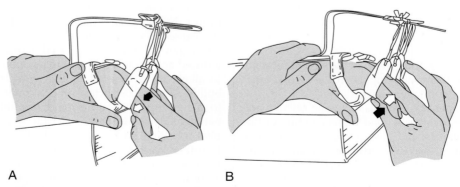

A   B

Fig. 17-22 Passive range-of-motion exercises being performed with the wrist supported. A force no greater than 2 lb of pressure is applied to the proximal phalanx of each MP joint for five repetitions each.

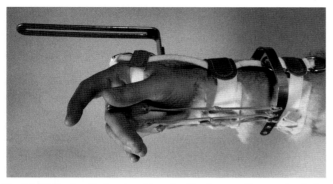

Fig. 17-23 Passive flexion is achieved with slings on the proximal phalanges attached volarly to the flexion outrigger, which is secured to the base of the high-profile hand splint. Passive flexion is applied for only 20 minutes at a time, usually three to six times daily in patients who demonstrate flexion limitation. Note: At the authors' facility, the low-profile design is used. Clinical judgment must be used to determine if attachment to the base of the dynamic extension orthosis or use of a separate volar based dynamic flexion orthosis should be used. This is usually determined by the patient's ability (or lack of ability) to safely remove/replace the dynamic extension orthosis, as well as the weight of the combined dynamic orthosis.

that some patients reach their goals more rapidly than others. Properly applied therapy can provide a better result for the patient.

Many types of orthoses are available for postoperative MP therapy. Historically, the dynamic extension and the dynamic flexion splints have been the standard for postoperative treatment in combination with an extensive therapeutic exercise program for gaining extension and flexion and for encouraging proper mechanical and rotational motions at the MP joint. Both the high-profile dynamic orthosis and the low-profile design are commonly used as well as custom-fabricated outriggers. There has been considerable debate about the advantages and disadvantages of the high-profile dynamic orthosis versus the low-profile design. Swanson strongly advocated the use of the high profile design. He felt it provided for more supination at the index finger, which is crucial for pad-to-pad opposition with the thumb. Swanson also recommended the use of the high-profile dynamic orthosis for the postoperative management of implant resection arthroplasty in the following cases: for patients demonstrating weak flexion strength, the high-profile requires less force to initiate and maintain motion; in patients requiring index supination because for pronation deformities, the high-profile *force couple* design provides greater index finger supination during range of motion. The advantages of the low-profile design are better cosmesis and ease of patient dressing.[10] Even though the low-profile design is significantly less cumbersome than the high-profile design, it is the experience of this therapist that it is perceived as being very cumbersome by patients for whom significant bilateral involvement makes it difficult to manage the splint components for compliance with performing home exercises and for performing basic routine occupational activities such as self-care and meal preparation. In addition, some patients have significant difficulty managing the initially intensive and demanding therapeutic regimen and frequent splinting adjustments that are an integral component of dynamic splinting after MP arthroplasty and may require frequent

trips to therapy for adjustments. The low-profile dynamic design has been the standard at this institution. It has been used successfully for many years and is therefore the most familiar to this therapist. There have been improvements made in the design of the commercially available low-profile outriggers that have provided more precise adjustments for controlling deviation and rotational motions at the MP and for providing a more optimal line of pull during dynamic flexion and extension.

Current practice appears to show a trend toward a postoperative program for MP arthroplasty that combines alternate static splinting in which the MPs are placed, alternately, in flexion and extension.[6a] The indications are that the static splints are more easily tolerated by patients, and the results are comparable. According to Wilson,[44b] "Early active mobilization was achieved more readily in the methods [they] adopted after 1979 . . ." which involve ". . . supervised active physiotherapy from the fourth post-operative day using a static resting splint"; additionally Wilson reports they have not used dynamic splinting for their postoperative treatment of MP arthroplasty since 1979. Another study by Thomsen[42b] was unable to prove that dynamic splinting produced significantly inferior results to static splinting, noting that "residual extension lag was significantly less . . . in the treated group" and "conclude[d] that postoperative dynamic splinting seems to be useful after replacement of MCP joint with silastic implants." However, although more comparison data and studies are needed, the advantages of a static, less complicated program are very appealing. It is especially advantageous for use with a certain population of patients for whom the dynamic splinting was a significant barrier for a variety of factors including lack of support at home, significant weight of the dynamic splint with all the components, mechanical difficulty with correctly removing/replacing parts of the dynamic splint during execution of home program for maintaining proper alignment at the MPs, and with poor compliance and failed appointments for postoperative management and adjustments of the dynamic components.

In short, the postoperative dynamic orthosis serves a variety of purposes. It provides adjustable tension to control alignment of the MP joint during the healing phase, while it limits motion to the desired plane and range during active exercises. It also assists flexor and extensor power to encourage desired finger motion following implant resection arthroplasty. The splint is generally worn day and night for about 6 to 8 weeks with night wear continued through 12 weeks. Postoperative static splinting seeks to stabilize and support the MPs with static splints while applying supervised early mobilization and alternating flexion and extension positioning to maintain full ROM during the healing (encapsulation) process.

Resources describing the fabrication and application of dynamic extension and flexion orthoses designed specifically for postoperative rehabilitation of the MP implant resection arthroplasties are not as readily available as are those for more commonly used orthoses. As an integral component to a successful outcome for an implant resection arthroplasty program, they are described in the following section. Details regarding the fabrication and application of the low-profile dynamic extension orthosis as well as the integration of the dynamic flexion components are presented. *Note:* Please refer to the third (prior) edition of this text for a detailed description of the high-profile dynamic extension orthosis as described by Swanson.

Method for assembly of low-profile dynamic extension orthosis

The low-profile dynamic extension orthosis splint (Fig. 17-24) is assembled and applied in much the same manner as the high-profile splint, but with very different components. Many of the principles are the same; however, the low-profile orthosis uses a pulley system and the longitudinal bars are attached to the fixed transverse bar via the adjustable pulleys. In contrast, the high-profile construction favored by Swanson featured a high-profile fixed longitudinal bar to which the transverse bar and the additional outriggers are attached (see Fig. 17-21). The thermoplastic base of the low-profile dynamic extension orthosis is custom fit dorsally and can be lined with closed cell foam padding if needed; however, this makes the orthosis more difficult to keep clean. Padding, if used, should be applied to the thermoplastic prior to conforming to the patient, as adding the padding after the splint is formed may result in pressure areas. Particular attention must be given to avoid pressure over any bony prominences or incisions and at orthosis or strap edges. If the patient has prominent bony protrusions, such as the ulnar styloid, padding is taped temporarily over the bony areas prior to shaping the base of the splint. When removed, a space remains between the bony area and the splint, which reduces the likelihood of pressure from the orthosis. As with the high-profile orthosis, the wrist should be positioned in near neutral. To obtain increased conformity and to reduce rotation and migration of the orthosis (this assumes no reconstruction was performed at the thumb), a thumb opening can be included at the distal–radial aspect and the plastic shaped and conformed around the base of the thumb. The orthosis should not restrict ROM of the thumb or the MP of the index. A thermoplastic should be selected that is as lightweight and durable as possible and that will allow reshaping as needed as the initial swelling subsides. Like the high-profile orthosis, it is trimmed to the correct length and the distal aspect shaped over the heads of the metacarpals with the correct oblique angle to conform to the descending angle of the phalanges.[4a] Care should be taken that there is conformity but also enough space over the MPs so that active motion is not impeded. Placement of the adjustable (latitudinal) outrigger should be determined, taking care to consider the desired line of pull and the best position to allow anticipated adjustments of the

longitudinal rod adjusters that will be attached. The upper latitudinal bar should correspond with the latitudinal line of the heads of the metacarpals and should be placed just proximal to them. Mark the desired placement on the dorsum of the orthosis.

For a seamless fit, the longitudinal rods at the bottom of the curved portion of the selected outrigger must be conformed to the dorsum of the thermoplastic splint, in the position selected. A second piece of the same type of thermoplastic material selected for the base is used to sandwich the longitudinal rods of the outrigger to the splint. To ensure less slippage of the outrigger as a result of the dynamic forces pulling distally, the ends should be bent slightly toward each other prior to sealing between the thermoplastic layers. This provides increased purchase of the plastic around the rods and is easily done using a wire bender. In addition, a bonding agent may be used for a more secure bond of the splinting material to reduce opportunity for separation and shifting of the outrigger. This is easily done at this stage, and can help avoid the need for time-consuming urgent repairs later should separation occur. The distal strap should be placed across the volar surface of the palm, proximal to the distal palmar crease and clearing the thenar eminence. Straps also are placed volarly across the distal and proximal forearm. Soft strapping material is used, with additional padding applied as needed to provide even pressure distribution and for patient comfort. The straps are applied snugly but should not cause pressure or constriction. The patient must be educated and trained to properly adjust the straps as appropriate.

The pulleys then can be placed on the outrigger bar in roughly the desired position over the corresponding metacarpal and the set screws only loosely applied. The rod adjusters are then slid individually into the pulleys, and adjustments are begun to align the direction of pull to 90 degrees, perpendicularly, over the center of the proximal phalanges. Choose the method for attaching the proximal ends of the tension line to the proximal aspect of the splint. This is the therapist's choice and may be springs or rubber bands attached to a D-ring or hook and loop tab. Small aluminum devices are available for adjusting the tension of the monofilament as well. The finger loops (which may be purchased or preassembled from soft strapping material) then are placed over proximal phalanges and trimmed to fit as appropriate so that they are not impeding motion. Thread the monofilament from the finger loops through the "pigtail" at the distal end of the adjuster rod and secure to the dorsum of the splint toward the proximal end. Make final adjustments to correct the line of pull to 90 degrees, perpendicular to the proximal phalanx, then make rotary adjustments as needed to accommodate for supination or pronation deformity and tighten the set screws. Mark the placement of the rods in the pulley with a permanent marker. Leaving enough length to allow for future adjustments, remove the rod and cut excess length off the proximal ends of the longitudinal rod adjustors with wire cutters. (*Caution: Cut under the cover of a towel and away from patient to avoid mishaps with flying debris.*) Replace the rods in the pulley and tighten the set screw. Place a dab of white glue on the cut end of the rod, and push the rubber protector cap over the end (these caps tend to fall off, and the patient may be cut or scratched on the exposed end; the glue helps keep the rubber caps intact). Complete the placement of the proximal end of

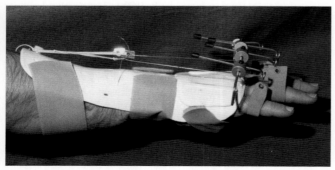

Fig. 17-24 Low-profile dynamic extension orthosis.

the tension line, marking the exact location if using hook and loop attachments. Hook and loop attachments allow changes to be made quickly; however, they can be adjusted by the patient, so patient education and compliance are important if this method of attachment is used. Correct placement of each tension line can be marked with a pen, and the patient can simply detach the hook and loop tab to easily perform the exercise program and reattach at the correct point when the exercise is completed. If there is bilateral involvement, the patient may have difficulty removing the loop from the finger, so compliance with the exercise program may be enhanced if the splint is less difficult to manage.

A lateral rod adjuster is placed at a 90-degree line of pull to the radial side of the middle phalanx of the index finger, to provide additional radial pull for controlling supination of the index finger. Keeping the mechanical principles and the encapsulation process in mind, this may need to be a static pull versus the dynamic pull provided by the rubber bands or springs, as greater stability is important at the index MP. Additional outriggers can be added as needed for positioning the thumb in abduction and for providing rotatory forces as needed for the digits. (See the section on the goals of dynamic orthoses used for postoperative care of MP resection arthroplasty.)

A dynamic flexion component can be added if at 3 weeks good extension has been achieved but flexion is poor. If expected extension has not been gained, a passive flexion component may be recommended. The dynamic flexion outrigger is assembled in the same manner as the extension component; however, it is fitted to a custom thermoplastic *volar* orthosis. Like the dorsal extension orthosis, the thumb can be included when forming the volar base for a more stable fit (assuming no reconstruction of the thumb has been performed). Again, take care not to impede ROM of the thumb or the MP joints. Slings are placed on the proximal phalanx of the digits, volarly, with the direction of pull towards the scaphoid bone. Adjustments in tension should be made accordingly. Dynamic flexion should be applied for only 20 minutes at a time, three to six times a day, but may be added more frequently if flexion limitations persist.

Treatment recommendations

Kits are available that include two sizes of outriggers to accommodate various widths across the heads of the metacarpals. Some also provide rod adjusters that allow more precise adjustments into horizontal, longitudinal, and vertical planes (e.g., Rolyan Adjustable Outrigger Kit from Sammons Preston Rolyan). The longitudinal rod adjuster allows adjustments to accommodate the changes that occur in the dynamic arc of motion as extensors strengthen. If the line of pull is not maintained at 90 degrees to the proximal phalanx, the forces will be altered, resulting in either jamming or distraction of the joint and a decrease in the rotatory force.[14] The Rolyan outrigger kit also has a third set screw on the pulley, which allows increased rod stability, and a force coupling unit for the index. A kit is also available for MP flexion.

Summary

Successful use of orthoses is made possible only through an integrated team approach including the patient, his or her significant others, and health care providers. It is important to note that the patient and the caregivers bring key physical, psychological, social and functional components to the orthotic process and should be considered the primary members of the team.[11]

Successful use of an orthosis in the treatment of arthritic hand deformities depends on many factors. The team of surgeons and therapists must determine which patients are suitable candidates for implant arthroplasty and which might be better served by nonoperative, supportive care. Surgeons must remember that operative intervention in the rheumatoid patient is palliative; joint replacement arthroplasty is not a cure.[20] When orthosis is indicated, the physician must determine the treatment goals of the orthosis and refer the fabrication of the orthosis to the appropriately trained therapist or orthotist.

The occupational therapist, as an expert in the adaptive use of the upper extremities in occupational performance tasks, has the major responsibility for the recommendation of appropriate orthoses, the testing and training in the use of orthoses for the upper extremities, and the selection, design and fabrication of thermoplastic.[11] To accomplish this, the occupational therapist must bring to the splinting process a knowledge of anatomy and biomechanics, skills in assessing function, and the ability to determine optimal intervention for each patient, wether it includes a splint or not.[4a] The therapist must be skilled in patient evaluation and orthotic fabrication techniques, have a thorough understanding of the disease process and treatment principles, and develop a good rapport with the patient.

Orthoses are often an integral component of occupational therapy for patients with physical dysfunction. Orthotics entails prescription, selection, design, fabrication, testing, and training in the use of these special devices.[11] Because it is both impossible and inappropriate to prescribe a single orthosis design for a particular diagnosis, occupational therapists create orthoses by adapting to individual patient variables. This generates a wide variety of orthosis configurations that are specifically designed to accomplish distinct therapeutic goals. It is therefore critical that therapists "thoroughly understand the exact purpose for the splint being prepared, the necessary mechanics to achieve it, and the available design options."[14] In addition, "the patient must understand the purpose of the orthosis, have an acceptance of the benefits that the orthosis can provide, and have the proper knowledge and ability to use the orthosis appropriately. When selecting the proper orthosis, the following principles outlined by Bennett must be understood.

(1) The device must serve a real need. Applying unnecessary apparatus can be as dangerous as not applying necessary apparatus. (2) The device prescribed must be of a design that can be constructed and, as necessary, repaired by [an experienced therapist or] orthotist. (3) The device must be as lightweight as possible but capable of standing up under expected wear. (4) The device must be reasonable in cost. (5) The device must be sufficiently simple that it can be applied by the patient or [caregiver]. (6) The device must be acceptable in appearance. (7) The device must in no way endanger the structural security of bodily segments through its use.[5]

It is only by adherence to these principles that optimum benefit for the patient with an arthritic hand lesion can be achieved.

Vendors of splints and splint supplies

Abledata
http://trace.wisc.edu

AliMed, Inc.
297 High Street, Dedham, MA 02026
800-225-2610, fax 800-437-2966

SIRIS splint, Silver Ring Splint Company
P.O. Box 2856, Charlottesville, VA 22902-286
800-311-7028, fax 888-456-8828
www.silverringsplint.com

North Coast Medical
18305 Sutter Blvd.
Morgan Hill, CA 95037-2845
877-213-9300
www.ncmedical.com

Sammons Preston Rolyan
P.O. Box 5071, Bolingbrook, IL 60440-5071
800-323-5547
www.sammonspreston.com

The following products are shown and/or mentioned in this chapter and are available from Sammons Preston Rolyan: Oval-Eight Splint, Freedom Arthritis Support, Rolyan Digi-Block Hand Exerciser, Swanson Hand Cone, Ezeform thermoplastic, Kay-Splint III thermoplastic, Rolyan Adjustable Outrigger Kit for MCP Flexion, and Rolyan Adjustable Outrigger Kit for MCP Extension, 90-degree wire bender, Sammons Preston Universal Bonding Agent, Rolyan Tension Adjustment Strips, Rolyan Tension-adjustable Connecting Pieces, and the individual components for fabrication of high-profile dynamic flexion/extension orthosis.

References

1. Alter S, Feldon P, Terrono AL: Pathomechanics of deformities in the arthritic hand and wrist. In Hunter JM et al., editor: *Rehabilitation of the hand and upper extremity, vol 2*, ed 5, Philadelphia, 2002, Mosby.
2. Arthritis Functional Hand Assessment, used in the Occupational Therapy Department at Rancho Los Amigos National Rehabilitation Center.
3. Backman C, Mackie H: The arthritis hand function test, *[AOTA] Physical Disabilities Special Interest Section Newsletter* 19:1–2, 1996.
4. Beckenbaugh RD, Linscheid RL: Arthroplasty in the hand and wrist. In Green DP, editor: *Operative hand surgery, vol. 1*, ed 3, New York, 1993, Churchill Livingstone, in collaboration with AB Swanson and G de Groot Swanson.
5. Bennett RL: Orthotics for function, *Phys Ther Rev* 36, 1956.
6. Brand PW, Hollister A: *Clinical mechanics of the hand*, ed 2, St. Louis, 1985, Mosby.
6a. Burr N, Pratt AL, Smith PJ: An alternative splinting and rehabilitation protocol for metacarpophalangeal joint arthroplasty in patients with rheumatoid arthritis, *J Hand Ther* 15(1):41, 2002.
7. Boozer J: Splinting the arthritic hand, *J Hand Ther* Jan:46, 1993.
8. Boozer JA, Sanson MS, Soutas-Litttle RW, Coale EH Jr, Pierce TD, Swanson AB: Comparison of the biomechanical motions and forces involved in high-profile versus low-profile dynamic splinting, *J Hand Ther* 7:171–182, 1994.
9. Buckner WS: Arthritis. In Pedretti LW, Early MB, editors: *Occupational therapy, practice skills for physical dysfunction*, ed 5, New York, 2001, Mosby.
10. Colditz JC: Low profile dynamic splinting of the injured hand, *Am J Occup Ther* 37:182, 1983.
11. Deshaies LD: Upper extremity orthoses. In Trombly CA, Radomski MV, editors: *Occupational therapy for physical dysfunction*, ed 5, Philadelphia, 2002, Lippincott Williams & Wilkins.
12. Feldon P, Millender LH, Nalebuff EA: Rheumatoid arthritis in the hand and wrist. In Green P, editor: *operative hand surgery, vol 2*, ed 3, New York, 1993, Churchill Livingstone.
13. Fess EE, Phillips CA: *Hand splinting principles and methods*, St. Louis, 1987, CV Mosby.
14. Fess EE, Kiel JH: Therapeutic adaptations, upper-extremity splinting. In Hopkins HL, Smith HD, editors: *Willard and Spackman's occupational therapy*, ed 8, Philadelphia, 1993, JB Lippincott.
15. Flatt EA: *Care of the arthritic hand*, St. Louis, 1983, CV Mosby.
16. Frisser RW: Splinting the rheumatoid arthritic hand. Current concepts in orthopaedics: a diagnosis related approach to splinting, Rolyan Medical Products, Bolingbrook, Ill, 1984.
17. Kirschenbaum D, Schneider LH, Adams DC, Cody RP: Arthroplasty of the metacarpophalangeal joints with use of silicone-rubber implants in patients who have rheumatoid arthritis, *J Bone Joint Surg* 75A:3–12, 1993.
18. Law M, Baptiste S, Carswell A, McColl MA, Polatajko H, Pollack N: *The Canadian Occupational Performance Measure*, ed 3, Ottawa, Ontario, Canada, 1998, CAOT Publications.
19. Loebl WY: Mobility of metacarpophalangeal joints in rheumatoid arthritis, *Hand* 5:165–169, 1973.
20. Lubahn JD, Wolfe, TL: Joint replacement in the rheumatoid hand: surgery and therapy. In Hunter JM et al., editor: *Rehabilitation of the hand and upper extremity, vol 2*, ed 5, St. Louis, 2002, Mosby.
21. Madden JW, Arem A, DeVore G: A rational postoperative management program for metacarpophalangeal implant arthroplasty, *J Hand Surg Am* 2:358–366, 1976.
22. Malick MH: Upper extremity orthotics. In Hopkins, Smith, editors: *Willard and Spackman's occupational therapy*, Philadelphia, JB Lippincott.
23. McCaffery M, Pasero C: *Pain: clinical manual, pain numerical rating scale*, St. Louis, 1999, Mosby.
24. McLaughlin HL, Baab OD: Carpectomy, *Surg Clin North Am* 31:451–461, 1951.
25. McMaster M: The natural history of the rheumatoid metacarpophalangeal joint, *J Bone Joint Surg* 54B:687–697, 1972.
26. Melvin JL: *Rheumatic disease in the adult and child: occupational therapy and rehabilitation*, ed 3, Philadelphia, 1989, FA Davis.
27. Melvin JL: *Rheumatic disease: occupational therapy and rehabilitation*, Philadelphia, 1982, FA Davis.
28. Moberg E: *Circulatory impairment in splinting: splinting in hand therapy*, New York, 1982, Thieme-Stratton.
28a. Nalebuff EA: The rheumatoid thumb, *Clin Rheum Dis* 10:589–607, 1984.
29. Nalebuff EA, Millender LH: Reconstructive surgery and rehabilitation of the hand. In Kelley WM et al., editor: *Textbook of rheumatology, vol II*, Philadelphia, 1981, WB Saunders.
30. Occupational Therapy Department of Rancho Los Amigos National Rehabilitation Center: *Upper extremity surgeries for patients with arthritis; a pre and postoperative occupational therapy treatment guide*, Rancho Los Amigos Hospital/The Professional Staff Association of the Rancho Los Amigos Hospital, Downey, Ca.
31. Phillips CA: The management of patients with rheumatoid arthritis. In Hunter JM et al., editor: *Rehabilitation of the hand*, St. Louis, 1990, CV Mosby.
32. *Postoperative care for patients with silastic finger joint implants (Swanson design): MCP and IP joints*. Compiled by Leonard J, Swanson A, deGroot Swanson G, Dow Corning Wright, Arlington, Tenn, 1985.
33. Rancho Los Amigos National Rehabilitation Center: *The Arthritis Hand Assessment, and Typical Day Assessment (rev 8/01)*. Occupational Therapy Department, Rancho Los Amigos National Rehabilitation Center, Downey, Ca.
33a. Rizio L, Belsky MR: Finger deformities in rheumatoid arthritis, *Hand Clin* 22:531–540, 1996.
33b. Shapiro JS: The wrist in rheumatoid arthritis, *Hand Clin* 12:477–498, 1996.
34. Stack HG, Vaughan-Jackson OJ: The zig-zag deformity in the rheumatoid hand, 3:67, 1971.
35. Swanson AB: *Flexible/implant resection arthroplasty in the hand and extremities: consideration for postoperative bracing and rehabilitation for flexible implant arthroplasty of the finger*, 1973, St. Louis, CV Mosby.
36. Swanson AB: Pathogenesis of arthritic lesions. In Hunter JM et al., editor: *Rehabilitation of the hand*, St. Louis, 1995, CV Mosby.
37. Swanson AB: Pathomechanics of deformities in hand and wrist. In Hunter JM et al., editor: *Rehabilitation of the hand*, St. Louis, 1995, CV Mosby.
38. Swanson AB: *Reconstructive surgery in the arthritic hand and foot*. Clinical symposium, Summit, NJ, CIBA Pharmaceutical Company, 1979.
39. Swanson, AB: *Treatment considerations and resource materials for flexible (silicone) implant arthroplasty*, 1985. Orthopedic Research Department, Blodgett Memorial Medical Center, Grand Rapids, Mich, 1985.

40. Swanson AB, Maupin BK, Gajjar NV, deGroot Swanson G: Flexible implant arthroplasty in the proximal interphalangeal joint of the hand, *J Hand Surg* 10(6 Pt 1):796–805, 1985.

41. Swanson AB, deGroot Swanson G, Leonard J: Postoperative rehabilitation program in flexible implant arthroplasty of the digits. In Hunter JM, Schneider LH, Mackin EJ, Bell JA, editors: *Rehabilitation of the hand*, ed 2, St. Louis, 1984, CV Mosby.

42. Swanson AB, et al.: Upper limb joint replacement. In Nickel VL, editor: *Orthopedic rehabilitation*, New York, 1982, Churchill Livingstone.

42a. Taliesnik J: Rheumatoid arthritis of the wrist, *Hand Clin* 5:257–277, 1989.

42b. Thomsen NOB, Boeckstyns MEH, Leth-Espensen P: Value of dynamic splinting after replacement of the metacarpophalangeal joint in patients with rheumatoid arthritis, *Scand J Plast Reconstr Surg Hand Surg* 37(2):113–116, 2003.

43. Vainio K: Surgery of rheumatoid arthritis, *Surg Ann* 6:309–335, 1974.

44. Vainio K: Vainio arthroplasty of the metacarpophalangeal joints in rheumatoid arthritis, *J Hand Surg* 14A:367–368, 1989.

44a. Wilson RL: Rheumatoid arthritis of the hand, *Orthop Clin North Am* 17: 313–343, 1986.

45. Wilson RL, Carlblom ER: The rheumatoid metacarpophalangeal joint, *Hand Clin* 5:223, 1989, In Hunter JM, et al., editors: *Rheumatoid arthritis, Rehabilitation of the Hand and Upper Extremity, vol 2*, ed 5, Philadelphia, 2002, Mosby.

45a. Wilson YG, Sykes PJ, Niranjan NS: Long-term follow-up of Swanson's silastic arthroplasty of the metacarpophalangeal joints in rheumatoid arthritis, *J Hand Surg* 18B:81–91, 1993.

45b. Wilton JC: *Hand splinting: principles of design and fabrication*, Philadelphia, 1997, Saunders.

46. Yasuda, Lynn Y: Rheumatoid arthritis and osteoarthritis. In Trombly CA, Radomski MV, editors: *Occupational therapy for physical dysfunction*, ed 5, Philadelphia, 2002, Lippincott Williams & Wilkins.

Chapter

18

Orthoses for brachial plexus injuries

Keith A. Bengtson and Alexander Y. Shin

Key Points
- Many brachial plexus injuries are surgically treatable.
- The ideal time for surgical reconstruction is 3 to 6 months after the injury.
- Older injuries may be treatable using free muscle transfers to power elbow flexion and finger function.
- Shoulder orthoses can be used to counteract glenohumeral subluxation.
- Dynamic or static wrist orthoses can provide added function in lower trunk brachial plexus injuries.

Injuries to the brachial plexus can result from a variety of etiologies, including birth injuries, penetrating injuries, falls, and motor vehicle trauma. Closed injuries produce the majority of brachial plexus injuries and often are the result of traction, compression, or a combination of both. Traction injuries occur when the head and neck are violently moved away from the ipsilateral shoulder, often resulting in an injury to the C5 or C6 roots or upper trunk. Traction to the brachial plexus can result from too violent arm movement. When the arm is abducted over the head with significant force, traction will occur within the lower elements of the brachial plexus (C8–T1 roots or lower trunk). Compression injuries to the brachial plexus occur between the clavicle and the first rib and can be secondary to expanding hematomas or malignancies.

The number of brachial plexus injuries that occur each year is difficult to ascertain. However, with the advent of more extreme sporting activities, more powerful motor sports, and the increasing number of survivors of high-speed motor vehicle accidents (secondary to the introduction of the airbag), the number of plexus injuries continues to rise in many centers throughout the world.[3,6,7,10–,11,12,23,24,32]

Demographically, a majority of patients with brachial plexus injury are males between 15 and 25 years of age.[2,3,24,44] The type and mechanism of injury to the plexus can effectively be summed up by Narakas' law of seven seventies.[54] Based on his 18+ years of experience with more than 1,000 patients with plexus injuries, Narakas has estimated that 70% of traumatic brachial plexus injuries occur secondary to motor vehicle accidents, and of the vehicle accidents, 70% involve motorcycles or bicycles. Of the cycle riders, 70% have multiple injuries. Overall, 70% have supraclavicular lesions, and of those with supraclavicular lesions, 70% have at least one root avulsed. If patients have a root avulsed, at least 70% of these patients with have avulsions of the lower roots (C7, C8, or T1). Finally, of patients with lower root avulsion, nearly 70% will experience persistent pain.

Evaluation of brachial plexus injuries often is performed after the acute life-threatening injuries are treated. Once and if the patient is cooperative, a thorough physical examination should be performed to determine if the lesion is preganglionic (i.e., the root is avulsed directly from the spinal cord proximal to the dorsal root ganglion) or postganglionic (avulsed or injured distal the dorsal root ganglion, within the trunk, divisions, cords, or terminal branches). The differentiation of preganglionic versus postganglionic injury has significant prognostic and therapeutic implications. Preganglionic injury indicates that avulsion of the nerve root has occurred *proximal* to the spinal root ganglion; complete motor and sensory loss in the involved root and denervation of the deep paraspinal muscles of the neck have occurred (Fig. 18-1). Specific clinical findings are pathognomonic for root avulsions. Rhomboid paralysis is indicative of a C5 avulsion, serratus anterior paralysis is consistent with C5, C6, and C7 avulsion, and Horner syndrome (ptosis, miosis, and anhidrosis) is pathognomonic for C8,

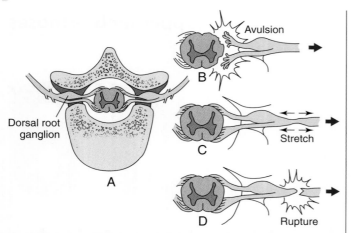

Fig. 18-1 Anatomy of the brachial plexus roots and types of injury. **A,** The roots are formed by the coalescence of the ventral (motor) and dorsal (sensory) rootlets as they pass through the spinal foramen. The dorsal root ganglion holds the cell bodies of the sensory nerves, whereas the cell bodies for the ventral nerves lie within the spinal cord. Three types of injury can occur: avulsion injuries pull the rootlets out of the spinal cord **(B)**; stretch injuries attenuate the nerve **(C)**; and ruptures result in a complete discontinuity of the nerve **(D)**. Injury to the nerve that occurs proximal to the dorsal root ganglion is called *preganglionic*; injury distal to the dorsal root ganglion is called *postganglionic*. (With permission from the Mayo Foundation.)

T1 avulsions (Fig. 18-2). Postganglionic injuries occur distal to the spinal ganglia and have a more favorable prognosis than do preganglionic injuries both for spontaneous recovery and for surgical reconstruction.

Historically, treatment recommendations for complete root avulsions have varied widely over the past 50 years, and the results of treatment have been fair to dismal. Following World War II, the standard approach was surgical reconstruction by shoulder fusion, elbow bone block, and finger tenodesis.[38] In the 1960s, transhumeral (above elbow) amputation combined with shoulder fusion in slight abduction and flexion was advocated.[31] The classic paper of Yeoman and Seddon[75] noted the tendency to become "one-handed" within 2 years of injury, which led to a dramatic reduction in successful outcomes regardless of the treatment approach. Their retrospective study revealed no "good" results from the primitive surgical reconstruction of that era but predominantly

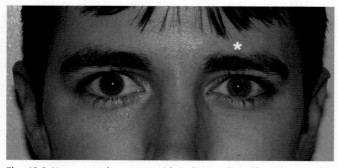

Fig. 18-2 Horner syndrome; asterisk indicates the affected eye. With avulsion of the T1 root, the first thoracic sympathetic ganglion is injured. The result is miosis (constricted pupil), ptosis (drooped lid), anhydrosis (dry eyes), and enophthalmos (sinking of the eyeball). This patient demonstrated miosis and ptosis after a lower trunk avulsion injury. (With permission from Mayo Foundation.)

"good" and fair" outcomes when amputation plus shoulder fusion were performed within 24 months of injury. They also noted that the loss of glenohumeral motion caused by brachial plexus injury limited the effectiveness of body-powered devices and that manual laborers seemed to accept hook prostheses much more readily than did office workers with similar injuries. Although these observations remain valid today, recent advances in brachial plexus reconstruction have yielded outcomes superior to historical results. A better understanding of the pathophysiology of nerve injury and repair as well as the recent advances in microsurgical techniques have allowed reliable restoration of elbow flexion in addition to useful prehension of the hand. The current advances in brachial plexus reconstruction, especially the microvascular reconstructive procedures, and the prosthetic/orthotic advances are the focus of this chapter.

Role of surgery

The two most important concepts in the surgical management of brachial plexus injuries are the understanding of the priorities of function restoration in the upper arm and the implication and timing of surgical reconstruction. The highest priority in restoration of the flail extremity is elbow flexion. This is followed by shoulder abduction, hand sensibility, wrist extension and finger flexion, wrist flexion and finger extension, and intrinsic function of the hand.

Timing of reconstruction or intervention depends on the mechanism of injury and the type of injury. Immediate exploration and primary repair of the injured portion of the brachial plexus is indicated in sharp open injuries. If the open injury is secondary to injury from a blunt object with avulsion of the nerve, the ends of the lacerated nerve should be tagged and a delayed repair performed 3 to 4 weeks later to excise the zone of nerve injury. Gunshot wounds should be observed, as a majority of these injuries are neurapraxic in nature. Early exploration and reconstruction (between 3 and 6 weeks) are indicated in cases where there is a high suspicion of root avulsion. Routine exploration (between 3 and 6 months) typically is performed in patients with partial injuries and partial paralysis in whom there is a suspicion for root avulsion. Delayed exploration is performed after 6 months, whereas late exploration is performed after 12 months. Delayed or late surgery often precludes successful direct repair or neurotization, as the time for the nerve to regenerate to the target muscles is greater than the survival time of the motor endplate after denervation.

In the most ideal situation, evaluation of the brachial plexus by electrodiagnostic studies should be performed by 3 to 4 weeks after injury, followed by computed tomographic (CT) myelography to evaluate the status of the cervical roots. The role of magnetic resonance imaging in the evaluation of the injured brachial plexus continues to evolve. It is best used for visualizing the dorsal and ventral rootlet but has been less accurate than CT myelography in determining root avulsion.[13,25,53] We prefer CT myelography; in our practice, it is the most sensitive and specific test for determining root avulsion injuries (Fig. 18-3). During the early postinjury course, consultation with a pain management team and hand therapist should be initiated as soon as possible to address the severe neuritic pain and prevent joint contractures.[43,47,50,51,54,61,62,72–75]

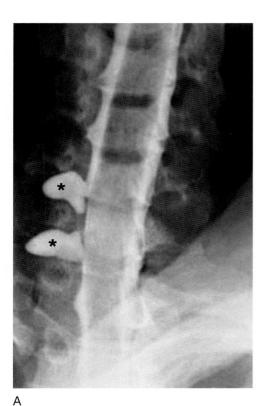

A

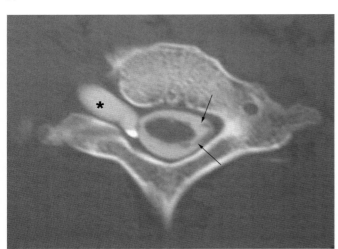

B

Fig. 18-3 Myelography and computed tomographic (CT) myelography can be instrumental in determining the level of nerve injury. If a pseudomeningocele is present, the likelihood of a nerve root avulsion is greater. Demonstrated in the myelogram (**A**; note asterisks) are multiple root avulsions that can be further evaluated by CT (**B**; note asterisk). (With permission from Mayo Foundation.)

Treatment

Several broad categories of surgical treatment of brachial plexus injuries include primary nerve repair, interposition nerve cable grafting, tendon/muscle transfers, neurotization, and free functioning muscle transfers. Tendon and muscle transfers should be delayed until it is evident that further recovery is unlikely. Primary repair is indicated in acute

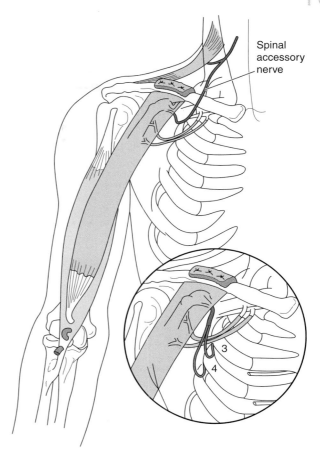

Fig. 18-4 A free gracilis muscle transfer can be used for elbow flexion. The proximal end of the gracilis is secured to the clavicle. Vascular inflow and outflow occur via the thoracoacromial trunk, and the muscle is powered by the spinal accessory or intercostal motor nerves. Distally the gracilis tendon is woven into the biceps tendon. (With permission from Mayo Foundation.)

sharp lacerations, whereas interposition nerve cable grafting is indicated in postganglionic injuries less than 6 months old. *Neurotization* refers to restoration of function by transfer of a functional but less important nerve to the distal but more important denervated nerve and is indicated for preganglionic lesions less than 6 months old. *Free functioning muscle transfer* refers to transplantation of a muscle and its neurovascular pedicle to a new location and neurotizing of the motor nerve to the flap (Fig. 18-4). Free functioning muscle transfers are indicated for delayed (between 3 and 6 months) or late presentations (>12 months)

Nerve grafts

Sources of donor nerve grafts include the sural nerves, ipsilateral cutaneous nerves, lateral cutaneous nerves of the thigh, saphenous nerve, and ulnar nerve (if C8 and T1 are avulsed). The size mismatch between the plexus and the individual nerve often requires use of multiple strands of nerves bundled together. Often these nerve segments are cabled together with fibrin glue and then sewn in place. In patients with complete brachial plexus avulsions, the ulnar nerve can be harvested as a vascularized nerve graft based on the superior collateral ulnar artery and can be effectively used as a free

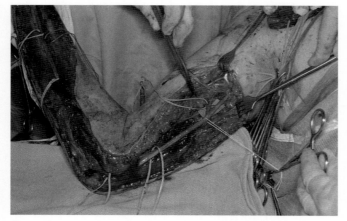

A

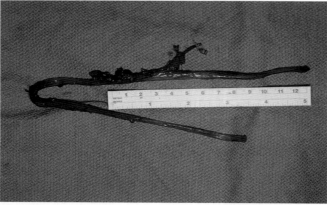

B

Fig. 18-5 With C8 and T1 avulsion, the ulnar nerve is unrepairable and can be used as a vascularized nerve graft, either as a pedicled graft or a free vascularized graft as is illustrated here. (With permission from Mayo Foundation.)

vascularized interposition nerve graft from neurotization sources to the median nerve (Fig. 18-5).

Neurotization

Intercostal nerves can be harvested from the third, fourth, fifth, and sixth ribs and can be effectively used to provide motor nerves to targeted muscles or sensation to injured sensory nerves.[15,19,30,37,48,52,66,71,75] Each intercostal nerve has a motor and sensory branch and can be easily harvested and neurotized to the target nerves (Fig. 18-6). Each intercostal nerve contains approximately 1,300 myelinated axons, so typically two to three intercostal nerves are used together. Occasionally the intercostal nerve requires elongation with a nerve graft because the distance to reach the target nerve/muscle is too long. The greatest disadvantage to using a nerve graft is that two lines of coaptation must be crossed. The advantage of using a nerve graft is that the intercostal nerve can be transected more proximally where the number of motor fibers is greater.

The spinal accessory nerve (cranial nerve XI) also can be used as a donor nerve.[4–6,15,16,23,24,27–29,37,48,52,64,66,71] The terminal branch of the spinal accessory nerve can be easily

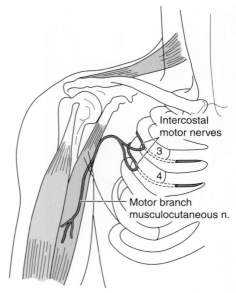

Fig. 18-6 Neurotization for elbow flexion with intercostal nerves. The motor branches from the intercostal nerves can be easily harvested and neurotized to the motor branch of the musculocutaneous nerve to the biceps. (With permission from Mayo Foundation.)

harvested and has approximately 1,700 myelinated axons. It is an excellent donor nerve for the suprascapular or axillary nerve to restore shoulder stability or neurotize a free functioning muscle transfer (Fig. 18-7).

The ipsilateral phrenic nerve can be used; however, prior to its use the diaphragmatic and pulmonary function must be assessed.[15,52,66] Hemidiaphragmatic paralysis is an absolute contraindication to phrenic neurotization. Patients with severe chest injury or multiple fractured ribs must be carefully evaluated with respect to pulmonary function because harvest of the phrenic nerve can further jeopardize

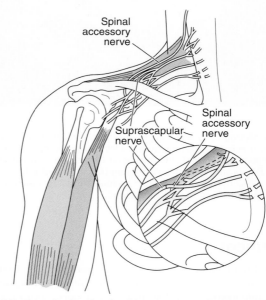

Fig. 18-7 Neurotization for shoulder abduction with the spinal accessory nerve can be performed in the supraclavicular exposure. The terminal branch of the spinal accessory nerve is used, thereby preserving some trapezius function. (With permission from Mayo Foundation.)

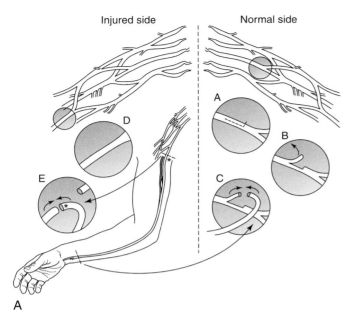

Injured side   Normal side

A

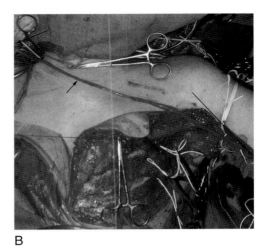

B

Fig. 18-8 Contralateral C7 (or as we prefer a hemicontralateral C7) nerve transfer via a vascularized ulnar nerve graft (in cases of complete C5-T1 avulsions) can be used to bring a large number of motor axons into the injured side. **A**, The contralateral hemi-C7 transfer can effectively be used with a vascularized ulnar nerve graft to reinnervate the median nerve for finger flexion and sensation. **B**, Clinical example of the vascularized ulnar nerve reaching across the chest to the contralateral C7. (With permission from Mayo Foundation.)

pulmonary function. Simultaneous intercostal nerve and phrenic nerve harvest results in early postoperative restriction of pulmonary function.[35] Phrenic nerve harvest is contraindicated in young infants and in patients with any diaphragm paralysis. The phrenic nerve is best suited for neurotizing the suprascapular nerve.

One advance associated with a controversial donor nerve is use of the uninjured contralateral C7 root. Its use was first described by Gu et al.[36] in 1992 and then by Chuang et al.[18] in 1993. These authors reported that transaction of the uninjured contralateral C7 did not produce significant functional loss. By elongating the C7 root from the contralateral side with a vascularized ulnar nerve graft to the ipsilateral median nerve, the contralateral C7 root can be used to neurotize the median nerve or lateral cord. Use of the anterior superior portion of C7 also has been reported and has lessened morbidity compared to use of the entire contralateral C7 root (Fig. 18-8).[68] Donor site morbidity is minimal, initially resulting in digital paresthesias in the C7 distribution and mild weakness of pectoralis, triceps, and/or wrist extension.[18,34,68] Over a period of 3 to 6 months, the paresthesias diminish, as does the motor weakness. Typically functional loss is limited to a reduction of sensibility of the index finger and some reduction in force of the triceps and finger extension.

Use of portions of an ipsilateral functioning nerve was described by Oberlin et al.[56,57] In patients with loss of the musculocutaneous nerve but preserved ulnar nerve function (i.e., upper trunk injury or C5-6 avulsions), several fascicles of ulnar motor nerves can be transferred to the biceps motor branch of the musculocutaneous nerve at the midhumerus level without significant loss of distal motor or sensory function to the ulnar nerve mediated muscles of the hand (Fig. 18-9). This is possible because individual ulnar nerve fascicles at this level are mixed, containing extrinsic and intrinsic motor fibers as well as sensory fibers. The results are excellent, and donor site morbidity is very low.

Other donor nerve sources for neurotization include the cervical plexus, long thoracic nerve, hypoglossal nerve, and nerve root stumps of postganglionic avulsions at the root-trunk level.

Free functioning muscle transfer

Advances in microsurgical techniques have led to innovations in surgical reconstruction of the upper extremity following brachial plexus injury. Reinnervation of the biceps and shoulder musculature using both nerve grafting and transfer techniques has resulted in reliable restoration of elbow flexion and shoulder abduction when surgical intervention occurs within 6 to 9 months of injury.[17–19,41,42,48,49,55,63,67,71] In many instances, however, delay in treatment or complete avulsion of the brachial plexus limits the surgeon's reconstructive options.

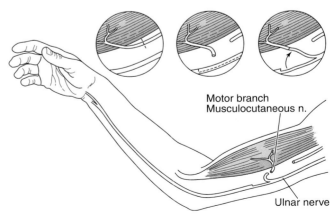

Motor branch
Musculocutaneous n.

Ulnar nerve

Fig. 18-9 When the ulnar nerve is normal (i.e., upper trunk injury, sparing C8 and T1) a fascicle can be transferred to the motor branch of the biceps to obtain elbow flexion. (With permission from Mayo Foundation.)

Free functioning muscle transfer refers to moving a muscle and its motor nerve to a donor site. The number of available extraplexal donor nerves is limited, and timing of reconstructive procedures becomes critical. Despite favorable results reported for early nerve grafting and transfer techniques, attempts at restoring function to long-standing denervated muscle have not been generally successful.[19,49,63,67] This has resulted in the use of free functioning muscle transfers in conjunction with extraplexal motor nerve transfer to restore function in the setting of brachial plexus avulsions or when time from injury to surgery is more than one year.[1,22,24,26,28,45,46] Free muscle transfers provide reliable elbow flexion when treatment delay prevents direct graft or biceps neurotization and proximal muscle strength is insufficient to allow tendon transfers.[1,9,26,24,29,41] In this method, the circulation of the transferred muscle is restored with microsurgical technique, vessels are anastomosed, and the motor nerve is neurotized with one of the nerves described above. Within several months, the transferred muscle begins to become innervated by the donor nerve, eventually gains independence, and begins to function. A variety of muscles can be transferred for function, including the latissimus dorsi (thoracodorsal nerve), rectus femoris (femoral nerve), and gracilis (anterior division of the obturator nerve). Of these muscles, the gracilis has become one of the most commonly used for brachial plexus reconstruction because of its proximally based muscle neurovascular pedicle, which allows earlier reinnervation, and its length, which can reach into the forearm for hand reanimation. The gracilis can be used for restoration of biceps function, especially if presentation is delayed (Fig. 18-10),[16,27] or as a double muscle transfer in the novel and revolutionary Doi procedure for restoration of elbow flexion, wrist extension, and finger flexion in the acute setting.[22–24]

Role of orthoses and prostheses

Shoulder support

The vast majority of brachial plexus injuries involve denervation of the shoulder's supporting musculature. A weak shoulder girdle allows subluxation of the glenohumeral joint. The shoulder joint is inherently unstable because of the very small contact surface between the head of the humerus and the glenoid fossa. Although the capsule and ligaments play a supporting role in joint stability, the majority of support is provided through active contraction of the supraspinatus muscle. Therefore, significant weakening of the supraspinatus leads to shoulder subluxation. This subluxation apparently causes pain by applying traction to the soft tissues of the shoulder, such as the supporting ligaments and upper extremity nerves. Historically, one of the goals of orthoses in brachial plexus injuries has been to support the weight of the upper limb and thus ease the traction forces on the shoulder. Secondarily, such support may assist in edema control.

A shoulder sling is the most readily available and well-known device used to support the arm. Unfortunately, a simple sling often is uncomfortable where the strap drapes over the opposite shoulder and neck area, and it may be a biomechanically unsound method for protecting against shoulder subluxation. Additionally, contractures are encouraged by holding the upper limb with the elbow flexed and the shoulder adducted and internally rotated.

In an excellent discussion on the biomechanics of controlling shoulder subluxation, Cool[21] suggests that the only reasonable point of upward force transmission is at the elbow joint. In order to transmit an upward force on the humerus, he suggests using a fulcrum point at the level of the proximal forearm. With this fulcrum, the downward weight of the hand, wrist, and distal forearm acts like a teeter-totter to push upward on the elbow and humerus. Using this paradigm exposes the simple sling as an inefficient method for exerting an upward force on the humerus because the simple sling exerts its force along the whole length of the forearm, wrist, and hand rather than on a single fulcrum point (Fig. 18-11).

The easily available alternative to the simple sling is the hemisling. The hemisling consists of two small 4- to 6-inch cradles attached by a long strap (Fig. 18-12). One cradle holds the proximal forearm and the other the wrist and hand. Ideally, the proximal forearm cradle acts as the fulcrum point described by Cool.[21] The weight of the hand, wrist, and distal forearm exert an upward force on the humerus. However, this concept relies on a certain amount of friction as the strap passes over the shoulder and neck. With friction, greater force can be maintained on the proximal forearm cradle than on the hand/wrist cradle. If there is free movement of the strap at the shoulder and neck, then the two forces equalize, and the situation is similar to the simple sling where the upward force is transmitted throughout the length of the forearm, wrist, and hand. Shoulder caps have been suggested to hold the weight of the arm using a cuff over the upper arm. The upward force on the arm is supplied by friction between the cuff and the upper arm. This is not an ideal situation with an insensate limb.

The two remaining devices that have attempted to address this problem are much more complex. The proximal forearm fulcrum can be established from above using some type of shoulder cap or from below using a support from the pelvic crest. This latter hip cap or pelvic support was popularized in California by Schottstaedt and Richards in the 1950s.[8,59,65] This device is sometimes referred to as a *gunslinger splint*. Clearly, this was a large and cumbersome device. A hip cap was attached be a belt on the waist and rested on the pelvic crest. A solid bar extended from the hip cap to the proximal forearm of the injured side. This bar could hold the humerus in neutral adduction or up to 45 degrees of abduction. Unfortunately, the hip cap tended to shift out of alignment whenever the wearer changed position from standing to sitting and back again. No mention of the hip cap device was found in the literature after 1978.

The alternative to the hip cap is the shoulder cap (Fig. 18-13). The shoulder cap applies the fulcrum to the proximal forearm from above. This is a refinement of the sling and hemisling designs. The shoulder cap fits snugly over the acromioclavicular joint region and is held in place by a strap that fits under the contralateral axilla. The cap can be kept from sliding medially either by extending the cap laterally over the deltoid or by a second strap under the ipsilateral axilla if necessary. Sometimes the two axillary straps are held together by a separate chest belt. Unlike the hemisling, the suspending straps are held in place by more than friction. As such, the suspending straps can exert their force on the proximal

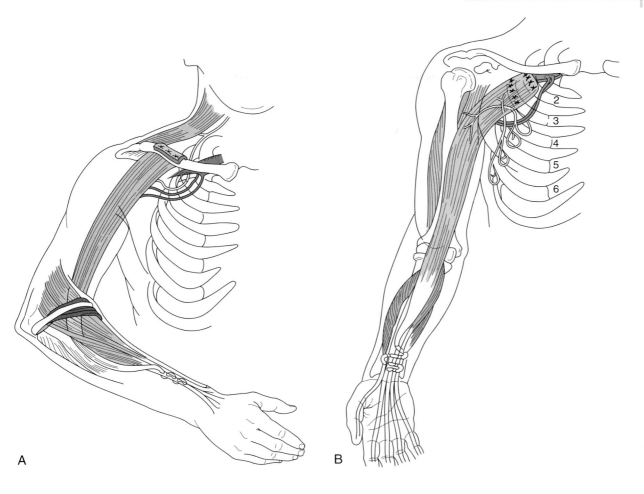

A

B

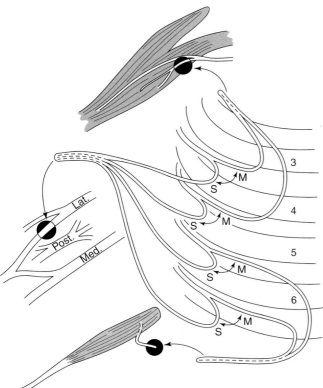

C

Fig. 18-10 A, Stage I Doi free gracilis muscle transfer. In the first stage, the brachial plexus is explored, and a free functioning gracilis is harvested and neurotized by the spinal accessory nerve and anastomosed to the thoraco-acromial trunk. The gracilis is attached proximally to the clavicle, routed distally under the brachioradialis and flexor carpi ulnaris pulley, and woven into the wrist extensors. **B, C,** Stage II Doi free gracilis muscle transfer. The second stage is performed 2 months after the first stage. A second gracilis muscle and motor and sensory intercostal nerves are harvested from beneath the third to sixth ribs. The gracilis is attached proximally to the second rib and neurotized with two of the intercostal motor nerves. The sensory intercostal nerves are neurotized to the median nerve for palmar sensation. The vascular supply occurs via the thoracodorsal artery and vein. The remaining two motor intercostals are used to neurotize the triceps. (With permission from Mayo Foundation.)

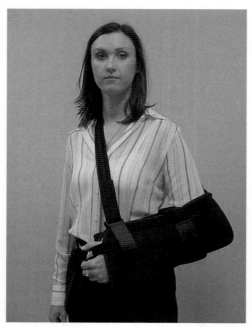

Fig. 18-11 Standard sling.

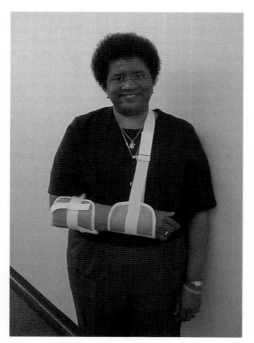

Fig. 18-12 Hemisling.

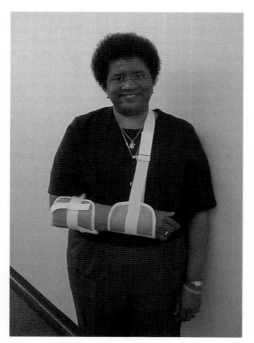

Fig. 18-13 Wilmer carrying orthosis with arm trough.

forearm in a more stable manner.[21,32,33,73] Unfortunately, one-handed patients may have difficulty donning and doffing such a device because it has more straps and adjustments. Newer designs have addressed this problem with fewer straps and an adjustable locking device at the elbow.

In the end, the decision must be made between an imperfect simple device (the hemisling) and a more stable complicated device (the shoulder cap). The hemisling has the advantages of cost and ease of donning and doffing. The shoulder cap offers the advantages of more comfort and greater stability. The

patient must decide whether or not he or she is willing to spend the extra money and the considerable more time in donning, doffing, and adjusting the shoulder cap device.

Shoulder and elbow support

Many brachial plexus injuries primarily involve the upper and middle trunks of the plexus (C4-7 nerve root distributions). These patients have paralysis or weakness of the shoulder girdle musculature as well as the elbow joint. Elbow flexion is affected more often than elbow extension. If the lower trunk or lower nerve roots (C7, C8, and T1) are preserved, then patients retain control of hand and wrist movements and possibly of elbow extension (triceps). These patients need support of the shoulder and elbow without encumbering the wrist and hand.

The elbow can be controlled by a ratchet device, a cable-powered device, or even a myoelectric device.[58] The ratcheted elbow locks the elbow in five different positions and is placed in position by either the opposite arm or by leveraging it against a table or other object.[32,33,73] A cable-controlled elbow is similar to an above-elbow amputation prosthesis and is powered by protraction/retraction of the opposite shoulder. If the triceps is intact, then elastic tubing or springs can be used to suspend the forearm from a shoulder cap in an antigravity fashion.[40] This allows active extension against the elastic bands with the intact triceps. Flexion is achieved passively by the elastic bands.

Unfortunately, allowing the elbow to move results in loss of control of glenohumeral subluxation. Therefore, the shoulder remains subluxed and must withstand the added weight of the orthosis. Historically, the hip cap design addressed this problem. However, the hip cap had many problems and is rarely used. A variation on the hip cap or gunslinger splint is the balanced forearm orthosis.[20] This nonmobile orthosis attaches to a table edge, chair armrest, or directly onto a wheelchair. The forearm and hand rest in a trough that moves freely on a set of mobile arms. Use of this device is limited to the situation where the patient is in a fixed position for long periods of time, such as sitting at a dinner table or work desk.

Flail arm

Many cases of brachial plexopathy involve damage to the whole plexus resulting in a completely flail arm. In such cases, an orthosis can be chosen to immobilize and protect the arm or to restore some amount of function to the arm. Orthoses that immobilize and protect the arm are essentially modifications to the shoulder immobilizers discussed above. Many patients choose to use a simple sling or a hemisling. In general, these options work quite well but may not control subluxation as well as possible. The alternative is the shoulder cap, which must be attached distally to a forearm trough in order to establish the fulcrum point for controlling subluxation. In the case of the flail arm, the trough usually extends all the way to the fingertips in order to control edema and provide protection to the whole extremity (Fig. 18-14). Generally, the wrist is positioned in 20 to 30 degrees of extension, the metacarpophalangeal joints in 60 degrees of flexion, and the interphalangeal joints in 10 degrees of gentle flexion.

Another goal of prosthetics in brachial plexus injury is adding function to the affected limb. Designs have largely borrowed from those used for proximal upper limb amputation, with power supplied by an intact trapezius muscle shrug or from the opposite arm. The distal prosthesis then encompasses rather than replaces the distal upper limb. This is termed a *functional arm orthosis* (FAO). Historically, the Schottstaedt-Richardson design was used in the polio population. The device incorporated multiple controls for the shoulder, elbow, and terminal device. The hand was bypassed from a functional standpoint, and a standard prosthetic terminal device was attached directly to the forearm cuff. These FAOs were powered by the opposite shoulder and even by a foot cable. Support for the shoulder and the weight of the FAO were provided by a pelvic cap.[8,59,65] The polio population probably was better suited for these devices than brachial plexus patients because the polio patients had intact sensation in the affected limb.

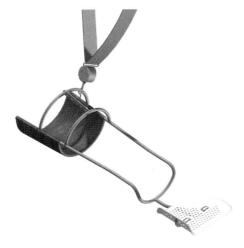

Fig. 18-14 Wilmer carrying orthosis with hand support for flail limb.

More contemporary FAOs are supported by a shoulder cap and have a simpler design. Wynn Parry has suggested an FAO for the flail arm that consists of a shoulder cap, a ratcheted elbow joint that locks into five different positions, and a forearm trough that is fitted with an artificial hand appliance.[73] The distal appliance is powered by protraction and retraction of the opposite shoulder.

Unfortunately, this approach has many drawbacks. Most significant is the problem of prosthetic weight. As mentioned earlier, the patient already has problems with subluxation of the shoulder secondary to the traction weight of the denervated upper limb. The added weight of the prosthesis compounds this difficulty because control of shoulder subluxation is sacrificed by incorporating a mobile elbow. Another difficulty with this approach is the insensate upper limb. Most brachial plexus injuries severely compromise sensation to the upper limb. Skin breakdown can be a severe and insurmountable problem. First, the area where the prosthesis contacts the skin must be examined regularly to ensure that areas of pressure ulceration do not develop. Second, any functional use of the limb must be tempered by the possibility of damage to the extremity. Not only may the extremity lack protective sensation, it also may lack proprioception to monitor speed and angle of movement.

Ultimately, one must determine how the FAO is to be used. If the FAO will used as a permanent device allowing for bimanual function, then the orthosis must be fitted to the patient as soon as possible after injury. As with upper extremity prosthetic use, the earlier the patient learns to use the FAO, the more likely he or she will use the device in the long term. If the patient learns to become one-handed, then he or she will be unwilling to accept use of the FAO. Perry et al.[59] reported on seven patients with complete plexus injuries who were fitted with FAOs supported by a pelvic cap or gunslinger device. The patients reported some pain relief with use of the device. However, once the pain remitted, the patients discarded use of the brace. The longest period that the FAO was worn was 2.5 months. Wynn Parry[73] suggests a much better compliance rate with FAOs using a shoulder cap support. On follow-up of 200 patients fitted with a flail arm FAO, he reported that 60% of patients were "regularly using the splint for work, hobbies, or both." However, a subsequent abstract by Chu et al.[14] reported that externally powered FAOs were "singularly unsuccessful."

Another philosophy is to use the FAO as a temporary device. In this case, the orthosis is used strictly during the recovery period until function returns.[69] The goals of using the brace are to (1) enhance healing of the brachial plexus, (2) relieve pain, (3) maintain motor function, (4) prevent elbow deformity, and (5) maintain bimanual activities.[8] After 18 to 24 months of recovery, the brace is discarded. Others suggest use of a whole series of orthoses, changing the type of brace used as the patient recovers strength in various muscle groups.[33] This approach requires close follow-up and multiple visits for splint assessment and refitting. Whether this approach affects long-term outcome is unclear.

Hand and wrist support

The lower trunk of the brachial plexus is less commonly injured. Patients with this injury may have preservation of shoulder and elbow function with loss of wrist and hand

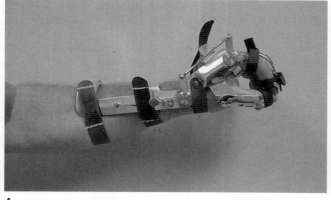 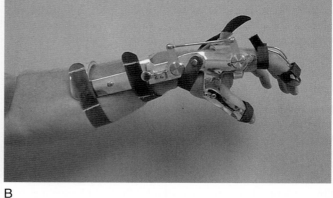

A   B

Fig. 18-15 Hinged wrist tenodesis splint for finger flexion and grasping.

control. In these cases, the principles of shoulder support and functional enhancement do not apply. Rather, these patients require some form of orthosis to stabilize the wrist and restore grip and pinch functions. If the patient has preservation of wrist extension (C7), then a tenodesis splint is appropriate (Fig. 18-15). This orthosis harnesses the power of wrist extension and applies it to finger and thumb flexion. Many designs using hinges or small cables are available. In most cases, sensory loss is limited to the ring and small fingers, so protective sensation and proprioception are not an issue.

Amputation with prosthetic fitting

Clearly, the orthotic options for severe brachial plexus injuries have many drawbacks, and many patients choose not to use these FAOs. Because of these drawbacks, many authors have advocated a more controversial approach that involves amputation of the involved limb above or below the elbow with immediate prosthetic fitting.[39,44,60,62,70] Unfortunately, in order to ensure compliance with the prostheses, the amputation must take place fairly soon after the initial injury. However, the sooner this irreversible step is taken, the less opportunity is available for assessing for any possible neurologic recovery. The preferred window of opportunity for brachial plexus reconstructive surgery is the 4- to 6-month period following injury. However, the optimal time for upper extremity prosthetic fitting is less than 2 months postinjury.[44] Therefore, the decision regarding amputation would have to be made before adequate assessment of possible neurological recovery has been made. This appears to be an insurmountable problem.

One misconception held by many patients is that amputation of a painful upper extremity after brachial plexus injury will relieve the neuropathic pain associated with the problem. Unfortunately, no studies have shown any benefit in pain control following amputation in this population.[60] Therefore, it must be made clear to the patient that such an amputation is not a treatment for pain.

Conclusion

Use of orthoses for brachial plexus injuries is in a state of flux. As the surgical treatment improves, the need for these orthoses becomes more limited. Most of the orthoses discussed in this chapter are of historical interest only. The engineering and biomechanical principles involved in these orthoses, however, are significant, especially when trying to solve the same biomechanical problems using surgical procedures rather than orthoses. In prescribing these devices, one must be aware of the significant costs involved in both therapist's time and splint fabrication.

References

1. Akasaka Y, Hara T, Takahashi M: Free muscle transplantation combined with intercostal nerve crossing for reconstruction of elbow flexion and wrist extension in brachial plexus injuries, *Microsurgery* 12:345–351, 1991.
2. Allieu Y: Evolution of our indications for neurotization. Our concept of functional restoration of the upper limb after brachial plexus injuries, *Chir Main* 18:165–166, 1999.
3. Allieu Y, Cenac P: Is surgical intervention justifiable for total paralysis secondary to multiple avulsion injuries of the brachial plexus? *Hand Clin* 4:609–618, 1988.
4. Allieu Y, Cenac P: Neurotization via the spinal accessory nerve in complete paralysis due to multiple avulsion injuries of the brachial plexus, *Clin Orthop* 237:67–74, 1988.
5. Allieu Y, Chammas M, Picot MC: Paralysis of the brachial plexus caused by supraclavicular injuries in the adult. Long-term comparative results of nerve grafts and transfers, *Rev Chir Orthop Reparatrice Appar Mot* 83:51–59, 1997.
6. Allieu Y, Privat JM, Bonnel F: Paralysis in root avulsion of the brachial plexus. Neurotization by the spinal accessory nerve, *Clin Plast Surg* 11:133–136, 1984.
7. Azze RJ, Mattar Junior J, Ferreira MC, Starck R, Canedo AC: Extraplexal neurotization of brachial plexus, *Microsurgery* 15:28–32, 1994.
8. Barber LM: Combined motor and peripheral sensory insufficiency, *Phys Ther* 58:287–294, 1978.
9. Berger A, Flory P-J, Schaller E: Muscle transfers in brachial plexus lesions, *J Reconstr Microsurg* 6:113–116, 1990.
10. Brandt KE, Mackinnon SE: A technique for maximizing biceps recovery in brachial plexus reconstruction, *J Hand Surg* 18A:726–733, 1993.
11. Brunelli G: Direct neurotization of severely damaged muscles, *J Hand Surg* 7A:572–579, 1982.
12. Brunelli G, Monini L: Direct muscular neurotization, *J Hand Surg* 10A(6 Pt 2):993–997, 1985.
13. Carvalho GA, Nikkhah G, Matthies C, Penkert G, Samii M: Diagnosis of root avulsions in traumatic brachial plexus injuries: value of computerized tomography myelography and magnetic resonance imaging, *J Neurosurg* 86:69–76, 1997.
14. Chu DS, Lehneis HR, Wilson R: Functional arm orthosis for complete brachial plexus lesion, *Arch Phys Med Rehabil* 68:594, 1987.
15. Chuang DC: Neurotization procedures for brachial plexus injuries, *Hand Clin* 11:633–645, 1995.
16. Chung DC, Carver N, Wei FC: Results of functioning free muscle transplantation for elbow flexion, *J Hand Surg* 21:1071–1077, 1996.

17. Chuang DC, Lee GW, Hashen F, Wei FC: Restoration of shoulder abduction by nerve transfer in avulsion brachial plexus injury: evaluation of 99 patients with various nerve transfers, *Plast Reconstr Surg* 96:122–128, 1995.

18. Chuang DC, Wei FC, Noordhoff MS: Cross-chest C7 nerve grafting followed by free muscle transplantations for the treatment of total avulsed brachial plexus injuries: a preliminary report, *Plast Reconstr Surg* 92:717–725, 1993; discussion 726–727.

19. Chuang DC, Yeh MC, Wei FC: Intercostal nerve transfer of the musculocutaneous nerve in avulsed brachial plexus injuries: evaluation of 66 patients, *J Hand Surg* 17A:822–828, 1992.

20. Chyatte SB, Long II C, Vignos PJ: The balanced forearm orthosis in muscular dystrophy, *Arch Phys Med Rehabil* 46:633–636, 1965.

21. Cool JC: Biomechanics of orthoses for the subluxed shoulder, *Prosthet Orthot Int* 13:90–96, 1989.

22. Doi K: New reconstructive procedure for brachial plexus injury, *Clin Plast Surg* 24:75–85, 1997.

23. Doi K, Kuwata N, Muramatsu K, Hottori Y, Kawai S: Double muscle transfer for upper extremity reconstruction following complete avulsion of the brachial plexus, *Hand Clin* 15:757–767, 1999.

24. Doi K, Muramatsu K, Hattori Y, et al: Restoration of prehension with the double free muscle technique following complete avulsion of the brachial plexus. Indications and long-term results, *J Bone Joint Surg* 82A:652–666, 2000.

25. Doi K, Otsuka K, Okamoto Y, Fujii H, Hattori Y, Baliarsing AS: Cervical nerve root avulsion in brachial plexus injuries: magnetic resonance imaging classification and comparison with myelography and computerized tomography myelography, *J Neurosurg* 96(3 suppl):277–284, 2002.

26. Doi K, Sakai K, Fuchigami Y, Kawai S: Reconstruction of irreparable brachial plexus injuries with reinnervated free-muscle transfer. Case report, *J Neurosurg* 85:174–177, 1996.

27. Doi K, Sakai K, Ihara K, Abe Y, Kawai S, Kurafuji Y: Reinnervated free muscle transplantation for extremity reconstruction, *Plast Reconstr Surg* 91:872–883, 1993.

28. Doi K, Sakai K, Kuwata N, Ihara K, Kawai S: Double free-muscle transfer to restore prehension following complete brachial plexus avulsion, *J Hand Surg* 20A:408–414, 1995.

29. Doi K, Sakai K, Kuwata N, Ihara K, Kawai S: Reconstruction of finger and elbow function after complete avulsion of the brachial plexus, *J Hand Surg* 16A:796–803, 1991.

30. Dolenc VV: Intercostal neurotization of the peripheral nerves in avulsion plexus injuries, *Clin Plast Surg* 11:143–147, 1984.

31. Fletcher I: Traction lesions of the brachial plexus, *Hand* 1:129–136, 1969.

32. Frampton VM: Management of brachial plexus lesions, *J Hand Ther* April:115–120, 1988.

33. Frampton VM: Management of brachial plexus lesions, *Physiotherapy* 70:388–392, 1984.

34. Gu YD, Chen DS, Zhang GM, et al: Long-term functional results of contralateral C7 transfer, *J Reconstr Microsurg* 14:57–59, 1998.

35. Gu YD, Ma MK: Use of the phrenic nerve for brachial plexus reconstruction, *Clin Orthop* 323:119–121, 1996.

36. Gu YD, Zhang GM, Chen DS, Yan JG, Cheng XM, Chen L: Seventh cervical nerve root transfer from the contralateral healthy side for treatment of brachial plexus root avulsion, *J Hand Surg* 17B:518–521, 1992.

37. Hattori Y, Doi K, Fuchigami Y, Abe Y, Kawai S: Experimental study on donor nerves for brachial plexus injury: comparison between the spinal accessory nerve and the intercostal nerve, *Plast Reconstr Surg* 100:900–906, 1997.

38. Hendry HAM: The treatment of residual paralysis after brachial plexus lesions, *J Bone Joint Surg* 31B:42, 1949.

39. Hoffer MM, Braun R, Hsu J, Mitani M, Temes K: Functional recovery and orthopedic management of brachial plexus palsies, *JAMA* 246:2467–2470, 1981.

40. Kohlmeyer K, Weber C, Yarkony G: A new orthosis for central cord syndrome and brachial plexus injuries, *Arch Phys Med Rehabil* 71:1006–1009, 1990.

41. Krakauer JD, Wood MB: Intercostal nerve transfer brachial plexopathy, *J Hand Surg* 19A:829–835, 1994.

42. Leechavengvongs S, Witoon CK, Uerpairojkit C, Thuvasethakul P, Ketmalasiri W: Nerve transfer to biceps muscle using a part of the ulnar nerve in brachial plexus injury (upper arm type): a report of 32 cases, *J Hand Surg* 23A:711–716, 1998.

43. Leffert R: Rehabilitation of the patient with a brachial plexus injury, *Neurol Clin* 5:559–568, 1987.

44. Malone JM, Leal JM, Underwood J, Childers SJ. Brachial plexus injury management through upper extremity amputation with immediate postoperative prostheses, *Arch Phys Med Rehabil* 63:89–91, 1982.

45. Manktelow RT: Functioning muscle transplantation. In Manktelow RT, editor: *Microvascular reconstruction: anatomy, applications and surgical techniques*, 1986, Springer-Verlag.

46. Manktelow RT, Zuker RM, McKee NH: Functioning free muscle transplantation, *J Hand Surg* 9A:32–39, 1984.

47. Meredith J, Taft G, Kaplan P: Diagnosis and treatment of the hemiplegic patient with brachial plexus injury, *Am J Occup Ther* 35:656–660, 1981.

48. Merrell GA, Barrie KA, Katz DL, Wolfe SW: Results of nerve transfer techniques for restoration of shoulder and elbow function in the context of a meta-analysis of the English literature, *J Hand Surg Am* 26:303–314, 2001.

49. Mikami Y, Nagano A, Ochiai N, Yamamoto S: Results of nerve grafting for injuries of the axillary and suprascapular nerves, *J Bone Joint Surg* 79B:527–531, 1997.

50. Millesi H: Brachial plexus injuries: management and results, *Clin Plast Surg* 11:115–120, 1984.

51. Millesi H: Trauma involving the brachial plexus. In Omer G, Spionner M, editors: *Management of peripheral nerve problems*, Philadelphia, 1980, WB Saunders.

52. Nagano A, Yamamoto S, Mikami Y: Intercostal nerve transfer to restore upper extremity functions after brachial plexus injury, *Ann Acad Med Singapore* 24(4 suppl):42–45, 1995.

53. Nakamura T, Yabe Y, Horiuchi Y, Takayama S: Magnetic resonance myelography in brachial plexus injury, *J Bone Joint Surg Br* 79:764–769, 1997.

54. Narakas A: The treatment of brachial plexus injuries, *Znt Orthop* 9:29–36, 1985.

55. Narakas A, Hentz VR: Neurotization in brachial plexus injuries: indication and results. *Clin Orthop* 237:43–56, 1988.

56. Oberlin C, Alnot JY, Comtet JJ: Vascularized nerve trunk grafts. Technic and results of 27 cases. *Ann Chir Main* 8:316–323, 1989.

57. Oberlin C, Beal D, Leechavengvongs S, Salon A, Dauge MC, Sarcy JJ: Nerve transfer to biceps muscle using a part of ulnar nerve for C5-C6 avulsion of the brachial plexus: anatomical study and report of four cases. *J Hand Surg Am* 19:232–237, 1994.

58. Ogce F, Ozyalcin H: A myoelectrically controlled shoulder-elbow orthosis for unrecovered brachial plexus injury, *Prosthet Orthot Int* 24:252–255, 2000.

59. Perry J, Hsu J, Barber LM, Hoffer MM: Orthoses in patients with brachial plexus injuries, *Arch Phys Med Rehabil* 55:134–137, 1974.

60. Ransford A, Hughes S: Complete brachial plexus lesions, *J Bone Joint Surg* 59B:417–420, 1977.

61. Robinson C: Brachial plexus lesions. Part I: management, *Br J Occup Ther* 49:147–150, 1986.

62. Rorabeck C: The management of the flail upper extremity in brachial plexus injuries, *J Trauma* 20:491–493, 1980.

63. Ruch DS, Friedman AH, Nunley JA: The restoration of elbow flexion with intercostal nerve transfers, *Clin Orthop* 314:95–103, 1995.

64. Samardzic M, Grujicic D, Antunovic V, Joksimovic M: Reinnervation of avulsed brachial plexus using the spinal accessory nerve, *Surg Neurol* 33:7–11, 1990.

65. Schottstaedt E, Robinson G: Functional bracing of the arm, *J Bone Joint Surg* 38A:477–499, 1956.

66. Songcharoen P: Brachial plexus injury in Thailand: a report of 520 cases, *Microsurgery* 16:35–39, 1995.

67. Songcharoen P, Mahaisavariya B, Chotigavanich C: Spinal accessory neurotization for restoration of elbow flexion in avulsion injuries of the brachial plexus, *J Hand Surg Am* 21:387–390, 1996.

68. Songcharoen P, Wongtrakul S, Mahaisavariya B, Spinner RJ: Hemi-contralateral C7 transfer to median nerve in the treatment of root avulsion brachial plexus injury, *J Hand Surg Am* 26:1058–1064, 2001.

69. Stanwood J, Kraft G: Diagnosis and management of brachial plexus injuries, *Arch Phys Med Rehabil* 52:52–60, 1971.

70. Van Laere M, Duyvejonck R, Leus P, Claessens H: A prosthetic appliance for a patient with a brachial plexus injury and forearm amputation: a case report, *Am J Occup Ther* 31:309–312, 1977.

71. Waikakul S, Wongtragul S, Vanadurongwan V: Restoration of elbow flexion in brachial plexus avulsion injury: comparing spinal accessory nerve transfer with intercostal nerve transfer, *J Hand Surg* 24A:571–577, 1999.

72. Wynn Parry CB: Brachial plexus injuries, *Br J Hosp Med* 32:130–139, 1984.

73. Wynn Parry CB: Rehabilitation of patients following traction lesions of the brachial plexus, *Clin Plast Surg* 11:173–179, 1984.

74. Wynn Parry CB: The management of injuries to the brachial plexus, *Proc R Soc Med* 67:488–490, 1974.

75. Yeoman PM, Seddon HJ: Brachial plexus injuries: treatment of the flail arm, *J Bone Joint Surg* 43B:493–500, 1961.

Chapter

19

Functional bracing of selected upper limb fractures

Loren L. Latta and Augusto Sarmiento

Key Points

- Closed fractures in segments of the body with two long bones experience the maximum and final shortening at the time of injury.
- Functional fracture bracing is predicated on the premise that physiologically induced motion at the fracture site is conducive to osteogenesis; therefore, immobilization of joints adjacent to the fracture and rigid fixation of fragments are detrimental to fracture healing.
- Soft-tissue compression is essential for maintenance of fracture alignment and stabilization of the fragments.
- Minor shortening, angulation, and rotation are not complications in most diaphyseal fractures but are simply inconsequential deviations from normal.
- Adjustable functional fracture braces are well accepted for treatment of the majority of humeral fractures and for isolated ulnar diaphyseal fractures. They also can be useful for selected displaced Colles fractures.

Functional fracture bracing is a philosophy of fracture care predicated on the premise that rigid immobilization of fractured limbs is unphysiologic and detrimental to fracture healing and that physiologically induced motion at the fracture site enhances osteogenesis.[6,21,25]

After extensive human and animal experimentation,[10,16,19,20–22,25] we concluded that, contrary to popular belief, closed fractures in the two segments of the body with two long bones experience the maximum and final shortening at the time of injury.[21,22,25,26] For example, a closed fracture of the tibia and fibula or of both bones of the forearm that demonstrates an initial shortening of 0.5 cm does not shorten any further after introduction of graduated weight-bearing ambulation or active use of the injured extremity. This fact contradicts the long-held perception that weight bearing on a fractured extremity causes additional and progressive shortening.

We initially emphasized the role of functional fracture bracing in the care of many different fractures and under a wide variety of circumstances. However, experience gained over the years prompted us to recommend its use for fewer types of fractures, not only because of failure to attain consistent satisfactory results with some of them but because of the great progress being made with other methods of treatment, particularly closed intramedullary nailing of long bone fractures.

Functional bracing can be accomplished with the wide variety of materials and devices available today. This chapter does not attempt to cover all the possible ways in which the philosophy of functional bracing can be achieved. We focus on the most recent developments and the most recent orthotic designs. The most easily applied devices are fully prefabricated orthoses.

Functional bracing is predicated on the premise that physiologically induced motion at the fracture site is conducive to osteogenesis; therefore, immobilization of joints adjacent to the fracture and rigid fixation of fragments are detrimental to fracture healing.[6,26] It also is based on the realization that anatomical restoration of alignment is not necessary in the management of most diaphyseal fractures. Minor shortening, angulation, and rotation are not functional complications but simply inconsequential deviations from normal.

Functional bracing of diaphyseal humeral fractures

Rationale

The most widely accepted treatment of the majority of humeral fractures is functional bracing.[1,3–5,7,17,23,28,30–32]

The humeral diaphysis tolerates well the minor posttraumatic deviations. As a matter of fact, the tolerance is greater than it is with most other long bones. Fifteen degrees of varus angulation is cosmetically difficult to detect in most instances. In heavy or flabby people, 25 to 30 degrees may be aesthetically acceptable, without compromise of function.

Not all diaphyseal humeral fractures are suitable for functional bracing. Other methods of treatment, such as internal fixation in the form of plating or intramedullary nailing or external fixation, are more appropriate under certain circumstances.

In order for a patient with a humeral fracture to truly benefit from bracing, he or she must be able to assume the erect position, cooperate with the physician, and be capable of adjusting the brace or have someone available who can provide that service on a regular basis. These are requirements because dependency of the extremity is necessary for restoration of adequate alignment of the fragments (Fig. 19-1) and because, during the early days, the brace must be adjusted several times daily as swelling decreases and muscle atrophy takes place.

Indications and contraindications

The majority of closed humeral diaphyseal fractures can be treated with functional bracing. Patients who cannot follow instructions or for other reasons cannot perform early passive exercise routines, which are crucial for a good outcome, should not be braced. These individuals include patients with multiple injures who are confined to bed for extended periods of time and those with insensitive arms. Patients with major open wounds cannot be managed early with braces and require other means of care until soft-tissue healing is sufficiently improved, after which the brace can be applied. The presence of an associated radial palsy does not preclude functional bracing.

The level of the diaphyseal fracture is not important. The brace does not need to cover the fracture site itself because its effectiveness is dependent on compression of the surrounding soft tissues. However, fractures of the surgical or anatomical neck of the humerus and those with distal intraarticular involvement require other therapeutic approaches.

Management

Patients with closed, isolated low-energy produced fractures of the humeral diaphysis rarely require hospitalization. One of the most typical closed, low-energy mechanisms of injury is a rotational force. In most instances these fractures do very well with functional bracing. The high velocity and high energy of the injury may cause comminution and/or segmental fracture. Most of these fractures also do well with functional bracing. However, if the trauma is severe and significant swelling or pain seems to be disproportional, in-hospital observation is desirable because of the possibility of developing a muscle compartment syndrome. This condition, if diagnosed, requires close attention and early surgery. In the absence of signs and symptoms suggestive of a possible compartment syndrome, the patient with a closed fracture of the humerus should have the injured extremity stabilized in either an above-the-elbow cast or a coaptation splint that leaves the forearm and hand exposed. In either case, a collar and cuff must be applied for additional comfort and to minimize distal edema.

It is of the utmost importance for the patient to relax the shoulder at this time. Ordinarily, the patient is apprehensive about the possibility of experiencing pain during application of the brace and unconsciously shrugs the shoulder. If the brace is fit while the shoulder is elevated, it is very likely that a varus deformity at the fracture site will occur upon relaxation of the musculature.

Once the cast or coaptation splint is applied, the patient should begin exercises of the hand and pendulum exercises of the shoulder. Because the first attempts to actively carry out pendulum exercises of the shoulder likely will be associated with pain, it is best for the patient to hold the injured extremity with the nonaffected hand. In this manner, the patient swings the arm in a circular manner as well as in alternate directions of adduction and abduction and forward and backward motions. These exercises are best conducted while leaning forward. The exercises soon can be conducted in an active manner. The sling should be used while the patient is in the recumbent position and during the early stages of healing. It can be gradually discontinued. Most patients may discard the sling once the elbow reaches full extension.

Open fractures associated with major soft-tissue damage and significant displacement between the fragments require surgical debridement of the wound and some type of stabilization. In these instances, external fixation or plating often is the treatment of choice. Many prefer plating when the fracture is associated with a proven laceration of a major nerve or artery injury. Intramedullary nailing also may be an appropriate treatment under those circumstances, although the complication rate from nailing is high. However, if the soft-tissue damage is not major and there

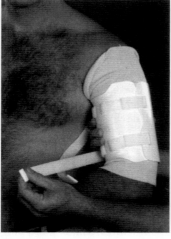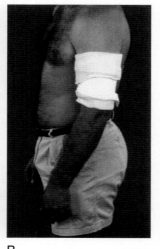

A   B

Fig. 19-1 Photographs of the humeral brace being applied **(A)** and demonstrating the range of elbow extension allowed **(B)**.

is no vertical distraction between the main fragments, functional bracing can be used effectively.

The presence of separation between the fragments in an axial direction suggests major damage to the surrounding musculature and might lead to nonunion. This is most likely to occur with transverse fractures. At times, the axial distraction between the major fragments disappears spontaneously within a short period of time, suggesting that the soft-tissue damage was not significant. In those instances, functional bracing usually renders good clinical results. Distraction usually is greater when nerve damage is present. Fractures of the humerus associated with brachial plexus injuries have a guarded prognosis. Nonunion is common. Surgical stabilization may be the treatment of choice.

Subluxation of the shoulder is common following the initial immobilization. It is best managed by active flexion and extension of the elbow. Because both flexor and extensor muscles have attachments on the scapula and distal humerus, their contraction forces the humeral head into the glenoid.

Most closed fractures with associated radial palsy can be treated with functional bracing in anticipation of spontaneous recovery. This is true especially if nerve palsy develops immediately after the injury. A dorsal cock-up wrist splint usually is not necessary if no contraindications exist for early gradual extension of the elbow. Once the elbow is extended, the partially paralyzed wrist spontaneously extends, preventing the development of a flexion–contracture of the joint.

If the palsy appears later, the prognosis is more guarded and suggests encroachment of the nerve by the forming callus. Magnetic resonance imaging (MRI) and electrical studies should be conducted to rule out the possibility of serious pathology. If pathology is identified, surgical exploration is necessary. Following repair of the nerve, the fractured humerus should be stabilized with either an external fixator or a plate.

Manipulation of a diaphyseal fracture of the humerus is strongly criticized because of the danger of producing nerve damage. Most angular deformities correct spontaneously as the brace compresses the soft tissues and the weight of the arm assists in improving alignment (Fig. 19-1). Most angular deformities are physiologically and cosmetically tolerated. In rare cases when an unacceptable deformity persists, a surgical intervention is required.

Brace application

In most instances, it is possible to exchange the cast for a functional brace between the end of the first and second post-injury weeks. This period of time usually is required for the subsidence of acute symptoms and the development of the patient's ability to perform the necessary exercises.

Whenever possible, the cast should be removed with the patient sitting on a high table. The brace is applied in the same position. After the arm is cleansed, a layer of stockinette is carefully rolled over the extremity, extending from just below the elbow to the level of the acromion process (Fig. 19-1). The appropriate size of brace is selected by measuring the length of the upper arm from approximately 1 inch below the axilla to 1 inch above the lateral condyle of the humerus.

The brace is applied to the arm and tightened to compress the soft tissues. The stockinette can be reflected back over the proximal and distal edges of the brace.

The brace should not press superiorly against the axilla because it will produce discomfort and sufficient pressure to lacerate the skin and force the patient to hold the arm in an abducted position. A varus angular deformity then occurs.

The collar and cuff are applied holding the elbow at 90 degrees. Exercises similar to those carried out during the cast immobilization period should continue. At first, the exercises should be passively assisted with the opposite hand. As soon as the patient realizes that the passive motion of the shoulder is not associated with pain, he or she should begin to combine the passive motion with active contraction of the biceps and triceps. The contraction of the flexors and extensors of the elbow assists in the correction of rotary deformities. This is possible because the two muscle groups have attachments to the proximal and distal fragments of the fracture. The malrotation of the bones at the time of the injury is accompanied by a parallel coiling of the muscles. Once they contract, they correct the rotary bony deformity.[21]

The brace must be adjustable, otherwise maintenance of firm compression on the soft tissues surrounding the fractured humerus is not possible. The snug fit of the brace provides comfort to the patient and permits the continued use of the injured extremity in a gradually progressive manner.

The brace should extend from approximately 1 inch below the axilla to approximately 1 inch above the humeral epicondyles. It does not necessarily have to extend above and below the fracture site. The important thing is the compression of the soft tissues around the fracture site. The sleeve should not extend over the acromion or the epicondyles of the humerus. The sleeve should not be suspended with a harness over the shoulder.

The proximal extension over the acromion does not add to the effectiveness of the sleeve. However, it can do harm by wrongly suggesting that in this manner the sleeve does not displace distally and provides greater stabilization to the fractured humerus. The extension of the brace over the epicondyles is another exercise in futility because in order for the condyles to prevent its distal slippage, a significant amount of pressure over the skin would be necessary, which might lead to pain and pressure sores.

Patient instructions

The patient should be instructed to continue pendulum exercises with the arm held in the sling, to be followed by similar exercises with the elbow in extension at a later date. Only after this time can the sling be temporarily discontinued. The sling should be worn only at night and discontinued once clinical and radiological stability have been achieved.

The exercises of the extremity should not be limited to the shoulder and elbow; they should include the hand and wrist. In this manner swelling is decreased. The arm must hang loosely at the side of the body so that gravity forces can assist in correcting the angular deformities. Leaning on the elbow should be strongly discouraged because it produces angular deformities. This may occur during the initial period of cast immobilization but more likely after application of the brace.

As atrophy takes place and swelling decreases, the brace has a ready tendency to slip distally. This slippage not only can produce irritation of the antecubital space but can result in loss of compression of the soft tissues. *This compression is essential for the maintenance of fracture alignment and stabilization of the fragments.* Therefore, it is important to use adjustable braces. As swelling subsides and muscle atrophy experiences recovery, the need for frequent adjustment of the brace decreases. The patient should be instructed to remove the brace for hygiene after bathing. The brace should be removed, the stockinette replaced with clean dry stockinette, and the brace reapplied.

Active abduction and elevation of the arm should be avoided until early radiographic evidence of healing is seen. Therefore, only passive exercises and active exercises that do not call for strong contraction of the abductors and elevators of the shoulder should be conducted. Once intrinsic stability at the fracture occurs, active elevation and abduction should be conducted. Physical and/or occupational therapy, if prescribed, should be limited to the exercises described previously.

Discontinue use of brace and follow-up

The brace is permanently discontinued when clinical and radiological evidence of union is documented (Fig. 19-2). The absence of pain and the presence of osseous bridging of the fragments indicate union. Patients should continue to exercise their joints and to rebuild the musculature of the arm. Strenuous exercises, such as sporting activities that require maximum force, should be introduced gradually. Failure to follow such protocol can result in refracture.

Expected outcome

Eventual return of normal motion of the shoulder and elbow joints should be expected in the overwhelming majority of instances. If a major deformity at the fracture site becomes permanent as a result of inappropriate use of the brace and extremity, a permanent limitation of motion of the elbow may result. Deformities of this degree are preventable and are more likely to develop in transverse nondisplaced fractures. Some loss of external rotation should be expected in many instances but usually disappears with continued use of the extremity.

Complications

Nerve palsy

Late onset of radial nerve palsy is rare but has been reported. It suggests entrapment of the nerve in the healing callus. Management of this complication may be surgical. MRI studies should help confirm the diagnosis of bony entrapment. Exploration of the nerve is necessary. Late palsy can be seen following manipulation of a fracture, performed in an attempt to improve fracture alignment. *We strongly discourage manipulation of diaphyseal humeral fractures and recommend unencumbered hanging of the arm at the site of the body.* In the unlikely event that gradual increase of exercises fails to create an acceptable alignment, surgery probably is the treatment of choice.

Malalignment

Most angular deformities encountered with functional bracing of humeral shaft fractures are varus deformities. This is particularly true for fractures below the middle third of the diaphysis. Proximal fractures may develop valgus angulation. The humeral diaphysis tolerates, functionally and cosmetically, angular deformities of degrees that cannot be tolerated by most other long bones. Arms with either large musculature or excessive adipose tissue camouflage deformity quite well. Loss of the "carrying angle" of the elbow is very common, particularly in fractures of the distal third of the bone. Because women are more likely to have valgus elbows, a varus deformity of 15 of 20 degrees is difficult to recognize.

Anteroposterior deformities can develop and are more likely to be seen in transverse nondisplaced fractures. A delay in reaching extension of the elbow may aggravate an angulation with an anterior apex. The "stiff elbow" creates abnormal stresses at the fracture site when the arm finally hangs over the side of the body.

Delayed and nonunion

It is not always easy to say with precision when a fracture is likely to develop nonunion. In other long bone fractures, it is

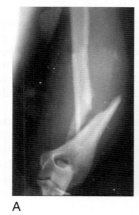 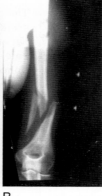 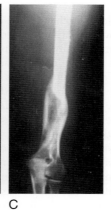

A B C

Fig. 19-2 Composite photograph of radiographs obtained shortly after the injury demonstrating varus angulation **(A)**, after application of the brace and introduction of compressive and gravity forces **(B)**, and upon completion of healing **(C)**.

not uncommon to see fractures demonstrate no evidence of clinical or radiologic union for long periods of time and still observe eventual healing. The humerus seems to behave differently. A humeral diaphyseal fracture that demonstrates frank motion at the fracture site 2 to 2.5 months after the injury is not likely to unite spontaneously. Such motion is of greater diagnostic significance than is the absence of peripheral callus. We have observed fractures with no radiologically demonstrable callus 2 months after the initial injury, but without gross motion at the fracture site, eventually heal solidly.

Fractures associated with peripheral nerve injury are the fractures most likely to develop nonunion, particularly if the injured nerve affects the function of the flexors and extensors of the elbow. As a rule, these fractures demonstrate initial axial separation between the fragments. This is an ominous sign. Axial distraction between fragments also can indicate major soft-tissue damage that requires earlier active use of the surrounding musculature. Failure to see a rapid correction of the distraction often calls for surgical intervention.

Skin problems

Allergic reaction to the stockinette or plastic brace is extremely rare. Its occurrence calls for the application of local medications or the discontinuation of the bracing technique. Because the brace can be easily removed and reapplied, daily hygienic measures prevent irritation or maceration of the skin.

Refracture

The likelihood of refracture of long bones that heal with peripheral callus is extremely rare. The strength of the bone at the level of the fracture is greater than before the fracture occurred.

If a new injury occurs, a fracture would be located either above or below the original fracture. When a diaphyseal fracture is treated with methods that produce rigid immobilization of the fragments, the strength of this bone is significantly less than that of the remaining bone, so refractures are more likely to occur.

Muscle weakness and limited range of motion

It is not unusual for diaphyseal humeral fractures treated with functional braces to heal with associated limitation of motion of the shoulder. In almost all instances, the limitation is temporary. Continued use of the extremity restores full range of motion. Loss of external rotation is the most common limitation. It is likely that the internal rotation position of the shoulder during the early stages of healing results in capsular contracture. The early conduct of pendulum exercises expedites recovery of motion. Passive exercises are replaced with active exercises within a few days as dictated by symptoms. Most patients are able to perform the exercises with ease within a few days.

Weakness of the surrounding arm musculature is inevitable, regardless of the method of treatment. Early use of the extremity prevents significant weakness. In our experience, most patients can begin to combine passive exercises with active exercises soon after the brace is applied. These exercises should apply to the flexors and extensor of the elbow.

Active contraction of these muscles not only prevents long-lasting muscle atrophy but assists in the correction of the frequently seen subluxation of the glenohumeral joint. Contraction of the flexors and extensor of the elbow also assist in the correction of rotary deformities created by the parallel coiling of the fractured fragments and the surrounding musculature.

Leaning on the elbow and active elevation or abduction of the shoulder should be forbidden. The resulting forces can produce a varus deformity. This varus deformity is more likely to occur if the fracture is transverse and even more so if the fragments are in contact with one another. If the fracture is comminuted or oblique, weight bearing provokes elastic pistoning between the fragments, a motion that is conducive to osteogenesis. The patient does not have to sleep in the sitting position; all that is needed is suspension of the arm in the sling. Regaining extension of the elbow is most desirable in preference to flexion because spontaneous gain of flexion is anticipated with performance of the necessary activities of daily living. Regaining extension early is important because once full extension of the elbow is reached, the patient can discontinue use of the sling and walk with the swing of the arm in a normal way. The weight of the distal arm can further assist in improving the ubiquitous varus angulation seen in humeral diaphyseal fractures.

Extension of the elbow eliminates the fulcrum effect created by the chest when the arm rests over protruding muscular tissues or large breasts. It is well known that large-breasted women have a greater tendency to develop varus deformities as a result of the alleged fulcrum effect.

Low-velocity, gunshot-produced fractures usually are associated with some comminution. The associated degree of soft-tissue pathology usually is mild. Therefore, healing of these fractures occurs at a pace comparable to that of closed fractures. Often the lateral displacement of the comminuted fragments enlarges the diameter of the bone at the level of the fracture. This enlarged diameter spontaneously decreases from the compression of the soft tissues by the functional sleeve and the gravity effect at the fracture site.

Functional bracing of diaphyseal ulnar fractures

Rationale

Plating of isolated ulnar fractures is a popular method of treatment, but the overall reported results are mixed. Postoperative infection is low, and nonunion and implant failure do not occur with great frequency. However, refracture is not uncommon, and the cost of surgical treatment remains higher and not totally free from surgical and anesthetic complications.

The popularity of surgical plating came from the observation that nonunion was occasionally encountered when the limb was immobilized in a cast that extended from the head of the metacarpals to just above the elbow. Such a long cast had been used to accommodate the long-held premise that joints above and below a fracture required immobilization. Today, such a practice has been proven flawed, and evidence that freedom of motion of joints and physiologically induced motion at the fracture site are beneficial has replaced that earlier concept.

The high rate of success with functional bracing of isolated ulnar fractures makes it difficult to justify the routine plating of these fractures.[2,3,11,13,15,24,27,32,33] However, open surgery is the treatment of choice for certain conditions.

Because isolated ulnar fractures usually are the result of direct blows over the forearm, the most common displacement of fragments is in a radial deviation. Because the damage caused by such an injury to the stabilizing interosseous membrane is minimal, the displacement of the fragments usually is mild.[8] Shortening is not possible because the intact radius prevents such a development. When the forearm is placed in a relaxed attitude of supination, the angular deformity tends to improve. In any event, the residual angulation does not result in a noticeable loss of pronosupination.[29] As a matter of fact, in our view the surgical trauma produced at the time of plate fixation is more likely to create a greater degree of limitation of motion. A synostosis between the two bones is a complication we have not observed with the use of functional braces.

Initial angular deformity in a volar direction usually is mild and the clinical consequences rarely of any significance. Major angular deformity may be seen in severe open fractures associated with significant amount of soft-tissue damage. These fractures may require stabilization with external fixators or plates. Their functional prognosis is guarded.

Indications and contraindications

Most isolated diaphyseal fractures of the ulna are the result of a direct blow over the forearm, and in most instances the fracture is of a closed type. When a fracture of the ulna diaphysis occurs after a fall on the outstretched hand, an associated dislocation of the radial head is almost always present. This condition, known as a *Monteggia fracture*, is a clear indication for surgical intervention because of the difficulties encountered in maintaining a manually achieved reduction.[8] Isolated ulnar fractures close to the radioulnar joint that show significant angulation might require surgical fixation if the deformity persists after application of the brace.

These observations suggest that the majority of isolated ulnar fractures can be successfully treated with functional braces that permit early use of the extremity without the need for preventing pronosupination of the forearm and flexion and extension of the elbow and wrist.

Low-grade open fractures can be treated in this manner after appropriate debridement of the injured soft tissues. More severe open fractures associated with major soft-tissue damage may require stabilization with external fixators until the condition of the area is satisfactory and the area is free of infection. At that point, internal fixation and bone grafting may be indicated.

Acute management

Closed fractures

In order to provide relief from the acute pain that accompanies any fracture, we prefer to stabilize the arm in an above-the-elbow cast that holds the elbow in a position of 90 degrees of flexion and the forearm in a relaxed attitude of supination. The position of relaxed supination is more likely to place the fragments in the most anatomical alignment. In addition, it helps to restore earlier pronosupination of the forearm. Routine daily activities call for the use of pronation more

frequently than supination, so patients, by necessity, pronate their forearm and regain the initially lost motion. In the case of a permanent loss of motion of the forearm, it is best to lose the last few degrees of pronation rather than supination. The shoulder girdle, through an inconspicuous motion of flexion and abduction, compensates for that loss. A comparable inconspicuous mechanism for the loss of supination and internal rotation does not exist.

The long arm cast is not always necessary. If the energy of the injury was moderate and the accompanying pain and swelling are not significant, a below-the-elbow cast or splint may suffice. In some instances, the functional brace can be applied initially.

When a cast or splint is used initially, it is held in place for no more than 1 week. After that time, most patients experience only minimal to moderate discomfort. Those who use their fingers from the outset are more likely to achieve quicker relief from pain. This is something important to keep in mind when dealing with bilateral fractures.

Open fractures

Open diaphyseal fractures produced by low-energy injury rarely demonstrate significant displacement between the fracture fragments. The intact radius and interosseous membrane prevent major displacement. In open fractures resulting from high-energy injuries and associated with major soft-tissue damage, the displacement between the fragments may be significant due to damage to the stabilizing interosseous membrane. These fractures require appropriate debridement of the wound and, not infrequently, stabilization with plates or external fixators. Less severe fractures can be managed with functional braces as soon as the wounds begin to show healthy signs of healing. The presence of an open wound does not preclude the use of braces because they are removable and permit cleansing of the wound and frequent dressing changes.

Initial immobilization

In the acute stages of the injury, the patient should be immobilized in a padded cast and given a sling for comfort. In most instances, the initial above-the-elbow cast is more comfortable than the below-the-elbow cast.

Brace application and function

At the end of the first week, the cast can be removed and the brace applied. A sling or a collar and cuff also are applied in order to eliminate the pain that the dependent arm likely will produce.

The brace ("sleeve") permits unencumbered use of the arm because the brace does not extend over the elbow or wrist. It simply limits pronosupination (Fig. 19-3). The ulna fracture brace, or sleeve, must be adjustable to allow its frequent removal and reapplication for hygienic purposes and to ensure maintenance of its desirable snugness against the soft tissues. Hook-and-loop straps are best for this purpose. Circular casts that cannot be adjusted slip distally as swelling subsides and atrophy of the musculature takes place. The brace should be short enough to allow free motion of the wrist and elbow, regardless of the location of the fracture. Rigid immobilization of fragments is not necessary.

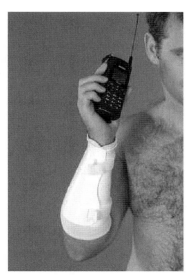

Fig. 19-3 Ulnar brace, which allows for unencumbered motion of the elbow and wrist while limiting pronosupination of the forearm.

The brace probably accomplishes nothing more than provision of comfort and protection to the arm from inadvertent forceful contact with hard objects.

Use of cotton stockinette under the brace is preferable, extending from just above the wrist to just below the elbow. It can be washed and replaced as often as necessary. The patient's forearm should be held in a relaxed attitude of supination during application of the brace. The snugness of the brace should not be too great because distal swelling can occur as a result of the tourniquet-like effect of the brace.

The ulnar brace, as in the case of the humerus and tibia, can be custom made or prefabricated. It can be made of casting material or of plastics.

Patient instructions

Patients are encouraged to use the extremity to the maximum degree allowed by pain. In most instances, the pain present at the time of application of the brace is only moderate. In our opinion, the early introduction of function results in more rapid disappearance of acute symptoms and faster healing.

The brace should be adjusted frequently during the first few days in order to maintain the desirable compression of the soft tissues and to prevent distal displacement of the sleeve over the wrist. The brace can be removed for hygienic purposes as often as necessary, and the collar and cuff permanently discontinued as soon as the systems subside.

Flexion and extension of the elbow are rapidly regained. Pronation and supination require a longer period of time because such motions are more painful. In a few instances we have treated with functional braces patients who had sustained bilateral isolated ulnar fractures. Their recovery was rapid and uneventful.

Brace removal and follow-up

The brace is permanently discontinued as soon as the symptoms subside. We do not believe the brace is necessary after that time, regardless of the degree of healing seen on radiographs.

Patients should avoid prolonged dependency of the injured extremity because of the likely possibility of development of distal edema. Frequent tightening of the fist and wrist active exercises assist in preventing and correcting this problem.

The patient can temporarily remove the brace in order to perform active pronosupination of the forearm when the degree of discomfort permits it. Most patients seem to be able to do so after wearing the brace for 1 to 2 weeks. Washing of the forearm can be done as often as desired.

Expected outcome

When the healing is complete, usually the patient has full range of motion of the elbow. The motion of the wrist may be slightly limited for an additional few weeks, particularly when the fracture was located close to the wrist joint. Permanent loss of pronation and supination is found in a small percentage of patients, particularly those with fractures located in the proximal third of the bone. The overall functional results are most gratifying.

Managing complications

We are not aware of any complications that can be directly traced to the brace other than possible allergic reaction to the stockinette or the plastic material of the appliance. Increased angulation at the fracture site is extremely rare. The intrinsic stability of the fracture provided by the interosseous membrane ensures that the original displacement will remain unchanged. Infection is unrelated to bracing treatment.

Synostosis

Synostosis is extremely rare when forearm fractures are treated with functional braces. Perhaps the early introduction of function prevents the building of a bridge between the two bones. Synostosis is more common following plate fixation. Fractures associated with head injuries are known to develop heterotopic bone. We observed one such instance of synostosis following an isolated ulnar fracture. This complication requires surgical excision of the bony bridge. The prognosis is not always good because a residual limitation of motion usually persists.

Malalignment

Because most fractures occur from a direct blow over the forearm, the degree of displacement of the fragments usually is minor. The associated damage of the interosseous membrane also is minimal, which explains the mild displacement. The direction of the blow dictates the displacement of the fragments, which in most instances is toward the intact radius. In this instance, damage to the interosseous membrane is the mildest. When the displacement of fragments is either dorsal or volar, soft-tissue damage is greater. Shortening does not occur due to the intact radius.

Delayed and nonunion

Most isolated ulnar fractures demonstrate radiological union within 2 to 2.5 months. Most of these fractures demonstrate large peripheral callus, indicating the beneficial effect of motion at the fracture site (Fig. 19-4). However, in some instances a gap between the fragments remains for a longer

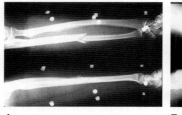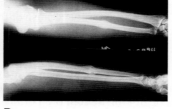

A   B

Fig. 19-4 Composite photograph of radiographs of fracture of the ulna stabilized in an ulnar brace **(A)** and fracture solidly united **(B)**.

period of time, suggesting a delayed union or a nonunion. If the associated symptoms are minimal or nonexistent, skillful neglect is the most appropriate approach. Eventually, radiological healing becomes apparent. Failure to achieve painless bony union calls for surgery and possibly a grafting procedure.

Skin problems

Allergic reactions to the stockinette of plastic material are rare. Poor hygiene is the most likely cause of skin irritation. Frequent removal of the brace and washing of the arm and hand, which are possible and recommended from the very outset, prevent skin problems. If present, they probably are due to excessive perspiration and a reaction to heat.

Refracture

Diaphyseal fractures that are treated with functional braces usually heal with peripheral callus. Under those circumstances the likelihood of refracture is minimal. The new bone at the level of the fracture is stronger than prior to the fracture. The thinning of the bony cortices, frequently seen under plates, does not occur. Management of a new fracture, if it were to occur, would not differ from the original one. Activities that require extreme force, such as strenuous athletic actions, may create a new fracture.

Poor grip and range of motion

It is logical to expect a temporary weakness of grip in all patients who sustain diaphyseal ulnar fractures. However, because the period of inactivity is relatively short, the resulting muscular weakness is mild and the recovery is rapid. The same applies to the residual limitation of motion. Some patients demonstrate a mild loss of pronation of the forearm, but inconspicuous compensation occurs with mild flexion and internal rotation of the shoulder, a mechanism similar to that used by below-the-elbow amputees who pronate the terminal device in same manner. The limitation of pronation detected at the time the brace is permanently discontinued improves with return to normal activities without the hindrance of the brace.

Functional casting and bracing of Colles fractures

Rationale

Functional casting and bracing of Colles fractures were first developed upon recognition of the high frequency of

redislocation of fragments following closed reduction. This observation led to studies that allowed us to conclude that the traditionally recommended position of pronation of the forearm was contributing to the complication. The contraction of the brachioradialis muscle—the only muscle with attachment to the distal radial fracture—was being encouraged by the position of pronation because this muscle functions as a flexor of the elbow when the forearm is in pronation. Electromyographic studies confirmed the clinical and anatomical observation.[12] Other muscular structures overlying the facture site can be deforming forces, but not to the extent the brachioradialis muscle is.

Indications

Loss of reduction of Colles fractures is observed primarily in comminuted fractures, especially in those with an associated initial dislocation of the radioulnar joint. Even after adequate reduction of the radial fracture and of the dislocation, recurrence of the deformity often occurs. These fractures are best managed surgically, preferably using plates and screws. Fractures in which the angle of inclination of the most radial fragment is rather vertical also are prone to recurrence of displacement as the brachioradialis exerts an opposed force.

Management

Following the initial reduction of the displaced Colles fracture, an above-the-elbow cast holding the forearm in a relaxed position of supination is the best means of initial stabilization. It provides greater comfort during the most acute period, facilitates finger motion, permits better radiological evaluation of the reduction, and ensures greater stability of the

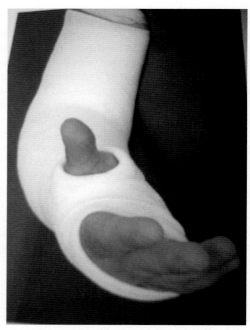

Fig. 19-5 Photograph of a Colles cast holding the forearm in a relaxed attitude of supination and the wrist in slight volar flexion and ulnar deviation.

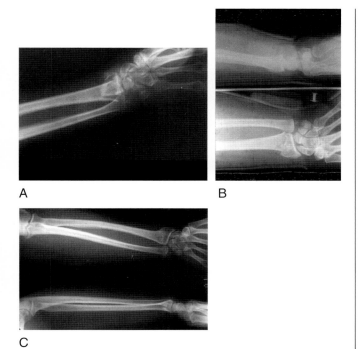

A B

C

Fig. 19-6 Radiographs of **(A)** displaced extraarticular, Colles fracture, **(B)** after reduction in a Colles brace (Munster design), which allows for slightly limited motion of the elbow, prevents pronosupination, but permits flexion of the wrist, **(C)** fracture healed with no change in alignment.

radioulnar joint. A few days later, the above-the-elbow cast can be replaced with a Munster-type cast, which allows almost complete flexion and extension of the elbow but prevents pronosupination of the forearm (Fig. 19-5).

Outcome

Clinical research has been conducted to determine the efficacy of stabilization of the forearm in relaxed pronosupination as well as to the fractures most likely to benefit from such protocol. We observed that extraarticular Colles fractures that do not show initial displacement do well in most instances regardless of the method of stabilization. Intraarticular fractures without radioulnar dislocation do best when stabilized in supination (Fig. 19-6).[14,18,19,24]

References

1. Balfour GW, Mooney V, Ashby ME: Diaphyseal fractures of the humerus treated with a ready-made fracture brace, *J Bone Joint Surg* 64A:11, 1982.
2. Bruggemann H, Kujat R, Tscherne H: Funkionelle frakturebehandlung nach sarmiento an unterschenkel, unterarm und oberarm, *Orthopaede* 12:143, 1983.
3. Ekkernkamp A, Kayser M, Althoff M: Knozept der funktionellen therapie am beispiel des frischen geschlossenen oberarmschaftbruches, *Zentralbl Chir* 114:788, 1989.
4. Ekkernkamp A, Muhr, G: Indikation und technik der funktionellen knochenbruchbehandlung oper-und unterarm. Unfallmed landesver, Gewerblich, GEW BG, 1985.
5. Hackstock H, Helmreich M: Isolierte bruche des ellenschaftes-behandlung mit sarmiento brace, *Verbandtechnik* 2:6, 1989.
6. Latta LL, Sarmiento A, Tarr RR: The rationale of functional bracing of fractures, *Clin Orthop Rel Res* 146:28–36, 1980.
7. McMaster WC, Tivnon MC, Waugh TR: Cast brace for the upper extremity, *Clin Orthop Rel Res* 109:126, 1975.
8. Moore TM, Lester DK, Sarmiento A: The stabilizing effect of soft-tissue constraints in the artificial Galeazzi fractures, *Clin Orthop Relat Res* 194:189, 1985.
9. Naver L, Aalberg JR: Humeral shaft fractures treated with a ready-made fracture brace, *Arch Orthop Trauma Surg* 106:20, 1986.
10. Park S-H, O'Conner K, McKellop H, Sarmiento A: The influence of active shearing compression motion on fracture healing, *J Bone Joint Surg* 80A:868–878, 1998.
11. Pollock FH, Pankovich AM, Prieto JJ, Lorenz M: The isolated fracture of the ulnar shaft: treatment without immobilization, *J Bone Joint Surg* 65A:339, 1983.
12. Sarmiento A: The brachioradialis as a deforming force Colles' fractures, *Clin Orthop Relat Res* 38:86, 1965.
13. Sarmiento A, Cooper JS, Sinclair WF: Forearm fractures. Early functional bracing: a preliminary report, *J Bone Joint Surg* 57A:297, 1975.
14. Sarmiento A, Pratt GW, Berry NC, Sinclair WF: Colles' fractures: functional bracing in supination, *J Bone Joint Surg* 57A:311–317, 1975.
15. Sarmiento A, Kinman PB, Murphy RB, Phillips JG: Treatment of ulnar fractures by functional bracing, *J Bone Joint Surg* 58A:1104, 1976.
16. Sarmiento A, Schaeffer J, Beckerman L, Latta LL, Enis J: Fracture healing in rat femora affected by functional weight bearing, *J Bone Joint Surg* 59A:369, 1977.
17. Sarmiento A, Kinman PB, Galvin EG, Schmitt RH, Phillips JG: Functional bracing of fractures of the shaft of the humerus, *J Bone Joint Surg* 59A:596, 1977.
18. Sarmiento A, Zagorski JB, Sinclair WF: Functional bracing of Colles' fractures: a prospective study of immobilization in supination versus pronation, *Clin Orthop Rel Res* 146:175–187, 1980.
19. Sarmiento A, Mullis DL, Latta LL, Alvarez RR: A quantitative, comparative analysis of fracture healing under the influence of compression plating vs. closed weight-bearing treatment, *Clin Orthop Rel Res* 149:232, 1980.
20. Sarmiento A, Latta L, Zilioli A, Sinclair WF: The role of soft tissues in the stabilization of tibial fractures, *Clin Orthop Rel Res* 105:116–129, 1974.
21. Sarmiento A, Latta LL: *The closed functional treatment of fractures*, Heidelberg, 1981, Springer-Verlag.
22. Sarmiento A, Latta LL, Tarr RR: Principles of fracture healing—part II: the effect of function on fracture healing and stability. In *AAOS Instructional Course Lectures, vol. XXXIII*, St. Louis, 1984, Mosby.
23. Sarmiento A, Horowitch A, Aboulafia A, Vangsness CT: Functional bracing of comminuted extra-articular fractures of the distal third of the humerus, *J Bone Joint Surg* 72B:283, 1990.
24. Sarmiento A, Abramzadeh E, Brys D, Tarr R: Angular deformities and forearm function, *J Orthop Res* 10:121–133, 1992.
25. Sarmiento A, Latta LL: *Functional fracture bracing*, Heidelberg, 1995, Springer-Verlag.
26. Sarmiento A, McKellop H, Llinas A, et al: Effect of loading and fracture motions on diaphyseal tibial fractures, *J Orthop Res* 14:80–84, 1996.
27. Sarmiento A, Latta LL, Zych GA, McKeever P, Zagorski JB: Isolated ulnar shaft fractures treated with functional braces, *J Orthop Trauma* 12:420–424, 1998.
28. Sarmiento A, Zagorski JB, Zych GA, Latta LL, Capps CA: Functional bracing for the treatment of fractures of the humeral diaphysis, *J Bone Joint Surg* 824A:478–486, 2000.
29. Tarr RR, Garfinkle A, Sarmiento A: Effects of angular and rotational deformities of both bones of the forearm, *J Bone Joint Surg* 66A:65, 1984.
30. Wasmer G, Worsdorfer O: Functional management of humeral shaft fractures with Sarmiento cast bracing, *Unfallheilkunde* 87:309, 1984.
31. Zagorski JB, Latta LL, Zych GA, Finnieston AR: Diaphyseal fractures of the humerus: treatment with prefabricated braces, *J Bone Joint Surg* 70A:607, 1988.
32. Zagorski JB, Zych GA, Latta LL, McCollough NC: Modern concepts in functional fracture bracing: upper limb. In *AAOS Instructional Course Lectures, vol. XXXVI*, Chicago, 1987, AAOS.
33. Zych GA, Zagorski JB, Latta LL: Treatment of isolated ulnar fractures with prefabricated fracture braces, *Clin Orthop* 219:1944, 1987.

Protective equipment to the upper limb in sport

Letha Y. Griffin, James Kercher, and James L. Shoop

Key Points

1. Protective equipment attempts to (1) decrease motion of certain body parts, (2) support and/or compress an area of prior injury, (3) reduce friction between surfaces, and/or (4) absorb energy of a direct low, dispersing the force over a large area.

2. To be effective, protective equipment must be properly fitted, well-maintained, and made of durable, lightweight material that is reasonably priced and appropriately designed.

3. Materials used to make protective orthoses include elasticized and cloth wraps and tapes, rigid thermoplastic materials, open- and closed-cell foam pads and splints, and pneumatic devices.

4. Orthoses for the upper limb in sport can typically be divided into protective devices and restraining devices.

5. Gloves in sport are used for protection, to increase grip, and to provide warmth in cool and cold situations.

Orthoses for the upper extremity in sport are used to protect normal anatomy from increased forces or to protect injured anatomy from normal forces. Protective equipment attempts to (1) decrease motion of certain body parts, (2) support and/or compress an area of prior injury, (3) reduce friction between surfaces, and/or (4) absorb energy of a direct blow, dispersing the force over a larger area.[16]

To be effective, protective equipment must be properly fitted, well maintained, and made of a durable, lightweight material that is reasonably priced and appropriately designed for the designated task. Proper fitting of equipment is essential, as the most expensive, expertly designed and fabricated equipment, if too big or too small, loses its effectiveness.[21] For recreational sport, style is also a concern. For example, wrist guards and helmets for rollerbladers became more acceptable to youngsters when manufacturers started making them in bright colors and had them signed by well-known bladers. The effectiveness of protective equipment was demonstrated in a study comparing the injury rate in American football players to New Zealand rugby players. The injury rate in football players utilizing protective equipment was approximately one third that of rugby players who wore no protective equipment.[12]

The thickness and density of material used for protective equipment determine impact resistance. Low-density materials, such as felt, foam rubber, and Pelite (Durr-Fillauer, Montgomery, AL), may be lighter and more comfortable to wear, but they absorb little energy and therefore are not appropriate in situations where high forces must be dissipated by deformation of the protective material. Materials often used for high-load situations include thermomoldable plastics (e.g., Orthoplast, Johnson & Johnson Orthopedics, New Brunswick, NJ; Aquaplast, WFR/Aquaplast Corp., Wyckoff, NJ; Polyflex, Smith & Nephew, Menomonee Falls, WI), fiberglass, and plaster. If padding is required to protect against repeated insults, a material that is resilient (i.e., resumes its preinjury shape following deformation) may be required.

Fabricators of protective equipment frequently use composite materials. Soft, lower-density, absorbent materials can be layered with a dense material for greater force absorption. Protective equipment that covers joints not only should be soft to the skin but also must be flexible enough to not limit joint motion. Protective equipment, designed to protect an area of prior injury, may need to incorporate hinges or check-rein straps to limit motion.

Suspension of a protective wrap or pad is critical because migrating pads offer limited protection at best and can cause injury if they impede function. Hook and loop or tape strips are frequently used to secure protective equipment. Tacky skin compounds (e.g., Tuf-Skin, Cramer Products, Gardner, KS; M-Tac, Mueller, Prairie du Sac, WI) can be applied to the skin to prevent migration of the tape or pad.

Materials such as neoprene (DuPont Dow Elastomers LLC, Louisville, KY) or elasticized tape or wrap also can be used where slippage is a problem. However, neoprene does not "breathe" as does the nylon Lycra trilaminated wear used in BioSkin braces (Cropper Medical, Ashland, OR) or the nylon polyethylene weave used in CoolFlex fabric for Drytex braces (DJ Orthopaedics, Vista, CA) and, therefore, may be less comfortable in warm weather.

Allergic reactions to any orthotic materials can occur. Protective devices should be applied only to clean, dry skin. With few exceptions, athletes should be cautioned to remove sport orthotic devices daily in order to clean the device as well as their skin.

Materials used to make protective orthotics

A variety of materials are available for use in the construction of protective devices for sport. The following is a brief overview of some of the more commonly used materials.

Wraps and tapes

Wraps and tapes are both strips of material. However, tapes have an adhesive backing and wraps do not. Both are extensively used in sport.

Elastic wraps or tapes (e.g., Coban, 3M Healthcare, St. Paul, MN; Elastikon, Johnson & Johnson Orthopaedics, New Brunswick, NJ; Conform, Tyco Health Group LLP, Mansfield, MA; Lightplast, Beiersdorf, Wilton, CT) are made to stretch and, like cloth wraps and tapes, are frequently used for compression, support, and protection of the musculoskeletal system. These materials are also effectively used to secure pads and other protective devices. In general, elastic wraps and tapes are more expensive than cloth wraps or tapes.

Cloth-backed tape is available in a variety of widths (0.5–3 inches). When ordering tape, consider tape grade, adhesive mass, and winding tension. The higher-grade tape has greater strength, which results from an increased number of threads per inch in both the vertical and longitudinal dimensions.[1]

The application of cloth-backed tape for support is an art. Principles of taping include the following:

1. Tape only at room temperature.
2. An underwrap (a thin porous foam wrap to protect the skin) can be used.
3. Shaving prior to tape application is generally recommended so that tape removal is easier and less painful.

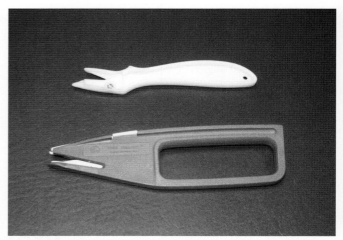

Fig. 20-1 Example of tape cutters. (Note the protected tips designed to avoid cutting the skin when removing tape.)

4. Circumferential taping should be avoided in areas that may swell. Successive strips of tape should generally be avoided.
5. Overlap tape by about one third. Avoid gapes between tape strips because skin can be pinched and blistering may occur.
6. For most areas, multiple tape strips are preferred over continuous taping.

To remove tape, tape cutters (Fig. 20-1) are recommended in lieu of scissors because they have protective tips to avoid cutting the skin and are made to slide easily under the tape's edge.

Rigid thermoplastic materials

Rigid thermoplastic materials include plastics, elastomer or rubberlike materials, or a combination of these two. Orthoplast, Multiform (Alimed, Dedham, MA), Aquaplast, Polyfoam (Smith & Nephew), Polyflex, and Ezetoy (Smith & Nephew) are common thermoplastic materials used to make rigid splints.[19] Plastic is more conforming than rubberlike materials and is used for smaller splints (e.g., those used for the finger). Both materials come in conveniently sized solid or perforated sheets.

To make a splint from thermoplastic materials, typically a pattern is first fashioned from paper, which can be easily folded when custom fitting it to the area. Using this pattern, the appropriately shaped piece of thermoplastic material can be cut, softened with heat (typically 150°–180°F)* either by immersing it in a hydrocollator or by using a heat gun and molded to the body part. The fabricated brace can be securely attached to the athlete by hook-and-loop straps, elastic webbing, or elastic or cloth tape, or it can be incorporated into the pockets of the uniform (Fig. 20-2). Prefabricated splints from these materials are available. When designing protective pads, one must be certain that the material selected for fabrication is permitted by the sport.

---

*Higher temperature thermoplastics do not become malleable until heated to 325–350°F and are typically made over plastic molds. These materials can be clear and are used on nasal and face masks (e.g., W-Clear [Smith & Nephew Roylan Inc., Nenomonee Falls, WI]).

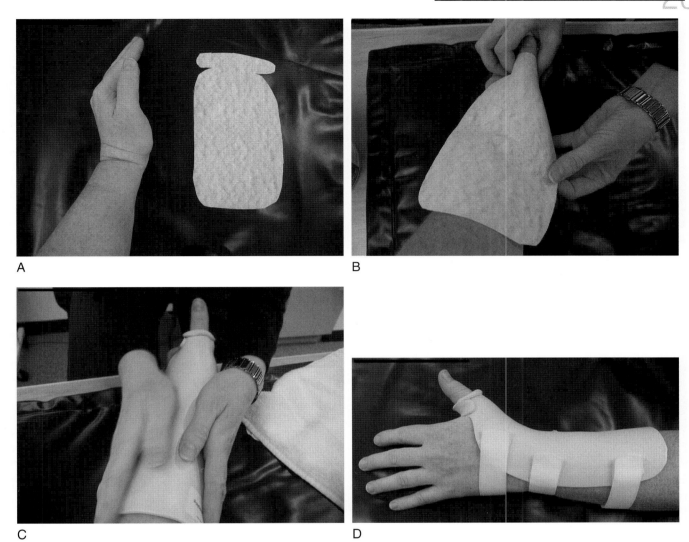

Fig. 20-2 Fabricating a custom-fitted orthosis from a thermomoldable material. **A,** Pattern is sized and cut. **B,** The pattern is used to fashion the orthosis from a piece of thermoplastic material. **C,** The orthosis is heat softened and molded to the athlete, taking care to not burn the athlete when applying the heated orthosis. **D,** The fabricated brace is secured to the athlete.

Governing bodies for sport typically determine the materials that are to be used. Regulations may vary depending on the sport, the age of participants, and the level of competition. The National Federation of High Schools (NFHS, Indianapolis, IN) and the National Collegiate Athletic Association (NCAA, Indianapolis, IN) may have additional rules. Splints and pads should protect the athlete but should not be able to be used as a weapon against the opponent, nor should they provide an unfair advantage to the athlete.

Open-cell and closed-cell foam pads and splints

Semirigid splints can be made from thermoplastic polyethylene closed-cell foams (e.g., Plastazote, Zotefoams, Walton, KY; Nickleplast, Alimed; Aliplast, Alimed) or from ethylene vinyl acetate (EVA) foam. Because these materials are less ridged than heat moldable plastic and rubberlike materials, they are permitted by most sport ruling bodies. Prefabricated splints

made from these materials also are available. EVA foam is a softer, more resilient material than polyethylene foams. Polyethylene foams are firmer and more resistant to heat. Both products have a fine uniform closed-cell structure, can absorb high energy, are poor water absorbers yet good thermal insulators, have a broad working temperature, provide good weather and chemical resistance, and have excellent buoyancy characteristics. Both can be molded for pressure distribution and protection and can be laminated with a closed-cell cushion-type material (e.g. Pelite, Durr-Fillauer, Montgomery, AL; Volara, Voltek, LLC., Lawrence, MA).

Open-cell foams, like foam rubber, are lower-density materials. The cells are connected and therefore allow for air passage. These materials can cushion and absorb fluids, but they are not good shock absorbers because they deform quickly with impact.

Silicone elastomer (Smith & Nephew or Dow Corning Corp., Midland, MI) is a liquid-type material that reinforces gauze bandages. When activated by a catalyst, it forms a soft splint material that can be used for casts and splints when more rigid materials such as plastic and rubberlike (elastomer) combinations or

273

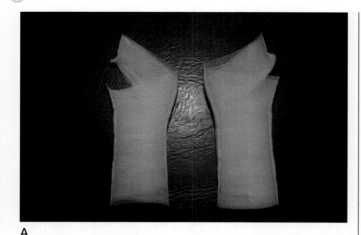

A

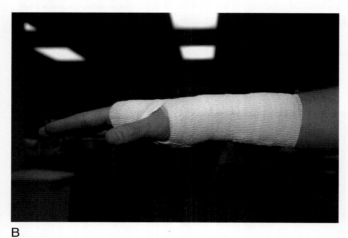

B

Fig. 20-3 Bivalved soft splint. The splint is taped to the athlete for protection during practice and play. It can be used in sports where a splint fashioned from more rigid material is not permitted. The athlete can wear the more rigid splint when not participating in sport.

polyethylene or EVA foams are not permitted by the sport.[3,4] Soft casting tape (e.g., 3M Healthcare) also can be used for this purpose (Fig. 20-3). After the splint is fashioned and allowed to harden, the device is bivalved so that, if needed, it can be replaced with a more rigid cast/splint for everyday uses. The softer splint is taped in place for play, practice, and competition.

Pneumatic devices

Air-filled braces and pads have gained in popularity in the last decade, but their use is limited because of problems with deflation and punctures. Pneumatic splints are used following trauma to immobilize injured extremities. Air pockets have been added for support in ankle braces, tennis elbow counterforce devices, and other protective orthosis.

Examples of protective equipment
Shoulder

Pads for protection
Tackling, checking, and violent ground contact leave the shoulder extremely susceptible to injury. Sports such as football, hockey, and lacrosse require the use of shoulder pads to help protect the sternum, clavicle, shoulder, and scapula. Significant improvements in shoulder pads design have been made over the last 25 years. Currently, pads are made of high-impact, plastic outer shells to deflect collision forces and an inner lining composed of open-cell or closed-cell foam or air dispersion pads to absorb force. They are lightweight and flexible to permit adequate range of motion (ROM) of the shoulder and neck, yet they provide sufficient protection of the chest, back, and shoulder girdle.

Football pads provide the player with greater protection than do hockey or lacrosse shoulder pads (Fig. 20-4). Attachments such as rib and back plates, biceps pads, and neck rolls add further levels of protection (Fig. 20-5). To decrease the incidence of injury and improve comfort, manufactures have added ventilation systems (e.g., Temperature Management System, Williams Sports Group, Jacksonville, FL). While on the sidelines, players connect small air hoses to their pads and can circulate cooled air through ventilation channels in the interior of the pads.

In football, shoulder pad selection is position specific. Offensive and defensive skill positions generally require smaller pads for greater glenohumeral mobility. However, receivers, running backs, and quarterbacks often require greater coverage of the chest, ribs, and back because these areas may be targeted by the opponent. Increased protection is required for tight ends, fullbacks, and linebackers, but not at the expense of mobility. Linemen exposed to constant contact impact have the least requirements for shoulder mobility and require the greatest amount of protection. Despite the differences in shoulder pads, the same fitting principles apply. Padding should cover the lateral extent of the shoulder; cups and flaps should cover the deltoid; straps should be snug to minimize movement; and the neck opening should not constrain the arms when they are fully abducted (Fig. 20-6). Ancillary padding for the acromioclavicular (AC) joint can be used as standalone devices or used in conjunction with shoulder pads to help protect the area following injury or to help protect the area from injury. The most basic supplemental protection to the AC joint is a doughnut pad placed over the joint, often made from dense foam (Fig. 20-7, *A*). This device can be worn with shoulder pads or as a standalone pad in sports in which a hard-shell orthosis is prohibited (e.g., wrestling). Shoulder injury pads (Adams USA, Cookeville, TN; Fig. 20-7, *B*) are commercially available lightweight pads that can be worn to elevate shoulder pads and thus provide additional capacity for force dispersion. However, these pads can interfere with proper fitting of the standard shoulder pads causing migration. Rather than purchase a prefabricated plastic shell shoulder pad, a custom pad can be constructed from moldable thermoplastic material. Care must be taken when making the splint to create a dome over the AC joint so that the pad does not contact the joint itself. The pad is held in place with tape or a strap.

Restraining devices
AC joint injury and glenohumeral joint instability are prevalent not only in athletes participating in contact sports but also among those who participate in gymnastics, basketball, racquet, and overhead throwing sports. Following the acute management of the injury, the athlete often can return to sport with the use of bracing and augmented padding. Taping provides stabilization of the AC joint, and off-the-shelf braces are

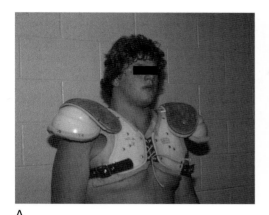

A

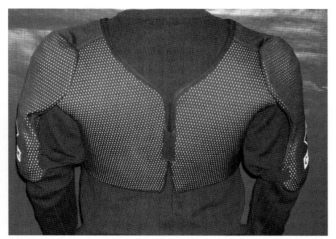

B

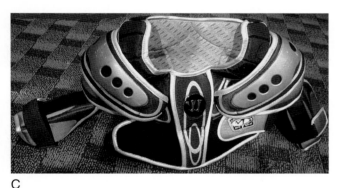

C

Fig. 20-4 Note the more protective football shoulder pads in comparison to pads used for hockey and lacrosse. **A,** Football shoulder pads. **B,** Hockey shoulder pads. **C,** Lacrosse shoulder pads.

malleable for protecting this area. Anterior glenohumeral joint instability secondary to an acute dislocation or repetitive trauma is difficult to treat with tape or sports orthoses. Moreover, return to play with bracing should only follow a full rehabilitation program. Although the pathology of the condition is multifactorial, it is known that abduction and external rotation of the glenohumeral joint is a vulnerable position.[2,6] Therefore, it may be impractical for overhead athletes who depend on abduction and external rotation for performance to play in a brace that restricts this motion. The brace is best used by hockey players and football linemen,

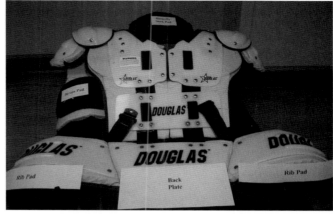

Fig. 20-5 Football shoulder pads with attached rib and back plates, biceps pads, and neck roll, all of which can be added to the basic pad for extra protection.

who can perform their sport with limited range of shoulder motion.

Several types of braces prevent recurrent episodes of glenohumeral instability. Three commonly used shoulder stabilizing braces designed to facilitate controlled ROM are the Denison-Duke Wyre harness (CD Denison Orthopaedic Appliance, Baltimore, MD), the SAWA shoulder brace (Brace International, Atlanta, GA), and the Shoulder Subluxation Inhibitor (Boston Brace International, Avon, MA; Fig. 20-8). The Sully brace (Saunders Group, Chaska, MN) and OmoTrain (Bauerfeind USA, Kennesaw, GA) are lighter-weight, stabilizing orthotics that permit a wider ROM and, therefore, can be used by athletes performing overhead throwing activities (e.g., basketball; Fig. 20-9). In football a variety of attachments to the shoulder pads (e.g., Simply Stable Shoulder Stabilizer, Trulife Group, Poulsbo, WA) are used (Fig. 20-10). These devices have a brachial cuff that is affixed to the shoulder pads via a strap. Few studies have tested these devices. One study found that none of the braces restricted active shoulder abduction and external rotation to preset limits due to deformation of pliable materials and loosening during repetitive motion.[20] However, these braces maintained the advantage of restricting vulnerable

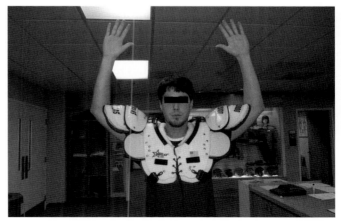

Fig. 20-6 Football shoulder pad. (Note that the neck opening does not constrain the arms when they are fully abducted.)

275

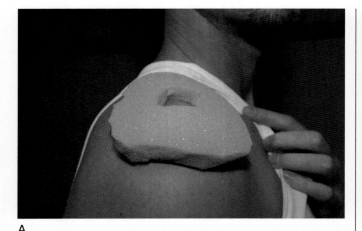

A

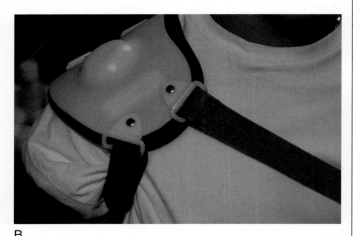

B

Fig. 20-7 Pads for protection. **A,** Doughnut pad worn with shoulder pads or as a standalone pad to protect the AC joint. **B,** Commercial shoulder injury pads, which elevate the shoulder pad to provide additional capacity for force dispersion. (With permission from Adams USA, Cookeville, TN.)

positions by adding stability to the shoulder in positions of abduction and external rotation.[20]

Elbow

The elbow joint is vulnerable to injury in both contact and noncontact sports. Overhead throwing and racquet-type sports place the elbow at risk for acute or chronic ligamentous injury and inflammation. Contact sports can result in a variety of injuries to the elbow, ranging from soft-tissue abrasions and contusions to dislocations. For this reason, many types of commercially available pads and orthotic devices are available to protect and stabilize the elbow.

Pads for protection

The most basic protective/supportive device is the elbow sleeve, which typically is constructed from elasticized cotton or Neoprene. Sleeves provide minimal protection from impact but do provide warmth and compression to the elbow joint. Football players wear such sleeves while playing on turf fields to avoid turf burn. These sleeves may also provide ball carriers with extra grip on the football when the ball is tucked under the arm.

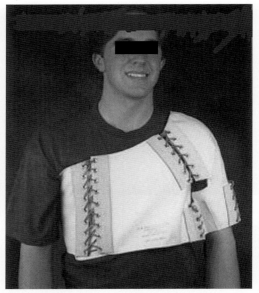

A

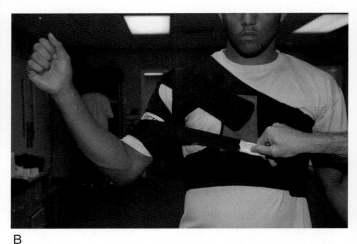

B

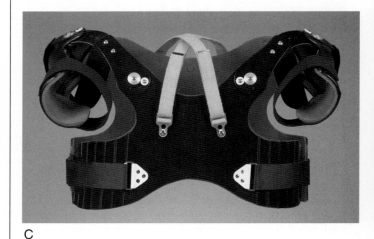

C

Fig. 20-8 Three commonly used shoulder stabilization braces. **A,** Denison-Duke Wyre harness. (With permission from CD Denison Orthopaedic Appliance, Baltimore, MD.) **B,** Sawa shoulder brace. (With permission from Brace International, Atlanta, GA.) **C,** Shoulder subluxation inhibitor. (With permission from Boston Brace International, Avon, MA.)

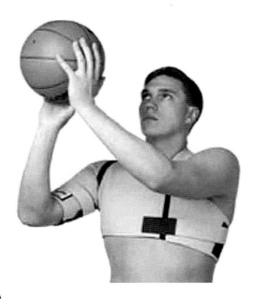
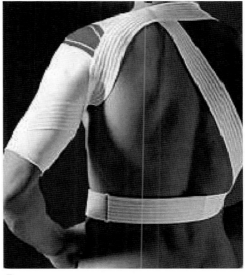

A   B

Fig. 20-9 Two lighter-weight stabilization shoulder braces that permit a wider range of motion. **A,** Sully brace. (With permission from Saunders Group, Chaska, MN.) **B,** OmoTrain. (With permission from Bauerfeind USA, Kennesaw, GA.)

Hockey and most lacrosse leagues require elbow pads to provide the athlete protection from blows from the sticks. These pads may consist of high-impact plastic cups to protect the olecranon and distal humerus as well as dense foam padding over the proximal forearm. They typically are incorporated into a pull-on sleeve or fit into pockets in the uniform (Fig. 20-11). Inline skaters also wear an impact shield over the olecranon area but, in general, do not use additional padding for the distal humerus and proximal forearm. Less protective but less expensive and more malleable foam padding to cover the olecranon can be used to protect contusions or abrasions in a variety of other contact sports.

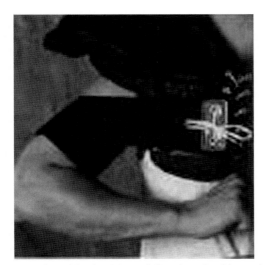

Fig. 20-10 Simply Stable Shoulder Stabilizer is a shoulder pad attachment that provides anterior arm protection. (With permission from Trulife Group, Poulsbo, WA.)

Restraining devices

Hyperextension of the elbow usually results from an acute injury during contact sports as well as falls during skateboarding, inline skating, and mountain biking. The typical mechanism of injury is a fall on the outstretched hand. The spectrum of injury can encompass mild sprains to frank ligamentous instability. Once fully rehabilitated, athletes can generally return to play with supportive devices.

Hyperextension taping using check-rein supports and valgus taping can be used to provide support for athletes with mild injuries. Circumferential tape anchors are placed at the distal humerus and proximal forearm. Check-rein supports are next connected to the anchoring strips using nonelastic tape over the cubital fossa with the elbow in flexion. The check reins then are overwrapped at the anchors, and a figure-of-eight elastic wrap can be added (Fig. 20-12).

More extensive injuries, such as those resulting from dislocations, may require supports with greater stability and additional ROM constraints. Hinged elbow braces can have a single medial hinge or have hinges both medially and laterally to protect against both varus and valgus stresses. Hinges can be open or enclosed in a protective sleeve and may provide full or limited ROM depending upon the need (Fig. 20-13).

Counterforce braces

Repetitive stress at the elbow joint can result in inflammation of tendons that originate from the medial and lateral epicondyles of the distal humerus. Lateral epicondylitis, commonly termed *tennis elbow*, involves inflammation of the common extensor tendons as they arise from the lateral epicondyle. Athletes who play racket sports, as well as those involved in baseball, javelin, golf, squash, and weightlifting, are predisposed. Medial epicondylitis resulting from inflammation of the origin of the flexor-pronator mass is less common than

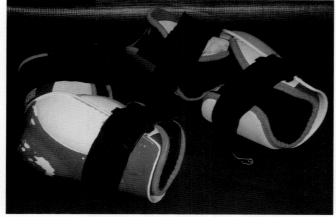

A

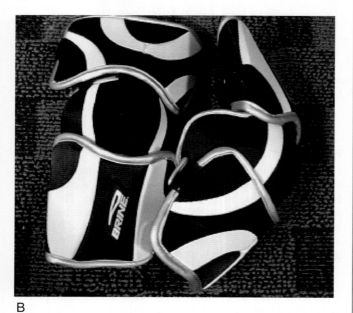

B

Fig. 20-11 Lacrosse elbow pad used to provide protection from stick blows. **A**, Lacrosse. **B**, Hockey.

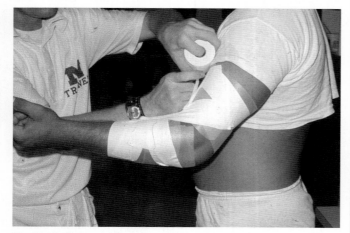

Fig. 20-12 Elbow taped to prevent hyperextension.

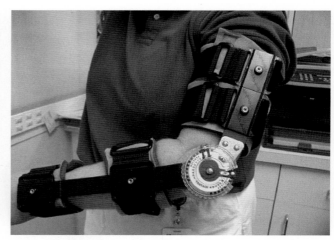

Fig. 20-13 Hinged elbow brace with a dial lock to limit motion.

lateral epicondylitis but is classically related to golf and bowling, hence the name *golfer's* or *bowler's elbow*. Racquet sport athletes, swimmers, and weightlifters also may develop medial epicondylitis. Treatment of these injuries includes a variety of activities. Exercise, ice massage, and other modalities are used to decrease inflammation and increase circulation to promote healing. An orthotic device, either a proximal forearm strap or a pull-on sleeve, also may be recommended. These devices, referred to as *counterforce braces* (Fig. 20-14), typically incorporate a pad placed over the muscle belly just below its origin of the epicondyle. The mechanism of action of these braces is thought to be counterpressure distal to tendon origin thereby relieving stress on the origin. Although there is debate on the validity of this proposed mechanism of action, most studies have found counterforce braces to be helpful in decreasing pain.[7]

Forearm and wrist

Protective pads

A variety of pads made of dense, closed-cell or open-cell foam are available to protect the forearm. They can be held in place with tape, elasticized tape, or a sleeve. Football linemen traditionally wear these pads for protecting the dorsal forearm during blocking; however, the game has evolved such that blocking now involves the use of the hands, eliminating the need for forearm protection. To fend off kicks and punches, participants in martial arts wear guards composed of a foam or plastic shield, attached to the forearm with hook-and-loop straps. Archers wear a reinforced leather or plastic orthotic on the volar distal forearm of the bow arm to protect the forearm from the bowstring as it moves forward after the release (Fig. 20-15).

Supports to dissipate force or limit motion

Athletes often subject the wrist or radiocarpal joint to repetitive dorsiflexion and compressive forces. Weightlifters, gymnasts participating in vault, beam, pommel horse, and floor exercises, cheerleaders, as well as football players who deliver blows with their hands often use wrist support to limit wrist dorsiflexion. Basic stabilization of the wrist can be achieved

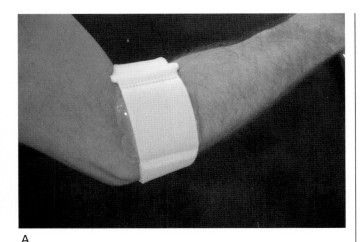

A

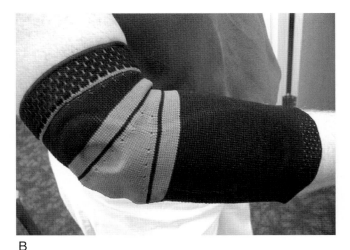

B

Fig. 20-14 Counterforce braces for lateral or medial epicondylitis. **A,** Strap. **B,** Sleeve.

with taping or a variety of Neoprene or elastic wraps, which provide support and compression while limiting dorsiflexion and palmar flexion (Fig. 20-16).

Support also can be achieved through use of dorsal wrist extension block splints fabricated from rigid or semirigid thermomolded materials and secured to the wrist with tape to prevent migration. To increase power and accuracy by minimizing wrist motion during ball release, bowlers use a wrist splint that includes a dorsal extension to the hand to minimize extension of the wrist and the ulnar three digits (Fig. 20-17).

Snowboarders, skateboarders, and in-line skaters use braces that incorporate rigid volar splints to minimize the incidence and severity of injuries from falls.[9]

Hand

Protective padding

Gloves in sport are used to provide protection, to increase grip, or to provide warmth in cold weather. Gloves with varying degrees of padding are used during contact sports. For example, lacrosse and hockey gloves extend over the wrist and are heavily padded on the dorsal aspect of the glove,

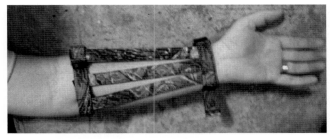

Fig. 20-15 Protective forearm pad for archery.

with the palmer aspect composed of leather to maintain tactile sensation and increase grip on the stick (Fig. 20-18). Hockey goalies wear two different types of gloves for blocking and catching. Catcher gloves resemble baseball mitts and are worn on the non-stick hand. Catcher gloves have an oversized catching area, with a molded thumb area padded on the dorsal aspect of the glove and the palmar aspect composed of leather to maintain tactile sensation and increase grip on the stick (Fig. 20-19). Blocker gloves are worn on the stick hand and have a padded leather or synthetic leather palm to hold the stick, but they also have a wide, rigid blocking pad on the dorsum to deflect shots (Fig. 20-19).

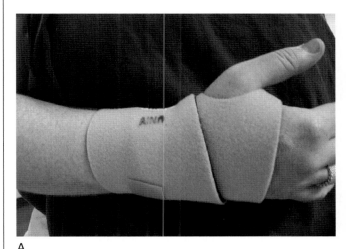

A

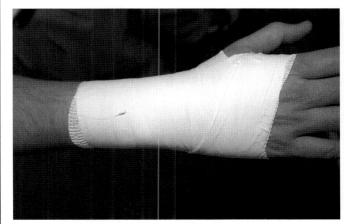

B

Fig. 20-16 Wrist wrap. **A,** Neoprene. **B,** Tape.

279

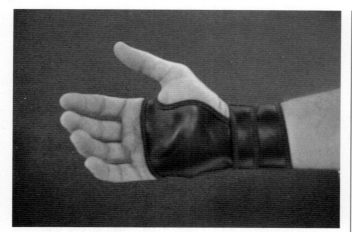

Fig. 20-17 Bowler's wrist splint.

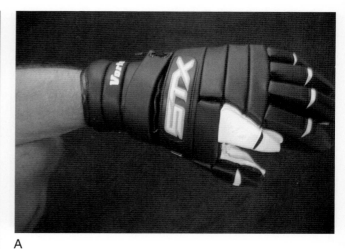

A

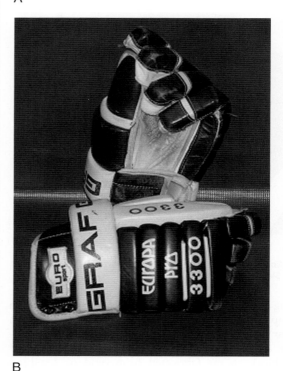

B

Fig. 20-18 Protective gloves used in contact sports are heavily padded on their dorsal aspect. **A,** Lacrosse gloves. **B,** Hockey gloves.

Football linemen's gloves are full-fingered gloves with padding over the bony prominences dorsally as well as over the thenar and hypothenar eminences. Linemen's gloves are generally less bulky than those used for hockey and lacrosse to improve grip strength while maintaining position and tactile sensation of the hands. Football running backs, receivers, and defensive players use thin gloves with a leather palm to help maintain grip, prevent abrasions, and provide warmth during cold games (Fig. 20-20).

Cyclists, during long-distance rides, wear a glove padded in the palm to prevent neuropathies resulting from compression of the medial and ulnar nerves in this area (Fig. 20-21). Compression of the ulnar nerve as it enters the hand through the Guyon canal results in handlebar palsy or ulnar neuropathy. Median neuropathy or carpal tunnel syndrome from compression of the median nerve in the carpal tunnel is less common in cyclists. Cyclist's gloves are generally lightweight and have vented fingerless gloves to keep the hands cool. Additionally, handlebar padding, correct seat height, and grip position help to prevent these disorders, which initially present as numbness and tingling in the fingertips.

Handball gloves protect the hand from the force of the ball, which can travel at speeds up to 55 miles per hour. These gloves are generally made of leather and are made with or without padding (Fig. 20-22). Experienced handball athletes tend to prefer less padding in order to maintain ball control.

Boxing gloves are designed as a mitten with the thumb separate. These gloves help to prevent fractures of the hand as well as trauma to the opponent's face. The three basic types of boxing gloves are competition gloves, sparring/training gloves, and bag gloves (Fig. 20-23). Typically the hand is prewrapped with tape to make the hand more rigid. Most professional and amateur boxing matches use 8- or 10-ounce gloves. However, during a match the weight of these gloves may double after they become wet with perspiration and water is doused on the boxer between rounds.[17] Training gloves are similar to competition gloves but are generally softer and contain more padding. Heavier-weight boxers use 16- to 18-ounce gloves, whereas lighter-weight boxers use gloves in the 12- to 14-ounce range. Some recommend that boxers train with heavier gloves to promote arm strength and endurance. Bag gloves are generally lighter weight and used for protection while training on the heavy bag.

Although boxing gloves initially were designed for protection, some have advocated a return to barehanded boxing because they believe that the weight of the glove transmits more force during blows, increasing the severity of injuries.[18]

Ski gloves should be warm and waterproof to protect the wearer from the elements as well as offer good flexibility to maintain hand dexterity while gripping the ski pole. Ski gloves are gauntlet-style gloves extending above the wrist to protect against lacerations from the ski edge and to prevent snow from getting under the gloves when skiing in deep powder.[13] Ski gloves are of two basic styles: mittens or gloves. By keeping the fingers together, mittens are warmer because there is less surface area for heat exchange. However, this advantage is offset by the loss of finger dexterity.

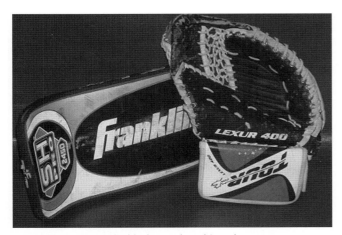

Fig. 20-19 Hockey goalie blocker and catching gloves.

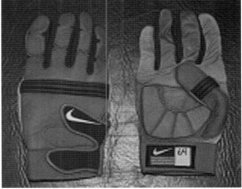

A

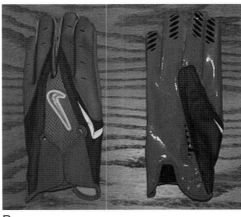

B

Fig. 20-20 Football gloves are designed differently for various positions. **A**, Linemen's gloves are less bulky than hockey or lacrosse gloves. **B**, Running back, receivers, and defensive players wear thin gloves with a leather palm to help maintain grip.

Novice skiers may have difficulty maintaining grip on the ski poles with mittens.

A variety of ski gloves have reinforced thumb guards to help prevent ulnar collateral ligament injuries, which can result from a retained pole producing a radially directed force on the abducted thumb.[15] Prophylactic or postinjury protection can be accomplished with the use of check-rein tape placed between the thumb and index finger (Fig. 20-24) or by use of thumb spica taping (Fig. 20-25).

Baseball players use a variety of gloves that are position specific (Fig. 20-26). Baseball catchers wear well-padded leather mitts to protect the palm from repeated trauma from the impact of high velocity pitches. The ulnar artery is particularly vulnerable because it can be crushed against the hook of the hamate, resulting in thrombosis, aneurysm formation, or hypothenar hammer syndrome. Hypothenar hammer syndrome is a reflex vasospastic disorder resulting from repeat blunt trauma to the ulnar artery leading to digital ischemia.[14] Fielder's gloves are well padded, similar to catcher's mitts, but have fingers in them for better ball control. The fingers of outfielder's gloves are generally longer than those of infielder's gloves, but both are sewn together to provide greater containment for a high-velocity ball. First basemen's gloves are made with a deeper pocket than are other infielders' gloves. Baseball batting gloves contain a leather palm to decrease slips on the bat due to poor grip or perspiration on the hands as well as minimize vibration from the bat during contact with the ball. Batters also require padding to protect their palms during sliding.

Soccer goalies wear gloves to increase grip and protect the hand (Fig. 20-27). The palm of a soccer goalie glove is composed of latex. Smooth latex generally provides the best grip; thicker and textured latex palms are more durable but sacrifice tactile sensation. For protection against hyperextension injuries to the fingers, some goalies prefer a glove that incorporates a semirigid extension block to the dorsal aspect of the gloves fingers.

Golfer's gloves are made of lightweight soft leather or synthetic leather and are worn on the lead hand to increase grip and absorb perspiration while maintaining flexibility. (The lead hand is the left hand in a right-handed golfer and vice versa for a left-handed golfer.)

Splints to protect and support injured fingers

Athletic injuries to the fingers can result from excessive axial, compressive, or rotational forces, or from overloads to the tendons during grasping activities. Finger injuries commonly seen in sport for which orthosis are prescribed include the following:

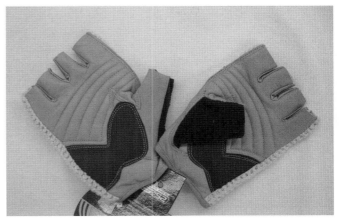

Fig. 20-21 Cyclist's gloves are padded in the palm to prevent neuropathies.

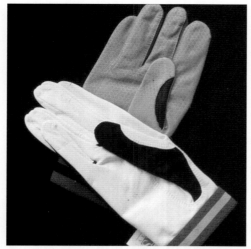

Fig. 20-22 Handball gloves are made of leather and may or may not have padding.

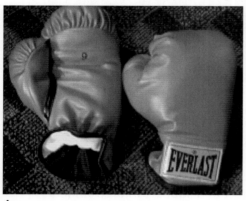

A

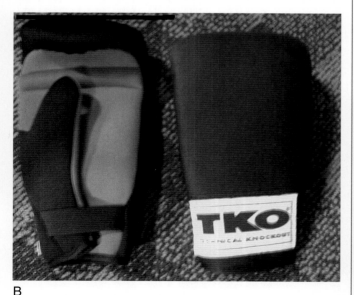

B

Fig. 20-23 Boxing gloves. **A,** Competition gloves. **B,** Bag gloves.

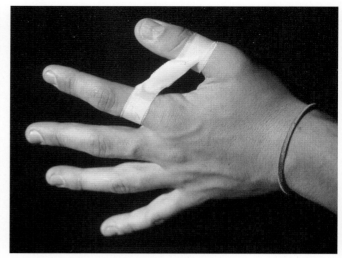

Fig. 20-24 Check-rein taping of the thumb.

Phalangeal or metacarpal fractures
Central slip disruptions of the proximal interphalangeal
  (PIP) joint (boutonnière deformity)
Volar plate avulsions of the PIP joint (swan neck deformity)
Collateral ligament sprains of the metacarpophalangeal
  (MCP) joints or interphalangeal joints
Extensor tendon avulsions of the distal phalanx (mallet,
  baseball, or drop finger)

Avulsion of the terminal extensor tendon at its insertion on the distal phalanx, otherwise known as *mallet finger, drop finger,* or *baseball finger,* is especially common not only in baseball but also in volleyball and basketball (Fig. 20-28). The mechanism of this injury is forced flexion of the extended distal interphalangeal (DIP) joint. These injuries can be managed with the DIP joint splinted in mild hyperextension, provided the avulsed fracture does not disrupt more than one third of the articular surface.[11] Foam padded aluminum splints can be cut to length and placed on the volar surface of the distal finger, permitting ROM at the PIP joint while maintaining slight hyperextension at the DIP joint. Commercially available, premolded splints (stack splints) also are available (Fig. 20-29). These types of splints should be worn 24 hours per day.[10] Care must be taken with all

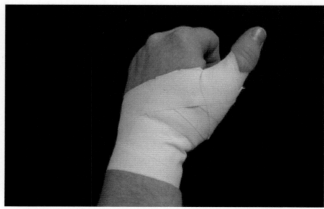

Fig. 20-25 Thumb spica taping.

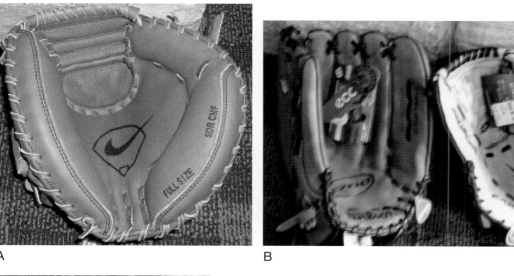

A

B

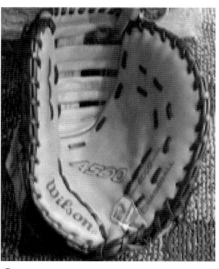

C

Fig. 20-26 Baseball gloves. **A,** Catcher's mitt is well padded. **B,** Fielder's glove is padded but has fingers unlike the catcher's mitt. (Note the longer fingers on outfielder's glove compared with the shorter fingers of infielder's glove.). **C,** First baseman's glove has a deep pocket compared with the infielder's glove.

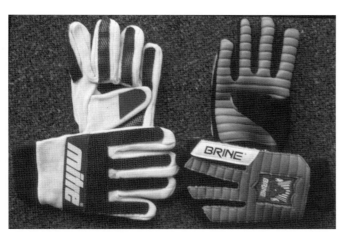

Fig. 20-27 Soccer goalie gloves.

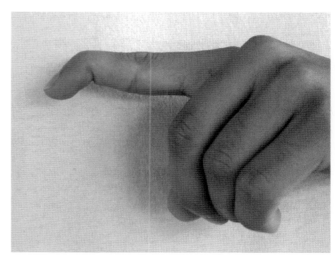

Fig. 20-28 Mallet finger.

283

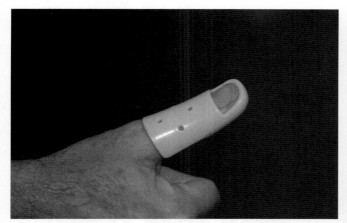

Fig. 20-29 Splints for distal interphalangeal joint injury (mallet finger).

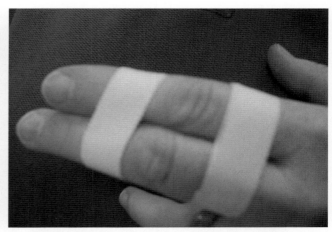

Fig. 20-31 Buddy taping for fingers can be used following collateral ligament injuries of the metacarpophalangeal or proximal interphalangeal joint.

splints to keep the skin beneath the splint clean and dry to prevent skin irritation.

Hyperextension of the PIP joint can result in injuries to the volar plate. The volar plate is a ligamentous structure forming the floor of the joint. Mild volar plate sprains can be managed with buddy taping until pain-free ROM occurs. More severe injuries, such as those associated with dislocations, are treated with a dorsally placed extension block splint with the PIP in slight flexion.[5] This type of splint permits early flexion to decrease the incidence of stiffness following the injury. The splint can be removed after 2 weeks to begin active ROM. Buddy taping should be used on initial return to sport. When the finger is taped, the DIP and PIP joints should remain free of tape to improve motion. It is important to

ensure that there is no neurovascular compromise following taping. Commercially available tandem finger straps can be be used to serve the same function (Fig. 20-30).

Collateral ligament injuries result from ulnar or radially directed forces to the MCP or PIP joints. These injuries can be managed initially with splinting in 30 degrees of flexion for several weeks, followed by buddy taping (Fig. 20-31). The injured finger should be buddy taped to the finger adjacent to the injury (i.e., an ulnar collateral ligament injury to the ring finger should be buddy taped to the small finger). Ulnar collateral ligament injuries to the thumb as discussed in the skier's section frequently can be managed with a fiberglass or thermomoldable rigid or semirigid cast or splint.

Boutonnière deformities or central slip avulsions of the PIP joint result in extension of the MCP and DIP joints with flexion of the PIP joint (Fig. 20-32). The typical mechanism of injury is forced flexion of the PIP joint or volar dislocation of the joint. Stable injuries can be managed with the PIP

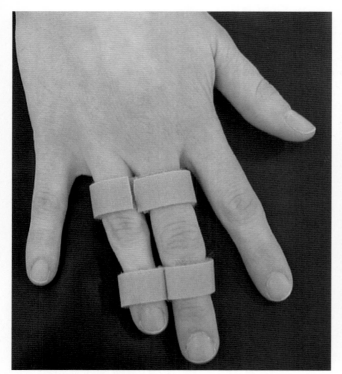

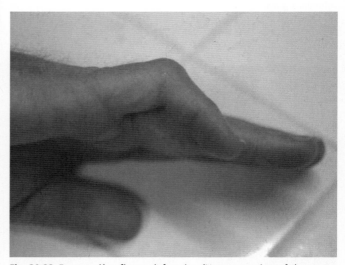

Fig. 20-32 Boutonnière finger deformity. (Note extension of the meta-carpophalangeal and distal interphalangeal joints with flexion of the proximal interphalangeal joint.)

Fig. 20-30 Tandem finger straps.

splinted in extension for 4 weeks, using aluminum foam or custom-molded thermoplastic splint.[8]

Acknowledgments

The authors thank Tanya Maxwell, MS, L/ATC, for photographic assistance in preparation of the manuscript and Charlene Corbett for manuscript preparation.

References

1. Andrews JR, Wilk KE: Shoulder injuries in baseball. In Andrews JR, Wilk KE, editors: *The athlete's shoulder*, New York, 1994, Churchill Livingstone.
2. Baker C, Wibe J, Whitman C: Arthroscopic evaluation of acute initial anterior shoulder dislocations, *Am J Sports Med* 18:25–28, 1990.
3. Bassett F, Malone T, Gilchrist R: A protective splint of silicone rubber, *Am J Sports Med* 7:358–360, 1979.
4. Bergfeld JA, Weiker GG, JT Andrish, et al: Soft playing splint for protection of significant hand and wrist injuries in sports, *Am J Sports Med* 10:293–296, 1982.
5. Browner: Fractures and dislocations of the hand. In Browner, Jupiter J, Levine A, Trafton P, editors: *Skeletal trauma: Basic science, management, and reconstruction*, Philadelphia, 2003, Saunders.
6. Buss DD, Lynch GP, Meyer CP, et al: Nonoperative management for in-season athletes with anterior shoulder instability, *Am J Sports Med* 32:1430–1433, 2004.
7. Chan HL, Gabriel YF: Effect of counterforce forearm bracing on wrist extensor muscles performance, *Am J Phy Med Rehabil* 82:290–295, 2003.
8. Graham TJ, Mullen DJ: Athletic injury of the adult hand. In DeLee JC, Drezs DJ, editors: *Orthopaedic sports medicine, principles and practice. Central slip disruption*, Philadelphia, 2003, WB Saunders.
9. Hagel B, Pless B, Goulet C: The effect of wrist guard use on upper-extremity injuries in snowboarders, *Am J Epidemiol* 162:149–156, 2005.
10. Lairmore JR, Engber WD: Serious, often subtle, finger injuries: avoiding diagnosis and treatment pitfalls, *Phys Sportsmed* 26:57–69, 1998.
11. Lubahn JD, Hood JM: Fractures of the distal interphalangeal joint, *Clin Orthop Relat Res* 327:12–20, 1996.
12. Marshall SW, Waller AE, Dick RW, et al: An ecologic study of protective equipment and injury in two contact sports, *Int J Epidemiol* 31:587–592, 2002.
13. Match RM: Laceration of the median nerve from skiing, *Am J Sports Med* 6:22–25, 1978.
14. Mueller LP, Mueller LA, Degreif J, Rommens PM: Hypothenar hammer syndrome in a golf player: a case report, *Am J Sports Med* 28:741–745, 2000.
15. Rettig AC: Athletic injuries of the wrist and hand: part ii: overuse injuries of the wrist and traumatic injuries to the hand, *Am J Sports Med* 32:262–273, 2004.
16. Roberts WO: Shielding a bruise: how to make a simple protective pad, *Phys Ssportsmed* 26:77–78, 1998.
17. Ryan AJ (moderator), Litel GR, Lundberg GD, et al: The medical aspects of boxing: a round table, *Phys Sportsmed* 13:56–74, 1985.
18. Ryan AJ: Eliminate boxing gloves, *Phys Sportsmed* 11:49, 1983.
19. Schulz LA, Busconi BD, Pappas AM: Protective equipment. In Pappas AM, Walzer J, editors: *Upper extremity injuries in the athlete*, New York, 1995, Churchill Livingstone.
20. Weise K, Sitler M, Tierney R, Swanik K: Effectiveness of glenohumeral-joint stability braces in limiting active and passive shoulder range of motion in collegiate football players, *J Athl Train* 39:151–155, 2004.
21. Wichmann S, Martin D: Bracing for activity, *Phys Sportsmed* 24:88–94, 1996.

Suggested readings

Anderson M, Hall S, Hitchings C, editors: *Fundamentals of sports injury management: protective equipment*, Media, PA, 1995, Williams & Wilkins.

DeCarlo MS, Malone KN, Gerig BH, Hunker MH: Protective devices for the shoulder complex. In Hawkins RJ, Misamore GW, editors: *Shoulder injuries in the athlete*, New York, 1996, Churchill Livingstone.

Griffin LY, editor: *Preventing injuries: athletic training and sports medicine*, Park Ridge Ill, 1991, American Association of Orthopaedic Surgeons.

Hwang I-K, Kim K-J: Shock-absorbing effects of various padding conditions in improving efficacy of wrist guards, *J Sports Sci Med* 3:23–29, 2004.

Pettrone FA: *Symposium: upper extremity injuries in athletes. American Academy of Orthopaedic Surgeons*, St. Louis, 1986, CV Mosby.

Saliba E, Foreman S, Abadie R: Protective equipment considerations. In Zachazewski JE, Magee DJ, Quillen WS, editors: *Athletic injuries and rehabilitation*, Philadelphia, 1996, WB Saunders.

Soos TH: Taping the injured athlete. In Kulund DN, editor: *The injured athlete*, Philadelphia, 1982, Lippincott.

The effectiveness of abduction shoulder orthoses on limiting anterior translation of the glenohumeral joint: a cadaveric study of comparison of abduction orthoses. *Clin J Sport Med* 10:230–231, 2000.

Orthoses for overuse disorders of the upper limb

Mary C. Burns and Michael W. Neumeister

Key Points

- Lateral epicondylitis, cubital tunnel syndrome, carpal tunnel syndrome, de Quervain tenosynovitis, trigger finger (stenosing tenosynovitis), and basilar joint arthritis represent overuse disorders of the upper limb.

- The anatomy, symptoms, and conservative splinting options for these overuse disorders are reviewed.

- A global approach to conservative treatment of overuse conditions is necessary, with orthoses used in conjunction with other treatment options such as nonsteroidal antiinflammatory drug, steroid injections, ergonomic modifications of work activities and the workplace, and exercise.

Our hands are the masters of many functions, ranging from delicate touches to forceful grips. We use our hands to lift, pull, push, pinch, and grasp. The hand is an instrument needed for building, communicating, feeding, and expressing emotion. Whereas a closed fist denotes anger, an open palm offers comfort and empathy. The blind use their hands to read, and the deaf to talk. Our hands are unique tools required to perform all aspects of our activities of daily living. The many daily tasks in our lives can impart a demanding burden upon the hand and upper extremity. Repetitive motion, improper posture, and poor mechanics can lead to cumulative trauma disorders characterized by inflammation, pain, limited movement, nerve compression, and ultimately impaired function.

This chapter focuses on the conservative orthotic management of overuse disorders of the upper extremity. Many of these conditions will also require other conservative treatments, including, but not limited to, nonsteroidal

antiinflammatory drug (NSAIDs), steroid injections, ergonomic modifications of work activities and the workplace, exercise, or modalities such as paraffin, hot pads, ice packs, iontophoresis, or ultrasound. Although a global approach to conservative treatment of these conditions is necessary and orthoses will be used in conjunction with other treatment options, this chapter discusses only the appropriate splints to be used with these overuse conditions.

In order to determine the type of splint necessary for any condition, it is important to understand the general goals of splinting. The ultimate purpose of orthosis in the upper extremity is to relieve pain and improve functional range of motion. Some of the general goals of splinting include (a) providing rest for a specific joint, (b) relieving tension from healing structures, (c) protecting and properly positioning edematous structures, (d) maintaining proper joint alignment and tissue length to prevent soft-tissue contracture, and (e) providing maximum functional use of the extremity while it is splinted. It is necessary for the physician and therapist to fully understand the anatomy of the involved structures and the anatomical implications of splinting to avoid pressure areas and compression of surrounding nerves and to prevent further inflammation of surrounding structures. If all of these factors are taken into consideration, splinting can be an effective option for conservative management of these nontraumatic conditions.

Lateral epicondylitis
Anatomy and symptoms

Lateral epicondylitis, or *tennis elbow*, is a very common condition of the lateral elbow. Patients generally present to the clinic with pain and localized tenderness of the extensor origin and lateral epicondyle of the humerus. Onset may be acute or insidious. Generally, the patient complains of increased pain with wrist extension or with gripping. In severe cases, the patient may complain of pain with lifting very light objects. Activities requiring full elbow extension and forearm pronation aggravate the discomfort. The pain of lateral epicondylitis often is accentuated by extreme wrist flexion from passive stretch of the extensor carpi radialis brevis (ECRB) muscle or by active contraction of the wrist extensors. The pain may not be isolated to the lateral epicondyle but actually may radiate proximally or distally.[9,11,26,27] Lateral epicondylitis is believed to be a tendinosis of the origin of the ECRB. Although the specific etiology is unknown,[2] it is postulated that microtears at the origin of the common extensor muscle mass, involving the extensor digitorum communis, extensor carpi radialis longus, supinator, and ECRB, are the likely precipitating factor for this condition. Many investigators believe that these small tears are caused by overuse and repetitive injury and strain of the common extensor origin at the lateral epicondyle. The instigating injury is the result of forced flexion of the wrist and fingers during extensor muscle contraction. Such mechanisms are seen with racquet sports where backhand volleys are required. As these microtears try to heal, continued use of the upper extremity causes continued strain and reinjury to the muscle origins.[10,26,27] This can lead to degeneration and possible avascularity at the muscle origin, which in turn leads to chronic inflammation causing the injured areas to remain weak and painful.

Splinting lateral epicondylitis

The primary goal of splinting lateral epicondylitis is to decrease the pain and inflammation at the origin of the ECRB. Several splints have been described in the literature.[2] One of the most common splints used is the wrist cock-up splint (Fig. 21-1). This rigid orthosis maintains the wrist in extension to offload the extensors of the forearm and promote healing at the muscle origin.[10] The appropriate posture of the wrist in the splint has been described in various positions, ranging from 0 to 45 degrees of extension.[4,10] Janson et al.[10] compared three types of wrist orthosis—dorsal wrist splint, volar wrist splint, and semicircumferential wrist

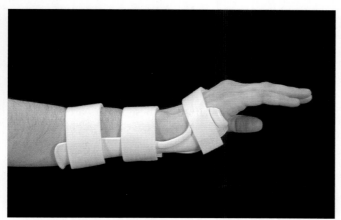

Fig. 21-1 Wrist cock-up splint with wrist positioned in extension to relieve tension on the wrist extensors.

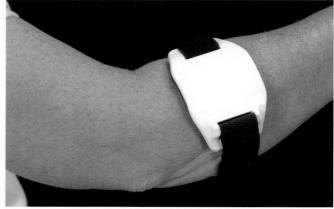

A

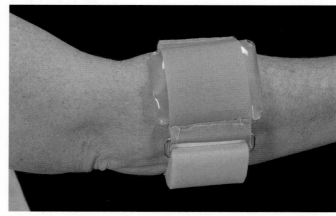

B

Fig. 21-2 A, Band-It™ (Pro Band Sports Industries) forearm band has medial and lateral supports, making it effective for both lateral and medial epicondylitis. **B,** Aircast® pneumatic armband (Northcoast Medical; Smith & Nephew Rolyan). Meyer et al.[17] showed the greatest reduction in EMG activity of the wrist extensors with this counterforce brace.

design—varying the amount of wrist extension and then evaluating muscle limitations by surface electromyography (EMG). The semicircumferential splint showed the greatest change in EMG electrical activity of the extensor muscles: a 6% decrease. The authors concluded that this reduction of electrical activity was comparable to the reduction of electrical activity of the wrist extensors seen while a proximal forearm counterforce brace was worn. Based on these findings, combined with the limited functional use while a rigid wrist orthosis was worn, the authors did not recommend wrist splinting. Clinically, we have found that compliance with a rigid wrist splint is poor because of the device's functional limitations.

The forearm support band or counterforce brace (Fig. 21-2) is a common splint prescribed for lateral epicondylitis. The counterforce brace decreases the force of the muscle contraction by inhibiting muscle expansion and reducing tension at the musculotendinous unit proximal to the band.[17] The counterforce brace essentially changes the functional origin of the extensor mass to a site distal to the radial head. This may assist in resting the origin of the common extensor tendon to permit healing.[9,17]

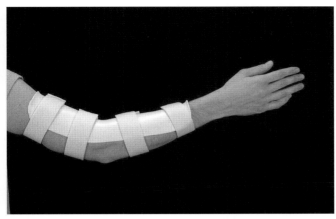

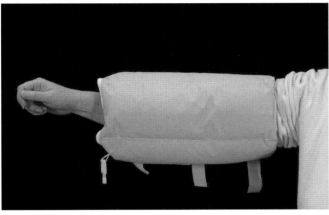

Fig. 21-3 A, Custom splint, fit with the elbow in approximately 45 degrees of flexion, prevents elbow flexion, reducing pressure on the ulnar nerve at night. **B,** Posey Soft Splint™ (J.T. Posey Co.). Soft splint prevents elbow flexion while sleeping.

Several designs of forearm bands are on the market. Both standard and Aircast® counterforce braces showed reduced EMG activity of the extensor muscles, with the greatest reduction of EMG activity seen with the Aircast® band (Fig. 21-3).[17] Further studies are needed to determine recommended wearing time and amount of pressure with application, but it is generally agreed that the counterforce brace should be worn for painful activities during the day and removed for any periods of inactivity. The brace typically is applied approximately 2 cm distal to the lateral epicondyle. It should be fit with a comfortable amount of pressure while the muscles are relaxed so that maximum contraction of the wrist extensors is prohibited. Potential complications with use of the counterforce brace include compression of the radial nerve or the anterior interosseous nerve, edema, and venous congestion. Clinically, we have found more positive compliance with the counterforce brace because it leaves the hand completely free for functional use.

In acute cases of painful lateral epicondylitis, an initial trial of complete immobilization may be necessary. An example is a long arm splint with the elbow in 90 degrees of flexion, the forearm neutral, and the wrist positioned in comfortable extension.[27] The other splinting methods previously described can be initiated once the acute pain has been relieved to a functional level.

Cubital tunnel syndrome

Anatomy and symptoms

Ulnar nerve compression at the medial elbow is known as *cubital tunnel syndrome*. The cubital tunnel is a fibroosseous tunnel at the elbow situated between the humerus and ulnar heads of the flexor carpi ulnaris. The cubital tunnel is bordered laterally by the ulnohumeral collateral ligament and anteriorly by the medial epicondyle. The roof of the cubital tunnel, known as Osborne's, is a fibrous band confluent with the two heads of the flexor carpi ulnaris starting just proximal to the medial epicondyle.[22]

The most common symptoms of cubital tunnel syndrome are paresthesias presenting as numbness and tingling of the ring and small fingers, especially notable at night. Patients may complain of tenderness or a sharp pain at the medial epicondyle or directly over the ulnar nerve. They may describe a vague, sometimes sharp, radiating pain down the ulnar forearm and into the hand. Symptoms may increase with provocative positions of elbow flexion or repetitive flexion/extension. Late stages or severe cubital tunnel syndrome may present with motor weakness and/or muscle atrophy of ulnar innervated muscles, causing a decrease in pinch and grip strength. Ulnar clawing and intrinsic muscle wasting may be present in late stages of cubital tunnel.

Prolonged elbow flexion or repetitive elbow flexion and extension can be a major causative factor to cubital tunnel symptoms. Apfelberg and Larson[1] described the condylar groove, where the ulnar nerve passes, as rounded and spacious during extension and flattened and triangular with elbow flexion, causing increased pressure on the ulnar nerve. Rayan et al.[21] showed that elbow flexion produces a significant rise in pressure at the condylar groove, and pressure increases further at the cubital tunnel when elbow flexion is combined with shoulder elevation.[22,24] Many patients experience an increase in symptoms at night because their elbows are flexed during sleep. Other potential causes of cubital tunnel syndrome include elbow injury and inflammation, and direct trauma or pressure to the ulnar nerve. Ulnar nerve subluxation or traction also may cause symptoms.

Splinting cubital tunnel syndrome

Patients with mild symptoms and no motor changes generally respond well to conservative splinting. The primary goal of splinting for this condition is to decrease pain and paresthesias. Immobilization with the elbow in extension decreases the stretch on the ulnar nerve and prevents repetitive motion that can promote an inflammatory response within the cubital tunnel. An elbow pad can be used during the day to protect the ulnar nerve from trauma or direct pressure.[24]

Night splinting is essential to prevent sleeping with the elbow flexed beyond 90 degrees. Splints for wear at night can be a custom-fit device or an off-the-shelf type

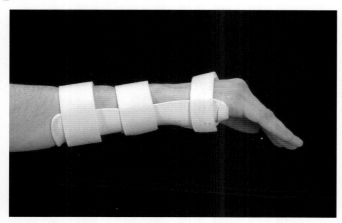

Fig. 21-4 Custom volar wrist splint with wrist positioned in neutral for treatment of carpal tunnel syndrome.

pillow splint. Full elbow extension allows for the least amount of pressure on the ulnar nerve; however, most patients will not be able to tolerate immobilization in full extension. Therefore, a custom splint should be fit with the elbow in comfortable extension, anywhere between 30 and 60 degrees of flexion.[3] The splint is generally fit anteriorly to avoid direct pressure on the nerve at the posterior medial elbow (Fig. 21-3). In our clinic, we have found this type of splint to be effective, yet the rigidity of the splint makes compliance questionable. For the elbow we tend to use a soft splint known as the Posey Soft Splint™ (Fig. 21-4) The Posey soft splint is a filled with polystyrene beads. The splint is easily applied with hook-and-loop closures and prevents elbow flexion. This splint is bulkier than the custom splint, but it is not rigid, is lighter and more comfortable, and improves patient compliance.

Carpal tunnel syndrome
Anatomy and symptoms

Carpal tunnel syndrome is the most common compression neuropathy of the upper extremity. The carpal tunnel is a small narrow space in the volar wrist that houses the median nerve, flexor pollicis longus, four flexor digitorum profundus tendons, and four flexor digitorum superficialis tendons as they course through the forearm into the hand. The tunnel is formed by the concave arch of the carpal bones and the transverse carpal ligament, which extends from the scaphoid tuberosity and trapezium radially, and attaches to the pisiform and the hook of the hamate on the ulnar side of the hand. The carpal tunnel has a defined space with little room for expansion. An increase in the volume of the contents of the tunnel will have a detrimental compressive effect on the tendons and median nerve, resulting in symptoms of carpal tunnel syndrome. Numerous causes of median neuropathy include inflammatory synovitis, trauma, repetitive flexion/extension, and autoimmune and endocrine disorders (Table 21-1).

The symptoms of carpal tunnel syndrome include numbness and tingling, paresthesias, or pain and burning typically in the radial three and a half digits of the hand. It is very common for patients to complain that the symptoms are worse at night. During sleep, the wrist often is flexed, increasing the pressure on the median nerve in the carpal tunnel. As pressure on the median nerve progresses, patients may begin to complain of daytime symptoms, which appear to be aggravated by forceful, repetitive hand motion. Patients also may have radiating pain along the volar forearm to the shoulder or neck. Late stages of carpal tunnel syndrome may cause weakness of thumb abduction, opposition, and a reduction in fine motor skills.

Several studies have shown increased pressure in the carpal tunnel with the wrist flexed or extended. A neutral wrist position appears to cause the least amount of intracarpal pressure, reducing compression on the median nerve.[23,24] Carpal tunnel pressure appears to be increased more with active range of motion of the wrist and digits rather than with passive range of motion.[23] Repetitive hand and wrist movements tend to be a major causative factor in carpal tunnel syndrome. Other causes of carpal tunnel syndrome are prolonged wrist flexion or extension, acute trauma, ergonomic factors, external pressure on the carpal tunnel, and pregnancy.

Splinting carpal tunnel syndrome

Splinting the wrist for carpal tunnel syndrome remains the standard of care even though varying rates of success have been reported in the literature.[15,23,24] Generally, a trial of conservative treatment and splinting is recommended before surgical options unless a patient presents with late-stage carpal tunnel syndrome, including muscle atrophy or continuous sensory impairment. Patients who present with mild symptoms will have the best response to conservative splinting.

Goals of splinting for carpal tunnel syndrome include immobilizing the wrist to prevent flexion of the wrist. Reducing wrist motion may help to decrease inflammation, which may be causing increased pressure on the median nerve. An increase in pressure within the carpal tunnel has been demonstrated with either wrist flexion or extension; therefore, splinting of the wrist in a neutral position is recommended. Mild symptoms of short duration may be relieved with night splinting only. Mild to moderate symptoms during the day or with minimal activity may require full-time splinting. Our general recommendation is to wear a wrist immobilization splint at night and during the day with any activity that increases symptoms. Increased symptoms with specific activities may indicate poor posturing and excessive pressure on the median nerve.

Several splints are commercially available. Conversely, custom-fit orthoses can be made for individual patients. Because external pressure can cause increased pressure on the median nerve, any custom volar splint must be molded such that pressure is evenly distributed over the wrist and forearm (Fig. 21-4). Many commercially available splints are circumferential with a volar metal stay, which often must be adjusted to ensure that the wrist is in a neutral position (Fig. 21-5). We commonly use a splint called the *Carpal Lock® carpal tunnel syndrome splint*

(Fig. 21-6, *A*) This is a dorsal-based splint that prevents any external pressure over the carpal tunnel. Narrow straps through the palm leave the palmar surface free, which is ideal for people who work while wearing their splint (Fig. 21-6, *B*).

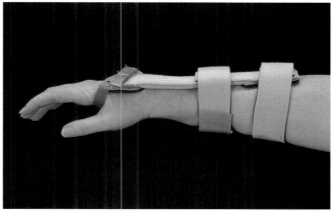

A

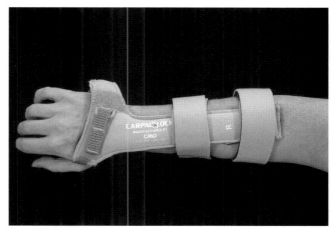

B

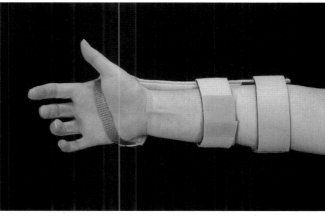

C

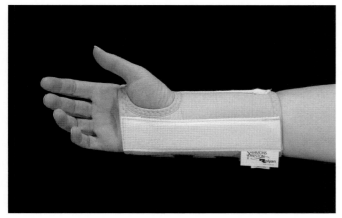

Fig. 21-5 Rolyan (Sammons Preston) prefabricated wrist splint with volar metal stay. This splint fits nicely, proximal to the distal palmar flexion crease, allowing full MP flexion.

Fig. 21-6 A, Lateral view of the Carpal Lock® wrist splint holding wrist in neutral. **B,** Dorsally based Carpal Lock splint prevents any pressure over volar wrist. **C,** Narrow strap across the palm leaves hand free for functional use.

De Quervain tenosynovitis

Anatomy and symptoms

de Quervain tenosynovitis was first described in 1895 as a stenosing tenosynovitis of the abductor pollicis longus (APL) and the extensor pollicis brevis (EPB) as the tendons course through the first dorsal compartment of the wrist.[12,25] The first dorsal compartment is a tunnel that houses the APL and the EPB; however, in a percentage of the population these two tendons occupy their own space separated by a fibrous septum within the first dorsal compartment. This septation is found more commonly in patients with de Quervain disease than in the general population. Approximately 70% of patients with de Quervain disease have a separate fibroosseous compartment of the EPB tendon.[13,25]

The most common cause of de Quervain tenosynovitis appears to be overuse or repetitive stress of the wrist and hand causing inflammation of the tendons or hypertrophy of the flexor retinaculum. Repetitive stretching or contractions of the EPB or APL tendons may result in increased friction and persistent inflammation, which in turn may cause fibrous thickening of the tendon sheath leading to the development of stenosis.[12] Less common causes of de Quervain tenosynovitis are acute injuries and direct trauma.

Patients may present to the clinic with radial wrist pain. Palpation reveals tenderness over the radial styloid and the first dorsal compartment. Pain often radiates distally to the thumb or proximally up the distal forearm, especially with radial or ulnar deviation of the wrist. The Finkelstein test is commonly used to diagnose de Quervain disease. When the patient is asked to fully flex and adduct the thumb with the wrist in ulnar deviation, he or she may experience sharp pain in the first dorsal compartment because the tendons are simultaneously stretched and compressed over the radius in an already inflamed melieu.[13] Resisted thumb extension may reproduce pain in the radial wrist, and visible swelling might be present.

Splinting de Quervain tenosynovitis

As with most overuse syndromes, splinting de Quervain tendonitis is most effective in the early stages. Wearing splints in the acute phase can help reduce pain. Primary goals of splinting this condition are to reduce inflammation, to minimize glide of the APL and the EPB tendons in the first dorsal compartment, and to reduce forceful exertion of these muscles. This is typically accomplished by splinting the wrist in neutral to slight extension with the thumb radially abducted. The thumb interphalangeal (IP) joint can be left free.

To prevent wrist ulnar deviation and thumb flexion, a rigid thermoplastic splint can be custom fit (Fig. 21-7). For patients with severe symptoms, the splint should be worn at all times. Patients with mild symptoms may not want to wear a rigid splint during the day because functional use will be significantly limited. In this situation, a soft support can be used during the day to allow for functional use. The patient is advised to wear the rigid splint at night while using the soft support during the day. We commonly use the soft splint know as the Comfort Cool™ thumb CMC restriction splint (Northcoast Medical; Fig. 21-8). This neoprene splint is lined with terry cloth for comfort. Full functional use of the hand is allowed because the device has no rigid supports;

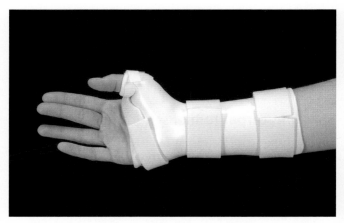

Fig. 21-7 Custom splint with wrist neutral to slightly extended, thumb in comfortable radial abduction, and thumb IP joint free for treatment of de Quervain tenosynovitis.

however, the extra carpometacarpal (CMC) support strap naturally causes the CMC joint to rest in abduction when the hand is not in use. The circumferential design provides gentle compression, which may aid in reducing pain and decreasing edema. This splint is also ideal for CMC arthritis [see section on basilar joint arthritis (CMC arthritis)].

Trigger finger (stenosing tenosynovitis)

Anatomy and symptoms

An inflammation of the flexor tendon sheath of the digits can cause a common problem known as *trigger finger* or *stenosing tenosynovitis*. Tendons of the fingers glide through fibroosseous canals bordered by the phalanges dorsally and the flexor sheath volarly. Each sheath has a series of thickenings, known as *pulleys*, which maintain the tendons juxtaposed to the phalanges to prevent bowstringing of the tendons during active flexion of the finger. There are five annular and three cruciform pulleys. The A1 pulley is the most proximal and represents the entrance to the finger's fibroosseous canal. Overuse or repetitive trauma, especially with direct pressure in the

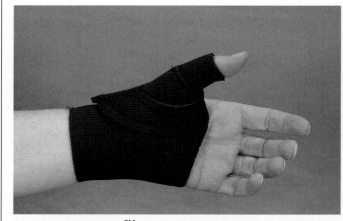

Fig. 21-8 Comfort Cool™ thumb CMC restriction splint (Northcoast Medical). This neoprene splint, with additional CMC support strap, allows the CMC to rest in comfortable abduction when not in use. Soft splint allows for increased functional use over rigid custom splint.

palm, can cause inflammation and thickening at the A1 pulley. Significant swelling and constriction of the tendon sheath inhibit friction-free gliding through the pulley system. Many authors site the discrepancy between the size of the pulley canal and tendon volume as a precipitating factor of decreased tendon glide.[8] The anatomical location of pathology of the triggering tendon usually is the hypovascular area beneath the A1 and A2 pulleys, most commonly the A1 pulley.[8] Blood flow and nutrition also can be further compromised, which may result in a nodule forming distal to the A1 pulley. This nodule significantly limits the ability of the tendon to glide through the A1 pulley during flexion. The nodules in the tendon rub forcefully at the proximal and distal edges of the A1 pulley, causing additional inflammation and pain as well as the sensation of clicking or popping in the finger. The clinician refers to this as *triggering*. With the digit in full flexion and a nodule proximal to the A1 pulley, the extensors may not be strong enough to pull the enlarged tendon through the pulley, resulting in a digit that locks in flexion. Initially, this locking digit may be passively extended but may progress to a completely locked position.

Trigger finger may present initially as a slight stiffness of the affected digit, especially in the morning. As the condition progresses, patients may complain of mild swelling and a "clicking" or "popping" of the digit with digital range of motion. This "popping" may occur with initiation of extension from a flexed position or initiation of flexion from an extended position. To patients this "clicking" or "popping" appears to originate from the proximal IP joint, but in actuality it will be palpated volarly, over the A1 pulley at the MCP joint. Pain may be present in chronic cases. With palpation the examiner may be able to detect inflammation and thickening of the flexor sheath.[12,13]

Splinting trigger finger

Splinting for trigger finger is designed to restrict tendon glide through the A1 pulley and to restore normal tendon glide by reducing inflammation of the tendon sheath. Patel and Bassini[18] reported a 77% success rate with splinting in patients whose symptoms were present for 6 months or less. Evans et al.[8] reported a 73% success rate if symptoms were present for less than 4 months. Thumb splinting for triggering produces less favorable results, and splinting for multiple digit involvement also may have limited success.[8,13,18]

According to Evans et al.,[8] altering the mechanical pressures at the A1 pulley and encouraging differential tendon gliding can reverse the pathological state of the flexor tendon sheath and tendon. They recommend a hand-based splint that immobilizes the MP joints in extension and leaves the IP joints free (Fig. 21-9). This type of splint will relieve pressure on the proximal pulley system, reducing friction between the tendon and pulley system. This in turn allows the inflamed tissues to rest.[8] Leaving the IP joints free allows for hook fisting yet limits full flexor tendon glide through the A1 pulley. Although Evans et al.[8] recommend that MP joints be splinted in full extension, Patel and Bassini[18] and Eaton[7] recommend splinting the MP joints in 10 to 15 degrees of flexion because patients can tolerate this position much better. This type of splint can be worn at night; however, Eaton[7] further recommends wearing a complete immobilization splint at

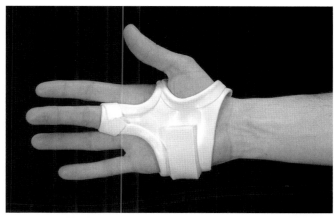

Fig. 21.9 Custom hand-based splint for trigger finger with MP joint immobilized in extension and IP joints free to allow tendon glide. Adjacent fingers can be included as needed.

night with the proximal IP joints in 15 to 20 degrees of flexion and the MP joints splinted at no more than 10 to 15 degrees of flexion. This position will draw the tendons distally and prevent tendon friction through the pulley at night. This in turn should reduce inflammation in the tendon sheath, allowing tendons to glide more easily in the morning.

Eighty percent of triggering occurs in the long and ring fingers.[8,14] The thumb is another common site for flexor triggering, but the results of thumb splinting have been less favorable, possibly due to the anatomical differences of the thumb flexor system.[8,13,18] If a trial of splinting will be used for thumb triggering, a hand-based splint with the MP and IP joints extended is the splint of choice.

Basilar joint arthritis (CMC arthritis)
Anatomy and symptoms

The most common arthritis of the hand is located at the base of the thumb at the CMC joint, also known as the *trapeziometacarpal joint*. The trapezium has four articulations in the hand, with the trapeziometacarpal articulation being the primary site of mobility of the thumb. The lesser articulations for the trapezium are associated with the scaphoid, trapezoid, and radial facets of the index metacarpal. This four-joint complex is commonly referred to as the *basilar joint complex*. The trapeziometacarpal joint is simply the basilar joint.[20] The trapeziometacarpal joint is the primary joint for symptomatic osteoarthritis of the thumb.

Osteoarthritis is a joint disorder that involves destruction of the articular cartilage and osteophyte formation, subchondral cysts, bone eburnation, loss of joint space, and deformity. Osteoarthritis can be caused by any condition that alters the shape of the articulating surface of the joint or ligamentous supports of surrounding soft tissues.[16] The forces encountered at the distal fingertip during pulp to pulp pinch are amplified at least 12 times by the time they reach the thumb CMC joint.[6] The trapeziometacarpal joint has limited bony constraints and relies on soft tissue for stability. This anatomical arrangement results in large contact stresses within the joint, with limited available surface area to transmit effective load.[20] Strenuous occupations requiring repetitive lateral pinch and grip activities cause significant load at

293

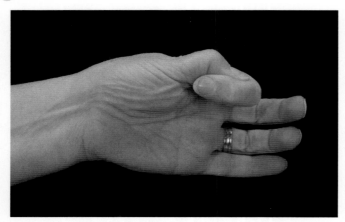

Fig. 21-10 Dorsal subluxation of the base of the first metacarpal alters biomechanical forces distally, which can cause the MP joint of the thumb to collapse into hyperextension with pinch.

the CMC joint. This constant loading on the joint makes the trapeziometacarpal joint susceptible to degenerative joint changes.

The CMC joint permits flexion, extension, and abduction and adduction of the thumb; together this is referred to as *circumduction*. Active pinching and the forces transmitted to this joint cause the dorsal part of the joint capsule to become attenuated, resulting in increased laxity. This increased laxity of the joint allows for dorsal subluxation of the first metacarpal on the trapezium. Pelligrini[19] described the natural progression of the pathogenesis of basilar joint arthritis, noting that with inflammation and joint destruction, the volar oblique (or "beak") ligament that keeps the first metacarpal in the adducted position attenuates and permits subluxation of the first metacarpal radially off the trapezium. Colditz[5] described the thenar muscle involvement in this process. When the thenar muscles contract, the first metacarpal flexes forward. As the metacarpal flexes forward, the laxity in the dorsal capsule combined with active pinch causes the proximal end of the metacarpal to shift dorsally while the distal end of the metacarpal tilts toward the palm. The proximal end of the metacarpal shifting on the trapezium combined with cartilage destruction in the joint can cause pain associated with basilar joint arthritis.

As the thumb CMC joint subluxates dorsally, the biomechanics of the thumb are altered distally. These altered forces can cause the MP joint of the thumb to collapse into hyperextension (Fig. 21-10).[5] The classic deformity of basilar joint arthritis is CMC adduction, MP hyperextension, and IP flexion. Poole and Pellegrini[20] suggest that recent observations bring into question whether hypermobility and MP hyperextension laxity of the thumb MP joint are a causative factor of CMC arthritis rather than merely a secondary manifestation of CMC joint subluxation as conventionally taught.

Symptoms of CMC arthritis may begin with mild stiffness or decreased range of motion secondary to cartilage degeneration and osteophyte formation. Patients generally seek medical attention when they begin to experience pain and a decrease in function. The pain may radiate proximally or distally and generally increases with pinching activities. The CMC joint may be tender to palpation. Characteristic of basilar joint arthritis is the finding of crepitance while the patient performs a grind test. This test is performed by axially

loading the basilar joint while rotating the metacarpal on the trapezium. Crepitance usually is accompanied by significant pain with the grind maneuver. Distraction of the basilar joint may reveal capsular tenderness.[16] Visual examination may reveal a protrusion or square appearance at the base of the thumb.[16] This prominence at the base of the radial thumb results from dorsal subluxation of the metacarpal off the trapezium. This is known as the *shoulder sign.* Pain patterns are similar to that of de Quervain syndrome, but a positive grind test may help to differentiate the two diagnoses.

Splinting basilar joint arthritis

The primary goal of splinting basilar joint arthritis is to stabilize the base of the first metacarpal and to inhibit CMC joint motion during grip and pinch activities. Minimizing dorsal subluxation of the first metacarpal should reduce pain and inflammation and help to increase functional use. Splinting basilar joint arthritis will not change or heal the involved structures; however, splints will help to increase function with less pain and may help to slow down the degenerative process.

In the past, the standard splint used for this condition was a long opponens splint. This splint stabilizes the CMC joint in abduction, minimizing the palmar tilting of the metacarpal while allowing IP motion of the thumb. The splint allows the ligaments and muscles to remain in a resting position and maximizes the joint space. This is the position of maximum stability based on ligament and bony constraints.[16] It now has been reported that a short opponens splint with the wrist and MP joint left free is more effective for pain relief than a long opponens splint that crosses the wrist and MP joints.[28]

Colditz[5] described a hand-based splint that leaves the thumb MP and IP free for active pinching. This splint is custom molded and stabilizes the CMC joint in palmar abduction. The thumb is free to allow tip to tip and lateral pinch while minimizing dorsal subluxation of the first metacarpal (Fig. 21-11). The only functional limitation with this splint is mildly limited functional grip due to the rigid material in the palm; however, Colditz reported good patient compliance and significant pain relief with this splint.

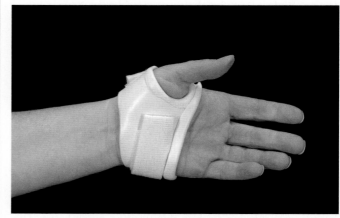

Fig. 21-11 Colditz[5] design splint for CMC arthritis supports the CMC joint while leaving MP and IP joints of the thumb free for functional use.

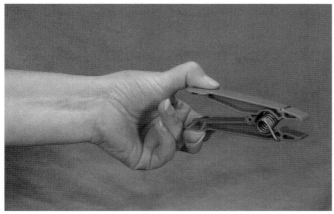

A

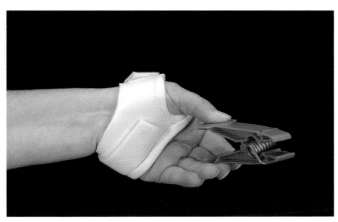

B

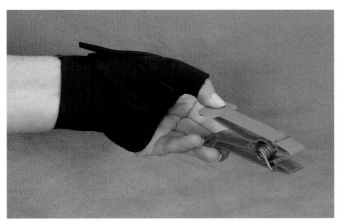

C

Fig. 21-12 A, Pinching a clothespin without support can cause increased pain. Note dorsal subluxation at the base of the first metacarpal, palmar tilt at the distal end of first metacarpal, and MP hyperextension. **B,** Colditz[5] design splint stabilizes the carpometacarpal joint during active pinch, reducing pain and allowing for normal flexion forces at the IP joints. **C,** Comfort Cool™ thumb CMC restriction splint also provides these stabilizing forces.

Proper fabrication of this splint is imperative for a successful outcome. Molding the splint with the patient touching the tip of the thumb to the tip of the index finger but not actively pinching will ensure that the patient will have pinching abilities once the splint is completed. A gentle pressure applied over the thenar muscles palmarly while applying a gentle counterpressure dorsoradially at the base of the first metacarpal will prevent the metacarpal from tilting forward and subluxating off the trapezium. This in turn should reduce pain with pinching activities.[5] Have the patient pinch a clothespin both with and without the splint (Fig. 21-12, *A*) The patient should note an immediate reduction of pain with pinching, which demonstrates proper fit and provides positive reinforcement for increased compliance.

An excellent soft neoprene splint that has been proven effective for CMC arthritis is the Comfort Cool™ thumb CMC restriction splint. This splint (as described earlier for use with de Quervain tenosynovitis) is lined with terrycloth for comfort and is easily applied. An extra strap provides CMC support to help prevent dorsal subluxation of the first metacarpal. Functional use with this splint is greatly increased compared to most rigid splints (Fig. 21-12, *B*).

Weiss et al.[28] completed a study comparing the custom-fit, Colditz design splint with the Comfort Cool™ neoprene splint for CMC arthritis. They showed that both of these splints help to stabilize the CMC joint, which can lead to pain reduction at the first CMC joint. This study reported greater radiographic stability with the custom thermoplastic splint but statistically decreased CMC joint subluxation with the Comfort Cool™ splint. Neither splint significantly changed the ability to generate pinch strength; however, pinch strength was greater with the Comfort Cool™ splint than with the custom-molded splint or with no splint at all. Seventy-two percent of their subjects chose the Comfort Cool™ neoprene splint over the Colditz design thermoplastic splint because of ease of application, pain reduction, comfort, and appearance. This study shows that although the degenerative arthritic process cannot be halted, splinting can be an effective option for decreasing pain with functional use.

Conclusion

Each musculotendinous unit and each joint of the upper extremity is subject to overuse disorders. Repetitive cumulative trauma, forceful muscle contractions, poor biomechanics, and undesirable posture put the finely tuned balance and biomechanical interplay of our upper extremities at risk. Surgery can offer solutions to a number of these overuse conditions but should be used only after conservative measures with orthoses, rest, therapy, and appropriate antiinflammatory drugs have been tried. Proper orthoses are paramount to the care and treatment of many of the afflictions encountered by our limbs.

References

1. Apfelberg DB, Larson SJ: Dynamic anatomy of the ulnar nerve at the elbow, *Plast Reconstr Surg* 51:79–81, 1973.
2. Barkholder CD, Hill VA, Fess EE: The efficacy of splinting for lateral epicondylitis: a systematic review, *J Hand Ther* 17:181–199, 2004.
3. Blackmore SM: Therapists management of ulnar nerve neuropathy at the elbow. In Mackin EJ, Callahan AD, Skirver TM, Schneider LH, Osterman AL, Hunter JM, editors: *Rehabilitation of the hand and upper extremity vol 1*, ed 5, St. Louis, 2002, Mosby.
4. Cannon NM, Beal BG, Walters KJ, et al: *Rehabilitation Center of Indiana: diagnosis and treatment manual for physicians and therapists*, ed 4, Indianapolis, IN, 2001, The Hand Rehabilitation Center of Indiana.

5. Colditz JC: The biomechanics of a thumb carpometacarpal immobilization splint: design and fitting, *J Hand Ther* 13:228–235, 2000.
6. Cooney W, Lucca M, Choa E, Linshield R: The kinesiology of the thumb trapeziometacarpal joint, *J Bone Joint Surg* 63A:1371, 1981.
7. Eaton RG: Entrapment syndrome in musicians, *J Hand Ther* 5:91–96, 1992.
8. Evans RB, Hunter JM, Burkhalter WE: Conservative management of the trigger finger: a new approach, *J Hand Ther* 2:59–68, 1988.
9. Fedorczyk JM: Therapists management of elbow tendonitis. In Hunter, Mackin, Callahan, editors: *Rehabilitation of the hand and upper extremity vol 2*, ed 5, 2002.
10. Jansen CW, Olson SL, Hasson SM: The effect of a wrist orthosis during functional activities on surface electromyography of the wrist extensors in normal subjects, *J Hand Ther* 10:283–289, 1997.
11. Johnson SL: Therapy of the occupationally injured hand and upper extremity, *Hand Clin* 9:289–298, 1993.
12. Kirkpatric WH, Lisser S: soft tissue conditions: trigger fingers and deQuervain's disease. In Hunter, Mackin, Callahan, editors: *Rehabilitation of the hand: surgery and therapy vol 11*, ed 4, 1995.
13. Lee MR, Nasser-Sharif S, Zelouf DS: Surgeons and therapists management of tendinopathies in the hand and wrist. In Mackin EJ, Callahan AD, Skirver TM, Schneider LH, Osterman AL, Hunter JM, editors: *Rehabilitation of the hand and upper extremity vol 1*, ed 5, St. Louis, 2002, Mosby, pp. 931–953.
14. Linder-Tons S, Ingell K: An alternative splint design for trigger finger, *J Hand Ther* 11:206–208, 1998.
15. Mansivias JJ, Bucher PA, Monsvias DB: Nonsurgically treated carpal tunnel syndrome in the manual worker, *Plast Reconstr Surg* 94:695–699, 1994.
16. Melvin JL: Therapists management of osteoarthritis in the hand. In Hunter, Mackin, Callahan, editors: *Rehabilitation of the hand and upper extremity vol 2*, ed 5, 2002.
17. Meyer NJ, Pennington W, Haines B, Daley R: The effect of the forearm support band on forces at the origin of the extensor carpi radialis brevis: a cadaveric study and review of literature, *J Hand Ther* 15:179–184, 2002.
18. Patel MR, Bassini L: Trigger fingers and thumb: when to splint, inject or operate?, *J Hand Surg* 17A:110–113, 1992.
19. Pelligrini VDJr: Osteoarthritis of the thumb trapeziometacarpal joint: a study of the pathophysiology of the articular cartilage regeneration part 1: anatomy and pathology of the aging joint, *J Hand Surg* 16A:967, 1991.
20. Poole JU, Pellegrini VD: Arthritis of the thumb basar joint complex, *J Hand Ther* 13:91–107, 2000.
21. Rayan GM, Jensen C, Duke J: Elbow flexion test in the normal population, *J Hand Surg* 17A:86–89, 1992.
22. Rayan GM: Proximal ulnar nerve compression: cubital tunnel syndrome, *Hand Clin* 8:325–336, 1992.
23. Rempel D, Maojilovic R, Levinsohn DG, Bloom T, Gordon L: The effect of wearing a flexible wrist splint on carpal tunnel pressure during repetitive hand activities, *J Hand Surg* 19A:106–110, 1994.
24. Sailer SM: The role of splinting and rehabilitation in the treatment of carpal and cubital tunnel syndrome, *Hand Clin* 12:223–241, 1996.
25. Stern PJ: Tendinitis, overuse syndromes and tendon injuries, *Hand Clin* 6:467–476, 1990.
26. Wadsworth TG: Elbow tendonitis. In Hunter, Mackin, Callahan, editors: *Rehabilitation of the hand and upper extremity vol 2*, ed 5, 2002.
27. Weiss S, Falkenstein N: Lateral epicondylitis: the therapist approach to conquering pain. *Exploring hand therapy* (DVD and outline), established 1997. www.handtherapy.com.
28. Weiss S, LaStayo P, Mills A, Bramlet D: Splinting the degenerative basal joint: custom made or prefabricated neoprene? *J Hand Ther* 17:401–406, 2004.

Suggested readings

Colditz JC: Antomic consideration for splinting the thumb. In Hunter, Mackin, Callahan, editors: *Rehabilitation of the hand and upper extremity*, 2, ed 5, 2002.

Jacobs ML, Austin N: *Splinting the hand and upper extremity: principles and process*, Philadelphia, 2003, Lippincott, Williams & Wilkins.

Johnson SL: Therapy of the occupationally injured hand and upper extremity, *Hand Clin* 9:289–298, 1993.

Muller M, Tsui D, Schnurr R, Biddulph-Deisroth L, Hard J, MacDermid JC: Effectiveness of hand therapy interventions in primary management of carpal tunnel syndrome: a systematic review, *J Hand Ther* 17:210–228, 2004.

Weiss AC, Sachar K, Gendrau M: Conservative management of carpal tunnel syndrome: a re-examination of steroid injection and splinting, *J Hand Surg* 19A:410–415, 1994.

Lower limb orthoses

This section brings to the readers a collection of chapters that have significant clinical relevance to the day-to-day lower limb orthotic practice. Experienced authors and talented teachers willingly gave of their time to create this content.

Section 4 has three major themes: biomechanics of the ankle and foot, knee, and hip; shoe modifications; and consequences of brace application to the lower limb joints. These subsections provide the reader with the knowledge infrastructure essential to all brace prescriptions. The authors provide clear and concise reviews of the sometimes complex but indispensable concepts for sound prescription of orthotic devices.

Diagnostic-specific subsections emphasize orthotic management of the upper motor neuron syndrome, with chapters on stroke, traumatic brain injury, and spinal cord injury. Differentiation of the treatment methods for each diagnostic grouping is important because it takes into consideration the necessary approach to provide an acceptable and successful orthotic prescription for the patient and to understand the potential side effects of the interventions as they relate specifically to each patient.

Chapters focus on the care of patients with lower motor neuron syndrome and other orthopedic needs, orthotic management of the neuropathic and/or dysvascular patient, orthoses for patients with postpolio syndrome, and devices for patients with complications after joint replacement or sports-related injuries.

The two postpolio syndrome chapters present different approaches, one from Europe and the other from the United States. We elected to have some overlap in the postpolio syndrome chapters because of the great need for clinicians who can effectively deal with the presenting problems of this population as well as the impact of aging.

These chapters should provide the fundamental clinical concepts applicable to most problems in the lower limbs that are amenable to orthotic management and serve as a solid guide to the management of patients with specific disorders.

It has been a pleasant challenge to work with all of the chapter authors and the other editors of this book as well as the editorial staff, to whom I am thankful for their help and collaboration in completing this project. I wish to thank my wife, Rosa, and my children, Alina, Arie, and Gabriel, for their patience and support during the many long nights and weekends required to complete this project.

Alberto Esquenazi

Section

2

Lower limb orthoses

Chapter

22

Biomechanics of the hip, knee, and ankle

Barry Meadows, Robert James Bowers, and Elaine Owen

Key Points
- Orthoses exert direct and indirect biomechanical effects.
- In normal gait the shank (lower leg) is inclined in mid-stance.
- Appreciation of segment kinematics can facilitate clinical reasoning and problem solving.
- External extension moments at the knee and hip are crucial to stability in mid and terminal stance.
- The effect of shortened biarticular muscles on kinematics and kinetics should be considered.
- Neurological conditions are very sensitive to small changes in the biomechanical features of orthoses and footwear.
- Orthoses must be dynamically "tuned" to optimize kinematics and kinetics.
- Footwear is an integral part of lower limb orthotic prescription.

When considering orthotic treatment of the lower limbs, an understanding of the biomechanical principles that underpin static and dynamic control of the joints and segments is an essential component of clinical reasoning. This understanding can facilitate the setting of biomechanical goals and the identification of interventions that are likely to achieve these goals. Understanding the biomechanics of the lower limb is easier if the topic is divided into manageable portions. Rather than attempting to describe the requirements of control at all joints and segments in all three planes, this chapter focuses on fundamental biomechanical principles, illustrated using clinical examples, which the reader can apply to any problems encountered in his or her own clinical practice.

Basic biomechanical principles

Statics

Action–reaction

Newton's third law tells us that *for every action, there is an equal and opposite reaction*. This means that when an orthosis applies forces to the body, equal and opposite forces are being applied by the body to the orthosis. When thinking about how an orthosis functions, it is essential to consider where and how it must apply corrective forces. However, when considering the structural requirements of the orthosis, it is necessary to think the other way round, that is, to appreciate how the body is applying forces to the orthosis. Failure to do so may result in deformation or structural failure of the device.

Pressure

Although a force may be considered as being applied at a single point, in clinical practice forces are applied over as large an area as possible in order to reduce pressure. Pressure is defined as force divided by area:

$$P(pressure) = F(force)/A(area).$$

Moments and levers

In most instances, the function of an orthosis is to resist or control *angular* motion at a joint; for example, knee flexion, hyperextension, varus, or valgus. Orthoses do this by applying a system of *linear* forces, each "pushing" on a different part of the body in a specific direction. The required control of angular motion results from the fact that some of these linear forces are applied at a distance from the joint's center of rotation. A force acting at a distance from a joint center creates a "turning effect," known as a *moment*. The magnitude of the moment is calculated using the following equation:

$$M(moment) = F(force) \times D(distance).$$

In this equation, the distance D (known as the *lever arm*) is defined as the *perpendicular* distance from the joint center to the line of action of the force (Fig. 22-1). Therefore, an orthosis that applies oblique, rather than perpendicular, forces will be less effective in generating the required moment because the lever arm will be smaller.

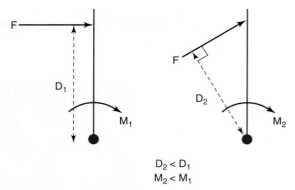

Fig. 22-1 Force (F) acting at distance (D₁) applies a moment (M₁). If the same force F acts obliquely, the lever arm is reduced (D₂), applying a smaller moment (M₂).

The creation of moments is the *critical function of most lower limb orthoses.* Increasing the lever arm is a clinically useful strategy because it enables the required moment to be generated while reducing the size of the applied force. Reducing the *force* reduces the *pressure* to which the tissue is subjected, with consequent benefits in terms of comfort and tissue viability. Pressure can also be reduced by increasing the *area* over which the force is applied. Increasing *both* the lever arm *and* the area over which force is applied maximizes function and comfort. In practice, of course, the lever arm is limited by the length of the anatomical segments involved or by other anatomical considerations such as tissue intolerance to pressure.

Equilibrium

In order to work successfully, an orthosis must apply a system of forces that have been set up to balance each other, creating a state of *equilibrium.* This equilibrium relates not only to the forces but also to the moments created by these forces. To control angular motion at a joint, the minimum number of forces required is three, the so-called *three-point force system* (Fig. 22-2). Two of the forces in this system must be applied on the "concave" side of the joint, and these two forces must be balanced by the third force on the opposite side, which should be located as close as possible to the center of joint rotation. A state of equilibrium is illustrated in Fig. 22-3. Mathematically this state is expressed as follows:

$$F_2 = F_1 + F_3.$$

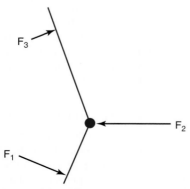

Fig. 22-2 A minimum of three forces is required for control of angular motion at a joint.

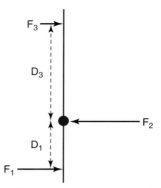

Fig. 22-3 The three-point force system is set up to be in equilibrium so that forces and moments balance.

Changing the magnitude of any one force in the system inevitably influences the magnitude of at least one of the others. If F_1 is increased, F_2 must also increase unless F_3 is decreased. However, the moments must also balance as expressed by the following equation:

$$F_1 \times D_1 = F_3 \times D_3.$$

If F_1 increases, then F_3 *also must* increase. Clinically, therefore, it is important to recognize that it is impossible to alter one force in a three-point force system without inevitably influencing the other two forces in the system.

In Figure 22-3 the three forces in the system are parallel to each other; however, this is not always the case. For example, the forces in the system that control ankle plantarflexion clearly are not parallel to each other, but they act in the same plane and still are in equilibrium (Fig. 22-4). This mechanical principle is known as a *triangle of forces.* From a practical point of view, in order to balance the other two forces and to "complete the triangle," the force F_2 applied on the dorsum of the foot cannot act in a horizontal direction but must act diagonally downward. To be effective, any ankle strap should be attached in the direction in which this force is required to act.

Shared overlapping force systems

Because three is the minimum number of forces required to control rotation at a joint, one might reasonably assume that control of two joints requires forces to be applied at six places.

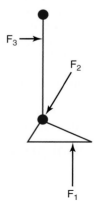

Fig. 22-4 The three-point force system applied by an AFO to control ankle plantar flexion.

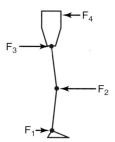

Fig. 22-5 Forces can be "shared" when controlling adjacent joints.

However, if the two joints are adjacent to each other, some of these forces may be "shared." This is seen when flexion at the knee and hip must be controlled simultaneously, for example, when using a standing frame, where two superimposed three-point force systems exist (Fig. 22-5). Forces F_1, F_2, and F_3 control knee flexion, while forces F_2, F_3, and F_4 control hip flexion. Thus, while each joint is indeed subject to a three-point force system, only four forces, strategically located, are sufficient to control adjacent joints.

In the above example, the force systems act in the same plane, but this is not always the case. For example, in the valgus foot, the systems that control hindfoot eversion (coronal plane) and forefoot abduction (external rotation in the transverse plane) share a common force (F_3) at the lateral calcaneus (Fig. 22-6).

Dynamics

These descriptions of static biomechanics are relevant to almost all situations involving orthoses. However, the treatment of locomotor disorders also necessitates consideration of the dynamic aspects of gait, including the accelerations and decelerations of the limb segments, particularly at specific instances of the gait cycle (Fig. 22-7).

One example is the inertial effect associated with accelerating and decelerating the mass of the lower limb segments when initiating and terminating swing. Here the distal masses of the orthosis and shoe become significant. The larger the mass to be accelerated or decelerated (or the higher the required acceleration and deceleration, as seen in faster walking), the greater the muscle forces required. From a practical point of view, in *most* circumstances it is beneficial to minimize the mass of distally applied orthoses or footwear, in order to reduce the demand on the neuromuscular system.

Another clinically significant example occurs in midstance in normal gait when deceleration of the forward movement of the shank (lower leg) is coupled with acceleration of forward

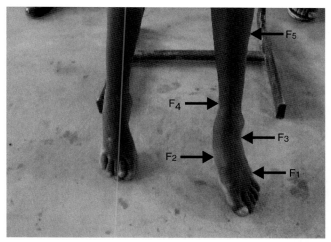

Fig. 22-6 Forces F_1, F_2, and F_3 control forefoot abduction; forces F_3, F_4, and F_5 control hindfoot eversion. Force F_3 is shared by both force systems.

movement of the thigh. The influence of orthosis and footwear design on these movements are considered later.

Kinematics and kinetics

As well as controlling deformity, orthoses are often used to influence either motion of an individual joint or patterns of locomotion. The branch of mechanics that studies motion is known as *kinematics*. The branch of mechanics concerned with the effects of forces on motion is called *kinetics*. Consideration of both of these branches is relevant to understanding the biomechanical aspects of orthotic management of the lower limb.

Ground reaction force and moments

Due to gravity, the weight of the body acts vertically downward on the ground. In accordance with Newton's third law, an equal and opposite force must act upward from the ground on the foot. This is known as the *ground reaction force* (GRF). Obviously there is no GRF during swing phase. The GRF has a *point of application* on the foot, a *magnitude*, and a direction, or *line of action* (Fig. 22-8). In static situations these all remain constant, with the magnitude equal to body weight. However, in dynamic situations such as locomotion (as will be seen later) they typically vary in a repetitive fashion. When the line of action of the GRF lies at a distance from the center of rotation of a joint, it creates an "external moment." As we know, the greater the perpendicular

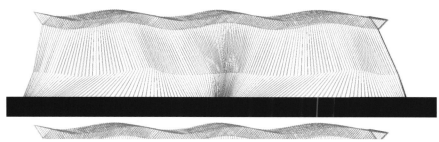

Fig. 22-7 During normal locomotion, the shank and thigh segments flow through patterns of motion, with the shank reclined at initial contact flowing to inclined in late stance. Note that in midstance the forward motion of the shank slows down, indicated by the cluster of lines.

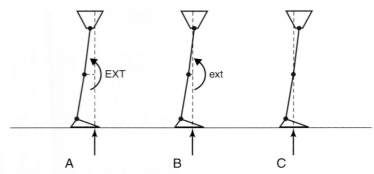

Fig. 22-8 Ground reaction force (GRF) and external moments. **A,** GRF line of action in front of knee with large lever arm resulting in large external knee extension moment. **B,** GRF line of action closer to knee with smaller lever arm resulting in smaller external knee extension moment. **C,** GRF line of action passes through knee resulting in no external knee moment

distance of the line of action of the GRF to the joint center (the "lever arm"), the greater the external moment will be. If the GRF is aligned close to the joint center, the external moment is smaller. If the GRF passes through the joint center, then no external moment is generated.

The presence of an external moment tends to cause motion at a joint and usually (but, as we shall see, not always) requires the generation of an opposing internal muscle moment to create equilibrium or to control this motion. The greater the external moment, the greater the required internal moment likely will be. In static situations, the internal and external moments will be equal and opposite and therefore in equilibrium. However, in dynamic situations, such as locomotion, it may be necessary for the moments generated by the muscles to be slightly greater or less than the external moments in order to control angular motion at the joints.

During a gait cycle the GRF alignment may pass from one side of the joint center to the other, "switching" moments from, for example, flexion to extension (Fig. 22-9). This implies transfer in neuromuscular demand. For example, the switch from an external plantarflexion moment to an external dorsiflexion moment at the ankle during midstance requires a switch from dorsiflexor activity to plantarflexor activity.

However, the external moment sometimes creates a desirable effect at a joint, reducing or even removing the need for muscle activity. For example, a paraplegic patient fitted with knee–ankle–foot orthoses (KAFOs) can achieve hip stability in standing by contriving to align the GRF posterior to the hip joints. At the end of joint range, the internal flexion moment required to balance the external extension moment may be generated (passively) by structures such as the ligaments or joint capsule. A dynamic example can be seen in the late stance phase of gait, when posterior alignment of the GRF to the hip extends and stabilizes the joint without the need for hip extensor activity (Fig. 22-9). This mechanism contributes to the energy efficiency of gait.

The exact magnitude of the external and internal moments (which are mutually dependent) generated at the joints is influenced by the accelerations and inertial effects of the individual limb segments.[39] For simplicity, the following discussion of gait ignores these influences. In clinical practice, consideration of the external moments resulting from GRF alignment and their modification by various forms of clinical intervention described later in this chapter can be a successful strategy.[3,17,27,34,35]

Application of biomechanical principles to normal and pathological gait

An appreciation of the biomechanical features of normal gait is an essential prerequisite to orthotic management of the lower limb. This chapter focuses on some important observations about normal gait biomechanics, which determine optimal prescription and design of lower limb orthoses. The normal gait of children and adults has been excellently described in depth.[10,13,31,32,38] The reader must be clear about the names of each of the phases and subdivisions of the gait cycle and the movements and forces that occur in each of these subdivisions in order to fully understand the concepts that will be discussed.[32]

Normal gait has been defined as a highly controlled, coordinated, repetitive series of limb movements whose function is to advance the body safely from place to place with a minimum expenditure of energy.[11] Five attributes of normal walking have been described: foot clearance in swing, adequate step length, prepositioning of the foot at initial contact, stability in stance, and conservation of energy.[11] If we are to replicate these attributes with orthoses, we must understand how they are achieved in normal gait and the extent to which they are interrelated. For example, joint stability is fundamental to stance phase, but it is also a prerequisite for achieving adequate step length in the contralateral leg, which in turn facilitates prepositioning of the swing foot at initial contact.

Most texts on normal gait and modern gait analysis focus on the kinematics of the joints, measured as angles between two adjacent segments. Typical graphs for hip, knee, and ankle kinematics then can be produced (Fig. 22-10). However, understanding and giving equal consideration to the kinematics of the *segments* of the body is key to achieving optimal design of lower limb orthoses (Fig. 22-10). Movement of the segments can be measured relative to the vertical or the horizontal.[1,13,39] Measurement of the segment relative to the vertical can be expressed as degrees of incline (leaning forward from the vertical) or recline (leaning backward from the vertical).

Observations of joint kinematics

Normal gait

Kinematic graphs (Fig. 22-10) show the minimum and maximum excursions at all three major joints of the lower limb and

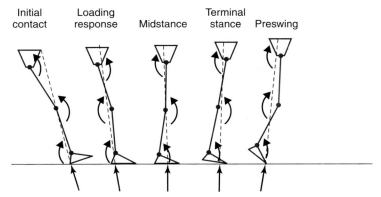

Fig. 22-9 In stance phase, the ground reaction force (GRF) is aligned as closely to as many joints as possible, minimizing the external moments and thus minimizing the biomechanical demand on the neuromuscular system. At times the GRF alignment passes from one side of the joint to the other, "switching" the moment.

their timing in the gait cycle. In the sagittal plane, maximum ankle dorsiflexion occurs in terminal stance, and the ankle is still dorsiflexed when the contralateral leg reaches initial contact. Knee extension is greatest in stance at initial contact and again in terminal stance at 40% gait cycle. At some times in the gait cycle movements are fast, such as knee flexion during preswing and initial swing and ankle plantarflexion in preswing. At other times movements are slow, such as hip flexion in terminal swing and ankle dorsiflexion in terminal stance. At terminal stance the ankle becomes stiffened, which is vital for the production of stability in stance.[32]

Pathological gait

Pathological gait potentially has joint kinematic deviations in all three planes and in all phases of the gait cycle. In the transverse plane there can be either excessive or insufficient rotations at hip, knee, ankle, and foot joints as well as in the pelvis, thigh, shank, and foot segments. In the coronal plane there can be excessive or insufficient pelvic obliquity, hip abduction or adduction, knee varus or valgus, or foot inversion or eversion. In the sagittal plane at the ankle and foot there can be excessive or insufficient plantarflexion or dorsiflexion. At the knee and hip there can be excessive or insufficient extension or flexion. Excessive extension occurs only rarely at the hip. More commonly there is excessive hip flexion, or insufficient hip extension, which may occur in combination with any abnormality at the knee and ankle. Inability to extend the hip may compromise the attainment of a stabilizing external extension moment at this joint. Orthoses should be designed so that they facilitate hip extension while minimizing other joint deviations.

Observations of segment kinematics

Normal gait

The limb segments follow typical movement patterns in all three planes during the gait cycle.[1,13,39] Figure 22-7 shows segment kinematics in the sagittal plane. In stance phase the thigh and shank move from a reclined to an inclined position, passing through vertical. The exact angle at any time can be determined by measuring the angle of the segment relative to the vertical. In the case of the shank this has been called the *shank angle to floor*,[27] but the more accurate term *shank to vertical angle* (SVA) is used here. Forward

progression of the shank is facilitated by the three rockers, which require movement at the ankle for the first and second rockers and at the metatarsophalangeal joints for the third rocker.[32]

The segments always move in a forward direction, but the angular velocity of the segments is not uniform throughout the gait cycle.[1,13,39] In particular, the shank slows during its movement into forward inclination in midstance.[1,30,13] While the shank is slowing, the thigh moves from a reclined to an inclined position at an angular velocity that is faster than that of the shank.[1,13,39] The slowing of the movement of the shank and the 10 to 12 degrees of incline adopted by the shank segment at this time are highly significant for the production of stability in stance, as this position places the center of knee joint over the center of the base of support, the foot, which is

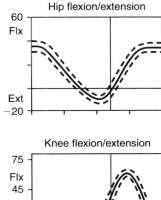

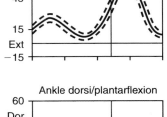

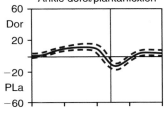

Fig. 22-10 Joint kinematic graphs for hip, knee, and ankle.

303

horizontal at this time.[23,27] This position is vital for conservation of energy as it shortens the stance limb and lowers the vertical excursion of the center of mass at the time when it otherwise would be at its highest position.[13]

In normal barefoot gait the inclination of the shank in midstance is produced by ankle dorsiflexion. When walking in footwear that has heels, the amount of dorsiflexion needed to achieve an inclined SVA at midstance decreases according to the pitch of the footwear.[19]

Pathological gait

Pathological gait potentially includes segment kinematic deviations in all planes and subdivisions of the gait cycle.

In the transverse plane there can be excessive or insufficient rotations at the pelvis, thigh, shank, and foot segments. A final "foot progression angle" that is excessively rotated relative to the line of progression of walking will reduce the effectiveness of orthotic interventions by compromising GRF alignment in the sagittal plane. Assessment of all the factors that influence the foot progression angle is essential so that they can be corrected in the orthosis where possible.[8]

In the sagittal plane the angles of incline or recline of the segments may be excessive or insufficient. The accelerations and decelerations of segment movement may be abnormal. The shank may fail to slow its forward movement during midstance, or it may slow but in an insufficiently or excessively inclined position.[17,27,33] In addition the shank can arrest or reverse its forward movement.[33] If shank kinematics is disrupted in these ways, stability in stance is compromised, with resultant abnormal compensatory segment kinematics proximally. The most common deviation affecting the thigh segment is the inability to achieve an inclined position.

Orthoses need to be designed so that they replicate normal or near-normal shank and thigh kinematics.

Observations of GRF kinetics

Normal gait

The GRF has three components: its point of application, its magnitude, and its line of action. In the stance phase of normal gait the point of application progresses along the foot, and the magnitude and the line of action vary through the gait cycle. Figure 22-11 displays the sagittal plane component of the GRF through one gait cycle, often called the *butterfly diagram*. During early and late stance the magnitude of the GRF is greater than body weight but in midstance is less than body weight as a result of the downward and upward accelerations of the body center of mass.[32] In normal gait the magnitudes of the two peaks are approximately equal. The fact that the GRF exceeds body weight in terminal stance indicates that body weight is being supported and propulsion is being generated successfully.

Pathological gait

In pathological gait the point of application, the magnitude, and the line of action of the GRF all can be abnormal in all planes. A common feature is that the magnitude of the first peak of the GRF is excessively high in early stance, but the second peak in terminal stance is insufficient. In this situation, the GRF is less than body weight and the limb is not supporting body weight sufficiently to remain fully

functional as a support (unless external support is being utilized, e.g., canes, crutches, or walking frame). As a consequence the contralateral limb may make heavy contact with the floor, thus generating an excessive first peak of the GRF.[17]

Orthoses must be designed so that they enhance stability in terminal stance in order to achieve a sufficient second peak of the GRF and, as a result, the contralateral first peak will not be excessive.

Observation of interactions between kinematics and kinetics

Normal gait

The segments move in ways that align the knee and hip joints closely to the GRF so as to minimize lever arms and produce sufficient (but not excessive) moments, making gait efficient.[32] The alignment of the GRF relative to the joints varies throughout the gait cycle (Fig. 22-9). In the sagittal plane the direction of the external moment switches at all joints during the gait cycle, once at the ankle (from a plantarflexion to a dorsiflexion moment early in midstance) and once at the hip (from a flexion moment to an extension moment late in midstance). However, at the knee there are three switches. During loading response the moment switches from extension to flexion, in midstance it switches back again to extension, and during preswing it swings back to flexion.

In the sagittal plane, once the GRF has aligned itself anterior to the knee and posterior to the hip, external knee and hip extension moments are created, producing stability in stance. Thus stability in the hip and knee is a consequence of GRF alignment rather than muscle activity. This critical alignment of the GRF is possible only with an inclined shank and thigh. In addition, only a narrow range of shank inclination in midstance will allow the occurrence of the necessary kinematic, and therefore kinetic, changes. This range probably is 7 to 15 degrees inclined, relative to the vertical, with the optimum position 10 to 12 degrees inclined.[27]

The "stiffness" of the ankle during terminal stance facilitates normal kinetics in two ways. First, it ensures that the point of application of the GRF is anteriorly located on the foot, with consequent anterior alignment at the knee. Second, it produces heel rise as the body falls forward, which further inclines the shank and consequently the thigh.[32] The rise of the heel also raises the body center of mass, at a time when it otherwise would be nearing its lowest in the gait cycle, thus conserving energy. As the thigh further inclines, the extension lever arm of the GRF at the hip increases. This in combination with the large magnitude of the GRF generates a large external hip extension moment. At the same time, the GRF is producing an external knee extension moment and the combination of the two provides the strong stabilizing external moments needed for stability in terminal stance.[17,27]

Pathological gait

Pathology can result in abnormal neurology, muscle weakness, muscle stiffness, muscle shortening, and bone and joint deformities, leading to joint, segment, and GRF misalignment. When the segments are misaligned, inevitably the GRF also is misaligned relative to the joints, resulting in

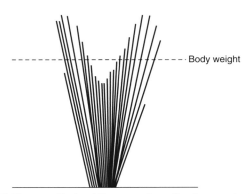

Fig. 22-11 The magnitude of the ground reaction force varies throughout stance, being greater than body weight during loading response and terminal stance.

abnormal lever arms and moments that destabilize or excessively stabilize the joints.

In the coronal plane the GRF may be excessively medially or laterally aligned relative to the hip, knee, ankle, or foot.

An example in the sagittal plane is an inability to incline the shank and thigh segments appropriately to allow the GRF to align itself anterior to the knee and posterior to the hip for stability (Fig. 22-12). This GRF alignment cannot be achieved if the shank is either insufficiently or excessively inclined in midstance.[27] If the shank is insufficiently inclined (or vertical), excessive knee extension moments are created and the production of hip extension moments is difficult. If the shank is excessively inclined, knee extension moments cannot be created. Even if the shank is in optimal alignment, the thigh must achieve a slightly inclined position for the GRF to be aligned anterior to the knee and posterior to the hip. In pathological gait this may not be possible.

The aim of biomechanical interventions should be to optimize segment kinematics to normal if this is appropriate for the patient or as near to normal as possible depending on the pathological condition. This in turn will facilitate appropriate alignment of the GRF relative to the joints and modify lever arms and moments. Orthoses must be designed so that they neither understabilize nor overstabilize joints, which would lead to instability or restrict required movement.

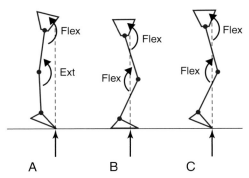

Fig. 22-12 A, Ankle plantarflexion combined with an insufficiently inclined shank in midstance results in an origin of the ground reaction force (GRF) at the forefoot at initial contact, with consequent abnormal GRF alignment at the knee and hip and generation of excessive external knee extension moment and hip flexion moment. **B, C,** Excessively inclined shank (with or without ankle dorsiflexion) results in inappropriate alignment of the GRF at the knee and hip resulting in creation of external flexion moments.

Observations of musculotendinous units

Normal gait

The body has unijointed, bijointed, and trijointed muscles. Examples are psoas and soleus (unijointed), the long hamstrings and rectus femoris (bijointed), and the gastrocnemius (trijointed). They have appropriate length, strength, and stiffness[15, 16] for their function, and they are neurologically activated at appropriate times through the gait cycle to fulfill a concentric, isometric, or eccentric role.

Pathological gait

Muscles in pathological gait may have abnormalities of length, strength, or stiffness. They may be working concentrically when eccentric work or no activity is required. Particular problems may arise in bijointed and trijointed muscles when they are either truly or dynamically (functionally) short. Movement occurring at one joint may "steal" the vital length needed for movement at another joint. An example of this is a flexed hip "stealing" hamstring length from the knee, preventing full extension. The effect at the knee is amplified because of the difference in lever arms of the muscle pull at the hip and knee, which has a ratio of 3:1 at initial contact.[37] For example, 10 degrees of hip flexion will reduce knee extension by 30 degrees.

Orthoses must be designed so that they take into account the length, strength, and stiffness of musculotendinous units, particularly the bijointed and trijointed muscles.

Application of biomechanical principles to orthoses

An orthosis achieves its biomechanical effects on the body in two ways. First are the direct biomechanical effects, which can be defined as "what the orthosis does to the joints and limb segments contained within the orthosis." Second are the indirect biomechanical effects, both kinetic and kinematic, which can be defined as "how the orthosis influences the rest of the body" (i.e., the joints and segments outside the orthosis).

Direct biomechanical effect of orthoses

Control of joint angulation in a single anatomical plane requires a system comprising a minimum of three corrective forces. In addition to maximizing lever arms and the area of force application, to be successful these forces must be applied in a way that respects the underlying anatomy. For example, in the case of a knee orthosis to prevent flexion, the biomechanical requirement is application of a posteriorly directed force at the level of the knee joint, countered by two anteriorly directed forces at the top and the bottom of the leg, as far apart as possible. However, because the patella is intolerant to pressure, the middle force should be split and applied above and below the bone. Having successfully avoided the patella, it remains mechanically important for the forces to be applied as close as possible to, that is, *immediately* above and below, the joint center rather than some distance away. It should be noted that splitting this force above and below the patella does not change the system from a three-force to a four-force system, as the net effect of the split force still is equivalent to that of a single force at the joint.

Another way that orthoses account for the underlying anatomy is by ensuring that the area of the orthosis applying the corrective force to the body is carefully shaped to match as closely as possible the contour of the underlying skeletal structures. For example, the section of any orthosis that applies force to the fifth metatarsal shaft to control forefoot abduction (external rotation), an alignment deviation commonly seen in conjunction with hindfoot (subtalar joint) pronation, must be carefully shaped to match the underlying bone contour rather than the contour of the overlying soft tissue. Preloading of soft tissue is a biomechanical concept that ensures that forces are applied to the body in an acceptable manner, without the creation of high-pressure areas.

Indirect biomechanical effect of orthoses

In weight bearing, the GRF is always present. In addition to the direct forces being applied to the limb by the orthosis, there also are indirect effects generated by the interaction of the limb with the GRF.

Lower limb orthoses usually are used with footwear. When weight bearing, the role of the footwear becomes at least equal to that of the orthosis because footwear design is so highly influential on the kinematics of the segments and joints and on the point of application, magnitude, and line of action of the GRF throughout the gait cycle. Although the footwear can manipulate the segment and joint kinematics and GRF advantageously if appropriately designed, it also can have adverse effects if poorly designed. To emphasize the importance of the footwear in the total orthotic prescription, it may be useful in clinical notations to include a reference to it, for example, "AFO footwear combination" (AFOFC) rather than simply "an AFO."[6,17]

If an orthosis and footwear can modify the kinematics of the segments to become close to normal, then the GRF and the moments generated also will approximate to normal (Fig. 22-13).[3,17,27] However, if the segment kinematics remains abnormal as a result of inappropriate design of the orthosis and/or the footwear, then, as in pathological gait, combinations of external moments may destabilize or

excessively stabilize the proximal joints. A focus on segment kinematics during the gait cycle, starting with the shank, is an effective approach to orthotic prescription and problem solving.[25-27] This is most clearly relevant in the use of AFOs but also applies, albeit to a lesser extent, in the use of knee–ankle foot orthoses and hip–knee–ankle foot orthoses.

As an example, consider how a fixed AFOFC can be used to normalize gait. In the presence of pathology, deviations of shank kinematics in the sagittal plane may result in excessive or insufficient incline or recline during the gait cycle. In addition, the shank can arrest its forward movement or reverse its movement.

When using an AFOFC, it can be useful to think about the stance phase of the gait cycle in terms of three rather than the usual five subdivisions of normal gait: entrance to midstance, midstance, and exit from midstance.[27,28] Whatever the gait abnormality, the shank kinematics within each of the three subdivisions needs to replicate normal, as closely as possible, through AFOFC design. Normal shank kinematics requires a slowing of the angular velocity of the shank in an inclined position of 10 to 12 degrees incline relative to the vertical at midstance. During entrance to midstance, the shank must move from the reclined position at initial contact to the midstance position, with an appropriate angular velocity. During exit from midstance, the shank must continue to further inclination with an appropriate angular velocity.

It is tempting to think that normal shank kinematics inevitably requires an AFO with ankle joints. However, even when a fixed AFO is indicated, although the ankle joint kinematics by definition cannot be normal, it still is possible to replicate near-normal *shank* kinematics. Success is dictated mainly by two biomechanical factors: the design of the AFO and the design of the footwear.[2,6]

The AFO must be designed to be strong enough to resist plantarflexion (which would result in insufficient shank inclination) or dorsiflexion (which would lead to excessive shank inclination) as required.

The ankle in the AFO must be held at an appropriate angle. The knee must be permitted to extend in midstance and terminal stance and again in terminal swing, so the AFO must not "steal" muscle length from the knee by holding the ankle in a position that is more dorsiflexed (or less plantarflexed) than can be achieved with the knee fully extended.[20,21,29] Other considerations for this choice are the stiffness of the calf muscles, the length at which the gastrocnemius and soleus muscles can produce maximal muscle power, the length and stiffness of the dorsiflexors, the triplanar requirements of the bones and joints of the foot, and the gait pattern[29]

When accepting a plantarflexed ankle angle in the AFO, the beneficial effect at the knee may be amplified. The ratio of the lever arms of the muscle pull at the ankle and at the knee is approximately 3:2 at 40% gait cycle when knee extension should be at its maximum.[36] Therefore, an increase in plantarflexion of only 6 degrees can result in an increase in knee extension of 9 degrees.

The AFO may be designed to either fix or leave free the metatarsophalangeal joints. This will influence the ability of the orthosis to control shank inclination in exit from midstance, whether excessive or insufficient. Fixing the metatarsophalangeal joints will prevent the use of anatomical third

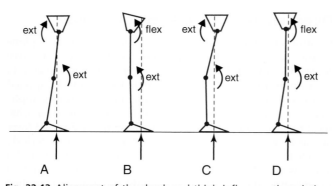

Fig. 22-13 Alignment of the shank and thigh influences the relationship of the ground reaction force to the proximal joints, thereby influencing external moments. During terminal stance *both* the shank and the thigh must be inclined in order to enable appropriate generation of external extension moments at knee and hip joints **(A)**. Vertical shank and thigh **(B)**, vertical shank with inclined thigh **(C)**, and inclined shank with vertical thigh **(D)** result in external knee and hip moments with inappropriate magnitudes and/or direction.

rocker so that shank kinematics in terminal stance is controlled by footwear design.[28]

No AFO design will control shank kinematics if the footwear design is not appropriate for the specific shank kinematic abnormality. Footwear design considerations are the pitch of the footwear ("heel–sole differential"), the design of the heel, the stiffness of the sole, and the design of the sole profile.[17,27] The pitch of the footwear and the angle of the ankle in the AFO combine to dictate the alignment of the AFOFC when standing with the weight equally distributed between heel and sole.[7,17,27] This has been called the shank angle to floor of the AFOFC,[23,27] but the more accurate term shank to vertical angle (SVA)[2,18,26] of the AFOFC is used here. The SVA of the AFOFC significantly influences the shank inclination at midstance, and any SVA can be achieved with any angle of the ankle in the AFO.[20,21,22,27] The design of the heel, the stiffness of the sole, and the design of the sole profile influence the kinematics of the shank during entrances and exits from midstance.

In midstance in normal gait, the SVA is about 10 to 12 degrees inclined.[27] Regardless of whether the observed deviation of the shank segment at this time is insufficient or excessive incline, the aim of the intervention with the AFOFC is to place the shank in a position that is as near normal as possible, so the SVA of the AFOFC needs to be approximately 10 to 12 degrees inclined. In some pathological situations, particularly those of neurological origin, the optimal SVA may be greater or less than the normal inclination.[17,23,27]

The importance of footwear sole design for the control of shank kinematics can be seen when trying to control excessive shank inclination in midstance and exit from midstance. Control of the anatomical joints within the orthosis, by direct forces alone, will not necessarily control shank kinematics. Suppose that, in an effort to control excessive shank inclination at midstance and exit from midstance, an AFO has been correctly designed to prevent ankle dorsiflexion and extension of the metatarsophalangeal joints. The shank can still incline excessively if the footwear that is combined with the AFO has a rounded sole profile, as is the case with most commercial footwear. The solution to this problem lies in the design of the sole profile. The optimum position and design of the rocker on a thick stiff sole, whether rounded or point loading with an appropriate toe spring angle, often influence shank kinematics in midstance and exit from midstance.[12,17,24,27] Failure to recognize the biomechanical contribution of the footwear may result in a less than optimal or even detrimental outcome.

The design of the AFO and footwear exerts influence not only through its effect on the joints and shank kinematics but also through its effect on kinetics. It manipulates the point of application, magnitude, and line of action of the GRF and its relationship to the joints. This modifies the external lever arms and moments at the ankle, knee, and hip.[3,17,27,35]

The GRF can be aligned in front of the knee and behind the hip only when the thigh is inclined (Fig. 22-13). This inclination of the thigh in midstance should occur in conjunction with an inclined shank to allow production of the appropriate stabilizing external extension moments at the knee and hip. The optimum SVA of an AFOFC for stabilization of knee and hip by means of external extending moments often is 10 to 12 degrees inclined. However, depending on the pathology, the optimum SVA may lie somewhere within a larger range of

7 to 15 degrees inclined and for the individual leg likely is critical to within a few degrees.[17,23,27] By correctly aligning the GRF to create external extension moments at the hip and knee, an appropriately aligned AFOFC can facilitate production of a second peak of the GRF that exceeds body weight,[15,17] which may be a crucial biomechanical objective in some patients.

Ankle joints are clinically appropriate in some situations. When mechanical ankle joints are used, the segment kinematic requirements throughout the gait cycle should be considered. In cases of insufficient shank inclination, an ankle joint that resists or prevents plantarflexion may be indicated; in cases of excessive shank inclination, an ankle joint that resists or prevents dorsiflexion may be indicated. In normal gait, contraction of the plantarflexors during terminal stance stiffens the ankle and ensures appropriate GRF alignment relative to the foot, knee, and hip. A fixed ankle AFO design or a jointed AFO that blocks dorsiflexion mimics normal ankle stiffness at this time if the patient cannot achieve it. When mechanical joints are used, the same beneficial consequences for kinetic alignment can occur if appropriate shank and joint kinematics are achieved throughout the gait cycle.

"Tuning" of the AFOFC often is necessary to optimize gait, either by adding or removing heel or sole height to change the SVA or by adjusting the characteristics of the footwear to influence entrance and exit from stance.[3,17,27] In an adult, an increase in Heel-Sole Differential (HSD) of just 5 mm will increase the SVA of an AFOFC by about 2 degrees. If the knee is straight at this time, the hip will move forward approximately 30 mm, facilitating GRF alignment (Fig. 22-14).

Tuning may be particularly appropriate for patients with neurological conditions and for growing children in whom the primary neurology often produces secondary skeletal conditions that may deteriorate over time if not well managed.[17,25–27] The kinetics often are unpredictable in patients with neurological conditions,[14] and clinical experience indicates that these conditions are very sensitive to small changes of perhaps only a few degrees in the alignment of an orthosis or to small changes to the design of the footwear. These patients often have only a small window of opportunity

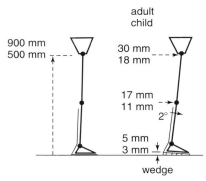

Fig. 22-14 Use of a heel wedge will increase the shank to vertical angle of an AFO footwear combination, thereby advancing the knee and hip joints. For example, a 5-mm heel wedge applied to an adult typically will result in approximately 2 degrees of increased inclination. This will advance the hip joint by about 30 mm. This may facilitate the alignment of the ground reaction force behind the hip joint, creating an external extension moment.

within which the biomechanical design parameters can achieve optimal function.

The tuning process can be difficult when gait is observed at normal speed. Slow-motion video recording can assist in the interpretation of kinematic features, for example, to confirm that the thigh inclines in late stance. If available, a system that allows visualization of the GRF adds kinetic information, which in some patients is crucial to enable normal, or as near normal as possible, GRF alignment.[34,35]

Combined direct and indirect biomechanical effects of orthoses

One example of the combined direct and indirect biomechanical effects of an orthosis can be seen in the treatment of knee hyperextension in stance phase. An appropriate approach may be use of a knee orthosis to apply a three-point force system directly to the knee to prevent hyperextension. The forces applied by such an orthosis may be high, perhaps intolerably so. However, if the hyperextension is caused in part by excessive anterior alignment of the GRF with respect to the knee, perhaps as a result of limited dorsiflexion range, accommodation of the plantarflexion contracture by use of a sufficiently high heel may enable realignment of the GRF relative to the knee joint. This reduces this component of the problem and consequently reduces the magnitude of the forces required from the orthosis.

Relevance of biomechanical principles to total patient management

If the biomechanics can be optimized, then the resultant improvements in kinematics and kinetics not only will have an immediate effect on gait, joints, and muscles but also may provide a therapeutic biomechanical environment that may contribute to long-term benefits.

Maintenance of adequate hip and knee range of motion is a major determinant of whether patients remain ambulant and whether they achieve a near-normal gait. One factor in the development of hip and knee contractures is abnormal GRF alignment in midstance and terminal stance. Once established, these contractures preclude the ability to achieve the desired GRF alignment, thus perpetuating the problem. The net result is an inability to generate an adequate second peak of the GRF, resulting in instability in midstance and terminal stance. As a consequence, the terminal swing phase in the contralateral leg and the swing phase in the ipsilateral leg may be compromised.

If a situation can be created where segment kinematics and kinetics are near normal, then the hip and knee joints may be able to move through a near-normal range of motion. This repetitive lengthening of the hamstrings, gastrocnemius, and hip flexors may minimize the risk of developing muscle and joint contractures and even may help to reduce existing contractures.

Because achieving the desired biomechanical situation using orthotic intervention alone may not be possible, use of additional forms of intervention to facilitate the attainment of kinematic and kinetic objectives may be necessary.

These interventions include physiotherapy to increase joint range, medication to reduce muscle stiffness, and surgery to modify lever arms.

Normalizing the kinetics of gait may have benefits for neurologically impaired patients. It has been postulated that the introduction of normal moment switching at a joint has a potential motor learning effect and that permanent changes in gait may be possible.[4,5] The possibility of such motor learning effects makes for exciting opportunities for orthotic interventions.

Optimum design and tuning of orthoses can turn what was a negative cycle of poor kinematics and kinetics into a positive cycle, which reinforces itself with all the consequent positive effects on bones, musculotendinous units, and neurology.

References

1. Borghese NA, Bianchi L, Lacquaniti F: Kinematic determinants of human locomotion, *J Physiol* 494:863–879, 1996.
2. Bowers RJ, Meadows CB: Case study—the effects of a solid ankle-foot orthosis on hemiplegic gait. In: *Conference proceedings. International Society for Prosthetics and Orthotics (ISPO) 11th World Congress (2004)*, Hong Kong, 2004, ISPO.
3. Butler PB, Nene AV: The biomechanics of fixed ankle foot orthoses and their potential in the management of cerebral palsied children, *Physiotherapy* 77:81–88, 1991.
4. Butler PB, Thompson N, Major RE: Improvement in walking performance of children with cerebral palsy: preliminary results, *Dev Med Child Neurol* 34:567–576, 1992.
5. Butler PB, Farmer SE, Major RE: Improvement in gait parameters following late intervention in traumatic brain injury: a long term follow up report of a single case, *Clin Rehabil* 11:220–226, 1997.
6. Condie DN, Meadows CB: Ankle-foot orthoses. In Bowker P, Condie DN, Bader DL, Pratt DJ, editors: *Biomechanical basis of orthotic management*, Oxford, 1993, Butterworth and Heinemann.
7. Cook TM, Cozzens B: The effects of heel height and ankle-foot-orthoses configuration on weight line location: a demonstration of principles, *Arch Phys Med Rehabil* 30:43–46, 1976.
8. Cusick BD, Stuberg WA: Assessment of lower-extremity alignment in the transverse plane: implications for management of children with neuromotor dysfunction, *Phys Ther* 72:3–15, 1992.
9. Damiano DL, Quinlivan ME, Owen BF, et al: What does the Ashworth scale really measure and are instrumented measures more valid and precise, *Dev Med Child Neurol* 44:112–118, 2002.
10. Gage JR: Gait analysis in cerebral palsy. In: *Clinics in developmental medicine no. 121*, London, 1991, MacKeith Press.
11. Gage JR, DeLuca PA, Renshaw TS: Gait analysis: principles and applications. Emphasis on its use in cerebral palsy, *J Bone Joint Surg* 77A:1607–1623, 1995.
12. Hullin MG, Robb JE, Loudon IR: Ankle-foot orthosis function in low-level myelomeningocele, *J Pediatr Orthop* 12:518–521, 1992.
13. Inman VT, Ralston HJ, Todd F. *Human walking*, Baltimore, 1981, Williams & Wilkins.
14. Kerrigan DC, Deming LM, Holden M: Knee recurvatum in gait: a study of associated knee biomechanics, *Arch Phys Med Rehabil* 77:645–650, 1996.
15. Khodadadeh S, Patrick JH: Forceplate studies of cerebral palsy hemiplegic patients, *J Hum Mov Stud* 15:273–278, 1988.
16. Lieber RL: Skeletal muscle structure, function, and plasticity. In: *The physiological basis of rehabilitation*, ed 2, Baltimore, 2002, Lippincott Williams & Wilkins.
17. Meadows CB. *The influence of polypropylene ankle-foot orthoses on the gait of cerebral palsied children*, PhD Thesis, Glasgow, 1984, University of Strathclyde.
18. Meadows CB, Bowers RJ, McLachlan P, et al: Case study—the effect of solid ankle-foot orthoses on the gait of a patient with facioscapulohumeral dystrophy. In: *Conference proceedings. International Society for Prosthetics and Orthotics (ISPO) 11th World Congress*, Hong Kong, 2004, ISPO.
19. Murray MP: Gait as a total pattern of movement, *Am J Phys Med* 46:290–333, 1967.
20. Nuzzo RM: High-performance activity with below-knee cast treatment. Part 1: mechanics and demonstration, *Orthopedics* 6:713–723, 1983.

21. Nuzzo RM: High-performance activity with below-knee cast treatment. Part 2: clinical application and the weak link hypothesis, *Orthopedics* 6:817–830, 1983.

22. Nuzzo RM: A simple treatment of genu recurvatum in ataxic and athetoid cerebral palsy, *Orthopedics* 9:123–127, 1986.

23. Owen E: Shank angle to floor measures of tuned "ankle-foot orthosis footwear combinations" used with children with cerebral palsy, spina bifida and other conditions, *Gait Posture* 16 (suppl 1):S132–S133, 2002.

24. Owen E: The point of "point-loading rockers" in ankle-foot orthosis footwear combinations used with children with cerebral palsy, spina bifida and other conditions, *Gait Posture* 20S:S86, 2004.

25. Owen E: Tuning of ankle-foot orthosis combinations for children with cerebral palsy, spina bifida and other conditions. In: *Proceedings of ESMAC Seminars*, Warsaw, 2004, European Society for Movement Analysis of Children and Adults.

26. Owen E, Bowers R, Meadows CB: Tuning of AFO-footwear combinations for neurological disorders. In: *Conference proceedings. International Society for Prosthetics and Orthotics (ISPO) 11th World Congress*, Hong Kong, 2004, ISPO.

27. Owen E. *"Shank angle to floor measures" and tuning of "ankle-foot orthosis footwear combinations" for children with cerebral palsy, spina bifida and other conditions*, MSc thesis, Glasgow, 2004, University of Strathclyde.

28. Owen E: A clinical algorithm for the design and tuning of ankle-foot orthosis footwear combinations (AFOFCs) based on shank kinematics, *Gait Posture* 22S:S36–S37, 2005.

29. Owen E: Proposed clinical algorithm for deciding the sagittal angle of the ankle in an ankle-foot orthosis footwear combination, *Gait Posture* 22S:S38–S39, 2005.

30. Perry J: Kinesiology of lower extremity bracing, *Clin Orthop Relat Res* 102:18–31, 1974.

31. Perry J: Normal and pathological gait. In: *American Academy of Orthopaedic Surgeons (1985) atlas of orthotics: biomechanical principles and applications*, ed 2, St. Louis, 1985, Missouri.

32. Perry J. *Gait analysis. Normal and pathological function*, Thorofare, NJ, 1992, Slack Inc.

33. Simon SR, Deutsch SD, Nuzzo RM, et al: Genu recurvatum in spastic cerebral palsy, *J Bone Joint Surg* 60A:882–894, 1978.

34. Stallard J: Assessment of the mechanical function of orthoses by force vector visualisation, *Physiotherapy* 73:398–402, 1987.

35. Stallard J, Woollam PJ: Transportable two-dimensional gait assessment: routine service experience for orthotic provision, *Disabil Rehabil* 25:254–258, 2003.

36. Stewart C, Roberts A, Jonkers I: Gastrocnemius: a three joint muscle, *Gait Posture* 20S:S65–S66, 2004.

37. Stewart C, Jonkers I, Roberts A: Estimates of hamstring length at initial contact based on kinematic gait data, *Gait Posture* 20:61–66, 2004.

38. Sutherland DH, Olshen RA, Biden EN, Wyatt MP: The development of mature walking. In: *Clinics in developmental medicine no. 104/105*, London, 1088, MacKeith Press.

39. Winter DA. *Biomechanics and motor control of human movement*, ed 2, New York, 1990, John Wiley & Sons.

Chapter

23

Biomechanics of the foot

Andrew Haskell and Roger A. Mann

Key Points

- The walking cycle is divided into a stance phase and swing phase, and the stance phase foot progresses through heel strike, flat foot, heel rise, and toe off.
- At initial ground contact the hindfoot everts and the transverse tarsal joint becomes supple allowing the foot to partially absorb the energy of impact.
- During heel rise and toe off the foot becomes rigid by both passive and active mechanisms.
- The oblique axis of the subtalar joint links axial rotation of the leg and hindfoot inversion/eversion.
- The function of the various leg muscles is related to the position of their tendons in relation to the axis across which they exert a force and to the muscle bellies' cross sectional area.

The biomechanics of the foot and ankle during gait describes a complex mechanism of energy transfer from the ground to the body and back from the body to the ground that allows a mode of bipedal motion unique to humans. Normal biomechanics minimizes energy expenditure and reduces stress on the bones, joints, and soft tissues of the lower extremities. Abnormal biomechanics contribute to most of the clinical problems affecting the foot and ankle. Orthopedic surgeons must have an intimate knowledge of this subject to make appropriate clinical decisions, such as placement of the ankle or the foot when carrying out an arthrodesis or proper application of a shoe lift or arch support.

At the most basic level, the biomechanics of the foot and ankle describes the means by which the foot is converted from a flexible shock absorber to a rigid lever. The main function of the foot at initial ground contact is to absorb impact and adapt to the ground. The shape of the hindfoot joints and

the integrity of the supporting ligamentous tissue allow this largely passive mechanism. During lift-off, on the other hand, the foot is converted from a flexible to a rigid structure by both passive and active mechanisms. When these mechanisms in the foot fail to function properly, the relationship of the foot to the ground is altered, which increases stress on one or more of the joints in the foot and ankle, leg, or pelvis.

This chapter discusses the mechanics by which energy is absorbed at the time of initial ground contact and the mechanisms by which the foot is converted to a rigid lever at the time of lift-off. The biomechanical implications of various surgical procedures on the foot are discussed.

Nomenclature

Depicting dynamic biomechanical events in text form relies on a commonly recognized set of terms that describe three-dimensional motions. Unfortunately, when reading the literature pertaining to the biomechanics of the foot and ankle, nomenclature can become quite confusing. Several terms are used to describe separately the hindfoot and forefoot, and some terms represent motions in more than one joint.

In this discussion, the motion at the ankle is described as *dorsiflexion* and *plantarflexion*. Subtalar motion is described as *inversion (varus)* and *eversion (valgus)*. Transverse tarsal motion is *adduction* and *abduction* and is carried out with the foot parallel to the ground with the hindfoot held in neutral position. The posture of the forefoot is described as *forefoot varus* or *forefoot valgus*, depending on whether the lateral (varus) or medial (valgus) border of the foot is in a more plantarflexed position.

The terms *pronation* and *supination* represent a combination of movements of the foot. When the foot is pronated, there is dorsiflexion of the ankle, eversion of the subtalar joint, and abduction of the transverse tarsal joint. When the foot is supinated, there is plantarflexion of the ankle joint, inversion of the subtalar joint, and adduction of the transverse tarsal joint.

Walking cycle

The walking cycle describes the repetitive nature of gait. By convention it begins and ends with heel strike of the same foot. The walking cycle is divided into a *stance phase*, in which the foot is on the ground, and a *swing phase*, in which the foot is off the ground and swinging forward. Normally, stance phase consumes approximately 60% of the walking cycle and swing phase 40% (Fig. 23-1). The stance phase is further divided into two periods of double-limb support and one period of single-limb support. The initial period of double-limb support begins with initial ground contact and ends with toe-off of the opposite limb at 12% of the cycle. Single-limb support then occurs until 50% of the cycle, when the opposite foot strikes the ground, entering the second period of double-limb support. This is shortly followed by lift-off at 62% of the cycle, which initiates the swing phase.

The stance phase can be further divided into various events that occur during a normal walking cycle. Following initial ground contact at 0%, the foot flat is achieved by 7%, and opposite toe-off occurs at 12%. Heel rise of the stance foot begins at 34% of the cycle, which is when the swing leg passes by the stance leg. Opposite heel strike occurs at 50% of the cycle and lift-off of the stance leg at 62%, which initiates the swing phase.

Careful observation of the events of a walking cycle is an important part of the physical examination and may reveal underlying pathology. A patient with spasticity or tight heel cords may make initial ground contact with the toes rather than the heel. Foot flat should occur by 7% of the cycle but may be delayed if an equinus contracture or severe spasticity is present. Early heel rise may occur in patients with spasticity, or delayed heel rise may occur in patients with weakness

in the calf or an elongated Achilles tendon. Occasionally the entire stance phase is prolonged because of significant dysfunction of the lower extremity.

Weight-bearing forces

As we walk, equal and opposite forces are created at the interface between the foot and the ground. One way to measure these forces is a force plate, which consists of load cells applied in orthogonal directions to a suspended platform. In this way, the overall vertical force, fore and aft shear, and medial–lateral shear can be directly measured during the gait cycle. At heel strike, the initial impact against the ground creates a vertical force of approximately 80% of body weight (Fig. 23-2). This rapidly rises to an initial peak of approximately 115% of body weight, representing the transfer of weight to the stance foot at opposite side toe-off. During this initial peak the body's center of gravity is accelerating upward in a sinusoidal pattern as the body moves over the extended leg. As the center of gravity reverses direction, there is a relative unloading of the foot and a corresponding dip in the vertical force curve to approximately 80% of body weight. A second peak of about 110% of body weight occurs when the heel rises and weight moves over the metatarsal heads. This counteracts the downward motion of the body's center of gravity. The vertical force against the ground rapidly falls after opposite heel strike. It reaches zero at the time of toe lift-off, indicating that the toes are lifted from the floor rather than forcefully push off the floor. The magnitude of the force against the ground can vary.

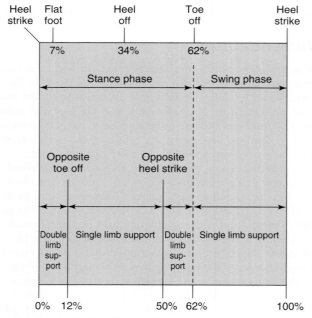

Fig. 23-1 Events of the walking cycle.

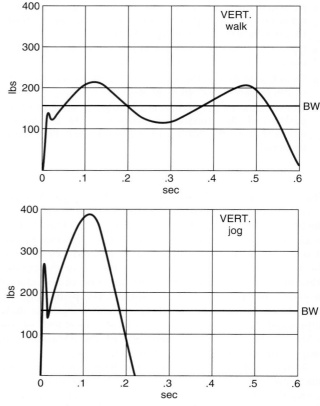

Fig. 23-2 Vertical force curve for walking compared to curve for jogging. Note the markedly increased loading that occurs during jogging.

superior temporal, spatial, and measurement resolution. These arrays can be built into a shoe insert or arranged as a grid on the floor, so they can be used in a variety of in vitro and in vivo studies. In this way, the pressures experienced by discrete points on the foot can be analyzed during gait. This type of study reveals a large initial force against the heel, which rapidly passes from the heel to the metatarsal area (Fig. 23-3). The foot usually is on the ground for approximately 620 ms. By approximately 300 ms all of the force is concentrated in the metatarsal region, after which it is transferred distally to the toes, particularly the hallux.

Anatomical basis of foot and ankle biomechanics

The unique anatomy of the human foot is well suited for bipedal gait. This section describes the separate components that make up the foot and ankle complex and relates their anatomy to the means by which the foot is converted from a flexible shock absorber to a rigid lever during walking. Understanding the functions and interconnections of the various anatomical structures during normal gait helps the orthopedist identify and treat pathology arising from altered biomechanics.

Ankle joint

The axis of the ankle joint passes just distal to the tip of each malleolus and can be estimated by placing one finger on each malleolus. Anthropometric studies demonstrate that although the tibial plafond is parallel to the floor, the angle between the axis of the ankle joint and that of the long axis of the tibia is tilted medially about 80 degrees (Fig. 23-4).[6] Comparing the long axis of the foot with the ankle axis, the foot is slightly internally rotated. In relation to the axis of the knee, the ankle axis is externally rotated approximately 20 to 30 degrees. These axes vary slightly from person to person, so when carrying out an ankle arthrodesis it imperative that the rotation of the operated extremity match that of the opposite side.

The motion that occurs at the ankle joint is that of dorsiflexion and plantarflexion. Dorsiflexion is most accurately

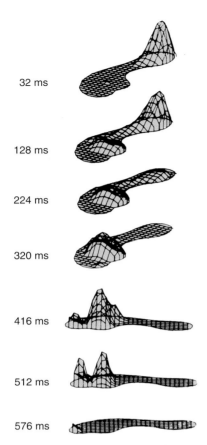

32 ms

128 ms

224 ms

320 ms

416 ms

512 ms

576 ms

Fig. 23-3 Force plate analysis. (From Clarke TE: *The pressure distribution under the foot during barefoot walking,* PhD thesis, University Park, Penn, 1980, Pennsylvania State University.)

A person walking slowly exerts less force than when walking quickly and much less than when jogging or running.

Measuring plantar pressures on discrete points of the foot can be accomplished using a variety of devices. The Harris mat and optical pedobarograph largely have been supplanted by arrays of miniature pressure transducers, which have

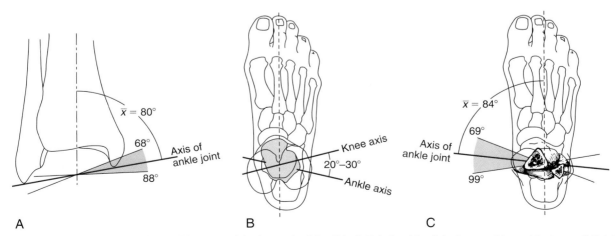

A   B   C

Fig. 23-4 A, Angle between the axis of the ankle joint and the long axis of the tibia. **B,** Relationship of the knee, ankle, and foot axes. **C,** Relationship of the ankle axis to the longitudinal axis of the foot.

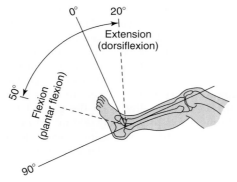

Fig. 23-5 Range and type of motion in the ankle joint.

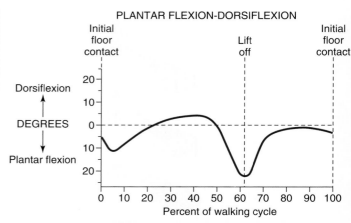

Fig. 23-6 Normal rotation of the ankle joint during one walking cycle.

assessed when the calcaneus is placed in line with the tibia and the head of the talus is covered by the navicular. This places the foot in neutral position (Fig. 23-5). Passively, dorsiflexion is approximately 20 degrees and plantarflexion 50 degrees, although a great deal of variation exists among individuals. Figure 23-6 shows the normal rotation that occurs at the ankle joint during walking.

Subtalar joint

The axis of rotation of the subtalar joint is oblique to both the sagittal and transverse planes. In the transverse plane, it deviates approximately 23 degrees medially from the long axis of the foot. In the sagittal plane, it deviates approximately 40 degrees superiorly to the horizontal plane (Fig. 23-7).[1,7] There is a significant degree of variation in the axis of the subtalar joint from individual to individual.

The motion that occurs in the subtalar joint is that of inversion and eversion. Inversion is movement of the heel in an inward direction, and eversion is movement outward (Fig. 23-8). The range of motion of the subtalar joint includes inversion of approximately 30 degrees and eversion about 10 degrees, although there is significant variation from individual to individual. During normal walking, eversion occurs at the time of initial ground contact until about 15% of the stance phase, after which progressive inversion occurs until the time of toe-off. The magnitude of eversion during the stance phase is about 8 degrees in individuals with a normal foot and 12 degrees in individuals with flat

foot (Fig. 23-9).[16] In individuals with a cavus foot, the degree of subtalar motion is less than that observed in normal feet.

Inman[6] believed that the axis of the subtalar joint permitted it to function as an oblique hinge-type mechanism. This oblique hinge mechanism permits rotatory motion to be passed back and forth between the lower extremity and foot (Fig. 23-10). Specifically, transverse plane rotation in the tibia is linked distally with hindfoot eversion/inversion and farther distally into transverse tarsal joint rotation (forefoot varus/valgus). Normal function of the subtalar joint requires normal function of the talonavicular and calcaneocuboid joints. If normal motion cannot occur in either of these joints, the motion in the subtalar joint is significantly restricted. Similarly, when subtalar joint motion cannot occur, increased stress is placed on the ankle joint proximally and the talonavicular joint distally. When subtalar stiffness is long-standing, degenerative arthrosis or a ball-and-socket ankle joint may result (Fig. 23-11), and changes in the talonavicular joint may occur (Fig. 23-12).

Transverse tarsal joint

The transverse tarsal joint consists of the talonavicular and calcaneocuboid joints. The transverse tarsal joint should be considered an integral part of the subtalar joint, because for normal motion to occur in the transverse tarsal and subtalar

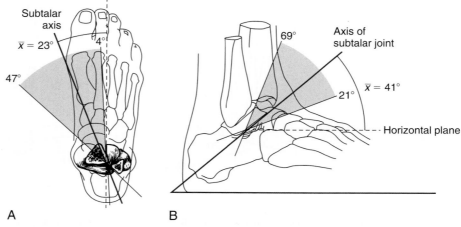

A   B

Fig. 23-7 Subtalar axis in the transverse plane (A) and the horizontal plane (B).

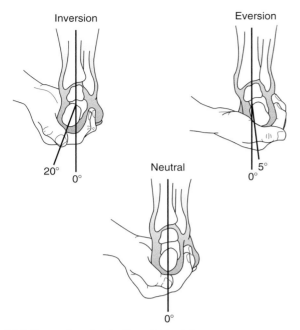

Fig. 23-8 Types of motion in the subtalar joint.

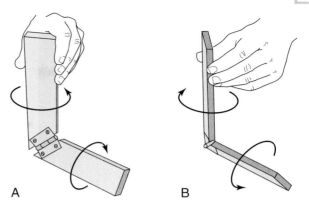

Fig. 23-10 Analogy of the subtalar axes to an oblique hinge. **A,** Outward rotation of the upper stick results in inward rotation of the lower stick. **B,** Inward rotation of the upper stick results in outward rotation of the lower stick.

joints all three joints must function in a normal manner. The transverse tarsal joint motion has been studied by Elftman,[3] who demonstrated that when the axes of the talonavicular and calcaneocuboid joints are parallel to one another, there is flexibility in the transverse tarsal joint, but when the axes are nonparallel, there is rigidity (Fig. 23-13). When the subtalar joint is in an everted position, the transverse tarsal joint axes are parallel, and the transverse tarsal joint is flexible. This is the observation at the time of initial ground contact (heel strike) when impact absorption is desirable. In the last half of the stance phase, a progressive inversion occurs in the subtalar joint, which results in the axes becoming nonparallel. This results in rigidity of the transverse tarsal joint and allows the forefoot to act as a rigid lever.

Metatarsophalangeal joints

The motion that occurs in the metatarsophalangeal joints is that of dorsiflexion and plantarflexion. The degree of this motion is extremely variable from individual to individual, but normally there is approximately 60 degrees of

dorsiflexion and 20 degrees of plantarflexion. During normal gait, dorsiflexion of the metatarsophalangeal joints is a passive mechanism that results from the body moving forward over the fixed foot. Plantarflexion during the gait cycle usually does not occur. As the metatarsophalangeal joints passively dorsiflex during the last half of the stance phase, the plantar aponeurosis is pulled distally, which depresses the metatarsal heads and elevates the longitudinal arch.

Metatarsal break

The metatarsal break describes the oblique axis of the four lateral metatarsophalangeal joints in the transverse plane (Fig. 23-14). This axis passes from medial to lateral at an angle of about 62 degrees to the longitudinal axis of the foot.[7] As the foot rises up onto the metatarsal heads during late stance, the obliquity of this axis enhances the external rotation of the lower extremity, which secondarily brings about inversion of the subtalar joint.

Plantar aponeurosis

The plantar aponeurosis arises from the tubercle of the calcaneus and passes distally to insert into the proximal phalanx of each of the toes. When inserting into the great toe, it surrounds the sesamoid bones (Fig. 23-15). During gait, the

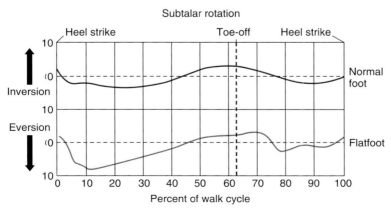

Fig. 23-9 Subtalar joint rotation.

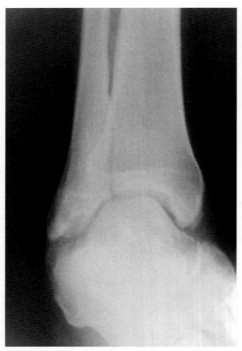

Fig. 23-11 Ball-and-socket ankle joint in a patient with a congenital abnormality of the subtalar joint that did not permit subtalar motion to occur. The resulting transverse rotation, which normally would be absorbed in the subtalar joint, was passed to the ankle joint, which in turn adopted an abnormal configuration to compensate for the loss of subtalar joint motion.

plantar aponeurosis plays an important role in the transition from a supple to a rigid foot. As the body passes forward across the foot during the gait cycle, the metatarsophalangeal joints are passively dorsiflexed. The plantar aponeurosis, which is attached to the base of the proximal phalanges, is drawn forward over the metatarsal heads and at the same time depresses them. This results in elevation of the longitudinal arch and provides considerable stability to the arch structure.[5] Pulling the aponeurosis distally also assists in inversion of the calcaneus because of the medially based origin. This powerful mechanism is most functional at the level of the first metatarsophalangeal joint and becomes less functional

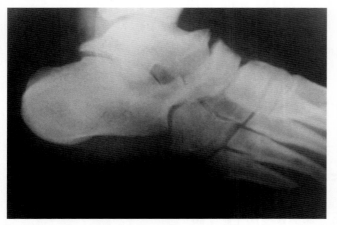

Fig. 23-12 Beaking and alteration of the head of the talus secondary to loss of normal function in the transverse tarsal joint area. This, in turn, was secondary to a calcaneonavicular coalition.

moving laterally toward the fifth metatarsophalangeal joint. If this mechanism is destabilized by loss of the metatarsal head or base of the proximal phalanx of the great toe, significant weakness results in the foot, and the stabilization of the longitudinal arch is significantly impaired.

Talonavicular joint

The articulating surface of the talonavicular joint is not shaped like a simple ball-and-socket joint but rather like an elliptical paraboloid with differing radii of curvatures in the transverse and sagittal planes. As force is applied across the joint, during the last half of stance phase the joint becomes increasingly stable. Conversely, when there is diminished force across the joint, such as observed at initial ground contact, there is flexibility within this joint (Fig. 23-16).

Transverse plane rotation

During gait, the entire lower segment, which consists of the pelvis, femur, and tibia, undergoes rotation in the transverse plane.[15] This is linked to rotation of the foot by the oblique axis of the subtalar joint. At heel strike, calcaneus eversion is transmitted proximally across the ankle joint and results in internal rotation of the remainder of the lower segment (Fig. 23-17). This forms part of the impact absorption mechanism of the lower extremity. In the last half of the stance phase, progressive external rotation occurs in the lower extremity, which is initiated by external rotation of the pelvis as the swing leg is moved forward ahead of the stance leg. The external rotation is transmitted distally to the femur and tibia and across the ankle joint and then is translated by the subtalar joint into inversion. Subtalar joint inversion helps to bring about stabilization of the longitudinal arch via the transverse tarsal joint. The function of the plantar aponeurosis and the functional axis of the metatarsal break accentuate this external rotation. The magnitude of the rotation that occurs increases moving distally from the pelvis to the tibia.

Muscle function versus joint axes

The muscles of the lower extremity play a vital role in foot and ankle biomechanics. The different muscle groups act in a carefully synchronized sequence to decelerate the foot after heel strike, to control the forward motion of the tibia after foot flat, and to continue to load the metatarsal heads after heel rise. Active inversion also helps lock the transverse tarsal joints, making the foot rigid during the latter part of the stance phase.

The function of a muscle is associated with its position relative to the axis across which it exerts a force and to the muscle belly's cross-sectional area. The greater the distance a muscle is from the axis of rotation, the greater its leverage; conversely, the closer a muscle is to the axis of rotation, the lesser its leverage (Fig. 23-18). The axes of the subtalar and ankle joints are shown in Figure 23-19. Muscles posterior to the ankle axis result in plantarflexion, and muscles anterior to the ankle result in dorsiflexion. The muscles lateral to the subtalar joint axis bring about eversion, and those medial to it bring about inversion. Looking at the figure, note that the muscles of the posterior calf are significantly greater in number and in mass than those anterior to it. This apparent

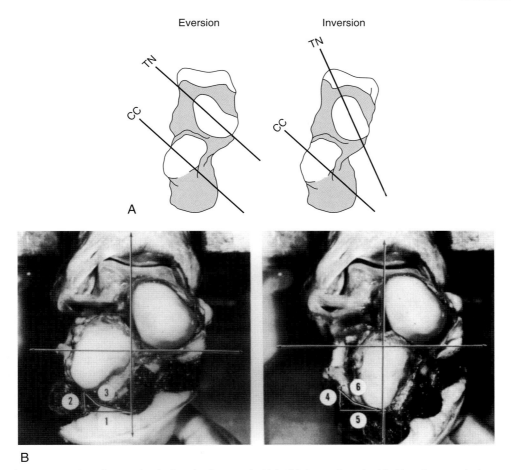

Eversion   Inversion

Fig. 23-13 A, Axes of rotation in the talonavicular (TN) and calcaneocuboid (CC) joints. When the hindfoot is everted, these axes are parallel, so relatively free motion in the transverse tarsal joint is permitted. When the hindfoot is inverted, the axes are divergent, so there is restriction of motion in the transverse tarsal joint and hence greater stability. **B,** Anatomical model of the hindfoot showing the relationship between talus and calcaneus. *Left,* Valgus position of os calcis involving abduction *(1),* extension *(2),* and pronation *(3). Right,* Varus position of calcaneus involving flexion *(4),* adduction *(5),* and supination *(6).* When calcaneus is in valgus position, the transverse tarsal joint is mobile. When calcaneus is in varus position, the transverse tarsal joint is locked. (From Sarrajian SK: *Anatomy of the foot and ankle,* Philadelphia, 1993, JB Lippincott.)

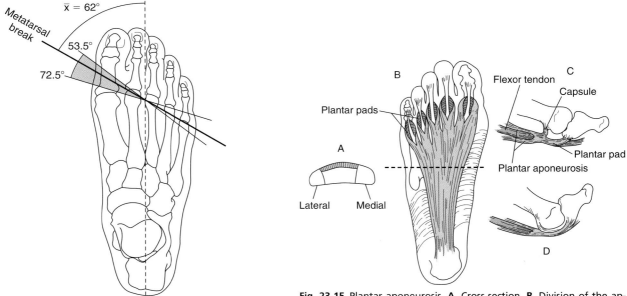

Fig. 23-14 Metatarsal break in relation to the longitudinal axes of the foot.

Fig. 23-15 Plantar aponeurosis. **A,** Cross-section. **B,** Division of the aponeurosis around the flexor tendons. **C,** Components of the plantar pad and its insertion into the base of the proximal phalanx. **D,** Toes in extension with the plantar pad drawn over the metatarsal head.

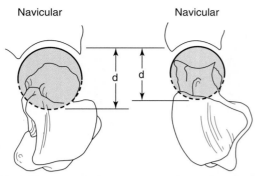

Fig. 23-16 Relationship of the head of the talus to the navicular, left superior and right lateral views. Note the different diameters of the head of the talus.

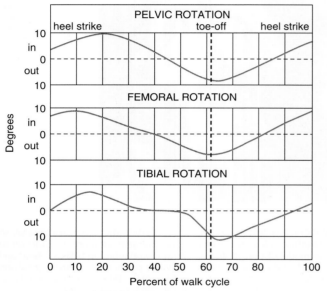

Fig. 23-17 Transverse plane rotation.

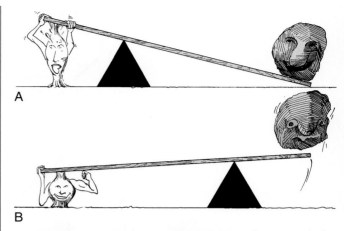

Fig. 23-18 **A**, The closer the muscle is to the axis of rotation, the less leverage it has to effect rotation about the axis. **B**, A muscle far from the rotation has a longer arm and hence can exert greater movement across the axis.

imbalance is kept in check by the proper function of the central nervous system, which enables coordinated function of these muscles to occur. After a head injury, stroke, or neuromuscular disorder, a significant deformity about the foot and ankle can occur because of the resultant muscle imbalance.

The main function of the anterior calf muscles, the tibialis anterior, and to a lesser extent the extensors of the toes is to control plantarflexion, which occurs following initial ground contact by an eccentric contraction (Fig. 23-20). Following foot flat, the anterior compartment muscles cease to function until about the time of lift-off, when the muscles once again become functional. This time, a concentric or shortening contraction brings about dorsiflexion of the ankle joint, which provides clearance of the foot during the swing phase of gait. If the anterior tibial group fails to function, a foot drop occurs that results in a steppage type of gait. A steppage gait is one in which increased flexion of hip and knee provides adequate toe clearance given the lack of dorsiflexion at the ankle joint.

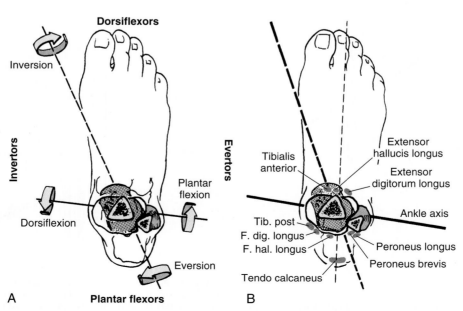

Fig. 23-19 **A**, Rotation about the subtalar and ankle axes. **B**, Relationship of the various muscles about the subtalar and ankle axes.

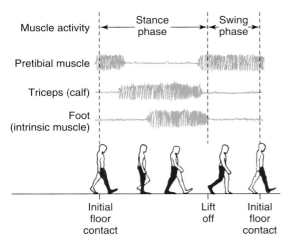

Fig. 23-20 Phasic electromyographic activity of the leg and foot muscles during normal gait.

The posterior calf muscles function during the stance phase of gait. These muscles become active as a group, following foot flat. The calf muscles then undergo an eccentric contraction until approximately 40% of the gait cycle, when plantarflexion of the ankle joint begins (Fig. 23-20). The muscle then undergoes a concentric or shortening contraction, bringing about plantarflexion of the ankle joint and inversion of the hindfoot, which ceases just before toe-off. The main function of the posterior calf in the first half of the stance phase is to control the forward movement of the tibia over the fixed foot.[11,14] If this muscle group fails to function, the support of the stance limb is inadequate, which results in a shortened step length on the contralateral limb.

The intrinsic muscles of the foot are active during the stance phase of gait and continue their activity until the time of toe-off.[8] These small muscles probably help with the functioning of the plantar aponeurosis and the stabilization of the metatarsophalangeal joints and toes. However, by nature of their small size they probably do not play a significant role compared to the plantar aponeurosis in the stability of the longitudinal arch.

Mechanics of walking

Thus far the forces against the ground and the function of the various joints of the foot and ankle have been discussed. This section correlates the various isolated facts and describes the function of the foot and ankle through a complete walking cycle.

At heel strike, the foot passively absorbs some of the impact of ground contact. The forces exerted against the ground exceed body weight during normal walking. Extrapolating for a 150-lb individual walking 1 mile, approximately 63 tons of force must be dissipated per foot per mile. This gives an indication of the amount of force that is dissipated at ground contact. The only muscles below the knee functioning at the time of initial ground contact are the anterior compartment muscles, which work to control plantarflexion of the ankle joint, helping to absorb energy. When the foot strikes the ground, it literally collapses and is restrained only by the shape of its articulations and their ligamentous support.

The events that occur at initial ground contact are as follows:

1. Heel pad striking the ground
2. Controlled ankle joint plantarflexion
3. Eversion of the calcaneus, which results distally in parallel axes of the transverse tarsal joint, thereby making the joint flexible, and proximally in enhancement of internal rotation of the lower extremity

All of these mechanisms result in absorption of the impact against the ground. This impact absorption can be further enhanced by soft shoe material, as opposed to hard leather heels and soles.

The events that occur at the time of toe-off are dynamic in nature and consist of the following:

1. Progressive external rotation of the tibia
2. Subtalar joint inversion
3. Transverse tarsal joint axes made nonparallel, resulting in locking of the joint
4. Dorsiflexion of the metatarsophalangeal joints, resulting in the plantar aponeurosis elevating the longitudinal arch
5. Seating of the talonavicular joint

To appreciate better the mechanisms that occur, one can look at the function of the foot in the sagittal and transverse planes. Sagittal plane activities include the following:

1. Ankle joint motion
2. Metatarsophalangeal joint motion
3. Plantar aponeurosis function
4. Intrinsic muscle function
5. Configuration of the talonavicular joint

Following initial ground contact, rapid plantarflexion of the ankle joint is mediated by eccentric contraction of the anterior compartment muscles. This muscle function initially controls the plantarflexion of the ankle joint and then probably helps to advance the tibia forward over the fixed foot. Progressive dorsiflexion of the ankle joint begins following foot flat until approximately 40% of the gait cycle. As this dorsiflexion occurs, it is controlled by an eccentric contraction of the posterior calf muscles. At 40% of the gait cycle when the force across the ankle joint is maximal,[13] plantarflexion of the ankle joint begins as a result of a concentric contraction of the posterior calf musculature (Fig. 23-21). This muscle function ceases at approximately 50% of the gait cycle, after which

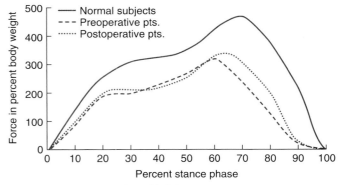

Fig. 23-21 Forces across the ankle joint.

319

the remainder of the plantarflexion is passive until the time of lift-off. During the swing phase, the anterior compartment muscles become active, bringing about dorsiflexion at the ankle joint.

The metatarsophalangeal joints play a passive role until the body moves across the fixed foot and plantarflexion of the ankle joint begins. Following these occurrences, there is progressive dorsiflexion of the metatarsophalangeal joints until the time of lift-off. The main function of dorsiflexion is to activate the mechanism of the plantar aponeurosis, which results in plantarflexion of the metatarsal heads and elevation of the longitudinal arch. The intrinsic muscles of the foot are functioning during this time to stabilize the metatarsophalangeal joints and then cease functioning after toe-off. The force analysis shown in Figure 23-3 demonstrates this weight transfer from the metatarsal area to the toes.

The talonavicular joint at initial ground contact is somewhat unstable, but the stability of the joint increases progressively as increasing force is placed across the joint in the last half of stance phase. The elliptical paraboloid shape of the joint aids in the progressive stability of the joint.

Transverse plane mechanisms include the following:

1. Rotation of the lower extremity, particularly the tibia
2. Subtalar joint motion
3. Transverse tarsal joint motion
4. Function of the metatarsal break

At the time of initial ground contact, internal rotation occurs in the lower extremity. This is a passive event, the magnitude of which is controlled by the degree of rotation permitted by the joints of the foot and their ligamentous support. Inward rotation reaches a maximum at the time of foot flat, after which progressive external rotation begins and reaches its peak at the time of toe-off. The rotation at the time of initial ground contact begins with collapse of the subtalar joint into eversion, which results in an internal rotation force proximally up the lower extremity. Subsequent external rotation probably is mediated from proximal to distal starting at the pelvis, with the rotation transmitted through the femur and across the knee and ankle joints to the subtalar joint. The progressive external rotation of the lower extremity helps to bring about inversion of the subtalar joint.

The rotation of the subtalar joint at the time of initial ground contact is one of eversion, which is a passive motion brought about by the loading of the hindfoot by the body. The magnitude of this rotation is mediated by the joints of the foot and their ligamentous support. An individual with a flat foot generally has a greater degree of eversion following ground contact than a person with a normal foot or cavus foot. Progressive inversion of the subtalar joint reaches a maximum at the time of toe-off. The progressive inversion is brought about by progressive external rotation that occurs in the leg above, but it is significantly enhanced by the function of the plantar aponeurosis and the metatarsal break. The plantar aponeurosis, as it becomes more functional in depressing the metatarsal heads, also brings about inversion of the calcaneus; this is further enhanced by the obliquity of the metatarsal break. Precisely what percent of the internal rotation can be attributed to the external rotation of the tibia, plantar aponeurosis, and metatarsal break has not been

determined, but these three mechanisms work in concert to bring about the final stabilization of the longitudinal arch.

The transverse tarsal joint functions in association with the subtalar joint.[9] At the time of initial ground contact, when the subtalar joint is everted, the joint axes of the calcaneocuboid and talonavicular joints are parallel to one another. This results in unlocking of the transverse tarsal joint. In the last half of the stance phase, the subtalar joint is inverting, and the joint axes are nonparallel, producing marked stability of the joint. The stability of the transverse tarsal joint is further enhanced by the seating of the talus into the navicular, the complete inversion of the subtalar joint, and the function of the plantar aponeurosis and the intrinsic muscles.

The model shown in Figure 23-22 points out these various mechanisms, all of which are functioning simultaneously but have been described individually.

During a full gait cycle, at the time of initial ground contact the foot is loaded, which results in plantarflexion of the ankle joint, eversion of the subtalar joint, internal rotation of the tibia, and unlocking of the transverse tarsal joint. This mechanism provides for maximum energy absorption. In the last half of the stance phase, increasing stability of the foot is brought about by external rotation of the lower extremity, progressive inversion of the subtalar joint, locking of the transverse tarsal joint, and function of the plantar aponeurosis mediated by dorsiflexion of the

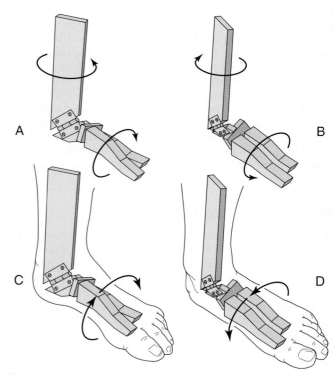

Fig. 23-22 Mechanism by which rotation of the tibia is transmitted through the subtalar joint into the foot. **A,** Outward rotation of the upper stick results in inward rotation of the lower stick. Thus, as seen in **C,** outward rotation of the tibia causes inward rotation of the calcaneus with elevation of the medial border of the foot and depression of the lateral border. **B,** Inward rotation of the upper stick results in outward rotation of the lower stick. Thus, as seen in **D,** inward rotation of the tibia causes outward rotation of the calcaneus with depression of the medial side of the foot and elevation of the lateral side.

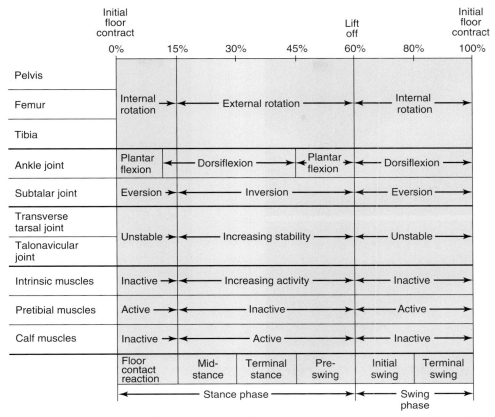

	Initial floor contract				Lift off				Initial floor contract
	0%	15%	30%	45%	60%	80%	100%		
Pelvis									
Femur	Internal rotation →	← External rotation →			← Internal rotation →				
Tibia									
Ankle joint	Plantar flexion	← Dorsiflexion →		←Plantar flexion→	← Dorsiflexion →				
Subtalar joint	Eversion →	← Inversion →			← Eversion →				
Transverse tarsal joint	Unstable →	← Increasing stability →			← Unstable →				
Talonavicular joint									
Intrinsic muscles	Inactive →	← Increasing activity →			← Inactive →				
Pretibial muscles	Active →	← Inactive →			← Active →				
Calf muscles	Inactive →	← Active →			← Inactive →				
	Floor contact reaction	Mid-stance	Terminal stance	Pre-swing	Initial swing	Terminal swing			
	← Stance phase →				← Swing phase →				

Fig. 23-23 Complete walking cycle. Note the rotations that occur in the various segments and joints as well as activity in the foot and leg musculature.

metatarsophalangeal joints. This mechanism produces a rigid foot for the time of toe-off (Fig. 23-23).

Surgical implications of the biomechanics of the foot

When performing operative procedures around the foot and ankle, the biomechanics of the foot must always be considered. In particular, increased stress on an adjacent joint results when an arthrodesis is carried out. This has long-term implications and must be carefully considered in the surgical decision making. As a general rule, performance of a corrective osteotomy or tendon transfer rather than an arthrodesis is preferable to avoid the added stress on adjacent joints. Likewise, use of an orthotic device should always be considered when feasible.

Ankle joint fusion

An ankle arthrodesis is commonly performed for a painful affliction of the ankle joint. Following an ankle arthrodesis with elimination of dorsiflexion and plantarflexion, increased stress is placed on the subtalar and transverse tarsal joints. An in vitro analysis revealed that following ankle fusions, approximately 50% of dorsiflexion and 70% of plantarflexion were eliminated. However, this means that the remaining 50% of dorsiflexion and 30% of plantarflexion occur at other joints (Fig. 23-24). Arthrosis present in the subtalar or transverse tarsal joints following an ankle fusion means the possibility of persistent pain. Long-term follow-up shows that after ankle fusion, the majority of patients develop hindfoot arthritis that worsens clinical outcome.[2,4] This concept must be taken into account when considering a fusion.

The alignment of the ankle fusion is extremely important. If the foot is not placed into a plantigrade position, abnormal stresses are applied to the foot and knee, resulting in patient dissatisfaction. An ankle undergoing fusion should be placed into a neutral dorsiflexion–plantarflexion position, into 3 to 5 degrees of valgus, and the degree of external rotation should equal that of the opposite side. Shortening should be kept to a minimum.

Plantarflexion of 5 to 10 degrees should be considered if the patient requires knee stability because of loss of quadriceps muscle function. Fixing the foot in equinus provides a back knee thrust that helps stabilize the knee joint. In the absence of this condition, it is important that the joint not be placed into equinus to prevent pressure against the posterior portion of the knee joint. Placing the ankle joint into excessive dorsiflexion increases the stress on the heel, which may be a problem, particularly in the patient with an insensate foot. When performing a pan-talar arthrodesis, however, slight dorsiflexion probably is beneficial because it permits the individual to roll over the foot more easily than when the ankle is placed in neutral. The varus–valgus alignment is critical. Surgical fusion of the ankle into excessive varus results in instability of the subtalar joint because the weight-bearing line passes lateral to the axis of the subtalar joint.

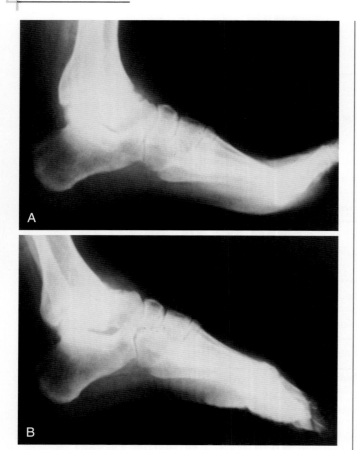

A

B

Fig. 23-24 Compensatory motion in the transverse tarsal and subtalar joints after an ankle arthrodesis. **A,** Full dorsiflexion. **B,** Full plantarflexion. Note the motion occurring in the joints distal to the ankle joint to compensate for loss of ankle motion.

The varus alignment also results in locking of the transverse tarsal joint, producing a rigid foot and a vaulting type of gait pattern. Sometimes the patient compensates by walking with the leg in external rotation. Fusing an ankle into excessive valgus applies stress along the medial side of the knee joint.

Subtalar joint fusion

When arthrodesis of a subtalar joint is performed, biomechanical principles indicate that the joint be placed in 5 to 7 degrees of valgus. In this way, the transverse tarsal joint is kept parallel (unlocked), which permits increased flexibility through the midtarsal area. If the subtalar joint is placed into varus, the transverse tarsal joints are nonparallel (locked), resulting in increased rigidity of the forefoot. A rigid forefoot results in a vaulting gait pattern or external rotation of the leg as a compensatory mechanism. The varus position also results in increased stress along the lateral aspect of the foot, and a diffuse callus may develop beneath the fifth metatarsal area.

Transverse tarsal joint fusions

Arthrodesis of the talonavicular joint or calcaneocuboid joint often significantly eliminates pain caused by arthrosis or deformity. However, it also results in loss of motion of

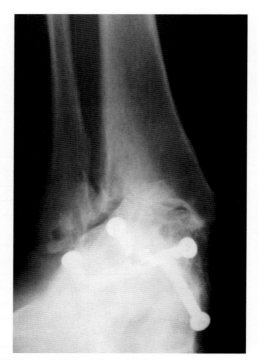

Fig. 23-25 Degeneration of the ankle joint.

the subtalar joint because the subtalar joint complex, which includes the subtalar and transverse tarsal joints, requires motion in each of the joints for full motion to occur. With elimination of motion at the talonavicular joint, essentially all of the subtalar joint motion is eliminated. If the calcaneocuboid joint is fused, about one third of subtalar and talonavicular joint motion is eliminated. Therefore, when performing a fusion through the transverse tarsal joint, it is essential that the hindfoot be placed into 5 to 7 degrees of valgus so that a plantigrade foot results.

Triple arthrodesis

The triple arthrodesis combines the fusion of the subtalar and transverse tarsal joints. This is an excellent procedure and one that is used to create a plantigrade foot. Following this fusion, approximately 13 degrees of dorsiflexion and 16 degrees of plantarflexion are eliminated. However, normal function of the subtalar joint (torque conversion from the tibia above into the calcaneus below) also is eliminated, which places increased rotational stress on the ankle joint. Several studies have demonstrated that in the years following a triple arthrodesis, arthrosis occurs at the ankle joint as an unfortunate sequela of this procedure in a certain percentage of cases (Fig. 23-25).[10,12] The alignment of the triple arthrodesis is critical and follows the principles used for the subtalar and transverse tarsal joints. However, two other factors must be considered. Forefoot abduction–adduction must be corrected back to neutral through the transverse tarsal joint as well as correction of any varus or valgus deformity of the forefoot. In essence, all the joints must be aligned to create a plantigrade foot.

Tarsal and metatarsal fusions

Fusions involving the tarsal and metatarsal joints one, two, and three result in some degree of stiffness of the forefoot, which usually does not cause any significant problem for the patient. The stiffness can be a factor if one of the metatarsals is fused in a plantarflexed position, which might result in a plantar callosity beneath the plantarflexed metatarsal head. Techniques such as tendon interposition may allow preservation of the mobile fourth and fifth metatarsocuboid joints. If the fusion mass includes the fourth and fifth metatarsocuboid articulation, the articulation between the cuboid and lateral cuneiform should be spared if possible because dorsiflexion–plantarflexion motion occurs in this joint.

Metatarsophalangeal joint arthrodesis

When carrying out a first metatarsophalangeal joint arthrodesis, the joint should be placed into approximately 15 degrees of valgus and 10 to 15 degrees of dorsiflexion in relation to the ground. This is approximately 25 to 30 degrees of dorsiflexion in relation to the first metatarsal shaft, which is inclined plantarward about 15 degrees. The rotation of the great toe also must be taken into account to ensure that the pad is placed flat on the ground and the toenails are aligned in the same plane. Proper alignment diminishes the stress placed on the interphalangeal joint.

In the patient whose first metatarsophalangeal joint has undergone arthrodesis, high-speed motion picture gait studies have demonstrated that as pressure is exerted against the great toe, the foot comes off the ground sooner than in the foot that has full dorsiflexion of the metatarsophalangeal joints.

Tendon transfers

The main consideration for a tendon transfer about the foot and ankle is to attempt use of a muscle that is working in the same phase as the nonfunctional one. The advantage of a phasic transfer is that the muscle naturally contracts at the same time of the walking cycle as the muscle it is replacing. A nonphasic transfer is one in which a muscle that normally works in the stance phase is transferred anteriorly to function as a swing phase muscle. Although muscles involved in nonphasic transfers can be trained, most of the literature indicates that eventually these procedures tend to function more as a tenodesis and do not actually provide active motor function. The other main principle in carrying out a tendon transfer is that for a tendon transfer to work successfully, the joint over which the tendon acts should have a normal or near-normal range of motion. If a joint contracture exists, the tendon transfer is unable to function.

Plantigrade foot

A plantigrade foot is one in which the foot is placed on the ground such that the center of gravity passes along the plantar aspect of the foot in a normal manner. At times, however, the foot posture may be altered because of either a congenital abnormality or an acquired problem. An example of a congenital abnormality is an untreated clubfoot. An example of an acquired problem occurs in a patient with a ruptured posterior tibial tendon or posttraumatic condition with significant distortion of the bony architecture. For the foot to function efficiently, it should be placed flat on the ground in near-normal alignment. Proper alignment at the time of surgery, particularly when carrying out an arthrodesis, has been discussed previously in the sections on surgical fusion.

To observe whether the foot is in a normal plantigrade position, the foot must be placed into what is termed *neutral alignment*. This is achieved by placing the calcaneus in line with the long axis of the tibia or in up to 5 degrees of valgus; centering the navicular over the head of the talus; and placing the metatarsal heads so that they are perpendicular to the long axis of the tibia. In this manner, the foot is in neutral alignment and is plantigrade. A malalignment of the foot can occur because of an abnormal posture of the hindfoot, forefoot, or both.

When the calcaneus is in neutral position and the medial side of the forefoot is more plantarflexed than the lateral, the forefoot is in a valgus position (Fig. 23-26). In this situation, the first metatarsal is more plantarflexed than the fifth metatarsal. From a clinical standpoint, this occurs most frequently in the patient with Charcot-Marie-Tooth disease or

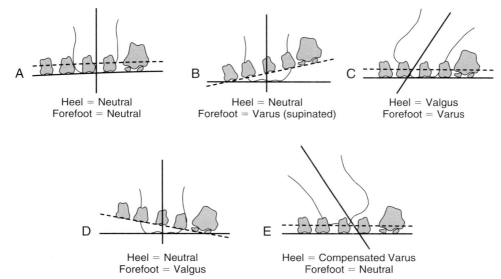

A Heel = Neutral
Forefoot = Neutral

B Heel = Neutral
Forefoot = Varus (supinated)

C Heel = Valgus
Forefoot = Varus

D Heel = Neutral
Forefoot = Valgus

E Heel = Compensated Varus
Forefoot = Neutral

Fig. 23-26 Foot alignment.

a cavus foot deformity. When an individual with a fixed fore-foot valgus configuration takes a step, the calcaneus must rotate into a varus position for the foot to remain plantigrade. Conversely, when the lateral border of the foot is more plantarflexed than the medial border, the condition is called forefoot varus. Under these circumstances, the calcaneus moves into a position of valgus with weight bearing. This is seen most frequently in the patient with a long-standing rupture of the posterior tibial tendon.

When a deformity is flexible, an orthotic device can be used to support and realign the foot, holding it in a plantigrade position. If the heel is in a neutral position, the orthotic device must support the forefoot either on the medial side for a varus deformity or on the lateral side for a valgus deformity so that the foot presents as plantigrade a posture to the ground as possible. At times, however, the deformity involves mainly the hindfoot, in which excessive varus or valgus is present. Under these circumstances, some type of medial or lateral heel support to realign the hindfoot is required, along with possibly a forefoot post (support) to obtain as planti-grade a foot as possible. As a general rule, the orthotic device should be made of a semiflexible material that has adequate padding to help absorb the forces at the time of initial ground contact.

References

1. Close J, Inman V: The action of the subtalar joint, *Univ Calif Prosthet Devices Res Rep* 11, 1953.
2. Coester LM, Saltzman CL, Leupold J, Pontarelli W: Long-term results following ankle arthrodesis for post-traumatic arthritis, *J Bone Joint Surg Am* 83A:219–228, 2001.
3. Elftman H: The transverse tarsal joint and its control, *Clin Orthop Relat Res* 16:41–46, 1960.
4. Fuchs S, Sandmann C, Skwara A, Chylarecki C: Quality of life 20 years after arthrodesis of the ankle. A study of adjacent joints, *J Bone Joint Surg Br* 85:994–998, 2003.
5. Hicks JH: The mechanics of the foot. II. The plantar aponeurosis and the arch, *J Anat* 88:25–30, 1954.
6. Inman V: *The joints of the ankle*, Baltimore, 1976, Williams & Wilkins.
7. Isman R, Inman V: Anthropometric studies of the human foot and ankle, *Bull Prosthet Res* 10–11:97, 1969.
8. Mann R, Inman VT: Phasic activity of intrinsic muscles of the foot, *J Bone Joint Surg Am* 46:469–481, 1964.
9. Manter J: Movements of the subtalar and transverse tarsal joints, *Anat Rec* 80:397, 1941.
10. Saltzman CL, Fehrle MJ, Cooper RR, Spencer EC, Ponseti IV: Triple arthrodesis: twenty-five and forty-four-year average follow-up of the same patients, *J Bone Joint Surg Am* 81:1391–1402, 1999.
11. Simon SR, Mann RA, Hagy JL, Larsen LJ: Role of the posterior calf muscles in normal gait, *J Bone Joint Surg Am* 60:465–472, 1978.
12. Smith RW, Shen W, Dewitt S, Reischl SF: Triple arthrodesis in adults with non-paralytic disease. A minimum ten-year follow-up study, *J Bone Joint Surg Am* 86A:2707–2713, 2004.
13. Stauffer RN, Chao EY, Brewster RC: Force and motion analysis of the normal, diseased, and prosthetic ankle joint, *Clin Orthop Relat Res* 127:189–196, 1977.
14. Sutherland DH: An electromyographic study of the plantar flexors of the ankle in normal walking on the level, *J Bone Joint Surg Am* 48:66–71, 1966.
15. Sutherland DH, Hagy JL: Measurement of gait movements from motion picture film, *J Bone Joint Surg Am* 54:787–797, 1972.
16. Wright DG, Desai SM, Henderson WH: Action of the subtalar and ankle-joint complex during the stance phase of walking, *J Bone Joint Surg Am* 46:361–382, 1964.

Chapter

24

Shoes and shoe modifications

Dennis J. Janisse

Key Points

- When fitting the shoe, be sure to fit the shoe to the foot, not the foot to the shoe.
- Efficient function and success of most lower limb orthotic devices depend greatly on appropriate footwear.
- Rocker soles are simple modifications that can restore lost motion, aid in propulsion, and improve gait.
- Be sure the shoe is appropriate for the patient's level and type of activity.
- Relasting a shoe can help to avoid the need for custom shoes or mismated shoes.

With few exceptions, the efficient function of virtually all lower extremity orthotic devices depends heavily on appropriate footwear.[15] The efficacy of an assistive device can be greatly enhanced through good footwear selection and/or shoe modifications. If a patient is unable to find a shoe to accommodate his or her ankle–foot orthosis (AFO), the brace is rendered useless. To complicate matters, many people are accustomed to purchasing and wearing ill-fitting shoes. Of note is a study by the AOFAS Women's Footwear Committee of 356 women, which found that nearly 90% wore improperly fitting shoes.[4] This chapter explores shoe anatomy and construction techniques; discusses shoe selection and the importance of proper shoe fit; and explains some of the most common shoe modifications and their corresponding indications for use.

Anatomy of a shoe

Choosing the proper footwear for use with or as an assistive device requires a basic understanding of shoe anatomy and construction. This section describes the parts of the shoe and lays the groundwork for future discussion. The following shoe components are common to all shoes; specific features individual to special shoes are excluded.

The most important parts of the shoe are illustrated in Figure 24-1. The terms used to describe parts of the upper include (1) *toe box*—part of the shoe that covers the toes; (2) *vamp*—part of the upper that covers the instep; (3) *counter*—section of the shoe anterior to the heel; (4) *tongue*—piece that covers the dorsum of the foot; and (5) *throat*—section where the tongue meets the vamp. The two basic types of throat openings are the blucher and the balmoral; one common variation is the modified balmoral (Fig. 24-2).

Figure 24-3 depicts a cross-section of the shoe. It illustrates the different layers of the sole: (1) *insole*—layer of sole closest to the foot; (2) *midsole*—layer directly below the insole that adds extra support, stability, and comfort to the shoe (not all shoes have a midsole); (3) *outsole*—bottommost part of the sole that comes into contact with the ground; (4) *foot bed*, some shoes have an additional removable foot bed inside the shoe, on top of the insole, for added comfort; and (5) *shank*—bridge between the heel and the ball area of the shoe; the shank portion of the shoe may be reinforced with a steel shank, a strip of spring steel between the outsole and insole.

Shoe construction

The two main components of interest in shoe construction are (1) the technique used to attach the sole to the upper, which can be accomplished in a number of ways depending on the type of shoe and its intended use; and (2) the shoe materials used in the construction of both the upper and the sole.[12]

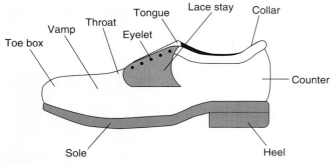

Fig. 24-1 Most important parts of a shoe.

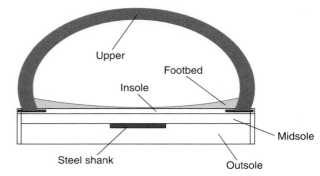

Fig. 24-3 Cross-section of a shoe.

Sole attachment techniques

The manner in which a sole is attached to the upper defines some of its functional properties and its appearance and can affect the fit of the shoe. Six major types of sole attachment techniques are considered (Fig. 24-4).

The *Goodyear welt* takes its name from the Goodyear sole-stitching machine that was invented in the late 1880s.[17] This technique is distinguished by its prominent use of a welt. A welt is a narrow strip of flat leather that is chain stitched to both the upper and the insole. The outsole then is lock stitched to the welt. Use of this technique yields a strong and structurally sturdy shoe. In order to provide a flat tread surface, the space between the insole and outsole is filled with

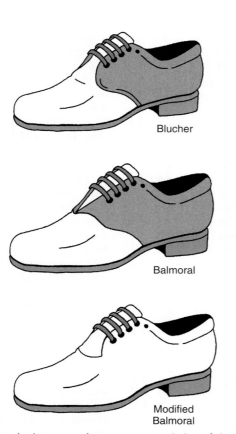

Fig. 24-2 Two basic types and one common variation of throat openings: the blucher, the balmoral, and the modified balmoral.

ground cork or some other lightweight material. Shoes constructed with a Goodyear welt tend be less flexible and not as lightweight as other types. The Goodyear welted shoe lends itself to the attachment of a metal bracing system better than any other type of shoe.

The *Littleway* and *McKay* are two different attachment techniques wherein the upper is fastened to the sole via staples and the outsole then is attached with either lock stitches (Littleway) or chain stitches (McKay).[17] This construction leads to the formation of a very flexible shoe, such as a moccasin or deck shoe.

In the *stitchdown* process, the upper is flanged outward and then stitched directly to the outsole. This is a simple construction technique and is quite cost effective. The stitchdown may or may not utilize a welt or midsole.

With the *cement* method, the upper is attached to the insole using a strong glue or cement. In a manner similar to that used in the Goodyear welt construction, the space between the insole and the outsole if filled with material. These types of shoes are lightweight and flexible. Many athletic shoes use this type of sole attachment.

Sliplasting is a technique whereby the upper is sewn to an insole made of a similar material. The outsole then is attached through a cementing process. Sliplasted shoes can be quite flexible and provide maximum shock absorption. Many athletic shoes, such as running shoes and court shoes, are constructed using sliplasting.

With *injection molding*, shoes are manufactured using a heat-sealing process. The outsole is made from a thermoplastic, which liquefies when heated. Using a special machine, the hot liquid plastic is injected into a form and heat sealed to the upper, rapidly hardening and forming an outsole. These types of shoes are fairly inexpensive to make, but they typically are not available in a wide range of sizes and widths and are not easy to modify or attach braces to. For injection-molded and unit bottom cemented soles, most manufacturers do not use a separate bottom for each last width. Typically, two or three different widths of uppers are used per unit bottom width.

Shoe construction materials

Dozens of base materials and literally hundreds of variations of those base materials are used in the manufacture of shoes. In this section, discussion is limited to general categories of materials found in shoes used in conjunction with orthoses and with or as assistive devices.

Upper materials

Upper materials are important because they affect the way the shoe fits, feels, and performs as well as the longevity of the shoe. Cowhide, or leather, is one of the most commonly used materials. Leather probably is the most durable upper material. It is easily stretched or modified.

Deerskin is significantly softer than leather. It stretches easier and is generally more accommodative but is not nearly as durable as leather. It scuffs easily and is hard to keep looking nice.

Some shoe uppers are formed with a lining that is heat moldable. These types of uppers can be molded to an individual foot. They are an especially useful alternative to custom shoes in patients with severe forefoot deformities who otherwise would not need custom shoes.

Shoe uppers are also frequently made of man-made materials such as fabric, nylon, canvas, and plastic. Uppers made of man-made materials sometimes are more durable than uppers made of leather or deerskin but generally are difficult to stretch or modify. A recent development in shoe upper technology is the use of elastic materials (e.g., neoprene) that will easily stretch around deformities.

Sole materials

Materials used in the construction of shoe soles vary greatly and have significantly different properties with regard to weight, durability, shock absorption and attenuation, flexibility, and support. The following is an examination of a handful of the most commonly used soling materials.

Leather at one time was the soling material of choice. Nowadays, it is reserved primarily for high-end men's and women's dress shoes. Leather soles are extremely durable. They tend to be stiff and heavy and offer little or no shock absorption. They can be slippery in wet conditions. Leather soles do allow for relatively simple attachment of AFOs.

Hard rubber is a great alternative to leather, especially when attaching an AFO, because it does not become slippery when wet. When used on welted shoe, a hard rubber outsole presents no real obstacle to attaching an AFO.

Crepe is a rubber compound that contains additives that give it a cellular structure. Crepe-soled shoes typically offer a great combination of shock absorption and traction. A shoe with a crepe sole still can have an AFO attached to it, although it is not as easy as with a leather- or rubber-soled shoe. Crepe outsoles are lightweight and lend themselves well to being modified. Crepe is the most commonly used material in after-market shoe modifications.

Vibram is a dense microcellular rubber. It has many of the good qualities of crepe but is more durable and can be even lighter and more shock absorbing than crepe. Vibram is used in work boots, hiking boots, walking shoes, and even stylish dress shoes.

Ethylene vinyl acetate (EVA) is used in the manufacture of almost every type of shoe today. This popular material is a blend of ethylene and acetate. It is shock absorbing, moldable, lightweight, and flexible. It is seen in the manufacture of foot beds, insoles, midsoles, and outsoles.

Shoe shape

The most important adage in shoe fitting is "Fit the shoe to the foot, not the foot to the shoe."[3,8,10,13,18] Both the shape of the sole and the shape of the upper must be considered. Some shoes have pointed toe boxes; others have rounded, or oblique, toe boxes. Some shoes are wide in the shank area whereas others are very narrow. Shoes that are considered to be *in-depth shoes* have extra room throughout the shoe, an extra deep toe box, and one or more removable foot beds. There are nearly as many variations of shoe shapes as there are foot shapes.

Lasts

The shape of a shoe is determined entirely by the last upon which it is made. Each differently shaped last produces a differently shaped shoe. The last is a solid, three-dimensional plastic or wooden model. If a shoe is made to be available in multiple true widths, then the manufacturer must use a different last for each size and width combination. The exorbitant cost of manufacturing the large number of lasts necessary to make shoes in multiple widths is a primary deterrent to many popular shoe companies producing shoes that are available in different widths. A last is measured at as many as 10 points, including the heel-to-toe measurement, heel-to-ball measurement, and circumferential measurements at the ball, waist, instep, and heel.[17] Each time one of these measurements increases, the other measurements increase proportionally to create larger lasts. Different style shoes made on different lasts, even shoes made by the same company, fit differently.[17]

Sizes and widths

As variable as last shape is from manufacturer to manufacturer, shoe sizing is just as confusing. There is little or no regulation of sizing in the footwear industry.[5,17] The most widely used scale in U.S. shoe manufacturing is the "common" scale, but what value the manufacturers choose as their baseline size is up to the individual manufacturer. To compound matters, the system itself makes little sense and could be considered archaic.

The shoe sizing system currently used by the majority of U.S. shoe manufacturers today is an evolution of a system developed in England in the mid-1300s AD by King Edward II. King Edward declared that three barleycorns, plucked from the center of the ear and laid end to end, would equal 1 inch. He decreed that 39 barleycorns would be equal to the size of the largest man's foot, or 13 inches, thereby a size 13. Going backward from size 13, each size would equal one barleycorn, or approximately ⅓ inch. A child's size 0 was equal to the width of a man's knuckles, or 13 barleycorns (Edward decided that when an infant's foot was equal to the width of a man's knuckles, the time was appropriate for the infant to begin wearing shoes). After going up 13 sizes (or barleycorns) the sizes start over. Therefore, a baby's foot (13 barleycorns) plus all 13 sizes of children's shoes (13 more barleycorns) plus 13 sizes of men's shoes (another 13 barleycorns) equals the length of 39 barleycorns, or a men's size 13.[7,17]

Until the Civil War, mass-produced shoes were not available in "lefts" and "rights"; they were straight lasted shoes that could be worn on either foot.[7] Twenty years later, Edwin Simpson of New York introduced a variation on the scale that, for the first time, included widths and half-sizes.[19]

In the American system, a women's shoe size is the same as a man's shoe size plus 1½. So in theory, a shoe that is a men's size 9 should be the same length as a women's size 10½.

Depending on the manufacturer, as the width of the shoe increases by one width (e.g., from an A to a B), the total interior girth (or the girth of the last) at the ball of the foot increases by ³⁄₁₆ to ¼ inch.

Many other sizing system are in use around the world. In most of Europe (except for the United Kingdom), shoes are sized according to the Continental, or Euro, scale. The Euro scale evolved from a French scale called *Paris points*. One Paris point equals ⅔ cm. The system begins at 0 cm and increases. There are no half sizes. The Euro scale is a unisex metric system whereby each shoe size is ⅔ cm, less than an American full size but more than an American half-size. To review, a US men's size 9 equals a US women's size 10½ equals a Euro size 43.[17]

Australia, Japan, Korea, Mexico, Russia, and the United Kingdom all use their own unique systems for sizing shoes.

Shoe selection

The three primary considerations for shoe selection are (1) shoe shape and fit; (2) purpose, duration, and level of activity for which the shoe will be used; and (3) ease with which the shoe can be modified. Secondary considerations are upper material selection based on patient's level of protective sensation; cost and insurance coverage or lack thereof; and lifestyle considerations such as fashion consciousness or workplace dress codes.

The first objective when choosing a shoe is proper fit. This can be a challenge if the patient is using foot orthoses or a molded AFO that is to be worn inside the shoe. These extra devices may consume a lot of space inside the shoe and must be considered. If a bulky device is being used unilaterally, the shoes may need to be mismated. Regardless, the shape of the shoe must be appropriate for the shape of the patient's foot. If no off-the-shelf shoe fits the patient's foot as is, the shoe may need to be modified to fit. If the shoe cannot be modified enough to fit, use of a custom shoe may be necessary.

Once shoes that do not match the foot shape have been ruled out, the next criterion to consider is the purpose or function the shoes will be asked to serve or perform. If the patient is fully ambulatory, then the shoe should be able to provide adequate support and control and have an outsole that will be durable. If the patient is essentially nonambulatory and footwear will be used only to protect the feet and aid in transferring, then a lightweight flexible shoe may be appropriate. If the patient will need to use some additional device, the shoe needs to have enough room to accommodate the device. This typically means a shoe with a deep toe box, high counter, blucher opening, and removable foot bed.

For athletic patients, activity-specific shoes are a necessity. One pair of sports shoes will not be appropriate for every activity. For example, running shoes are designed for forward motion. They have rocker soles and ample padding in the forefoot and hindfoot and often are designed to control excessive pronation. Therefore, running shoes are completely inappropriate for playing tennis, which requires lateral stability and a wide flat base of support. Similarly, it would be uncomfortable, if not outright detrimental, for a patient to attempt jogging in a basketball shoe that is flat on the bottom and lacks sufficient shock absorption under the heel and ball of the foot.

The modifiability of a shoe is an important consideration when discussing orthotic devices. With the constant development of new and better adhesives and techniques, there is nary a shoe that cannot be modified. It is merely a matter of the degree of difficulty with which a shoe can be modified and the practitioner's level of ambition. However, there are some shoes to which attachment of a metal AFO is not possible or is extremely difficult. If the prescription and/or the goal of the treatment plan will require shoe modifications, then the sole material and method of construction must be given serious contemplation, as well as the overall quality of the shoe. Shoes that are designated for attachment to braces must be durable; simply put, they must be worth the effort and cost of attaching the brace to them.

Off-the-shelf shoes

It is generally accepted that there are seven basic types of shoes; the rest are considered variations of these basic styles.[17] The seven basic shoe types are as follows: (1) *boot*—any footwear that extends proximal to the ankle; (2) *clog*—thick, wooden-soled, backless, slip-on shoe; (3) *oxford*—low-cut shoe fastened with laces; (4) *moccasin*—oldest form of shoe, low-vamp loafer, originally made entirely of one piece of leather; (5) *mule*—backless shoe or slipper with low or no heel; (6) *sandal*—shoe with an upper consisting of an arrangement of straps; and (7) *pump*—thin-soled, slip-on shoe with varying heel heights.

For orthotics and prosthetics, the two shoe types most frequently used are the boot and the oxford. Shoes that have emerged from the oxford family tree include today's modern walking, running, athletic and lace-up comfort, dress, and in-depth shoes.

In-depth shoes

In-depth shoes are the most prevalent shoes used in, with, or as assistive devices. In-depth shoes are designed with an extra ¼ to ⅜ inch of depth throughout the shoe compared to "regular"-depth counterparts.[11] Combined with the fact that in-depth shoes have removable foot beds, this type of shoe provides ample room to accommodate a molded AFO or custom foot orthosis. Traditionally, in-depth shoes have been a basic oxford style shoe, available in men's and women's styles and in multiple sizes and widths. They are made from a variety of materials, with leather being the most common. Three subcategories of in-depth shoes warrant discussion for orthotic use: athletic shoes, moldable shoes, and lace-to-toe shoes.

Athletic shoes

A large percentage of athletic shoes today are being manufactured with removable foot beds and therefore have enough extra internal volume to be considered in-depth shoes. Many patients, especially younger patients, find athletic shoes to be more socially acceptable than traditional in-depth shoes. In addition, athletic shoes usually have lightweight, shock-absorbing soles and strong, supportive counters. Most walking and running shoes are made with a significant rocker sole.

Moldable shoes

Some in-depth shoes are specially designed to be molded to an individual foot. They have uppers made of a soft leather, or deerskin, laminated to an internal lining of soft, heat-moldable polyethylene foam. The upper can be heated and stretched in localized areas. It will retain its shape, accommodating moderate to severe deformities, such as hallux valgus, hallux varus, hammer toes, claw toes, and rheumatoid nodules. Moldable shoes can be reheated and remolded as the need arises. Because of the softness of the inner foam lining and the fact that they are moldable, these shoes perform quite well for patients who have diminished sensation in their feet.

Lace-to-toes shoes

Shoes with a lace-to-toe, or surgical, opening have lace stays that extend all the way to the front of the shoes. This shoe has a blucher throat opening and is available as an oxford or a boot. The advantage to this type of shoe is that the shoe can be unlaced and completely opened from the top, and the patient can gently set the foot down into the shoe and close the shoe over the foot. It is especially useful for patients who lack flexibility because of trauma or fusions, have loss of motor control, or need to use a solid ankle, molded AFO. These shoes accommodate severe deformities better than traditional in-depth shoes. Many off-the-shelf in-depth shoes can be modified to become lace-to-toe shoes.

Indications

Use of off-the-shelf shoes is preferable to custom shoes whenever possible. Because off-the-shelf shoes are available in so many shapes, styles, sizes, and widths and can be modified by varying degrees, they can fit most foot shapes and accommodate most deformities. The shoes may need to be mismated, that is, one size on one foot and a different size on the other foot, but as long as the shoe fits the patient's foot and adequately accounts for the space consumed by the orthotic device, an off-the-shelf shoe is preferred. Cosmesis plays a large role in patient compliance; invariably, a patient will accept an off-the-shelf shoe or even an extensively modified off-the-shelf shoe before he or she will accept a custom-molded shoe. Also, off-the-shelf shoes, even when modified, are generally much more cost effective than custom shoes.

Custom shoes

Custom-made shoes are constructed using a cast or model of the patient's foot.[1] Custom shoes can be molded around the model or carefully handcrafted to look like regular shoes. As a rule, custom shoes are quite expensive and often have significant delay in delivery time because construction is labor intensive.

Indications

Custom shoes should be used only when all off-the-shelf options have been exhausted. They are necessary in rare cases where the deformities are so severe that no other type of shoe will work. For example, a muscle flap may be too bulky to be appropriately accommodated in an off-the-shelf shoe. Other cases where custom shoes may be used are patients with diabetic Charcot deformity, clubfoot deformity, or severely advanced Charcot-Marie-Tooth disease.

Custom shoes may be helpful in cases where the difference in foot size and width from left to right is so great that mismating of off-the-shelf shoes is not possible, as in patients with postpolio syndrome.

Custom shoes can be used to disguise extreme modifications that otherwise would be especially cosmetically unappealing. One example is a large leg-length discrepancy where the necessary buildup can be hidden inside the custom shoe as opposed to being added to the outsole on an off-the-shelf shoe.

Basic shoe fitting principles

Once the proper model of shoe has been selected based on foot shape and desired function, the next step is actually fitting the shoe, that is, finding the proper size. The shoe fitter is concerned with three measurements: (1) *overall foot length*, which ensures that the shoe is long enough, (2) *arch length* (heel to ball), which ensures that the widest part of the foot rests comfortably in the widest part of the shoe, and (3) *width*, which ensures that the shoe is wide or narrow enough to fit the foot correctly.[5] Both feet should be measured because they may be different.[3,16,18] Feet should be measured both non–weight bearing and weight bearing because the structural foot changes seen with weight bearing needed to be accounted for.

These measurements are obtained using a foot-measuring device; the most common are the Ritz stick and the Brannock device.[7,17,21] Remember that regardless of the device used, the resulting measurement is a measurement of foot size only, not necessarily shoe size. Shoe size, as discussed previously, depends entirely on the individual manufacturer. The foot size is merely the starting point. A competent shoe fitter is intimately familiar with how each different shoe style in his or her inventory fits and corresponds to the measurement derived from a particular measuring device. This knowledge and experience are imperative because they are the only guides available for properly fitting a three-dimensional shoe based on a two-dimensional measurement.[2] Although the American shoe sizing scale provides us with nearly 300 size–width combinations, there still are significant variables to navigate due to the differences in lasts and manufacturers.[17]

Guidelines for achieving proper fit[11,12,17]

1. Measure both feet. Feet should be measured each time a pair of shoes is purchased because feet tend to change significantly over the course of a lifetime.
2. Check the fit of *both* shoes while weight bearing.
3. Check that the ball of the foot is resting in the widest part of the shoe.

4. Check for correct toe length. When weight bearing, there should be approximately ⅜ to ½ inch between the end of the longest toe (not necessarily the great toe) and the end of the shoe. This allows adequate toe room and allows for a bit of necessary heel movement throughout gait.
5. Check for proper width. The upper material should not be stretched taut over the dorsum of the foot.
6. Check for a snug, but not tight, heel fit.
7. Check that proper fit over the instep has been achieved by an appropriately high vamp. The laces should have room for adjustment.
8. The patient should walk in the shoes before agreeing to purchase them or have them modified. The shoes must feel comfortable to the patient (provided the patient has adequate sensation to make this determination).

Shoe fit should be checked periodically, in much the same way as the fit, usage, and wear of an AFO or foot orthosis are monitored. Proper shoe fit can be the key to a successful outcome with use of a shoe–orthosis system. Improper shoe fit is often the culprit when the system fails or the patient refuses to wear the device as a result of discomfort.

Shoe modifications

A shoe can be modified in many different ways. The upper can be modified to aid in donning and doffing of shoes and devices. The soles can be modified to accommodate deformities, give additional support or control, and improve function and ease of ambulation.

Modifiability

The modifiability of a shoe is an important, and frequently overlooked, consideration in shoe selection. Given the vast and constantly growing array and availability of materials, adhesives, and pedorthic equipment, the shoe that cannot be modified is a rare find. Some shoe constructions lend themselves better to specific sole and upper modifications, so the key then is determining which shoe is best suited to which type of modification, all the while factoring in the practitioner's or technician's level of hand skills, competency, and proficiency. To achieve the best outcome, the shoe chosen should effectively and efficiently accommodate the desired modification while being as cosmetically pleasing to the patient as possible.

The practitioner should remember that a significant number of shoe manufacturers have responded to the needs and requests of orthotists, pedorthists, and their patients and now produce a wide variety of socially acceptable shoes designed to accommodate feet with deformities and special needs. Many shoes commercially available today have, from the factory, many of the features required by orthotic patients, such as a long shank, wide midfoot, rocker soles, flares, without the need for modification. In many cases, there is a shoe that does not require modification or that *once modified* may work well.

Many shoes, especially athletic shoes, are constructed without a true midsole. Shoes with a midsole are some of the simplest to modify because they offer a solid platform and stable, sturdy construction. Shoes with a midsole are simple to deconstruct and often have an EVA sole. EVA is easy to grind and accepts traditional adhesives with little or no preparation, a quality not shared by many of the materials used in injection molding.

Many running shoes and walking shoes come equipped from the factory with some degree of rocker sole, which sometimes can eliminate the need for modification. An increasing number of walking, running, work, and comfort shoes have special shock absorbing systems built into their soles, systems consisting of separate or connected air- or gel-filled bladders or even springs. Some running shoes and cross-trainers utilize medial and/or lateral plastic or graphite reinforcement bars and walls.

In the past, therapeutic or "orthopedic" shoes tended to be heavy because of their sturdy and supportive construction and their thick, stiff soles. To combat this issue of heavy weight, many soles today have hollow pockets or holes divided by a series of baffles. Some shoes also feature hidden depth. Hidden depth means that the foot bed actually is set down into the sole, giving the appearance of a lower toe box while maintaining the additional depth traditionally associated with therapeutic footwear. All of these features must be considered when a shoe must be modified.

Preparing a shoe for brace attachment

In the past, it was generally accepted that a metal AFO could be attached only to a shoe with a leather or hard rubber sole, a Goodyear welt, and a separate heel. By most standards, this still is the easiest type of shoe to which an AFO can be attached but by no means is the only type. An AFO can be attached to virtually any shoe that has a steel shank. If a shoe does not come from the factory with a steel shank, one can be added. Almost all types of athletic shoes, in-depth shoes, and even crepe-soled casual or dress shoes can be strengthened enough to handle the addition of an AFO.

The procedure for preparing a nontraditional shoe for brace attachment is fairly straightforward. The technician first carefully cuts off all but ⅟16 to ⅛ inch of the existing outsole. After determining exactly which type of AFO will be attached, the proper steel shank is added. Speaking in general terms, a regular shank is used with a free ankle motion AFO, and an extended shank is used with a fixed ankle joint. The shank will need to be extended and reinforced if the AFO system uses a dorsiflexion stop. Next, a thin midsole (⅛–³⁄16 inch) is cemented to the entire bottom of the shoe. Great care must be taken to maintain the original shoe shape once the outsole has been removed so that the original outsole can be replaced after the AFO has been secured to the shoe.[12]

Patients are more inclined to accept a metal bracing system if the shoe is cosmetically appealing.

Rocker soles

The rocker sole is one of the most commonly prescribed shoe modifications.[6] As the name suggests, the basic function of a rocker sole is to rock the foot from heel strike to toe-off without requiring the shoe to bend. The rocker sole can be used to enhance and ease forward propulsion. It also can be used to offload areas of high plantar pressure, reduce bending forces, and replace or restore lost motion due to injury or deformity. The actual shape of the rocker sole depends on the patient's specific foot problems and the desired biomechanical effect of the rocker sole.

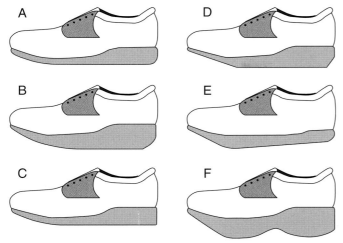

Fig. 24-4 Six major types of rocker soles.

Two terms relevant to the discussion of rocker soles are (1) *midstance*, the middle portion of the rocker sole that is in contact with the ground during stance phase; and (2) *apex*, the high point of the rocker sole, located at the distal end of the midstance. If the rocker sole is being asked to offload an area of plantar pressure, then the apex must be proximal to the pressure area.

In general, rocker soles are custom made for each patient; however, for the purpose of discussion they can be categorized as the following six basic types (Fig. 24-4).[11]

Mild rocker sole (A) The mild rocker sole is the most basic, popular, and widely used of all rocker soles. It is characterized by a mild rocker angle at both the heel and toe.

This type of rocker can effectively be used to reduce pressure under the metatarsal heads and can assist gait by easing and increasing forward propulsion. It can reduce enough motion at the first metatarsophalangeal joint, mitigating the pain associated with early hallux rigidus. The mild rocker can be used to replace some of the motion lost due to use of a rigid toe plate or extended steel shank. This type of rocker is a common feature of walking and running shoes.

Heel-to-toe rocker sole (B) A heel-to-toe rocker sole typically is thicker than a mild rocker sole and has a more severe rocker angle at both the heel and the toe. It is designed to significantly aid in propulsion at toe-off. It also decreases heel-strike forces on the calcaneus, talus, and tibia, and it reduces the need for ankle motion.

A heel-to-toe rocker sole is appropriate for a patient who has undergone an ankle or triple arthrodesis. It can replace motion lost due to use of a solid ankle AFO. This type of rocker sole is contraindicated for patients who are experiencing balance and/or proprioception issues because this rocker sole has the shortest midstance.

Toe-only rocker sole (C) The toe-only rocker sole has a significant rocker angle at the toe, with only a very mild rocker angle at the heel. The midstance on this shoe extends all the way to the posterior end of the sole. The main use for this rocker sole is to increase weight bearing proximal to the metatarsal heads. It provides a stable midstance and reduces the need for toe dorsiflexion on toe-off.

Indications for this type of sole include hallux rigidus and metatarsal head ulcers associated with diabetic neuropathy.[9] This rocker sole is suitable for patients with balance and/or proprioception problems.

Severe-angle rocker sole (D) This rocker sole, sometimes referred to as a *Carville rocker*, has a severe rocker angle at the toe and no heel rock. The purpose of the severe rocker sole is to eliminate weight-bearing forces on the forefoot. This type of rocker sole is contraindicated for patients that are experiencing balance and/or proprioception deficits.

Negative heel rocker sole (E) This rocker sole has a mild heel rocker angle and a significant toe rocker angle. What distinguishes this rocker sole is that the end result places the patient's heel at the same height as, or lower than, the ball of the foot in stance phase.

The purpose of a negative heel rocker sole is either to accommodate a foot fixed in such a position or to relieve forefoot pressure by shifting the weight-bearing forces to the hindfoot and midfoot. Because additional material usually is not needed in the fabrication of a negative heel rocker sole, it is a good modification for patients who feel unstable with the normal height of other rocker soles or in higher-heeled shoes. A word of caution regarding use of the negative heel rocker sole: inability to attain the necessary ankle dorsiflexion (i.e., tendo-Achilles contracture, severe ankle arthritis, ankle fusion, or AFO) will cause discomfort and imbalance and may actually increase pressure on the problem area(s).

Double rocker sole (F) This type of rocker sole is essentially a mild rocker sole from which the middle section of sole has been removed, thereby giving the appearance of two rocker soles: one at the forefoot and another under the hindfoot.

This rocker is indicated for use when the desire is to unload the midfoot area, as with a Charcot midfoot or a prominent base of fifth metatarsal head in a cavus foot. Whereas all other rocker soles tend to increase plantar pressure at the midfoot, the double rocker sole will not.[6]

Wedges and flares

A flare is an extension, either medially or laterally, of the sole that provides stabilization. The flare can be added at the heel only, or it can run the entire length of the shoe. A flare is not designed to correct deformity, only to control side-to-side motion.

Indications for a flare include a patient with a posttraumatic foot in whom the heel is fixed in varus and the patient who feels unstable. A lateral heel flare will act as an outrigger, give the foot a wider base of support, and decrease the patient's sensation that the ankle is "rolling" laterally.[20]

A wedge is used to help correct flexible deformities of the hindfoot and/or forefoot. A shoe with a medial wedge has more material under the medial border of the foot than the lateral border and vice versa. A medial heel wedge also can be used to ease the pain of posterior tibial tendonitis. A wedge is contraindicated for fixed deformities.

Elevations

Elevations can be used for a variety of reasons. They can be used to compensate for an acquired or congenital limb-length discrepancy. Elevations also can be used to offset the limb-length discrepancy created by an AFO, cast, or walker boot. When added to the contralateral shoe of a patient using a fixed ankle AFO, it can ease the swing phase of the affected foot.

Elevations can be applied either under the heel only or under the whole bottom of the foot. They can be applied internally or added to the outsole.

A heel-only elevation is appropriate for accommodating a fixed equinus position or alleviating strain on the Achilles tendon. A buildup less than ½ inch can be added inside the shoe. Any higher and the patient will have difficulty keeping the shoe from slipping off the heel. A buildup of ½ inch or more should be added externally.

A heel-only buildup greater than ½ inch is contraindicated for any other purposes than that discussed in the previous paragraph because of the gait problems it creates as well as the risk of promoting the development of a tendo-Achilles contracture.

A buildup that extends from heel to ball with a functional rocker angle at the toe is the more practical way to compensate for a limb-length discrepancy. Buildups can be added to virtually any shoe. Careful attention should be paid so that as the height of the elevation increases, so does the width of the base of shoe in order to provide mediolateral stability.[14]

Relast

Relasting a shoe is one way to avoid using custom shoes for patients with severe deformities, such as a fixed flatfoot deformity or Charcot midfoot. The modification involves removing the outsole and widening the shank area of the shoe. This usually is achieved by cutting through the midsole and insole, opening the shank area wide enough to accommodate the patient's foot, and filling in the space with a semi-rigid material (Bock foam, rigid crepe, or viscoelastic polymer).

It is important to remember that the most a shoe can be widened is ¾ to 1 inch, and that as the width of the midfoot increases, the depth of the shoe decreases proportionally and may affect the length as well.

Extended rigid shanks

An extended rigid shank is traditionally a strip of spring steel that is placed between layers of outsole, extending from the heel to the medial toe of the shoe. Although steel still is the most commonly used material, shanks available today are made from carbon fiber of varying rigidities. An extended rigid shank is most commonly used in conjunction with a rocker sole, sometimes making the rocker sole more effective. An extended rigid shank eliminates or reduces bending stresses in the midfoot and forefoot. It can aid propulsion at toe-off and add to the overall strength, structure, and stability of the shoe.

The extended rigid shank is indicated for hallux rigidus, metatarsalgia (with a rocker sole), Charcot midfoot (reduce bending forces on midfoot), and limited ankle motion.

Cushion heel

A cushion heel is a wedge of shock-absorbing material that is added between the heel and the sole of a shoe. The purpose of a cushion heel is to provide the maximum amount of shock absorption and attenuation on heel strike while maintaining a stable stance phase.

A cushion heel is indicated for patients after ankle fusions or following a calcaneal fracture. It also is indicated for patients with persistent shin splints.

Fiberglass counters

Another type of stabilization technique consists of reinforcing the counter of the shoe with fiberglass. The inside of the counter is lined with fiberglass and then covered with moleskin or another thin, soft material. This type of stabilization is not visible when the shoe is worn, so cosmetic acceptance of this modification is high. The shoe should be slightly broken in before this modification is performed.

Indications for fiberglass counters include flexible posterior tibial tendon dysfunction, varus or valgus heels, and pes cavus feet.

Upper modifications

The upper of the shoe can be modified in several ways. A blucher opening can be extended to the end of the shoe, turning a regular oxford shoe into a lace-to-toe shoe. Lace-up shoes can be converted to hook-and-loop closures, and vice versa. Sometimes the posterior collar of a shoe is extended proximally so that the collar better grips the heel. For prominent hammer toes or bunions, the leather over the painful prominence may be cut out and replaced with soft deerskin of the same color. Finally, leather or deerskin shoes can always be stretched to fit the foot better.

Conclusion

The use of appropriate, properly fitting shoes is absolutely essential to the success of any foot orthosis or AFO. Factors to consider when selecting a shoe are shape, fit, and function. The construction of the shoe is important when considering the function and the modifiability of a shoe. Many off-the-shelf shoes are available and most can be modified, thereby limiting the need for custom shoes and increasing the patient's perception of social acceptability, which ultimately may lead to better compliance.

References

1. Davis A. Custom shoe therapy. In Janisse DJ, editor: *Introduction to pedorthics*, Columbia, Md, 1998, PFA.
2. Decker W, Albert S: *Contemporary pedorthics*, Seattle, Wash, 2002, Elton-Wolf.
3. Foltz-Gray D: Get square with your feet, *Arthritis Today* 15:58–60, 2001.
4. Frey C, Thompson F, Smith J, Sanders M, Horstman H: American Orthopedic Foot and Ankle Society women's shoe survey, *Foot Ankle* 14:78–81, 1993.
5. Janisse DJ: The art and science of fitting shoes, *Foot Ankle* 13:257–262, 1992.
6. Janisse D, Brown D, Wertsch J, Harris G: Effects of rocker soles on plantar pressures and lower extremity biomechanics, *Arch Phys Med Rehabil* 85:81–86, 2004.
7. Janisse DJ, Wertsch J, Del Toro D: Foot orthoses and prescription footwear. In Redford J, Basmajian J, Trautman P, editors: *Orthotics: clinical practice and rehabilitation technology*, Kansas City, 1995, Churchill Livingstone.
8. Janisse DJ: Picking the shoe to fit the occasion. In Hantula R, editor: *The best of diabetes self management*, New York, 2002, DSM Books.
9. Janisse DJ: Pedorthic care of the diabetic foot. In Janisse DJ, editor: *Introduction to pedorthics*, Columbia, Md, 1998, PFA.
10. Janisse DJ: Prescription insoles and footwear, *Foot Ankle* 12:41–61, 1995.
11. Janisse DJ: Proper shoe fit: appendices A and B. In Janisse DJ, editor: *Introduction to pedorthics*, Columbia, Md, 1998, PFA.

12. Janisse D: The shoe in rehabilitation of the foot and ankle; pedorthics in the rehabilitation of the foot and ankle. In Sammarco GJ, editor: *Rehabilitation of the foot and ankle*, St. Louis, 1995, Mosby-Year Book.

13. Johnson JE: Prescription footwear. In Sammarco GJ, Cooper PS, editors: *Foot and Ankle Manual*, ed 2, Baltimore, 1998, Williams & Wilkins.

14. Marzano R: Fabricating shoe modifications and foot orthoses. In Janisse DJ, editor: *Introduction to pedorthics*, Columbia, Md, 1998, PFA.

15. Michaud TC: *Foot orthoses and other forms of conservative foot care*, Newton, Mass, 1997, Thomas C Michaud.

16. Rossi WA: The high incidence of mismated feet in the population, *Foot Ankle* 4:105–112, 1983.

17. Rossi WA, Tennant R: *Professional shoe fitting*, New York, 1984, National Shoe Retailers Association.

18. Tremaine DM, Awad EM: *The foot and ankle sourcebook*, ed 2, Los Angeles, 1998, Lowell House.

19. *When the shoe fits course textbook*, New York, 1996, National Shoe Retailers Association.

20. Wu K: *Foot orthoses: principles and clinical applications*, Baltimore, 1990, Williams & Wilkins.

21. Zamosky I, Redford JB: Shoes and their modifications. In Redford JB, editor: *Orthotics etcetera*, ed 3, Baltimore, 1986, Williams & Wilkins.

Chapter

25

Foot orthoses

Miguel Mojica

Key Points

- Shoe wear is a central component of the general function of the foot orthosis.
- Complete evaluation of all aspects of foot function will improve overall outcomes.
- Selection of the appropriate impression-taking technique plays an essential role in the fit of the custom foot orthosis.
- Selection of materials for the foot orthosis involves an understanding of material characteristics, desired shoe wear, and established orthotic objectives.
- Established biomechanical needs dictate the components and shape of the foot orthosis.

Foot orthoses are devices that are confined to the foot only and do not encompass the ankle. This form of support primarily covers the plantar surface and benefits the foot only upon weight bearing. The foot must be positioned and held on the orthosis for the device to be effective in achieving its goals. For this reason the foot orthosis is most commonly placed inside a closed shoe, and the structure of the shoe becomes an integral part of the orthosis. When the primary objective of the orthosis cannot be achieved within the confines of the shoe, many times the design is extended to encompass the ankle and is classified as an ankle–foot orthosis.

The benefit of a foot orthosis is subject to much discussion and controversy.[7] Instrumentation has been used to conduct studies measuring its direct effects on the foot. Quantifying its indirect effects on proximal joints has proven to be difficult, so little sound research is available. As technology improves, research likely will show the functional benefits of foot orthoses providing the necessary documentation for

insurance coverage. In the United States, the Medicare health care system presently funds foot orthoses only when they are used for treatment of patients with diabetes. Even without clear documentation on the effectiveness of foot orthoses, these devices are commonly prescribed for treatment of various foot/ankle pathologies, and many individuals profess their benefits.

This chapter reviews evaluation, impression-taking techniques, orthotic designs, materials, components, and applications of foot orthoses.

Evaluation

As with all orthotic treatment, success begins with a complete evaluation of the patient's condition. In designing the foot orthosis, important physical findings must be collected to maximize the benefits of the orthosis. Some important aspects include examination of skin condition, foot shape, range of motion (ROM), muscle strength, dynamic performance, and shoe wear patterns. The following sections review each of these aspects in more detail.

Skin condition provides some insight into the cause of the problem and assists with orthotic design selection. Callus formation is a result of repetitive pressure. The location of the callus on the plantar surface pinpoints areas of high stress when weight bearing. This information is used when designing the orthosis to dissipate the stress in these areas. Callus forms not only on the plantar surface but on any stressed area. The lack of width and depth of the shoe's toe box may result in excessive pressure over the dorsum of the foot. In some cases, callus formation is the source of discomfort and patient education will be important in controlling callus buildup. Dry cracking skin may be the result of a systemic condition. Delicate fragile skin will require softer materials in

335

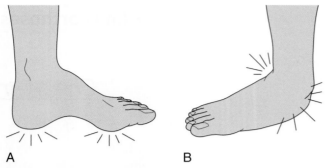

A   B

Fig. 25-1 A, Cavus foot tends to be less flexible, resulting in added pressure under the heel and the metatarsal heads. **B,** Planus foot tends to be too flexible, resulting in poor joint alignment with added pressure of the anatomical medial arch support structures and possible lateral malleolus impingement.

the construction of the orthosis. Corrective forces applied by the orthosis must be limited to protect skin integrity. Sensation is an important factor in protecting the overall integrity of the foot, and any deficit in its normal function must be noted. Diminished or complete absence of sensation will require a more accommodative and protective approach by using an orthosis made of softer materials. Careful examination of the skin is essential in preventing complications and providing optimum orthotic treatment.

Shape of the foot (cavus or planus) is a good predictor of potential problems that commonly present (Fig. 25-1).[3] Cavus feet usually are less flexible, resulting in decreased shock-absorbing capabilities. This deficit in the mechanics of the foot results in excessive pressure on the ball of the foot and the heel. Severe cavus deformities also result in pressure on the base and the head of the fifth metatarsal. At initial contact and loading response, the cushioning effect that occurs through pronation when the talonavicular joint and the calcaneocuboid joint axis are congruent is lost. The foot remains stiff throughout stance phase, with normal performance through the latter part of stance when a rigid toe lever is necessary for normal push-off.[10] In contrast, the planus foot usually is flexible and presents with problems related more to poor alignment of the joints of the foot and ankle. With the foot in the pronated position the calcaneus remains everted, the talus is plantarflexed, and the forefoot is abducted.[8] Stress is placed on the supporting structures of the medial arch, and severe pronation may result in stress being placed on the lateral malleolus. Through the stance phase the foot acts relatively normal during initial contact and loading response as the foot absorbs the shock, but additional effort is necessary to achieve the rigid toe lever necessary for the latter part of stance phase. Although there is a potential for the mentioned deformities to develop, many individuals are asymptomatic and never require professional treatment. The general shape of the foot has an effect on how the foot responds to different supportive approaches.

To completely assess foot function, ROM in the foot and the ankle must be determined. The hindfoot, midfoot, and forefoot are assessed in both the open and closed chain environment to determine if any limitations or excesses are present. Emphasis is placed on the closed chain, when the role of the foot is most important. Normal subtalar joint ROM permits the foot to operate naturally moving from pronation at the beginning of stance to supination during the

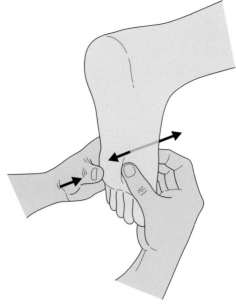

Fig. 25-2 While ensuring that the subtalar joint is in neutral alignment, one method for evaluating foot function is to dorsiflex the fifth ray to lock the midfoot joint and assess alignment of the calcaneus and mobility of the first ray.

latter part of stance phase.[10] If limitations exist, the foot will not perform normally throughout the stance phase. Several techniques are available to determine subtalar neutral. Whatever the method used, the clinician should develop consistency in finding this position. With the foot held in a subtalar neutral position,[15] the fifth metatarsal is dorsiflexed to lock the midfoot joint (Fig. 25-2). In this position, note the alignment of the calcaneus to the long axis of the tibia, documenting any significant abnormalities. Also note the flexibility and position of the first ray. Some research findings point to the importance of first ray stability.[12] If the foot is viewed as a three-legged stool, a flexible first ray represents an instability in the stool (Fig. 25-3). Following this same concept, the foot will have a greater tendency to pronate and/or more stress will be placed on the second metatarsal to stabilize the foot. If the first ray is stable, its alignment with all the metatarsals should be noted to determine if some

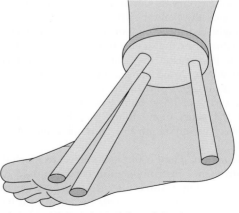

Fig. 25-3 When considering the stability of the foot, a common comparison is a three-legged stool, stressing the importance of first ray stability.

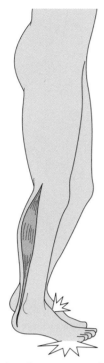

Fig. 25-4 A limitation in dorsiflexion range of motion will add pressure under the metatarsal heads and increase bending stress to the midfoot joint as early as midstance.

compensation is required to distribute the weight evenly across the heads. True ankle ROM must be determined to ensure that the foot can perform normally during gait (see Chapter 23 for a review of ROM examination and anatomy). In normal gait the ankle dorsiflexes 5 to 10 degrees. Significant limitations to this range will change the normal biomechanics of the foot, resulting in some compensatory changes (Fig. 25-4). Under these circumstances more pressure is placed on the metatarsal heads during the late part of midstance, with additional stress placed on the midfoot. Inspection of the metatarsophalangeal (MTP), proximal interphalangeal (PIP), and distal interphalangeal (DIP) joint ROM of the toes will reveal existing complications as well as the development of hammer toe or claw toe deformities.

Manual muscle testing of the major muscle groups surrounding the foot and ankle provides important information regarding weaknesses that may be the source of foot complications. The ankle dorsiflexors work as an antagonist to the plantarflexors, assist with toe clearance through swing, ensure heel contact at the beginning of stance phase, and prevent foot slap at loading response.[10] Weakness of this group usually requires an ankle–foot orthosis to compensate for the lost function. Roles of the plantarflexor muscle group include antagonist to the dorsiflexors, weight acceptance during midstance, and stability of the toe lever during terminal stance.[14,16] Absence of this muscle group warrants use of an ankle–foot orthosis with a solid ankle or dorsiflexion stop. Inversion and eversion strength play an important role in hindfoot and midfoot function. Weakness in the function of the inverters and everters will result in mediolateral instability. One significant role of these groups is to ensure good alignment and stability in preparation for initial contact and loading response. To resist excessive varus or valgus

tendencies during loading response, heel wedges and posts can be added to the foot orthosis.[5,9,13] Attention should focus on the function of the posterior tibialis given its importance in medial longitudinal arch stability and plantarflexion.[2] During the muscle testing process, discomfort could be a sign of injury to the muscle, attachment points, or tendons. Muscle imbalances at the MP, PIP, and DIP joints result in the development of toe deformities and should be noted. To ensure successful orthotic treatment, manual muscle testing of the foot and ankle should be performed to determine the most appropriate orthosis to be prescribed.

The most important role of the foot is weight bearing during ambulation. Therefore, the evaluation should include observation of foot function during weight bearing and walking. Some important observations related to foot function include the amount of time spent on each extremity, ankle motion, calcaneal motion, pronation and supination, and tibial internal and external rotation. Findings should be compared to normal gait[10] and any abnormalities documented. Identifying the phase of gait at which the pain or problem is present allows the clinician to isolate the problem and to examine any deficits present during that stage.

Wear patterns on the shoe provide important information related to foot performance while walking. Abnormal sole wear should be noted as well as any significant displacement of the upper hindfoot or forefoot on the sole. If the shoes are rubber soled, the location of any visible height reduction due to compressive forces must be documented. Examination of the integrity of the medial and lateral walls of the shoe assists in identifying a tendency for excessive pronation or supination through the gait process. A comparison between the amount of time the shoe has been worn and the condition of the shoe helps to determine the amount of wear that the foot orthotic will undergo.

Impression-taking techniques

Flexibility of the foot helps determine two important aspects of treatment: the primary orthotic treatment approach and the method that will be used for impression taking. If the foot is flexible, the option for the corrective approach to treatment is viable. Other aspects to be considered when taking the corrective approach include sensation of the foot and the potential effect on the surrounding joints. The amount of flexibility and the ease of holding the foot in the desired position will determine the impression-taking process. The slipper cast technique provides the clinician with the most control of the foot and its joints during the procedure (Fig. 25-5).[17] This process entails placing the patient in a prone position with the involved limb flexed at the knee or with the foot hanging off the end of the plinth. This position provides the clinician with the most optimum view for correctly aligning the forefoot and hindfoot. A plaster splint is used to cover the plantar surface, with access to palpate and keep the subtalar joint in a neutral position while the fifth metatarsal is dorsiflexed, locking the midfoot joint. Positioning the patient in the prone position is the only drawback to using this technique. Some individuals will not be able to place themselves in this position. A circumferential wrap with a cutting strip can be used with the patient in a sitting position (Fig. 25-6). With this technique subtalar neutral alignment relies more on visual inspection because of coverage over the dorsum of the foot

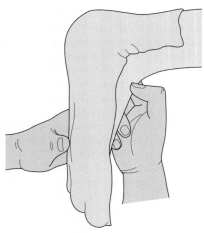

Fig. 25-5 One method of impression taking is the slipper cast technique. This method allows easy access for palpating the talonavicular joint and easy manipulation of forefoot alignment.

that impedes palpation of the talonavicular joint. A foam impression block can be used to take an impression of the flexible foot (Fig. 25-7).[17] The impression usually is taken with the patient in a sitting position, knee flexed, and the foot placed on a flat surface. The negative impression is taken by pushing the foot into a foam block. The difficulty with this procedure involves the ability to press the foot in the foam deep enough, achieve the desired forefoot alignment, and end with the subtalar joint in neutral. Palpation of the talonavicular joint is possible throughout the process, which is one advantage to this procedure. Eliciting help from the patient may risk distortion or poor alignment of the impression and should be avoided. This technique of impression taking is optimum when the deformity is mild or the deformity is rigid. A learning curve should be expected prior to successful utilization of this method of impression taking. When the deformity of the foot is rigid, a corrective approach cannot be taken. In this case the orthotic objective is to accommodate the deformity, which requires accurate identification of how the weight is borne on the foot. The easiest method for achieving this objective is to ask the patient to step into the foam impression block. Taking a good impression for

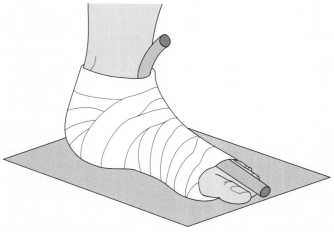

Fig. 25-6 A circumferential wrap can be used to take an impression of the foot. Subtalar joint alignment relies more on visual inspection with limited access for palpating the talonavicular joint.

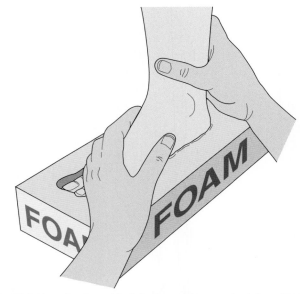

Fig. 25-7 Use of a foam block is the quickest method for taking an impression of the foot. Although it is the quickest method, a learning curve is required to consistently achieve a good impression of the hypermobile foot.

fabrication of a custom orthosis is one of the most important components of treatment. Care should be taken to evaluate the flexibility of the foot, which will help select the best method of impression.

Design

An attempt to organize and classify foot orthoses can be difficult. Foot orthoses are prescribed for many purposes, and any combination of materials can be used to construct orthoses. Classification methods that are consistently used involve categorizing the devices according to their primary purpose. A second method involves categorizing the devices according to the materials used and the rigidity of the final products. With the first method, foot orthoses are categorized as corrective, supportive, or accommodative. This method can cause some confusion because the orthoses are categorized according to the intent of the treatment and not primarily by the materials used. Therefore, a single material can fall into different categories depending on the purpose of the orthosis. With the second method, foot orthoses are categorized as rigid, semirigid, or soft. The problem with this method is the lack of a clear and reliable measurement guide for when an orthosis moves from one category to another. For example, how much flexibility is required before a rigid orthosis is moved into the semirigid category? In an attempt to prevent some of this confusion, this section reviews the basic shapes of orthoses, and the following section reviews the materials and how they can be applied to accomplish different therapeutic goals.

When designing a foot orthosis, size and shape will provide some benefits and limitations. If the orthosis is designed full length, all three components of the foot are encompassed and can have an affect on the hindfoot, midfoot, and forefoot (Fig. 25-8). The toe box of the shoe should have sufficient depth to accommodate the thickness of the orthosis. The full length ensures that the orthosis stays in place. Interchanging between

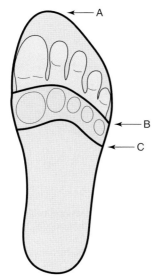

Fig. 25-8 Many lengths and configurations of trim lines are used to accomplish different objectives with foot orthoses. The most common designs have the distal edge end of the foot orthosis full length *(A)*, at the sulcus of the toes *(B)*, or just proximal to the metatarsal heads *(C)*.

shoes is limited to basically the same shoe design to prevent sizing complications when moving the orthosis from shoe to shoe. Extending the distal edge of the orthosis to the sulcus of the toes still allows for some control of the three components of the foot. However, the transition of the orthosis to the shoe insole under the toes now becomes an issue. Toe box depth is still a concern, but the orthosis can be moved more easily to a variety of shoes without experiencing fitting problems. Finally, the distal edge of the orthosis can extend just proximal to the metatarsal heads. This design limits direct effects on the midfoot and the hindfoot. Indirectly some of the weight can be shifted proximally to the metatarsal heads, thereby relieving some pressure. Forefoot posting under the lateral or medial pillar cannot be accomplished unless an extension is added. This design allows more room in the toe box, and the orthosis can be used with a wide variety of shoes. The length of the orthosis allows the device to migrate in the shoe and may present difficulty with consistent placement. Both shoe design and orthotic objectives play significant roles in determining the length of the orthosis.

Materials

Before decisions regarding the type and amount of materials to be used for fabrication are made (Fig. 25-9), an appropriate top layer or interface must be selected. Second, if cushioning is an objective, a material must be added to provide this function. Finally, the degree of support necessary will determine which material will provide structure to the orthosis. Although room in the shoe determines the amount of

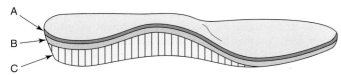

Fig. 25-9 Top layer *(A)*, shock-absorbing component *(B)*, and supportive component *(C)*.

materials, three layers should be considered the limit. The following section provides some information about the decision process and some of the characteristics of the more commonly used materials.

The top layer comes in direct contact with the foot or linings such as socks or nylons. Materials with a low coefficient of friction will help decrease sheer stress. Leather with a finish is thin and malleable but will require occasional replacement because of wear; it also absorbs moisture. Synthetic material such as vinyl is more resilient with a low coefficient of friction, but vinyl will crack over time and will need replacement. Nylon also provides a good finish but usually is adhered to a base material that will add some thickness to the orthosis. Nylon can detach from the base layer over time and will need replacement. Foams can be used as a top layer to provide cushioning and are relatively resilient. A closed-cell foam should be used to prevent the absorption of perspiration. Foam materials produce more friction but will provide a soft pliable surface. These materials are thicker and require more space in the shoe. When selecting materials for the top layer, consideration of durability and the effect of shear stresses on the plantar surface are key to providing a comfortable and effective orthosis.

When the objective of the orthosis is to provide cushioning, a foam material should be used in the construction of the orthosis. Thermoformable foam materials come in many densities and rigidities, thereby providing an array of options. Each has its advantages and disadvantages. Many substances and fabrication processes are used to produce thermoformable sheet foam that can be used in any combination when constructing the orthosis. These materials can be considered in two extreme groups: rigid and soft.

Some of the more rigid materials made of rubber, foam plastic, and cork are commonly used as a base material to provide structural stability to the orthosis. Two methods that provide more support are increasing the density of the material and increasing the thickness of the material. Rigid materials are ideal when a combination of support and shock absorption is needed. For example, if the orthosis will be used in repetitive impact activities such as sports, rigid material will provide support to the structures of the foot and shock absorption as well. If grinding equipment is available, rigid material is easy to modify by removing and adding as needed to customize the fit and function of the orthosis. Using rigid material has some drawbacks. The orthosis will be relatively thick and have limited durability. More space is needed to comfortably accommodate the orthosis and the foot. However, some casual and athletic shoes with ¼-inch removable insoles provide ample room for use of this orthosis design. Depending on the density and thickness, the material will compress and lose its contour after long-term use. With this in mind, follow-up care should be scheduled to ensure that the structural integrity of the orthosis is not lost.

Softer thermoformable foams are incorporated into the design of the orthosis when comfort and protection of the skin are the primary objectives. Some common materials in this group are Plastazote, Pelite, and Ali-plast. These materials are available in different densities and thicknesses that allow customization of the amount of cushioning in the orthosis. The thermoformable qualities of the material produce a moldable effect that responds to pressure. Depending on the material's density, an imprint of the foot can be seen on the material after use. One advantage of this effect is that pressure is dissipated over wider surfaces, reducing the possibility of skin breakdown. A second advantage is that this effect provides detail on how the weight is borne on the feet, so necessary adjustments can be made to dissipate the high-impact areas. Softer thermoformable foams also provide a degree of shock absorption. The material can be used when managing insensate feet.[1] Some of the disadvantages of this material are the limited durability, lack of long-term rebound, and the link between its benefit and material thickness. The softer the material, the easier it will be to scar and tear. Care must be taken to not damage the material and shorten the life of the orthosis. Along the same concept, this material initially provides good cushioning and shock absorption, but time and repeated impact will compress the material and decrease its benefits. The thickness of the material adds height to the orthosis, and shoes with some overall depth are needed to accommodate the thickness. Periodic replacement of the complete orthosis or a layer of material may be necessary when the softer foams are used.

Materials that are not heat formable yet provide some cushioning and shock absorption provide a positive benefit to the foot orthosis.[11] Some of the more common materials in this group are Poron, PPT, and neoprene. The most important attribute of these materials is their ability to resist permanent deformation. The rebound capability is high, providing a long-term shock-absorbing benefit. This prevents the need to consistently replace the material if cushion against impact is one of the primary objectives of the orthotic treatment plan. This type of shock-absorbing material is commonly included as a component of the orthosis in a variety of combinations to ensure that the cushioning effect is not sacrificed with the fatigue of the surrounding materials.

All custom foot orthoses need some structural stability that will maintain the shape and intended support. Vacuum formable foams will fill this need to a point. Other materials that achieve this requirement are laminates and thermoplastics. Rigid materials of this type are used when maximum support is required, durability is an issue, or shoe wear sets a space limitation. Laminated materials will provide the thinnest and most supportive orthosis available. Rigid materials must be used when prevention of motion and bending stresses on the foot are the objective. For example, a hallux rigidus can be managed with a rigid extension that encompasses the first MTP joint. Another reason for incorporating laminated or thermoplastic materials in the orthosis is to increase durability for high activity, constant interchanging of shoe wear, or an individual's excessive weight. These materials last longer and prevent the need for frequent orthosis replacement. Finally, if the plan is to use the orthosis in dress shoes, the material can be made thin and still provide some stability. Because the material is strong the areas underneath the arch support do not need filling, which keeps the orthosis thin. A disadvantage to using laminated and thermoplastic materials is that some of the materials are not easily adjustable short of increasing the thickness in specific areas. Attempts to heat and mold the material will risk the durability of the orthosis due to fatigue or delamination. Another issue to consider in the overall treatment scheme is the lack of shock absorbance by rigid materials. Adding a component of padding will thicken the orthosis but may cause problems in tighter shoes. The more

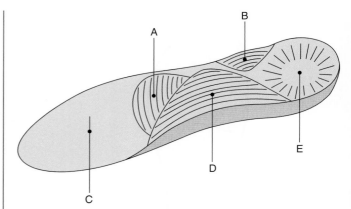

Fig. 25-10 Metatarsal pad *(A)*, lateral longitudinal arch support *(B)*, toe bed *(C)*, medial longitudinal arch support *(D)*, and heel bed *(E)*.

rigid materials provide benefits, but their drawbacks must be considered as well.

Components of the foot orthosis

The medial longitudinal arch support is one of the most important aspects of the foot orthosis (Fig. 25-10). The support lies under the medial aspect of the foot, extending from the calcaneus to a point just proximal to the head of the first metatarsal. The widest portion of the support extends just medial to the base of the fifth metatarsal. Its purpose is to prevent excessive pronation of the foot by providing external support to the medial longitudinal arch. Support of this arch decreases stress on all the supporting structures of the medial arch.

The metatarsal pad is a common addition to the foot orthosis. This support starts at a point close to the center of the plantar surface and extends just proximal to the metatarsal heads. The pad supports the transverse arch of the foot; the width usually extends from the first to the fifth metatarsal and narrows toward the proximal end of the support. This pad is primarily used to decrease the pressure from under the metatarsal heads by shifting the weight onto the shafts of the metatarsals. Another benefit is mild expansion of the space between the metatarsal heads. This pad is commonly prescribed to assist with managing metatarsalgia and neuromas that develop between the metatarsal heads.[4] Blending of this pad into the medial longitudinal arch support improves the comfort.

The lateral longitudinal arch support is not commonly discussed but is a part of the orthosis. This arch support is under the lateral portion of the foot, starting from the calcaneus and extending to a point just proximal to the head of the fifth metatarsal. This support is narrower than the medial and provides external support to the lateral longitudinal arch. The lateral arch of the foot is lower in height and is more rigid.[6] These characteristics make it less prone to problems. With external support of this arch, care must be taken to have a relief for the base of the fifth metatarsal. This arch support can be accentuated to assist with treatment of problematic cavus feet. Another benefit of this support is that it provides resistance to a varus tendency in the hindfoot.

The heel bed of the foot orthosis is an integral component. The shape of the bed can be designed as flat, concave, deep, or shallow. The deeper the bed, the more control the orthosis

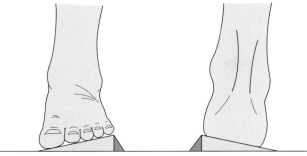

Fig. 25-11 Wedges can be incorporated into the foot orthosis to provide inversion and eversion corrective forces full length or to target the hindfoot or midfoot only.

will have on the calcaneus. If the bed is shaped with more of a concavity, pressure will be distributed more evenly under the heel.

Wedges and posts that span the entire length or cover only particular sections can be added to the bottom of the orthosis (Fig. 25-11). These additions are prescribed to compensate for rigid varus or valgus deformities of the hindfoot and forefoot or to provide some resistance to flexible varus or valgus tendencies in the forefoot and hindfoot.[8] In the case of severe pronation, if the medial arch support cannot be tolerated, a full-length medial wedge can be added to invert the entire foot and decrease the stretching of the medial support structures and compression of the lateral structures surrounding the ankle. When wedges and posts are used, care must be taken to ensure that medial/lateral stress is not applied to joints proximal to the ankle.[5,9,13]

Conclusion

Much has been written regarding foot orthoses. This chapter briefly reviewed some of the basic points of this orthotic intervention. In a majority of lower limb orthoses the foot will be encompassed and issues related to function and the required support will be addressed. An understanding of foot biomechanics and functional anatomy is an important foundation to treatment of the lower limb. When managing the foot, an organized approach to evaluation should be taken to focus the treatment and produce successful outcomes.

References

1. Brand PW: Management of sensory loss in the extremities. In Omar GE, Spinner M, editors: *Management of peripheral nerve problems*, Philadelphia, 1980, W. B. Saunders.
2. Coetzee JC, Castro MD: The indications and biomechanical rationale for various hindfoot procedures in the treatment of posterior tibialis tendon dysfunction, *Foot Ankle Clin* 8:453–459, 2003.
3. Esterman A, Pilotto L: Foot shape and its effect on functioning in Royal Australian Air force recruits. Part 1: prospective cohort study, *Military Med* 170:623–628, 2005.
4. Hayda R, Tremaine MD, Tremaine K, et al: Effect of metatarsal pads and their positioning: a quantitative assessment, *Foot Ankle Int* 15:561–566, 1994.
5. Johanson MA, Donatelli R, Wooden MJ, Andrew PD, et al: Effects of three different methods on controlling abnormal subtalar pronation, *Phys Ther* 74:149–158, 1994.
6. Kapandji IA: *The physiology of the joints: volume two, lower limb*, ed 5, New York, 1987, Churchill Livingstone.
7. Landorf KB, Keenan A: Efficacy of foot orthoses: what does the literature tell us? *J Am Podiatr Med Assoc* 90:149–158, 2000.
8. Michaud TC: *Foot orthoses and other forms of conservative foot care*, Baltimore, 1993, Williams & Wilkins.
9. Nester CJ, Van der Linden ML, Bowker P: Effect of foot orthoses on kinematics and kinetics of normal walking gait, *Gait Posture* 17:180–187, 2003.
10. Perry J: *Gait analysis, normal and pathological function*, Thorofare, NJ, 1992, Slack.
11. Pratt DJ: Medium term comparison of shock attenuating insoles using a spectral analysis technique, *J Biomed Eng* 10:426–428, 1988.
12. Roukis TS, Landsman AS: Hypermobility of the first ray: a critical review of the literature, *J Foot Ankle Surg* 42:377–390, 2003.
13. Sasaki T, Yasuda K: Clinical evaluation of the treatment of osteoarthritic knees using a newly designed wedged insole, *Clin Orthop Relat Res* 221:181–187, 1987.
14. Simon SR, Simon SR, Mann RA, Hagy JL, Larsen LJ: Role of the posterior calf muscles in normal gait, *J Bone Joint Surg Am* 60:465–472, 1978.
15. Sobel E, Levits SJ: Reappraisal of the negative impression cast and subtalar joint position, *J Am Podiatr Med Assoc* 87:32–33, 2000.
16. Sutherland DH: An electromyographic study of the plantar flexors of the ankle in normal walking on the level, *J Bone Joint Surg Am* 48:66, 1966.
17. Wu KK: *Foot orthoses: principles and clinical applications*, Baltimore, 1990, Williams & Wilkins.

Chapter

26

Lower limb orthoses

John W. Michael

Key Points

- Lower limb orthoses are among the most commonly prescribed biomechanical devices intended to assist individuals with neuromuscular deficits.

- Orthoses can be rationally and succinctly prescribed by specifying the functional outcome desired in biomechanical terms.

- Ankle–foot orthoses can be designed with sufficient mechanical lever arms to effectively control the ankle complex and to influence the knee joint indirectly.

- The recent development of stance control knee joints has eliminated several drawbacks associated with knee–ankle–foot orthoses that lock the knee throughout gait.

- Limited scientific evidence regarding the use of lower limb orthoses is available.

Lower limb orthoses, with their many variations, are among the most commonly prescribed biomechanical devices intended to assist individuals with neuromuscular deficits.[15] The preponderance of lower limb devices in clinical use reflects both the strong desire by most individuals with a physical disability to achieve independent mobility in the community and the fact that present orthotic technology often does a reasonably effective job of restoring gross physical functions such as walking and standing. For athletes, subtle interventions with foot orthoses sometimes overcome small physiologic deficits that otherwise might impede performance. Therefore, lower limb orthoses are applicable to enhance function for many biomechanical deficits, both large and small.

Custom footwear and modifications to commercial footwear are extremely important aspects of orthotic and pedorthic practice. Not only can shoe adaptations successfully treat many simpler problems, but they also can significantly enhance the effectiveness of orthotic management when more proximal devices are required.[9] The shoe and its functions are discussed in more detail in Chapter 24.

Foot orthoses

Foot orthoses (FOs) are the foundation for lower limb management. Not only are they suitable for treating many of the basic problems encountered in daily practice, but each and every more proximal orthosis (e.g., ankle–foot orthosis [AFO], knee–ankle–foot orthosis [KAFO], hip–knee–ankle–foot orthosis [HKAFO]) is first and foremost an FO. In general, the FO portion should be used to manage as many deficits as possible, relying on more proximal designs *only* when an FO alone is insufficient. This approach is the most cost effective and enhances patient acceptance because most FOs are "invisibly" contained within the footwear.

Conceptually FOs usually are divided into three broad categories[33]:

1. Accommodative or soft devices
2. Intermediate or semirigid devices
3. Corrective or rigid devices

Accommodative FOs typically are used to "cradle" and protect rigidly deformed, insensate, or dysvascular feet. They can be made from a variety of soft or flexible materials. Minor complaints, such as mild metatarsal pain, may respond to over-the-counter (OTC) or prefabricated inserts of resilient materials. Significant problems most often are managed with custom-molded FOs.

Intermediate FOs made of semirigid materials are popular clinically because they can be fabricated from multiple layers of materials of slightly different densities to provide graduated degrees of control, thereby enhancing client acceptance. OTC, prefabricated, or modular intermediate FOs may suffice for mild problems such as metatarsalgia without ulceration. These somewhat generic devices also may be suitable for a clinical trial to verify the effectiveness of orthotic management in a given case. Chronic conditions as well as moderate and severe problems, including all feet with a history of ulceration or sensory limitation, typically require custommolded devices to ensure the most meticulous fit.

Corrective FOs made of rigid materials can be extremely difficult to fit successfully and require meticulous attention to detail.[2] A weaning period of several weeks is commonly recommended for client acceptance. Most orthotists and pedorthists reserve the use of rigid materials for easily correctable, flexible deformities such as mild ankle valgus, and for subtle control of a nearly normal foot with slight biomechanical deficits, such as slight excess pronation in a distance runner.

Remember that the foot is a dynamically changing organ during the gait cycle, whereas the FO is a relatively static device. A thorough understanding of foot and ankle biomechanics, in addition to careful follow-up and adjustments, is essential for long-term success with this modality. Few hypotheses regarding the use of FOs have been investigated in controlled studies, so much of the variance encountered is based on clinical experience and judgment.

Ankle–foot orthoses

Ankle–foot orthoses (AFOs) can be designed with sufficient mechanical lever arms to effectively control the ankle complex and to influence the knee joint indirectly, making them applicable for the management of more extensive disabilities than can be managed with FOs. Successful use of electronic AFOs based upon electrical stimulation of weak or paralyzed muscles has been reported with increasing frequency in recent decades.[13] In the United States, commercial versions of orthoses that incorporate neuromuscular electrical stimulation (NMES) recently have become clinically available.[31]

When a mechanical AFO is desired, the clinician must choose from among metal alloy devices, plastic devices, and a hybrid assembly incorporating both materials. In most cases, such technical decisions are best left to the orthotist and patient, who can take the time to fully discuss the various advantages and disadvantages of each approach. In general, plastic or hybrid plastic/metal systems predominate in North America because of the greater degree of client acceptance and circumferential control they offer.[18] Carbon fiber composite AFOs that are thinner, lighter, and stronger than thermoplastic devices are now available. Composite AFOs have been very well accepted by patients and offer improvements in range of ankle motion and push-off characteristics.[7] Unfortunately, funding restrictions continue to prevent many good candidates from having access to the most modern orthotic technology and effectively discourage the development of more advanced future orthoses.

The older-style metal and leather orthoses usually are reserved for selected applications, including the following:

- Satisfied previous wearers
- Unusually large or heavy individuals
- When minimal contact with the leg is desirable

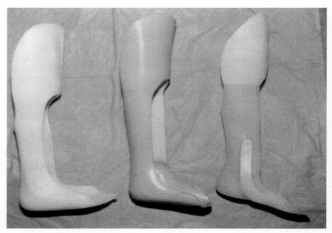

Fig. 26-1 Plastic AFO, with a rigid ankle set to accommodate various heel heights, uses floor reaction forces to reduce knee flexion in the latter half of the stance phase.

Minimal contact designs are sometimes best for persons with fluctuating edema and for heat-sensitive individuals who cannot tolerate the more intimately fitting plastic contours.[23] Some clinicians prefer metal systems for growing children because of their adjustability for growth, but many others believe that plastic or hybrid devices are just as versatile in this regard.[24] One of the most significant factors in material selection is client (or parent) preference, which largely determines acceptance and therefore should predominate over all moot points in the final decision.

Functionally, all orthotic devices including AFOs must achieve one or more fundamental goals, such as[4] (1) control of motion, (2) correction of deformity, and (3) compensation for weakness. Figure 26-1 illustrates one common application of *control of motion:* a rigid, plastic AFO with the ankle locked in slight dorsiflexion and a well-padded anterior proximal segment to stabilize the tibia. This design, first reported in 1969 by the Israeli orthotist Saltiel, is often colloquially termed a *floor reaction AFO*[28] because the extended, rigid forefoot section accentuates the knee *extension* moment at midstance and thereby prevents tibial collapse that otherwise would result from weak or absent gastrocnemius–soleus strength. This illustrates one of the critical treatment principles of orthotic management: *The orthosis may indirectly affect remote body segments, and this characteristic can be used therapeutically.* The sagittal plane biomechanics of this AFO at midstance are shown in Figure 26-2.

Orthoses can be rationally and succinctly prescribed based on the biomechanical function desired.[19] The plastic floor reaction AFO with ankle locked in slight dorsiflexion usually is applicable when the patient has a paralyzed ankle–foot complex but good or better quadriceps and balance. Examples of pathologies that could result in this clinical picture include myelodysplasia, spinal cord injury, peripheral nerve injury, poliomyelitis, and gastrocnemius–soleus trauma or dysfunction.

One of the more common lower limb deficits is a flaccid equinus, which may result from many causes, including Charcot-Marie-Tooth disease, cerebrovascular accidents with mild residual symptoms, muscular dystrophy, and peroneal palsies of various types. The orthotic options to *compensate for*

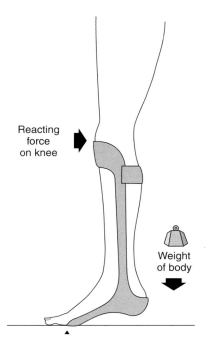

Fig. 26-2 Biomechanics of the floor reaction AFO, from the original illustration by Saltiel. In late stance, the extended forefoot plate contacts the floor and creates a knee extension moment via the well-padded anterior contours.

pretibial compartment *weakness* or paralysis definitively (Fig. 26-3) include the following:

1. Bilateral 2-inch heel lifts
2. Piano wire AFO
3. Metal alloy dorsiflexion assist AFO
4. Flexible plastic AFO
5. Peroneal NMES

A functionally based prescription, such as "orthosis to compensate for weakened pretibial musculature," ensures that the orthotist considers all available alternatives before determining the optimum solution for a particular patient.[23] A more restrictive prescription, such as "prefabricated plastic AFO to provide dorsiflexion assist," is appropriate only if that is the sole desirable solution—and all others are automatically ruled out.

The first alternative, which in some instances might be supplied by the 2-inch heels typical of cowboy footwear, prevents the plantarflexed forefoot from dragging in swing phase because the boot stabilizes the flaccid foot, and the heel height lengthens both legs sufficiently for clearance of a plantarflexed foot. This simple option may be acceptable in some instances as long as the affected leg has sufficient mediolateral ankle stability.

The next two choices are essentially spring-loaded metal devices attached to the client's shoes. Use of a caliper box and removable stirrups with the dorsiflexion assist AFO allows shoe interchange (as does the spring wire AFO), but the cost and inconvenience of modifying all shoes should not be underestimated. The chief advantage of the metal systems is the limited contact with the leg, which must be balanced against the bulk, weight, and maintenance required for such mechanical solutions.

The fourth option (flexible plastic AFO) may be either prefabricated or custom molded. The device can be made from thermoplastics, carbon fiber composites, or silicone elastomer. In general, prefabricated solutions are applicable for short-term use by patients who retain protective sensation (e.g., mild iatrogenic palsy from cast application) as long as the limb contours are within normal limits. Deformed limbs, insensate limbs, and definitive long-term applications generally require custom-made devices to ensure long-term comfort and success.

The fifth option (NMES) recently has become commercially available in the United States. Although the biomechanical result (increased toe clearance during swing) is similar among all AFO designs, potential additional benefits from electronic AFOs[30] include the following:

- Strengthening of the weakened muscle group
- Inhibition of spasticity in the antagonist muscle group
- Short-term "carryover" permitting ambulation without any orthosis

Various elastic slings available for management of temporary flaccid equinus have been omitted from the discussion because such OTC items usually are intended as "therapy training equipment" to facilitate gait retraining and therefore are not commonly provided for long-term outpatient use. This discussion also has excluded the compensatory steppage gait characterized by excessive hip flexion, which is a common *adaptation* to untreated flaccid equinus that does not correct the underlying biomechanical gait abnormality.

Note that all the devices discussed in this section offer similar function: compensation for weakness by the creation of an ankle dorsiflexion force. The particular orthosis selected for an individual patient must take into consideration a variety of additional criteria, including ease of donning, weight, cost, cosmesis, and durability.

Correction of flexible deformities is so common in lower limb orthotic management that it has become a sine qua non for effective treatment: reduce all flexible deformities to a neutral or balanced position.[3] This usually is accomplished by careful positioning of the affected limb during the casting or digital scanning procedure. Such careful alignment markedly reduces the floor reaction moments trying to collapse the limb segment further under weight bearing, lowers the magnitude of stabilizing force necessary, and results in a more comfortable device, thus enhancing long-term acceptance.[5]

Correction of more rigid deformities is feasible only in selected cases where the cause is short term and primarily soft tissue related. Figure 26-4 illustrates an example of a bilateral hybrid AFO designed to allow ambulation as well as to help reduce the plantarflexion contractures caused by a hypertonic gastrocnemius following a traumatic brain injury. Many other pathologies that result in spastic contractures can present a similar biomechanical challenge.

Initially the ankle joints were set to accommodate the full contracture, and the plastic foot and tibial shells held the limb securely, eliminating clonus. External wedges of a lightweight material were added to the plantar surface of the orthosis so that the tibia-to-floor angle simulated slight dorsiflexion, which allowed ambulation without the painful hyperextension moment at the knee that occurred during barefoot walking.

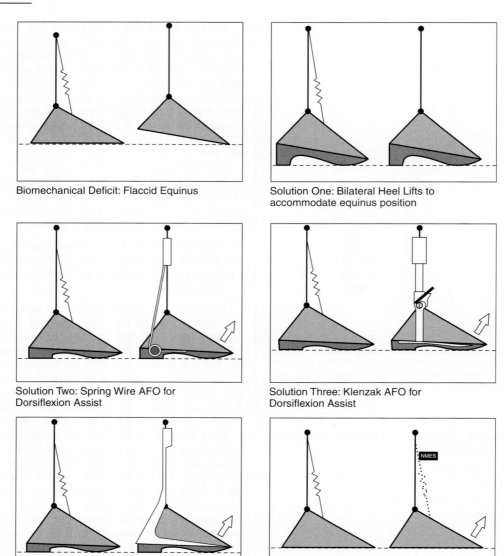

Biomechanical Deficit: Flaccid Equinus

Solution One: Bilateral Heel Lifts to accommodate equinus position

Solution Two: Spring Wire AFO for Dorsiflexion Assist

Solution Three: Klenzak AFO for Dorsiflexion Assist

Solution Four: Molded Plastic AFO for Dorsiflexion Assist

Solution Five: Functional Electrical Stimulation for Dorsiflexion Assist

Fig. 26-3 Matrix depicting different potential orthotic solutions for treatment of flaccid equinus.

Over time, neurological recovery, pharmacological treatment, and physical therapy mobilization decreased the spasticity, making the deformity less rigid. By incrementally readjusting the ankle joints, the orthosis then was used to maintain the limb in a less deformed attitude, 24 hours per day, to consolidate the gains made during daily treatments.

Slices of the wedge material were removed over time to restore the proper tibia-to-floor attitude as the ankle attitude approached neutral. Ultimately the patient was discharged as a community ambulator with her ankles held in slight dorsiflexion by the orthoses, which now fit comfortably inside conventional athletic footwear.

This case example illustrates two important additional treatment principles: (1) application of low-level, tolerable forces over an extended period may result in significant biological changes; and (2) the tibia-to-floor angle can be varied independently of the ankle–foot attitude to facilitate gait.

The matrix shown in Figure 26-5 summarizes typical motion control options available at the ankle and provides examples of both metal and plastic AFOs that offer such function. This graphic summary is intended to help the reader visualize how these common options work mechanically. Much like the ingredients in a recipe, these simple options (when properly and creatively combined) create a result that is more effective than just the sum of the individual parts. This is the clinical art of orthotic practice.

On rare occasions, orthoses are prescribed to offer an additional function: partial axial unweighting of more distal limb segments.[27] Figure 26-6 depicts an AFO designed to fully unload the calcaneus, bilaterally. Such devices can be used to protect hindfoot fractures, recalcitrant heel ulcerations, and similar pathologies. Figure 26-7 shows a hybrid system with metal uprights and ankle joints sometimes used to unload the ankle–foot complex partially during the consolidation phase of neuropathic (Charcot) arthropathy.[21]

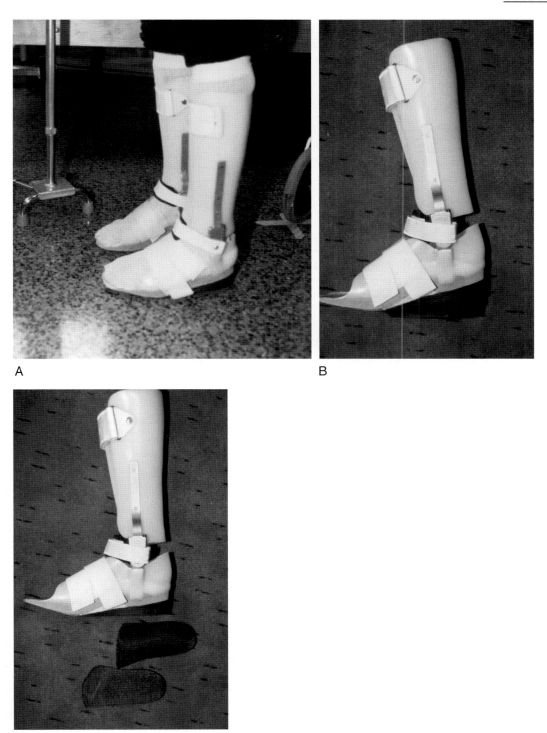

A

B

C

Fig. 26-4 A, Bilateral hybrid AFOs combine the intimate secure fit of custom-molded plastic shells with the ease of adjustment of metal double-action ankle joints. **B, C,** As the patient improves over time, the ankle joint is adjusted to maintain the improved posture, and the compensating wedge is reduced accordingly.

Orthotic Ankle Control Options

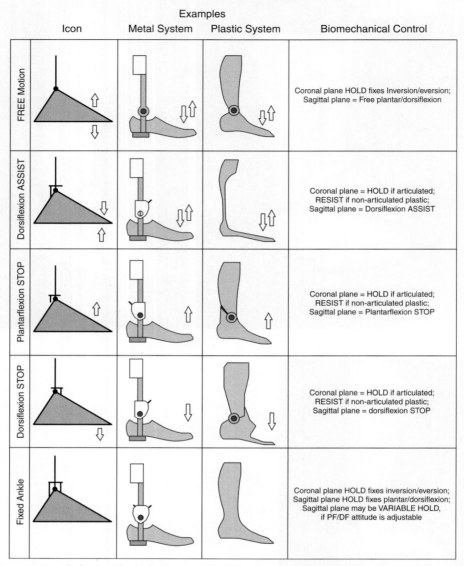

Fig. 26-5 Ankle joint components and plastic orthosis designs provide various biomechanical controls in the sagittal and coronal planes.

Knee–ankle–foot orthoses

As noted in the introduction, simpler orthoses enjoy a much higher long-term acceptance rate than do more complex devices. Therefore, a knee–ankle–foot orthosis (KAFO) should not be prescribed unless there is a compelling reason to do so. The most common justification for a KAFO is the need for direct control of the knee complex that cannot be accomplished in another fashion, *in addition to a need for suspension or for ankle or foot control.*[20] Obviously, if knee control alone is the objective, the simpler KO (see section on knee orthoses) may suffice if suspension and rotary stability can be achieved without incorporating the foot into the orthosis.

Figure 26-8 illustrates key types of available orthotic knee joints and offers examples of typical applications. When combined with the plethora of ankle controls available, literally scores of orthoses can be constructed from these basic mechanical elements. Prescribing orthotic management on a functional basis allows the physician to direct the team's efforts while allowing the knowledgeable orthotist to consider all available permutations before selecting the preferred approach.

Figure 26-9 shows a metal KAFO designed for a polio survivor with a flail leg from the hip distally. The offset knee joints are held in extension during late stance by loading on the anterior proximal thigh band. The individual's biological knee is allowed to go into slight recurvatum, which is sufficient to stabilize it via floor reaction forces that occur when the dorsiflexion stop inside the orthotic ankle joint applies force to the extended steel shank placed inside the sole of the shoe. This biomechanical result is shown in Figure 26-10.

The biomechanics during loading response are crucial, and the biomechanics for this KAFO are shown in Figure 26-11. The resistance from a mild plantarflexion resist spring allows the foot to descend to the floor in a controlled manner, replacing the function of the pretibial muscles.

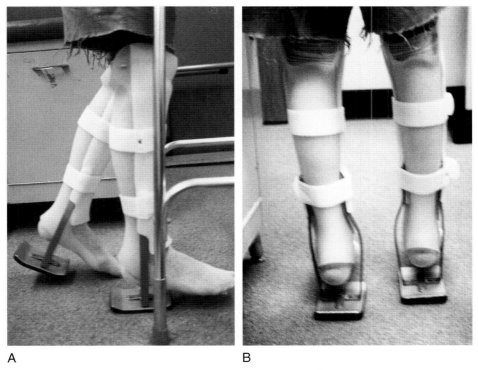

A   B

Fig. 26-6 Custom-designed AFOs with patten bottom extensions used successfully to protect calcaneal fractures until healing was complete.

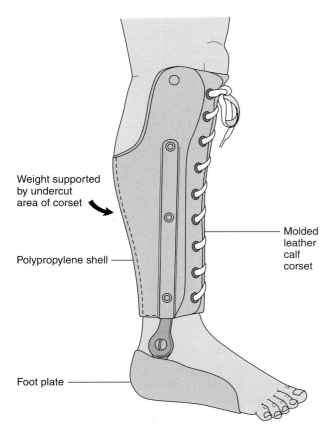

Weight supported
by undercut
area of corset

Polypropylene shell —

Foot plate —

— Molded
leather
calf
corset

Fig. 26-7 One type of AFO designed to partially unload the ankle–foot complex.

The orthotist must carefully analyze the resultant forces throughout the device to anticipate and deal with their effect.[32] Had a rigid plantarflexion stop been provided instead, as depicted in Figure 26-12, the resulting knee flexion moment during loading response would cause the orthotic knee joint to flex, and the individual might fall. To prevent this, a manually locked or stance control knee mechanism would be required for the same biomechanical reason.

The development of a number of stance control knee joints suitable for use in orthoses has eliminated several of the major drawbacks associated with locking the knee throughout gait. Stance control orthoses permit many individuals with significant knee paresis or paralysis to walk safely because the knee is mechanically stabilized during weight bearing but is free to flex during swing phase. Particularly for individuals who retain significant hip flexor or extensor strength, the ability to have more normal swing phase kinematics seems to result in a gait that not only is more normal but also is more energy efficient. Clinical acceptance and reliability of this new biomechanical option has been encouraging, with successful reports of both unilateral and bilateral applications. Figure 26-13 shows the use of a stance control KAFO for walking outdoors.

The variety of knee lock mechanisms available should generally be reserved for those cases where a stance control knee component will not suffice. For example, persistent knee spasticity may interfere with release of stance control joints, making a locked knee the only option. Figure 26-14 illustrates one locked knee design intended to facilitate limited ambulation despite bilateral paralysis of the lower limbs. The fixed ankle with adjustable joints, combined with specially reinforced shoes, provides a solid base of support. Careful adjustment into a slightly dorsiflexed attitude, combined with the

	Example	Biomechanical Control	Typical Clinical Application
Single Axis	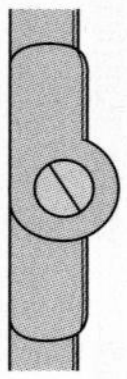	Coronal plane HOLD stabilizes genu varum/valgum; Sagittal plane = FREE flexion-extension; Integral hyperextension stop	Mild to moderate genu varum or genu valgum
Offset	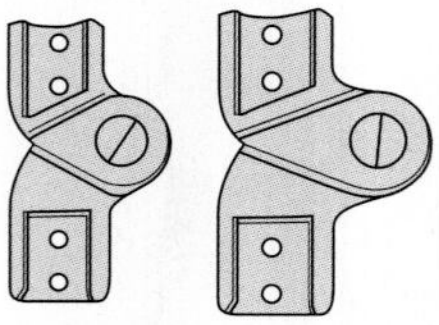	Coronal plane HOLD stabilizes genu varum/valgum; Sagittal plane = FREE flexion-extension; Integral hyperextension stop	Moderate to severe genu recurvatum
Polycentric	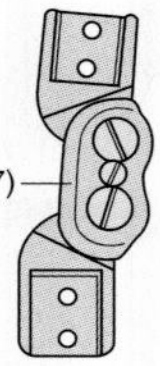 (7)	Coronal plane HOLD stabilizes genu varum/valgum; Sagittal plane = FREE flexion-extension; Integral hyperextension stop	Self-suspending knee orthoses, to reduce "pistoning" on the leg
Stance Control	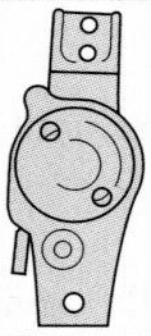	Coronal plane HOLD stabilizes genu varum/valgum; Sagittal plane = No knee flexion under weight bearing; FREE flexion-extension when un-weighted; Integral hyperextension stop	Knee extensor paralysis or paresis
Lock	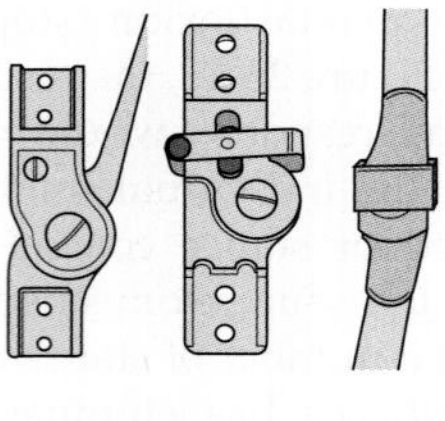 Bale Wedge Ring	Coronal plane HOLD stabilizes genu varum/valgum; Sagittal plane = **removable** HOLD in full extension during stance and swing phase of gait; Can be released for sitting; Integral hyperextension stop	Knee extensor paralysis or paresis, when stance control is not feasible
Lock + Variable Flexion	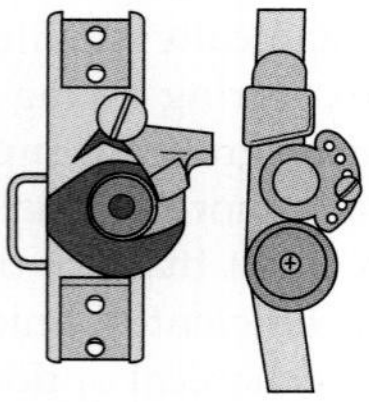	Coronal plane HOLD stabilizes genu varum/valgum; Sagittal plane = **removable** HOLD in full extension during stance and swing phase of gait; Can be released for sitting; Integral, adjustable extension stop	Spastic paralysis with reducible knee flexion contracture

Fig. 26-8 Orthotic knee joint options. Knee joint components provide various biomechanical controls in the sagittal and coronal planes.

locked knee mechanisms and therapy training to teach the patient to extend the hips and hang on the hip ligaments, results in hands-free balance. Ambulation for limited distances is possible using crutches, at least for the young or vigorous individual. This type of KAFO bears the eponym Scott-Craig after the Colorado rehabilitation hospital that popularized its application.[29]

Knee orthoses

Knee orthoses (KOs) originally were rarely prescribed. Their application was limited to isolated knee pathologies, typically varus or valgus angulation secondary to advanced arthritic destruction of the condylar area (Fig. 26-15). To unload the painful condyle as well as to resist further progression of deformity, extensive bracing with long moment arms

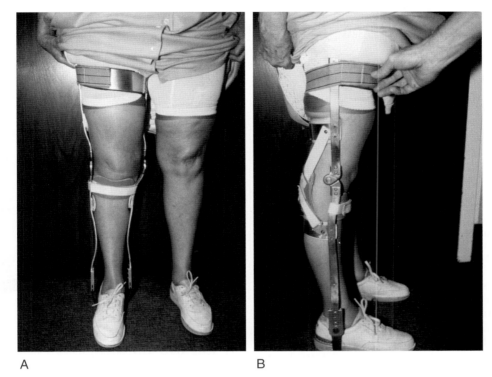

A   B

Fig. 26-9 Metal KAFO designed to control genu recurvatum and flaccid equinus in a flail leg.

is required. In this instance, the need for self-suspension was met by careful contouring to the deformed limb, supplemented with a supracondylar indention similar to the prosthetic suspension technique. In the past decade, researchers have investigated the ability of specific KO designs to unload the medial or lateral compartment of the arthritic knee joint.[8]

The Lenox Hill brace was developed in the 1970s and gradually became the first widely accepted KO for sports applications.[25] In the decades that followed, literally hundreds of self-suspending KOs with medial and lateral hinges have been marketed. The original custom-molded designs gradually have been supplanted in many cases with prefabricated and even OTC variants. Many have only superficial biomechanical differences; some are made of poor-quality materials; and none has been convincingly demonstrated to be globally "superior" to any other variant.

Indications for sports KOs remain equivocal other than for nonoperative applications in which surgery has been refused or is not feasible.[1] Prophylactic application to prevent injuries has not been shown definitively to be effective, and some fear transfer injuries to adjacent joints. Despite numerous studies, the role of KOs for sports activities has not yet been completely elucidated.[14]

Hip orthoses

Hip orthoses (HpOs) may be prescribed for isolated problems in the acetabular region, which may be the result of (1)

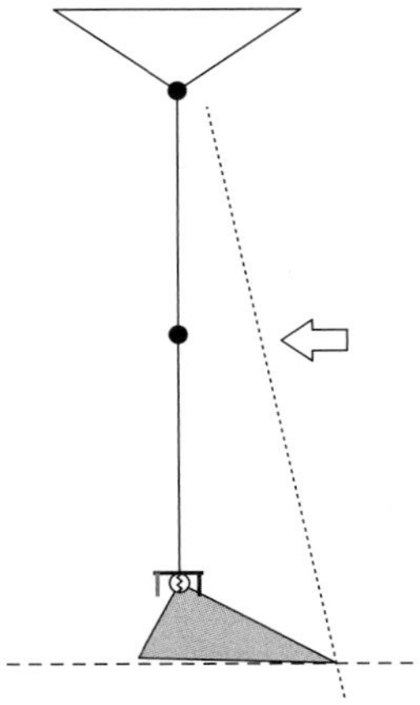

Fig. 26-10 KAFO biomechanics in late stance. An extended steel shank inside the sole of the shoe creates an extension moment at the knee.

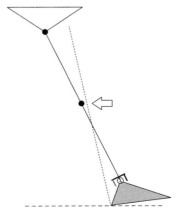

Fig. 26-11 KAFO bimechanics during loading response. With an articulated ankle joint that permits plantarflexion, a slight knee extension moment is generated that helps stabilize the limb.

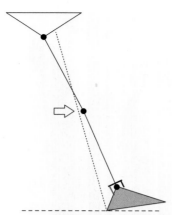

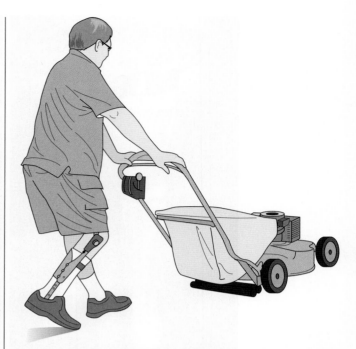

Fig. 26-12 KAFO biomechanics during loading response. When plantarflexion is blocked, a significant knee flexion moment is generated. If the limb is flail, then the knee will collapse unless a stance control or locked knee joint is provided.

Fig. 26-13 KAFO incorporating stance control knee joints provides weight-bearing stability without interfering with swing phase knee flexion, providing greater midswing toe clearance than KAFOs with a locked knee. This facilitates walking both indoors and on uneven surfaces such as a lawn. (From Horton's Technology, Inc.)

dysplastic disorders, (2) traumatic injury, or (3) surgical procedures (total hip replacement). A variety of devices are available to treat infantile developmentally dysplastic hips, with generally good clinical results. The prefabricated soft (Pavlik) harness is one of the most common HpOs.[26] A variety of custom-made HpOs were formerly used to treat Legg-Calvé-Perthes disease in adolescence, based on the containment theory, which states that if the femoral head is maintained in the acetabulum during the active phase of the disorder, a more congruent head results. Controlled studies have not supported the efficacy of this form of treatment.[11]

The most common application of the HpO in adults is for postoperative protection of total hip replacement, particularly after revisions that are unstable. Devices that incorporate an extensive hemishell at the hip (technically called *lumbosacral HpOs*) are believed to provide the most effective biomechanical control.[16] Note that no orthosis has yet been developed that can fully protect the at-risk hip, particularly with an uncooperative or incoherent client. Under such circumstances, the HpO at best decreases the risk of dislocation.

Definitive HpO applications are rare. Figure 26-16 shows one example of a young man with total loss of adductor power secondary to one of the muscular dystrophies. This custom-made HpO prevented the progressive abduction that otherwise would have immobilized him (with his legs abducted maximally) after just a few steps, while allowing free sagittal plane motion.

Hip–knee–ankle–foot orthoses

Hip–knee–ankle–foot orthoses (HKAFOs) are most commonly prescribed for pediatric patients, who often do remarkably well even with complex devices.[24] HKAFOs are selectively recommended for adults with bilateral paralysis from spinal cord injuries, who tend to abandon more involved orthoses after the first year because of the tremendous energy required to ambulate despite bilateral paralysis.[6] Unilateral applications of HKAFOs are rare, except for short-term use to provide protected ambulation after hip arthroplasty.

One of the most common HKAFOs uses a mechanical linkage to couple flexion of one hip with extension of the other, which permits a reciprocal step-over-step gait. One example

of such an HKAFO is illustrated in Figure 26-17. Colloquially referred to as *reciprocating gait orthoses*, these HKAFOs are used for a variety of pathologies that result in paraplegia, including spinal cord injury and myelodysplasia.[12] A review of the use of KAFOs and HKAFOs for ambulation found very limited scientific evidence to guide clinical decision-making about these devices.[10]

Compound orthoses

Devices that cross more than five body segments can be considered *compound* orthoses, composed of two (or more) primary devices. The terminology reflects this perspective as two or more individual orthoses; the device pictured in

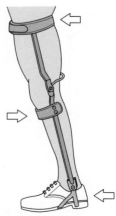

Fig. 26-14 Bilateral KAFO with locked knee and adjustable solid ankle is one approach to paraplegic standing and walking. This design was popularized by Craig Rehabilitation Hospital in Colorado.

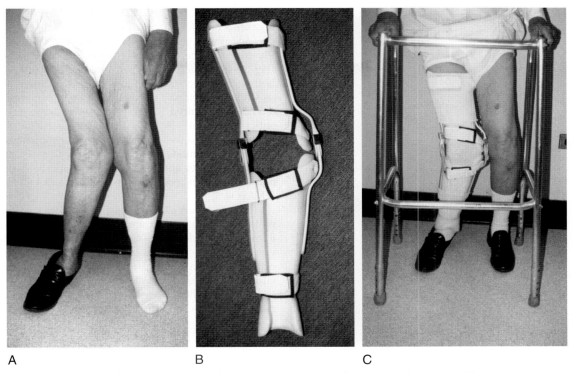

A   B   C

Fig. 26-15 Custom-designed KO designed to unload the lateral compartment to relieve pain and prevent further progression of osteoarthritic deformity. Note the extended lever arms on the thigh and shin, which significantly lower the pressure per unit area, enhancing comfort despite the strong corrective forces required in response to the marked genu valgum deformity.

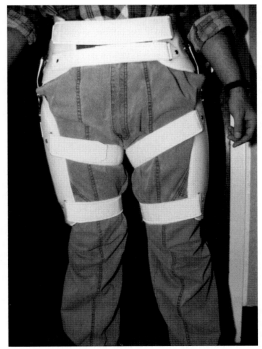

Fig. 26-16 Bilateral hinges connect the lateral thigh panels to the pelvic section on this hip orthosis, controlling the amount of abduction while permitting free motion in the sagittal plane.

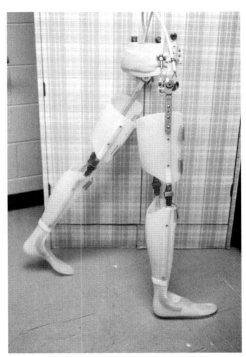

Fig. 26-17 HKAFO that links hip extension on one side with hip flexion on the contralateral side. This permits a reciprocating foot-over-foot gait as well as the option to swing to or swing through.

353

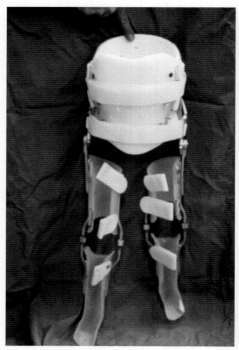

Fig. 26-18 Compound orthosis consisting of a plastic TLSO for control of paralytic scoliosis plus bilateral HKAFOs to allow paraplegic gait. Children often tolerate such involved bracing and usually are able to ambulate reasonably well for short distances.

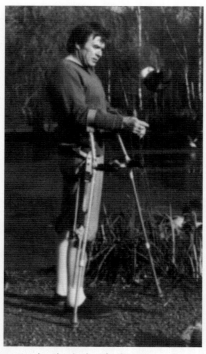

Fig. 26-19 Compound orthosis that facilitates a reciprocal gait. The hip and knee joints are mechanically linked for coordinated locking/unlocking. Powerful pressurized gas struts provide an extension assist at each knee to help the person with paraplegia arise from a chair more easily.

Fig. 26-18 is described as a thoracolumbosacral orthosis (TLSO) plus HKAFO. Such extensive bracing occasionally is successful with young adults who are extremely motivated, as illustrated by the Advanced Reciprocal Gait Orthosis (ARGO) (Fig. 26-19), which is designed to assist the adult paraplegic in both ambulating and arising from/sitting down in a chair.[17]

Children typically do well with such complexity. Even if a TLSO is required full time for scoliosis management and superincumbent HKAFOs are used daily for ambulation, youngsters often wear such compound orthoses without complaint and ambulate reasonably well with a reversed walker. However, as they approach adulthood, most will prefer to use a wheelchair for independent mobility and will abandon the HKAFOs.[22]

The most complex orthosis involving the lower limbs, which could be termed a *cervicothoracolumbosacral HKAFO + bilateral shoulder–elbow–wrist–hand orthosis*, theoretically would provide full body control. Although an articulated orthosis of such complexity is presently a bionic myth, miniature implanted electrical stimulation devices with wireless controls and other technologies currently under development may make such complex interventions feasible in the future.

References

1. Albright JP, Saterbak A, Stokes J: Use of knee braces in sport: current recommendations, *Sports Med* 20:281–301, 1995.
2. Anthony RA: *The manufacture and use of functional foot orthoses*, New York, 1991, Karger.
3. Bowker P: The biomechanics of orthoses. In Bowker P, Condie DN, Bader DL, Pratt DJ, editors: *Biomechanical basis of orthotic management*, London, 1993, Butterworth-Heinemann.
4. Bunch WH, Keagy RD: *Principles of orthotic treatment*, St. Louis, 1976, CV Mosby.
5. Carlson JM, Berglund G: An effective orthotic design for controlling the unstable subtalar joint, *Orthot Prosthet* 33:39, 1979.
6. Coughlan JK, et al: Lower extremity bracing in paraplegia: a follow-up study, *Paraplegia* 1:25, 1980.
7. Desloovere K, Molenaers G, Van Gestel L, et al: How can push-off be preserved during use of an ankle foot orthosis in children with hemiplegia? A prospective controlled study, *Gait Posture* 24:142–151, 2006.
8. Draganich L, Reider B, Rimington T, Piotrowski G, Mallik K, Nasson S: The effectiveness of self-adjustable custom and off-the-shelf bracing in the treatment of varus gonarthrosis, *J Bone Joint Surg* 88A:2645–2652, 2006.
9. Edwards CA: *Orthopaedic shoe technology: II. Clinical conditions requiring orthopaedic footgear*, Muncie, Ind, 1985, Ball State University Press.
10. Fatone S: A review of the literature pertaining to KAFOs and HKAFOs for ambulation. Proceedings: knee-ankle-foot orthoses for ambulation, *J Prosthet Orthot* 18(suppl):137–168, 2006.
11. Herring JA, Kim HT, Browne R: Legg-Calve-Perthes disease. Part II: prospective multicenter study of the effect of treatment on outcome, *J Bone Joint Surg Am* 86:2121–2134, 2004.
12. Katz DE, Haideri N, Song K, Wyrick P: Comparative study of conventional hip-knee-ankle-foot orthoses versus reciprocating-gait orthoses for children with high-level paraparesis, *J Pediatr Orthop* 17:377–386, 1997.
13. Kralf A, Acimov K, Stanic U: Enhancement of hemiplegic patient rehabilitation by means of functional electrical stimulation, *Prosthet Orthot Int* 17:107, 1993.
14. Kramer JF, Dubowitz T, Fowler P, Schachter C, Birmingham T: Functional knee braces and dynamic performance: a review, *Clin J Sport Med* 7:32–39, 1997.
15. Lehmann JL: Lower limb orthotics. In Redford JB, editor: *Orthotics etcetera*, ed 3, Baltimore, 1986, Williams & Wilkins.
16. Lima D, Magnus R, Paprosky WG: Team management of hip revision patients using a post-op hip orthosis, *J Prosthet Orthot* 6:20, 1994.
17. Lissens MA, et al: Advanced reciprocating gait orthosis in paraplegic patients, *Eur J Phys Med Rehabil* 3(suppl 4):147, 1993.
18. *Lower-limb orthotics*, New York, 1986, New York University Medical Center Staff, Prosthetics & Orthotics.
19. McCollough NC: *Biomechanical analysis systems for orthotic prescription*. In: Bunch WH, Keagy R, Kritter AE, Letts M, Lonstein JE, et al, eds: *Atlas of*

orthotics: biomechanical principles and application, ed 2, St. Louis, 1985, CV Mosby.

20. Merritt JL: Knee-ankle-foot orthotics: long leg braces and their practical applications, *Phys Med Rehabil State Art Rev* 1:67, 1987.
21. Michael JW, Isbell MA, Harrelson JM: Orthotic management of diabetic neuropathic arthropathy, *J Prosthet Orthot* 4:55, 1991.
22. Michael JW: KAFOs for ambulation: an orthotist's perspective, *J Prosthet Orthot* 18(suppl):187–191, 2006.
23. Michael JW: Orthotic treatment of neurological deficits. In Good DC, Couch JR, editors: *Handbook of neurorehabilitation,* New York, 1994, Marcel Dekker.
24. Michael JW: Pediatric prosthetics and orthotics, *Phys Occup Ther Pediatr* 10:123, 1990.
25. Nicholas JA: The five-one reconstruction for anteromedial instability of the knee: indications, technique, and the results in fifty-two patients, *J Bone Joint Surg Am* 55:899, 1973.
26. Pavlik A: The functional method of treatment using a harness with stirrups as the primary method of conservative therapy for infants with congenital dislocation of the hip, *Clin Orthop Relat Res* 281:4, 1992.
27. Rose GK: *Orthotics principles and practice,* London, 1986, Heinemann Medical Books.
28. Saltiel J: A one-piece laminated knee locking short leg brace, *Orthot Prosthet* 23:68, 1969.
29. Scott BA: Engineering principles and fabrication techniques for the Scott-Craig long-leg brace for paraplegia, *Orthot Prosthet* 25:14, 1971.
30. Stein RB: *Historical overview of FES.* Presented at 2007 Annual Meeting of the American Academy of Orthotists & Prosthetists, San Francisco, CA, Thursday, March 22, 2007.
31. Weber DJ, Stein RB, Chan KM, et al: BIONic WalkAide for correcting foot drop, *IEEE Trans Neural Syst Rehabil Eng* 13:242–246, 2005.
32. Wiest DR, et al: The influence of heel design on a rigid ankle-foot-orthosis, *Orthot Prosthet* 33:3, 1979.
33. Wu KK: *Foot orthoses,* Baltimore, 1990, Williams & Wilkins.

Lower limb orthoses for persons with spinal cord injury

Ross S. Chafetz, Therese E. Johnston, and Christina L. Calhoun

Key Points

- For individuals with spinal cord injury, the three main goals of orthotic use are to (1) protect/maintain joint integrity, (2) encourage normal orthopedic development, and (3) assist with upright mobility.

- Prescription of (hip)–knee–ankle–foot orthoses [(H)KAFOs)] for upright mobility requires a multidisciplinary client-centered approach that focuses on the patient's goals and motivations for upright mobility.

- Orthotic prescription of (H)KAFOs depends on patient goals and sagittal/transverse upright stability.

- Although (H)KAFOs for upright mobility can be used for functional activities, the wheelchair generally is the primary mode of mobility for patients with complete motor loss at L2 and above (American Spinal Injury Association classification).

- Technological advances that combine orthoses with surface or implanted functional electrical stimulation are promising for upright mobility.

Approximately 11,000 individuals in the United States sustain a spinal cord injury (SCI) every year. Between 220,000 and 285,000 individuals currently are living with an SCI.[35–38,47,114] The average age at injury is 38 years; 78% of SCIs occur in men.[35–38,47] An estimated 54.1% of injuries occur in individuals between 16 and 30 years old.[36,114,121] Primary causes of SCI include motor vehicle accidents, military- or paramilitary-related injuries, violence, sports, and falls.[2,114,121]

The spinal cord is the bidirectional conduit between the brain and the rest of the body; therefore, it provides a means of travel for motor and sensory information. When the spinal cord is injured, sensory and motor signals cannot move across the site of injury. As a result, an individual will present with impairments in volitional motor control, strength, and sensation that limit functional mobility and the performance of daily tasks. Because the injury presentation will depend on the specific neural structures affected in the spinal cord, it is critical that the level of injury determination is standardized and clearly defined, especially when discussing the use of orthoses as a treatment intervention.

Pathophysiology

Level of injury

The most accepted and consistent means of SCI classification and measure of impairment is the International Standards for Classification of Spinal Cord Injury, written by the Neurological Standards Committee of the American Spinal Injury Association (ASIA).[3] This examination allows a clinician to systematically examine the dermatomes and myotomes in order to determine the spinal cord segments affected by injury.

The sensory examination requires that 28 key dermatomes, C2 through S4–5, be tested for sensitivity to pin prick and light touch on both sides of the body. Appreciation of pin prick and light touch are scored on a three-point scale, where 0 is absent, 1 is impaired (partial or altered appreciation), and 2 is normal. The external anal sphincter is assessed for sensation and is graded as being present or absent.

For the motor examination, a consensus of experts paired key motions with specific myotomes. Levels included muscles corresponding to myotomes C5–T1 in the upper limbs and L1–S1 in the lower limbs. Strength is graded on a six-point scale as follows: 0 is total paralysis, 1 is palpable or visible contraction, 2 is movement through the full range of motion (ROM) in a gravity eliminated position, 3 is movement through the full ROM against gravity, 4 is movement through the full ROM with moderate resistance, and 5 is movement through the full ROM with full resistance. The external anal sphincter is tested and graded based on the absence or presence of contraction around the examiner's finger.

A very important but often misunderstood concept from the ASIA examination is the distinction of incomplete from complete SCI. A patient is classified as having an incomplete SCI if partial preservation of sensory and motor function is found below the neurological level and must include the lowest sacral segment (S4–S5).[3,93] A person is classified as having a complete injury if he or she has no sensory or motor function in the lowest sacral segment. The definitions have changed since the Frankel Classification, so caution should be taken when comparing studies conducted before and those after 1996.[3,44,93]

Following the examination, a motor and sensory score and level are determined for both sides of the body. The sensory level is the highest dermatome intact to light and sharp/dull touch. The level at which the patient scores a 3/5 on manual muscle test and 5/5 for superior levels is the motor level. When considering lower limb bracing, motor level is the most pertinent.

Current issues

For individuals with SCI, the three main goals of orthotic use are to (1) protect/maintain a bone or joint, (2) assist with function, and (3) encourage normal orthopedic development in children.

Protecting and/or maintaining a joint with an orthosis is the least controversial of goals. For example, if during the time of the injury a patient fractures the femur, then utilization of a knee immobilizer or fracture brace to protect the injured area is appropriate. For long-term maintenance of a joint, an orthosis can prevent contractures. In the early stages of an injury, a patient typically is in spinal shock and presents with flaccid lower limbs (hypotonicity).[5] The foot falls into the plantarflexed position combined with inversion, producing an equinovarus position. As the patient emerges from spinal shock, typically 1 to 3 months after an injury, tone gradually intensifies. As tone increases, the lower limbs will experience muscle spasms into an extensor synergy, typically hip internal rotation, knee extension, ankle plantarflexion, and foot inversion. Therefore, there is a tendency both before and after spinal shock for the ankle to be in equinovarus. In a relatively short period of time, a patient can develop a plantarflexion contracture, which has detrimental effects on future transfers, ambulation, wheelchair positioning, and dressing. To prevent a plantarflexion contracture, the ankle should be held in a neutral position, which is easily accomplished using a prefabricated antifootdrop orthosis (Fig. 27-1).[137,138] Regardless of the type of orthosis used, it must be well padded, and the feet must be checked frequently for pressure areas. Loss of sensation resulting from SCI places all patients who wear orthoses at high risk for developing pressure ulcers. Once the orthosis is removed, any redness should

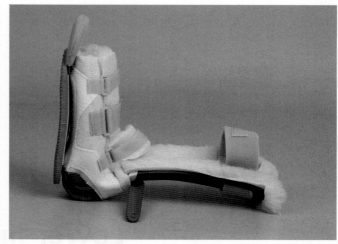

Fig. 27-1 Antifootdrop orthosis. For nighttime use, this orthosis maintains the foot in a neutral position. Its padding and design reduce the risk of pressure areas, particularly at the heel.

resolve after 20 minutes. With routine findings on skin examinations, wearing time is gradually increased.

For children with SCI, orthoses are vital for promoting normal bone alignment during growth. Areas that can indirectly impact the lower limb and frequently require orthotic interventions are the hips and spine. A level pelvis is vital for maintenance of an erect stable position for functional activities in sitting and for adequate distribution of sitting pressures for prevention of skin breakdown.[17,41,80] From 80% to 98% of children injured before the age of skeletal maturity develop scoliosis.[88,91] Early bracing of the spine may delay the age at which surgical intervention is required, and curves less than 20 degrees reduce the possibility of requiring a surgical fusion.[99] Prescribing a thoracolumbosacral orthosis (TLSO) may serve several functions, including maintaining skeletal alignment that prevents the rapid progression of scoliosis, distributing seated pressures, providing trunk stabilization during functional activities, assisting with breathing, and increasing stability during upright mobility during ambulation.[17,33,91,94,112,139] Of note, although a TLSO may aid in some activities, it has been shown to interfere with activities such as dressing, transfers, and wheelchair propulsion.[22]

In addition to scoliosis, hip subluxation/dislocations in injured children are a concern.[128,160] In a review of 62 patients, McCarthy et al.[98] found that 93% of patients injured before age 11 years had at least one hip subluxed or dislocated, compared to 9% of patients older than 11 years. Poor development of the hip results from a combination of decreased muscle tone, which is necessary for maintaining femoral head positioning, poor acetabular development resulting from the absence of weight bearing and muscle pull, and, for patients with spasticity, the constant positioning of the hip in adduction and internal rotation. To facilitate proper femoral head/acetabular positioning while supine, an abduction pillow can be used to maintain hip abduction.[19] When sitting in the wheelchair, a patient should be positioned with the pelvis facing forward and the femurs in slight abduction, which can be facilitated by use of an abduction pommel. Similarly, when sitting upright or playing on the floor, children should be encouraged to circle sit and to avoid side sitting.[57] Side sitting encourages a windswept deformity with one limb maintaining an adducted and internally rotated position, which encourages subluxation of the femoral head.

The most controversial use of lower limb orthoses, also referred to as (hip)–knee–ankle–foot orthoses [(H)KAFOs], in patients with SCI is for functional mobility. Frequently, the primary goal of an acutely injured individual is to "walk again." After an injury, patients must quickly come to the realization that the ability to stand and achieve mobility ("walking") is significantly reduced, if not impossible. Being upright and returning to mobility symbolize recovery or the "appearance of recovery" to many patients. When presenting the options of bracing for upright mobility to a patient, it is the responsibility of the health care provider to discuss their use to ensure that the patient's expectations are realistic.[102,155,161,162] Although no evidence indicates that being upright promotes neurological recovery, some evidence indicates that (H)KAFOs have perceived psychological, social, and possible physiological benefits.[21,42,76–78,86,96,132,152,155]

To guide clinicians who work with patients having SCI, the American Paraplegia Society has created clinical practice guidelines based on outcomes studies and expert clinical judgments for patients with motor complete SCI at 1 year after injury.[26] These outcome-based practice guidelines, available through the Paralyzed Veterans Association, should be used by clinicians throughout their practice. The guidelines suggest using a stander for individuals with injuries above T1. For injuries at T1 and below, either a stander or orthoses for therapeutic or functional activities are an option.[26]

Walking patterns

The walking pattern a patient hopes to achieve plays an important role in orthotic selection. The two main walking patterns are reciprocal stepping (step to/step through) and swing through/swing to.[5,146] In the former, patients move each limb independently; in the latter, patient move both lower extremities simultaneously. Depending on the patient's physical condition, either pattern can be accomplished with a standard walker, rolling walker, or crutches. In a step-to/step-through pattern, the patient shifts weight laterally and uses body position or the mechanics of a brace to advance the contralateral limb. For a swing-through/swing-to pattern, the patient lifts the entire body weight and uses momentum and body positioning to simultaneously advance both legs.

Types of orthoses
Ankle–foot orthosis

For upright mobility, the ankle–foot orthosis (AFO) is an option for patients who have retained or recovered substantial leg strength. The patient should have sufficient active hip flexion to advance the legs and a 4/5 or greater quadriceps muscle grade. When a patient has decreased dorsiflexion strength, an AFO will prevent the patient from dragging the toes on the ground and reduce the amount of hip flexion required to clear the limbs during the swing phase of gait. With weakened quadriceps, the patient may require an AFO

with anterior band or a solid AFO set in 2 to 5 degrees of plantarflexion. This type of AFO has a rigid ankle, full-length footplate, and an anterior shell or broad anterior band. This AFO is sometimes referred to as a *ground* or *floor reaction orthosis*. As the patient moves from foot flat to the midstance phase of gait, the ground reaction force on the brace creates an extension moment at the knee. The advantage of this brace is that the patient can stabilize the knee in stance phase without having to use a knee–ankle–foot orthosis (KAFO). If a patient has sufficient knee strength, then a pair of articulating AFOs may be prescribed. This orthosis has an adjustable ankle joint that allows dorsiflexion, increasing ease of functional activities such as ascending stairs, squatting, and moving from sitting to standing. A wide variety of ankle components can assist, resist, prevent, or allow ankle motion, both plantarflexion and/or dorsiflexion.

Knee–ankle–foot orthosis

A KAFO is used to provide stability at the knee and ankle while indirectly affecting hip stability through ground reaction forces. It typically is prescribed for individuals who have little to no quadriceps strength. A KAFO consists of leather or thermoplastic thigh and calf bands attached to metal uprights joined by a footplate. The most common KAFO is the Scott-Craig KAFO or a variant of the Scott-Craig KAFO.[89,136] In a patient with paraplegia, maximal stability in standing with a KAFO is achieved with the ankle positioned in neutral or dorsiflexion, the knees locked in extension, and the hips passively positioned in extension. In this position, sometimes referred to *parastance*, an extension moment is created at the hips, which prevents the individual from folding forward while hip extension is passively maintained by the anterior capsular ligaments of the hip (Fig. 27-2).[5,133,146] However, when the patient ambulates, the hips transition through flexion, and crutches or other assistive aids are essential for stability.

Hip–knee–ankle–foot orthosis

A hip–knee–ankle–foot orthosis (HKAFO) is an orthosis whose components stabilize or lock the hip, knee, and ankle. The typical HKAFO is a pair of KAFOs linked above the hip with either a pelvic band, lumbosacral orthosis, or TLSO. An individual may require a hip component because of the level of injury; hip flexion, knee flexion, or ankle plantarflexion contractures; poor balance; or decreased motor control. The hip section provides significant stability in the transverse plane and, if the hip joints are locked, also provides sagittal plane stability. When the hips are locked, individuals will commonly use a swing-to or swing-through gait.[133] Some patients are able to unlock the hips to achieve a reciprocal gait pattern using body positioning and weight shifting. A hip guidance orthosis (HGO), also known as the Orthotic Research and Locomotor Assessment Unit (ORLAU) Parawalker, is an example of an HKAFO with free-moving hip joints that allow a reciprocal gait pattern.[18,130,131,152]

A reciprocating gait orthosis (RGO) is an HKAFO that uses a mechanical system that connects the two sides of the brace by an isocentric bar (IRGO), double cable (LSU RGO from Louisiana State University), or single push/pull cable system (advanced RGO [ARGO] developed by Hugh

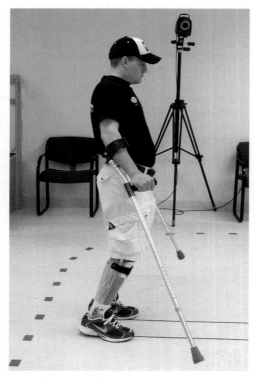

Fig. 27-2 Parastance. With bilateral ankles in dorsiflexion and knees locked in extension, the patient can maintain hip extension by passive "hanging" on the anterior capsule of the hip.

Steeper Ltd.).[40,70,109,167] Regardless of the mechanism, the patient achieves a reciprocal gait by shifting body weight forward and laterally while extending the hips and upper trunk. In theory, the hip extension of the weight leg enables the orthosis mechanism to advance the unweighted leg. Unlike a swing-through gait that requires users to lift body weight plus the weight of the orthosis, the RGO relies on weight shifting and orthotic mechanics for mobility. Although it has been suggested that RGOs are less energy demanding than standard (H)KAFOs, the evidence is not conclusive.[27,157,165] Furthermore, some authors have questioned the usefulness of the linkage system in driving the hip into flexion during the swing-through phase of gait; but they do suggest that the RGO system may increase stability by limiting hip flexion of the stance leg or bilateral hip collapse during double support.[28,29,62]

Two orthoses in development that have expanded on the basic RGO are the hip and ankle linked orthosis (HALO) and the stance control orthosis (SCO).[46,127] The HALO is a cable system that links both ankle joints with a medial hip joint. The linkage of the ankles by way of a pulley system results in assistance of the swinging leg when the contralateral ankle is flexed. The design maintains parallel alignment of the feet to the ground, reducing the need for excessive pelvic rotation.[46] The SCO has knee joints, thus providing stability during stance but free motion of the knee during swing through. The developers of the SCO suggest combining their design with the IRGO concept in an attempt to decrease the energy required during gait for the SCI population.

Progressive upright mobility bracing

Initially, some individuals are unable to achieve a parastance with KAFOs alone and therefore require an (H)KAFO, such as an RGO. Eventually, as strength, coordination, or balance improves or contractures reduce, the hip component can be modified or removed, progressing the individual to less bracing. Having an RGO or HKAFO with a detachable superior section allows an individual to experience the advantage and disadvantage of the different gait patterns (swing through or reciprocal) without and with hip stabilization. After trying each option, the individual can decide what brace and gait pattern works best for him or her.[52,155,161,168]

Treatment recommendations

When considering orthoses for upright mobility, first and foremost the clinician must understand the patient's expectations and motivation. Expectations must be realistic. Patients, particularly those with higher-level injuries, should understand that the substitution of orthoses for upright mobility rather than utilization of a wheelchair is the exception rather than the rule.[43,56,90,129,155] Patients may accomplish limited indoor functional mobility with bracing and in most cases (with assistance and time) can continue to use upright mobility for therapeutic benefits.[43,90,124] Patients and caregivers must understand that upright mobility is not a treatment of spinal cord injury. During semistructured interviews before starting gait training, some caregivers have expressed the "hope" that using braces would "wake up" the spinal cord and promote recovery (personal communication, senior author). On the other hand, other interviewees did not expect neurological recovery but viewed upright mobility as another important step in the rehabilitation process. These patients/caregivers expressed to the coauthor (R.C.) that even if they did not have long-term use of the braces, at least they knew they could do it.

For patients who are interested in being upright for psychological and physiological benefits but are not interested in mobility, the most appropriate device may be a stander.[56,124,150] For children, several options are available. A custom stander, such as the L-frame (Fig. 27-3, *A*), can be ordered. The parapodium and swivel standers can provide the ability to be upright with limited mobility using a footplate or an oval bottom.[147,162] By using assistive devices, patients can move slowly, leaning their body to one side and rotating the trunk to the opposite side. The Rabbit, an appliance in which a patient is strapped into a stander and has large wheelchairlike wheels for mobility, is another option. (Fig. 27-3, *B*). For children and adults, standing can be accomplished with commercially available standers. These standers have either a seat into which the patient transfers or straps to secure the pelvis so that the patient can stand positioned directly from the wheelchair. A hydraulic pump on the side of the stander aids transition to the upright posture (Fig. 27-3, *B*).

To help the patient understand the limitations of custom orthoses for upright mobility, a thorough interview and physical examination are required. During the interview, the clinician should determine why the patient wants to be upright and what he or she hopes to accomplish. For example, consider an athletic patient with a T9 injury and no significant comorbidities. If this patient's goal is spontaneity of activities for short

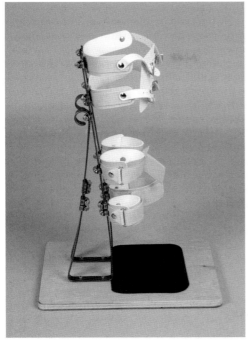

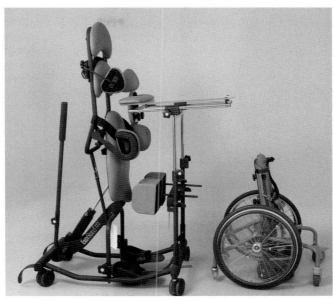

A   B

Fig. 27-3 A, Custom L-frame stander. **B**, Rabbit stander and adult stander. For the adult stander, the patient transfers on the standers seat and then uses the hydralic pump to transition to standing.

distances, using lightweight KAFOs that can be hidden under clothing may be appropriate. On the other hand, if the patient is interested in using the orthoses for limited function and prefers a reciprocating gait pattern, then a Parawalker or RGO may be more suitable. To ensure understanding of the pros and cons of orthosis use, patients should talk to peers who have used braces in the past. Videos will help patients visualize the different assistive devices used, gait patterns, and appearance of orthoses. Temporary adjustable KAFOs and/or trial ARGO are another option (Fig. 27-4).[134]

Once the patient's goals are understood, the physical examination will determine if the patient's expectations are reasonable and what orthosis will be necessary. In general, the higher the level of the injury, the more bracing is required. Orthopedic considerations that affect standing include scoliosis, pelvic

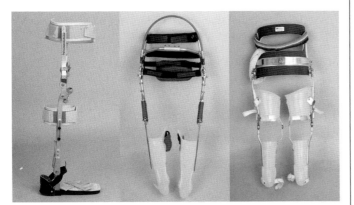

Fig. 27-4 *Left*, Trial adjustable KAFO. *Center*, Trial adjustable ARGO. The ARGO has a single bar connecting each KAFO section, a single cable for driving reciprocal gait, and hydraulic knee joints to assist with stand to/from stand. *Right*, Isocentric RGO.

obliquity, hip subluxation/dislocation, lower limb contractures, spasticity, and history of lower limb fractures. At each joint, ROM should approach normal. A hip flexion contracture greater than 30 degrees and/or knee contractures exceeding 20 degrees, which are not compensated by lumbar lordosis, will limit the patient's ability to achieve and maintain the upright position. At the ankle, up to 15 degrees of plantarflexion contracture can be compensated by a heel wedge and hyperextension at the hip or lumbar lordosis.

If orthopedic considerations are minimal, spasticity should be assessed next. Standing may reduce the severity of spasticity. In contrast, movement may trigger a patient's spasticity, preventing safe advancement of the lower limbs. If spasms are severe, antispasticity medications are an option.[1] Lastly, patients who have not been upright for many weeks are at risk for hypotension. A hypotensive patient can adjust to the upright position by graduated use of a tilt table and compressive elastic garments.

Orthotic management

The two types of braces for individuals with SCI at motor level L2 or above are (H)KAFOs (including RGOs) and KAFOs. Depending on the patient's goals and physical presentation, the type of orthosis and assistive devices will vary. During evaluation and fitting, it is best to consider stability in all planes.

Sagittal plane

At the foot, custom molding the device to the foot is best. Placing the orthosis in the shoes is cosmetically more appealing, allows the orthoses to be worn with a variety of shoes, and facilitates donning of the orthoses (Fig. 27-5). Care should be taken to ensure adequate arch support is provided to prevent

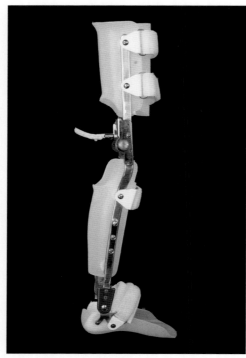

Fig. 27-5 KAFO with custom-molded shoe insert attached to dual-channel adjustable ankle with a bail lock at the knee.

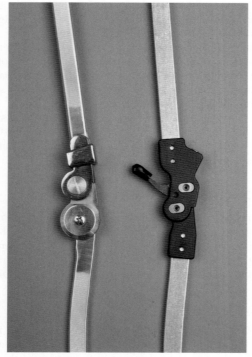

Fig. 27-6 Example of knee locks. *Left,* Drop lock is a metal sleeve that slips over the joint to lock into extension. *Right,* Step lock rachets into extension and is released by upward pressure on the lever.

excessive foot pronation. Without arch support, excessive pronation increases both forefoot and calcaneal valgus, increasing pressure on the head of the fifth metatarsal and the lateral calcaneous.[116] A second option is a steel stirrup riveted to the shoe. A third option, used primarily with the Parawalker and some pediatric RGOs, is a broad external footplate that attaches directly to the two metal supports. The broad base of support will increase standing stability. Because the device is worn external to the shoe, it can be donned and doffed with ease.[130,165] Regardless of the footwear, during initial training a small rocker sole can facilitate toe-off.

At the ankle, options range from a custom solid molded AFO to a variety of joints that attach metal uprights to the foot insert or stirrups. Although a solid AFO maximizes pressure distribution and stability, it minimizes motion of the ankle. Using adjustable ankle joints, dorsiflexion can be adjusted to aid in maintaining parastance. Furthermore, ankle adjustment can be made if the patients gains or loses ROM over time.[11] It has been suggested that special modifications to a patient's shoe may increase walking speed and step length.[153]

For sagittal stability at the knee, several options are available. The most common type of joint is a ring-type drop lock that the patient pushes down over the orthotic knee joint (Fig. 27-6, *left*). Another common lock is the Step Lock (Steplock OTS Corp., Weaverville, NC) which ratchets into position and is released with a lever (Fig. 27-6, *right*). A pawl lock automatically locks the knee when fully extended and is released by upward pressure. Some orthoses are made with the pawl locks attached by a metal "bail" behind the knee (Fig. 27-6).[141] Using the bail, patients can back up to a chair, apply upward pressure to the bail, and release the locks to allow sitting. With the bail some caution is necessary over tight trousers or adductor spasticity, which can accidentally trigger the unlocking mechanism. A mechanical locking mechanism is unnecessary in patients with sufficient quadriceps strength. A posteriorly offset knee join keeps the knee stable in standing because the orthotic joint axis is posterior to the anatomical knee axis. Caution is warranted with posteriorly offset knee joints because an improper weight shift or standing on a downgoing ramp can destabilize the knee. A more advanced knee joint with gas-filled struts is available with ARGOs.[70] This joint assists with the upward motion during sit-to-stand transfers and provides assistance with deceleration from standing to sitting (Fig. 27-4, *center*). New knee joints are being introduced into clinical use that allow for limited knee flexion during gait or have computers that control stability.[48,127,158]

At the hip, sagittal stability is required for patients who have hip flexion contractures and therefore are unable to achieve the parastance. As for the knee, the most common hip joint is a pair of drop locks attached to a pelvic band. If more trunk stability is required, a custom lumbosacral orthosis or TLSO section can be added. For patients with an RGO, a trunk section is necessary to engage the reciprocating mechanism in stance (Fig. 27-4, *right*). Although the hip component will increase standing stability, the addition of a hip section can make donning and doffing the brace cumbersome.[76] Abduction hinges with locks will control hip adduction and increase the ease of donning/doffing and bowel/bladder management (Fig. 27-7).

Transverse plane stability

Orthotic stability in the transverse plane typically is achieved by connecting the legs of the orthoses, which can be done at

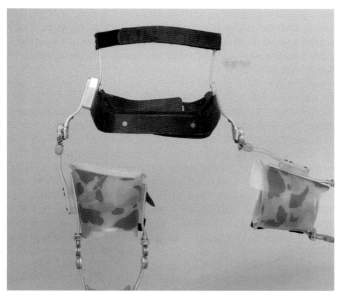

Fig. 27-7 HKAFO with bilateral abduction hinges (right side unlocked in picture) for ease of donning/doffing and bowel/bladder management.

or below the hip. The hip sections can be linked with a pelvic band for increased stability in the transverse plane. If sagittal stability at the hip is not an issue, the hip joints can remain unlocked, allowing a reciprocal gait pattern as in the HGO. Reported benefits of the HGO are its lateral stiffness, which prevents adduction during swing through of the free limb, and broad footplates, which encourage stability during double limb stance.[130,148] A patient with a hip obliquity due to scoliosis or hip subluxation will have difficulty

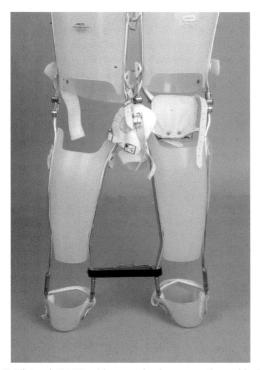

Fig. 27-8 Bilateral KAFO with spreader bar near the ankle joint to increase transverse plane stability.

maintaining parallel alignment of the lower limbs and thus may benefit from some type of connected hip section. It has been suggested that children, whose Y-ligaments are more pliable, may have trouble maintaining a stable parastance and would benefit from a pelvic section.[102] Transverse stability also can be achieved by linking each leg below the hip by using a spreader bar; however, a spreader bar does eliminate the possibility of a reciprocal gait (Fig. 27-8). For a reciprocal gait without transversing the hip, KAFO sections can be linked with a single medial hinge joint such as the walkabout orthosis (WO) or the Primewalk orthosis.[103–105,153]

Current research

Orthoses

An individual with an SCI who learns about bracing for ambulation frequently assumes that the braces will allow functional ambulation, replacing the wheelchair. Unfortunately, for most patients (particularly those with lesions above T12), this goal is unrealistic because of the physiological demands of ambulation with orthoses.[12,20,49,60,164] Gordon and Vanderwalde[49] conducted one of the first studies quantifying energy expenditure in neurologically impaired patients. They concluded that the high-energy costs are prohibitive for ongoing ambulation. They ended their study by concluding that "paraplegic ambulation ranges from moderate to hard work and must be judiciously prescribed." Confirming the decreased efficiency of paraplegic ambulation, Cerny[20] compared the energy required for level walking with KAFOs to wheelchair propulsion in patients with paraplegia. He found that subjects traveled at more than twice the velocity at a statistically lower physiological cost when using a wheelchair as compared to walking. Comparing published metabolic measures for paraplegic brace ambulation to noninjured subject walking, he found that velocity was half, with the rate of oxygen uptake increased by 50%. Furthermore, the respiratory quotient was 0.12 higher than normals, indicating increased dependency on anaerobic energy production. When compared to paraplegic wheelchair propulsion, the subject's heart rate, oxygen uptake, and respiratory quotient mirrored normal walking with only 2% to 6% increase. He confirmed earlier reports that the energy expenditure during paraplegic ambulation was nine times greater than that of normals.[24,101] Merkel et al.[101] found that for higher-level injury (C8–T3), energy per meter during ambulation was 25 times that of normals. Looking at more functional tasks with KAFOs, Miller et al.[107] compared energy expenditure of patients with SCI to normals while negotiating different architectural barriers found in a typical environment, such as ramps, stairways, narrow corridors, and multiple turns. They found that, depending on the task, the energy cost per meter was up to 15 times that of noninjured subjects. Their studies support what patients discover, namely, that functional mobility in a wheelchair is more efficient than walking with braces.[20,43,56,90,129,155]

More recent studies suggest that adding the hip component has reduced overall energy costs. Nene et al.[118,119] studied energy costs in 10 subjects with T4–9 spinal lesion who used the Parawalker (HGO) and compared their results to the published literature on KAFOs. They found that braces that crossed the hips increased the users' velocity of ambulation and reduced energy cost. Improvement in gait efficiency with HGOs may make ambulation a realistic active activity in patients with mid- to high-level injuries. In a comparison of HGO to RGOs, Banta et al.[8] found that HGOs produced a more efficient gait and a greater walking velocity. Whittle et al.[165] studied a group of 18 patients who trained with both HGOs and RGOs. Their report did not look at energy costs but rather a series of tasks and self-reported ease of use. At the end of the study, of the 16 patients, 12 chose to continue with their RGOs and 4 with the HGOs. Ease of donning and doffing was reported with use of HGOs, whereas the RGOs were preferred for their appearance and stability when standing. In another study comparing within the same patient, Katz et al.[79] compared the energy efficiency of patients with myelodysplasia who were using an HKAFO or an RGO. They found the mean oxygen cost was 1.5 mL/kg/m with the HKAFO and 0.73 mL/kg/m with the RGO. Patients were faster with the RGO than with the HKAFO (14.6 m/min and 11.9 m/min, respectively). Using braces in the community setting, several patients commented that the RGO was easier to manage on rough terrain. At the end of the study, seven of the eight subjects preferred to continue use of the RGO. In a comparison of the LSU RGO and the IRGO, Windchester et al.[167] examined energy cost using the physiologic cost index (PCI, calculated by dividing the difference between walking and resting heart rate by velocity). They found in four subjects with paraplegia that PCI was significantly lower for IRGO compared to RGOs and concluded that energy costs were lower for the IRGO.

Comparing IRGOs to the WO, Harvy et al.[53] also found lower metabolic demands with the RGOs. In their randomized cross-over study of 10 patients with complete T9–12 paraplegia, oxygen cost was essentially twice as much with the WO (range 3.95–4.91) compared to the IRGOs (range 1.6–1.8).[53] Furthermore, the IRGOs resulted in a faster more independent gait among patients.[55] Regardless of the advantages of the IRGOs over the WO, both orthoses were used mainly for therapeutic purposes only once every 1 to 2 weeks.[54]

It is clear from the literature that metabolic efficiency does necessarily translate to the primary outcome of long-term orthotic use. In addition to metabolic economy, the independence, cosmesis, reliability, and cost (as described by Stallard et al.[149]) are crucial to the successful design of an orthosis. A wide range of long-term orthotic use has been reported in the literature. Major et al.[92] reviewed the charts of 42 patients older than 16 years who were prescribed the Parawalker. Their cohort included patients with myelomeningocele and traumatic or acquired SCI. They found 59.5% compliance with the braces after 71 months. This finding supports a report by Moore and Stallard,[108] who found that Parawalker use at an average follow-up of 34.4 months was 64% in 50 adult patients with spinal lesions. This finding is similar to a previously reported study with a shorter follow-up period of 20 months that found 85% (17/20 patients) Parawalker use.[152] Franceschini et al.[43] examined the outcomes of 74 patients with SCI. In this multicenter study with much shorter follow-up of 6 months, reported orthosis use was 68%. The majority of patients reported using their orthosis for functional gait or therapeutic exercise. The authors found correlations between functional ambulation and age, level of lesion, stair climbing ability, duration of training, and lapse of orthosis use. They suggested that by discharge from the hospital, the patient

should use the orthosis 5 to 6 hours per day indoors and outdoors and should be able to climb some stairs.[43] Jaspers et al.[69] found a similarly high rate of use. In their report of 14 patients, 85% who were prescribed ARGOs continued their use after 3.3 years of follow-up.

Although these results are encouraging, lower proportions of use also have been reported.[25,42,43,56,61,106,129,132,150,155,161] Robb et al.[129] followed 22 patients with L3–4 and above paraplegia (mostly spina bifida) who were randomly prescribed either an RGO or an HGO. At 1 year, regardless of type of orthotic assigned, none of the participants were scored as wheelchair users on the Hoffner scale. At follow-up of all participants at 5 years, orthosis used dropped to 45%, and after another 5 years was 23%. Similar to previously published work, the HGO required fewer repairs than RGOs.[90] Using a mailed questionnaire, Eng et al.[42] found that 30% of respondents participated in some form of standing activity, mostly for therapeutic than for functional purposes. Subjective benefits of standing included a "feeling of well-being, looking others in their eye, reduction of spasticity, improved circulation, digestion, breathing, sleep, pain, and bowel/bladder function." Their reported outcomes may actually be lower as they had a response rate of only 35%.[42] In another study, 85 patients given an RGO from 1986 to 1993 were sent questionnaires regarding orthotic use. In this study, nonresponders or unreachable patients were classified as nonusers.[155] After a mean follow-up of 5.4 years, only 29% were classified as orthosis users. In this study, higher use was associated with function independence and age.[155] Scivoletto et al.[135] examined the outcomes of orthotic use based on social, physical, and psychological factors in patients with SCI who received gait training with RGOs. After 1 year, 56% of patients continued using their RGO. Similar to previous studies, they found associations with nonuse because of difficulty during functional activities such as donning/doffing, car transfers, outdoor ambulation, and stair climbing. Examining psychological outcomes, they found that nonusers had higher frequency values over the mean in the extroversion scale for the Eysenck Personality Questionnaire. This study underscores the importance of not only trying to make an orthosis more energy efficient but also exploring the expectations, motivations, and goals of the patients.[135]

Caution is warranted when comparing outcomes across studies. There is significant variation in orthosis designs, assistive devices, patient ages, caregiver support, gait patterns, and orthosis experience. Furthermore, it is unclear if the level of injury reported is for the highest level of neurological impairment or highest motor impairment.

Hybrid systems

In recent years, more attention has been given to the combination of functional electrical stimulation (FES) and (H)KAFO.[58,65,120,125,126] By stimulating key muscles, such as the hip flexors, leg advancement is an active rather than passive motion. The goal is to increase efficiency of walking and ease of transfers from sitting to standing, increase stability in stance, and improve incline ambulation while reaping the physiological benefits of muscle activation.[58,59,144]

In a series of 70 patients who trained with the RGO II hybrid (RGO with FES), Solomonow et al.[142,145] found significant physiological benefits marked by a reduction in spasticity, lower total cholesterol and low-density lipid profiles, and increased knee extensor torque. Trends toward improved cardiac output, stroke volume, and vital capacity also were noted. They concluded that use of the hybrid RGO II results in general improvement of physiological conditions when used 3 to 4 hours per week.[143] Also worth noting is continuation of use after discharge from training. Of the 70 subjects who started the study, 41 were contacted to assess use, utility, and impact on quality of life postdischarge. Approximately 80% of the 41 patients were considered regular users at follow-up. Main reasons for nonuse were lack of motivation, time, and family support, environmental barriers, and medical problems.[142,143]

Hirokawa et al.[58] examined the energy consumption of six patients with paraplegia while ambulating with an RGO, RGO with FES, or KAFO. They found that energy costs were lowest for the RGO with FES, followed by RGO alone and then KAFO. Although energy expenditure remained higher than with normal walking, they suggested that the addition of FES may "provide paraplegics a mode of independent ambulation superior to that of a wheelchair."[58] Syke et al.[154,156] studied energy expenditure in patients ambulating 5 minutes with an RGO with or without FES. They found that addition of FES during short-distance ambulation provided no substantial benefit in terms of energy expenditure or long-term use. Similarly, in a comparison of the Parawalker, RGO, and RGO with FES, Merati et al.[100] found that ambulation with the RGO with FES did not substantially decrease energy expenditure. Although no substantial reduction in energy expenditure was detected, they did find improvement of locomotion as a consequence of hemodynamic effects. At 4-year follow-up, only three RGO users continued with orthosis use.

Limited bracing with FES

Lower limb FES is another option for providing upright mobility for patients with complete and incomplete SCI. Use of FES has several advantages over use of (H)KAFO. When FES is used to enable standing, the knees start in a flexed position as opposed to being locked into extension as with the (H)KAFO. This reduces the lever arm and creates less force to be overcome by the upper extremities during sit-to-stand transfers. Children with motor complete SCI could stand up faster[15] and independently when using FES in combination with AFOs compared to (H)KAFOs only.[73] Johnston et al.[73] attributed this gain in speed and independence to decreased demand on the upper limbs when the transition was started in the flexed knee position. Using FES to stand from the wheelchair allows this transition in more confined areas because the feet remain close to the wheelchair. With (H)KAFOs locked into knee extension, the feet are farther from the wheelchair when the user begins to stand, which then requires more space for this task.[15] Another advantage of FES is that the user can sit in the wheelchair without concern for fit as a result of bulky (H)KAFOs.[73] FES uses the person's muscles to stand, which potentially provides a conditioning effect.

In addition to clinical requirements for successful upright mobility with (H)KAFOs, an important consideration with FES is the innervation status of the lower limb muscles of interest. FES requires that the lower motor neurons (LMNs) be intact in order to obtain a stimulated response.

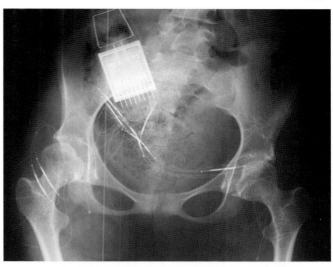

Fig. 27-9 Example of a completely implanted FES system (NeuroControl Corp., North Ridgeville, OH) consisting of an implanted control unit placed under the skin in the right abdomen. The electrode leads are tunneled under the skin to reach the targeted muscles.

The incidence of damage to the LMN increases as the level of injury progresses caudally in adults with SCI.[39,75] With injuries sustained to the spinal cord at the level of L1 and lower, the likelihood of damage to the LMN has been shown to be greater.[39,75] When a potential user is evaluated, the presence of spasticity is a clinical sign that the LMN is intact and that muscles likely are innervated. However, a test of the stimulated responses of targeted muscles should be performed. Diagnostic electromyographic testing can be conducted if questions about innervation status remain.

Most of the research on FES for upright mobility involves muscle stimulation with electrodes placed on the skin surface[16,85] or through percutaneous intramuscular electrodes[15,73,82,110,111,140] that are implanted directly into the muscle and exit at the skin surface. Collectively, this research has shown that upright mobility with FES is feasible and safe. More recently, completely implanted systems have been used in adults[30–32,72,83,84,159] and in children with motor complete SCI (Fig. 27-9).[13,73] Some studies have used AFOs in combination with FES.[13,31,72,73,84] Implanted electrodes provide the user with a more permanent system. An implanted system avoids the challenges of applying surface electrodes daily, caring for percutaneous electrodes, and managing multiple external cables between the stimulator and the electrodes. Another advantage of the implanted system is that it makes FES use more spontaneous as the radiofrequency antenna that communicates with the external controller can be easily worn throughout the day (Fig. 27-10). Although these systems have functional benefits, they require a surgical procedure with potential complications and at this time are available only as research devices.

FES for reciprocal walking

Systems designed to create a reciprocal walking pattern for individuals with motor complete SCI have used skin surface electrodes, percutaneous electrodes, and completely implanted FES systems. One surface stimulation system, the Parastep (Sigmedics, Fairborn, OH), is approved by the Food and Drug Administration (FDA) and is

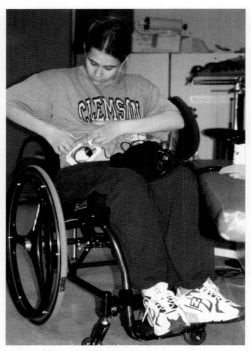

Fig. 27-10 Radiofrequency antenna is placed over the skin, directly over the site of the implanted control unit. This antenna enables communication between the internal and external components.

commercially available. Because functional outcomes with the Parastep are comparable to those of the (H)KAFO, it has been approved by the Centers for Medicare and Medicaid. The Parastep system provides a reciprocal walking pattern via stimulation to the gluteals and/or back extensors, the quadriceps, and the peroneal nerve to create a flexor withdrawal response. A microcomputer contained within a portable stimulation device provides the stimulation patterns required for gait.[16] The user activates the stimulation using push buttons on the walker.[85] The system is recommended for persons with neurologically stable complete SCI, adequate trunk control and upper body strength, and without a history of significant medical issues or irreversible contractures. Individuals with incomplete injuries who cannot extend their knees fully and can tolerate the sensation of stimulation also may be able to use the Parastep system.[51] The system is intended to be an alternative to a wheelchair and not a substitute. Individuals with primarily complete paraplegia can obtain independent ambulation with a walker with walking speeds of 0.03 to 0.4 m/s[16,67] and peak walking and standing times of 6 to 187 minutes.[81] The Parastep is associated with improvements in cardiovascular function,[16,67,68,113] lower limb blood flow,[113] muscle size,[16,81] lean tissue,[81] and stimulated muscle strength.[16] Changes in bone mineral density at the hip have not been observed.[117]

Percutaneous FES for reciprocal walking currently is available only in research applications. Studies using percutaneous FES for individuals with complete SCI have evaluated walking with an assistive device while stimulating from 8 to 24 muscles. In individuals with motor complete paraplegia, percutaneous FES for reciprocal gait is energy demanding[82] and allows walking speeds ranging from only 0.4 to 0.5 m/s.[82,83]

Other systems have used both 16-channel[84] and 18-channel systems[72] to achieve a reciprocal walking pattern with an assistive device. Despite the number of electrodes, subjects in both studies wore AFOs for standing and walking activities. Use of this system did allow one subject to ascend stairs using a reciprocal pattern.[72]

FES for swing-through and swing-to walking

Some studies have focused on achieving a walking pattern that more closely resembles typical gait. However, other studies have used fewer electrodes without attempting to mimic typical gait. Instead, these studies have focused on the use of FES to create the swing-through or swing-to pattern more typically seen when wearing an (H)KAFO. This swing-through/swing-to pattern may be more energy efficient. The goal of these systems typically has been short-distance ambulation.

The swing-through/swing-to walking pattern has been achieved using percutaneous and implanted systems, usually with the user wearing bilateral AFOs. Two studies have compared these systems to (H)KAFOs. Bonaroti et al.[15] reported that children and adolescents required equal or less assistance when walking with FES or (H)KAFO. Using this same system, Bonaroti et al.[14] showed that a child with paraplegia had a similar walking distance and energy cost (oxygen consumption divided by walking speed) when walking with FES and (H)KAFOs but that oxygen consumption was greater with FES. The child reported that he stopped walking with FES when he felt overall fatigue and stopped walking with (H)KAFOs because of upper limb pain.[14] In a later study, Johnston et al.[73] compared the functional use of an eight-channel completely implanted FES and bilateral AFO to the use of (H)KAFOs in children and adolescents with SCI and found overall similar results.

Finally, Johnston et al.[72] looked at swing-through gait in addition to reciprocal gait using an 18-channel implanted system. Young adult subjects could ambulate using a swing-through gait pattern for 39.3 to 251.1 m during a 6-minute walk test, far slower than a typical walking speed. The subjects preferred this walking pattern and therefore did not practice the reciprocal pattern sufficiently to become skillful with it.

FES for standing, transfers, and exercise

Another potential advantage of FES over traditional orthoses for individuals with complete SCI is that FES can be used more spontaneously during the day for short-duration functional activities, such as transfers and standing to perform functional activities. Although both FES and orthoses can provide exercise while walking, percutaneous and implanted FES systems have the advantage of providing exercise to individual muscles in a more traditional strengthening mode.

Moynahan et al.[110] studied functional home use of a percutaneous FES system that stimulated up to 11 muscles per leg and reported that participants used the FES system every 3 to 4 days. FES was used for exercise 51% to 84% of the time, with the remaining time used for functional activities, including reaching and other one-handed tasks. FES also was used to perform activities such as standing to play video games, doing laundry, cooking, and retrieving items from a car trunk.

Two studies compared the use of FES and (H)KAFOs during brief upright functional activities. The studies found that children and adolescents could complete the activities in at least equal time when they used FES compared to (H)KAFOs.[15,73] Bonaroti et al.[15] reported that two transfer activities (standing to reach a high object and transferring to a high surface) were significantly faster with a percutaneous FES system, likely because the knees did not have to be locked prior to standing as with (H)KAFOs and because of decreased demand on the upper extremities. Johnston et al.[73] reported differences in levels of assistance required when a completely implanted FES system versus (H)KAFOs was used. Several younger children could not stand from the wheelchair without assistance with (H)KAFOs but could with FES, providing them with more functional independence.

Johnston et al.[72] later examined similar short-term outcome measures in three participants implanted with an 18-channel FES system for standing and reciprocal or swing-through walking with bilateral AFOs. In addition to being able to complete short-duration functional activities, the participants could stand continuously for 16 to 34 minutes, providing the potential for longer-duration functional activities while standing.

Agarwal et al.[2] reported that adults with at least 1 year of experience with an eight-channel implanted FES system used it 2 to 4+ times per week for exercise and standing. The system helped with transfers, circulation, maneuvering in areas where the wheelchair did not fit, and ROM exercises. All subjects felt that their health had improved as a result of using the system and that the system was safe, reliable, and easy to use.[2] Davis et al.[30] reported that most subjects could stand with 90% of their weight on the lower limbs and that the system assisted with stand pivot transfers for individuals with higher-level injuries, thus decreasing the demand on the caregiver.

FES and incomplete SCI

Although most of the FES research has focused on the population with motor complete SCI, several studies have evaluated the ability of FES to impact function in individuals with incomplete SCI. Studies of FES in this population typically have used FES to augment the user's current gait pattern and have used both surface and percutaneous electrodes with or without supplemental orthoses. Improvements have been shown in muscle strength,[50,74] energy expenditure during walking,[50,74,87] walking speed,[74,87,151] walking distance,[87] step length,[87] and walking patterns[6,7,74,87] both with stimulation turned on and turned off. Various combinations of muscles were stimulated, ranging from a single channel of stimulation to multiple channels. Two commonly selected stimulation sites are the quadriceps femoris and the peroneal nerve to create a withdrawal reflex.[74,87,151]

Best practices

In general, comparing outcomes from different studies is difficult. In a review of 12 studies, Ijzerman et al.[63] found several threats to both internal and external validity that make comparing studies difficult, if not impossible. As they point out, many studies did not have control groups. Of the studies that used control groups, weaknesses were found in the test methodology, lack of statistical power, and variability in inclusion criteria (e.g., level of injury, motivation to

ambulation, orthosis design, age, etc.). The literature has demonstrated a large range (8%–85%) of orthotic use by individuals with SCI after discharge.[56,152] Because of the cost of bracing (up to $5,000 US, not including FES) and associated cost of gait training, some authors have questioned the utility of prescribing orthoses for upright mobility.[4,54,55,90,135] A stander or a standing wheelchair may accomplish the goal of maintaining the patient upright while improving compliance to being upright.[56,124,150] Others believe that in addition to the possible physiological benefits, the psychological benefits of upright standing warrant continued use of orthoses with or without FES.[21,42,76,96,97,115,132,152,155]

Although the purposes and the range of studies are broad, several themes are evident. First and foremost, (H)KAFOs and/or FES for upright mobility rarely replace a wheelchair as the primary means of mobility. Compliance tends to be higher for patients who can use their orthoses for functional purposes.[52,115,155] A substantial number of patients who continue orthosis use for upright mobility do so for the reported therapeutic benefit. The level of injury is inversely related to (H)KAFO use, which would be expected based upon the increased physiological demand.[24,61] More recently, some success with Parawalker use for higher-level injuries has been described.[118,219] Although studied less frequently in SCI, an inverse relationship between age and orthotic use has been suggested.[106,108,150,152,155,161] This pattern also has been noted in patients with myelodysplasia.[9,23,52,95,129,166] Other obstacles to brace use include difficulty donning/doffing, obesity, dependence on others for guarding assistance, and mechanical breakdown of the orthotics.[43,90,129,155,165] Donning and doffing of braces that extend above the hips are particularly difficult, and these braces may interfere with more complex situations, such as moving to/from a couch or car transfers.[76,108,135]

Emerging evidence shows that patients with SCI are at risk for chronic conditions of age due to inactivity, such as hypertension, cardiovascular disease, obesity, and diabetes.[10,34,45,64,66,122,123,163] Therefore, it is important for patients to find enjoyable physical activities that encourage exercise. For some patients, (H)KAFOs and/or FES may provide the opportunity for limited exercise doing an enjoyable activity. Equally important are the self-reported physiological benefits of bowel/bladder management, pressure relief, and spasticity reduction and the reported psychological benefits, such as looking at peers at eye level and feeling and looking more "normal."

- Orthoses are prescribed for stabilization after injury and to facilitate normal growth
- Anti-footdrop orthoses are commonly prescribed in the SCI population to prevent plantarflexion contractures
- In the SCI population, TLSOs can be prescribed for spine and pelvic stability[94,99,112,137,138]
- Orthoses are commonly prescribed to achieve therapeutic and in some cases functional upright mobility
- For C4–T3 motor levels, encourage use of stander for obtaining upright positioning[26,56,132,150]
- For C7–L1 motor levels, encourage use of either a stander and/or orthosis for upright mobility, generally for therapeutic exercise but for possible functional mobility[24,26,42,43,90,92,97,101,115]
- Higher-level injuries (C7–T10 motor levels) likely will benefit from a hip component, such as an HGO (Parawalker), RGO, or (H)KAFO[8,102,119]

- When prescribing any orthosis, encourage the patient to be realistic about goals for daily use of orthoses[132,135,155,161]
- The pediatric population has higher use of orthoses for upright mobility, but use most likely declines with age[9,129,155,162,166]
- During training, maximize independence in donning/doffing, ambulation, and stair climbing prior to discharge[97,115,135,149,155,167]
- Incorporating FES with an RGO or Parawalker may decrease energy cost during ambulation while providing physiological benefits[100,142,143,145]
- Advancements in surface, percutaneous, and implanted systems demonstrate promise for future independent ambulation[2,6,7,16,30,31,68,71,73,74,81-84,113,117,151,159]

References

1. Adams MM, Hicks AL: Spasticity after spinal cord injury, *Spinal Cord* 43:577–586, 2005.
2. Agarwal S, Triolo RJ, Kobetic R, et al: Long-term user perceptions of an implanted neuroprosthesis for exercise, standing, and transfers after spinal cord injury, *J Rehabil Res Dev* 40:241–252, 2003.
3. American Spinal Injury Association: International Standards for neurological classification of spinal cord injury, revised 2002. Chicago, 2002, American Spinal Injury Association
4. Atrice A: lower extremity orthotic management for the spinal cord injured client, *Top Spinal Cord Inj Rehabil* 5:1–10, 2000.
5. Atrice M, Gonter M, Griffin S, Morrison S: Traumatic spinal cord injury. In Umphred D, editor: *Neurological rehabilitation*, St. Louis, 1990, Mosby.
6. Bajd T, Kralj A, Stefancic M, Lavrac N: Use of functional electrical stimulation in the lower extremities of incomplete spinal cord injured patients, *Artif Organs* 23:403–409, 1999.
7. Bajd T, Stefancic M, Matjacic Z, et al: Improvement in step clearance via calf muscle stimulation, *Med Biol Eng Comput* 35:113–116, 1997.
8. Banta JV, Bell KJ, Muik EA, Fezio J: Parawalker: energy cost of walking, *Eur J Pediatr Surg* 1(suppl 1):7–10, 1991.
9. Bartonek A, Saraste H, Samuelsson L, Skoog M: Ambulation in patients with myelomeningocele: a 12-year follow-up, *J Pediatr Orthop* 19:202–206, 1999.
10. Bauman W, Spungen A: Disorders of carbohydrate and lipid metabolism in veterans with paraplegia or quadriplegia: a model of premature aging, *Metabolism* 43:749–756, 1997.
11. Ben M, Harvey L, Denis S, et al: Does 12 weeks of regular standing prevent loss of ankle mobility and bone mineral density in people with recent spinal cord injuries? *Aust J Physiother* 51:251–256, 2005.
12. Bernardi M, Canale I, Castellano V, Di Filippo L, Felici F, Marchetti M: The efficiency of walking of paraplegic patients using a reciprocating gait orthosis, *Paraplegia* 33:409–415, 1995.
13. Betz RR, Johnston TE, Smith BT, Mulcahey MJ, McCarthy JJ: Three-year follow-up of an implanted functional electrical stimulation system for upright mobility in a child with a thoracic level spinal cord injury, *J Spinal Cord Med* 25:345–350, 2002.
14. Bonaroti D, Akers J, Smith BT, Mulcahey MJ, Betz RR: A comparison of FES with KAFO for providing ambulation and upright mobility in a child with a complete thoracic spinal cord injury, *J Spinal Cord Med* 22:159–166, 1999.
15. Bonaroti D, Akers JM, Smith BT, Mulcahey MJ, Betz RR: Comparison of functional electrical stimulation to long leg braces for upright mobility for children with complete thoracic level spinal injuries, *Arch Phys Med Rehabil* 80:1047–1053, 1999.
16. Brissot R, Gallien P, Le Bot MP, et al: Clinical experience with functional electrical stimulation-assisted gait with Parastep in spinal cord-injured patients, *Spine* 25:501–508, 2000.
17. Brown JC, Swank SM, Matta J, Barras DM: Late spinal deformity in quadriplegic children and adolescents, *J Pediatr Orthop* 4:456–461, 1984.
18. Bulter PB, Major RE, Patrick JH: The technique of reciprocal walking using the hip guidance orthosis (HGO) with crutches, *Prosthet Orthot Int* 8:33–38, 1984.
19. Campbell J, Bonnett C: Spinal cord injury in children, *Clin Orthop Relat Res* 112:114–123, 1975.
20. Cerny K: Energetics of walking and wheelchair propulsion in paraplegic patients, *Orthop Clin North Am* 9:370–372, 1978.
21. Chafetz R: Bracing for success, *SCI Nurs* 19:196–198, 2002.

22. Chafetz R, McDonald C, Mulcahey MJ, et al: Timed motor test for wheelchair users: initial development and application in children with spinal cord injury, *J Spinal Cord Med* 27(Suppl 1):S38–S43, 2004.
23. Charney EB, Melchionni JB, Smith DR: Community ambulation by children with myelomeningocele and high-level paralysis, *J Pediatr Orthop* 11:579–582, 1991.
24. Clinkingbeard JR, Gersten JW, Hoehn D: Energy cost of ambulation in the traumatic paraplegic, *Am J Phys Med* 43:157–165, 1964.
25. Coghlan JK, Robinson CE, Newmarch B, Jackson G: Lower extremity bracing in paraplegia: a follow-up study, *Paraplegia* 18:25–32, 1980.
26. Consortium for Spinal Cord Medicine: *Outcomes following traumatic SCI: clinical practice guidelines for health care professionals*, Washington D.C., 1999, Paralyzed Veterans of America.
27. Cuddeford TJ, Freeling RP, Thomas SS, et al: Energy consumption in children with myelomeningocele: a comparison between reciprocating gait orthosis and hip-knee-ankle-foot orthosis ambulators, *Dev Med Child Neurol* 39:239–242, 1997.
28. Dall P, Granat M: The function of the reciprocal link in paraplegic orthotic gait, *J Prosthetcs Orthosis* 13:10–13, 2001.
29. Dall PM, Muller B, Stallard I, Edwards J, Granat MH: The functional use of the reciprocal hip mechanism during gait for paraplegic patients walking in the Louisiana State University reciprocating gait orthosis, *Prosthet Orthot Int* 23:152–162, 1999.
30. Davis JA Jr, Triolo RJ, Uhlir J, et al: Preliminary performance of a surgically implanted neuroprosthesis for standing and transfers: where do we stand? *J Rehabil Res Dev* 38:609–617, 2001.
31. Davis R, Houdayer T, Andrews B, Barriskill A: Paraplegia: prolonged standing using closed-loop functional electrical stimulation and Andrews ankle-foot orthosis, *Artif Organs* 23:418–420, 1999.
32. Davis R, Patrick J, Barriskill A: Development of functional electrical stimulators utilizing cochlear implant technology, *Med Eng Phys* 23:61–68, 2001.
33. Dearolf WW III, Betz RR, Vogel LC, Levin J, Clancy M, Steel HH: Scoliosis in pediatric spinal cord-injured patients, *J Pediatr Orthop* 10:214–218, 1990.
34. Dearwater SR, LaPorte RE, Robertson RJ, Brenes G, Adams LL, Becker D: Activity in the spinal cord-injured patient: an epidemiologic analysis of metabolic parameters, *Med Sci Sports Exerc* 18:541–544, 1986.
35. DeVivo MJ, Black KJ, Stover SL: Causes of death during the first 12 years after spinal cord injury, *Arch Phys Med Rehabil* 74:248–254, 1993.
36. DeVivo MJ, Go BK, Jackson AB: Overview of the national spinal cord injury statistical center database, *J Spinal Cord Med* 25:335–338, 2002.
37. DeVivo MJ, Shewchuk RM, Stover SL, Black KJ, Go BK: A cross-sectional study of the relationship between age and current health status for persons with spinal cord injuries, *Paraplegia* 30:820–827, 1992.
38. DeVivo MJ, Stover SL: Long-term survival and causes of death. In Stover S, Delisa J, Whiteneck G, editors: *Spinal cord injury: clinical outcomes from the model systems*, Gaithersburg, Md, 2004, Aspen Publication.
39. Doherty JG, Burns AS, O'Ferrall DM, Ditunno JF Jr: Prevalence of upper motor neuron vs lower motor neuron lesions in complete lower thoracic and lumbar spinal cord injuries, *J Spinal Cord Med* 25:289–292, 2002.
40. Douglas R, Larson PF, D'Ambrosia R, McCall RE: The LSU-reciprocation-gait orthosis, *Orthopaedics* 6:834–838, 1983.
41. Drummond D, Breed AL, Narechania R: Relationship of spine deformity and pelvic obliquity on sitting pressure distributions and decubitus ulceration, *J Pediatr Orthop* 5:396–402, 1985.
42. Eng JJ, Levins SM, Townson AF, Mah-Jones D, Bremner J, Huston G: Use of prolonged standing for individuals with spinal cord injuries, *Phys Ther* 81:1392–1399, 2001.
43. Franceschini M, Baratta S, Zampolini M, Loria D, Lotta S: Reciprocating gait orthoses: a multicenter study of their use by spinal cord injured patients, *Arch Phys Med Rehabil* 78:582–586, 1997.
44. Frankel HL, Hancock DO, Hyslop G, et al: The value of postural reduction in the initial management of closed injuries of the spine with paraplegia and tetraplegia. I, *Paraplegia* 7:179–192, 1969.
45. Garshick E, Kelley A, Cohen S, et al: A prospective assessment of mortality in chronic spinal cord injury, *Spinal Cord* 43:408–416, 2005.
46. Genda E, Oota K, Suzuki Y, Koyama K, Kasahara T: A new walking orthosis for paraplegics: hip and ankle linkage system, *Prosthet Orthot Int* 28:69–74, 2004.
47. Go B, DeVivo M, Richards J: The epidemiology of spinal cord injury. In Stover S, Delisa JA, Whiteneck GG, editors: *Spinal cord injury: clinical outcomes from the model systems*, Gaithersburg, Md, 1995, Aspen Publication.
48. Goldfarb M, Korkowski K, Harrold B, Durfee W: Preliminary evaluation of a controlled-brake orthosis for FES-aided gait, *IEEE Trans Neural Syst Rehabil Eng* 11:241–248, 2003.

49. Gordon EE, Vanderwalde H: Energy requirements in paraplegic ambulation, *Arch Phys Med Rehabil* 37:276–285, 1956.

50. Granat MH, Ferguson AC, Andrews BJ, Delargy M: The role of functional electrical stimulation in the rehabilitation of patients with incomplete spinal cord injury: observed benefits during gait studies, *Paraplegia* 31:207–215, 1993.

51. Graupe D, Kohn KH: Functional neuromuscular stimulator for short-distance ambulation by certain thoracic-level spinal-cord-injured paraplegics, *Surg Neurol* 50:202–207, 1998.

52. Guidera KJ, Smith S, Raney E, et al: Use of the reciprocating gait orthosis in myelodysplasia, *J Pediatr Orthop* 13:341–348, 1993.

53. Harvey LA, Davis GM, Smith MB, Engel S: Energy expenditure during gait using the walkabout and isocentric reciprocal gait orthoses in persons with paraplegia, *Arch Phys Med Rehabil* 79:945–949, 1998.

54. Harvey LA, Newton-John T, Davis GM, Smith MB, Engel S: A comparison of the attitude of paraplegic individuals to the walkabout orthosis and the isocentric reciprocal gait orthosis, *Spinal Cord* 35:580–584, 1997.

55. Harvey LA, Smith MB, Davis GM, Engel S: Functional outcomes attained by T9–12 paraplegic patients with the walkabout and the isocentric reciprocal gait orthoses, *Arch Phys Med Rehabil* 78:706–711, 1997.

56. Hawran S, Biering-Sorensen F: The use of long leg calipers for paraplegic patients: a follow-up study of patients discharged 1973–82, *Spinal Cord* 34:666–668, 1996.

57. Hinderer KA, Hinderer SR, Shurtleff DB: Myelodysplasia. In Campbell SK, Vander Linden DW, Palisano RJ, editors: *Physical therapy for children,* ed 2, Philadelphia, 2000, WB Saunders.

58. Hirokawa S, Grimm M, Le T, et al: Energy consumption in paraplegic ambulation using the reciprocating gait orthosis and electric stimulation of the thigh muscles, *Arch Phys Med Rehabil* 71:687–694, 1990.

59. Hirokawa S, Solomonow M, Baratta R, D'Ambrosia R: Energy expenditure and fatiguability in paraplegic ambulation using reciprocating gait orthosis and electric stimulation, *Disabil Rehabil* 18:115–122, 1996.

60. Huang CT, Kuhlemeier KV, Moore NB, Fine PR: Energy cost of ambulation in paraplegic patients using Craig-Scott braces, *Arch Phys Med Rehabil* 60:595–600, 1979.

61. Hussey RW, Stauffer ES: Spinal cord injury: requirements for ambulation, *Arch Phys Med Rehabil* 54:544–547, 1973.

62. IJzerman MJ, Baardman G, Hermens HJ, Veltink PH, Boom HB, Zilvold G: The influence of the reciprocal cable linkage in the advanced reciprocating gait orthosis on paraplegic gait performance, *Prosthet Orthot Int* 21:52–61, 1997.

63. Ijzerman MJ, Baardman G, Hermens HJ, Veltink PH, Boom HB, Zilvold G: Comparative trials on hybrid walking systems for people with paraplegia: an analysis of study methodology, *Prosthet Orthot Int* 23:260–273, 1999.

64. Imai K, Kadowaki T, Aizawa Y, Fukutomi K: Morbidity rates of complications in persons with spinal cord injury according to the site of injury and with special reference to hypertension, *Paraplegia* 32:246–252, 1994.

65. Isakov E, Douglas R, Berns P: Ambulation using the reciprocating gait orthosis and functional electrical stimulation, *Paraplegia* 30:239–245, 1992.

66. Jacobs P, Nash M: Exercise recommendations for individuals with spinal cord injury, *Sports Med* 34:727–751, 2004.

67. Jacobs PL, Mahoney ET: Peak exercise capacity of electrically induced ambulation in persons with paraplegia, *Med Sci Sports Exerc* 34:1551–1556, 2002.

68. Jacobs PL, Nash MS, Klose J, Guest RS, Needham-Shropshire BM, Green BA: Evaluation of a training program for persons with SCI paraplegia using the Parastep 1 ambulation system: part 2. effects on physiological responses to peak arm ergometry, *Arch Phys Med Rehabil* 78:794–798, 1997.

69. Jaspers P, Peeraer L, Van Petegem W, Van der Perre G: The use of an advanced reciprocating gait orthosis by paraplegic individuals: a follow-up study, *Spinal Cord* 35:585–589, 1997.

70. Jefferson RJ, Whittle MW: Performance of three walking orthoses for the paralysed: a case study using gait analysis, *Prosthet Orthot Int* 14:103–110, 1990.

71. Johnston TE: Implanted functional electrical stimulation for upright mobility in pediatric spinal cord injuries, *Advances in Clinical Neuroscience and Rehabilitation* 6:27–28, 2006.

72. Johnston TE, Betz RR, Smith BT, et al: Implantable FES system for upright mobility and bladder and bowel function for individuals with spinal cord injury, *Spinal Cord* 43:713–723, 2005.

73. Johnston TE, Betz RR, Smith BT, Mulcahey MJ: Implanted functional electrical stimulation: an alternative for standing and walking in pediatric spinal cord injury, *Spinal Cord* 41:144–152, 2003.

74. Johnston TE, Finson RL, Smith BT, Bonaroti DM, Betz RR, Mulcahey MJ: Functional electrical stimulation for augmented walking in adolescents with incomplete spinal cord injury, *J Spinal Cord Med* 26:390–400, 2003.

75. Johnston TE, Greco MN, Gaughan JP, Smith BT, Betz RR: Patterns of lower extremity innervation in pediatric spinal cord injury, *Spinal Cord* 43:476–482, 2005.

76. Kaplan L, Grynbaum B, Rusk H, Anastasia T, Gassier S: A reappraisal of braces and other mechanical aids in patients with spinal cord dysfunction: results of a follow-up study, *Arch Phys Med Rehabil* 47:393–405, 1966.

77. Kaplan PE, Gandhavadi B, Richards L, Goldschmidt J: Calcium balance in paraplegic patients: influence of injury duration and ambulation, *Arch Phys Med Rehabil* 59:447–450, 1978.

78. Kaplan PE, Roden W, Gilbert E, Richards L, Goldschmidt JW: Reduction of hypercalciuria in tetraplegia after weight-bearing and strengthening exercises, *Paraplegia* 19:289–293, 1981.

79. Katz DE, Haideri N, Song K, Wyrick P: Comparative study of conventional hip-knee-ankle-foot orthoses versus reciprocating-gait orthoses for children with high-level paraparesis, *J Pediatr Orthop* 17:377–386, 1997.

80. Kilfoyle R, Foley J, Norton P: Spine and pelvic deformity in childhood and adolescent paraplegia: a study of 104 case, *J Bone Joint Surg Am* 47:659–682, 1965.

81. Klose KJ, Jacobs PL, Broton JG, et al: Evaluation of a training program for persons with SCI paraplegia using the Parastep 1 ambulation system: part 1. Ambulation performance and anthropometric measures, *Arch Phys Med Rehabil* 78:789–793, 1997.

82. Kobetic R, Marsolais EB: Synthesis of paraplegic gait with multichannel functional neuromuscular stimulation, *IEEE Trans Rehabil Eng* 2:66–79, 1994.

83. Kobetic R, Triolo RJ, Marsolais EB: Muscle selection and walking performance of multichannel FES systems for ambulation in paraplegia, *IEEE Trans Rehabil Eng* 5:23–29, 1997.

84. Kobetic R, Triolo RJ, Uhlir JP, et al: Implanted functional electrical stimulation system for mobility in paraplegia: a follow-up case report, *IEEE Trans Rehabil Eng* 7:390–398, 1999.

85. Kralj A, Bajd T, Turk R, Krajnik J, Benko H: Gait restoration in paraplegic patients: a feasibility demonstration using multichannel surface electrode FES, *J Rehabil* 20:3–20, 1983.

86. Kunkel CF, Scremin AM, Eisenberg B, Garcia JF, Roberts S, Martinez S: Effect of "standing" on spasticity, contracture, and osteoporosis in paralyzed males, *Arch Phys Med Rehabil* 74:73–78, 1993.

87. Ladouceur M, Barbeau H: Functional electrical stimulation-assisted walking for persons with incomplete spinal injuries: changes in the kinematics and physiological cost of overground walking, *Scand J Rehabil Med* 32:72–79, 2000.

88. Lancourt JE, Dickson JH, Carter RE: Paralytic spinal deformity following traumatic spinal-cord injury in children and adolescents, *J Bone Joint Surg Am* 63:47–53, 1981.

89. Lehmann JF, Warren CG, Hertling D, McGee M, Simons BC, Dralle A: Craig-Scott orthosis: a biochemical and functional evaluation, *Arch Phys Med Rehabil* 57:438–442, 1976.

90. Lotta S, Fiocchi A, Giovannini R, et al: Restoration of gait with orthoses in thoracic paraplegia: a multicentric investigation, *Paraplegia* 32:608–615, 1994.

91. Lubicky JP, Betz RR: Spinal deformity in children and adolescents after spinal cord injury. In Betz RR, Mulcahey MJ, editors: *The child with a spinal cord injury,* Rosemont, Ill, 1996, American Academy of Orthopaedic Surgeons.

92. Major RE, Stallard J, Farmer SE: A review of 42 patients of 16 years and over using the ORLAU Parawalker, *Prosthet Orthot Int* 21:147–152, 1997.

93. Marino RJ, Ditunno JF Jr, Donovan WH, Maynard F Jr: Neurologic recovery after traumatic spinal cord injury: data from the model spinal cord injury systems, *Arch Phys Med Rehabil* 80:1391–1396, 1999.

94. Mayfield JK, Erkkila JC, Winter RB: Spine deformity subsequent to acquired childhood spinal cord injury, *J Bone Joint Surg Am* 63:1401–1411, 1981.

95. Mazur JM, Kyle S: Efficacy of bracing the lower limbs and ambulation training in children with myelomeningocele, *Dev Med Child Neurol* 46:352–356, 2004.

96. Mazur JM, Shurtleff D, Menelaus M, Colliver J: Orthopaedic management of high-level spina bifida. Early walking compared with early use of a wheelchair, *J Bone Joint Surg Am* 71:56–61, 1989.

97. McAdam R, Natvig H: Stair climbing and ability to work for paraplegics with complete lesions: a sixteen-year follow-up, *Paraplegia* 18:197–2003, 1980.

98. McCarthy JJ, Chafetz RS, Betz RR, Gaughan J: Incidence and degree of hip subluxation/dislocation in children with spinal cord injury, *J Spinal Cord Med* 27(suppl 1):S80–S83, 2004.

99. Mehta S, Betz RR, Mulcahey MJ, McDonald C, Vogel LC, Anderson CJ: Effect of bracing on paralytic scoliosis secondary to spinal cord injury, *J Spinal Cord Med* 27:S88–S92, 2004.

100. Merati G, Sarchi P, Ferrarin M, Pedotti A, Veicsteinas A: Paraplegic adaptation to assisted-walking: energy expenditure during wheelchair versus orthosis use, *Spinal Cord* 38:37–44, 2000.

101. Merkel KD, Miller NE, Merritt JL: Energy expenditure in patients with low-, mid-, or high-thoracic paraplegia using Scott-Craig knee-ankle-foot orthoses, *Mayo Clin Proc* 60:165–168, 1985.

102. Merrit JL, Yoshida MK: Knee-ankle-foot-orthoses: indications and practical applications of long leg braces, *Phys Med Rehabil* 14:395–422, 2000.

103. Middleton JW, Fisher W, Davis GM, Smith RM: A medial linkage orthosis to assist ambulation after spinal cord injury, *Prosthet Orthot* 22:258–264, 1998.

104. Middleton JW, Sinclair PJ, Smith RM, Davis GM: Postural control during stance in paraplegia: effects of medially linked versus unlinked knee-ankle-foot orthoses, *Arch Phys Med Rehabil* 80:1558–1565, 1999.

105. Middleton JW, Yeo JD, Blanch L, Vare V, Peterson K, Brigden K: Clinical evaluation of a new orthosis, the "walkabout," for restoration of functional standing and short distance mobility in spinal paralysed individuals, *Spinal Cord* 35:574–579, 1997.

106. Mikelberg R, Reid S: Spinal cord lesions and lower extremity bracing: an overview and follow-up study, *Paraplegia* 19:379–385, 1981.

107. Miller NE, Merritt JL, Merkel KD, Westbrook PR: Paraplegic energy expenditure during negotiation of architectural barriers, *Arch Phys Med Rehabil* 65:778–779, 1984.

108. Moore P, Stallard J: A clinical review of adult paraplegic patients with complete lesions using the ORLAU Parawalker, *Paraplegia* 29:191–196, 1991.

109. Motlock WM: Principles of orthotic management for child and adult paraplegia and clinical experience with the isocentric RGO, Proceedings, Seventh World Congress of ISPO, p. 28, 1992.

110. Moynahan M, Hunt M, Halden E: Evaluation of standing and ambulation: needs and outcomes. In Betz R, Mulcahey M, editors: *The child with a spinal cord injury*, Rosemont, Ill, 1996, American Academy of Orthopaedic Surgeons.

111. Mulcahey MJ, Betz RR: Upper and lower extremity applications of functional electrical stimulation: a decade of research with children and adolescents with spinal injuries, *Pediatr Phys Ther* 6:113–122, 1997.

112. Muller EB, Nordwall A: Brace treatment of scoliosis in children with myelomeningocele, *Spine* 19:151–155, 1994.

113. Nash MS, Jacobs PL, Montalvo BM, Klose KJ, Guest RS, Needham-Shropshire BM: Evaluation of a training program for persons with SCI paraplegia using the Parastep 1 ambulation system: part 5. Lower extremity blood flow and hyperemic responses to occlusion are augmented by ambulation training, *Arch Phys Med Rehabil* 78:808–814, 1997.

114. National Spinal Cord Injury Statistical Center. The annual statistical report for the shrine spinal cord injury units. Birmingham, AL, 2003.

115. Natvig H, McAdam R: Ambulation without wheelchairs for paraplegics with complete lesions, *Paraplegia* 16:142–146, 1978.

116. Nawoczenski DA: *Introduction to Orthotics: Rationale for Treatment*. In Nawoczenski D, Epler M, editors: *Orthotics in functional rehabilitation of the lower limb*, Philadelphia, 1997, WB Saunders.

117. Needham-Shropshire BM, Broton JG, Klose KJ, Lebwohl N, Guest RS, Jacobs PL: Evaluation of a training program for persons with SCI paraplegia using the Parastep 1 ambulation system: part 3. Lack of effect on bone mineral density, *Arch Phys Med Rehabil* 78:799–803, 1997.

118. Nene AV, Jennings SJ: Physiological cost index of paraplegic locomotion using the ORLAU ParaWalker, *Paraplegia* 30:246–252, 1992.

119. Nene AV, Patrick JH: Energy cost of paraplegic locomotion with the ORLAU ParaWalker, *Paraplegia* 27:5–18, 1989.

120. Nene AV, Patrick JH: Energy cost of paraplegic locomotion using the ParaWalker–electrical stimulation "hybrid" orthosis, *Arch Phys Med Rehabil* 71:116–120, 1990.

121. Nobunaga AI, Go BK, Karunas RB: Recent demographic and injury trends in people served by the model spinal cord injury care systems, *Arch Phys Med Rehabil* 80:1372–1382, 1999.

122. Noreau L, Shephard RJ: Spinal cord injury, exercise and quality of life, *Sports Med* 20:226–250, 1995.

123. Noreau L, Shephard RJ, Simard C, Pare G, Pomerleau P: Relationship of impairment and functional ability to habitual activity and fitness following spinal cord injury, *Int J Rehabil Res* 16:265–275, 1993.

124. O'Daniel WE Jr, Hahn HR: Follow-up usage of the Scott-Craig orthosis in paraplegia, *Paraplegia* 19:373–378, 1981.

125. Petrofsky JS, Smith JB: Physiologic costs of computer-controlled walking in persons with paraplegia using a reciprocating-gait orthosis, *Arch Phys Med Rehabil* 72:890–896, 1991.

126. Phillips CA, Hendershot DM: Functional electrical stimulation and reciprocating gait orthosis for ambulation exercise in a tetraplegic patient: a case study, *Paraplegia* 29:268–276, 1991.

127. Rasmussen AA, Smith KM, Damiano DL: Biomechanical evaluation of the combination of bilateral stance-control knee-ankle-foot orthoses and a reciprocating gait orthosis in an adult with a spinal cord injury, *J Prosthetics Orthotics* 19:42–47, 2007.

128. Rink P, Miller F: Hip instability in spinal cord injury patients, *J Pediatr Orthop* 10:583–587, 1990.

129. Robb JE, Gordon L, Ferguson D, Dunhill Z, Elton RA, Minns RA: A comparison of hip guidance with reciprocating gait orthoses in children with spinal paraplegia: results of a ten-year prospective study, *Eur J Pediatr Surg* 9(suppl 1):15–18, 1999.

130. Rose GK: The principles and practice of hip guidance articulations, *Prosthet Orthot Int* 3:37–43, 1979.

131. Rose GK, Sankarankutty M, Stallard J: A clinical review of the orthotic treatment of myelomeningocele patients, *J Bone Joint Surg Br* 65:242–246, 1983.

132. Rosman N, Spira R: Paraplegic use of walking bracing; a survey, *Arch Phys Med Rehabil* 55:310–314, 1974.

133. Schmitz T: Traumatic spinal cord injury. In O'Sullivan TJ, Schmitz TJ, editors: *Physical rehabilitation: assessment and treatment*. IV, Philadelphia, 2001, F.A. Davis.

134. Scivoletto G, Mancini M, Fiorelli E, Morganti B, Molinari M: A prototype of an adjustable advanced reciprocating gait orthosis (ARGO) for spinal cord injury (SCI), *Spinal Cord* 41:187–191, 2003.

135. Scivoletto G, Petrelli A, Lucente LD, et al: One year follow up of spinal cord injury patients using a reciprocating gait orthosis: preliminary report, *Spinal Cord* 38:555–558, 2000.

136. Scott BA: Engineering principles and fabrication techniques for the Scott-Craig long leg brace for paraplegics, *Orthot Prosthet* 25:14–19, 1971.

137. Scott OM, Hyde SA, Goddard C, Dubowitz V: Prevention of deformity in Duchenne muscular dystrophy: a prospective study of passive stretching and splintage, *Physiotherapy* 67:177–180, 1981.

138. Seeger BR, Caudrey DJ, Little JD: Progression of equinus deformity in Duchenne muscular dystrophy, *Arch Phys Med Rehabil* 66:286–288, 1985.

139. Shakhazizian KA, Massaglei T, Southard TL: *Spinal cord injury*, Philadelphia, 2004, WB Saunders.

140. Shimada Y, Sato K, Kagaya H, Konishi N, Miyamoto S, Matsunaga T: Clinical use of percutaneous intramuscular electrodes for functional electrical stimulation, *Arch Phys Med Rehabil* 77:1014–1018, 1996.

141. Shurr DG, Cook TM: *Prosthetics & orthotics*, Norwalk, Conn, 1990, Appleton & Lange.

142. Solomonow M, Aguilar E, Reisin E, et al: Reciprocating gait orthosis powered with electrical muscle stimulation (RGO II). Part I: performance evaluation of 70 paraplegic patients, *Orthopedics* 20:315–324, 1997.

143. Solomonow M, Aguilar E, Reisin E, Baratta RV, D'Ambrosia R: Evaluation of 70 paraplegic patients treated with the reciprocating gait orthosis powered by muscle stimulation, 1999, *Medscape Orthopaedics & Sports Medicine eJournal* at www.medscape.com/viewarticle/408503.

144. Solomonow M, Baratta R, Hirokawa S, et al: The RGO Generation II: muscle stimulation powered orthosis as a practical walking system for thoracic paraplegics, *Orthopedics* 12:1309–1315, 1989.

145. Solomonow M, Reisin E, Aguilar E, Baratta RV, Best R, D'Ambrosia R: Reciprocating gait orthosis powered with electrical muscle stimulation (RGO II). Part II: medical evaluation of 70 paraplegic patients, *Orthopedics* 20:411–418, 1997.

146. Somers MF: *Spinal cord injury: functional rehabilitation*, Saddle River, NJ, 2001, Prentice-Hall.

147. Stallard J, Lomas B, Woollam P, et al: New technical advances in swivel walkers, *Prosthet Orthot Int* 27:132–138, 2003.

148. Stallard J, Major RE: The influence of orthosis stiffness on paraplegic ambulation and its implications for functional electrical stimulation (FES) walking systems, *Prosthet Orthot Int* 19:108–114, 1995.

149. Stallard J, Major RE, Patrick JH: A review of the fundamental design problems of providing ambulation for paraplegic patients, *Paraplegia* 27:70–75, 1989.

150. Stauffer ES, Hoffer MM, Nickel VL: Ambulation in thoracic paraplegia, *J Bone Joint Surg Am* 60:823–824, 1978.

151. Stein RB, Belanger M, Wheeler G, et al: Electrical systems for improving locomotion after incomplete spinal cord injury: an assessment, *Arch Phys Med Rehabil* 74:954–959, 1993.

152. Summers BN, McClelland MR, Masri E: A clinical review of the adult hip guidance orthosis (ParaWalker) in traumatic paraplegia, *Paraplegia* 26:19–26, 1988.

153. Suzuki T, Sonoda S, Saitoh E, et al: Development of a novel type of shoe to improve the efficiency of knee-ankle-foot orthoses with a medial single hip joint (Primewalk orthoses): a novel type of shoe for Primewalk orthosis, *Prosthet Orthot Int* 29:303–311, 2005.

154. Sykes L, Campbell IG, Powell ES, Ross ER, Edwards J: Energy expenditure of walking for adult patients with spinal cord lesions using the reciprocating gait orthosis and functional electrical stimulation, *Spinal Cord* 34:659–665, 1996.

155. Sykes L, Edwards J, Powell ES, Ross ER: The reciprocating gait orthosis: long-term usage patterns, *Arch Phys Med Rehabil* 76:779–783, 1995.

156. Sykes L, Ross ER, Powell ES, Edwards J: Objective measurement of use of the reciprocating gait orthosis (RGO) and the electrically augmented RGO in adult patients with spinal cord lesions, *Prosthet Orthot Int* 20:182–190, 1996.

157. Thomas SS, Buckon CE, Melchionni J, Magnusson M, Aiona MD: Longitudinal assessment of oxygen cost and velocity in children with myelomeningocele: comparison of the hip-knee-ankle-foot orthosis and the reciprocating gait orthosis, *J Pediatr Orthop* 21:798–803, 2001.

158. Tokuhara Y, Kameyama O, Kubota T, Matsuura M, Ogawa R: Biomechanical study of gait using an intelligent brace, *J Orthop Sci* 5:342–348, 2000.

159. Uhlir JP, Triolo RJ, Kobetic R: The use of selective electrical stimulation of the quadriceps to improve standing function in paraplegia, *IEEE Trans Rehabil Eng* 8:514–522, 2000.

160. Vogel LC, Gogia RS, Lubicky JP: Hip abnormalities in children with spinal cord injury, *J Spinal Cord Med* 18:172, 1995.

161. Vogel LC, Lubicky JP: Ambulation in children and adolescents with spinal cord injuries, *J Pediatr Orthop* 15:510–516, 1995.

162. Vogel LC, Lubicky JP: Ambulation with parapodia and reciprocating gait orthoses in pediatric spinal cord injury, *Dev Med Child Neurol* 37:957–964, 1995.

163. Washburn R, Figoni S: Physical activity and chronic cardiovascular disease prevention in spinal cord injury: a comprehensive literature review, *Topics Spinal Cord Injury Rehabil* 3:16–32, 1998.

164. Waters RL, Lunsford BR: Energy cost of paraplegic locomotion, *J Bone Joint Surg Am* 67:1245–1250, 1985.

165. Whittle MW, Cochrane GM, Chase AP, et al: A comparative trial of two walking systems for paralysed people, *Paraplegia* 29:97–102, 1991.

166. Williams EN, Broughton NS, Menelaus MB: Age-related walking in children with spina bifida, *Dev Med Child Neurol* 41:446–449, 1999.

167. Winchester PK, Carollo JJ, Parekh RN, Lutz LM, Aston JW Jr: A comparison of paraplegic gait performance using two types of reciprocating gait orthoses, *Prosthet Orthot Int* 17:101–106, 1993.

168. Yngve DA, Douglas R, Roberts JM: The reciprocating gait orthosis in myelomeningocele, *J Pediatr Orthop* 4:304–310, 1984.

Chapter

28

Orthoses in total joint replacement

Dulcey Lima

Key Points

- Dislocation following total hip arthroplasty is a difficult clinical problem whose incidence varies depending on whether the procedure is primary or secondary.

- Although hip spica casts have been shown to be useful for preventing future dislocations so long as the femoral and acetabular components are well positioned, orthoses offer advantages in wound care, hygiene, and patient comfort.

- When treating a hip that dislocates in a posterior direction, a hip orthosis terminating proximal to the knee is typically sufficient.

- Patients who dislocate in an anterior direction often demonstrate global instability and are managed with a pelvic segment connected to a knee-ankle-foot orthosis to provide increased directional control and rotational stability.

- Patients at increased risk for dislocation may be managed with prophylactic bracing.

- Orthoses are rarely used following total knee replacement unless specific complications such as knee extensor weakness are present or when there is a need to stabilize the joint with a hinged knee orthosis or knee-ankle-foot orthosis.

- Knee-ankle-foot orthoses and bivalve cylinder knee orthoses are often used following knee arthrodesis after removal of the postoperative cast.

Primary total joint replacements of the hip and knee are reliable operations. They usually are successful in restoring function to patients with severe arthritis and other debilitating conditions. Although orthoses are rarely needed after primary surgical procedures of the hip and knee, some external support may be needed in cases involving revision or complicated primary surgery, surgical complications, or unusual pathology. This chapter presents orthotic approaches to the management of conditions that may require treatment with an orthosis following hip or knee arthroplasty. Orthotic intervention is described and protocols are provided for a variety of clinical indications.

Review of the literature

Several authors indicate that a hip dislocation in the early post-operative period in a hip with proper orientation and restored mechanics can be treated successfully with patient education and adjunctive bracing.[1,2,9,12] This group included a retrospective study of 80 patients managed with a hip orthosis to prevent dislocation following hip revision surgery.[7] The primary shortcoming of such studies is the lack of control groups, statistical analysis, and long-term outcomes. DeWal et al.[4] retrospectively reviewed 91 patients who dislocated for the first time and 58 patients who had a history of recurrent dislocation to determine if hip abduction orthoses were effective in reducing redislocations after a closed reduction. They found that patients fit with a hip abduction orthosis redislocated at the same rate as those who did not receive an orthosis.[4] The study had several limitations: no orthotic protocols were provided, the report did not state whether the patients who received hip orthoses had injuries of similar severity, and the report did not indicate whether the patients were wearing the orthosis at the time of the dislocation.[2] Differences in surgical procedures, prosthetic components, and types of hip orthoses used all can impact the dislocation rate and subsequent management with a hip orthosis. Clearly, long-term, controlled studies are needed to determine which patients may benefit from orthotic management following dislocation or as a means of preventing first-time dislocations in complicated cases.

New surgical procedures may have an impact on the dislocation rate. Constrained acetabular liners have significantly reduced the incidence of dislocation but are subject to premature wear and disruption. Many surgeons now use prosthetic components with larger articulating bearing surfaces to help prevent dislocation.[2] Surgical procedures now are being performed with smaller incisions, leaving the abductor muscles more intact and more able to provide hip stability. In addition, new hip resurfacing procedures are emerging, which replace the acetabular component and cap the head of the femur, leaving most of the head intact. This procedure, performed on younger patients, retains more bone and may help to prevent dislocation. Although early reports are promising, long-term study is needed to evaluate the impact of these new procedures on component longevity and resistance to dislocation.

Dislocation following hip surgery

Dislocation of a total hip prosthesis is a difficult clinical problem. The incidence of dislocation varies, depending on whether the procedure is a primary (1.7,[5] 3.9%,[13]. 7.2%[2]) or a revision arthroplasty (11.2%[2]–14.4%[13]). The rate of dislocation for these procedures is also linked to factors such as component selection,[2] prosthetic component orientation,[4,7,9] and surgical technique.[6,9,11] Dislocation rates were higher for patients with a history of dislocation, those with poor abductors or adductor spasticity, patients with anterior wall weakness or global instability, those with acetabular transplants, and patients with two or more surgeries on the affected side.[7]

It is important to understand the cause and direction of instability in order to provide appropriate orthotic management. Patients who dislocate with satisfactory

radiographic positioning of the prosthetic components often can be managed with a closed reduction of the hip and a hip orthosis to discourage motion that can lead to dislocation.[9] If the referring physician has not indicated the direction of dislocation, the orthotist should review the patient's activity at the time of the dislocation and clarify the instability with the physician.[7] Posterior dislocations occur 85% of the time and usually involve hip flexion, adduction, and internal rotation. Activities associated with posterior dislocation include sitting and reaching toward the uninvolved side, exiting a vehicle, reaching for an object on the floor, leaning over to apply shoes, or rising from a low chair, toilet seat, or soft cushion. Anterior dislocation is linked with external rotation and extension and often occurs during activities such as reaching up on a high shelf, extending hips and trunk to move back into bed, reaching behind the body while standing to put on a coat, or lying in bed with hips extended.[7] Anterior dislocations are also seen in patients diagnosed with hip dysplasia, who have excessive femoral anteversion.

Often physicians are able to reduce a dislocated hip with a closed reduction performed under local anesthesia. In cases where the pain is too severe or when efforts to reduce the hip are unsuccessful while the patient is awake, a closed reduction can be performed under general anesthesia. Once reduced, a total hip can be stabilized with an orthosis until the compromised soft tissue heals and creates scarring around the joint. This usually prevents further dislocations if the femoral and acetabular components are well positioned. In the past, hip spica casts have been shown to be useful for this purpose. Currently, orthoses offer several advantages over casts. Orthoses weigh less, which makes them easier to tolerate during ambulation. An orthosis can be carefully removed, providing access for wound care and hygiene. In addition, hip orthoses are widely available in adjustable, prefabricated models, facilitating immediate stabilization of the patient, limited in-patient hospitalization, and earlier return to activities (Fig. 28-1).[1,7]

Management of posterior dislocations

The hip orthosis used to treat a hip that dislocates in a posterior direction is generally proximal to the knee. A snugly fit pelvic band suspends the orthosis and provides an attachment point for the hip joint. A laterally placed, adjustable range of motion hip joint capable of controlling flexion, extension, abduction, and adduction attaches to a snug-fitting thigh cuff that holds the hip in 10 to 20 degrees of abduction and allows 0 to 70 degrees of flexion. This joint position combined with properly fitting pelvic and thigh components provides a kinesthetic reminder against excessive flexion, adduction, and internal rotation. Another study recommends that the hip be held in 0 to 10 degrees of flexion, externally rotated, and abducted 15 to 20 degrees for posterior dislocations.[9] Once properly fit, most patients ambulate with minimal support and can perform most activities of daily living while wearing the orthosis. The orthosis is worn under clothing to ensure protection in all positions, including toileting. Innovations include joints that abduct as the hip moves into greater amounts of flexion and rotational control incorporated into the hip joint mechanism. Internal and external continue to be the most difficult motions to control in an orthosis that ends proximal to the knee. When used to prevent another

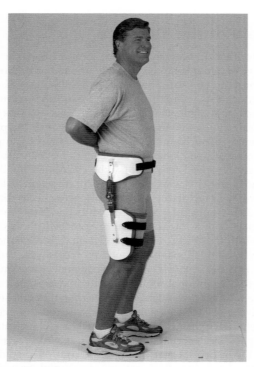

Fig. 28-1 Orthosis to prevent posterior dislocation is set to prevent specific ranges of hip flexion, adduction, and internal rotation. (Courtesy Orthomerica Products.)

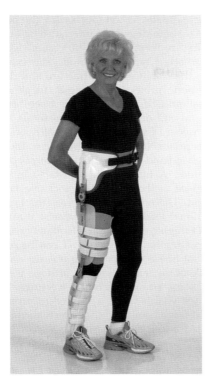

Fig. 28-2 Orthosis to prevent anterior dislocation limits hip extension and extends distally to the floor to maximize control of hip rotation. This orthosis can also be used to stabilize femoral fractures following total hip arthroplasty. (Courtesy Orthomerica Products.)

dislocation, the orthosis is worn at all times.[2,7,9,12] If radiographs demonstrate malposition or instability of either the femoral or acetabular prosthetic component, if an orthosis is not effective, and if the patient is a good candidate, surgery is generally performed to stabilize the hip.[9]

Management of anterior dislocations

When patients have anterior wall weakness or global instability, extension, rotation (usually external rotation), and abduction usually is the mechanism of dislocation. Extension range is blocked at −40 degrees, and flexion range is generally safe up to 70 degrees, unlike posterior dislocations where flexion is one component of dislocation.[7] Patients who dislocate in an anterior direction often demonstrate global instability due to acetabular insufficiency. To provide rotational control, a knee–ankle–foot orthosis (KAFO) rather than a simple thigh cuff is suspended from the pelvic band. Although this adds considerable bulk to the orthosis, it also provides increased directional control and stability. Patients who wear a hip–knee–ankle–foot orthosis (HKAFO) often need additional assistance to perform activities of daily living because the orthosis adds considerable bulk and motion restriction. Patients generally wear the orthosis at all times for 3 to 6 months. Often, fluoroscopy is used to determine the exact mechanism of dislocation. In conjunction with the physician, the orthotist should adjust the range of motion settings to address the patient's specific instability.[7]

In another study highlighting orthotic management of anterior dislocations, the author recommends setting the hip joint to allow flexion between 20 and 30 degrees and provide 0 to 10 degrees of internal rotation and 20 degrees of abduction.[9] For the most severe revision surgeries and patients with compromised bone, a custom lumbosacral orthosis and molded thigh cuff without a hinge on the affected side with thigh cuff and hinge on the contralateral side can be used in place of a prefabricated hip orthosis. Because anterior dislocations occur only 15% of the time and precautions are very different than those for posterior dislocations, the orthotist should educate other staff members about the positions that can place the patient at risk for dislocation in an anterior direction (Fig. 28-2).

Wearing time

Orthotic wearing time is impacted by factors such as the intrinsic stability of the hip joint, the patient's ability to follow hip precautions, reasons for wearing the orthosis, and rate of soft-tissue healing, which varies among patients. Depending on the reasons for the orthosis, patients may be advised by their physician to wear the orthosis at all times, only in bed, or when out of bed.

When worn to prevent a first posterior dislocation (such as after revision surgery), it is common for the patient to wear the orthosis for at least 8 to 12 weeks when out of bed. Longer periods of orthotic protection and full-time wear are indicated for patients with impaired soft-tissue healing, patients with a history of recurrent dislocations, patients who are at risk for dislocation in an anterior direction, or patients who are noncompliant with range of motion restrictions. If noncompliance is suspected, the orthotist or physician can wrap a few layers of fiberglass over the pelvic band and thigh cuff to discourage removal. The patient can wear a soft undershirt under the pelvic component to increase comfort. Patients with chronic hip instability who are poor surgical candidates may require permanent bracing to prevent dislocation.[1,7]

Prophylactic orthotic management to prevent a first dislocation

Revision patients are at increased risk for dislocation and have been shown to benefit from prophylactic treatment with a brace similar to the one described for treatment of a dislocated primary hip. Although some surgeons routinely brace all revision patients, many use prophylactic bracing only after revisions involving extensive soft-tissue dissection or in patients with identified risk factors for dislocation. Risk factors include patients who have undergone two or more surgeries on the affected side, are chronic dislocators prior to surgery, or have acetabular or other component insufficiency at the time of surgery.[7] Patients generally wear a standard hip orthosis for 8 weeks after surgery to provide support, limit motion that can lead to dislocation, provide a kinesthetic cue, and allow soft tissue to heal. Although most patients undergoing primary hip arthroplasty do not need prophylactic orthotic management, it should be considered in several cases. Indications include patients with hip dysplasia, those with poor bone quality, and patients unable to follow hip precautions. Patients with neuromuscular disease, such as Parkinson disease, spasticity secondary to cerebral palsy or cerebrovascular accident, or sensory neuropathy are at risk for recurrent dislocations, despite optimally positioned implants. Prophylactic orthotic management should be

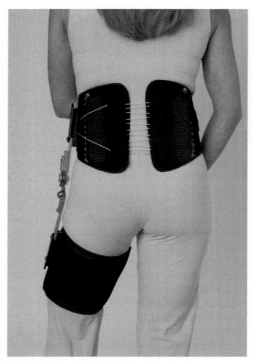

Fig. 28-3 Strong mesh fiber in the reinforced pelvic and thigh components provides more comfortable control for patients wearing this orthosis at all times. (Courtesy Orthomerica Products.)

considered in this population because hip flexion and adductor tone can lead to pain and dislocation.[7]

Patients undergoing acetabular transplants are prophylactically fit with an HKAFO with restricted extension and flexion range (−40 to 70 degrees), neutral hip alignment of the limb (no hip abduction or adduction), and free knee and ankle joints. The orthosis is worn at all times for 6 months until the soft tissue heals and there is bony integration of the component.[7]

The elderly, confused patient treated with an endoprosthesis for a femoral neck fracture is at particular risk for dislocation because of impaired cognition. Although some of these patients may benefit from a hip orthosis, a knee immobilizer has also been shown to be effective in this group. A knee immobilizer locks the knee in extension and prevents excessive hip flexion, especially in the elderly population.[2] The knee immobilizer can be easily removed when the patient is supervised, as in physical therapy, and therefore does not impede rehabilitation.[8] The knee immobilizer does not, however, help limit hip flexion when the patient is moved by hospital staff or family members and does not prevent adduction in any position. Any hip orthosis worn in bed should be well padded to improve comfort and compliance and prevent skin breakdown. Soft hip systems are available to provide more comfortable hip control for patients who must wear the orthosis full time and spend the majority of time in bed (Fig. 28-3).

Periprosthetic femoral fractures

Femoral fractures can occur during surgery when the femoral component is being positioned in the femur or after surgery, usually because of falls. When this occurs, the physician generally provides some degree of internal fixation of the fracture, including replacement of the stem with a longer component or other type of fixation. The surgeon is best able to judge the stability of the fracture and determine the degree of orthotic protection required. In general, orthotic stabilization should be considered for fractures that extend below the distal end of the femoral prosthesis and are associated with insecure fixation or poor quality bone.

The appropriate orthosis to stabilize these fractures includes a pelvic band and KAFO to control rotation all the way to the floor. A hinge with adjustable hip flexion and extension is used at the hip, with a lockable knee joint and free ankle joint. The orthosis must cross the knee and ankle because rotational loads pose the greatest threat to fracture stability, and a thigh cuff does not adequately control rotation of the lower extremity. A pelvic band can be omitted when patients are not obese and/or when fractures are located in the distal third of the femur. Such an orthosis is similar to the treatment of some primary femoral fractures. If additional protection from axial loading is needed to promote healing, a well-molded thigh component with ischial containment can be incorporated into the orthosis.

The duration of orthotic treatment must be determined for each patient based on radiographic and clinical findings that indicate fracture union. External support usually is required for at least 12 weeks but varies according to the fracture pattern, patient's age, patient's ability to follow postoperative instructions, and other factors associated with fracture healing.

Neurological complications

Femoral and sciatic nerve palsies are well-known complications of hip replacement surgery. The injury usually is secondary to nerve traction, contusion, or laceration. Motor deficits may resolve in a few days or months, or they may be permanent. When neurological deficits do not resolve by the time the patient is ready to leave the hospital, an orthosis can be used to provide stability during ambulation.

The most common neurological finding is paralytic equinus, which results from injury to the peroneal portion of the sciatic nerve. Decreased ankle dorsiflexion during swing impairs rehabilitation and often makes the patient's gait unsafe. Patients are at risk to lose dorsiflexion range of motion and have particular difficulty ambulating on uneven ground. Excessive ankle plantarflexion may create knee extension instability in stance, complicate forward progression, and effect balance, which may already be compromised in the elderly population. When there is fair dorsiflexion strength, a simple prefabricated ankle–foot orthosis (AFO) may be all that is required to support the foot and provide some dorsiflexion assist. In patients with complete motor loss to the dorsiflexors, a rigid AFO is required to control sagittal and coronal plane motion. Patients requiring long-term support benefit from a custom-molded device that can be inserted into various shoes. Other AFOs that can be considered include those with stirrups or calipers attached to an orthopedic shoe, although metal systems are seldom used now unless the skin is compromised. The selected orthosis should be worn until active dorsiflexion of the foot returns.

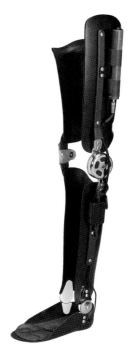

Fig. 28-4 For long-term use, a KAFO with stance control knee joints can promote a more normal gait pattern in active patients with knee flexion instability following knee arthroplasty. (Courtesy Becker Orthopedic.)

Femoral nerve injury during the surgical procedure affects the quadriceps, resulting in knee flexion instability. Some patients learn to lock their knee in extension by using their hip extensors while the foot is held in plantarflexion, but this gait deviation can lead to knee pain and instability on uneven ground. Patients with short-term knee extension instability are best managed in a custom-to-measure KAFO with knee locks and solid ankle so that the knee is stable for rehabilitation activities. Active patients requiring the orthosis for long-term use can benefit from a custom KAFO with stance control knee joints to allow free knee flexion in swing and stability in stance. Nerve recovery may be complete or incomplete, and any orthosis should be used until the knee is stable (Fig. 28-4).

Resection arthroplasty

Resection arthroplasty of the hip (girdlestone procedure) is performed rarely as a primary reconstructive procedure now that more components, surgical procedures, and medications are available to address joint salvage procedures. Currently, it is most commonly indicated for patients in whom hip replacements have failed because of unresolved infections[8] or severe bone loss, and who are not satisfactory candidates for revision total hip arthroplasty. After proximal femoral resection, the operated extremity tends to shorten. If shortening occurs, the patient may benefit from a shoe lift to provide more symmetrical alignment. Ambulation usually is limited due to the instability of the hip, but a tight-fitting compression orthosis with a trim line distal to the trochanter may provide some external support and stability for the affected side. This can be augmented with a thigh cuff and hip joint to provide additional alignment and stability for the limb.

Orthoses after knee replacement

Orthotic support is used infrequently after total knee replacement except in cases of surgical complications, inadequate bone integrity, or poor recovery after the surgery. The primary indications for orthotic management include weakness or injury to the extensor mechanism (i.e., avulsion of the patellar tendon), insufficiency of the medial collateral ligament, and loss of knee flexion or extension range of motion. In very complicated surgeries, salvage procedures for total knee arthroplasty, such as arthrodesis or resection arthroplasty, usually require orthotic treatment as part of postoperative management.

Extensor mechanism deficiency

Occasionally the quadriceps tendon or the patellar tendon is disrupted during or after knee replacement. Patients with severe weakness of the quadriceps because of neuromuscular disease and patients who are nonsurgical candidates for extensor mechanism repair may need orthotic management to prevent uncontrolled loss of knee extension during the stance phase of gait. If the weakness is permanent, it can be managed with either a stance phase KAFO with free knee motion during swing or a double-upright KAFO with appropriate locking mechanism.

A variety of stance control knee joints provide new options for patients with long-term knee flexion instability. Several joints are available that provide swing phase knee flexion and stance phase stability without locking the knee. A major benefit of the joints is a smoother gait pattern and less need for patients to think about whether their knee is stable with each step. The joints are quite expensive and are not appropriate for patients who need knee extension stability for a short time.

Another orthosis commonly used for patients with an unstable knee is a KAFO with drop or bail locks to provide stability in stance. The patient can unlock the knee joints for comfortable sitting. A disadvantage of these locks is that the lock stays engaged in swing phase, requiring circumduction of the leg and hip hiking to achieve adequate clearance. To assist with clearance of the involved side, a heel and sole lift can be added to the contralateral side. A posterior offset hinge can also be used without locks to achieve a more extended knee position in stance and allow free flexion during swing. More agile patients and those with some residual active knee extension may prefer this to the drop lock hinge, but the lack of a positive locking mechanism may be inadequate for safe ambulation on uneven surfaces. Surgical treatment usually is the treatment of choice for patients with knee flexion instability. Depending on the success of the repair, an orthosis to prevent knee collapse may be indicated. In this situation, a prefabricated knee orthosis with adjustable locking hinges for sagittal plane motion is indicated. Such a device allows the therapist or orthotist to increase the range of motion as healing progresses and extension strength improves.

Most patients achieve full range of motion after total knee arthroplasty, but occasionally restriction of motion in either extension or flexion range occurs. Preexisting range limitations can complicate surgical recovery, and therapy often is required during the recovery period to improve functional

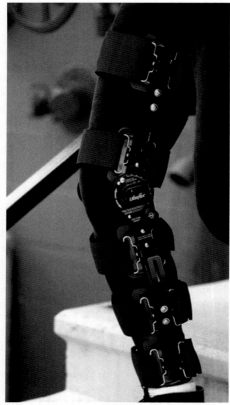

Fig. 28-5 Dynamic knee flexion or extension orthosis can be used to regain range of motion following knee replacement surgery. (Courtesy Ultraflex.)

range of motion. A knee orthosis designed to provide dynamic motion can be used to increase the range, maintain therapeutic gains, and improve function and stability (Fig. 28-5).[10]

Collateral ligament instability

Stability of the medial and collateral ligaments is an important factor in successful total knee surgery. Patients with knee valgus or varus soft-tissue instability can be managed with a hinged knee orthosis to help maintain the surgical correction and promote alignment. Depending on the patient's activity level, a functional knee orthosis can provide stability, especially when the orthosis is needed only to provide protection from valgus or varus forces temporarily.[3] Patients with severe coronal plane instability may require an orthosis that unloads the affected compartment or may benefit from a KAFO if the knee is globally unstable.

Arthrodesis and resection arthroplasty

When a total knee implant fails secondary to sepsis or severe bone loss, a knee arthrodesis (fusion) may be necessary. Prolonged casting is indicated after this procedure except when an intramedullary rod is used for internal fixation. The time to union can be as long as 12 months, so a custom-molded KAFO with knee locks usually is needed after the cast is removed. This support is helpful in

controlling edema, which can be problematic in these patients. The orthosis is discontinued when solid union of the arthrodesis is observed. Another infrequent complication after total knee arthroplasty is infection, and this may necessitate a resection arthroplasty. The failed components are removed, antibiotics are administered, and orthotic immobilization is used in the immediate postoperative period. One orthotic option is a total contact, custom-molded, bivalved knee orthosis with foam liner, which replaces the cast and allows skin inspection and hygiene. A second option for support and immobilization of the knee is a custom-to-cast or custom-to-measure KAFO with locked knee and well-padded ankle foot component to prevent distal migration. After this procedure, some patients will undergo a revision knee arthroplasty, and others will not have the components replaced. In the latter case, patients may require permanent bracing with a double-upright KAFO with knee locks to provide greater knee instability.

Summary

Orthotic support occasionally is required after total hip arthroplasty, primarily in cases of dislocations with satisfactory implant positioning or after hip revision surgery to prevent dislocation. In total knee replacement, an orthosis may be required in cases of significant postoperative instability or in salvage resection procedures for patients who are not candidates for further reconstruction procedures. In both situations, an orthosis is an adjunctive modality to enhance the patient's function, stabilize the hip or knee, and limit undesirable motion.

References

1. Bradford MS, Paprosky WG: Total acetabular transplant allograft reconstruction of the severely deficient acetabulum, *Semin Arthroplasty* 6:86–95, 1995.
2. Callaghan JJ, Heithoff BE, Goetz DD, et al: Prevention of dislocation after hip arthroplasty, *Clin Orthop Relat Res* 393:157–162, 2001.
3. Cameron HU, Harris WR: Acquired valgus instability after knee replacement, *Clin Orthop Relat Res* 154:216–219, 1981.
4. DeWal H, Maurer SL, Tsai P, et al: Efficacy of abduction bracing in the management of total hip arthroplasty dislocation, *J Arthroplasty* 19:733–738, 2004.
5. Khatod M, Barber T, Paxton E, et al: An analysis of the risk of hip dislocation with a contemporary total joint registry, *Clin Orthop Relat Res* 447:19–23, 2006.
6. Kwon MS, Kuskowski M, Mulhall KJ, et al: Does surgical approach affect total hip arthroplasty dislocation rates?, *Clin Orthop Relat Res* 447:34–38, 2006.
7. Lima D, Magnus R, Paprosky W: Team management of hip revision patients using a post-op hip orthosis, *J Prosthet Orthot* 6:20–24, 1994.
8. Masri BA, Salvati EA, Duncan CP: Revision hip replacement for the infected implant, *Bombay Hospital Journal* 38:3, 1996. Retrieved February 3, 2003 from www.bhj.org/journal/1996/3803_july/special_532.htm.
9. Morrey BF: Difficult complications after hip joint replacement, *Clin Orthop Relat Res* 344:179–187, 1997.
10. Mont MA, Seyler TM, Marulanda GA, et al: Surgical treatment and customized rehabilitation for stiff knee arthroplasties, *Clin Orthop Relat Res* 446:193–200, 2006.
11. Nishii T, Sugano N, Miki H, et al: Influence of component positions on dislocation, *J Arthroplasty* 19:162–166, 2004.
12. Padgett DE, Warashina H: The unstable total hip replacement, *Clin Orthop Relat Res* 420:72–79, 2004.
13. Phillips CB, Lingard GA, Kate JN: Incidence rates of dislocation, pulmonary embolism, and deep infection during the first six months after elective total hip replacement, *JBJS* 85:20–26, 2003.

Chapter

29

Knee orthoses for sports-related disorders

Brett William Wolters

Key Points

- Understanding of knee joint biomechanics is essential to the prescription of knee orthoses for sports-related disorders
- There are three different kinds of knee orthoses: prophylactic, functional, and rehabilitative
- Prophylactic knee braces attempt to limit the strain on the MCL and ACL through force reduction
- Functional knee braces are intended to protect patients with ACL-deficient or graft-reconstructed knees
- Rehabilitative knee bracing goals are to prevent excessive load on an injured or reconstructed ligament and to allow early return to activity

Knee injuries are common during participation in both contact and noncontact sports. As the number of individuals participating has increased, so has the number of knee injuries. The most commonly injured knee structures include the anterior cruciate ligament (ACL), posterior cruciate ligament (PCL), medial collateral ligament (MCL), lateral collateral ligament (LCL), and medial and lateral menisci. When these structures are injured, knee joint function and stability are compromised. Also, the protection provided by these structures is decreased, and the tibiofemoral and patellofemoral surfaces do not articulate properly. This can lead to pain and, eventually, advanced degenerative joint disease.

Knee braces have been used in each step of the injury process, including injury prevention, ligament rehabilitation after reconstruction, and treatment of functional instability of the knee joint. Because of the incidence of knee injuries in high-profile athletes and aggressive marketing campaigns by brace manufacturers, interest in knee braces has increased.

However, accurate unbiased information regarding the proper use of knee braces is difficult to find.

To offset some of the confusion, the American Academy of Orthopaedic Surgeons classified knee braces into three categories: (1) *prophylactic braces*, intended to prevent injury in a healthy individual; (2) *functional braces*, designed to provide stability to the unstable knee, and (3) *rehabilitative braces*, designed to allow protected range of motion during the rehabilitation or early postoperative period.[4]

Current braces are designed to recreate normal knee kinematics while accomplishing all of these goals. However, the effectiveness of these braces remains debatable. Players, coaches, trainers, therapists, and physicians remain confused because studies have shown beneficial, equivocal, and negative results of brace wear in each setting.

Knee joint biomechanics

The knee joint acts as a hinge, allowing flexion and extension in the sagittal plane of motion (Fig. 29-1). However, flexion and extension occur about a constantly changing center of rotation, called *polycentric rotation*.[42] This allows for a process called *femoral rollback*. As knee flexion starts in full extension, the femoral condyle begins to roll without sliding, and with further knee flexion sliding becomes more predominant. The knee joint also undergoes axial rotation during flexion and extension. Axial rotation occurs because of a differential radius of curvature between the medial and lateral femoral condyles, the convex shape of the medial tibial plateau, the concave shape of the lateral tibial plateau, and the ability of the MCL to stretch more rapidly than the lateral collateral ligament. As a result, when the knee joint continues to flex throughout the entire range of motion, there is inward rotation of the tibia, whereas the reciprocal is true with knee extension.

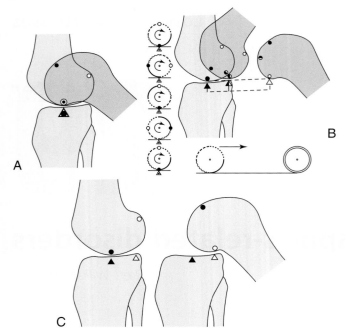

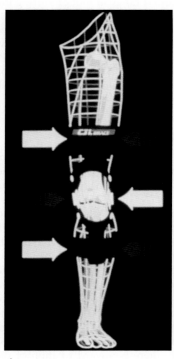

Fig. 29-1 A, With knee flexion there is pure sliding of the femur on the tibia. If the knee was restricted to pure sliding, then posterior femoral metaphyseal impinge would prohibit increased knee flexion angles. **B,** With knee flexion there is pure rolling of the femur on the tibia. If the knee was restricted to pure rolling, then both tibial and femoral contact points would change as the femur rolls on the tibia. The knee would dislocate with increased knee flexion. **C,** Actual knee motion involves both rolling and sliding. (From Scott WN: *The knee*, St. Louis, 1994, Mosby.)

Knee stability

The function of the knee motion also depends on the four major ligamentous structures of the knee, specifically the ACL, PCL, MCL, and LCL structures. Kapandji[50] described the dependence of knee stability on these structures as the four-bar linkage system. These ligaments are responsible for maintaining knee stability during femoral rollback and axial rotation of the knee joint. If the knee orthosis does not accommodate normal knee kinematics, range of motion may be limited, or the ligaments may be stressed leading to laxity.[38]

Brace design

Knee braces are designed to transfer load while allowing for normal knee motion (Fig. 29-2). This depends on the amount of leverage the knee brace can provide. Longer braces produce a greater amount of leverage; therefore, athletes typically select the longest brace that provides the best fit to the extremity.[18] The optimal position to apply the leverage depends on the goal of the knee brace. Prophylactic braces usually are designed with unilateral, single-hinge systems. Some newer designs have bilateral uprights and polycentric hinges. They are used to prevent MCL strain by applying leverage laterally on the femur and tibia to inhibit excessive valgus. Functional knee braces typically are designed with bilateral, polycentric hinge systems. These braces act to prevent recurrent instability in patients with ACL tears. They act by applying leverage to resist abnormal forward translation of the tibia on the femur.[35]

Off the shelf

Both off-the-shelf and custom-made designs have proven effective if the geometry of the brace matches the geometry

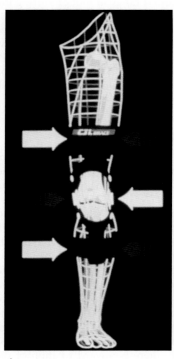

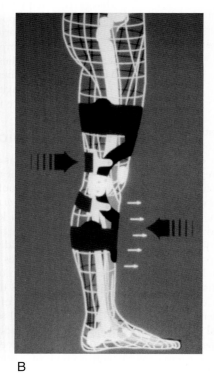

Fig. 29-2 Knee braces are designed to apply leverage to the extremity by preventing excessive varus/valgus forces and abnormal tibial translation. (From Goldberg B, Hsu JD: *Atlas of orthoses and assistive devices*, ed 3, St. Louis, 1997, Mosby.)

A   B

of the extremity.[12] Off-the-shelf knee braces are designed based upon the approximate geometry and length of the individual knee. Therefore, it is recommended that athletes try on different braces from different companies in order to determine the best fit.

Custom

Custom knee braces usually are cast molded or leg traced to match the shape of the brace to the geometry of the thigh, knee, and calf. Theoretically, custom designs more accurately recreate normal knee motion; however, studies have shown that even custom designs limit knee flexion in the swing phase of running compared to unbraced conditions.[54,55]

Ultimately, brace efficacy is dependent on how load is distributed across the limb. This is dependent on a number of factors, including geometry and mechanism of attachment, fabrication materials, and hinge design.[74]

Geometry and mechanism of attachment

The brace attaches to the extremity through the geometry of the femoral and tibial supports. The thigh and calf supports connect to the upright(s) while remaining contoured to the extremity. Tibial and femoral condylar padding have been shown to provide more contact.

The mechanism of attachment of the brace to the extremity usually is through strapping. The two types of strapping are elastic and nonelastic (or shell) designs. The flexible elastic straps are more comfortable, but leverage is lost with each muscle contraction. Theoretically, the shell design is an improvement because constant leverage can be applied, but they are less well tolerated because of their restrictive nature.

The number of straps and the strap arrangement determine how the load is distributed across the knee. Most braces have at least four straps. Some functional braces have more straps with larger surface areas to increase the amount of leverage applied. The most important strap is the suprapatellar strap because it maintains the position of the brace on the knee by preventing inferior migration of the brace.

Fabrication materials

Braces originally were fabricated from heavy steel and plastic. These braces weighed in excess of 5 lb. More recently, braces

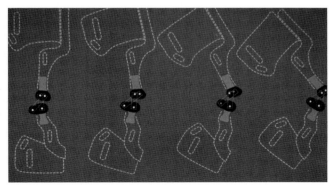

Fig. 29-3 Kinematic hinge designed to replicate femoral rollback with knee flexion. (From Goldberg B, Hsu JD: *Atlas of orthoses and assistive devices,* ed 3, St. Louis, 1997, Mosby.)

have been manufactured with composite lightweight materials, such as carbon fiber and aluminum, weighing less than 1 lb. These braces allow for less energy expenditure and a better fit for athletes while remaining quite durable.

Hinge design

In order for the knee brace to function properly, the knee hinge must recreate polycentric rotation and femoral rollback (Fig. 29-3). Simple unicentric hinges, as used in prophylactic braces, do not allow normal knee joint kinematics. Newer polycentric hinges, as used in functional braces with dual hinges, have been developed that more closely approximate normal knee kinematics.[24] Ultimately, optimal brace performance depends on placing the hinge(s) in correct relation to the femoral condyles.[74]

There is a great deal of debate on which factor is the most important. Based on mathematical models, some authors have found that the mechanical characteristics of the brace, the structural integrity of the brace, and the interaction of the brace with the limb during loading are the most important.[57] Others authors have suggested that hinge position is the most important.[94]

Brace design limitations

Many studies have shown that braced athletes have equivocal or negative efficacy compared to nonbraced athletes. This may reflect the limitations of the knee brace.

As previously stated, single-hinge knee braces have been criticized for prestressing ligaments and causing chronic ligamentous laxity, whereas double-hinge systems more accurately recreate normal knee motion and avoid these complications.[38] Braces have a tendency to migrate distally because the soft tissue consists of compressible materials. This limits the knee brace's ability to apply leverage. Authors recommend adequate sizing, tightening of straps, tape, or hook-and-pile fasteners, and shaving leg hair to decrease this potential for lost leverage.[74] Additionally, braces provide little control of axial rotation because they offer limited ability to resist translational loads. Because of the exposed metal, brace-induced injuries have been known to be inflicted on other players. Finally, braces have an endurance limit, such that repetitive cyclic loading of the components eventually may lead to plastic deformation and ultimate failure of the knee brace.[24]

Clinical relevance

Knee injuries compose a significant portion of the injuries seen in athletic training rooms, emergency departments, and physician offices. These include injuries to the ACL, PCL, and MCL.

The actual ACL injury rate to the knee remains quite low, approximately 80,000 per year annually in the United States.[29] The highest incidence appears to occur among 15- to 25-year-old athletes who participate in pivoting sports. Some studies have suggested that the rate of knee injuries, specifically ACL tears, may be increasing[88]; however, other authors have concluded that the injury rate remains unchanged.[1] Gender differences in the rate of knee injuries do exist. In fact, data suggest that collegiate female athletes participating in the same activity are two to eight times more likely to sustain an ACL injury than are males.[1,6] Some authors have suggested that delays in the treatment of these injuries may be associated with an increased risk of medial meniscus tears.[66]

The amount of force acting on the normal ACL depends upon the activity the knee is experiencing. Forces range between 400 N during normal daily activities to much higher forces during strenuous activity.[70,71] Although the ultimate strength of the ACL is age dependent, the average ultimate strength is 2,100 N.[97] Some researchers have attempted to use knee braces to limit the force experienced by the ACL in order to prevent injury. However, if the force exerted on the ACL is greater than its ultimate strength, an ACL rupture will still occur.

Approximately 30% of ACL injuries are thought to be due to direct contact between another player or object; the other 70% are believed to be the result of noncontact mechanisms, including pivoting and decelerating activity, "out of control play," and awkward landings.[40] Risk factors for noncontact injuries, including environmental, anatomic, hormonal, and biomechanical factors, have been suggested.

Because the ACL is composed of fibrocartilage, it does not have an intrinsic ability to heal itself.[45] ACL-deficient athletes often note a "giving way" or instability after attempts to return to sport because the ACL is the primary restraint to anterior tibial displacement. As a result of the functional instability, the secondary restraints of the knee are often injured.[23] Current recommendations for return to play in the ACL-deficient athlete mostly include surgical ACL reconstruction because of the repercussions of conservative management of the unstable knee. However, some have used knee braces to facilitate functional return to sport in an ACL-deficient knee and as an adjunct to surgical intervention in the postoperative rehabilitative period.

PCL tears represent approximately 3% to 37% of all knee ligament injuries, depending on the mechanism of injury.[22,67] A PCL injury is sustained as the result of contact (posterior force directed against a flexed knee) and noncontact (hyperextension) mechanisms.[44] No study has reported a trend toward an increasing incidence or gender difference in PCL injury. The PCL is the primary restraint to posterior tibial displacement and secondary restraint to external rotation.[19] With PCL rupture there is posterior subluxation of the tibia on the femur. This has been shown to result in increased contact pressures in the patellofemoral joint and medial femoral condyle.[60,87] Some older short-term studies have noted that patients with PCL injuries who are treated nonoperatively do well.[28,34,92,93] Other long-term studies have shown that the clinical and radiological incidence of degenerative joint disease increases in proportion to length of time after PCL injury to the knee.[22,26,52,75] Interestingly, the PCL has the intrinsic ability to heal itself because it is made of fibroblastlike cells.[83,84] This may allow for full functional recovery with proper nonoperative management. In some cases this may include the use of rehabilitative braces.[44] However, one must be aware that the PCL may heal in a lengthened position.[32]

The incidence of MCL injury is difficult to determine because of the wide spectrum of injury severity. Additionally, the ACL, PCL, or LCL may be injured concomitantly. Most injuries occur as a result of significant valgus stress applied to the lateral aspect of the knee, as the MCL is the primary medial restraint to valgus loading.[95] Then, with increasing stress, the ACL and PCL provide medial restraint.[36,77] The MCL also provides resistance to abnormal external tibial rotation.[41]

Because the MCL has an intrinsic ability to heal itself, treatment of isolated MCL tears for the past 25 years has been a conservative, nonsurgical approach. Knee braces are used frequently during rehabilitation to facilitate early range of motion while protecting the healing ligament. Some also have recommended a bilateral upright knee orthosis when returning to play.

Historical perspective

Historically, casting was used to treat knee injuries and fractures about the knee.[59] Unfortunately, some patients had residual knee stiffness and functional instability of the knee joint.[53] Knee orthoses originally were designed to treat congenital and acquired deformities around the knee, including genu varum and quadriceps paralysis in polio patients. More recently, Sarmiento[81] used knee orthoses in a rehabilitative setting to treat fractures about the knee while preventing loss of range of motion. In the 1960s and 1970s, physicians began using orthoses to treat athletes with functional knee instability from ACL injuries.[25] In the late 1970s, Anderson et al.[5] modified a rehabilitative brace, the Anderson Knee Stabler, to prevent recurrent injury to the medial collateral ligament. Physicians, coaches, and players then started to use these braces to prevent knee injuries.

In the mid-1980s, some of the negative aspects of brace wear began to emerge, and assumptions were made that knee braces were bad. More recent epidemiological studies have not shown any negative consequences of brace wear.

Currents issues regarding knee braces are multifaceted, including whether or not to wear a brace in a prophylactic, functional, or rehabilitative capacity and how long to wear these braces, whether the performance inhibition is worth the perceived decreased risk of injury, and whether an off-the-shelf or custom design is better.

Prophylactic braces

Prophylactic knee braces have been used mostly by football and lacrosse players to prevent MCL and ACL injury. The prophylactic knee braces attempt to limit the strain on the MCL and ACL by redirecting a lateral impact force away from the joint line to points more distal on the tibia or femur (Fig. 29-4).[33] There is a great deal of controversy surrounding the use of a prophylactic knee brace in sport.

Current research

Current research has attempted to document brace effectiveness more objectively. Biomechanical testing of surrogate limb models and cadaveric specimens have attempted to define the role of bracing in sports. However, these testing methods are limited by lack of active muscle contraction and poor soft-tissue compliance, both of which influence the measurement of strain on knee ligaments.[12]

Using a cadaveric model, Meyer et al.[65] compared a lateral, upright brace (Anderson Knee Stabler, Omni Scientific, Lafayette, IL) and a bilateral, nylon upright brace

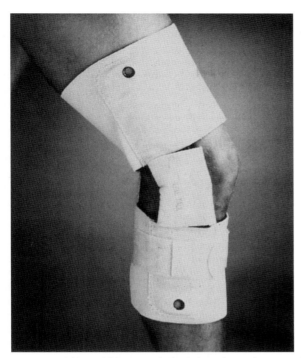

Fig. 29-4 McDavid lateral hinge prophylactic knee brace. (From Insall J, Scott W: *Surgery of the knee*, ed 3, Philadelphia, 2001, Churchill Livingstone.)

(AmPro, APO, Iowa City, IA) to a nonbraced condition under dynamic valgus loading. They found a decrease in load-induced MCL elongation with the AmPro (25.1%) and the Anderson Knee Stabler (18.3%) versus the unbraced knee. However, the knees were loaded at relatively slow speeds of 100 mm/s, which does not emulate actual game play environment.

Because of difficulty conducting cadaveric-based research, a number of scientists have developed surrogate knee models to test braces and their possible protective effects on ligaments. Surrogates are made of metal and polymeric components with ligament substitutes that are fabricated to emulate the shape and biomechanical properties of the human knee. Problems with these models include a lack of muscle tone and a variation in normal ligamentous structure.

Using a surrogate knee model in 10 knee braces, Liu et al.[58] found that only two braces, the Townsend (Townsend Design, Bakersfield, CA) and the Marquette Knee Stabilizer II (Vixie Enterprises I, Eugene, OR), effectively limited anterior tibial translation at 400 N. These braces were bilateral hinge, post, shell designs. Most other braces failed at forces less than 300 N.

France et al.[36] tested six different knee braces—DonJoy (dj Orthopaedics Inc., Vista, CA), Anderson Knee Stabler (Omni Scientific, Vista, CA), Stromgren (Stromgren, Hays, KS), Mueller (Mueller, Prairie du Sac, WI), Tru-Fit, and McDavid—for their ability to prevent MCL or ACL injury. They reported that braces were most effective for large-mass, low-velocity impacts with the hip and ankle fixed and the knee extended. Only the DonJoy, a unilateral upright, dual-hinged knee brace, provided an impact safety factor (ISF) > 1.50 more than 50% of the time for the MCL testing conditions. None of the braces protected the ACL at ISF > 1.50. Overall, they concluded that braces with the greatest stiffness and that were offset from the knee to prevent premature joint contact had the greatest ISF, but that none of the braces provided the level of protection necessary to prevent MCL or ACL injury at high-impact loads.

Paulos et al.[76] provided data from a surrogate limb model suggesting that bracing increased the impact duration, which protected the ACL more than the MCL. They concluded that bracing does provide some degree of protection to the ACL and MCL under direct lateral impact.

Brown et al.[17] found a direct relationship between tightness of the brace tension and the degree of relative MCL strain attenuation achieved. Daley et al.[27] used Brown's model to test the effectiveness of knee braces with varying hinge length and offset, upright length, breadth, thickness, and cuff surface area. They showed that the best design simulated the original Anderson Knee Stabler.

Others have criticized the surrogate limb model because it does not represent the ligamentous or soft-tissue structures seen in and around the normal knee. Thus, Erickson developed a hybrid of cadaveric and surrogate models that incorporated an artificial substitute for the human thigh and leg surface in the contracted muscle state while retaining the actual ligaments, muscles, and bones of the cadaveric specimens.

Erickson et al.[33] measured in vitro MCL and ACL strain values during dynamic loading in four unilateral, upright prophylactic knee braces (Anderson Knee Stabler, McDavid Knee Guard, DonJoy, SMI Preventive Knee Brace, and DePuy Knee Protector [BSN Medical, Charlotte, NC]). They found that the prophylactic brace was able to reduce the impact load at the point of contact and reduce the resulting lengthening in both the MCL and ACL. However, only the DonJoy brace significantly lowered the peak strain in the MCL at 30 degrees of knee flexion, whereas the McDavid brace significantly reduced the peak strain of the MCL at full knee extension. None of the braces decreased the amount of ACL strain from a valgus force.

Based on in vivo Hall data, Beynnon et al.[10] suggested that any protective effects on ACL strain relief are minor. They have concluded that under weight-bearing conditions, a prophylactic knee brace probably would not protect an ACL from injury during a rapid valgus stress at high speeds.

Current clinical studies have been challenged to directly test brace efficacy by measuring tibiofemoral translation and rotation. Most studies have indirectly measured brace effectiveness using the KT-1000, KT-2000, Genucom, and Stryker Knee Laxity Tests. These measurements appear to be inaccurate with the brace in place. Additionally, most studies have examined brace effectiveness at low loads and not at loads seen during athletic competition.

Beynnon et al.[12] loaded the knee while subjects were wearing three custom and four off-the-shelf braces and tested the Hall-effect strain behavior in the ACL. At low anterior shear loads, two braces provided some protection, but at higher anterior shear loads, no brace provided protection. Beynnon et al.[11] also showed that because of the compressive load across the knee produced during weight bearing, braces are not able to reduce ACL strain.

Any strain relief for the MCL provided by a unilateral, upright, off-the-shelf brace appears to be minor (20%–30%) based upon the surrogate knee model studies. However, prophylactic knee braces may be able to help prevent ACL injury caused by excessive medial opening at the time of valgus loading at low loads only. Some authors have suggested that clinical and laboratory knee bracing studies should address different levels of play (high school, college, and professional) and different types of sports (football, skiing, and soccer).[69]

Epidemiological studies

Early reports indicated that prophylactic knee braces prevented knee injuries in collegiate athletes. However, studies published in the mid-1980s detailed the negative effects of knee bracing.[80,91] Based on the results of a 2-year retrospective study, Teitz et al.[91] suggested that prophylactic knee bracing may result in an increased frequency and severity of MCL injury. They suggested that decreased agility and mobility caused the braced individuals to sustain more MCL injuries. However, they did not take string (starter and nonstarter) into account, and they used a variety of knee brace designs. Grace et al.[38] showed that brace type may be a more important factor. They suggested that use of a single-hinged brace caused prestressing of the collateral ligaments and accounted for the increased injury rates in some knee-braced individuals. Others reported that knee braces were not more or less likely to cause knee injuries.[8,37,47,63]

Because of the negative results reported in these studies, the American Academy of Orthopaedic Surgeons eventually released a position statement on the use of prophylactic braces, stating that these devices have not been shown to be effective for preventing knee injuries. Additionally, these devices may be associated with an increased frequency and severity of knee injury. This statement is now known to be a misguided suggestion. Since that time, other epidemiological studies have shown that knee bracing may prevent the number and severity of knee injuries in some athletes.

In 1990, Sitler et al.[86] reported their results of a 2-year prospective, randomized trial at the U.S. Military Academy on the incidence of knee injuries in intramural tackle football. They compared the results of individuals who wore the DonJoy Orthopedic Protector Knee Guard, a single, upright, double-hinged knee brace, to results of nonbraced individuals. They were able to control athletic shoe wear, playing surface, knee injury history, and brace assignment. They found a greater number of knee injuries in the control group (3.4 per 1,000 athlete exposure) versus the braced group (1.5 per 1,000 athlete exposure). There also was a trend toward a higher percentage of less severe MCL and ACL sprains (Fisher exact probability, 0.81) in the braced group. Some have addressed concerns that the study was conducted on players participating in intramural tackle football, which does not represent the intensity seen during intercollegiate play.[1]

In the late 1980s, the Big Ten Conference studied the effect of knee bracing on the incidence of MCL sprains in collegiate football players. Based on the results of the study, they determined that the likelihood of injury was dependent on the session (games or practices), string group (players or nonplayers), and position group (line, linebacker/tight end, or skill position). During practice, injury rates were equal for braced and nonbraced, line and linebacker/tight end positions, whereas the rate of injury was twice as high for skill players. During these conditions, players had a lower injury rate if they wore a brace. During games, all positions had an increased rate of knee injury, with line positions having the greatest risk. The rate of injury was found to be dependent on brace wear. If linemen and linebackers/tight ends wore a brace, they had a lower injury rate, whereas skill position players did not. Although the results were not statistically significant, the authors suggested a trend toward wearing braces and a decreased rate of knee injury. Most importantly, the study showed that there was no greater risk of injury to the knee in athletes wearing knee braces. A significant limitation of the study was that players in the study wore different brace designs. As shown previously, different brace designs may or may not have a protective effect on the MCL or ACL, which may have affected the final results of the study.[2,3]

In 1999, the Hunt Valley Consensus Conference on Prevention of Noncontact ACL Injuries was held to discuss ACL injury prevention. The attendees concluded that there was no evidence that knee braces prevented noncontact ACL injuries. They suggested that shoe-surface coefficient of friction and introducing training programs to enhance body control by activating protective neuromuscular responses were more important.[40] They based these recommendations on the fact that some authors had shown that technique modification decreased the incidence of ACL injuries from 1.15 to 0.15 injuries per team.[21] However, other authors have developed programs that address these neuromuscular strength and coordination deficits and have shown a 3.6 times lower incidence of ACL injury in trained athletes.[46] More recently, Yu et al.[98] suggested that knee braces may be able to prevent low knee flexion angles during landing, possibly reducing the risk of an ACL tear.

Braces may be effective in reducing the risk of sustaining an MCL sprain in male football players; however, epidemiological studies in other sports and in female players are necessary to determine their efficacy in these venues. Additionally, epidemiological studies have not addressed the ability of prophylactic knee braces to prevent an ACL tear. These studies would require a large, homogeneous population in order produce statistically significant information.

Clinical performance

Many athletes wear prophylactic knee braces in practice but not in games because they fear performance limitations. In fact, recent exercise physiology research has shown that brace wear does affect performance.

Houston et al.[48] noted a decrease in muscle performance and an increase in blood lactate concentration while wearing a brace. Zetterlund et al.[99] noted this performance inhibition was velocity dependent. Gender-specific differences may exist, as Sforzo et al.[82] noted no performance inhibition with a Stromgren dual-hinged knee brace in 25 male football players but did in 10 female collegiate lacrosse players.

Based on the work of Jerosch et al.[49] and Styf et al.,[89] researchers believe that knee braces cause premature muscle fatigue by reducing perfusion to the working muscles. Specifically, Styf et al.[89] tested the effect of functional braces, including two bilateral upright hinged braces (DonJoy Hinged Neoprene Knee Support and Omni II, Omni) and an elastic sleeve with semirigid stays (Bell-Horn Knee Sleeve, Bell-Horn, Philadelphia, PA). Resting muscle pressure and muscle relaxation pressures increased significantly in all testing conditions, whereas relaxation pressures returned to normal only after removal of the brace or the distal straps.

With regard to actual performance, Greene et al.[39] tested 30 collegiate football players on a 40-yard dash and four-cone agility drills using two functional knee braces with bilateral hinges (DonJoy Legend, DonJoy, Carlsbad, CA; and Breg Tradition, Breg Inc., Vista, CA) and four prophylactic knee braces with lateral-only hinges (OMNI-AKS 101W, OMNI Life Science, Springville, UT; McDavid Knee Guard, McDavid, Clarendon Hills, IL; models 1 and 2 of the Air Armor Knee and Thigh Protection System, Air Armor Inc., Scottsdale, AZ). The 40-yard dash times were significantly slower in the Air Armor 2, Breg, DonJoy, and McDavid groups than in the controls. In the four-cone agility test, only the Breg was significantly slower than controls. They suggested that braces do increase energy expenditure and restrict motion, but that experienced knee braced individuals may have fewer or no performance test effects. Greene et al. also noted limited brace efficacy after the brace migrated distally. Based on the results of their testing conditions, they concluded that all of the braces experienced some degree of inferior migration. Najibi and Albright[69] have suggested using hook-and-loop material to suspend the brace from the thigh portion of the athlete's pants to limit this inferior migration.

Functional braces

The majority of functional knee braces are designed to protect a patient with an ACL-deficient knee or to protect the ACL-reconstructed graft while returning to full activity (Figs. 29-5 and 29-6). Authors have reported that some functional knee braces are effective in protecting healing or ligament-deficient knees.[9,72] Other authors have reported patients continue to experience instability despite functional bracing.[23,90]

Current research

ACL-deficient knees have been shown to have less proprioception than normal knees.[14] Cook et al.[23] showed enhanced proprioception with brace wearing in the ACL-deficient knee, but others have shown that a functional brace does not alter electromyographic activity or change patterns of muscle firing.[15]

Wojtys et al.[96] compared patients with ACL-deficient knees in braced and unbraced conditions and found a 28% to 84% reduction in anterior tibial translation in braced individuals. Beynnon et al.[11] showed similar results in weight-bearing and non–weight-bearing conditions, but found that the braces offered no protection during transfer from non–weight-bearing to weight-bearing conditions. Additionally, the loads and speeds tested in these studies were substantially less than those seen during participation in sport.

With regard to clinical performance, some studies found that custom-made functional braces, including the Generation II and Lenox Hill braces, did not interfere with the performance of ACL-deficient knees.[61] However, long-term conservative management of ACL-deficient knees in skeletally immature patients has been shown to result in increased degenerative change and consistently fair and poor Lysholm

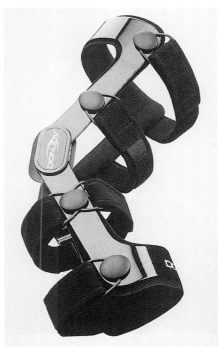

Fig. 29-5 The 4TITUDE, an example of an off-the-shelf anterior cruciate ligament functional brace. (From Insall J, Scott W: *Surgery of the knee*, ed 3, Philadelphia, 2001, Churchill Livingstone.)

scores. Without clinical support, authors have recommended functional bracing for sport participation until ACL reconstruction can be performed.[68] This recommendation seems to be highly controversial given the brace's limited ability to control knee motion at physiological conditions.

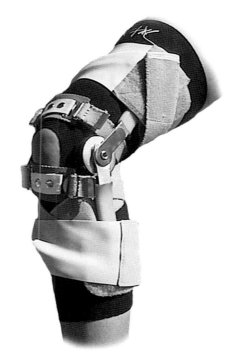

Fig. 29-6 The Lenox Hill, an example of a custom-made anterior cruciate ligament functional brace. (From Insall J, Scott W: *Surgery of the knee*, ed 3, Philadelphia, 2001, Churchill Livingstone.)

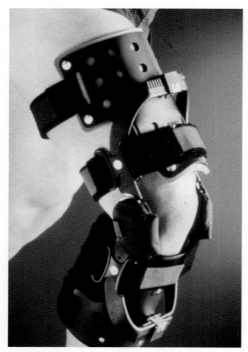

Fig. 29-7 Rehabilitation brace can provide rigid immobilization at selected angles and controlled motion during knee motion. (From Goldberg B, Hsu JD: *Atlas of orthoses and assistive devices*, ed 3, St. Louis, 1997, Mosby.)

DeVita et al.[30] and Knutzen et al.[55] showed that braces can increase the axial force on the knee, which has implications for patients with chondral defects and meniscal tears, possibly leading to accelerated osteoarthritis. Branch et al.[16] showed that bracing decreases quadriceps muscle function, which may explain the increased axial loads seen in previous studies. Others have suggested that patients involved in a hamstring strengthening program may show equivalent decreases in anterior tibial translation compared to results with bracing the ACL-deficient knee.[7]

Some ACL-deficient athletes subjectively benefit from the use of a functional knee brace. However, given the brace's limited ability to control translation and axial rotation at the physiological loads seen during strenuous exercise, most physicians recommend surgical ACL reconstruction. However, no prospective study has directly compared the two treatments.

Rehabilitative knee braces

Individuals with ligamentous injuries of the knee, including ACL, PCL, and MCL injuries, are managed with a variety of nonsurgical and surgical options. Knee braces have been used in each of these settings to facilitate return to play.

The goal of a rehabilitative brace is twofold: (1) to prevent excessive loads on the damaged or reconstructed ligament and (2) to allow early return to activity (Fig. 29-7).[12] Long rehabilitation braces are used because they best utilize leverage to prevent abnormal motion, but they are often cumbersome. Therefore, shorter intermediate braces are prescribed to allow early functional rehabilitation until quadriceps and hamstring strength has returned and the graft has incorporated. Although rehabilitative knee braces offer these benefits, early functional rehabilitation and improved surgical techniques have been shown to more effectively allow early return to activity. Therefore, recent studies have addressed the question: Do patients need a brace after reconstruction, and, if so, when can the brace be discontinued?

Current research

ACL

After ACL reconstruction, the graft must incorporate into the femur and tibia before the structural properties of the new ligament can function like the native ACL. Authors suggest that the period of time an ACL-reconstructed graft needs in order to incorporate is at least 3 months[19] and no greater than 8 months.[13]

DeVita et al.[31] showed that 3 weeks after an ACL reconstruction with bone–patella tendon–bone autograft, bracing decreased extensor moment and load on the ACL graft. Additionally, studies have shown that the knee joint suffers from a lack of proprioception after an ACL reconstruction.[85] Kuster et al.[56] showed a reduction in postural sway and increased ground reaction forces with the use of a compression knee sleeve and speculated that proprioception and muscle coordination are enhanced with use of a knee orthosis. Because knee braces have been shown to decrease strain on the ACL graft and enhance proprioception about the knee, authors have recommended their use.[12,31,58] Still others believe that a rehabilitation program emphasizing coactivation of the hamstrings, quadriceps, and gastrocnemius offers an equally good result.[73]

Recent epidemiologic research has been aimed at determining the need for wearing a brace postoperatively. Specifically, Risberg et al.[79] prospectively compared bracing to no bracing for 3 months after ACL reconstruction. They reported that at 3 months the braced group showed significantly improved Cincinnati knee scores and increased thigh atrophy. Otherwise, no differences between the groups were discovered when comparing KT-1000, range of motion, muscle strength, functional knee tests, patient satisfaction, and pain at 3 or 6 months. At 2-year follow-up, no evidence was seen that bracing increased or decreased future knee injuries.

In 2004, McDevitt et al.[64] compared use of a functional brace protocol for 1 year to use of a knee immobilizer for 3 weeks after isolated bone–patella tendon–bone ACL reconstruction in 100 military cadets. They found that many braced patients were noncompliant; in fact, 21 of 47 braced patients discontinued brace use 1 to 4 months prematurely. Most patients discontinued brace use because they believed the device interfered with performance. They found no difference with regard to range of motion, isokinetic testing, Lysholm score, International Knee Documentation Committee score, KT-1000, Lachman test, or pivot shift test. They noted a 6% reinjury rate in the unbraced group versus 4% in the brace group. The authors noted they would need 1,800 patients to detect any significant difference. Interestingly, 50% of the braced patients indicated they would use a knee brace in the future if they needed a revision ACL reconstruction. As a result of this study, the military academy changed their protocol to the following. Use a knee immobilizer for 3 weeks or discontinue use when good quadriceps strength is obtained, and brace only for subjective instability.

Other prospective, randomized trials reported similar results.[43,51] A meta-analysis in 1999 stated that no difference was seen with or without a brace.[62] Howell[48a] showed good results using hamstring autograft for ACL reconstruction and no brace postoperatively. Despite these studies, most athletes continue to wear a brace postoperatively.

MCL

Treatment of MCL sprains has evolved from a predominance of surgical treatment to nonsurgical treatment based upon the functional results of early protected range-of-motion protocols. Knee bracing has been the major factor allowing the use of these functional rehabilitation programs. Reider et al.[78] showed excellent results for treatment of grade III MCL sprains. They used two lateral knee hinged braces (McDavid Knee Guard and Anderson Knee Stabler) and the University of Wisconsin rehabilitation protocol to treat 35 isolated grade III MCL sprains. They found that 50% of the athletes returned to sport within 2 weeks and that most athletes chose to continue wearing the brace upon return to competition. However, no randomized trial has been published suggesting that use of a brace decreases the time to return to sport, and limited data suggest which brace is best.

PCL

Isolated acute PCL injuries are best treated conservatively. Specifically, acute grade I and II PCL tears have been shown to heal with bracing, protected weight bearing, and quadriceps muscle rehabilitation.[83] Although treatment of isolated, acute grade III PCL tears seems to be more controversial than treatment of grade I and grade II PCL tears, these injuries can be treated with a rehabilitative brace in full extension for 2 to 4 weeks, then gradual return to activity within 3 months. Harner and Höher[44] concluded that symptomatic chronic grade I and II injuries usually respond well to physical therapy. They do not recommend functional knee bracing for these chronic injuries, although they suggest that chronic grade III injuries are best treated with surgery.

Multiligament and LCL

A discussion of the treatment of multiligamentous and lateral collateral ligamentous knee injuries is beyond the scope of this chapter; however, such treatment remains extremely controversial.

References

1. Agel J, Arendt EA, Bershadsky B: Anterior cruciate ligament injury in national collegiate athletic association basketball and soccer: a 13-year review, *Am J Sports Med* 33:524–530, 2005.
2. Albright JP, Powell JW, Smith W, et al: Medial collateral ligament knee sprains in college football: Effectiveness of preventive braces, *Am J Sports Med* 22:12–18, 1994.
3. Albright JP, Powell JW, Smith W, et al: Medial collateral ligament knee sprains in college football: Brace wear preferences and injury risk, *Am J Sports Med* 22:2–11, 1994.
4. American Academy of Orthopaedic Surgeons: Knee braces. In Derz DJ, editor: *Seminar report*, Chicago, 1985, American Academy of Orthopedic Surgeons.
5. Anderson G, Zeman SC, Rosenfeld RT: The Anderson Knee Stabler, *Physician Sportsmed* 7:125–127, 1979.
6. Arendt E, Dick R: Knee injury patterns among men and women in collegiate basketball and soccer: NCAA data and review of literature, *Am J Sports Med* 23:694–701, 1995.
7. Bagger J, Raven J, Lavard P, Blyme P, Sorensen C: Effect of functional bracing, quadriceps and hamstrings on anterior tibial translation in anterior cruciate ligament insufficiency: a preliminary study, *J Rehabil Res Dev* 29:9–12, 1992.
8. Baker BE, VanHanswyk E, Bogosian SP, Werner FW, Murphy D: The effect of knee braces on lateral impact loading of the knee, *Am J Sports Med* 17:182–186, 1989.
9. Bassett GS, Fleming BW: The Lenox Hill brace in anterolateral rotatory instability, *Am J Sports Med* 11:345–348, 1983.
10. Beynnon BD, Fleming BC: Anterior cruciate ligament strain in-vivo: a review of previous work, *J Biomech* 17:182–186, 1998.
11. Beynnon B, Johnson R, Fleming B, et al: The effect of functional knee bracing on the anterior cruciate ligament in the weightbearing and nonweightbearing knee, *Am J Sports Med* 25:353–359, 1997.
12. Beynnon BD, Pope MH, Wertheimer CM, et al: The effect of functional knee-braces on strain on the anterior cruciate ligament in vivo, *J Bone Joint Surg Am* 74A:1298–1312, 1992.
13. Beynnon BD, Risberg MA, Tjornsland O, et al: Evaluation of knee joint laxity and the structural properties of the anterior cruciate ligament in the human. A case report, *Am J Sports Med* 25:203–206, 1997.
14. Beynnon B, Ryder S, Konradsen L, Johnson R, Johnson K, Renstrom P: The effect of anterior cruciate ligament trauma an bracing on knee proprioception, *Am J Sports Med* 27:150–155, 1999.
15. Branch TP, Hunter R, Donath M: Dynamic EMG analysis of anterior cruciate deficient legs with and without bracing during cutting, *Am J Sports Med* 17:35–41, 1989.
16. Branch TP, Hunter R, Reynolds P: Controlling anterior tibial displacement under static load: a comparison of two braces, *Orthopedics* 11:1249–1252, 1988.
17. Brown TD, Van Hoeck JE, Brand RA: Laboratory evaluation of prophylactic knee brace performance under dynamic valgus loading using a surrogate leg model, *Clin Sports Med* 9:519–525, 1990.
18. Burger RR: Knee braces. In Baker CL, Flandry F, Henderson JM, editors: *The Hughston Clinic sport medicine book*, Baltimore, 1995, Williams & Wilkins.
19. Butler DL, Grood ES, Noyes FR et al: Mechanical properties of primate vascularized vs. nonvascularized patellar tendon grafts; changes over time, *J Orthop Res* 7:68–79, 1989.
20. Butler DL, Noyes FR, Grood ES: Ligamentous restraints to anterior-posterior drawer in the human knee. A biomechanical study, *J Bone Joint Surg Am* 62:259–270, 1980.
21. Caraffa A, Cerulli G, Projetti M, Aisa G, Rizzo A: Prevention of anterior cruciate ligament injuries in soccer: a prospective controlled study of proprioceptive training, *Knee Surg Sports Traumatol Arthrosc* 4:19–21, 1996.
22. Clancy WG, Shelbourne KD, Zoellner GB, et al: Treatment of knee joint instability secondary to rupture of the posterior cruciate ligament: report of a new procedure, *J Bone Joint Surg Am* 65:310–322, 1983.
23. Cook FF, Tibone JE, Redfern FC: A dynamic analysis of a functional brace for anterior cruciate ligament insufficiency, *Am J Sports Med* 17:519–524, 1989.
24. Crawley PW: Post-operative knee bracing, *Clin Sports Med* 9:763–770, 1990.
25. Crawley PW, France EP, Paulos LE: The current state of functional knee bracing research: a review of the literature, *Am J Sports Med* 19:226–233, 1991.
26. Cross MJ, Powell JF: Long-term follow-up of posterior cruciate ligament rupture: a study of 116 cases, *Am J Sports Med* 12:292–7, 1984.
27. Daley BJ, Ralston JL, Brown TD, Brand RA: A parametric design evaluation of lateral prophylactic knee braces, *J Biomech Eng* 115:131–136, 1993.
28. Dandy DJ, Pusey RJ: The long-term results of unrepaired tears of the posterior cruciate ligament, *J Bone Joint Surg Br* 64:92–94, 1982.
29. Daniel DM, Fritschy D: Anterior cruciate ligament injuries. In DeLee JC, Drez D Jr, editors: *Orthopaedic sports medicine: principles and practice*, Philadelphia, 1994, WB Saunders.
30. Devita P, Hunter PB, Skelly WA: Effects of a functional knee brace on the biomechanics of running, *Med Sci Sports Exerc* 24:797–806, 1992.
31. Devita P, Lassiter T, Hortobagyi T, Torry M: Functional knee brace effects during walking in patients with anterior cruciate ligament reconstruction, *Am J Sports Med* 26:778–784, 1998.
32. Dowd GSE: Reconstruction of the posterior cruciate ligament, *J Bone Joint Surg Br* 86:480–491, 2004.
33. Erickson AR, Yasuda K, Beynnon B, Johnson R, Pope M: An in vitro dynamic evaluation of prophylactic knee braces during lateral impact loading, *Am J Sports Med* 21:26–35, 1993.

34. Fowler PJ, Messieh SS: Isolated posterior cruciate ligament injuries in athletes, *Am J Sports Med* 15:553–557, 1987.

35. France EP, Paulos LE: In vitro assessment of prophylactic knee brace function, *Clin Sports Med* 9:823–841, 1990.

36. France EP, Paulos LE, Jayaraman G, Rosenberg TD: The biomechanics of lateral knee bracing, part II: impact response of the braced knee, *Am J Sports Med* 15:430–438, 1987.

37. Garrick JG, Requa RK: Prophylactic knee bracing, *Am J Sports Med* 15:471–476, 1987.

38. Grace W, Skipper B, Newberry J, et al: Prophylactic knee braces and injury to the lower extremity, *J Bone Joint Surg Am* 70:422–427, 1988.

39. Greene DL, Hamson KR, Bay C, Bryce CD: Effects of protective knee bracing on speed and agility, *Am J Sports Med* 28:453–459, 2000.

40. Griffin LY, Agel J, Albohm MJ, et al: Noncontact anterior cruciate ligament injuries: risk factors and prevention strategies, *J Am Acad Orthop Surg* 8:141–150, 2000.

41. Grood ES, Noyes FR, Butler DL, et al: Ligamentous and capsular restraints preventing straight medial and lateral laxity in intact human cadaver knees, *J Bone Joint Surg Am* 63:1257, 1981.

42. Gunston FH: Polycentric knee arthroplasty: prosthetic simulation of normal knee movement, *J Bone Joint Surg Br* 5B:272, 1971.

43. Harilainen A, Sandelin J, Vanhanen I, et al: Knee brace after bone-tendon-bone anterior cruciate ligament reconstruction. Randomized, prospective study with two years follow-up, *Knee Surg Sports Traumatol Arthrosc* 5:10–13, 1997.

44. Harner CD, Höher J: Evaluation and treatment of posterior cruciate ligament injuries, *Am J Sports Med* 26:471–482, 1998.

45. Hefti FL, Kress A, Fasel J, Morscher EW: Healing of the transected anterior cruciate ligament in the rabbit, *J Bone Joint Surg Am* 73:373–383, 1991.

46. Hewett TE, Lindenfeld TN, Riccobene JV, Noyes FR: The effect of neuromuscular training on the incidence of knee injury in female athletes: a prospective study, *Am J Sports Med* 27:699–706, 1999.

47. Hewson GF Jr, Mendini RA, Wang JB: Prophylactic knee bracing in college football, *Am J Sports Med* 142:262–266, 1986.

48. Houston ME, Goemans PH: Leg muscle performance of athletes with and without knee support braces, *Arch Phys Med Rehabil* 63:431–432, 1982.

48a. Lawhorn KW, Howell SM: Principles for using hamstring tendon for ACL reconstruction. *Clin Sports Med* 26(4):567–585, 2007.

49. Jerosch J, Castro WH, Hoffstetter I, Reer R: Secondary effects of knee braces on the intracompartmental pressure in the anterior tibial compartment, *Acta Orthop Belg* 61:37–42, 1995.

50. Kapandji IA: *The physiology of the joints*, ed 5, London, 1987, Churchill-Livingstone.

51. Kartus J, Stener S, Kohler K, et al: Is bracing after anterior cruciate ligament reconstruction necessary? A two-year follow-up of 78 consecutive patients rehabilitated with or without a brace, Knee Surg Sports, *Traumatol Arthrosc* 5:157–161, 1997.

52. Keller PM, Shelbourne KD, McCarroll JR, Rettig AC: Nonoperatively treated isolated posterior cruciate ligament injuries, *Am J Sports Med* 21:132–136, 1993.

53. Kennedy JC: Complete dislocation of the knee joint, *J Bone Joint Surg Am* 45:889, 1963.

54. Knutzen K, Bates B, Hamill J: Electrogoniometry of post-surgical knee bracing in running, *Am J Phys Med* 62:172–181, 1983.

55. Knutzen K, Bates B, Schot P, et al: A biomechanical analysis of two functional braces, *Med Sci Sports Exerc* 19:303–309, 1987.

56. Kuster MS, Grob K, Kuster M, Wood GA, Gachter A: The benefits of wearing a compression sleeve after ACL reconstruction, *Med Sci Sport Exerc* 31:368–371, 1999.

57. Liggins AB, Bowker P: A quantitative assessment of orthoses for stabilization of the anterior cruciate ligament deficient knee, *Proc Inst Mech Eng [H]* 205:81–87, 1991.

58. Liu SH, Lunsford T, Gude S, Vangsness CT: Comparison of functional knee braces for control of anterior tibial displacement, *Clin Orthop Relat Res* 303:203–210, 1994.

59. Lucas-Championniere J: Treatment of fractures by massage and mobilization, *Br Med J* 2:1533–1534, 1912.

60. MacDonald PB, Miniaci A, Fowler PJ, Marks P: *Biomechanical of joint contact forces in the posterior cruciate deficient knee.* Paper presented at the 60th Annual Meeting of the American Academy of Orthopaedic Surgeons, February 18–23, San Francisco, California, USA.

61. Marans HJ, Jackson RW, Piccinin J, Silver RL, Kennedy DK: Functional testing of braces for anterior cruciate ligament-deficient knees, *Can J Surg* 34:167–172, 1991.

62. Martinek V, Friederich NF: To brace or not to brace? How effective are knee braces in rehabilitation?, *Orthopade* 28:565–570, 1999.

63. McCarthy P: Prophylactic knee braces: where do we stand?, *Phys Sportsmed* 16:102–115, 1986.

64. McDevitt ER, Taylor DC, Miller MD, et al: Functional bracing after anterior cruciate ligament reconstruction. A prospective, randomized, multicenter study, *Am J Sports Med* 32:1887–1892, 2004.

65. Meyer SJ, Brown TD, Jimenez BS, Brand RA: Benchtop mechanical performance of prophylactic knee braces under dynamic valgus loading: a cadaver study, *Iowa Orthop J* 10:1777–1780, 1989.

66. Millet PJ, Willis AA, Warren RF: Associated injuries in pediatric and adolescent anterior cruciate ligament tears: does a delay in treatment increase the risk of meniscal tear?, *Arthroscopy* 18:955–959, 2002.

67. Miyasaka KC, Daniel DM: The incidence of knee ligament injuries in the general population, *Am J Knee Surg* 4:3–8, 1991.

68. Mizuta H, Kubota K, Shiraishi M, et al: The conservative treatment of complete tears of the anterior cruciate ligament in skeletally immature patients, *J Bone Joint Surg Br* 77:890–894, 1995.

69. Najibi S, Albright JP: The use of knee braces, part 1: prophylactic knee braces in contact sports, *Am J Sports Med* 33:602–611, 2005.

70. Noyes FR, Butler DL, Grood ES, Zernicke RF, Hefzy MS: Biomechanical analysis of human ligament grafts used in knee-ligament repairs and reconstruction, *J Bone Joint Surg Am* 66:344–352, 1984.

71. Noyes FR, Grood ES, Butler DL: Clinical laxity tests and functional stability of the knee: biomechanical concepts, *Clin Orthop Relat Res* 144:84–89, 1980.

72. Noyes FR, Matthews DS, Mooar PA, Grood ES: The symptomatic anterior cruciate-deficient knee: Part II. The results of rehabilitation, activity modification, and counseling on functional disability, *J Bone Joint Surg Am* 65:163–174, 1983.

73. O'Connor JJ: Can muscle co-contraction protect knee ligaments after injury or repair, *J Bone Joint Surg Br* 75:41–48, 1993.

74. Paluska SA, McKeag DB: Knee braces: current evidence and clinical recommendations for their use, *Am Fam Physician* 61:411–424, 2000.

75. Parolie JM, Bergfeld JA: Long-term results of nonoperative treatment of isolated posterior cruciate ligament injuries in the athlete, *Am J Sports Med* 14:35–38, 1986.

76. Paulos LE, Cawley PW, France EP, et al: Impact biomechanics of lateral knee bracing: the anterior cruciate ligament, *Am J Sports Med* 19:337–342, 1991.

77. Paulos LE, Drawbert JP, France EP: Lateral knee braces in football: do they prevent injury? *Phys Sportsmed* 14:119–124, 1986.

78. Reider B, Sathy MR, Talkington J, Blynak N, Kollias S: Treatment of isolated medial collateral ligament injuries in athletes with early functional rehabilitation: a five-year follow-up study, *Am J Sports Med* 22:470–477, 1993.

79. Risberg MA, Holm I, Steen H, Eriksson J, Ekeland A: The effect of knee bracing after anterior cruciate ligament reconstruction. A prospective, randomized study with two years' follow-up, *Am J Sports Med* 27:76–83, 1999.

80. Rovere GD, Haupt HA, Yates CS: Prophylactic knee bracing in college football, *Am J Sports Med* 15:111–116, 1987.

81. Sarmiento A: A functional below-the-knee brace for tibial fractures. A report on its use in one hundred thirty-five cases, *J Bone Joint Surg Am* 52:295–311, 1970.

82. Sforzo GA, Chen NM, Gold CA, et al: The effect of prophylactic knee bracing on performance, *Med Sci Sports Exerc* 21:254–257, 1989.

83. Shelbourne KD, Davis TJ, Patel DV: The natural history of acute, isolated, nonoperatively treated posterior cruciate ligament injuries: a prospective study, *Am J Sports Med* 27:276–283, 1999.

84. Shelbourne KD, Jennings RW, Vahe TN: Magnetic resonance imaging of posterior cruciate ligament injuries: assessment of healing, *Am J Knee Surg* 12:209–213, 1999.

85. Shiraishi M, Mizuta H, Kubota K, Otsuka Y, Nagamoto N, Takagi K: Stabilometric assessment in the anterior cruciate ligament reconstructed knee, *Clin J Sports Med* 6:32–39, 1996.

86. Sitler M, Rya J, Hopkinson W, et al: The efficacy of a prophylactic knee brace to reduce knee injuries in football: a prospective, randomized study at West Point, *Am J Sports Med* 18:310–315, 1990.

87. Skyhar MH, Warren R, Ortiz GJ, Schwartz E, Otis JC: The effects of sectioning of the posterior cruciate ligament and the posterolateral complex on the articular contact pressure within the knee, *J Bone Joint Surg Am* 75:694–699, 1993.

88. Steinert KM: Increased incidence of anterior cruciate ligament tears in adolescent females, *Dartmouth Undergrad J Sci* 3:31–36, 2000.

89. Styf JR, Nakhostine M, Gershuni DH: Functional knee braces increase intramuscular pressures in the anterior compartment of the leg, *Am J Sports Med* 20:46–49, 1992.

90. Tegner Y, Lorentzon R: Evaluation of knee braces in Swedish ice hockey players, *Br J Sports Med* 25:159–161, 1991.

91. Teitz C, Hermanson B, Kronma R, et al: Evaluation of the use of braces to prevent injury to the knee in college football players, *J Bone Joint Surg Am* 69:2–8, 1987.

92. Torg JS, Barton TM, Pavlov H, Stine R: Natural history of the posterior cruciate ligament-deficient knee, *Clin Orthop Relat Res* 246:208–216, 1989.

93. Trickey EL: Rupture of the posterior cruciate ligament of the knee, *J Bone Joint Surg Br* 50:334–341, 1986.

94. Vailas JC, Pink M: Biomechanical effects of functional knee bracing: practical implications, *Sports Med* 15:210–218, 1993.

95. Warren F, Marshall J: The supporting structures and layers on the medial side of the knee, *J Bone Joint Surg Am* 61:56, 1979.

96. Wojtys EM, Kothari SU, Huston LJ: Anterior cruciate ligament functional brace use in sports, *Am J Sports Med* 24:539–546, 1996.

97. Woo S-L, Inoue M, McGurk-Burleson, et al: Treatment of medial collateral ligament injury. II: structure and function of canine knee in response to differing treatment regimens, *Am J Sports Med* 15:22–29, 1987.

98. Yu B, Herman D, Preston J, Lu W, Kirkendall D, Garrett W: Immediate effects of a knee brace with a constraint to knee extension on knee kinematics and ground reaction forces in a stop-jump task, *Am J Sports Med* 32:1136–1143, 2004.

99. Zetterlund AE, Serfass RC, Hunter RE: The effect of wearing the complete Lenox Hill derotation brace on energy expenditure during horizontal running at 161 meters per minute, *Am J Sports Med* 14:73–76, 1986.

Chapter

30

Orthotic management of the neuropathic and/or dysvascular patient

Richard B. Chambers, Nancy Elftman, and John H. Bowker

Key Points

- Care of the lower limb in the neuropathic and/or dysvascular patient requires the efforts of many professionals.
- The goal of treatment of the neuropathic and/or dysvascular limb is preservation of the patient's foot, especially as multiple studies have shown the increased energy demands of prosthetic ambulation that may preclude walking for the diabetic amputee with impaired cardiopulmonary reserve.
- The diabetic with a neuropathic ulcer should be treated with appropriate debridement and antibiotics if infection (often polymicrobial) is present. Orthotic devices alone do not compensate for lost sensation in the neuropathic limb, but when combined with an educated compliant patient and early intensive medical and surgical treatment, amputation can often be avoided.
- The patient with an ulcer caused by vascular insufficiency should be evaluated for possible vascular reconstruction. The members of the treatment team, which must include the patient, should work cooperatively to compensate for the deficits that accompany the neuropathic and/or dysvascular limb.

Loss of peripheral nerve function is closely associated with tissue loss because the neuropathic limb is threatened by delayed recognition of injury. Effective orthotic treatment can partially substitute for the missing link of sensation in the body's early warning system. Shoes, shoe inserts, and lower limb orthoses, in conjunction with use of substitute warning systems, such as vision and touch, can provide considerable protection to the neuropathic limb. In this manner,

orthotic treatment of the neuropathic foot can often prevent or greatly delay the need for amputation.

Peripheral neuropathy

Peripheral neuropathy can produce many combinations of sensory, motor, or autonomic loss of nerve function. The clinical result is frequently the same—ulceration—although the exact cause of an ulcer can vary. With sensory loss, acute or chronic skin trauma can go unrecognized for hours or days. Acute injury from penetration of the skin by a nail or chronic injury from a poorly fitting shoe are two common examples. Charcot joint degeneration may result in an ulcer beneath a bony prominence, or an ulcer may occur at the apex of an angular deformity such as a bunion (hallux valgus). Clawing of the toes, secondary to motor neuropathy of the intrinsic foot muscles, imperils ulcer-prone skin on the plantar surface of the metatarsal heads, dorsal surface of the proximal interphalangeal (PIP) joints, and toe tips. Autonomic nerve loss contributes to skin breakdown by producing dry, inelastic skin due to loss of oil and sweat glands. Although these structures cannot be restored, protection of these feet can be achieved with careful shoe fitting and foot monitoring.

The loss of sensation in peripheral neuropathy is symmetrical and equidistant from the spine in both arms and legs (Fig. 30-1). Therefore, the hands should be evaluated for neuropathy as well as the feet. Little attention has been paid to the "diabetic hand syndrome" in which the joints of the fingers and wrists exhibit limited joint mobility. This condition occurs in 30% to 50% of people who have had type 1 diabetes for more than 15 years. One sign of severe limited joint mobility is the inability to place pronated hands flat on

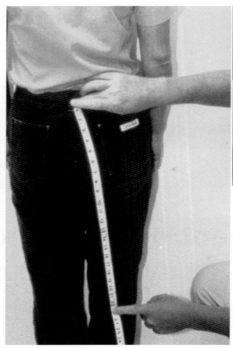
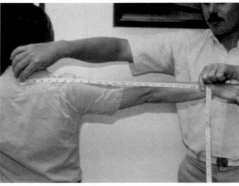

Fig. 30-1 Peripheral neuropathy affects all limbs symmetrically and equidistant from the spine, beginning with the feet and hands.

a table or to touch the palms together in the prayer position (Fig. 30-2). The skin is thick and cannot be "tented" on the back of the fingers.[24] Thenar atrophy and clawing of the fingers may be present. Hand deficits affect functions such as the ability to don and doff an orthosis and footwear.[4]

Bilateral testing for sensation is especially important for both the unilateral and bilateral amputee in order to map areas of insensitivity and to follow their progression. Neuropathy may affect a single nerve (mononeuropathy) due to nerve trauma or entrapment, but in most chronic diseases it presents as a polyneuropathy with uncomfortable paresthesias such as prickling, tingling, burning, and jabbing sensations.[44,47]

The most common disease processes resulting in peripheral neuropathy are as follows:

- Diabetes mellitus
- Spina bifida
- Hansen disease (leprosy)
- Lupus erythematosus

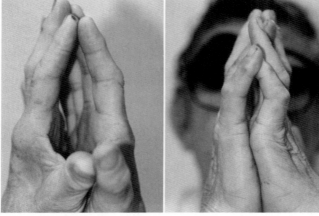

Fig. 30-2 Motor neuropathy of hands resulting in limited joint mobility.

- Acquired immune deficiency syndrome (AIDS)/human immunodeficiency virus (HIV)/AIDS-related complex (ARC)
- Cancer
- Multiple sclerosis
- Vascular disease
- Charcot-Marie-Tooth disease

The following substances and conditions can also cause peripheral neuropathy[8,9,27]:

- Alcoholism
- Arsenic
- Lead
- Steroids
- Gold
- Uremia
- Vitamin B deficiency
- Isoniazid (INH)

A high index of suspicion for neuropathy is useful when examining the feet of individuals with these conditions. Diabetes mellitus is the leading cause of peripheral neuropathy in the United States, with 54,000 amputations of the lower limb occurring yearly in a population of 14 million diabetics at an annual cost of $14 billion.[3,21,32,35,37,48]

Complaints of numbness, tingling, or burning night pain are common with neuropathy. The degree of sensory loss is difficult to quantify, but it is important to use an objective method of evaluation for initial detection as well as follow-up. Patients who are unable to detect a Semmes-Weinstein monofilament of 5.07 diameter (10g of force) pressed against their skin have loss of protective sensation and are at risk for foot injury without protective shoes and inserts. It is important to closely inspect the insensate foot, looking and feeling for areas of callused or atrophic skin vulnerable to breakdown, especially on weight-bearing surfaces. In addition, one should check for bony prominences related to claw toes, bunions, or Charcot fracture malalignment. Signs of concomitant dysvascularity, such as pulselessness, decreased hair growth, decreased skin temperature, or gangrene, indicate a high risk of eventual amputation if remedial steps are not taken.

Pressure on the skin can lead to ulceration and destruction of tissue in the neuropathic limb:

1. Ischemic necrosis is caused by moderate pressure (2–3 psi) over long periods of time. Local capillary circulation is interrupted, leading to skin death and ulceration. This is the mechanism of ulcer production at sites on the foot compressed by shoes that are too narrow and/or have a low toe box.
2. Inflammatory destruction occurs with repetitive moderate pressure (40–60 psi). Chronic inflammation develops and weakens the tissue, leading to ulceration. Breakdown over bony prominences occurs as a result of this mechanism.
3. Penetration occurs when a high pressure (600 psi) is suddenly applied to a small area of skin, as when stepping on a nail. Acute skin destruction also may be caused by heat or chemicals.

Infection abets the spread of tissue destruction. Once the skin is broken, bacterial invasion may cause the surrounding skin to become more vulnerable to even slight pressure, rendering it unsuitable for weight bearing.[11]

Recurrent ulceration is common over bony prominences, especially in weight-bearing skin. A newly healed ulcer is covered by thin, scarred skin that is likely to tear with stress. Skin adherent to bone has poor shock- and shear-absorbing qualities, making it vulnerable to breakdown. Protection of such skin areas is possible with careful shoe and insert construction.[10,12]

Charcot neuroarthropathy (Charcot joint)

Charcot joint is a relatively painless, progressive degenerative arthropathy of single or multiple joints associated with neuropathy, which can be periosteal and not cutaneous, so the skin surface may have intact sensation. There are several theories regarding the causes of Charcot joint:

1. Multiple microtraumas to the joints that cause microfractures. These fractures lead to relaxation of the ligaments and joint destruction.
2. Increased blood flow related to autonomic neuropathy, leading to osteolysis and bone reabsorption. Patients with Charcot joints usually have bounding pedal pulses.
3. Changes in the spinal cord leading to trophic (circulatory) changes in bones and joints.
4. Osteoporosis manifested by an abnormal brittleness of the bones leading to spontaneous fracture.[17]

Whatever the cause(s), Charcot neuroarthropathy can lead to radical changes in the shape and stability of affected joints. Its clinical stages, outlined in Table 30-1, should be followed and documented carefully, with management at each stage designed to minimize deformity. Treatment consists of casting in the neutral position for several months, followed by an orthosis such as a neuropathic walker, also known as a Charcot restraint orthotic walker. When the process becomes quiescent, the foot should be protected with appropriate shoes and inserts. If it does not become quiescent or recurs, a permanent ankle–foot orthosis (AFO) may be required.

Examination

The neuropathic limb with intact skin requires careful physical examination to identify deformities that may lead to ulceration in the future. Shoes and socks are removed from both feet at every visit to allow full visualization of calluses, bony prominences, and areas of skin inflammation or breakdown. Thickening of the skin (callus) is a response to increased local pressure or friction (shear).[14,45] Skin dryness is the result of autonomic neuropathy, in which sweat and oil production are decreased. Loss of hair growth may be indicative of vascular impairment. Motor neuropathy and Charcot neuroarthropathy often leave the foot deformed.

Joint stiffness increases the risk of ulceration by decreasing normal motion of foot joints during gait, thereby increasing

Table 30-1 Charcot neuroarthropathy (Charcot joint)[a]

Stage	Clinical Notes	Laboratory Test Results	Treatment Protocol
Acute/early stage (duration 1–2 months)	Limb usually painless, swollen, red, and 5°F–10°F hotter than contralateral limb	Unhealed fractures often radiographically present	Total-contact cast applied Cast changed in 5-7 days and followed in midstage
Advanced/midstage (6 months–1 year)	Warm with reduced swelling	Extensive bone demineralization and reabsorption	Changing of cast at 1- to 2-week intervals Casting important for retention of foot shape
Late stage and chronic	Complete bony healing, temperature equal to contralateral limb	Architectural distortion with shortening and widening of the joint[35]	Accommodate with splint, then shoes/inserts for midfoot to forefoot deformities Deformities of hindfoot or ankle require neuropathic walker or total-contact AFO Resultant bony deformities may require surgical intervention

[a]Stages of Charcot joint should be followed and documented carefully to reduce deformity.

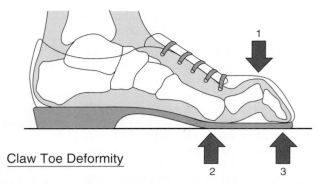

Claw Toe Deformity

Fig. 30-3 Clawing of toes makes skin over PIP joints more vulnerable to ulceration. *1*, Metatarsal heads have increased weight-bearing role. *2*, Dorsal callosity over PIP joint indicates increased contact with shoe. *3*, Toe tips become weight bearing, leading to nail problems.

foot–shoe contact pressures. It is important that the ankle have a dorsiflexion range of at least 10 degrees to allow ambulation without harm to midfoot joints or the great toe.[38] When the heel rises, the forces on the plantar surface of the metatarsal heads and toes can peak to 80% of body weight when walking and 275% when running. With limited motion in the metatarsophalangeal (MTP) joints, these forces can result in ulceration.[4,41,44]

Toe deformities

Toe deformities can lead to ulceration by contact with shoe surfaces or adjacent toes. Clawed toes are dorsiflexed at the MTP joints and plantarflexed at the interphalangeal (IP) joints. Excessive pressure occurs where the shoe makes contact with the metatarsal heads and toes (Fig. 30-3). Soft corns are hyperkeratotic lesions caused by pressure on the skin of tightly apposed toes in a moist environment.[14] These can be relieved with tube foam placed over the adjacent toes or lamb's wool between the toes (Fig. 30-4). Hypertrophy of

nails caused by fungus (onychomycosis) is common in the diabetic population. These nails tear shoe linings, creating rough surfaces that may abrade the toes.

The great toe should be carefully examined for deformity. An ankylosed IP joint can cause ulceration that is especially difficult to relieve. As the person thrusts the great toe into extension when ambulating, shoe contact can result in callus and discoloration on the distal end near the nail. Excessive great toe pronation causes a callus on its medial/plantar surface. Hallux rigidus, with greatly limited dorsiflexion of the first MTP joint due to degenerative arthritis, causes a callus on the plantar/medial aspect of the IP joint. This requires a rigid rocker-bottom shoe to allow rollover at the end of stance without excessive pressure at the IP joint. Hallux valgus (bunion) is a deviation of the great toe toward the lateral side of the foot, requiring a shoe that can be molded over the medial bony prominence of the bunion. The distal end of toe amputation sites may require similar protection from trauma.

Complications of the neuropathic foot

Several common complications are associated with care of the neuropathic limb. A sinus tract may persist when an ulcer, which appears to have healed, is merely covered with an excess of callus. This callus must be removed on a frequent basis to allow the ulcer to heal from its depths to the surface without trapping residual bacteria and necrotic tissue within. Another common occurrence in neuropathic feet is burns, often caused by spilling hot liquids or grease on poorly shod feet while cooking or by chemicals such as over-the-counter callus removers containing salicylic acid. Sources of thermal injury related to barefoot walking include the sun, hot beach sand, and floor furnace grids. Hot foot soaks and frost bite are other hazards. The insensitive foot cannot provide the warning signals necessary to prevent these injuries.

Dermatological conditions can affect the insensate limb. Necrobiosis lipoidica diabeticorum can be confused with

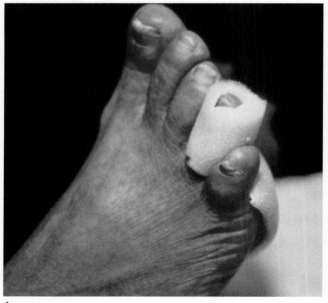

A

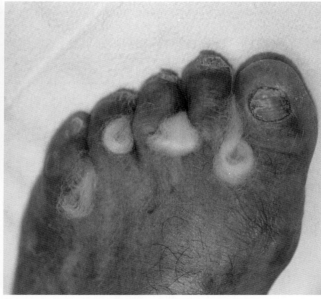

B

Fig. 30-4 Toe protection. To prevent maceration and breakdown from soft corns, toes can be spaced with tube foam **(A)** or lamb's wool **(B)**.

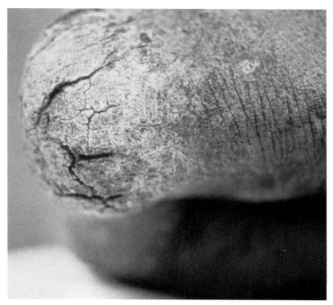

Fig. 30-5 Keratodermia plantaris. Loss of sweat and oil glands (autonomic neuropathy) can lead to keratin buildup and deep fissures, predominantly on heels.

venous stasis disease but does not require or respond to the extensive treatment required of the latter condition. The round, firm plaques of necrobiosis, which later ulcerate, are reddish brown to yellow and are seen three times more often in women than men.[34,49] They are common along the tibia and require only protective dressings until the ulcers heal. Plantar keratoderma is an excessive buildup of keratin following the loss of sweat and oil production in the skin associated with autonomic neuropathy. As a result, the entire margin of the heel pad undergoes diffuse thickening, followed by fissures that allow entrance of bacteria and subsequent infection (Fig. 30-5). Prevention includes reduction of keratin buildup by debridement and retention of skin moisture with

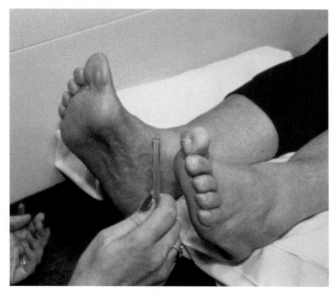

Fig. 30-6 Sensation testing. Semmes-Weinstein monofilament tip is placed on skin, pressed to bending point, removed, and patient response noted. Sensory loss in peripheral neuropathy occurs first in toes, then extends proximally over time.

the use of various creams.[14] *Pseudomonas* is a bacterium that produces a green pigment within a moist environment. Colonization of the skin by this bacterium is treated by exposing the limb to air. It is important to remember that more dermatological conditions in neuropathic diabetics are discovered by inspection than by patients' complaints of discomfort.[49]

Sensation

To assess the risk of ulceration in a neuropathic limb, the level of sensation must be determined. Because sensory loss can have a gradual, almost unnoticed onset, patient history can be misleading. Repeated quantitative measurements of sensation over time help assess progression of sensory impairment. Calibrated Semmes-Weinstein monofilaments, mounted on Lucite rods, provide a simple, quantitative method to determine sensory loss.[36] This is a single-point perception test in which the examiner presses the end of the monofilament against the skin until it bends, then removes it from the skin surface and notes the patient's response (Fig. 30-6). The monofilaments have reliability at the 95% confidence level.[6] They are used to categorize feet into those with normal sensation (4.17 diameter: $1g$ pressure); loss of protective sensation requiring protective footwear (5.07 diameter: $10g$ pressure); and no sensation (6.10 diameter: $75g$ pressure). Ulcer risk is proportional to the severity of sensory loss. Although Semmes-Weinstein monofilaments can be obtained in larger sets, researchers at the Hansen's Disease Center (Carville, LA) concluded that testing with the three sizes noted is sufficient for grading the insensitive limb. Use of the monofilament is not to be confused with testing for sharp/dull sensation.

Temperature

Areas of increased skin temperatures (hot spots) offer another physical sign that is helpful in detecting areas prone to ulceration.[5] Therefore, palpating the surface of the foot should be a part of every foot examination, including twice-daily self-examination for all patients with feet at risk for ulceration.[15] Temperature scanning/mapping of areas that commonly break down can be precisely done with surface-sensing devices (thermocouple or infrared) (Fig. 30-7). The infrared units allow

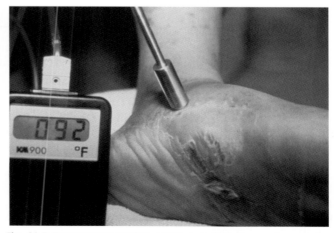

Fig. 30-7 Temperature testing. Using a surface temperature-sensing instrument, temperatures are recorded in predetermined areas and used for objective diagnostic as well as follow-up information.

ORTHOTIC FOOT EVALUATION FORM

PATENT _____ DIAGNOSIS _____

CODE _____ ORTHOTIST _____ DATE _____

INSENSITIVE FEET WITHOUT ULCERATION

CATEGORY	MONOFILAMENT RESPONSE	FOLLOW UP	PROTECTIVE SENSATION	INSERT	ULCER	DEFORMITY
A	+5.07 (10gm)	12 Mos.	Yes	Cushion	No	Yes/No
B	−5.07 (10gm)	6 Mos.	No	Molded	No	No
C	−5.07 (10gm)	4 Mos.	No	Molded	No	Yes
D	−5.07 (10gm)	3 Mos.	No	Molded	Yes	Yes/No
E	−6.10 (75gm)	2 Mos.	No	Molded	Yes/No	Yes/No

SKIN TEMPERATURE

○ WITHIN 3°

⊕ INCREASED TEMP + 3°

◉ INCREASED TEMP > +3°

⊖ DECREASED TEMP

ULCER GRADE

0 INTACT SKIN
1 SUPERFICIAL
2 TENDON OR BONE
3 ABSCESS OR OSTEO
4 FOREFOOT GANGRENE
5 FOOT GANGRENE

◌ DORSAL

○ OTHER

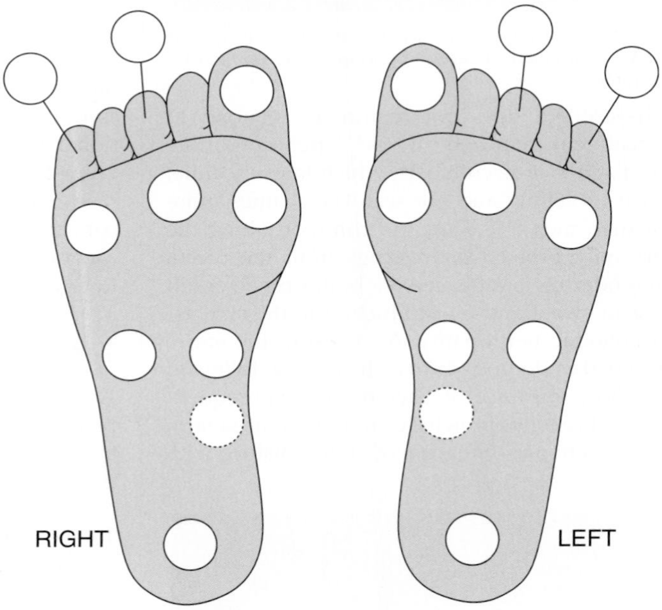

RIGHT   LEFT

_____

_____

_____

Fig. 30-8 A standard documentation form is important for recording sensation and temperature. Follow-up protocol is determined by the results of the evaluation.

recording of multiple readings, providing a rapid scan of the limbs. When one area definitely has a temperature 3°F (2°C) or more higher than adjacent areas, it can be assumed that there is an area of inflammation due to high pressure, Charcot neuroarthropathy (fracture/dislocation), or infection. This area must be immediately relieved of pressure until a definitive diagnosis has been made, allowing appropriate treatment to be instituted. On follow-up of the patient, the temperature differential should decrease as healing progresses. Vascular impairment should be suspected when one limb is significantly colder or distal portions of the foot show a drop in temperature.[12] It should be remembered, however, that the lower limbs normally become somewhat cooler from proximal to distal.[5]

Documentation

Continuity of documentation is essential to ensure high-quality care. This requires a standard form for initial assessment and future follow-up (Fig. 30-8). Tracing the outline of an ulcer on transparent radiological or other rigid film allows for a detailed record of healing progression. Providing the patient with a duplicate tracing to follow the progress of the ulcer may

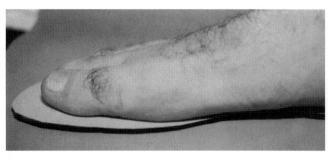
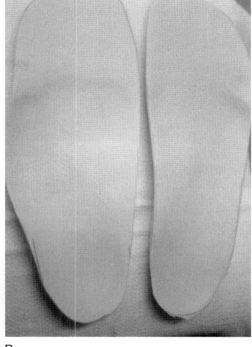

A   B

Fig. 30-9 Prescription by sensation. **A,** Patients with protective sensation require only properly fitting shoes and simple cushioning inserts. **B,** Neuropathic patients require depth shoes and custom accommodative insoles to protect weight-bearing surfaces of feet.

improve compliance. Photographs of an ulcer are important for visualizing reduction in its area and volume.

Prevention and patient education

It is an important responsibility to teach patients with insensate limbs practical methods to compensate for the lack of sensory feedback. Self-care begins with daily inspections of the feet using mirrors and magnifying glasses. The sensory-impaired patient must use sight and touch for self-examination, but the impaired vision and hand sensation of many poorly controlled diabetics will limit the accuracy of these examinations. For these patients, frequent foot checks by family members, friends, and medical caregivers may be required. Footwear and orthoses must be examined each day for foreign objects and wear.

Routine foot care

Patients should wash their feet each day with mild soap and water, then carefully dry them, especially between the toes. Application of an emollient cream will maintain skin flexibility but should not be put between the toes. Use of alcohol-based products, sun lamps, and sun exposure will cause excessive dryness. Remember that skin that is either too dry or too moist is vulnerable to ulceration. Direct damage to the skin can occur during removal of adhesive tape, especially when used repeatedly. When patients select footwear, they must not only choose the correct size but avoid shoes with stitching over the forefoot. Stitched areas do not mold to the foot but instead abrade the skin, especially in bony areas. Many foot care products, such as lotions with alcohol and callus removers, must not be used by neuropathic patients. There are occasional warnings on the labels of these salicylic acid-based callus removers to this

effect, but usually the print is too small to be read by a diabetic. Exercise programs promote good health, but high-impact activities such as running and jumping may increase the risk of ulceration by producing direct forces on the foot many times body weight.[20] Safe exercise programs for patients with insensate feet include swimming, cycling, and low-impact dancing. In general, walking should be done with slow, short steps.[22]

Orthotic treatment

Foot ulcers

The most important contribution of shoes and orthotic devices to the prevention of ulcers is the redistribution of forces that impact the foot. For vulnerable but intact skin, forces can be reduced by optimizing the shape and minimizing the stiffness of materials used to fabricate the shoe and insert (Fig. 30-9). When a patient has no ulcer (grade 0) and no deformity and can sense the 10g monofilament, he or she has protective sensation and usually does well with standard shoes of correct size and shape and a simple shock-absorbing pad. In other words, this patient will sense pain before damage occurs to the feet. The patient with no ulcer or deformity but without protective sensation requires depth shoes with a total-contact accommodative insert to redistribute pressures, thereby reducing forces on areas of potential breakdown. The insert can be molded to the patient or fabricated over a cast of the foot. The cast does not have corrective forces added, only accommodation (Fig. 30-10).

Shoes and inserts can be made to accommodate many minor common deformities, but more severe conditions require more complex orthotic treatment. For ulcerated skin, maximum pressure relief is desired. An outline of treatment by ulcer grade is given in Table 30-2. Orthotic treatment,

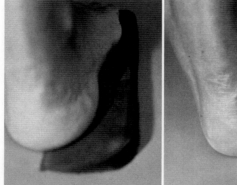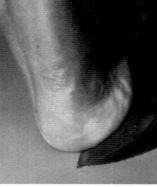

Fig. 30-10 Accommodation, not correction. **A,** Foot with normal sensation senses corrective wedge and moves body weight away from excess force. **B,** Neuropathic foot continues to bear weight over corrective force because of lack of sensation. Full weight bearing will cause breakdown of skin at site of corrective force.

including total-contact casting, is appropriate for ulcer grades 0 through 2, provided no significant infection is present. Higher grades imply the need for preorthotic surgery in the form of operative debridement or amputation.[47] Walking in a total-contact cast (TCC) decreases plantar pressures under an ulcer and its associated bony prominence by distributing weight-bearing pressures over the entire plantar surface of the foot. In addition, TCCs can shorten the duration of stance by forcing the patient to take smaller steps. They have been successful as a treatment for plantar ulcerations but require careful application, close follow-up, and patient compliance with walking limitations and scheduled appointments to minimize complications.[31] The average healing time for ulcers in insensate feet treated with a healing cast is 6 weeks.[7] This method has been used in patients with and without evidence of peripheral vascular disease.[42]

Attempts have been made to heal ulcers using a cast shoe molded of plaster. The initial cast must be changed in 3 days and then reapplied every 10 days. Healing of plantar ulcers in 39 days has been reported.[18] Some health care professionals are concerned that casting does not allow for daily wound inspections and dressing changes. Making a window in the cast should be avoided so that a secondary wound does not occur due to localized window edema and shear stresses.[10] Contraindications to use of a TCC include active infection with erythema and drainage, significantly hypotrophic skin with a thin, shiny appearance, and severe peripheral edema.[7] Use of shoes and orthotic devices to prevent or heal foot ulcers in insensate feet should always be integrated with other treatment modalities.

Charcot joint

The foot undergoing Charcot degeneration typically is swollen, erythematous, and excessively warm but relatively painless. A history of injury often is lacking. Radiologically, Charcot limbs may show multiple fractures/dislocations accompanied by extensive bone demineralization and reabsorption. Later stages reveal architectural distortion with shortening and widening of the foot.[34]

The foot joints most often involved with Charcot changes are as follows:

Tarsometatarsal	30%
Metatarsophalangeal	30%
Tarsal	24%
Interphalangeal	4%

Charcot neuroarthropathy is frequently misdiagnosed, often being confused with infection or other forms of arthritis, such as gout. The clinical presentations and laboratory tests for Charcot foot and osteomyelitis are so similar that the patient must be monitored closely to verify the diagnosis. The only difference on physical examination is the presence of an opening in the skin in the case of osteomyelitis and,

Table 30-2 Foot pathology*

Foot Pathology	Orthosis	Shoe/Orthosis	Comments
Claw toes	Accommodative inserts	Depth/leather soft toe box	Severe claw toes may require custom shoes
Grade 0 foot (with protective sensation)	Cushion insole	Shoes of correct size and width with shock absorption	Patient ceases weight bearing when pain begins, preventing further trauma
Grade 0 foot (without protective sensation)	Accommodative with reliefs for calluses and trauma	Depth shoes	Insert provides only accommodation and pressure relief
Grade 1 foot (superficial ulcer)	Accommodative insert/relief	ODS splint Weight-relief shoe Total-contact cast	ODS splint contains insert that can be adjusted Cast must be changed in 5–7 days, then every 1–2 weeks
Grade 2 foot (deeper ulcer)	Accommodative insert/relief	ODS splint	May require resection of underlying bony prominence to achieve healing to grade 0
Grade 3-5 foot	Not applicable	Not applicable	Medical/surgical intervention
Chronic heel ulcer or calcanectomy	Neuropathic walker Axial resist AFO	No shoe required Larger shoe to fit over orthosis	Relief in heel of integral insert; contralateral shoe lift Contraindicated for dysvascular patients

*Evaluation of deformity and correct accommodation. Shoes and inserts can be used for many deformities, but orthotic treatment is required for more severe conditions.

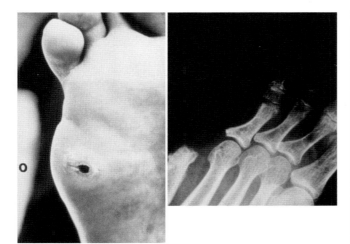

Fig. 30-11 Osteomyelitis. **A,** Obvious skin opening in area of bony involvement provides path for infection, indicating possible osteomyelitis. **B,** Radiograph shows bony deterioration of fifth metatarsal head, indicative of osteomyelitis.

possibly, a fever. Radiographically, osteomyelitis produces progressive bone destruction in contrast to the steady bony consolidation of Charcot neuroarthropathy provided the foot is immobilized (Fig. 30-11).[2,33]

Untreated Charcot joints may leave the patient with deformities that require surgical intervention, expensive custom footwear, or both. In the acute stage, the affected area of the foot is 5° to 10°F warmer than the same area of the contralateral foot. The affected foot usually does not have an ulceration (Fig. 30-12). To maintain bone alignment and prevent or minimize deformity, the Charcot foot should be promptly immobilized in a TCC. The duration of bone destruction, joint dissociation, and eventual bony consolidation vary with the individual, but average healing times in TCCs are as follows:

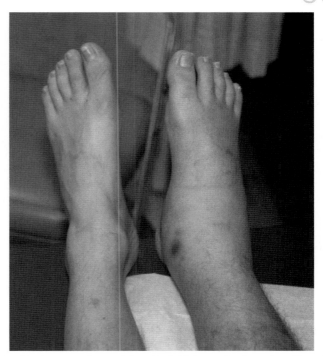

Fig. 30-12 Acute Charcot joint. On initial examination, the affected foot is red, hot, and swollen and has bounding pulses.

Hindfoot	12 months
Midfoot	9 months
Forefoot	6 months

The process can be monitored by checking joint stability and skin temperature over the affected joints at each cast change (Fig. 30-13). The casting program should be continued until the local temperature returns to within 3°F (2°C) of the

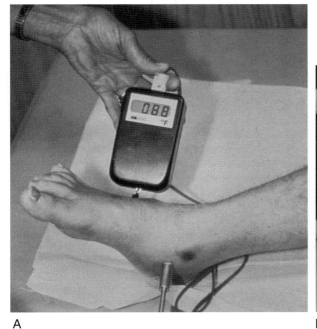

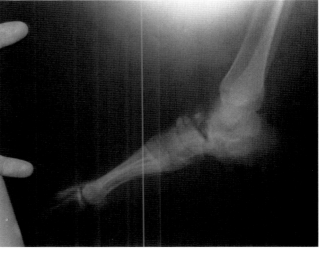

A   B

Fig. 30-13 Charcot joint evaluation. **A,** Using a thermometer, the affected foot may be found to be more than 5°F hotter than the unaffected foot. **B,** Verification by radiographs shows acute midtarsal joint destruction.

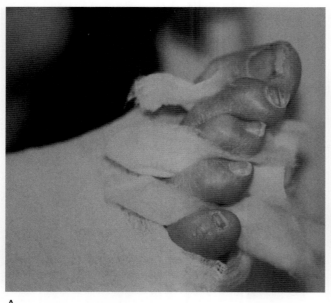

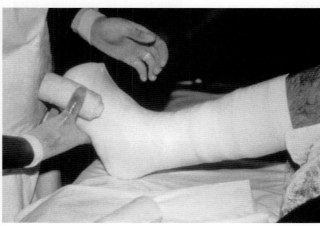

A

B

Fig. 30-14 Total-contact casting. **A,** Toes must be separated with cotton before cast is applied to increase toe room within cast and decrease risk of maceration. **B,** Leg is held in neutral position for casting.

uninvolved foot and all affected joints are clinically stable. Radiographs then will show bony consolidation in the region of the Charcot joint, which implies resolution of the process. Avoiding residual deformity and gaining joint stability with bony healing remain the main objectives of treatment. With prolonged cast immobilization in a position of neutrality (ankle at 0 degrees dorsiflexion and 0 degrees inversion/eversion, i.e., plantigrade), a useful foot is preserved even if little joint motion is present. When midfoot joints are affected, large plantar and medial bony prominences may cause the overlying skin to ulcerate on weight bearing. To prevent ulceration or to avoid recurrence of an ulcer healed by a total-contact cast, the prominence must be removed surgically. Arthrodesis of Charcot joints remains controversial and difficult to achieve.

Application technique for a TCC varies with different institutions. The healing cast originally was designed with minimal padding, but padded variations are used successfully. Most importantly, the cast should be applied by a skilled health care provider.

The Carville healing cast (TCC) is applied as follows (Fig. 30-14):

- Ulcer covered with thin layer of gauze
- Cotton placed between toes to prevent maceration
- Stockinette sleeve rolled onto foot and leg
- ⅛-inch felt over malleoli and anterior tibia
- Foam padding over toes
- Total-contact plaster shell carefully molded
- Shell reinforced with plaster splints
- Walking heel attached
- Fiberglass roll applied over plaster to reinforce the foot and ankle areas

The patient is instructed to limit ambulation time to 33% of his or her usual amount. The initial cast usually becomes loose in 5 to 7 days and must be replaced. New casts are applied every 2 to 3 weeks.[31] To allow thorough drying, the patient should not stand or walk in the cast for 24 hours after each application.[7]

Orthotic dynamic system splint

The orthotic dynamic system (ODS) splint was developed to combine the casting method of a TCC with a custom-molded insert that can be removed and modified as needed to adjust areas of relief (Fig. 30-15). With most of the advantages of the TCC, the following options were added with the ODS splint: daily inspection of the wound, allowing cleaning/dressings/debridement and adjustments to areas of excessive pressure

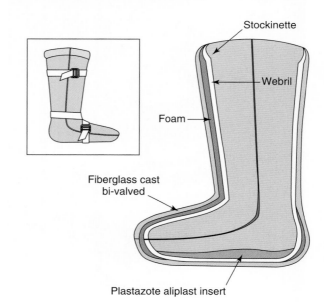

Fig. 30-15 Orthotic dynamic system (ODS) splint uses total-contact cast concept with incorporation of custom-molded insert. Removable insert is adjustable, which assists in pressure relief of affected areas.

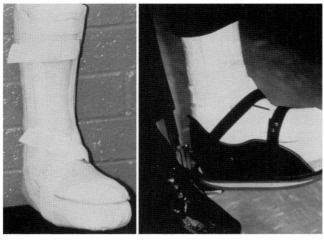

Fig. 30-16 Completed ODS splint is fitted with rocker-bottom cast shoe for ambulation.

and/or friction. To prepare the splint, a Plastazote/Aliplast insert is first molded to the plantar surface of the patient's foot with ¼-inch length added beyond the toes. A stockinette is placed on the leg, the insert is positioned, and another stockinette is applied to hold the insert in place. A padded total-contact fiberglass cast is applied. The cast is bivalved, straps are added, the edges are finished, and the insert is removed, modified to relieve the area of ulceration and replaced within the splint. The patient ambulates with the splint in a rocker-bottom cast shoe (Fig. 30-16). Limb volume is controlled by the patient with socks of varying thickness. The major disadvantage is that the patient can remove the splint at any time, making the validity of the entire treatment program dependent on the patient's compliance.

Nonremovable cast walker

Although TCCs have long been the "gold standard" for diabetic ulcer treatment, they have not been as widely accepted as hoped because of the expense of frequent cast changes and the likelihood of new ulcerations from the casts if they are not skillfully applied. A recent prospective, randomized, controlled trial compared ulcer treatment using a commercially available cast walker, made nonremovable by applying a roll of fiberglass tape, to total-contact casting. The cast walker was removed weekly, the wound examined and debrided, and the same device replaced, secured with a new roll of fiberglass tape. Healing rates within 12 weeks were equivalent to TCC, but the overall cost was less.[25]

Shoes

Shoes for the insensitive foot should have uppers formed of soft leather. They also must have adequate width across the ball of the foot and sufficient depth for an accommodative orthosis. When properly fit, the instep leather should not be taut, and the toe box should have sufficient space beyond the longest toe to prevent distal contact throughout the gait cycle. Soft leather gradually adapts to the conformation of the foot, retains its shape between wearings, and breathes and absorbs perspiration.[28] Because of loss of sensation, neuropathic patients should not depend on the feel of shoes for correct sizing or they will select a pair that is excessively tight. The shoe should have no stitching over the forefoot because stitched areas never mold to the foot but instead abrade the skin, especially over bony prominences.

Three tests determine the proper fit of shoes:

Length: Check for ½ to ¾ inch of space beyond the longest toe (Fig. 30-17).

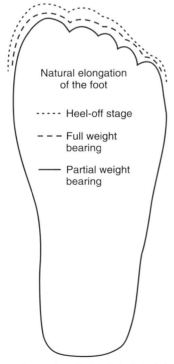

Natural elongation
of the foot

----- Heel-off stage

- - - Full weight
bearing

—— Partial weight
bearing

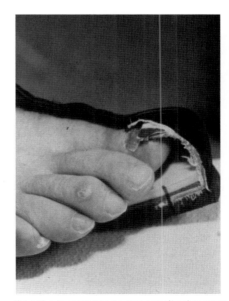

Fig. 30-17 Neuropathic foot requires a shoe that is ½ to ¾ inch longer than the longest toe to prevent distal contact during ambulation.

401

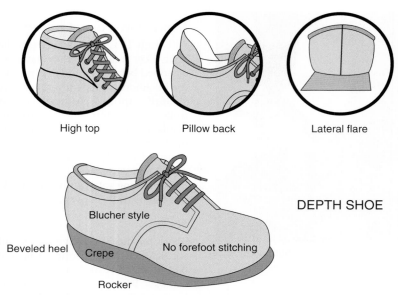

DEPTH SHOE

Fig. 30-18 Standard-depth shoes without stitching over the forefoot can be modified for the neuropathic foot. Additions include high top, pillow back, lateral flare, beveled heel, rocker sole, and stretching of leather as required.

Ball width: With the patient standing, pinch the vamp material of the shoe; if the leather cannot be pinched, it is too tight. The ball of the foot (metatarsal head level) should be located in the widest part of the shoe.[23]

Heel-to-ball length: Measure the distance from the posterior aspect of the patient's heel to the first and fifth metatarsal heads. Bend the shoe at the toe break and repeat the measurements on the shoe. They should be nearly the same.[30]

Lace shoes give the best stability but must be broken in slowly, beginning with 2 hours per day, then slowly adding time.[10] Cut-out sandals are not recommended for neuropathic persons because of the possibility of ulceration along the borders of the straps.[7] Likewise, the thong between the great and second toes of "flip-flop" sandals will ulcerate the web space.

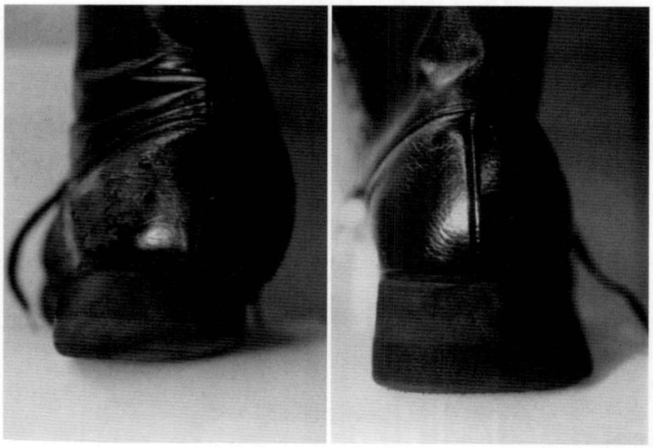

In general, sandals fail to protect the toes from common everyday trauma. Standard modifications of in-depth shoes (Fig. 30-18) for the neuropathic patient include stretching the toe box, padding the tongue, flaring the lateral soles to discourage varus instability (Fig. 30-19), and adding a shank/rocker bottom for a partial foot amputation, hallux rigidus, or decreased motion at the first MTP joint. A rocker bottom should also be added to the shoe when MTP joint extension is to be avoided.[10] Tapering the heel and toe of the standard depth shoe sole allows a more natural gait. To temporarily protect and accommodate a healing area over which bulky dressings are to be applied, a healing shoe lined with Plastazote is useful because it provides increased volume and adjustability. Socks for the neuropathic limb should have no mended areas or seams over bony prominences. A cotton/acrylic blend helps in the wicking of perspiration away from the foot.[19] The socks should be fully cushioned and have nonelastic tops. A partial foot requires a sock that conforms to the foot's shape without prominent seams or excess material at the distal end (Fig. 30-20).

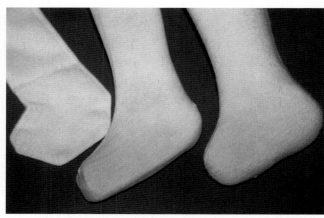

Fig. 30-19 Lateral flare. **A,** This is an extension of the lateral sole, not a wedge. **B,** Without the lateral flare, motor and sensory losses at the ankle lead to lateral instability and possible injury.

Fig. 30-20 Single-size partial foot sock accommodates Chopart disarticulation as well as distal transmetatarsal amputation without excess material at distal end.

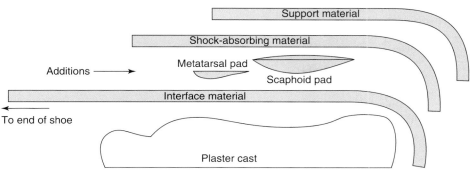

Fig. 30-21 Insert fabrication. Using a plaster model of the plantar surface, a composite insert is formed by first adding interface material that contacts the foot. Next a soft metatarsal or scaphoid pad is added, followed by a layer of shock-absorbing material. Final base/support material fills space between the foot contours and the inner surface of shoe sole.

Special socks for full or partial feet with silicone over high-stress areas are available.

Accommodative inserts

Treatment of the neuropathic foot requires accommodation of bony prominences, relief of pressure/shear forces, and shock absorption. An accommodative insert merely fills the spaces between the flat structural shoe insole and the foot contours without applying any corrective forces (Fig. 30-21). A semi-rigid insert will provide pressure relief and some cushioning.[29] A rigid insert or pad will apply corrective forces, likely causing skin breakdown in an insensate foot, and therefore is contra-indicated in neuropathic diabetics. If metatarsal or scaphoid pads are required, they must be of a soft durometer. Metatarsal pads are placed proximal to the metatarsal heads to transfer weight from the heads to the metatarsal shafts.

A closed-cell polyethylene foam insert can be provided immediately in the clinic. Most polyethylene foams can be heated and molded directly onto the patient's foot (Fig. 30-22).[10] The orthotist must never mold the insert material around the toes or create ridges that the toes will ride over as the patient ambulates. The disadvantage of using an insert composed of closed-cell polyethylene foam alone is its short life due to compaction with weight bearing. By combining two materials with different attributes (e.g., Plastazote and Poron or PPT) over a plaster model of the foot, a composite insert is created that can achieve the goal of accommodation while providing an effective life up to 1 year (Fig. 30-23).[39,40]

An insert with a Plastazote closed-cell foam surface in contact with the foot/sock can be an excellent diagnostic tool for follow-up. The self-molding property of this material allows deep impressions to form in areas of high pressure that should then be relieved. These areas should continue to be relieved in future inserts for that individual. Temperature can be used as a guide for evaluating the effectiveness of pressure relief. Areas of skin with excessive warmth after walking are still receiving undue pressure and/or shear forces. After the inserts have been modified, the temperature differential should decrease if the proper accommodation has been achieved. If the temperature has not decreased in these areas, the reliefs may require further enhancement, or an underlying complication such as Charcot arthropathy or infection must be investigated. All reliefs are applied on the surface in contact with the shoe and never the surface in contact with the foot. The surface in contact with the foot should always be unbroken without any edges that would apply shear forces to the foot.

Partial foot blocks

The partial foot amputee may require a block of material within the anterior part of the shoe to fill the void left by the amputation (Table 30-3). A forefoot block holds the shoe

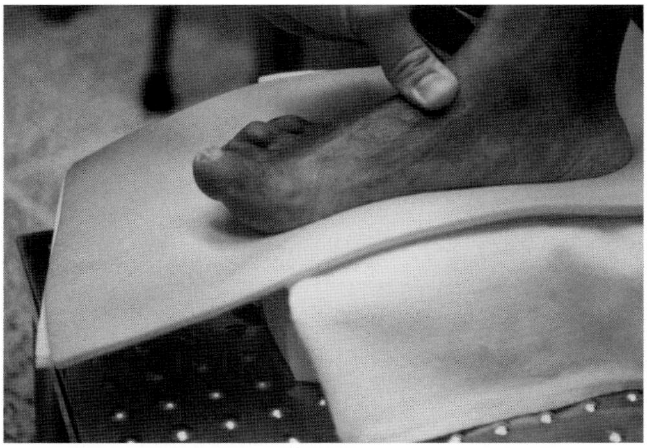

Fig. 30-22 Closed-cell polyethylene foam insert is molded directly onto patient's foot. Soft cushion, proximal to toes, is used to mold foot contours without leaving toe prints on surface.

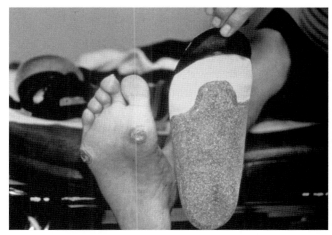

Fig. 30-23 Reducing specific pressures. Composite insert is designed to reduce forces on vulnerable areas, preventing future callus buildup that can lead to skin breakdown.

Table 30-3 Orthoses for the partial foot

Partial Foot	Orthosis	Shoe	Comments
First toe amputation	Accommodative insert with toe block	Depth shoe	Toe block reduces shear
Central toe amputation (2, 3, or 4)	Accommodative insert without toe block or spacer	Depth shoe	Constant low pressure of spacer may produce ulcers
Distal amputation of all toes or transmetatarsal	Accommodative insert with forefoot block	Short shoe Full-length shoe	Total-contact insert improves weight-bearing characteristics Patients, especially unilateral amputees, prefer full-length shoe for cosmesis
Lisfranc amputation	Accommodative with forefoot block	Shoe with shank, rocker bottom, and high top	Suspension is a concern for the short foot
Chopart amputation	Accommodative with forefoot block Neuropathic walker Total-contact AFO Limited prosthesis	Shoe with shank, rocker bottom, and high top No shoe required Larger shoe required Standard shoe to accommodate	Suspension is a concern for the short foot Custom AFO/boot

leather away from the distal end of the residual foot and discourages its distal migration or rotation (Fig. 30-24). A great toe amputation may require a block to hold the foot in a corrected position within the shoe (Fig. 30-25). No block or prosthetic toe is to be used for a central digit amputation. The chronic low pressures applied by a block to central digits can cause ischemic ulcerations on adjacent toe surfaces. All types of blocks must be slightly spaced from the amputation site and be an integral part of the insert, not added to an existing one (Fig. 30-26). Forefoot blocks should be augmented by a rigid rocker sole to prevent ulceration of the distal end.

Neuropathic walker

The neuropathic walker or Charcot restraint orthotic walker is an AFO consisting of anterior and posterior copolymer shells lined with closed-cell foam and fitted with a nonskid rocker sole. It is individually designed to provide total contact for weight redistribution and to reduce force through the Lisfranc joint or ankle (Fig. 30-27). This device is used frequently for 2 or 3 months after serial total-contact casting of a Charcot foot prior to depth shoe fitting. It also is indicated for permanent use by the patient with unstable Charcot changes in ankle and subtalar joints, repeated Charcot recurrence, and chronic ulcerations. The removable insert can be adjusted to redistribute weight-bearing areas on the plantar surface and to reduce pressure over chronic breakdown areas, such as the ankle malleoli, posterior heel, and bunions. Although the walker is easily donned and doffed and its rocker sole allows smooth ambulation, the contralateral shoe will need adjustment for height. The patient must be

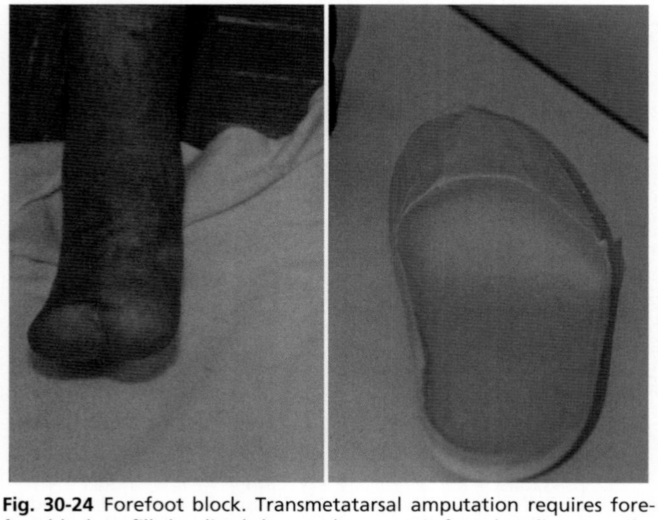

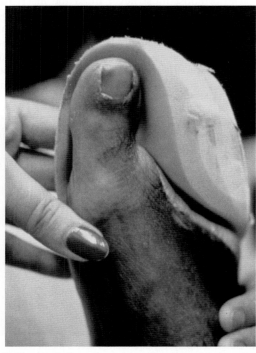

Fig. 30-25 Toe block. Resection of rays 2 to 5 requires insert with integral block to prevent migration or rotation of the foot within the shoe.

Fig. 30-24 Forefoot block. Transmetatarsal amputation requires forefoot block to fill the distal shoe and prevent it from bending over the distal end of amputation.

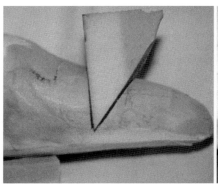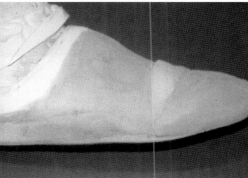

Fig. 30-26 Toe break in forefoot block. To reduce pressure on the distal end of the partial foot, a soft foam wedge can be added just proximal to the forefoot block.

instructed to check his or her skin daily for redness, excessive warmth, and possible breakdown. The temperatures of the plantar surface should be recorded for possible adjustment of insert pressures. Sock management is important for volume control in order to maintain a snug fit of the orthosis.

Total-contact AFO

The total-contact AFO, like the neuropathic walker, is used by the patient whose leg size is near normal. The orthosis, which fits inside a shoe, includes a removable custom insert and is lined with Plastazote (Fig. 30-28). The casting procedure is the same as for the neuropathic walker. The toes are open, and the anterior shell terminates at midfoot. Short leg walkers and orthopaedic walkers, traditionally used for immobilization of acute ligament/muscle strains and fractures, have been used by some clinics but fail to provide total contact.

Axial resist (patellar tendon-bearing) orthosis Axial resist (patellar tendon-bearing) designs are intended to decrease

forces on the plantar weight-bearing surface of the foot (Fig. 30-29). This design has also been used in plaster casting of tibial fractures. Considerable axial force from the knee region is transmitted to the cast, but it does not offer rotary stability. One study showed little effectiveness in reducing the load on the lower leg.[26] The patellar tendon-bearing AFO has been used successfully after calcanectomy, plantar skin graft, and heel ulceration. This orthosis is contraindicated in patients with vascular impairment because of potential popliteal constriction compromising arterial flow to the foot.

Prosthosis

A *prosthosis* is a device that combines features of a *prosthesis* and an *orthosis*. It is custom designed for the patient with a complicated amputation who is not a candidate for standard prosthetic management. A prosthosis can be a useful device for transfers and limb protection as well as ambulation. Each device is a creative design, with no two the same, unique to the individual and his or her needs.

Peripheral vascular disease

Peripheral vascular disease is a serious condition affecting millions of Americans. Of the 500,000 annual vascular-related ulcers in the United States, 70% are venous and 10% are arterial.

Fig. 30-27 Neuropathic walker (Charcot restraint orthotic walker) provides total contact to affected limb with adjustability for chronic plantar surface deformities. A patient with recurrent Charcot joint or chronic ulceration may require this orthosis instead of a shoe.

Plastazote lining

Copolymer shell

Removable Plastazote aliplast insert

Rocker sole

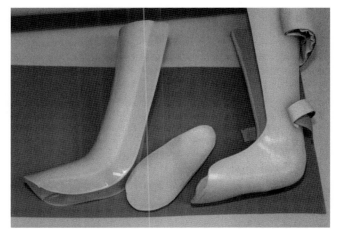

Fig. 30-28 Total-contact AFO consists of Plastazote-lined anterior and posterior plastic shells that are formed over a removable plantar insert. The orthosis is designed to fit within the shoe.

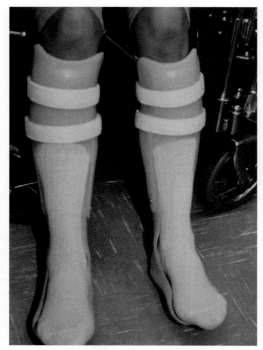

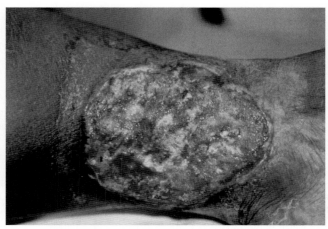

Fig. 30-31 Venous stasis ulceration. The medial distal leg and ankle are common sites of ulceration in venous stasis because of thin skin and close proximity of veins.

Fig. 30-29 An axial resist (patellar tendon-bearing) AFO is preferred when partially unweighting of the heel is required. This device is not recommended for dysvascular patients because of constriction in the area of the popliteal artery.

Venous stasis ulcers

Venous stasis ulcers have a better prognosis for healing than do arterial ulcers. In venous stasis ulceration, the valves within inelastic veins no longer help return blood to the heart against gravity, leaving blood to pool in the lower limbs (Fig. 30-30). The pooling interferes with perfusion of newly oxygenated blood into the soft tissues, and the vein

walls begin to leak fluid into the lower limbs. Venous stasis ulcers are commonly located in the anteromedial malleolar and pretibial areas. The ulcers are irregular in shape and surrounded by discolored skin. They may bleed when abraded.

Orthotic treatment of venous stasis and ulcers

Unna boot

Treatment of venous stasis ulcers begins with leg elevation and compression using elastic bandages or an Unna boot (Fig. 30-31).[16] The Unna boot is a semirigid dressing impregnated with gelatin, zinc oxide, and glycerin (Fig. 30-32). It protects the surrounding intact but vulnerable skin from the weeping exudate, especially distal to the ulcer site. The

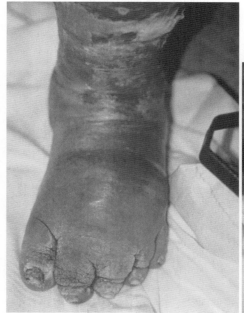

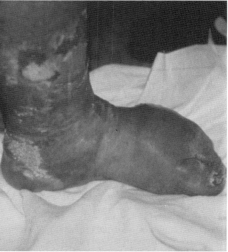

Fig. 30-30 Lower limb edema. Failure of venous return against gravity is shown by increased edema in the foot and lower leg.

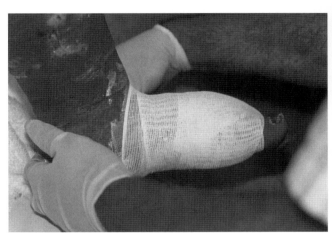

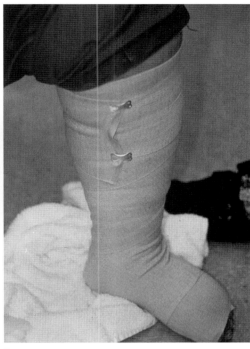

A   B

Fig. 30-32 Unna boot application. Venous stasis limb is wrapped with the Unna boot followed by elastic wrap. Tension on the wrap should gradually decrease from distal to proximal to promote return of fluid to the heart via lymphatics and veins.

Unna boot is applied wet, but when it dries it forms a stable porous mold that adheres to the skin. This treatment has been used for venous stasis for 100 years. It is a means for controlling edema when applied across a joint. The motion of the joint generates a pumping action.[13]

Pressure-graduated stockings

The lower limb with chronic venous stasis but no ulcer still has edema that must be controlled. The limb with moderate edema should be treated with pressure-graduated stockings as daily prevention, with an Unna boot and elastic wrap reserved for severe edema or during periods of skin breakdown. Elastic stockings, with pressure gradients that fall from distal to proximal, facilitate a venous pumping action which diminishes lower limb edema (Fig. 30-33). With pressure-graduated stockings, limb compression occurs in the calf (knee-length) or calf and thigh (hip-length). Compressing the foot provides a further assist to the venous system. Most patients do well with compression in the range of 30 to 40 mm Hg beginning at the foot and ankle. When prescribing these stockings for the neuropathic and/or dysvascular patient, it must be specified that they cover the toes and have no seams over bony prominences or zippers over the malleoli. Antiembolism stockings, in contrast, are designed for the nonambulatory, supine patient. They provide insufficient compression in the standing position and are therefore ineffective in supporting the pumping action required.

The health care practitioner must judge the potential compliance of neuropathic patients. Although they do not willfully neglect self-care activities, these patients often are unaware of the probable dangers of neglect.[41] Lack of awareness may be partly related to the tendency of most health care providers to focus on the immediate problem (i.e., neuropathic ulcer) and not teach self-care techniques adequately. The diabetic may also have other complications that adversely affect compliance in lower limb care. These include impaired vision from retinopathy and impaired smell from autonomic neuropathy, either or both of which compromise their ability to detect infection or other potential problems.

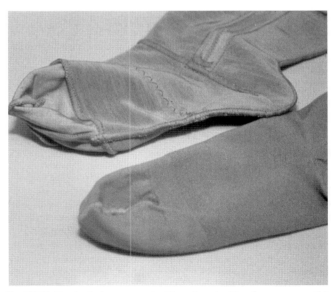

Fig. 30-33 Graduated-pressure stocking. Any stocking for a neuropathic limb should have a toe cover and no prominent seams in weight-bearing areas or zippers over susceptible malleoli. Pressure should be equal at the foot and ankle and should gradually decrease proximally.

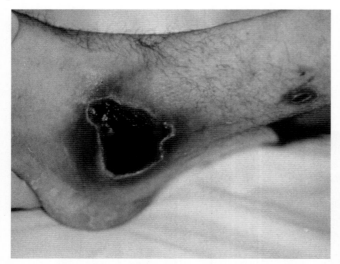

Fig. 30-34 Arterial (ischemic) ulceration. Arterial system failure shows as dark, well-demarcated necrotic areas of skin.

Arterial (ischemic) ulcers

The intimal wall of an artery usually is smooth; however, with the onset of atherosclerosis, platelets, calcium, and connective tissue are deposited on the intimal wall. Atherosclerosis leads to impaired circulation in the legs and is one of the most important causes of gangrene, leading to amputation.[1] In the early stages of atherosclerosis, the patient may experience muscle cramping (intermittent claudication) in the lower limb after walking a certain distance. As the disease progresses, claudication may appear during inactivity (rest pain).[35] Advanced arterial compromise can be noted as loss of hair growth, shiny atrophic skin, and cool skin over the toes.[34] Arterial ulcers can be located on toe tips, between toes, on the heel, the metatarsal heads, the side or sole of the foot, and over the lateral malleolus (Fig. 30-34). The ulcer looks "punched out" with a nonbleeding base and well-demarcated edges. The ulcer base may be pale red or black and necrotic. In patients with arterial insufficiency, the initial step in treatment is determining whether the person is a candidate for arterial reconstruction. Noninvasive tests, such as segmental Doppler determination of systolic blood pressure of the lower limbs compared to systolic pressure in the upper limbs or transcutaneous Po_2 measurements of the ischemic lower limb, are helpful. The ultimate treatment of ulcers caused by arterial insufficiency is vascular reconstruction.

Conclusion

Care of the lower limb in the neuropathic and/or dysvascular patient requires the efforts of many professionals. The goal of treatment of the neuropathic and/or dysvascular limb is preservation of the patient's foot, especially as multiple studies have shown the increased energy demands of prosthetic ambulation that may preclude walking for the diabetic amputee with impaired cardiopulmonary reserve. The diabetic with a neuropathic ulcer should be treated with appropriate debridement and antibiotics if infection (often polymicrobial) is present. Orthotic devices alone do not compensate for lost sensation in the neuropathic limb, but when combined with an educated

compliant patient and early intensive medical and surgical treatment, amputation can often be avoided. The patient with an ulcer caused by vascular insufficiency should be evaluated for possible vascular reconstruction. The members of the treatment team, which must include the patient, should work cooperatively to compensate for the deficits that accompany the neuropathic and/or dysvascular limb. Although the principles of treatment are simple and understandable, applying them consistently over a lifetime remains difficult.

References

1. Apelqvist J, Castenfors J, Larsson J: Prognostic value of systolic ankle and toe blood pressure levels in outcome of diabetic foot ulcer, *Diabetes Care* 12:373–378, 1989.
2. Ashbury A: Foot care in patients with diabetes mellitus, *Diabetes Care* 14(suppl 2):18–19, 1991.
3. Bamberger D, Stark K: Severe diabetic foot problems: avoiding amputation, *Emerg Decis* 3:21–34, 1987.
4. Barber E: Strength and range-of-motion examination skills for the clinical orthotist, *Prosthet Orthot* 5:49–51, 1993.
5. Bergtholdt HT: Temperature assessment of the insensate foot, *Phys Ther* 59:18–22, 1979.
6. Birke JA, Sims DS: Plantar sensory threshold in the ulcerative foot, *Br Leprosy Relief Assoc* 57:261–267, 1986.
7. Birke JA, Novick A, Graham SL, Coleman WC, Brasseaux DM: Methods of treating plantar ulcers, *Phys Ther* 71:116–122, 1991.
8. Bowker JH: Partial foot and Syme amputations: an overview, *Clin Prosthet Orthot* 12:10–13, 1988.
9. Bowker JH: Neurological aspects of prosthetic/orthotic practice, *Prosthet Orthot* 5:52–54, 1993.
10. Brand PW: Management of sensory loss in the extremities. In Omer GE Jr, Spinner M, editors: *Management of peripheral nerve problems*, Philadelphia, 1980, WB Saunders.
11. Brand PW: Neuropathic ulceration, *The Star* May/June:1-4, 1983.
12. Brand P: *Insensitive feet: practical handbook on foot problems in leprosy*, London, 1977, The Leprosy Mission.
13. Brenner MA: *Management of the diabetic foot*, Baltimore, 1977, Williams & Wilkins.
14. Cailliet R: *Foot and ankle pain*, Philadelphia, 1983, FA Davis.
15. Chan AW, MacFarlane IA, Bowsher D: Contact thermography of painful diabetic neuropathic foot, *Diabetes Care* 14:918–922, 1991.
16. Cherry G, Ryan T, Cameron J: Blueprint for the treatment of leg ulcers and the prevention of recurrence, *Wounds Compend Clin Res Pract* 3:1–15, 1991.
17. DeJong R: *The neurological examination*, New York, 1969, Harper & Row.
18. Diamond J, Sinacore D, Mueller M: Molded double-rocker plaster shoe for healing a diabetic plantar ulcer, *Phys Ther* 67:1550–1552, 1987.
19. Dwyer G, Rust M: Shoe business, *Diabetes Forecast* June:60–63, 1988.
20. Furman A: Give your feet a sporting chance, *Diabetes Forecast* April:17–22, 1989.
21. Fylling C: Conclusions, *Diabetes Spectrum* 5:358–359, 1992.
22. Graham C: Neuropathy made you stop, *Diabetes Forecast* Dec:47–49, 1992.
23. Hack M: Fitting shoes, *Diabetes Forecast* Jan: 63–67, 1989
24. Huntley AC: Taking care of your hands, *Diabetes Forecast* Aug:11–12, 1991.
25. Katz IA, Harlan A, Miranda-Palma B, et al: A randomized trial of two irremovable off-loading devices in the management of plantar neuropathic diabetic foot ulcers, *Diabetes Care* 28:555–559, 2005.
26. Lauridsen K, Sorensen CG, Christiansen P, et al: Measurements of pressure on the sole of the foot in plaster of Paris casts on the lower leg, *Prosthet Orthot Int* 13:42–45, 1989
27. Letts M: The orthotics of myelomeningocele. In: *AAOS: atlas of orthotics*, St. Louis, 1985, CV Mosby.
28. In Levin M, O'Neal L, Bowker JH, editors: *The diabetic foot*, ed 5, St. Louis, 1993, CV Mosby.
29. Lockard MA: Foot orthosis, *Phys Ther* 68:1866–1873, 1988.
30. McPoil TG Jr: Footwear, *Phys Ther* 68:1857–1865, 1988.
31. Mueller M, Diamond J, Sinacore D: Total contact casting in treatment of diabetic plantar ulcers, *Diabetes Care* 12:384–388, 1989.
32. Newman B: A diabetes camp for Native American adults, *Diabetes Spectrum* 6:166–202, 1993.

33. Newman LG, Waller J, Palestro CJ, et al: Unsuspected osteomyelitis in diabetic foot ulcers: diagnosis and monitoring by leukocyte scanning with indium in oxyquinoline, *JAMA* 266:1246–1251, 1991.

34. Olefsky J, Sherman R: *Diabetes mellitus: management and complications*, New York, 1985, Churchill Livingstone.

35. Olin J: Peripheral vascular disease, *Diabetes Forecast* Oct:78–81, 1992.

36. Omer GE Jr: Sensibility testing. In Omer GE Jr, Spinner M, editors: *Management of peripheral nerve problems*, Philadelphia, 1980, WB Saunders.

37. Pecoraro R, Reiber G, Burgess E: Pathways to diabetic limb amputation: basis for prevention, *Diabetes Care* 13:513–521, 1990.

38. Perry J: Normal and pathologic gait. In: *AAOS: atlas of orthoses and assistive devices*, St. Louis, 1997, CV Mosby.

39. Pratt DJ: Medium term comparison of shock attenuating insoles using a spectral analysis technique, *J Biomed Eng* 10:426–428, 1988.

40. Pratt DJ: Long term comparison of shock attenuating insoles, *Prosthet Orthot Int* 14:59–62, 1990.

41. Shipley D: Clinical evaluation and care of the insensitive foot, *Phys Ther* 59:13–22, 1979.

42. Sinacore D, Mueller M, Diamond J: Diabetic plantar ulcers treated by total contact casting, *Phys Ther* 67:1543–1549, 1987.

43. Thomas PK: *Clinical features and differential diagnosis: peripheral neuropathy*, Philadelphia, 1984, WB Saunders.

44. Thomas PK, Eliasson SG: *Diabetic neuropathy*, Philadelphia, 1984, WB Saunders.

45. Tiberio D: Pathomechanics of structural foot deformities, *Phys Ther* 68:1840–1849, 1988.

46. Tsairis P: Differential diagnosis of peripheral neuropathies. In Omer GE Jr, Spinner M, editors: *Management of peripheral nerve problems*, Philadelphia, 1980, WB Saunders.

47. Wagner FW Jr: A classification and treatment program for diabetic, neuropathic and dysvascular foot problems, *AAOS Inst Course Lect* 28:143–165, 1979.

48. Weingarten M: Commentary, *Diabetes Spectrum* 5:342–343, 1992.

49. Wilson J, Foster D: *Textbook of endocrinology*, Philadelphia, 1992, WB Saunders.

Chapter

31

Orthoses for persons with postpolio syndrome

Frans Nollet and Cornelis Th. Noppe

Key Points

- Postpolio syndrome (PPS) is highly prevalent among the large and aging population of polio survivors.

- PPS is characterized by late-onset new neuromuscular symptoms, especially new muscle weakness and/or abnormal muscle fatigability.

- PPS may be aggravated by degenerative disorders of the locomotory system, aging, and comorbidity.

- Management of PPS aims to restore the balance between decreasing physical capacity and the persistent demands of conducting activities of daily living.

- There is an urgent need for evaluative and comparative studies to provide evidence for selecting and providing the appropriate orthotic devices in polio subjects.

Pathophysiology

Many years after acute paralytic poliomyelitis, new neuromuscular symptoms may develop in a condition termed *postpoliomyelitis syndrome* or *postpolio syndrome* (PPS). In 2000 the diagnostic criteria were revised as follows[39]:

1. Confirmed history of paralytic poliomyelitis characterized by an acute illness with fever and usually asymmetrically distributed, flaccid paresis of a varying number of muscle groups. Evidence of motor neuron loss on neurological examination with signs of residual weakness, atrophy, loss of tendon reflexes, and intact sensation. Signs of denervation or reinnervation on electromyography (EMG).

2. Period of partially to fairly complete neurological recovery after acute paralytic poliomyelitis followed by neurological and functional stability for at least 15 years.

3. New or increased muscle weakness or abnormal muscle fatigability (decreased endurance), with or without generalized fatigue, muscle atrophy, or muscle and joint pain.

4. Symptoms usually have a gradual, but sometimes a sudden, onset and should persist for at least 1 year.

5. No other medical diagnosis explains the symptoms.

Population-based studies have demonstrated that the prevalence of new symptoms in prior polio patients is high. In these studies, new muscle weakness varied between 35% and 58% and new neuromuscular symptoms between 64% and 78%.[31,53,71] Risk indicators for the development of PPS are more severe initial polio paresis, better recovery from the acute polio, more severe residual impairments, contraction of acute polio at older age, number of years elapsed since acute polio, increasing age, and female gender.[31,36,53,64,71]

Paralytic poliomyelitis develops in 0.1% to 2% of polio virus infections when the virus invades the central nervous system and destroys the motor neurons in the spinal cord, causing an acute, usually asymmetrically distributed, flaccid paresis. After the acute paralytic phase, muscle function usually recovers partially to fairly completely due to extensive reinnervation of denervated muscle fibers through collateral sprouting of axons from motor neurons that survived the acute phase and regained their function. Motor units may increase five to eight times in size.[60] Strength also improves because of muscle fiber hypertrophy, with fiber areas increasing up to twice their normal size.[21,25] It is assumed that muscle fiber hypertrophy develops in response to the relatively high loads on paretic muscles in performing activities of daily living.[25] After the recovery phase, the severity and extent of residual paresis, with large intraindividual and interindividual variation, remain stable for decades.

The origin of PPS is unknown. The leading hypothesis is that excessive metabolic stress on remaining motor neurons over many years eventually causes premature degeneration of the nerve terminals that were newly formed through reinnervation.[69] The role of aging seems limited, as most PPS patients develop new symptoms in their 40s, an age range in which a physiological loss of motor neurons normally does not occur.[11] A persistent poliovirus infection seems unlikely, but this theory has proponents.[56] An immune-mediated hypothesis is not commonly accepted, but a study has shown increased intrathecal cytokine production in PPS patients.[24] The validity of the different hypotheses on the pathophysiological mechanisms underlying PPS remains uncertain.

No diagnostic tests for PPS are available. Laboratory tests are used to show evidence of prior polio paralysis and to exclude other diseases. EMG displays signs of reinnervation and denervation in both symptomatic and nonsymptomatic muscles. Muscle biopsy findings include type grouping of muscle fibers as the result of reinnervation and hypertrophy of muscle fibers as compensation for loss of muscle fibers.[12,15,25] Size and number of motor units diminish over time.[41,60] However, even with these investigations PPS cannot be distinguished from stable neuromuscular functioning following polio.

The central issue in PPS is the gradual loss of muscle function, that is, new weakness. It is important to realize that the effect on neurons in the acute phase of polio often was more widespread than clinically apparent, and paralytic and nonparalytic polio are not two distinctly different forms of polio virus infection. In 1961, Beasley[4] demonstrated in a large sample of polio patients that the degree of paresis showed a continuum from severe to normal, and that strength, especially in the larger lower extremity muscles, could be markedly reduced but remain undetected on clinical examination due to the upper limit in measurement range of manual muscle testing. (Note that manual strength testing can easily lead to overestimation of the individual's capacity for activities such as walking.) Modern imaging techniques have confirmed that loss of muscle mass may be present while manual muscle strength is objectively normal.[32] These observations are relevant to understanding that even patients without clinically detected weakness may retain residuals of their polio and can develop PPS later in life.[55]

A major complaint of patient with PPS is fatigue.[44] Fatigue may be associated with exertion, but often patients have the perception of general fatigue. Several causes of fatigue have been considered, such as impaired calcium kinetics. Altered calcium levels may account for disturbances in excitation–contraction coupling of actin and myosin filaments,[57] decreased capillary density, reduced oxidative and glycolytic enzyme potentials,[8] impaired voluntary muscle activation (possibly due to impaired reflex mechanism),[3,5] increased neuromuscular transmission defects in degenerating nerve terminals,[66] and degeneration of neurons of the reticular formation and basal ganglia.[10]

A systematic review of the course of functional status and muscle strength showed that muscle strength deteriorated slowly over years, and this effect was reported only in studies with follow-up of at least 4 years.[63] No prognostic factors could be identified, and the influence of comorbidity and aging is unknown. In another study of 38 subjects who were followed for 15 years, 31 reported progressive weakness during the study period.[58] All subjects showed a modest decline of strength and functioning of motor unit numbers. In this small group, no difference was found between symptomatic and asymptomatic subjects, and only the magnitude of neurological deficit at baseline was a prognostic factor for the development of new symptoms. In a study with 6-year follow-up of functional status, the severity of paresis at baseline was found to be the single prognostic factor for increasing problems with physical mobility over the study period.[47]

Historical perspective

One of the first descriptions of late-onset muscle weakness following poliomyelitis was made by Raymond[54] in 1875. Several cases have been reported since then. These early papers often described patients with rapidly progressive paresis.[46] At that time, little was known about the cause and transmission of acute polio, and the diagnosis of infantile paralysis was not always certain. This explains why an association between PPS and amyotrophic lateral sclerosis has been suggested in the past,[42] but the idea has been abandoned because of lack of supporting evidence.

PPS became generally recognized in the 1980s when large numbers of polio survivors of the polio epidemics in the 1940s and 1950s voiced new complaints as they grew older.[26] The diagnostic criteria of PPS have been adapted several times. Initially different forms of PPS were distinguished, such as postpoliomyelitis progressive muscle atrophy (PPMA).[15] PPMA was intended to classify cases in which strength loss and new atrophy were objectified with serial examinations. However, the ability to detect individual changes in strength is limited[28,43] given that the rate of decline in muscle strength is slow and has been found only in studies with long-term follow-up.[63] The current conclusion is that there is insufficient basis to classify subtypes of PPS.[39]

Between the end of the 19th century and the middle of the 20th century, when large polio epidemics swept across the western world, physicians were familiar with acute polio, the subsequent forms of recovery, and the treatment of residual impairments. Because of the disappearance of acute polio, much of that experience has been lost. Now the challenge is to treat large numbers of former polio patients who have new neuromuscular symptoms and functional deterioration many years after their acute polio infection.

Current issues

The nature and time course of PPS are still matters of debate. Although the symptoms and functional decline of PPS are recognized as common problems in many former polio patients, discussion continues on whether they signify a progressive loss of muscle function.[30] Some argue that degenerative disorders of the locomotory system are the main cause of the complaints reported by many patients with new neuromuscular complaints and therefore are not to be considered as signifying PPS. However, both joint degeneration and a decline in muscle function can occur simultaneously in the same individual and can negatively affect each other. Making the distinction between PPS and joint degeneration may be impossible in such cases. The ability to make such a distinction would be especially important if it were relevant to long-term prognosis or choice of treatment. The debate will continue as long as no diagnostic test for PPS is available. A better knowledge of the pathophysiological mechanisms of PPS is needed.

Another important issue is the lack of success of pharmacological treatment. A number of agents with different therapeutic actions have been investigated: human growth hormone and insulinlike growth factor-1, which promote protein synthesis in muscle cells and axonal sprouting; amantadine, bromocriptine, and selegiline, which are centrally acting dopaminergic agonists; high-dose prednisone, which has a strong antiinflammatory effect; and pyridostigmine, which improves neuromuscular transmission. No medication has been proven to increase strength or decrease fatigue in patients with PPS in a randomized controlled trial.[19,29,61,65] Reasons proposed to explain the failure of medications to show an effect include the slow progression of the disease, the heterogeneity of patients, and the variation in measurement.[16] Given these factors, relatively large study samples and long follow-up periods are required to reveal clinical relevant effects of pharmacological interventions or exercise programs.

Current research

Current research issues include the long-term changes in PPS and its prognostic factors, the continued search for the pathophysiology of PPS, the search for pharmacological treatment, the design and evaluation of rehabilitation regimens, and the further development and evaluation of orthotic devices and assistive technology.

Long-term prospective studies underway include use of age-matched controls and specific attention to potential prognostic factors such as aging and comorbidity.

Treatment recommendations

No curative treatment exists for PPS. Pharmacological treatment is available only for relief of symptoms such as pain. Management of PPS aims to restore the balance between decreasing physical capacity and the persistent demands of conducting activities of daily living. The leading concept in treatment is that symptoms of PPS, such as muscle pain, increased fatigue after physical activity, and delayed recovery following physical activity, signify that muscles are overused in conducting ordinary activities of daily living.[6,50] Support for the theory of chronic overuse of muscles has been provided by studies showing elevated levels of serum creatine kinase related to the distance walked during the previous day[68] and by studies showing a predominance of type I fibers in lower leg muscles supposedly due to fiber type transformation from chronic overload.[7] Also, PPS subjects have been found to recover more slowly from fatiguing exercise than do stable polio subjects.[2] Another factor said to contribute to symptoms is a poor cardiorespiratory condition,[18,49] but one study reported that the cardiorespiratory condition of polio subjects was not worse than that of healthy, comparably active subjects.[45] In this study, the reduced submaximal

performance capacity of the polio subjects appeared to be strongly correlated with the limited available muscle capacity, and movement economy was diminished compared with the control subjects. Lower concentrations of some oxidative enzymes in the muscles of polio subjects have been reported, whereas other oxidative enzymes within normal ranges have been reported.[8] The clinical significance of these findings has been debated.[48]

PPS patients are best treated with a multidisciplinary, specialized rehabilitative approach.[23] Because individuals show considerable differences in polio residuals, treatment is adjusted on a case-by-case basis and should be preceded by a thorough customized medical and functional evaluation. PPS is a diagnosis by exclusion, and other possible causes for the symptoms should be ruled out first. The most commonly encountered neuromuscular problems that can be managed effectively and should not be confused with PPS include radiculopathies and compression neuropathies, such as carpal tunnel syndrome, ulnar neuropathies at the wrist or elbow, and plexopathies. Compression of nerves may result from long-term use of wheelchairs, crutches, or braces, or from poor posture. Orthopedic disorders are common, especially pain from joint degeneration and joint instability, and distinguishing these symptoms from PPS may be difficult. Patients with significant joint pain may limit their physical activity, which can lead to disuse weakness and atrophy. It is important to recognize orthopedic problems as a possible cause for declining muscle function in patients with PPS because appropriate treatment of orthopedic problems may slow down or arrest that decline.

To reduce overuse and rebalance the capacities and demands, conservative management consists of three essential components: exercise, assistive devices, and lifestyle changes. Exercise can optimize cardiorespiratory fitness and may add to the patient's sense of well-being.[33,70] Exercise should be nonfatiguing and performed at submaximal levels to avoid overloading the limited muscle capacity. Exercise can improve muscle strength, especially when caused by disuse in muscle groups that are only moderately affected. Intensive strengthening exercises are not generally recommended, although they may occasionally be indicated. Functional training may be useful to improve the efficiency of ambulation.

Assistive devices (e.g., crutches, wheelchairs, and motorized scooters) and home adaptations (e.g., elevators and seating devices in the kitchen or shower) may be helpful. The need for these devices should be individually indicated and aim to reduce the physical strain of performing highly demanding activities of daily living.

Pacing of activities and taking rest intervals are of paramount importance to relieve symptoms. It has been shown that upper extremity complaints often result from overuse of shoulder and arm muscles.[35] Many PPS patients have successfully learned to deny their symptoms from childhood on in order to achieve a normal life.[40] Therefore, PPS patients may have great difficulty adapting their lifestyle to their decreasing abilities, and psychological support may be necessary.

Orthotic Management

Individuals with PPS may require leg orthoses for walking and standing if muscle weakness causes instability, falling, decreasing walking ability, or muscle pain caused by overuse.[38,52] Other indications for orthoses are (painful) joint degeneration and joint instability as a result of prolonged and biomechanically altered loading of hypoplastic and deformed joints that were formed during growth.

In patients with very severe weakness who walk mainly by stabilizing their joints passively in hyperextended positions, orthotic devices may be rejected because the resulting alteration in gait pattern can block these compensations sufficiently to reduce the patient's walking ability. These patients often exhibit very limited walking activity in daily life at an extremely high energy cost. The energy cost of walking has been shown to be strongly inversely related to the severity of polio pereses.[9]

An orthotic device may improve walking and standing, but will inevitably also have negative effects on functional abilities and may, for instance, interfere with transfers, stair climbing, sitting, and related activities such as car driving. Any device may also cause intermittent discomfort and have cosmetic implications. These consequences should all be discussed with the patient beforehand. It should also be realized that PPS patients may dislike braces because they are associated with memories of earlier use in childhood.

The most successful result is achieved in well-motivated patients with serious problems (such as increased falling and instability that hamper safe ambulation) who are walking regularly and who are able to adapt their gait pattern to the use of an orthosis.

Best practice

Regarding pharmacological treatment, the effects of pyridostigmine,[29,65] amantadine,[61] and high-dose prednisone[19] have been studied in randomized, placebo-controlled trials. Two studies with a sufficient number of patients showed no therapeutic effect of pyridostigmine on muscle strength or fatigue.[29,65] A study by Horemans et al.[29] showed only a small but positive effect of pyridostigmine on walking performance. These studies provide level I evidence that pyridostigmine is not effective in treating muscle strength or fatigue. The studies with amantadine and prednisone included a small number of patients and found no effect.

The effectiveness of muscle strengthening has been investigated only in small case series (level IV).[1,20,22,59] These studies showed improvement in strength with training programs that varied between 6 and 22 weeks and consisted of isokinetic, isometric, and endurance strengthening exercise with differing intensity and frequency. One randomized controlled trial (level I) in 10 PPS patients reported significant improvement in the muscular strength of hand muscles after isometric training.[13] However, these results cannot be generalized to larger muscle groups, as in the legs, which are loaded differently in daily life.

Evidence for the effectiveness of exercise on cardiovascular fitness is limited. Two randomized studies (level II) of ergometer cycle exercise[33] and aerobic training in upper extremities[37] showed that cardiovascular fitness improved significantly. In a nonrandomized controlled trial, aerobic walking exercise movement economy of walking improved, although cardiovascular fitness did not.[17]

The effectiveness of lifestyle modifications is not substantiated by results of randomized studies. One randomized controlled study of 22 postpolio patients did not show that lifestyle modifications in addition to exercise were more effective than exercise alone in resolving overuse symptoms.[34]

Improving old devices or prescribing new orthotic devices is reported to reduce overuse symptoms and improve walking ability in case series (level IV).[14,67] No controlled studies have compared different devices. New technologies such as carbon fiber orthoses and stance-control knee joints appear to be promising but have only been evaluated in case series (level IV). The outcomes in these studies (assessed as patient preferences and energy cost of walking) were in favor of the new technology.[6a,9a,27,30a,62] Figures 31-1 through 31-9 show examples of lightweight, high-strength, custom-made carbon fiber composite orthoses preferred by this population.

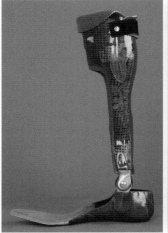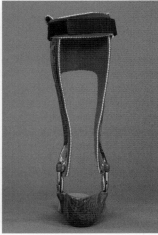

Fig. 31-1 Preimpregnated carbon composite ankle–foot orthosis with dorsiflexion stop hinges with posterior springs to enable ankle rocker in calf weakness. The anterior part of the footplate is flexible and made of Kevlar to enable forefoot rocker.

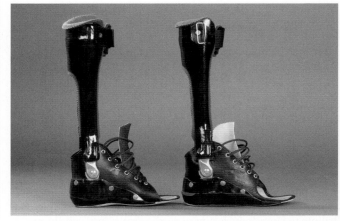

Fig. 31-2 Preimpregnated carbon composite ankle–foot orthoses with custom-made inner boots for severe and partially fixed foot deformities. Wearing comfort is enhanced by optimizing the distribution of forces applied to correct the foot in this manner.

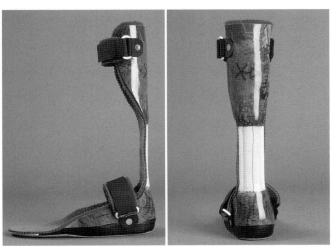

Fig. 31-3 Custom-made posterior leaf spring ankle–foot orthosis for calf weakness. The strength of the spring is determined by varying the number of layers of preimpregnated carbon to the layers of Kevlar.

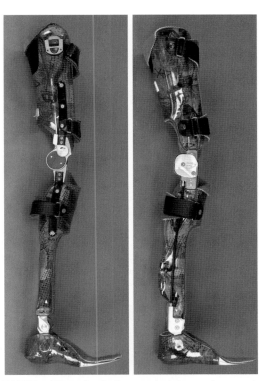

Fig. 31-5 KAFO with mechanically operated stance-phase control knee joints. The knee joint on the left side (Swing Phase Lock by Basko Healthcare/Fillauer) is controlled with a pendulum that moves by gravity. The knee joint on the right side (NeuroMatic by Fior & Genz) is controlled by ankle movement with a cable connection.

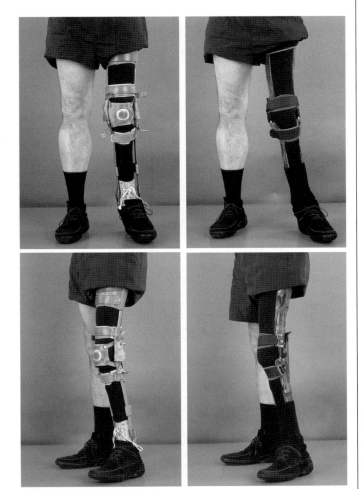

Fig. 31-4 Comparison between a metal and leather knee–ankle–foot orthosis (KAFO) and a preimpregnated carbon composite KAFO. Note the improvements in fitting, deformity correction, and use of normal shoes with the preimpregnated design.

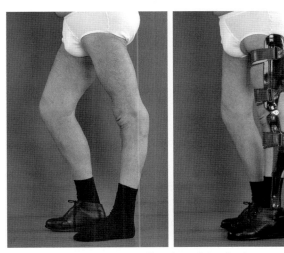

Fig. 31-6 A KAFO with an offset knee joint for hyperextension. To ensure stability in case of quadriceps weakness, the KAFO should allow some hyperextension. Alternatively, a stance-phase control or a locked knee joint can be applied.

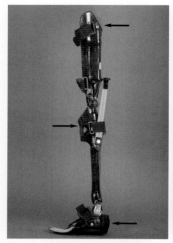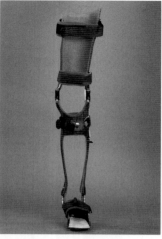

Fig. 31-7 KAFO with locked knee joints and ischial seat. The pretibial shell complements the seat because the three pressure points form one rigid three-point pressure system in the sagittal plane.

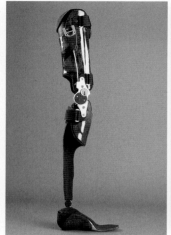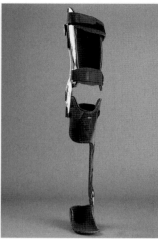

Fig. 31-9 KAFO with mechanical stance-phase control knee joint with a left-sided single upright.

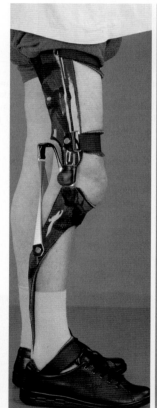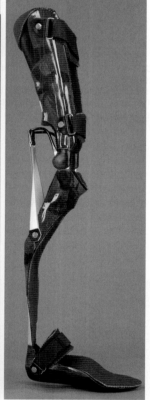

Fig. 31-8 KAFO with locked knee joints and posterior leaf.

Supporting evidence

- No drug has been proven effective in treating postpoliomyelitis syndrome.
- Several studies of limited quality (level IV) consistently show that strength training is effective in increasing muscle strength.
- Evidence (level II) indicates that exercise can improve cardiovascular fitness.

- Evidence on the effectiveness of lifestyle modifications in reducing the symptoms of postpoliomyelitis syndrome is insufficient.
- Evidence (level IV) that lightweight orthoses are subjectively beneficial for patients with postpoliomyelitis syndrome is limited.

References

1. Agre JC, Rodriquez AA, Franke TM: Strength, endurance, and work capacity after muscle strengthening exercise in postpolio subjects, *Arch Phys Med Rehabil* 78:681–686, 1997.
2. Agre JC, Rodriquez AA, Franke TM: Subjective recovery time after exhausting muscular activity in postpolio and control subjects, *Am J Phys Med Rehabil* 77:140–144, 1998.
3. Allen GM, Gandevia SC, Neering IR, et al: Muscle performance, voluntary activation and perceived effort in normal subjects and patients with prior poliomyelitis, *Brain* 117:661–670, 1994.
4. Beasley WC: Quantative muscle testing: Principles and applications to research and clinical services, *Arch Phys Med Rehabil* 42:398–425, 1961.
5. Beelen A, Nollet F, de Visser M, et al: Quadriceps muscle strength and voluntary activation after polio, *Muscle Nerve* 28:218–226, 2003.
6. Bennett RL, Knowlton GC: Overwork weakness in partially denervated skeletal muscle, *Clin Orthop Relat Res* 12:22–29, 1958.
6a. Bernhardt KA, Irby SE, Kaufman KR: Consumer opinions of a stance control knee orthosis, *Prosthet Orthot Int* 30:246–256, 2006.
7. Borg K, Borg J, Edstrom L, Grimby L: Effects of excessive use of remaining muscle fibers in prior polio and LV lesion, *Muscle Nerve* 11:1219–1230, 1988.
8. Borg K, Henriksson J: Prior poliomyelitis-reduced capillary supply and metabolic enzyme content in hypertrophic slow-twitch (type I) muscle fibres, *J Neurol Neurosurg Psychiatry* 54:236–240, 1991.
8a. Brehm MA, Beelen A, Doorenbosch CA, Harlaar J, Nollet F: Effect of carbon-composite knee-ankle-foot orthoses on walking efficiency and gait in former polio patients. *J Rehabil Med* 39:651–657, 2007.
9. Brehm MA, Nollet F, Harlaar J: Energy demands of walking in persons with postpoliomyelitis syndrome: relationship with muscle strength and reproducibility, *Arch Phys Med Rehabil* 87:136–140, 2006.
10. Bruno RL, Sapolsky R, Zimmerman JR, Frick NM: Pathophysiology of a central cause of post-polio fatigue, *Ann N Y Acad Sci* 753:257–275, 1995.
11. Campbell MJ, McComas AJ, Petito F: Physiological changes in ageing muscles, *J Neurol Neurosurg Psychiatry* 36:174–182, 1973.
12. Cashman NR, Maselli RA, Wollman RL, et al: Late denervation in patients with antecedent paralytic poliomyelitis, *N Engl J Med* 317:7–12, 1987.
13. Chan KM, Amirjani N, Sumrain M, et al: Randomized controlled trial of strength training in post-polio patients, *Muscle Nerve* 27:332–338, 2003.
14. Clark DR, Perry J, Lunsford TR: Case studies: orthotic management of the adult post polio patient, *Orthot Prosthet* 40:43–50, 1986.

15. Dalakas MC: Morphologic changes in the muscles of patients with postpoliomyelitis neuromuscular symptoms, *Neurology* 38:99–104, 1988.

16. Dalakas MC: Why drugs fail in postpolio syndrome: lessons from another clinical trial, *Neurology* 53:1166–1167, 1999.

17. Dean E, Ross J: Effect of modified aerobic training on movement energetics in polio survivors, *Orthopedics* 14:1243–1246, 1991.

18. Dean E, Ross J: Movement energetics of individuals with a history of poliomyelitis, *Arch Phys Med Rehabil* 74:478–483, 1993.

19. Dinsmore S, Dambrosia J, Dalakas, MC: A double-blind, placebo-controlled trial of high-dose prednisone for the treatment of post-poliomyelitis syndrome, *Ann N Y Acad Sci* 753:303–313, 1995.

20. Einarsson G: Muscle conditioning in late poliomyelitis, *Arch Phys Med Rehabil* 72:11–14, 1991.

21. Einarsson G, Grimby G, Stalberg E: Electromyographic and morphological functional compensation in late poliomyelitis, *Muscle Nerve* 13:165–171, 1990.

22. Ernstoff B, Wetterqvist H, Kvist H, Grimby G: Endurance training effect on individuals with postpoliomyelitis, *Arch Phys Med Rehabil* 77:843–848, 1996.

23. Gawne AC, Halstead LS: Post-polio syndrome: pathophysiology and clinical management, *Crit Rev Phys Rehabil Med* 7:147–188, 1995.

24. Gonzalez H, Khademi M, Andersson M, et al: Prior poliomyelitis: evidence of cytokine production in the central nervous system, *J Neurol Sci* 205:9–13, 2002.

25. Grimby G, Einarsson G, Hedberg M, Aniansson A: Muscle adaptive changes in post-polio subjects, *Scand J Rehab Med* 21:19–26, 1989.

26. Halstead LS, Rossi CD: New problems in old polio patients: results of a survey of 539 polio survivors, *Orthopedics* 8:845–850, 1985.

27. Heim M, Yaacobi E, Azaria M: A pilot study to determine the efficiency of lightweight carbon fibre orthoses in the management of patients suffering from post-poliomyelitis syndrome, *Clin Rehabil* 11:302–305, 1997.

28. Horemans HL, Beelen A, Nollet F, et al: Reproducibility of maximal quadriceps strength and its relationship to maximal voluntary activation in postpoliomyelitis syndrome, *Arch Phys Med Rehabil* 85:1273–1278, 2004.

29. Horemans HL, Nollet F, Beelen A, et al: Pyridostigmine in postpolio syndrome: no decline in fatigue and limited functional improvement, *J Neurol Neurosurg Psychiatry* 74:1655–1661, 2003.

30. Howard RS: Poliomyelitis and the postpolio syndrome, *BMJ* 330:1314–1318, 2005.

30a. Irby SE, Bernhardt KA, Kaufman KR: Gait of stance control orthosis users: the dynamic knee brace system, *Prosthet Orthot Int* 29:269–282, 2005.

31. Ivanyi B, Nollet F, Redekop WK, et al: Late onset polio sequelae: disabilities and handicaps in a population-based cohort of the 1956 poliomyelitis outbreak in The Netherlands, *Arch Phys Med Rehabil* 80:687–690, 1999.

32. Ivanyi B, Redekop W, de Jongh R, de Visser M: Computed tomographic study of the skeletal musculature of the lower body in 45 postpolio patients, *Muscle Nerve* 21:540–542, 1998.

33. Jones DR, Speier J, Canine K, et al: Cardiorespiratory responses to aerobic training by patients with postpoliomyelitis sequelae, *JAMA* 261:3255–3258, 1989.

34. Klein MG, Whyte J, Esquenazi A, et al: A comparison of the effects of exercise and lifestyle modification on the resolution of overuse symptoms of the shoulder in polio survivors: a preliminary study, *Arch Phys Med Rehabil* 83:708–713, 2002.

35. Klein MG, Whyte J, Keenan MA, et al: The relation between lower extremity strength and shoulder overuse symptoms: a model based on polio survivors, *Arch Phys Med Rehabil* 81:789–795, 2000.

36. Klingman J, Chui H, Corgiat M, Perry J: Functional recovery. A major risk factor for the development of postpoliomyelitis muscular atrophy, *Arch Neurol* 45:645–647, 1988.

37. Kriz JL, Jones DR, Speier JL, et al: Cardiorespiratory responses to upper extremity aerobic training by postpolio subjects, *Arch Phys Med Rehabil* 73:49–54, 1992.

38. Lord SR, Allen GM, Williams P, Gandevia SC: Risk of falling: predictors based on reduced strength in persons previously affected by polio, *Arch Phys Med Rehabil* 83:757–763, 2002.

39. March of Dimes Foundation: *Post-polio syndrome: identifying best practices in diagnosis & care*, White Plains, NY, 2002, March of Dimes.

40. Maynard FM, Roller S: Recognizing typical coping styles of polio survivors can improve re-rehabilitation, *Am J Phys Med Rehabil* 70:70–72, 1991.

41. McComas AJ, Quartly C, Griggs RC: Early and late losses of motor units after poliomyelitis, *Brain* 120:1415–1421, 1997.

42. Mulder DW, Rosenbaum RA, Layton DD: Late progression of poliomyelitis or forme fruste amyotrophic lateral sclerosis? *Mayo Clin Proc* 47:756–761, 1972.

43. Nollet F, Beelen A: Strength assessment in postpolio syndrome: validity of a hand-held dynamometer in detecting change, *Arch Phys Med Rehabil* 80:1316–1323, 1999.

44. Nollet F, Beelen A, Prins MH, et al: Disability and functional assessment in former polio patients with and without postpolio syndrome, *Arch Phys Med Rehabil* 80:136–143, 1999.

45. Nollet F, Beelen A, Sargeant AJ, et al: Submaximal exercise capacity and maximal power output in polio subjects, *Arch Phys Med Rehabil* 82:1678–1685, 2001.

46. Nollet F, de Visser M: Postpolio syndrome, *Arch Neurol* 61:1142–1144, 2004.

47. Nollet F, Ivanyi B, Beelen A, et al: Perceived health in a population based sample of victims of the 1956 polio epidemic in the Netherlands, *J Neurol Neurosurg Psychiatry* 73:695–700, 2002.

48. Nordgren B, Falck B, Stalberg E, et al: Postpolio muscular dysfunction: relationships between muscle energy metabolism, subjective symptoms, magnetic resonance imaging, electromyography, and muscle strength, *Muscle Nerve* 20:1341–1351, 1997.

49. Owen RR, Jones D: Polio residuals clinic: conditioning exercise program, *Orthopedics* 8:882–883, 1985.

50. Perry J, Barnes G, Gronley JK: The postpolio syndrome. An overuse phenomenon, *Clin Orthop Relat Res* 233:145–162, 1988.

51. Perry J, Clark D: Biomechanical abnormalities of post-polio patients and the implications for orthotic management, *Neurorehabilitation* 8:119–138, 1997.

52. Perry J, Fontaine JD, Mulroy S: Findings in post-poliomyelitis syndrome. Weakness of muscles of the calf as a source of late pain and fatigue of muscles of the thigh after poliomyelitis, *J Bone Joint Surg Am* 77:1148–1153, 1995.

53. Ramlow J, Alexander M, LaPorte R, et al: Epidemiology of the post-polio syndrome, *Am J Epidemiol* 136:769–786, 1992.

54. Raymond: Note sur deux cas de paralysie essentielle de l'enfance, *Gaz Med Paris* 225–226, 1875.

55. Rekand T, Karlsen B, Langeland N, Aarli JA: Long-term follow-up of patients with nonparalytic poliomyelitis, *Arch Phys Med Rehabil* 83:533–537, 2002.

56. Sharief MK: Poliovirus persistence in the postpolio syndrome, *Ann Neurol* 34:415–417, 1993.

57. Sharma KR, Kent-Braun J, Mynhier MA, et al: Excessive muscular fatigue in the postpoliomyelitis syndrome, *Neurology* 44:642–646, 1994.

58. Sorenson EJ, Daube JR, Windebank AJ: A 15-year follow-up of neuromuscular function in patients with prior poliomyelitis, *Neurology* 64:1070–1072, 2005.

59. Spector SA, Gordon PL, Feuerstein IM, et al: Strength gains without muscle injury after strength training in patients with postpolio muscular atrophy, *Muscle Nerve* 19:1282–1290, 1996.

60. Stalberg E, Grimby G: Dynamic electromyography and muscle biopsy changes in a 4-year follow-up: study of patients with a history of polio, *Muscle Nerve* 18:699–707, 1995.

61. Stein DP, Dambrosia JM, Dalakas MC: A double-blind, placebo-controlled trial of amantadine for the treatment of fatigue in patients with the post-polio syndrome, *Ann N Y Acad Sci* 753:296–302, 1995.

62. Steinfeldt F, Seifert W, Gunther KP: Modern carbon fibre orthoses in the management of polio patients: a critical evaluation of the functional aspects, *Z Orthop Ihre Grenzgeb* 141:357–361, 2003.

63. Stolwijk-Swuste JM, Beelen A, Lankhorst GJ, Nollet F: The course of functional status and muscle strength in patients with late-onset sequelae of poliomyelitis: a systematic review, *Arch Phys Med Rehabil* 86:1693–1701, 2005.

64. Trojan DA, Cashman NR, Shapiro S, et al: Predictive factors for post-poliomyelitis syndrome, *Arch Phys Med Rehabil* 75:770–777, 1994.

65. Trojan DA, Collet JP, Shapiro S, et al: A multicenter, randomized, double-blinded trial of pyridostigmine in postpolio syndrome, *Neurology* 53:1225–1233, 1999.

66. Trojan DA, Gendron D, Cashman NR: Anticholinesterase-responsive neuromuscular junction transmission defects in post-poliomyelitis fatigue, *J Neurol Sci* 114:170–177, 1993.

67. Waring WP, Maynard F, Grady W, et al: Influence of appropriate lower extremity orthotic management on ambulation, pain, and fatigue in a postpolio population, *Arch Phys Med Rehabil* 70:371–375, 1989.

68. Waring WP, McLaurin TM: Correlation of creatine kinase and gait measurement in the postpolio population: a corrected version, *Arch Phys Med Rehabil* 73:447–450, 1992.

69. Wiechers DO, Hubbell SL: Late changes in the motor unit after acute poliomyelitis, *Muscle Nerve* 4:524–528, 1981.

70. Willen C, Sunnerhagen KS, Grimby G: Dynamic water exercise in individuals with late poliomyelitis, *Arch Phys Med Rehabil* 82:66–72, 2001.

71. Windebank AJ, Litchy WJ, Daube JR, et al: Late effects of paralytic poliomyelitis in Olmsted County, Minnesota, *Neurology* 41:501–507, 1991.

Chapter

32

Orthoses for persons with postpolio sequelae

Thomas V. DiBello, Carolyn Kelley, Carlos Vallbona, and Teresa Kaldis

Key Points

- Poliomyelitis infection may present different symptoms in the acute, chronic, and late stages. The latter two are often referred to as postpolio paralysis (PPP) and postpolio syndrome (PPS).

- Due to the complex and variable presentation of PPP and PPS, this patient population benefits from a multidisciplinary treatment team and an individualized biomechanical prescription based on detailed physical evaluation and observational gait analysis.

- Modern orthoses used for PPP and for PPS are similar, emphasizing light weight and biomechanically functional design to enhance patient acceptance and community ambulation.

- An orthotic management algorithm based on prior experience with orthoses may be helpful in determining the specifics of the orthotic prescription for individual patients.

Management of the orthotic needs of patients with postpolio sequelae, including postpolio paralysis (PPP) and postpolio syndrome (PPS), is one of the more challenging tasks presented to orthotists. Beyond the unique characteristics of the disability created by the original onslaught of the disease, the patient with postpolio sequelae presents with completely overlapping and complicating factors that require careful assessment, evaluation, and implementation. The team approach is vital to effective management of this patient population. This chapter describes the process required for effective orthotic prescription, design, fabrication, and fitting.

Several theories exist on the cause of the new muscle weakness and atrophy commonly observed in this patient population. First, many of these individuals are aging and consequently have a significantly diminished neuromuscular system. Small losses that typically occur with normal aging may appear more pronounced because they represent loss of a greater percentage of the surviving nerve and muscle cells after poliomyelitis infection. Second, the neuronal sprouting and neuroplasticity that occurred during the acute recovery period may be more physiologically fragile and, therefore, place the patients at risk for premature aging and breakdown. In addition, the neuronal sprouting that occurred caused the development of giant motor units. The metabolic demand of these giant motor units is tremendous, as one cell body now is innervating many times more muscle cells than it had previously. If the physiological demand is too great for too long a time period, some of the neuronal sprouting will be pruned. There is some evidence of instability at the neuromuscular junction, which may cause muscular fatigue and less endurance.[35] Additionally, patients with muscle pain due to overuse may show elevated creatine kinase levels in their blood, indicating damage of the skeletal muscle at a cellular level.[9]

Historical perspective

Acute anterior poliomyelitis, also known as *infantile paralysis*, is a devastating infectious disease. After smallpox, it may become the second infectious disease completely eradicated from the planet. The infectious agent is the polio virus, of which there are three types: I, II, and III. The name *poliomyelitis* is derived from the Greek word *polio* (meaning gray) and *myelitis* (meaning infectious process of the spinal cord). As the prefix polio indicates, infection of the spinal cord occurs exclusively in its gray matter, which is populated by neurons. However, the polio virus also may affect the motor neurons of the cranial nerves, which are located in the brain.

Poliomyelitis is an old disease that initially caused paralysis mostly in children, but it also affected adults of various age groups, mostly young. The first record available of the poliomyelitis is a graphic representation of a paralyzed Egyptian priest, who is depicted with typical deformities of his right leg and seems to support himself by holding his left arm on a long staff, a sort of an orthotic device. The picture is engraved in the so-called *stella of Ruma*, which depicts a scene of the 18th Egyptian Dynasty (1580–1350 BC). Another old record is an Italian jar of the 15th century BC, which depicts a man with a deformed right leg and equinus deformity of the left foot who supports himself on a stick.

The first written description of a patient with a clinical picture resembling poliomyelitis is credited to Salzmann, who in 1734 reported on the history of a person who had contracted a paralytic condition during childhood but had a gradual recovery and partial cure. The patient died as an adult after 10 years of being psychologically upset, becoming an alcoholic and speaking of being tired of life and desiring to die. Postmortem examination of the body revealed "degenerated muscle bellies replaced by fatty and fibrous tissue."[32] If this person indeed had poliomyelitis, were his problems before death manifestations of what we now call postpolio syndrome? In 1789, Underwood described a case of "debility in the lower extremities," but whether the patient's weakness was actually due to another cause, perhaps a vertebral lesion due to tuberculosis (Fishbein et al., 1951), has been questioned.[10] Other extensive and creditable descriptions were made in the 19th century by the German physician Jacob Von Heine (1806–1879) and the Swedish physician Oskar Medin (1847–1928). For about a century, throughout Europe the disease had been referred to as the *Heine-Medin disease* rather than poliomyelitis because the simple mention of the word poliomyelitis created a lot of panic in the general population, especially during the frequent summer epidemics.

The disease is caused by any one of three types of virus and leads to permanent cross-immunity, although a few patients affected by one type of virus may contract a second episode with a different type.

The polio virus is transmitted to humans through contact with infected air droplets or ingestion of contaminated water or other liquids. Prior to the era of water sanitation, the virus was ubiquitous in public water supplies, and the majority of the population was exposed to the virus in early infancy. If the virus did not cause the paralytic disease, it likely conferred permanent immunity, as if it were a form of natural vaccination. However, as a result of water sanitation and other good hygienic practices in developed nations, chronic access to minute quantities of the virus became infrequent, and increasingly more people did not acquire natural immunity and thus became more susceptible to infection.

The polio epidemics of the 1930s, 1940s, and 1950s took a major toll in the United States, where it was estimated that as many as 40,000 to 50,000 new cases occurred every year. The advent of the Salk vaccine in 1955 (administered intramuscularly with a killed virus) and the Sabin vaccine in 1960 (administered orally with a live attenuated virus) eliminated the ravages of the epidemics, and increasingly fewer cases occurred in the United States throughout the 1960s and early 1970s.

Use of poliomyelitis vaccines throughout the world led to a rapid decline in the incidence of PPP in many countries. In the Americas, the last documented new case of polio infection occurred in Peru in 1991. Whenever a continent or a large area of the world does not have a single reported new case of polio for a period of 5 years, the disease is considered to have been eradicated in that continent or area. Accordingly, the whole continent of the Americas was declared free of polio in 1996. Subsequently, all other continents have been certified as free of polio with the exception of Africa and Asia, where as of May 2006, 309 new cases of polio were registered in Equatorial Africa, the Asian subcontinent, and Indonesia.

Although acute poliomyelitis has ceased to be a problem for most of the world, the sequelae of polio continue to create serious health problems in polio survivors. Some 30 to 50 years after an acute episode of the disease, patients who had contracted polio may begin to present new symptoms of weakness in formerly affected and formerly unaffected muscles, leading to a new form of disability now called *postpolio syndrome*.

The medical literature of the late 1800s contains at least three reports of patients who presented problems similar to those of our current PPS cases.[6,8,31] In the period from 1875 to 1975, approximately 200 cases were reported. However, the problem did not become readily apparent in the United States until the early 1980s, when numerous persons who had been affected with poliomyelitis during the epidemics of the 1930s, 1940s, and 1950s began to develop clear manifestations of PPS. It has been estimated that approximately 30% of the more than 1.5 million polio survivors in the United States are affected with the syndrome, but the real prevalence among survivors likely is much greater.

The majority of patients who survived the acute stage of poliomyelitis were left with important sequelae of PPP, mostly in the lower extremities but in some cases in the arms as well. It was customary to use ingenious devices such as crutches of different shapes and various types of footwear to compensate for the weakness of the ankle and other joints of the legs. These devices became known as *orthoses*. In addition, a variety of slings were developed for individuals who had major weakness of the arms. The early braces were made with leather and hard metal to provide support to a weakened leg, but the devices were heavy and bulky, and often they were not aesthetic. As a result, most young polio survivors were reluctant to use their prescribed braces and tended to discard the devices as soon as they recovered enough strength to walk by themselves in spite of permanent residual weakness.

Use of orthoses for persons with PPP proliferated considerably in the first half of the 20th century in the United States and in Europe. The prescription of orthoses for polio survivors required elaborate adaptations to each patient's needs given the scattered and asymmetrical paralysis typical of poliomyelitis. Use of off-the-shelf orthoses rarely was possible. The availability of new materials that are lighter than the traditional leather and steel used in older orthoses has made possible better customization of the newer devices described in this chapter, which are much more accepted by polio survivors than the older and heavier devices.

Many individuals who had recovered from the initial polio infection began to experience increased weakness in muscles known and not known to have sustained polio-related damage and presented for medical help in the 1970s and 1980s.[35] PPS has been described as a syndrome since the mid 1980s. From 25% to 70% of all polio survivors develop PPS. The median reported time from acute poliomyelitis to PPS is 35 years.[34]

Current issues

From the standpoint of orthotic management, the development of pain and weakness in the contralateral or "strong side" of the patient with PPS often results in the need for use of orthoses in individuals who for many years had been able to compensate for their weakness without any type of external assistive device. These patients often have difficulty accepting the need for an orthosis after so many decades of functioning without a brace.

Replacement of older heavier designs with newer, more lightweight orthoses that improve control, particularly in the transverse plane, in an effort to diminish energy expenditure in the PPS population can pose difficulties to longtime users of orthoses. Because patients with postpolio sequelae have intact and often heightened sensation, they may have difficulty accepting the different "feel" of today's lightweight, intimately fitting orthoses compared to the much heavier, less biomechanically secure braces they are accustomed to wearing. The required lifestyle changes necessitated by the onset of PPS along with the prescription of new orthoses also prove challenging for many patients.

Current research

Advances in technology have created more options in orthotic design and fabrication that adequately protect and assist paretic or paralyzed lower extremities in gait, standing, and transfers. The most commonly seen advance in orthotic fabrication is the use of plastic or carbon fiber materials. These materials act primarily to decrease the weight of the orthosis, but they also increase the level of mechanical control and/or support of the limb. Decreasing the weight by even a few grams or ounces can make a huge difference for a person with weakness. Patients should select the lightest-weight shoes they can find to decrease the overall weight and energy needed to move the affected limb. Excessive hip flexion during limb advancement is a frequently observed compensation. Increased weight on the limb, particularly distally, can greatly impact the person's ability to adequately clear the foot in swing.[13,27,35]

One of the technological advances in the area of treating PPS patients is the lightweight carbon fiber knee–ankle–foot orthosis (KAFO). Orthotists fabricate the orthosis with the lightest-weight materials available to increase patient acceptance. In a study of 14 patients with PPS and 14 age- and gender-matched healthy subjects, polio survivors had 28% lower walking speed, 9% higher energy consumption, and 40% higher energy cost.[4] Lower extremity muscle strength was significantly correlated with walking speed and energy cost. Five of the subjects wore unilateral KAFOs, one wore a unilateral ankle–foot orthosis (AFO), one wore bilateral AFOs, and six used canes with or without their orthoses.[4]

Heim et al.[13] conducted a pilot study examining the efficiency of lightweight carbon fiber KAFOs in the management of symptoms of people with PPS. Thirty subjects with PPS who wore metal and leather KAFOs participated in the study; 27 completed the study. Twenty-one of the 27 wore their custom-made carbon fiber KAFOs daily and reported that the devices were lighter weight, better fitting, and more aesthetic. The carbon fiber KAFOs weighed an average of 1,150 g compared to 1,720 g for the metal KAFOs (approximately one third heavier in weight). Eight of the 27 participants preferred the metal orthoses because of skin irritation, excessive sweating, and the inability to change the shape of the device after fabrication to accommodate weight gain or swelling in the carbon fiber orthosis. The participants reported other disadvantages of the carbon fiber orthoses, such as the exact fit required, greater manufacturing time (average 17.5 weeks), and greater expense.[13]

Another technological advance is the use of a stance control knee joint within KAFOs. These electronic or mechanical knee joints allow automatic locking during stance phase and automatic unlocking for knee flexion during swing phase.[12,17] Hebert and Liggins[12] performed a case study of a 61-year-old patient with PPS, comparing various gait parameters and the Physiological Cost Index (PCI) with use of a KAFO in either the stance control or locked mode. No significant changes were noted in velocity, cadence, stride length, or step length, or during toe-off. With the KAFO in locked knee position, the knee remained in approximately 6 degrees of flexion throughout all phases of gait. With the KAFO in stance control mode, the knee was in 17 degrees of flexion and progressed to 55 degrees of flexion at 75% of the gait cycle. Stance control mode decreased transverse plane pelvic rotation by 6 degrees and overall excursion through the entire gait cycle by 6 degrees. In stance control mode, vertical pelvic displacement was reduced from 67.0 ± 5.9 mm to 58.7 ± 5.6 mm. Lateral pelvic excursion also was reduced, from 128.8 ± 12.0 mm to 108.6 ± 11.0 mm. PCI was 0.447 at self-selected walking velocity of 49.2 m/min in stance control mode compared to 0.554 at a velocity of 49.7 m/min with a locked knee.[12]

Similarly, a pilot study was conducted of two participants with PPS and one with an incomplete spinal cord injury (SCI). All subjects demonstrated improved velocity, cadence, stride length, and step length while using the KAFO in stance control mode. Less hip hiking and lateral trunk flexion were observed. The two participants with PPS completed the obstacle course more quickly while using stance control. While walking for 5 minutes on a treadmill, the two participants with PPS had lower increases in heart rate in stance control than locked condition, and the participant with incomplete SCI experienced a lower treadmill-induced heart rate while using the stance control mode.[23]

Waring et al.[36] examined the effects of lower extremity orthotic management on gait, pain, and fatigue in individuals with PPS. Among 104 participants, they found that a new orthosis was more frequently prescribed for a previously braced limb or an additional device for a previously untreated limb for patients who had worn orthoses earlier in their lives than for those who had never worn orthoses (28/56 who had worn orthoses vs 9/48 who had not worn orthoses). Seventy-two percent of those who had undergone an ankle fusion required new orthoses. A follow-up questionnaire returned by 78% of participants showed that appropriate orthoses significantly improved fatigue, weakness, walking ability, perceived walking safety, and knee pain.[36]

The frequency and types of orthoses prescribed for individuals with postpolio sequelae were described in a retrospective study of 5,045 cases of postpolio infantile paralysis conducted in Saudi Arabia. A total of 3,280 lower extremity orthoses were supplied, including 730 AFOs, 1,518 KAFOs, and 1,032 hip–knee–ankle–foot orthoses (HKAFOs) or bilateral HKAFOs.[1] The number of individuals in this study who were polio survivors diagnosed with PPS is unclear.

In a retrospective study of 772 patients diagnosed with PPS seen at the in-house postpolio outpatient clinic between 1999 and 2005 at the Postpolio Outpatient Clinic at the Texas Institute for Rehabilitation and Research (TIRR), 337 either wore orthoses or were prescribed new orthoses. A total of 207 KAFOs (51.8%) and 191 AFOs (47.8%) either were worn by or prescribed for these patients. Of the KAFOs, 78 had been used for the patient's lifetime since onset of acute poliomyelitis (most with locked knees), 52 orthoses with posterior offset knee joints (one replacing lifetime locked knee joint) had been prescribed, 24 orthoses with stance control knee joints (two replacing lifetime-use locked knee joints) had been prescribed, and the rest had locked knees with drop/ring, bail, or cable release locks, or undocumented types of knee joints. Of the AFOs, 71 were rear entry ground reaction design with articulating ankle joint and dorsiflexion assist; 17 were rear entry ground reaction design with either solid or undocumented ankle joints; 29 were traditional solid ankle; 29 were posterior leaf spring design; eight were traditional articulating ankle with dorsiflexion assist, plantarflexion stop, or both; 32 were undocumented ankle joint; and three were supramalleolar design. Additionally, one Swedish knee cage and one knee brace designed to unload the femorotibial joint to slow joint deterioration were noted. Fifty-seven individuals (16.9%) wore bilateral devices.[18]

Orthotic management

Patient evaluation

Management of patients with postpolio sequelae requires a thorough history and clinical evaluation by the orthotist. The history should include a review of the patient's past orthotic management, surgical interventions, existing painful joints, vocational and nonvocational activities, along with the patient's description of how often he or she is falling or nearly falling and the circumstances surrounding those falls or near falls. Clinical evaluation should include assessment of basic manual muscle strength and passive range of motion, static alignment of the joints of the lower limb, overall posture of the patient, and careful observational gait analysis.[26]

Through the course of this initial evaluation, the orthotist must assess the patient's willingness to accept the device. Often patients with PPS have managed quite well without an orthosis for the majority of their lifetimes and are reluctant to use an orthotic device. Many perceive that use of an orthotic device signifies that a disease they had overcome has again reared its head and begun to control their lives.[34] Finally, it is important that the orthotist ask the patient what he or she hopes the device will do for him or her. If the patient's expectations are unrealistic, the orthotist must carefully define what the device can and cannot reasonably be expected to do for the patient. Unrealistic expectations can lead to disappointment that in turn leads the patient to dissatisfaction with or even abandonment of the device. With this information and the team's prescription for the orthotic design, the orthotist can begin the process of designing the optimal orthosis.

Design

Only a handful of basic designs are used in the management of the population with postpolio sequelae, including those with PPP and PPS. However, a large number of combinations and permutations of orthotic designs and components can improve the outcome of the devices for each patient. In all cases, a functionally optimal device that is as lightweight as possible should be the goal.

Ankle–foot orthoses

An AFO can be used to stabilize and protect the joints of the foot and ankle and provide swing phase clearance and stance phase stability. Secondarily, an AFO will have an impact on knee kinematics.[21,24,33] These devices are available in a variety of designs. The designs most commonly used in the management of the population with postpolio sequelae are discussed here.

Posterior leaf spring AFO The posterior leaf spring ankle–foot orthosis (PLS AFO) provides clearance of the foot through swing phase (Fig. 32-1). Its impact in stance phase is limited to mild control of ankle inversion or eversion and only mild resistance to tibial advancement. It permits smooth advancement from initial contact to loading response and eliminates "foot slap." As with the metal Klenzak dorsiflexion assist AFO (described below), this device is appropriate only for a narrow range of individuals with PPS and should be used only when good stance phase stability exists.[33]

Solid ankle AFO The plastic solid ankle AFO is designed to provide a high degree of control to the ankle–foot complex during stance (Fig. 32-2). In addition to good control of dorsiflexion, plantarflexion, and inversion and eversion of the ankle, it can control movement in the transverse plane.[21,24,33] With proper reinforcement, this design can be quite rigid. It protects the painful ankle that sometimes occurs in the PPS population as decades-old fusions begin to deteriorate. Use of this design often incorporates a rocker

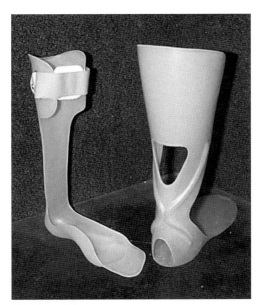

Fig. 32-1 Posterior leaf spring AFO.

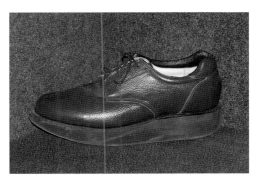

Fig. 32-3 Rocker sole.

sole on the shoe to smooth movements through early and late stance phase (Fig. 32-3). However, individuals with severe quadriceps weakness may feel unstable with the addition of the rocker sole. If used, careful attention to placement of the apex of the rocker is necessary.

Articulated ankle plastic AFO The plastic articulated ankle AFO incorporates a mechanical articulation at the ankle (Fig. 32-4). This allows movement fore and aft, permitting the anatomical ankle to move through a specific range of motion. A variety of ankle joint components can be used to provide dorsiflexion and plantarflexion control. The specific component chosen should provide the amount of movement necessary to satisfy the patient's needs in swing and stance.[24]

The existing ankle components do an excellent job of providing plantarflexion control but a much less effective job of controlling dorsiflexion. The stress of the dynamic transfer of weight to the stance side places high loads on these components as they attempt to control dorsiflexion. Unless a double action ankle joint of the type previously reserved for metal AFOs is incorporated into the design,[21] these other joint components should be reserved for lightweight or limited ambulation patients (Fig. 32-5).

Ground reaction AFO The ground reaction AFO is designed to provide a posteriorly directed force to the knee in stance by blocking forward tibial advancement (Fig. 32-6).[21] The ankle angle at which the orthosis is set must be carefully established so that the orthosis is in a few degrees of forward tilt when sitting in the shoe. When properly designed, this plastic device is quite rigid and can fully accept the entire weight of the patient without deformation. As in the solid ankle AFO, the rigid ankle of the ground reaction

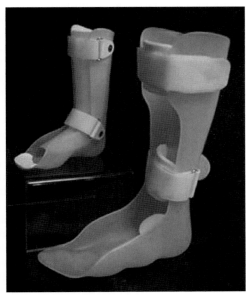

Fig. 32-2 Plastic solid ankle AFO.

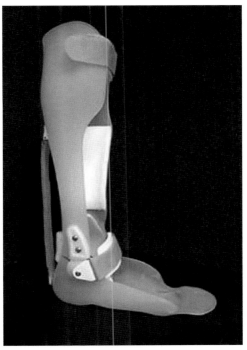

Fig. 32-4 Plastic articulated ankle AFO.

423

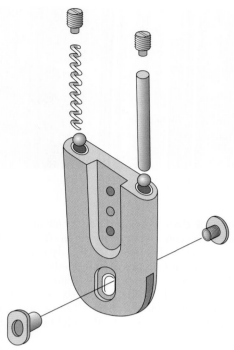

Fig. 32-5 Exploded double action ankle joint.

AFO protects the painful ankle and necessitates the use of a rocker sole on the shoe to smooth the patient's movement through stance.

Articulated rear entry ground reaction AFO The articulated ground reaction rear entry AFO is designed to incorporate the beneficial attributes of several designs (Fig. 32-7). The geometric shape of the plastic over the front of the leg gives it

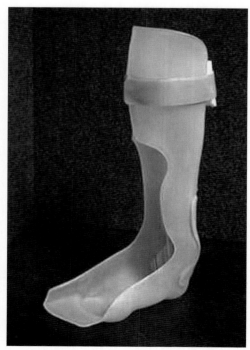

Fig. 32-6 Ground reaction AFO.

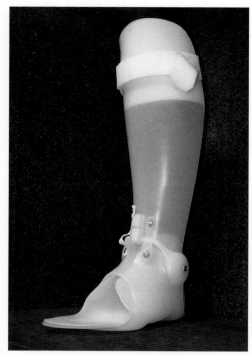

Fig. 32-7 Articulated ground reaction rear entry AFO.

significant resistance to the deforming forces that occur in stance phase without reinforcement. The dorsiflexion stop can be made adjustable. Incorporation of an elastic dorsiflexion assist and adjustable plantarflexion stop typically will allow 5 degrees of plantar flexion and engage the dorsiflexion stop at 5 to 10 degrees to permit swing phase clearance and good stance phase control without disruption of early or late stance phase rockers. Allowing smooth transition through these rockers can be especially important in this population in which balance is sometimes tenuous and decreasing energy expenditure in walking is essential.[26]

Metal double upright AFO This traditional design is useful for individuals with fluctuating edema or those who have worn a metal device for years and are unwilling to consider changing to a plastic orthosis (Fig. 32-8). In these cases, the design typically uses a double adjustable ankle joint. This permits the orthotist a nearly infinite range of adjustability. A pin or spring can be used in the posterior compartment to provide clearance of the foot in swing phase. The spring affords a smoother transition from initial contact to loading response and is the preferred choice when limited plantarflexion is not needed to stabilize the limb in stance.[24] The anterior compartment of the joint should utilize a pin, thereby controlling anterior tibial advancement in stance and creating a knee extension moment at heel-off. A spring in the anterior compartment is unable to effectively resist dorsiflexion as the patient's incumbent body weight is transferred to the stance side. In the past, many polio survivors were fitted with dorsiflexion assist devices designed with Klenzak joints at the ankle, which provided adequate swing phase clearance but no effective resistance to tibial advancement in stance (Fig. 32-9). With time, these individuals developed increased weakness in their plantarflexors and lost their ability to control the limb in stance.

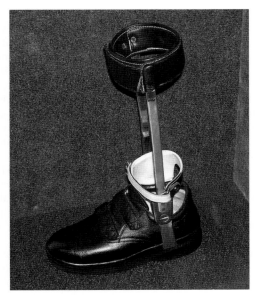

Fig. 32-8 Metal double upright AFO.

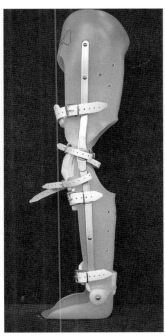

Fig. 32-10 Knee–ankle–foot orthosis.

The result was a shortened stance phase on the involved side and an exaggerated limp with overuse of the contralateral side. Therefore, the dorsiflexion assist design should be used cautiously in isolation and only in individuals who have strong plantarflexors. The treating orthotist must realize that the need may arise for more complex orthotic components as the patient's strength decreases.

Knee–ankle–foot orthoses

By crossing the knee, the KAFO extends the level of control proximally and is useful when buckling or hyperextension of

the knee occurs (Fig. 32-10). In the PPS population, it can be used effectively to partially deweight the limb through utilization of a quadrilateral or ischial containment design. This is particularly important in the segment of the PPS population that currently is wearing a KAFO of traditional design and whose chief complaint is contralateral side pain, fatigue, or increased weakness. By permitting the patient to more efficiently transfer his or her weight through the proximal brim of the KAFO,[2] the stance period of the involved side can be lengthened and reduce the stress on the contralateral untreated side.

Knee joints

Posterior offset Posterior offset knee joints can be used effectively when the patient presents with unilateral hyperextension of the knee (Fig. 32-11). Typically in the patient with hyperextension, the knee is not corrected fully to 180 degrees, but is set in a number of degrees of hyperextension that permits the patient to feel secure and safe in transferring his or her weight over the involved side. The amount of hyperextension at the knee is limited. thus reducing the stress on the posterior capsule of the knee. Remember that if the amount of hyperextension built into the orthosis is less than the patient can effectively balance on and transfer weight through, the knee will buckle. If that occurs, either a remake, increasing the amount of hyperextension, or use of a lock will be required.

Locking the knee on this type of patient should be avoided. The locked knee forces the patient to hike the hip and circumduct the leg, substantially increasing energy expenditure. Finding the correct angle of hyperextension in which to build the orthosis can be challenging. Too little will cause the knee to buckle, while too much will diminish the effectiveness of the device. A simple technique can be used to

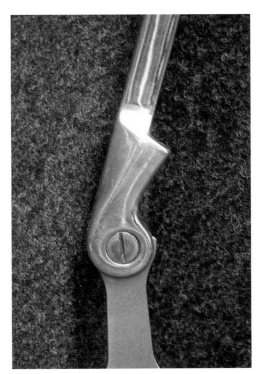

Fig. 32-9 Klenzak joint.

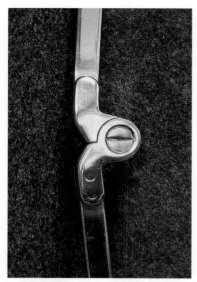

Fig. 32-11 Posterior offset knee joint.

determine the optimal angle. Holding a walker in front of him or her, position the patient with the back and the popliteal fossa of the involved knee against the wall. Assist the patient to slowly move his or her back closer to the wall, forcing the patient to straighten the knee. Simultaneously ask the patient if the knee feels as though it is about to buckle. When the patient reaches the point where he or she feels the knee has become unstable, reverse the movement until the patient feels secure again and note the angle of the knee. If the orthosis is built at this angle plus 5 degrees of additional hyperextension, the patient should have a successful outcome.

Drop (ring) lock The drop lock knee joint is one of the strongest knee locking mechanisms currently available. It is commonly used in the population with postpolio sequelae when lower extremity weakness includes significant weakness of the quadriceps (Fig. 32-12). It is designed to keep the knee locked anytime the patient is standing. When

the leg is pushed into a fully extended position, the rings will drop downward and engage over the joint preventing it from bending. Unlocking the knee requires the patient to fully extend the knee and then pull the rings proximally to disengage the locks. Because some patients have difficulty balancing while bending over to disengage the locks, in the past the medial joint lock in this type of joint occasionally was eliminated to permit easier unlocking of the device. However, this practice is strongly discouraged because too much torque is placed on the single lateral lock and may result in catastrophic failure of the joint or sidebar. A ball retainer can be added to assist the patient in unlocking the knee by holding up one ring while the patient disengages the other. Conversely, the ball retainer can increase the difficulty of the sit-to-stand transition because the patient must bend forward to manually lock both sides.

Bail and lever locks The bail or lever lock is designed to permit simultaneous locking and unlocking of both the medial and lateral knee joints (Fig. 32-13). Its application mirrors that of the ring lock but may be more convenient for the wearer. A proximally directed force will cause the bail to rise and disengage both locks simultaneously. The drawback is that a bail lock can be inadvertently disengaged when bumped, causing a sudden unlocking of the knee and a possible fall. The development of the cable locking mechanism resolves the problem of inadvertent disengagement and enables the simultaneous unlocking and locking of the joints without the danger to the wearer. The cable locking system is preferable in the aging PPS population in which a fall can be quite debilitating. It has the additional advantage of eliminating the need for the wearer to bend forward to unlock the knee joints, a difficult task when poor muscle strength or poor balance exists.

Adjustable flexion and extension ring lock knee joints These joints are designed to accommodate individuals

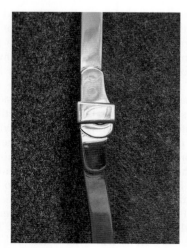

Fig. 32-12 Drop lock knee joint.

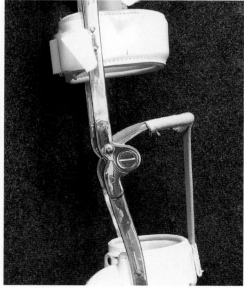

Fig. 32-13 Bail or lever lock.

with knee flexion contractures and can be adjusted to match the flexion angle of the patient's knee (Fig. 32-14). The ring lock then will drop when the desired angle is achieved.

Stance control knee joints Stance control knee joints are designed to provide the patient with a stable knee during stance phase and an automatically free knee during swing (Fig. 32-15). The advantages of this joint over a locked knee are a reduction in hip hiking and circumduction in swing seen in traditional locked knee KAFOs resulting in lower energy consumption.[16,12] The knee joints operate using a variety of mechanisms ranging from electronic switch activation with a microprocessor control to a simple mechanical switch. These knee joints are a good option for polio survivors with unilateral involvement that previously would have required a locking knee. The patient should be relatively contracture free and have the ability and motivation to work through a training period that some have likened to the early training of a patient with a transfemoral prosthesis.

All of the current designs can be used successfully when matched with the appropriate candidate as described by the manufacturer's recommendations. The orthotist must be thoroughly familiar with each manufacturer's specific requirements along with the appropriate training techniques. Careful patient assessment is of utmost importance in the application of this technology. The patient must have both the ability and the willingness to return for follow-up appointments as well as possible physical therapy gait training.

Proximal thigh section designs

Standard thigh section The standard thigh section is useful in the PPS population only when the patient is a limited ambulator or when he or she is wearing a bilateral KAFO (Fig. 32-16). In these cases, the need to transfer body weight

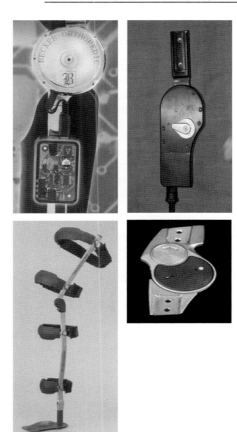

Fig. 32-15 Stance control knee joints.

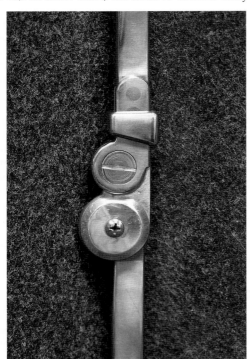

Fig. 32-14 Adjustable flexion and extension ring lock knee joint.

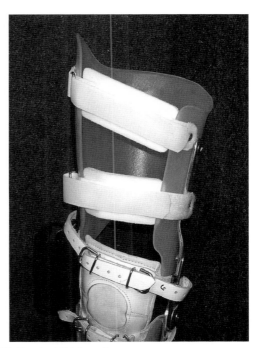

Fig. 32-16 Standard thigh section.

over the involved limb is limited, and this simpler design is quite appropriate.

Quadrilateral and ischial containment thigh sections The quadrilateral or ischial containment thigh section is designed to permit partial transfer of the patient's weight through the KAFO during stance phase (Fig. 32-17). This weight shift, however small, permits the patient to extend the stance side period on the involved side. This brings more effective balance to the patient's gait as the resultant stance period on the contralateral side shortens, thus reducing the stress and strain on the stronger of the patient's legs.

Miscellaneous components

These components can be used in combination with any of the designs described.

Molded inner boot Many different types of orthopedic procedures are performed on the feet and ankles of the pediatric PPS population. For some individuals, these procedures resulted in very bony, deformed feet and ankles. These joints can be difficult to effectively and comfortably control. A polyethylene molded inner boot can be used with good success to overcome the problem of discomfort (Fig. 32-18). This device encompasses the foot and ankle in a soft flexible plastic and then is supported by the rigid foot and ankle section of the orthosis. Its total-contact fit reduces pressure without compromising control.

Metal and leather AFO or KAFO For many polio patients, their first exposure to orthoses during the worldwide polio epidemic consisted of traditional metal and

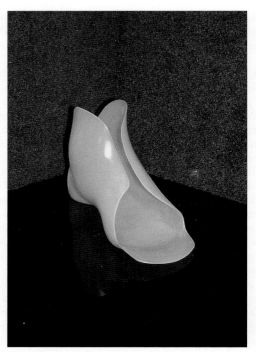

Fig. 32-18 Molded inner boot.

leather AFOs and KAFOs. Although some patients continue to wear these designs because of an unwillingness to try newer designs and materials, others do so because the devices do an effective job of satisfying their functional needs. The primary disadvantage of these designs is the limited contact of the rigid bands with the limb. This limited contact reduces the amount of control possible with the device, particularly in the transverse plane. In addition, it can result in limb deformation within the orthosis. To determine if a new design using newer materials can improve the patient's function or comfort, the clinician must assess the existing device and its appropriateness in light of today's technology.

Other materials Titanium and steel can be substituted for aluminum when increased strength is needed because of the patient's weight or activity level. Laminated and pre-impregnated carbon fiber materials can be substituted for thermoforming plastics to increase strength and stiffness without increasing weight. As in patients with a lower limb paralysis, device weight is very important in the PPS population. Keeping the device as lightweight as possible is of utmost importance. Because of its lighter weight, titanium is preferable to steel when aluminum is not appropriate.

Orthotic management algorithm

Management of the population with postpolio sequelae requires a thorough understanding of the current concepts of the etiology of the disorder. Unlike other types of lower limb paralysis, the patient with postpolio sequelae retains his or her sensation, proprioception, and ability to balance

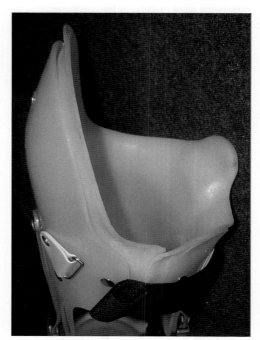

Fig. 32-17 Quadrilateral or ischial containment thigh section.

over the stronger limb.[29] As a result, many patients with post-polio sequelae have developed very complex methods to compensate for limb weakness. By substituting other stronger muscles or abnormally positioning the joints of the limb, they create enough stability to support their body weight for short periods. They minimize the period spent in stance and transfer weight to the stronger of the lower limbs. Consequently, any orthosis that is applied will disrupt the delicate balance that has become second nature to these patients. This must be carefully assessed by the orthotist and given careful consideration when designing the orthosis.

In orthotic management of patients with postpolio sequelae, utilization of orthotic components and designs can be illustrated with some of the most common patient presentations. As these typical presentations are discussed, remember that this patient population presents some unique challenges. Consequently, in addition to a complete and thorough evaluation, careful consideration must be given to the following points.

- Patients who have never worn a brace or who discontinued its use at a young age often consider being brace-free a sign of success and achievement. It signifies that they have "beaten the disease" and require no form of external device for ambulation. Being brace-free was a psychologically significant and important aspect of their recovery. These patients frequently have difficulty accepting that an orthosis now may be necessary.
- Similarly, for patients who have depended on an orthosis for many years and have become accustomed to the device and all of its characteristics, the idea that a new design utilizing newer materials and techniques often is difficult to accept.[31]

In all cases, patients have developed certain gait compensations that result in their ability to continue ambulation in spite of muscle and/or limb weakness. Compensations or adjustments in the normal mechanism of gait have become subconscious and automatic to polio survivors, and the new orthosis will disrupt these compensations.[7] The orthotist must thoroughly understand and assess the impact the new device will have upon the patient's gait, explain in advance the impact to the patient, receive his or her acceptance of it, and prepare the patient for the challenges it may present and the adjustments that it will require. It is necessary to discuss the impact the device will have upon his or her activities of daily living. Depending upon the type of device prescribed and designed, activities such as working the pedals in a car or walking up and down ramps or stairs may require modification. The patient must be made aware of these possibilities in advance if the patient is to accept the orthosis. Ultimately, however, acceptance is dependent upon the team and the orthotist's ability to prescribe, design, and fit a device that the patient perceives to be helpful. If the orthosis assists in some quantifiable way, that is, it relieves pain, improves stability, decreases the incidence of falls, or reduces energy consumption, most likely it will be accepted. The patient then will be willing to make the adjustments necessary to make the orthosis a part of his or her daily routine.

Following is the orthotic management algorithm we use, with general orthotic recommendations for some of the most common presentations. The orthotic recommendations are purposely general, and the specific design and components selected should be based upon the assessment, evaluation, and device characteristics already described.

- Type 1: No previous orthosis wear. Painful joints exist in the lower extremity of one limb, typically the weaker limb, but may affect both limbs. Abnormal body mechanics result in the potential for additional joint damage.

  ○ Goal: Restrict or eliminate painful joint motion.

    ■ Evaluate leg-length discrepancy.

      • Apply appropriate lift up to 80% of the difference in leg lengths.

  ○ Possible Orthotic Solutions

    ■ AFO with appropriate motion control components at the ankle.
    ■ KAFO–drop (ring) lock knee joint design. Indicated when severe quadriceps and/or gluteus maximus weakness is present, no hyperextension exists, and patient complains of knee buckling.
    ■ KAFO–posterior offset knee joint design, no lock. Indicated when knee hyperextension is present. Reduces hyperextension without eliminating stance stability.
    ■ KAFO–stance control knee joint. Indicated when some hip flexor and quadriceps strength exist, and the patient has sufficient balance ability to shift weight.
    ■ Tune orthosis and shoe combination to ensure smooth movement through stance phase rockers.

- Type 2: Discontinued orthosis wear in childhood or adolescence. Stronger leg is becoming fatigued more quickly or becoming painful, or patient is tripping and falling more often.

  ○ Goal: Stabilize weaker side and reduce stress on stronger side.

    ■ Evaluate leg-length discrepancy.
    ■ Apply appropriate lift up to 80% of the difference in leg lengths.

  ○ Possible Orthotic Solutions

    ■ AFO–ground reaction, articulated with dorsiflexion stop, dorsiflexion assist, and plantarflexion stop.
    ■ KAFO–on weaker side with ischial or quadrilateral thigh section, drop (ring) lock, or posterior offset knee joint, depending on the presence of hyperextension and a double action ankle joint that will utilize a spring posteriorly and a pin anteriorly.

      • Consider stance control knee joint when the patient has fair-to-good hip flexors, poor-to-fair quadriceps, and sufficient balance control.

■ Tune orthosis and shoe combination to ensure smooth movement through stance phase rockers.

- Type 2A: Unilateral painful knee with hyperextension greater than 15 degrees.

  ○ Goal: Reduce pain by decreasing hyperextension to less than 15 degrees.

    ■ Evaluate leg-length discrepancy.

      • Apply appropriate lift up to 80% of the difference in leg lengths.

  ○ Possible Orthotic Solutions

    ■ AFO–rarely effective in this type of early stance phase hyperextension.

    ■ KAFO–with posteriorly offset knee joint designed to permit only enough hyperextension to eliminate pain without causing instability, rigid anterior thigh section and posterior leaf spring type ankle, providing swing phase clearance with minimal resistance to tibial advancement.

    ■ Tune orthosis and shoe combination to ensure smooth movement through stance phase rockers.

- Type 3: Long-term unilateral orthosis wearer with painful knee, hip, or sacroiliac joint on the stronger contralateral side.

  ○ Goal: Improve body mechanics in an effort to reduce repetitive stress to the affected joints.

    ■ Shift weight bearing through the orthosis to the weaker side and shorten stance period on the sound side to reduce both Trendelenburg hip movement and the period of weight bearing on the stronger limb.

  ○ Possible Orthotic Solutions

    ■ Evaluate leg-length discrepancy.

      • Apply appropriate lift up to 80% of the difference in leg lengths.

    ■ AFO–ground reaction, articulated with dorsiflexion stop, dorsiflexion assist, and plantarflexion stop.

    ■ KAFO–ischial containment or quadrilateral thigh control and locked knee.

      • Consider stance control knee joint when patient has fair-to-good hip flexors, poor-to-fair quadriceps, and good balance control.

    ■ Tune orthosis and shoe combination to ensure smooth movement through stance phase rockers.

- Type 3A: Painful knee on stronger side secondary to overuse syndrome, with grade three or higher muscle strength above and below the knee and a contralateral limb that is significantly weaker.

  ○ Goal: Stabilize the affected knee through stance.

    ■ This is the limb the patient primarily depends upon through stance, and the orthotist should reduce movement only enough to reduce pain.

■ Evaluate leg-length discrepancy.

  • Apply appropriate lift up to 80% of the difference in leg lengths.

■ AFO–ground reaction design with dorsiflexion stop, dorsiflexion assist, and plantarflexion stop.

■ KAFO–with ischial containment or quadrilateral thigh section, drop (ring) lock knee joints.

■ KAFO–stance control knee joints and double action ankle joints with springs in the posterior channel and pins in the anterior channel.

■ Tune orthosis and shoe combination to ensure smooth movement through stance phase rockers.

- Type 4: Long-term bilateral orthosis wearer. Possible painful joints within or above orthosis, labored gait with increased tripping and falls, and increased fatigue, pressure, and/or pain from the orthosis itself.

  ○ Goal: Reduce or eliminate pain or discomfort within the orthosis and/or the joints above it.

    ■ Evaluate leg-length discrepancy.

      • Apply appropriate lift up to 80% of the difference in leg lengths.

    ■ Evaluate current orthoses.

      • Suggest improved design where deficiencies in function, components, weight, and/or cosmesis exist.

      • Recommend more aggressive bracing when appropriate.

      • Tune orthosis and shoe combination to ensure smooth movement through stance phase rockers.

This orthotic management algorithm is depicted as a flow chart in Fig. 32-19.

These recommendations are intended to be broad. Management of contractures and complicated foot deformities can require special attention as outlined. The specifics of each patient and his or her presentation and clinical signs ultimately will determine the optimal orthotic design. Provision of the orthotic device must include "tuning" of the orthosis and shoe combination. The angle at which the ankle is set may require modification of the shoe to permit a smooth movement through stance. Often a rocker sole, rocker heel, or both can be used to achieve this goal. The rocker heel will smooth out the transition from initial contact to loading response while the rocker sole will permit a smoother transition from midstance to toe-off.

The patient must be trained on the use of the device. In nearly all patients with postpolio sequelae, the goal is to shift the patient's weight over the orthosis, normalize stance phase mechanics, and reduce the asymmetry between the stance period from side to side. Additional training with a physical therapist may be necessary, especially when the patient has difficulty accommodating the changes in gait pattern due to fear or not trusting the device, learning how to address uneven terrain, or utilizing the stance control knee joint feature to its fullest extent.

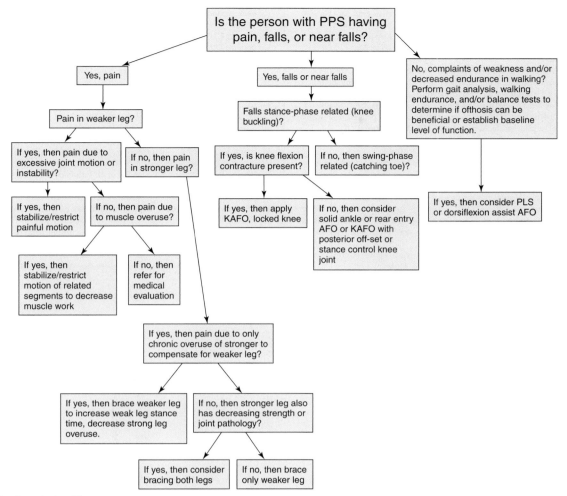

Fig. 32-19 Treatment algorithm.

References

1. Al-Turaiki, Mohammed HS: Poliomyelitis and orthotic management at Riyadh Medical Rehabilitation Centre: a retrospective study, *Journal of Orthotics and Prosthetics* 1:76–81, 1989.
2. Anderson E: The axial loading on a static knee-ankle-foot orthosis, *Journal Med Eng Technol* 1:100–102, 1977.
3. Bodian D: Virus and host factors determining the nature and severity of lesions and of clinical manifestations: Poliomyelitis, Proceedings of the 2nd International Poliomyelitis Conference, Philadelphia, 1952, Lippincott.
4. Brehm M, Nollet F, Harlaar J: Energy demands of walking in persons with postpoliomyelitis syndrome: relationship with muscle strength and reproducibility, *Arch Phys Med Rehabil* 87:136–140, 2006.
5. Bruno RL: *The polio paradox: what you need to know*, New York, 2002, Warner Books.
6. Carriere M: Des amytrophies spinales secondaire: contribution a l'etude de la diffusion des lesions irritaves du syteme nerveu, *These de Montpeleliere*, France, 1875.
7. Clark DR, Perry J, Lunsford TR: Case studies—orthotic management of the adult post polio patient, *Orthot Prosthet* 1:43–50, 1986.
8. Cornil V, Lepine R: Sur un cas de paralysie generale spinale anterieure subaige, suivi d'autopsie, *Gaz Med Paris* 4:127–129, 1875.
9. Ernstoff B, Wetterqvist H, Kvist H, Grimby G: Endurance training effect on individuals with postpoliomyelitis, *Arch Phys Med Rehabil* 77:843–848, 1996.
10. Fishbein M, Salmonsen EM, Hektoen L: *A bibliography of infantile paralysis, 1789–1949, with selected abstracts and annotations*, Philadelphia, 1951, Lippincott.
11. Harrington ED, Lin RS, Gage JR: Use of the anterior floor reaction orthosis in patients with cerebral palsy, *Orthot Prosthet* 4:34–42, 1984.
12. Hebert JS, Liggins AB: Gait evaluation of an automatic stance-control knee orthosis in a patient with postpoliomyelitis, *Arch Phys Med Rehabil* 86:1676–1680, 2005.
13. Heim M, Yaacobi E, Azaria M: A pilot study to determine the efficiency of lightweight carbon fibre orthoses in the management of patients suffering from post-poliomyelitis syndrome, *Clin Rehabil* 11:302–305, 1997.
14. Hislop HF, Montgomery J: *Daniels and Worthingham's muscle testing: techniques of manual examination*, ed 2, Philadelphia, 2002, WB Saunders.
15. Hurmuzlu Y, Basdogan C, Stoianovici D: Kinematics and dynamic stability of the locomotion of post-polio patients, *J Biomed Eng* 118:405–411, 1996.
16. Irby SE, Bernhardt KA, Kaufman KR: Gait of stance control orthosis users: the dynamic knee brace system.
17. Jerrell ML: Stance control orthoses: revolutionizing patient care, *O P Business News* 12:24–32, 2003.
18. Kelley C, DiBello T: Retrospective chart review of orthoses worn or prescribed for individuals with post-polio syndrome. Preliminary unpublished findings, Texas Woman's University, 2006.
19. Klein MG, Whyte J, Esquenazi A, et al: A comparison of the effects of exercise and lifestyle modification on the resolution of overuse symptoms of

the shoulder in polio survivors: a preliminary study, *Arch Phys Med Rehabil* 83:708–713, 2002.

20. Kriz JL, Jones DR, Speier JL, et al: Cardiorespiratory responses to upper extremity aerobic training by postpolio subjects, *Arch Phys Med Rehabil* 73:49–54, 1992.

21. Lin RS: Ankle foot orthoses. In Lusardi M, Nielsen C, editors: *Orthotics and prosthetics in rehabilitation*, Woburn, Mass, 2000, Butterworth-Heinemann.

22. Lin RS, Moore TJ: Orthoses for postpolio syndrome. In Goldberg B, Hsu J, editors: *Atlas of orthoses and assistive devices*, ed 2, St. Louis, 1997, Mosby.

23. McMillan AG, Kendrick K, Zabel R, et al: Stance control orthosis to improve functional gait: a pilot study, *Neurol Rep* 26:209, 2002(abstract).

24. Michael J: Lower limb orthoses. In Goldberg B, Hsu J, editors: *Atlas of orthoses and assistive devices*, ed 2, St. Louis, 1997, Mosby.

25. Nolet F, Beelen A, Prins MH, et al: Disability and functional assessment in former polio patients with and without postpolio syndrome, *Arch Phys Med Rehabil* 80:136–243, 1999.

26. Perry J: *Gait analysis-Normal and pathological function*, Thorofare, NJ, 1992, Slack Incorporated.

27. Perry J, Mulroy SJ, Renwick SE: The relationship of lower extremity gait and strength parameters in patients with post-polio syndrome, *Arch Phys Med Rehabil* 74:164–169, 1993.

28. Perry J: Normal and pathological gait. In Goldberg B, Hsu J, editors: *Atlas of orthoses and assistive devices*, ed 2, St. Louis, 1997, Mosby.

29. Phillipi AF, Leffler CT, Leffler SG, et al: Glucosamine, chondroitin, and manganese ascorbate for degenerative joint disease of the knee and low back: a randomized, double blind, placebo-controlled pilot study, *Mil Med* 164:85–91, 1999.

30. Prithan C, Craik R, Cook T: Orthotic management of the late postpolio patient, *Orthot Prosthet* 1:50–59, 1979.

31. Rida A: A dissertation from the early eighteenth century, probably the first description of poliomyelitis, *J Bone Joint Surg Br* 44-B(3):735–740, 1962.

32. Sarno A, Lehneis HR: Prescription considerations for plastic below-knee orthoses, *Arch Phys Med Rehab* 11:503–510, 1971.

33. Sarno JE, Lehneis HR: Prescription considerations for plastic below-knee orthoses, *Arch Phys Med Rehab* 11:503–510, 1971.

34. Silver JK: *Post-polio syndrome: a guide for polio survivors and their families*, New Haven, Conn, 2001, Yale University.

35. Smith LK, Kelley C: The postpolio syndrome. In Umphred DA, editor: *Neurological rehabilitation*, ed 4, St. Louis, 2001, Mosby.

36. Waring WP, Maynard F, Grady W, et al: Influence of appropriate lower extremity orthotic management on ambulation, pain, and fatigue in a post polio population, *Arch Phys Med Rehabil* 70:371–375, 1989.

37. Williams KA, Petronis J, Smith D, et al: Effect of Iyengar yoga therapy for chronic low back pain, *Pain* 115:107–117, 2005.

38. Witt DC, Brinkhaus B, Jena S, et al: Acupuncture in patients with osteoarthritis of the knee: a randomized trial, *Lancet* 366:136–143, 2005.

39. Young GR: Energy conservation. In Halstead LS, editor: *Managing post-polio: a guide to living well with post-polio syndrome*, Washington, DC, 1998, NRH Press.

Chapter

33

Lower limb orthoses for persons who have had a stroke

Elizabeth Condie and Robert James Bowers

Key Points

- All orthotic intervention must be based on clearly identified objectives.
- The most useful type of lower limb orthosis in stroke rehabilitation is the ankle–foot orthosis (AFO)
- Control of stance phase is an important function of an AFO.
- The maximum angle of dorsiflexion of the AFO is limited by the length of the gastrocnemius.
- Articulated AFOs are only appropriate when gastrocnemius length and ankle range of motion are adequate.
- The angle of tibial inclination in the AFO is critical for control of knee hyperextension and second rocker.
- Early use of AFOs as a therapeutic aid to stroke rehabilitation should be considered.

Stroke: "A clinical syndrome (a collection of symptoms and signs) of focal (or global) disturbance of cerebral function, lasting no more than 24 hours or leading to death, with no apparent cause other than of vascular origin."

This definition, published by Aho et al.[2] on behalf of the World Health Organization (WHO), is the broadly accepted standard definition of stroke. The definition is generally considered to include all cases of cerebral infarction, primary intracerebral hemorrhage, and subarachnoid hemorrhage.[39] A stroke may also involve the cerebellum and/or brain stem.

Pathophysiology

Pathological type

Intracerebral hemorrhage and cerebral infarction are the two major pathological types of stroke, with cerebral infarction leading to 81% of strokes.[5] The third acute cerebrovascular disease, subarachnoid hemorrhage, may or may not result in a clinical stroke.

Although the pathological type of stroke is of clinical significance and influences immediate medical management, it is only a crude predictor of disability and handicap, which are important determinants of medium- and long-term health care needs.[24]

The system of classification of stroke used in the Oxfordshire Community Stroke Project is widely used (Table 33-1).[5]

Epidemiology

Many authors have commented on the difficulty of obtaining accurate data on the mortality rate, incidence, and prevalence of stroke.[7,39,40] However, according to WHO estimates, 15 million people suffer strokes each year, and five million are left permanently disabled.[3] An estimated 5.5 million deaths from stroke occurred worldwide in 2002, of which approximately 20% to 25% occurred within the first month of stroke and 30% to 40% within the first year.[30]

Wide geographic and age-related variations are noted, with stroke predominantly a disease of the elderly. Overall prevalence rate is 6 to 8 per 1,000 persons; however, the rate rises to 40 to 70 per 1,000 persons 65 years and older.[16]

A consequence of age-related prevalence coupled with the fact that most populations are aging is that the *number* of stroke survivors will increase even if the incidence does not.[43]

The cost of stroke is enormous. The American Heart Association estimated that for 2003 in the United States alone, the total cost, including nursing home bills, was $59 billion US.[4]

Table 33-1 Oxfordshire community stroke project classification of subtypes of cerebral infarction[5]

Lacunar infarct (LACI)	Pure motor stroke, pure sensory stroke, sensorimotor stroke, or ataxic hemiparesis
Total anterior circulation infarct (TACI)	Combination of new higher cerebral dysfunction (e.g., dysphasia), homonymous visual field defect, and ipsilateral motor and/or sensory deficit of at least two areas (out of face, arm, and leg)
Partial anterior circulation infarct (PACI)	Only two of the three components of a TACI, or with higher cerebral dysfunction alone, or with a motor/sensory deficit more restricted than those classified as LACI (e.g., confined to one limb)
Posterior circulation infarct (POCI)	Any of ipsilateral cranial nerve palsy with contralateral motor and/or sensory deficit, bilateral motor and/or sensory deficit, disorder of conjugate eye movement, cerebellar dysfunction, or isolated homonymous visual field defect

Clinical features

Some commonly encountered features of stroke are as follows:

1. Changes in resting tone (increase *or* decrease)
2. Spasticity
3. Weakness or paralysis
4. Postural deficit
5. Loss of proprioception
6. Sensory deficit
7. Neglect
8. Cognitive, emotional, intellectual impairment

The first five clinical features, often in combination with one or all of the others, lead to loss of coordinated patterns of movement. This, in turn, leads to considerable difficulty with walking, loss of independent mobility, and significant reduction in functional ability.

Historical perspective

Historically, the rehabilitation community has been resistant to the use of orthoses in the treatment of persons who have suffered a stroke. This has been particularly true among therapy professionals who have been trained in certain neurological and neurodevelopmental approaches and believe that use of orthoses will in some way interfere with normal physiological recovery of patients. There now is growing acceptance of the use of orthoses, both for the lower and the upper limb, as an adjunct to therapy.

In situations where orthoses *have* been used, all too commonly they were considered at a late stage in the rehabilitation process, almost as a last resort. However, this also is changing with recognition of the benefits of early intervention. Orthoses used in the past were constructed from metal and leather and often poorly designed from a biomechanical point of view. Current good orthotic practice dictates that custom-fabricated plastic orthoses best meet the needs of patients and that traditional metal and leather designs should be consigned to history.

Key issues of today

- What is the optimal timing of orthotic intervention?
- What are the benefits of early use of orthoses?
- How can the practice of health care professionals around the world be influenced to include routine consideration of selective use of orthoses for patients with stroke?

Current research

In 2003 the International Society for Prosthetics and Orthotics (ISPO) commissioned a systematic review of current research activity in orthotics in preparation for an international consensus conference on the orthotic management of stroke patients. A report of the conference, including recommendations, was published in 2004.[13] In this review, Morris[27] concluded that "despite technological development, on the whole there remains a dearth of unbiased clinical research regarding the effectiveness of orthotic intervention for stroke with most studies reporting small numbers of subjects, short follow-up periods and often lacking an adequate control for comparison. The poor methodological basis for much of the clinical evidence leaves us prone to errors in interpretation. . . ."

Findings of the conference agreed that, according to the grading system proposed by Shekelle et al.,[37] weak evidence at level C (cross-sectional surveys or case reports) supported the beneficial effects of ankle–foot orthoses (AFOs) on the energy cost of gait, walking speed and cadence, step length, gait symmetry, weight bearing through the affected leg, control of equinus and varus, and hyperextension of the knee. No evidence supporting the view that AFOs could improve spasticity was found.[8]

In a 2004 systematic review of physiotherapy (physical therapy) and functional outcomes after stroke, Van Peppen et al.[42] found that there was "no or insufficient evidence in terms of functional outcomes for (the use of) orthotics and assistive devices."

The consensus conference sought to address these clear deficiencies in research evidence by including recommendations for research in its published report (Table 33-2). This conference also expressed concern at the inconsistent terminology used both within and between professional groups.

Table 33-2 Recommendations for research in orthotics

Agree on standard terminology and definitions
Clearly define biomechanical design, materials, and components
Perform well-controlled, multidisciplinary, multicenter research
Use "good practice points" in consensus conference report as basis for priority research

Adapted from Condie E, Campbell J, Martina J: Report of a consensus conference on the orthotic management of stroke patients, Copenhagen, 2004, ISPO.

It held the view that unless and until an agreed *"lexicon"* of terms was developed and implemented internationally, then establishing large-scale, multicenter trials would be difficult.

Treatment recommendations

Functional deficit/biomechanical deficit

Regardless of the causes and precise pathology of stroke, detailed analysis of the biomechanical and functional effects on the patient is essential to the planning of appropriate treatment strategies.

Specifically, for the lower limb and trunk, knowledge of the kinetics and kinematics of normal gait will allow the clinician to identify abnormal patterns (or components) of stroke gait and motion (see Chapter 22).

Commonly, the justification for prescribing an AFO is to address the problem of a "dropped foot." However, this group of patients faces many more significant challenges to mobility than simple swing phase equinus. Although it is true that in the early stages of recovery after stroke the foot and ankle often are flaccid, leading to difficulty clearing the toes during swing phase, the picture commonly changes over time to one in which the foot and ankle adopt a more typical position of persistent plantarflexion and supination. Many of the most significant gait problems facing stroke survivors occur in the stance phase of gait and are related to the abnormal biomechanical situation.

Although the population of stroke survivors is not homogeneous, a number of commonly encountered gait problems can be identified. Hemiparetic gait can be characterized as slow and stiff, with a reduction in both cadence and step length.[34] Poor coordination of movement leads to primary and compensatory gait deviations and a considerable increase in energy cost.[23]

Hemiparetic gait is markedly asymmetrical, with the step length of the affected limb greater than that of the unaffected side, while the duration of stance is shorter and that of swing longer on the affected side. This situation is associated with difficulty in bearing weight through the affected limb.[29,35] Initial contact of the foot on the ground typically occurs with the lateral forefoot because of tone-induced equinovarus deformity. Persistence of supination throughout stance affects both ankle stability and balance. Knee hyperextension in mid to late stance is common, and tibial progression in second rocker is impeded by the abnormally plantarflexed position of the foot. In swing, hip and knee flexion and ankle dorsiflexion are reduced or absent, with hip circumduction used to aid ground clearance.[33]

Further complications of hemiparetic gait arise due to abnormal alignment of the ground reaction force (GRF) relative to the joints of the lower limb, leading to altered moments and increasing the demand on a damaged neuromuscular system. Any treatment that can achieve realignment of the GRF and reduce this demand likely will improve mobility and function. In addition to realigning the joints to correct deformity, realignment of the GRF is fundamental to orthotic management.

Principles of assessment

Effective treatment of stroke depends on accurate assessment of deficits, knowledge of the range of treatments available, and setting realistic objectives or goals with involvement of the patient, family, and caregivers. The assessment process, at its optimum, is interdisciplinary in nature should include consideration of balance and posture and passive range of motion of the joints. However, muscle length and the effects of tone and spasticity are of equal, and arguably more, importance.

For example, gastrocnemius shortening is commonly encountered following stroke.[28,38,41] As a result of the shortening, passive range of dorsiflexion in the affected leg is greater when the knee joint is flexed than when the knee is extended. Failure to consider this condition when providing an orthosis may lead to a situation in which the foot is dorsiflexed to a position that is inconsistent with the length of the gastrocnemius. The result of this inappropriate dorsiflexion may be prevention of full knee extension in terminal stance and, consequently, persistence of an external hip flexion moment at this important stage of gait (see Chapter 22). The maximum desirable angle of dorsiflexion in the orthosis is dictated by the length of the gastrocnemius.

The team with responsibility for assessment must be experienced and skilled in observational gait analysis. More sophisticated instrumented gait analysis systems can be used according to local availability and are a prerequisite for surgical procedures.[20]

Setting objectives

When considering any orthotic intervention after a stroke, the prescription of an orthosis should be based upon clearly defined objectives. One objective may be to assist the therapist in the rehabilitation of the patient, with the orthosis acting as an "extra pair of hands" to improve postural alignment.

Some objectives may be highly specific, such as improving swing phase ground clearance, stance phase weight bearing, and stability, or controlling or preventing deformity, such as equinovarus at the foot and ankle or hyperextension at the knee. Objectives can be established only after thorough physical and neurological assessment, gait analysis, and identification of biomechanical deficits.

Orthotic management alone will not successfully address all problems. For example, a patient with an equinovarus deformity at the foot and ankle and weak knee extensors may also present with a flexion contracture at the hip, which contributes to an external flexion moment at this joint. The provision of an AFO to control foot, ankle, and knee problems may be the ideal orthotic solution; however, physiotherapy to increase hip extension range *prior* to orthotic fitting almost certainly would optimize the function of the orthosis. Similarly, medication that can modify muscle tone or reduce hyperreflexia may be beneficial in improving limb kinematics.

In summary, a combination of several treatment modalities may be appropriate, and these modalities may change as the patient's condition changes. It follows that assessment and objective setting should not be one-off events. Rather, they should be viewed as a continuous process with regular opportunities to modify and revise goals.

It is beyond the scope of this chapter to provide details of the therapeutic effects of functional or therapeutic electrical stimulation or the indications for pharmacological or surgical treatment; however, a brief description of physiotherapy treatment is given here.

Physiotherapy

Physiotherapy (also known as *physical therapy*) is often perceived as one of the key disciplines in organized stroke care.[22] Traditionally, techniques or treatments based on neurological or neurodevelopmental approaches, such as Bobath (prevention of abnormal movements, facilitation of normal movement)[6] and Brunnstromm (use of abnormal synergies, incorporating them into functional activities), were used.[10] Other techniques that gained a following included motor relearning,[12] proprioceptive neuromuscular facilitation (PNF),[21] and conductive education.[14]

These, and many other techniques, have been used for many years with the broad aims of improving or restoring motor control, walking ability, activities of daily living, and social functioning.

Despite the widespread use of such interventions, a study in the United Kingdom found that treatment selection all too often was determined by clinicians' experience working with patients rather than by basic training, theory, or findings reported in the literature.[15] High-quality research into the effectiveness of these interventions has been slow to emerge. A systematic review on the "impact of physical therapy on functional outcomes after stroke" concluded that no or insufficient evidence for functional outcome with many of the therapeutic techniques was found. However, evidence was found with task-oriented exercise training, particularly when applied intensively and early after stroke.[42]

Some therapists and physicians have used orthoses in the management of stroke patients, sometimes providing the device themselves, at other times obtaining them from an orthotist. This use of orthoses for both the upper and lower limbs has been recognized as a treatment option for many years; however, there is widespread variation in the nature of orthotic intervention, not just between countries but also between centers at a local level.

In particular, there is no agreed upon "best practice" in terms of selection of patients suitable for orthotic fitting, orthotic design, and timing of orthotic intervention. Evidence regarding these issues is lacking in the scientific literature, and few high-quality studies have measured the effectiveness of orthoses. This acknowledged lack of evidence led in 2003 to the organization of the international consensus conference on the orthotic management of stroke patients. The unanimous conclusion of the expert group of participants (45 professionals from 15 countries) was that "the use of orthoses, both for the lower and upper limb *should* be considered in the management of patients with stroke."

Orthotic management

The decision about which orthosis to use in any given circumstance is confusing to many clinicians. The range of available options is extensive, and some of the published research is unclear, providing inadequate details about the design characteristics of the orthosis being studied. Such poor information prevents the reader from drawing adequate conclusions and does not inform confident decision-making. Some of the available literature reports on research into orthoses that have been inappropriately prescribed or poorly fitted.

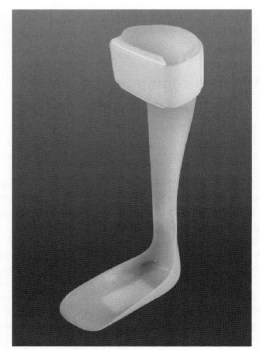

Fig. 33-1 Posterior leaf spring AFO.

Other studies use well-designed orthoses, but the studies are methodologically flawed.[27]

Prefabricated orthoses

A range of proprietary (off-the-shelf) orthoses is available, including a variety of "ankle braces." However, these devices are only effective in providing control in the coronal plane.[1,11] Some prefabricated plastic AFOs are available but are of limited value. They should be used only as temporary evaluation devices or in cases requiring early mobilization before a custom orthosis can be provided.[13]

Many prefabricated AFOs are made in the style of a posterior leaf spring (PLS). This orthosis has highly specific prescription criteria (Fig. 33-1): isolated weakness of the dorsiflexor muscles, no significant problem of tone or spasticity, no significant mediolateral subtalar joint instability, and no requirement for orthotic influence on the knee and/or hip.[13] These very specific prescription criteria exclude many stroke patients, who have increased tone, knee hyperextension, hip flexion and retraction, and supination deformity of the foot.

Clearly, care must be taken when using any prefabricated orthosis as an evaluation tool because its function may be markedly different from that of a custom-fabricated AFO. Use of a readily available but biomechanically inappropriate evaluation orthosis may easily mislead the clinician to draw the conclusion that orthotic treatment is of little or no value, when a biomechanically appropriate orthosis of an alternative design could be extremely useful.

Custom-fabricated AFOs

A trained orthotist should be responsible for the design and fitting of a custom-fabricated AFO based on thorough assessment of the biomechanical deficit and clearly identified

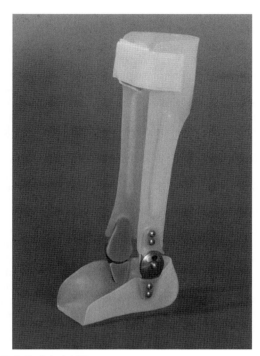

Fig. 33-2 Articulated AFO.

functional goals. Some AFOs have mechanical ankle joints that allow or assist motion in one direction while preventing or limiting motion in another (Fig. 33-2). Others rely on the characteristics of the plastic to create the desired degree of flexibility or rigidity to achieve control.

Control of the foot and ankle

The most commonly encountered deformity at the ankle–foot complex is equinus with varus (supination), although excessive uncontrolled dorsiflexion and valgus (pronation) also can be seen.

Equinus control

Following a stroke, foot equinus can cause problems either in swing phase alone or in both swing and stance. The orthotic solutions to foot equinus are as different as the problems caused.

Equinus associated with low tone

Flaccid paralysis of the dorsiflexors, in the absence of any significant increase in plantarflexor tone, results in a dropped foot that is a problem only in swing phase. This leads to difficulty clearing the ground with the affected leg, with adoption of compensatory strategies such as vaulting or circumduction. Initial contact of the foot on the ground will be made with the forefoot, with foot-flat occurring as the foot is dorsiflexed by body weight. Orthotically, this situation can be easily managed with a PLS orthosis (Fig. 33-1). An alternative is an articulated AFO in which the mechanical ankle joint either acts as a plantarflexion-resisting spring or incorporates a stop, blocking plantarflexion at an appropriate angle (typically 90 degrees). Alternatively, the flexibility of the plastic PLS orthosis is controlled by adjusting the trim line at the ankle to provide adequate resistance

to plantarflexion. Allowing plantarflexion to occur in a controlled fashion, rather than blocking it completely, is beneficial in reestablishing first rocker but may be inappropriate in the presence of knee hyperextension, as indirect orthotic control of recurvatum using an AFO relies on prevention of stance phase plantarflexion.

Equinus associated with high tone

More common than the flaccid dropped foot is equinus associated with a significant increase in plantarflexor tone, leading to difficulties not only in swing but also in stance. Once again, initial contact is made with the forefoot, but in this case, rather than the foot dorsiflexing under body weight to achieve full plantar surface contact with the ground, the foot remains plantarflexed and is able to make full contact only at the expense of persistent knee extension, or hyperextension, which can be regarded as a secondary, acquired deformity.

Hypertonic equinus control using articulated AFO

In this case, the foot clearly requires a greater degree of equinus control from the orthosis. Many clinicians will be tempted to use an orthosis with an ankle joint that stops, rather than resists, plantarflexion. However, this type of joint, which is designed to allow dorsiflexion, can be inappropriate in the case of plantarflexor shortening, whether true or dynamic.[18] Free-dorsiflexion ankle joints are of benefit only in the presence of adequate dorsiflexion range, more specifically gastrocnemius length. No evidence in the literature indicates that gastrocnemius length can be increased by allowing free dorsiflexion in an orthosis. The only way this dorsiflexion can occur in the presence of a short gastrocnemius is for the knee to go into early and excessive stance phase flexion. If a treatment objective is passive stretch of the gastrocnemius, a better strategy is to utilize extension of the knee in late stance. In this case, the orthosis should be designed to block dorsiflexion.

Hypertonic equinus control using one-piece plastic AFO

A better alternative to an articulated AFO with plantarflexion stop is a one-piece plastic AFO with sufficient stiffness to overcome the high plantarflexion moment caused by the hypertonus. Adequate stiffness can be ensured by selecting a suitably stiff plastic, such as homopolymer polypropylene, with anterior trim lines, perhaps incorporating reinforcements of carbon composite material. An ankle strap almost certainly will be required to maintain the position of the foot in the orthosis. Extending the sole of the orthosis to the end of the toes is recommended in the presence of tonic toe flexion reflex. Any plantarflexion contracture can be accommodated by wedging the orthosis under the heel to achieve an appropriate anterior inclination of the tibia so that stance phase progression is not impeded and knee hyperextension is controlled (Fig. 33-3).

Dorsiflexion control

Paralysis of the plantarflexors can lead to uncontrolled and excessive dorsiflexion in late stance and, in the presence of quadriceps weakness, may contribute to knee instability. The orthotic requirement is to block dorsiflexion (or, more accurately, tibial progression) at an appropriate angle. This can be achieved by either using ankle joints with a dorsiflexion stop or constructing a one-piece plastic AFO that is rigid enough to

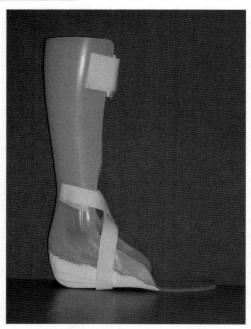

Fig. 33-3 One-piece plastic AFO with ankle strap, full-length sole piece, and accommodation for plantarflexion contracture

counter the considerable dorsiflexion moment in late stance. Material choice and thickness are critical factors, and a stiff plastic such as homopolymer polypropylene, perhaps reinforced with carbon composite inserts, will be suitable. Alternatively, an orthosis entirely constructed from carbon composite can be used (Fig. 33-4).

Supination (varus) control

Traditionally, orthotic control of the varus (supinated) foot has been attempted using a metal and leather AFO

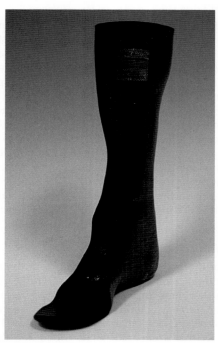

Fig. 33-4 Carbon fiber AFO.

with a T-strap stitched to the lateral side of the shoe and fastened around the medial upright of the orthosis. However, hindfoot supination is a complex triplanar deformity that commonly presents in conjunction with triplanar deformity at the midtarsal joint. Attempting to control such complex triplanar deformities in this way is simplistic and only partially effective at best as the foot commonly distorts within the shoe. A close-fitting plastic AFO that applies the appropriate corrective forces to control both the subtalar joint and the midtarsal joint is required. Inclusion of ankle joints in an orthosis may be detrimental to the intimacy of fit such that control of moderate-to-severe varus is compromised; therefore, ankle joints are not recommended in this situation.

Pronation (valgus) control

Orthotic control of the valgus (pronated) foot traditionally has been addressed using a conventional metal and leather AFO with a medially attached T-strap tightened around the lateral upright of the orthosis. This is a simplistic and inadequate approach to the management of complex triplanar deformity of the subtalar and midtarsal joints. A close-fitting plastic AFO that applies the appropriate corrective forces likely will be more successful.

Control of the knee

Knee hyperextension control

Knee hyperextension following stroke is common and should not be ignored.[13] The problem can be addressed orthotically in a variety of ways. The most obvious solution is use of an orthosis that structurally bridges the joint, such as a knee orthosis or knee–ankle–foot orthosis (KAFO).

Knee orthoses are rarely of value in this patient population because knee instability typically coexists with deformity or instability at the foot and ankle and requires concurrent treatment.

A KAFO may be a better option because it can address simultaneously the problems of the knee and the ankle–foot. If a KAFO is to be used, locking the knee joints may not be necessary, with reliance instead on the inherent limitation in their extension range (typically 180 degrees). This will be appropriate only in patients with sufficient quadriceps strength to stabilize the knee against unwanted flexion.

Indirect control of knee hyperextension

Even significant knee hyperextension can be satisfactorily controlled using an AFO that prevents plantarflexion in stance. A number of authors have reported on the importance of the angle of dorsiflexion in the orthosis if knee hyperextension is to be controlled. Lehmann et al.[23] successfully used a metal solid AFO set in 5 degrees of dorsiflexion. Miyazaki et al.[26] found that a dorsiflexion angle of 7 degrees ensured good results, whereas Oshawa et al.[31] recommended 10 degrees. From the evidence in the literature, it appears that some angle of dorsiflexion is necessary to normalize the external moment about the knee, the essential element in the control of recurvatum. However, this is an oversimplification. It is the angle of inclination of the tibia relative to the ground in stance that is the important factor, rather than the angle of dorsiflexion per se.[32] If the AFO must be made in plantarflexion because of a contracture, the appropriate angle of tibial inclination still can be achieved by varying the heel height of the footwear or by using heel wedges.

Knee flexion control

Uncontrolled knee flexion due to weakness of the quadriceps, the plantarflexors, or a combination of the two clearly places the patient at considerable risk for falling. For more severely affected patients, a KAFO may be the best and safest device for transfer or ambulation. A KAFO also may be helpful in the early stages of rehabilitation, improving postural alignment and enabling better weight bearing through the affected limb. Reduction of the KAFO prescription to an AFO may be possible after reassessment of the patient's requirements.[19]

One of the main reservations about the use of KAFOs in the stroke population has been the need to lock the mechanical knee joint in order to provide knee stability, with the consequent increase in the energy cost of walking. Recent improvements in orthotic knee joint design have resulted in the development of a range of joints that are locked in stance phase but unlocked in swing, similar to some prosthetic knee mechanisms. These innovations may lead to improvements in gait efficiency, but evidence is not yet available.

Indirect control of knee flexion

An AFO can provide indirect control of knee flexion. In this case, the requirement is to block dorsiflexion and thereby manipulate the GRF such that it passes in front of the knee center, creating an extension moment at the critical stage of stance. This principle was used in the design of the floor reaction orthosis (FRO), an AFO whose primary objective is control of knee flexion by virtue of preventing ankle dorsiflexion, but it applies equally to any AFO used for this purpose. The angle at which dorsiflexion is blocked is critical and over the years has proved somewhat controversial. Although the original FRO design stipulated that the ankle must be held in a position of plantarflexion, this alignment causes difficulty with tibial progression in stance phase.[36] Glancy and Lindseth[17] concluded that the best gait pattern is achieved when the ankle is held in 5 degrees of dorsiflexion. Ultimately, the alignment of the ankle joint is of considerable importance and is best determined for each patient individually. Double-adjustable metal ankle joints can be incorporated into the orthosis to allow for "fine-tuning" of ankle alignment. Optimization of third rocker by footwear modification, such as the addition of a rocker sole, can facilitate switching of the ground reaction vector from extension to flexion in preswing.

Knee valgus and varus

Valgus and varus instability of the knee are not commonly seen in stroke patients but may be present as a preexisting deformity. If encountered, the orthotic solution likely is a KAFO rather than a knee orthosis because of the likelihood of coexisting ankle–foot deformity.

Control of the hip

Hip flexion/retraction

Direct control of the hip using either a hip orthosis or a hip–knee–ankle–foot orthosis is impractical in the stroke population, and in our experience these devices are never used.

A more pragmatic approach to the commonly encountered problems of flexion and retraction may be use of an AFO to control the sagittal plane alignment of the ankle, thereby manipulating the GRF and modifying its relationship with the hip. Following stroke, the GRF typically is aligned far anterior to the hip joint, contributing to the abnormal position and kinematics of the joint. Evidence is lacking on the use of an AFO to influence the hip joint in this way in the stroke population, although a paper presented at the ISPO World Congress in Hong Kong in 2004 provided some supporting data from early research results.[9] It seems reasonable to assume that evidence of this effect on the orthotic management of cerebral palsy reported in the literature may be extrapolated to stroke patients.[25]

Best practice

The ISPO Consensus Conference on Orthotic Management of Stroke Patients[13] agreed upon the following "best practice" points and, where appropriate, allocated a grade of recommendation (A, B, C, or *) according to the system proposed by Shekelle et al.[37]

	Grade of Recommendation
Indications for nonarticulated AFO	
Poor balance, instability in stance	*
Inability to transfer weight onto affected leg in stance	C
Moderate-to-severe foot abnormality; equinus valgus or varus, or combination	C
Moderate-to-severe hypertonicity	*
As above, but with mild recurvatum or instability of the knee	C
To improve walking speed and cadence	C
Indications for articulated AFO	
Dorsiflexor weakness only	*
In presence of passive or active range of dorsiflexion	*
To control knee flexion instability only, articulated AFO with dorsiflexion stop	*
To control recurvatum only, articulated AFO with plantarflexion stop	*
To improve walking speed and cadence	B
Indications for posterior leaf spring AFO	
Isolated dorsiflexor weakness	*
No significant problem with tone	*
No significant mediolateral instability	*
No need for orthotic influence on the knee or hip	*
Indications for prefabricated AFO	
As a temporary evaluation orthosis	*
In case of need for early mobilization before provision of a custom orthosis	*
No problematic increased tone	*
No significant mediolateral instability	*
Benefits of providing an AFO for use in weight bearing as soon as the patient is medically stable	
Encourages balanced standing	*

Continued

Provides ankle stability	*
Promotes postural alignment	*
Maintains range of motion at the ankle	*
Supports early mobilization	*
Indications for use of a KAFO	
Poor standing balance, instability, and weight transference	*
Moderate-to-severe genu recurvatum uncontrolled by AFO	*
Recommendations applicable to all lower limb orthoses	
Alignment of orthosis at terminal stance/preswing is critical and influences step length, gait symmetry, speed, and energy consumption	C
Contracture at any lower limb joint may limit the effectiveness of an orthosis	*

References

1. Aggett T: An investigation into the effects and use of the air-stirrup brace with subjects following stroke, *Neurorehabil Neural Repair* 13:38, 1999 (abstract).
2. Aho K, Harmsen P, Hatano S, et al: Cerebrovascular disease in the community: results of a WHO collaborating study, *Bull WHO* 58:113–130, 1980.
3. *The Atlas of Heart Disease and Stroke*, 2004. Retrieved October 7, 2005 from http://www.who.int/cardiovascular-diseases/resources/atlas/en/.
4. American Heart Association: *Heart disease and stroke statistics—2003 update*, Dallas, Tex, 2003, American Heart Association.
5. Bamford J, Sandercock P, Dennis M, et al: A prospective study of acute cerebrovascular disease in the community: the Oxfordshire Community Stroke Project 1981-1986, 11: incidence, case fatality rates and overall outcome at one year of cerebral infarction, primary intracerebral haemorrhage and subarachnoid haemorrhage, *J Neurol Neurosurg Psychiatry* 53:16–22, 1990.
6. Bobath B: *Adult hemiplegia: evaluation and treatment*, ed 3, Oxford, 1990, Butterworth-Heinemann.
7. Bonita R, Stewart A, Beaglehole R: International trends in stroke mortality; 1970-1985, *Stroke* 21:989–992, 1990.
8. Bowers RJ: Non-articulated ankle-foot orthoses. In Condie ME, Campbell J, Martina JD, editors: *Report of a consensus conference on the orthotic management of stroke patients*, Copenhagen, 2004, ISPO.
9. Bowers RJ, Meadows CB: Case study: the effects of a solid ankle foot orthosis on hemiplegic gait (abstract). In Boone D, editor: *Proceedings of the 11th World Congress of the International Society for Prosthetics and Orthotics*, Hong Kong, 2004, ISPO.
10. Brunnstrom S: *Movement therapy in hemiplegia*, London, 1970, Harper and Row.
11. Burdett RG, Borello-France D, Blatchly C, et al: Gait comparison of subjects with hemiplegia walking unbraced, with ankle-foot orthosis and with air-stirrup brace, *Phys Ther* 68:1197–1203, 1988.
12. Carr JH, Shepherd RB: *A motor relearning programme for stroke*, ed 2, London, 1987, Heinemann.
13. Condie E, Campbell J, Martina J: *Report of a consensus conference on the orthotic management of stroke patients*, Copenhagen, 2004, ISPO.
14. Cotton E, Kinsman R: *Conductive education for adult hemiplegia*, Edinburgh, 1983, Churchill Livingstone.
15. Davidson I, Waters K: Physiotherapists working with stroke patients, *Physiotherapy* 86:69–80, 2000.
16. Feigen VL, Lawes CMM, Bennett DA, Anderson CS: Stroke epidemiology: a review of population-based studies of incidence, prevalence and case-fatality in the late 20th century, *Lancet Neurology* 2:43–53, 2003.
17. Lindseth RE, Glancy J: Polypropylene lower-extremity braces for paraplegia due to myelomeningoceli, *J Bone Joint Surg Am* 56(3):556-563, 1974.
18. Hoy DJ, Karas Reinthal, MA: Articulated ankle foot orthosis designs. In Condie ME, Campbell J, Martina JD, editors: *Report of a consensus conference on the orthotic management of stroke patients*, Copenhagen, 2004, ISPO.
19. Kakurai S, Akai M: Clinical experiences with a convertible thermoplastic knee-ankle-foot orthosis for post-stroke hemiplegic patients, *Prosthet Orthot Int* 20:191–194, 1996.
20. Keenan M-A: Recommended reading list, lower limb surgery for stroke patients. In Condie ME, Campbell J, Martina J, editors: *Report of a consensus conference on the orthotic management of stroke patients*, Copenhagen, 2004, ISPO.
21. Knott M, Voss D: *Proprioceptive neuromuscular facilitation: patterns and techniques*, New York, 1968, Harper and Row.
22. Langhorne P, Legg L, Pollok A, et al: Evidence-based stroke rehabilitation, *Age Ageing* 31(suppl 3):17–20, 2002.
23. Lehmann JF, Price R, Condon SM, De Lateur BJ: Gait abnormalities in hemiplegia: their correction by ankle-foot orthoses, *Arch Phys Med Rehabil* 68:763–771, 1987.
24. Mant J, Wade D, Winner S. Stroke. Retrieved October 7, 2005 from http://hcna.radcliffe.radcliffe–Oxfordcom/stroke.htm.
25. Meadows CB: *The influence of polypropylene ankle-foot orthoses on the gait of cerebral palsied children*, PhD thesis, Glasgow, UK, 1984, University of Strathclyde.
26. Miyazaki S, Yamamoto S, Kubota T: Effect of ankle-foot orthosis on active ankle moment in patients with hemiparesis, *Med Biol Eng Comput* 35:381–385, 1997.
27. Morris C: Current research in orthotics. In Condie ME, Campbell J, Martina J, editors: *Report of a consensus conference on the orthotic management of stroke patients*, Copenhagen, 2004, ISPO.
28. O'Dwyer NJ, Ada L, Neilson PD: Spasticity and muscle contracture following stroke, *Brain* 119:1737–1749, 1996.
29. Olney SJ, Richards C: Hemiparetic gait following stroke. Part I: characteristics, *Gait and Posture* 4:136-148, 1996.
30. Olsen TS: Stroke: understanding the problem. In Condie ME, Campbell J, Martina J, editors: *Report of a consensus conference on the orthotic management of stroke patients*, Copenhagen, 2004, ISPO.
31. Oshawa S, Ikeda S, Tanaka S: A new model of plastic ankle-foot orthosis (FAFO (II)), *Prosthet Orthot Int* 16:104–108, 1992.
32. Owen E: *Shank angle to floor measures and tuning of ankle-foot orthosis footwear combinations for children with cerebral palsy, spina bifida and other conditions*, MSc thesis, Glasgow, UK, 2004, University of Strathclyde.
33. Perry J: *Gait analysis: normal and pathological function*, Thorofare, NJ, 1992, Slack, Inc.
34. Richards CL, Malouin F, Dumas F, Tardif D: Gait velocity as an outcome measure of locomotion after stroke. In Craik RL, Oatis CA, editors: *Gait analysis: theory and applications*, St. Louis, 1995, Mosby.
35. Ryerson S, Levit K: *Functional movement reeducation*, New York, 1997, Churchill Livingstone.
36. Salteil J: A one-piece laminated knee locking short leg brace, *Orthot Prosthet* 23:68–75, 1969.
37. Shekelle PG, Woolf SH, Eccles M, Grimshaw J: Clinical guidelines: developing clinical guidelines, *BMJ* 318:593–596, 1999.
38. Sinkjaer T, Magnussen I: Passive, intrinsic, and reflex-mediated stiffness in ankle extensors of hemiparetic patients, *Brain* 117:355–363, 1994.
39. Sudlow CLM, Warlow CP: Comparing stroke incidence worldwide: what makes studies comparable?, *Stroke* 27:550–558, 1996.
40. Sudlow CLM, Warlow CP: Comparable studies of the incidence of stroke and its pathological types, *Stroke* 28:491–499, 1997.
41. Thilmann AF, Fellows SJF, Ross HF: Biomechanical changes at the ankle joint after stroke, *J Neurol Neurosurg Psychiatry* 54:134–139, 1991.
42. Van Peppen RPS, Kwakkel G, Wood-Dauphines, et al: The impact of physical therapy in functional outcomes after stroke: what's the evidence?, *Clin Rehabil* 18:833–862, 2004.
43. Warlow CP, Dennis MS, van Gijn J, et al: *Stroke: a practical guide to management*, ed. Oxford, 2001, Blackwell Science.

Assessment and orthotic management of gait dysfunction in individuals with traumatic brain injury

Alberto Esquenazi

Key Points

- Understanding normal and pathological gait is imperative to appropriately prescribing lower limb orthoses that will address the patients' functional deficits

- Understanding the timing and functional impact of the gait deviations will facilitate appropriate orthotic prescriptions

- Both molded and metal orthoses have a role in the management of patients with residual dysfunction from traumatic brain injury

Most survivors of a brain insult have the potential for return of significant function and resumption of useful lives. The average age at which an injury occurs is bimodal, with a peak between 16 and 24 years and another later in life between 65 and 70 years. The incidence is higher in men. Life expectancy for patients who survive the first month after traumatic brain injury (TBI) is fairly long, particularly in the younger group. At least 70% of hemiplegic patients regain the ability to walk.[3] Basic treatment principles are often waived on the erroneous assumption that the patient will not survive. For example, a patient whose fractures are left untreated because it is believed he or she will not survive poses a much greater treatment problem in later periods of recovery. Many patients will develop other complications due to injury to the central nervous system and polytrauma, such as spasticity, muscle overactivity, incoordination, and development of heterotopic ossification.

Abnormal bone formation near proximal limb joints may take years to mature, and clinical experience dictates that surgical removal be delayed until maturity of the new bone has been reached.

This chapter discusses the factors affecting ambulation and possible orthotic interventions in patients after a brain injury.

Some features of normal gait control should be considered before discussing the different types of abnormal ambulation in patients with upper motor neuron. Normal gait involves a cyclic, highly automated, stereotypic movement pattern with rhythmic alternating motion of the trunk and extremities. In normal individuals, cycle-to-cycle variation of the details of the movement is relatively low.[18] Locomotor action patterns are symmetrical and involve the entire body. In healthy subjects, gait is a skill that is mastered in a relatively uniform way. The three main functional goals of human ambulation are (1) to move from one place to another, (2) to move safely, and (3) to move efficiently. The gait of the patient after a TBI frequently is neither safe nor energy efficient.[17] Compensatory movements necessary for ambulation produce abnormal or exaggerated vertical and horizontal displacements of the center of gravity. Impaired balance, sensory and visual deficits, and foot drag all can contribute to loss of balance, falls, and increased anxiety regarding ambulation and its accompanying risks.[16] Cardiopulmonary fitness and joint range of motion may be impaired because of decreased intensity and frequency of exercise and ambulation, particularly early in the rehabilitation process.

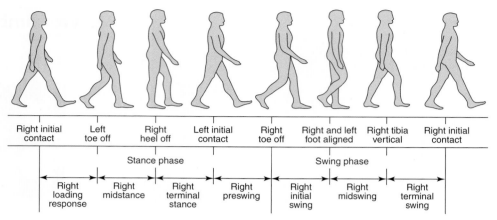

| Right initial contact | Left toe off | Right heel off | Left initial contact | Right toe off | Right and left foot aligned | Right tibia vertical | Right initial contact |

Stance phase | Swing phase

| Right loading response | Right midstance | Right terminal stance | Right preswing | Right initial swing | Right midswing | Right terminal swing |

Fig. 34-1 Gait cycle.

Normal locomotion

From the clinical standpoint, an understanding of the events occurring during the walking cycle is important so that pathologic locomotion can be correlated to cause and effect and precise timing during gait. Some basic terminology is reviewed here to help identify the components and events of the gait cycle.[2,5,14] From the perspective of one limb, the gait cycle has two basic components: *stance phase*, during which the limb is in contact with the ground, and *swing phase*, during which the limb is off the ground. The stance phase can be subdivided into one event and four functional subphases: (1) initial contact, (2) loading response, (3) midstance, (4) terminal stance, and (5) preswing. The swing phase can be subdivided into three functional subphases: (1) initial swing, (2) midswing, and (3) terminal swing.[2] A *stride* is one complete gait cycle and can be defined as the time from initial contact of one foot until the next initial contact of the same foot. *Double support* is the period of time during which both feet are in contact with the ground. *Single support* is the period when only one foot is in contact with the ground and is the equivalent to the swing period of the contralateral limb. *Step length* is the distance covered in the direction of progression during one step. The *step period* is the time measured from an event in one foot to the subsequent occurrence of the same event in the other foot (Fig. 34-1).

Step time and step length are fairly symmetrical for normal individuals and are important treatment indicator parameters in the patient population.

Gait can be studied through the collection of a wide range of information. The variables that can be recorded can be grouped into the following categories: (1) temporal and stride measures, (2) kinematics, (3) kinetics, and (4) electromyography (EMG).

Temporal and spatial descriptive measures

In order to characterize gait, some basic output variables regarding temporospatial structure and sequencing of the stance and swing phases can be measured. These data can be obtained by measuring the distances and timing involved in the floor contacts of the feet. In the Gait and Motion Analysis Laboratory (GMAL), a device called the Gait Mat II is used to extract this type of information. A left and right "footprint record" is obtained, and a printout is generated that provides information about average and standard deviation of walking velocity, cadence, stance, and swing times for each side as well as stride lengths, step lengths, and base of support. Comparison of right and left parameters can be used to determine the extent of unilateral impairment or the effect of intervention.[14]

Kinematics

Kinematics provides a description of movements without regard to the forces generating them. The earlier techniques were photographic and cinematographic. Other techniques include the use of accelerometers and electrogoniometers. Modern systems use high-speed video/film recording with retro-reflective markers or, as in the GMAL, specialized optoelectronic apparatus in which active optical sources (e.g., infrared-emitting diodes) attached to the subject serve as markers. Time coincidence between controller illumination and camera reception uniquely identifies each light-emitting diode. Once the kinematic information is available as coordinate data, it can be processed and displayed as graphs or stick figures that demonstrate the gait sequence in the imaged plane (Fig. 34-2). Joint angles can be computed and displayed as a function of time or as a percentage of the stride period. Velocities and accelerations can be calculated. Video is a good alternative when instrumenting the subject is unacceptable.

Kinetics

Kinetic analysis deals with the forces, moments, and mechanical energies that develop during the course of walking. Ground reaction forces are generally measured using a triaxial force platform. Ideally, as in our laboratory, four platforms adjacent to one other should be used so that the forces transmitted through the contact surface for each foot can be recorded independently and simultaneously during sequential steps. The measured ground reaction forces are often normalized to body weight or expressed in Newtons. In the GMAL at MossRehab, the ground reaction force vector is visualized and superimposed in real time on the video image of the walking subject using laser optics. This is a useful tool that does not require patient instrumentation

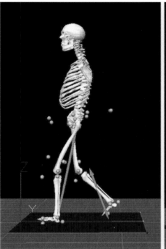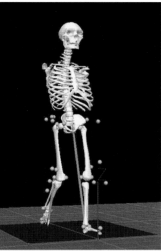

Fig. 34-2 Graphic representations of anatomical figure showing anterior posterior and lateral views of the gait sequence and line of force. (Data generated using CODA CX1, Charnwood Dynamics Ltd., UK, and C-Motion Software, Ontario, Canada.)

and facilitates determination of the effect of bracing or shoe modifications during walking.

Lower limb orthoses

Orthoses are devices applied to the external surface of the body part to achieve one or more of the following goals: (1) relieve pain, (2) immobilize musculoskeletal segments by limiting/directing joint motion, (3) reduce axial load, (4) prevent or correct deformity, and (5) improve function. Overall, orthoses can be divided into two major categories: corrective and accommodative devices. *Corrective devices* are meant to improve the position of the limb segment by stretching a contracture or correcting the alignment of skeletal structures.[1] *Accommodative devices* are meant to provide additional support to already deformed joints and or tissues, to prevent further deformity, and ultimately to improve function. Orthoses can be further classified as *static* or *dynamic*. Dynamic orthoses permit movement of the involved joint(s) while controlling the direction or alignment of the movement and, at times, providing a substitute power source for weak muscles. The spectrum of orthotic devices available is broad, ranging from a simple plastic device applied across one joint to a much more complex device that is made of a variety of materials and crosses multiple joints.[1]

Knowledge of the disease or disorder in question, functional anatomy, medical comorbidities, biomechanics, orthotic components, materials, and recognition of the anticipated functional outcome are essential for proper orthotic prescription.

The orthotic components chosen depend on which functions they fulfill, but most orthoses consist of three basic elements: interface components, structural components, and joints. In orthoses of newer design, such as the plastic ankle–foot orthosis (AFO), differentiating the joints from the structural and interface components may be impossible.[18]

The shoe is an integral part of any lower limb orthosis that includes the foot; it serves as the foundation for the device and directly impacts its function. Correct shoe fit must take

into consideration size while the patient is standing because the configuration of the foot changes with weight bearing and can be altered by spasticity and contractures.

The choice of materials in the fabrication of orthoses is expanding rapidly; a more detailed review can be found in other sections of this text. Factors that dictate the type of material used in orthotic fabrication include the length of time the orthosis will be used, the magnitudes of forces applied across the orthosis, and the amount of axial weight loading. Three primary material groups (thermoplastics, metals, and composite materials) are used for the fabrication of orthoses in the TBI population. Thermoplastics offer the benefits of light weight, total contact, adjustable flexibility, ability to reshape or remold, and more cosmetic appearance. Metal orthoses often have the advantage of increased durability and, in the hands of a skilled orthotist, built-in adjustability. The advent of newer materials, such as carbon composites and extruded plastic materials, make available the advantages of maximal tension strength, lightweight design, and ease of adjustability.

A complete orthotic prescription should specify the joints the device encompasses and suggest the desired biomechanical alignment and materials of fabrication. When the orthosis is ready, it should be evaluated both off and on the patient to ensure proper fit and function. When these characteristics are achieved, appropriate training of the patient and family on device use should begin. In the majority of patients after TBI, orthotic management, if possible, is best accomplished with use of plastic molded orthoses. They provide more intimate contact, with better distribution of the controlling/corrective forces over a larger area. These devices tend to be more cosmetic and hence better accepted by the patient. The patient is allowed to exchange shoes as long as constant heel height is maintained to avoid altering the dynamic alignment of the device. Plastic materials are lighter and easier to clean than the traditional metal and leather designs. Lack of sensation and fluctuating edema are relative contraindications to the prescription of plastic molded orthoses. If the patient has adequate visual perception, minimal cognitive impairment, and good social support, he or she can compensate for these deficits and receive the added benefits provided by plastic braces. The availability in recent years of a variety of adjustable ankle joints that can be attached to plastic orthoses has eliminated a major disadvantage of these devices.[6,13] Adjustments to the biomechanical alignment and fit must be made by an orthotist.

Metal/leather orthoses continue to have a definite place in the treatment of the TBI patient. In most areas, patients are being transferred to rehabilitation programs much earlier than in the past, and the length of stay in the rehabilitation programs has decreased significantly. Predicting the final rehabilitation outcome of these patients early in their rehabilitation program may be difficult. The ability to adjust the biomechanical alignment of the orthosis with simple tools or to convert a controlling force into an assistive one in order to respond to the patient's needs is an important advantage. Proper biomechanical alignment of any orthosis is critical to the optimization of ambulation.[11] Joint malalignment (lack of congruence between orthotic and anatomical joints) creates a discrepancy in motion that ultimately may produce pain, skin breakdown, and other preventable problems, and can and does prevent a borderline walking patient from becoming a functional ambulator. Some patients with better recovery may be able to compensate for inadequate orthotic prescription or alignment, but this ability does not diminish the importance of appropriate orthotic prescription and fit.

Pathological gait in TBI

The mechanism of TBI can produce varied patterns of presentation of residual dysfunction. Head trauma frequently is the result of a high-velocity accident with a coup–countercoup effect of the brain shearing against the rough inner surface of the skull. Multiple injuries are common, and initial diagnosis is difficult. Lifesaving resuscitation efforts often detract from complete examination, resulting in 11% of patients with missed fractures or dislocations and 34% of patients with missed peripheral nerve injuries. The resulting upper motor neuron syndrome and residual dysfunction can affect one side of the body (hemiparesis), two limbs (paraparesis), three limbs, or all four limbs (quadriparesis). According to the presentation, disturbances of the temporal, spatial, kinematic, kinetic, and possibly EMG patterns of gait occur and are well documented.[7,14]

Although differences occur from patient to patient, some generalities have been demonstrated, including decreased walking velocity with shorter stride length, shorter stance time, and increased swing time for the involved limb.[3,14,15] A decrease in weight bearing on the involved limb has been noted as well as a decrease in single support time. The unaffected limb has increased stance time. Stance phase abnormalities include forefoot first or flat foot initial contact rather than heel first. In addition, ankle inversion may occur, causing the lateral border of the foot to contact the ground and producing instability during weight bearing. Incomplete knee extension may be noted, but more commonly hyperextension of the knee is observed, with continued equinovarus deformity of the ankle during midstance. Limited or missing heel contact may be present. During terminal stance, terminal contact can occur early or late, and the pelvis may drop on the contralateral side.[1]

Inadequate hip and knee flexion during the initial swing phase may result in toe drag. During midswing, insufficient ankle dorsiflexion is a major problem. Inability to perform coordinated hip flexion and knee extension during terminal swing produces a shortened step length, which may be further complicated by an ankle held in plantarflexion.[11]

From the functional perspective and to facilitate assessment, gait dysfunction can be categorized on the basis of timing with respect to the gait cycle. During stance phase, an abnormal base of support and limb instability may make walking unsafe, energy inefficient, and possibly painful. Inadequate limb clearance and limb advancement during the swing phase interfere with safety and energy efficiency. A comparison of normal gait patterns to patterns exhibited by individuals with hemiplegia demonstrates differences in temporal, kinetic, and kinematic factors and muscle activation patterns across multiple joints. In order to properly identify and evaluate the gait problems of the TBI patient, the clinician must be able to understand what the problem is, when and where it is present, and, if possible, why it occurs. Knowledge of the orthotic devices available to correct the problem, the anatomic limitations of the patient, and a thorough medical,

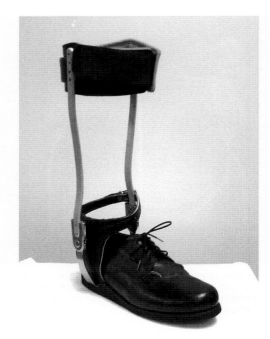

Fig. 34-3 Double adjustable AFO with plantarflexion and ankle inversion strap attached to an orthopedic shoe.

cognitive, and social history are needed to determine the most appropriate orthotic intervention.[3]

Abnormal base of support

Equinovarus deformity is the most common pathological lower limb posture seen in the TBI population. This abnormal posture results in an unstable base of support during stance phase. Contact with the ground occurs with the forefoot first, and weight is borne primarily on the lateral border of the foot. This position is maintained during the stance phase. Heel contact may be limited or missing. Limitation in dorsiflexion prevents forward progression of the tibia over the stationary foot, causing knee hyperextension and interference with terminal stance and preswing where lack of propulsive phase is noted.[8] The lack of an adequate base of support results in instability of the whole body. For this reason, correction of the abnormal ankle–foot posture by orthotic means or, if these fail, by chemodenervation or surgical methods is essential. During the swing phase, a sustained plantarflexed and inverted posture of the foot may result in a limb clearance problem. Use of an AFO to control the abnormal posture of the ankle during stance and swing phase should be attempted. An ankle inversion strap or pad should be used to assist in controlling the ankle inversion attitude. The orthosis preferentially is attached to an orthopedic shoe, and the orthotic ankle should include a plantarflexion stop to control ankle plantarflexion during swing and stance phases (Fig. 34-3).[12] If ankle clonus is triggered during stance phase, a dorsiflexion stop should be used as well to prevent the stretch response triggering this phenomenon. The stop should be set just before the clonus appears. When cognition and sensation are not impaired or adequate social support exists for supervision, use of a molded plastic AFO (molded AFO) with inversion control buildup and/or strap is preferred, casted whenever possible in calcaneo neutral position (Fig. 34-4).

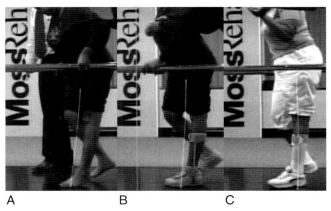

Fig. 34-5 **A**, Equinovarus foot posture. Effect of AFO (**B**) or molded AFO in combination with a heel lift (**C**) on control of ankle equinovarus and knee hyperextension. Red line represents line of force and relationship to knee joint center under each condition.

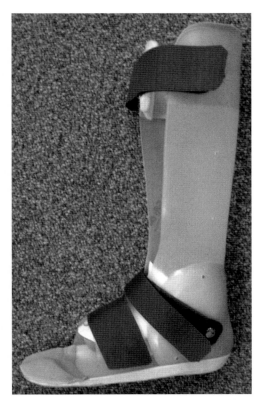

Fig. 34-4 Molded plastic AFO with inversion control buildup and forefoot strap cast in calcaneo neutral position.

A molded AFO with a long plastic footplate and soft padding in combination with a forefoot strap and an extra-depth shoe with high toe box can be used as an option to accommodate abnormal flexed toe posture.[6]

Limb instability

Knee flexion during early stance phase results in limb instability. In TBI patients this problem interferes with transfer and gait training. It is more commonly observed in the early phase of recovery, when flaccidity and weakness affect the lower limbs. The patient is unable to control the knee flexion moment during early stance phase and is unable to walk without assistance. External means of knee control can be provided by a knee–ankle foot orthosis (KAFO), knee orthosis, or molded AFO that provides knee stability (based on the biomechanical design) during early stance, permitting the patient to maintain limb stability and safely ambulate.[11]

A KAFO with off-set or stance control knee joints, a molded AFO set in a few degrees of plantarflexion, or a shoe with a solid ankle-cushion heel provides varying degrees of knee stability by positioning the ground reaction force anterior to the knee mechanism during stance phase. It is critical that a knee extensor strengthening program be encouraged and maintained during the early phases of the rehabilitation program, as knee weakness is promoted by the muscle disuse that can result from orthotic intervention.[6]

Knee hyperextension present during stance phase is commonly produced by spasticity of the ankle plantarflexors, plantarflexion contracture, lack of motor control, or, less likely in the TBI population, compensation for knee extensor weakness. This abnormal posture of the knee prevents adequate contralateral limb advancement, with resultant shortening of step length. Orthotic management of this problem includes use of an AFO with limited plantarflexion or, if an ankle plantarflexion contracture is present, the combination of an AFO and a modified shoe with a heel lift (Fig. 34-5). These two options will limit the knee hyperextension and will preclude knee collapse if the brace alignment is appropriate. The deformity also can be corrected by decreasing ankle plantarflexor spasticity, if present, with oral antispasticity drugs, chemodenervating agents, or surgery.

Hip flexion during stance phase is a less frequently seen gait deviation. When it occurs, trunk instability and significant disruption of ambulation present. This problem is common in the early stage of recovery with flaccidity or in patients with significant flexor spasticity of the trunk or hips. Use of a locked external hip joint attached proximally to a pelvic belt (or, for more severe cases, a lumbosacral corset) and distally to a thigh section has been useful for providing orthotic control of this gait deviation. With this intervention, hip hiking and trunk lean to the opposite side or a contralateral shoe lift will be needed as compensation to facilitate limb advancement and clearance during the swing phase.

Limb clearance

During the swing phase, limb clearance and advancement occur. When limb clearance is insufficient, limb advancement usually is compromised. In the TBI population, the most common causes of limb clearance problems are lack of appropriate hip flexion, knee flexion, and ankle dorsiflexion. The clinician must recognize the importance of coordinated lower limb motion during the swing phase to achieve this task.

At this time, no mechanical external orthotic intervention addresses lack of hip flexion. Electrical stimulation directly to the hip flexors has many potential problems with existing technology. Functional electrical stimulation with an indwelling wire electrode to the iliacus may be helpful in retraining and strengthening this muscle group. Stimulation of the hamstrings or the sural nerve at the foot to elicit a flexor

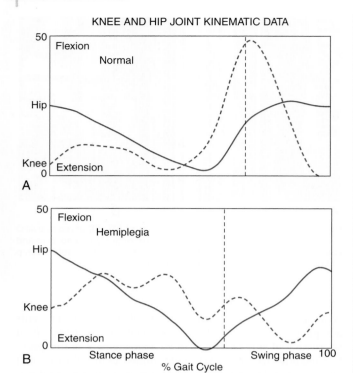

KNEE AND HIP JOINT KINEMATIC DATA

Fig. 34-6 **A**, Graph illustrating normal knee and hip range of motion during slow walking (normal). **B**, Stiff knee gait pattern in a patient with hemiplegia. Vertical hashed lines indicate swing phase. (Data generated with CODA CX1, Charnwood Dynamics Ltd.)

withdrawal has been attempted in research work, with some reported improvement.[5] This problem effectively prevents physiologic "shortening" of the limb, producing a toe drag during the swing phase. Training in the use of compensatory walking techniques, such as hip adduction and external rotation to advance the limb, should be considered. A shoe lift to produce functional lengthening of the contralateral limb or use of a thigh corset with a waist belt to prevent lengthening by gravity of the affected limb can be attempted.[7]

Total joint displacement and synchronization of motion between the involved joints are essential to produce adequate limb clearance during walking. Stiff knee gait pattern is commonly seen in this patient population. The patient's inability to adequately flex the knee creates a large moment of inertia, which increases the energy required to initiate the swing phase of the involved limb.[19] The patient then must utilize ipsilateral hip and trunk and contralateral limb compensatory motions. Even if the ankle–foot system is in an appropriate position, early swing toe drag is evident and can be corrected only by generating knee flexion or increasing the contralateral limb length as suggested. One possible explanation for this problem can be found using the dynamic poly-EMG, which in some cases demonstrates increased activity in the quadriceps muscles. Lack of forward momentum because of decreased walking speed or an ankle equinus posture is another possible cause of this problem. Electrical stimulation applied directly to the hamstrings or in the form of a nociceptive stimulus delivered to the sural nerve in the preswing phase when maximal hip extension occurs has been attempted (Fig. 34-6).[4]

Abnormal hip adduction

Increased hip adduction can interfere with ipsilateral and contralateral limb advancement and with other activities of daily living (e.g., perineal hygiene). Overactivity of the adductor musculature or power imbalance of the hip abductor and adductor muscle groups is the most common cause of this problem. Because many patients may use the hip adductors to compensate for lack of hip flexion during limb advancement, the clinician must be certain that elimination of adductor muscle activity by chemodenervation or surgery does not render the patient nonambulatory. Orthotic interventions such as use of a thigh corset attached to a waistband through an external hip joint that limits adduction can be attempted.

Incomplete knee extension

Another common gait deviation in this patient population is incomplete knee extension, seen during the late swing and early stance phases, that frequently results from hamstring spasticity. This problem interferes with ipsilateral limb advancement, as the knee is flexed and is unable to "reach" the ground easily. As a decrease in functional height occurs, contralateral limb clearance is affected, requiring increased compensatory hip and knee flexion to avoid foot drag.

Pelvic retraction

Pelvic retraction is another problem affecting the involved limb during the gait cycle that interferes with limb advancement. The main outcome of this problem is a shortened contralateral step length because of limited hip extension. Pelvic retraction and incomplete knee extension currently are not amenable to orthotic intervention.

Summary

Basics of gait and orthotic intervention as they apply to the patient with a brain injury have been reviewed and the potential use of surgical or pharmacologic intervention noted, where appropriate. The majority of patients who survive a traumatic brain injury and other brain insults achieve limited ambulation. Use of orthoses, shoe modifications, and other types of interventions in an attempt to optimize functional capabilities of patients and encourage improved functional level and quality of life is indicated.

References

1. American Academy of Orthopedic Surgeons: *Atlas of orthotics*, St. Louis, 1985, CV Mosby.
2. Bampton S: A guide to the visual examination of pathological gait. In: *Temple University-Moss Rehabilitation Hospital, Rehabilitation Research and Training Center #8*, 1979.
3. Condie E, Campbell J, Martina JD, editors: *Report of a consensus conference on the orthotic management of stroke patients*, Copenhagen, 2004, ISPO.
4. Craik R, Cozzens B, Miyazaki S: Enhancement of swing phase clearance through sensory stimulation. In: *Proceedings of the 4th Annual Conference on Rehabilitation Engineering. Chicago, Rehabilitation Engineering Society of North America*, 1981.
5. De JB, Saunders MB, Inman VT, Eberhart HD: Major determinants in normal and pathological gait, *J Bone Joint Surg* 35A:543–558, 1953.
6. Esquenazi A, Wikoff E, Hirai B, et al: Effects of a plantar flexed plastic molded ankle foot orthosis on gait pattern and lower limb muscle strength.

In: *Proceedings of the VI World Congress of the International Society for Prosthetics and Orthotics*, 1989.

7. Finch L, Barbeau H: Hemiplegic gait: new treatment strategies, *Physiother Can* 38:36–40, 1986.

8. Fuller DA, Keenan MA, Esquenazi A, Whyte J, Mayer N, Fidler-Sheppard R: The impact of instrumented gait analysis on surgical planning: treatment of spastic equinovarus deformity of the foot and ankle, *Foot Ankle Int* 22:738–743, 2002.

9. Inman VT, Ralston HJ, Todd F: *Human walking*, Baltimore, 1981, Williams & Wilkins.

10. Glenn MB, Whyte J: Nerve blocks. In Glenn MB, Whyte J, editors: *The practical management of spasticity in children and adults*, Malvern, Penn, 1990, Lea & Febiger.

11. Gok H, Kucukdeveci A, Altinkaynak H, Yavuzer G, Ergin S: Effects of ankle-foot orthoses on hemiparetic gait, *Clin Rehabil* 17:137–139, 2003.

12. Katz DI, White DK, Alexander MP, Klein RB: Recovery of ambulation after traumatic brain injury, *Arch Phys Med Rehabil* 85:865–869, 2004.

13. Miyazaki S, Yamamoto S, Kubota T: Effect of ankle-foot orthosis on active ankle moment in patients with hemiparesis, *Med Biol Eng Comput* 35:381–385, 1997.

14. Ochi F, Esquenazi A, Hirai B, Talaty M: Temporal-spatial features of gait after traumatic brain injury, *J Head Trauma Rehabil* 14:105–115, 1999.

15. Ofluoglu D, Esquenazi A, Hirai B: Temporal-spatial parameters of gait after obturator neurolysis in patients with spasticity, *Am J Phys Med Rehabil* 82:832–836, 2003.

16. Olney S, Monga T, Costigan P: Mechanical energy of walking of stroke patients, *Arch Phys Med Rehabil* 67:92–98, 1986.

17. Peat M, Dubo H, Winter D, et al: Electromyographic temporal analysis of gait: hemiplegic locomotion, *Arch Phys Med Rehabil* 57:421–425, 1976.

18. In Redford JB, editor: *Orthotics. Physical medicine and rehabilitation: state of the art review*, Philadelphia, 1987, Hanley & Belfus.

19. Winter DA: Pathologic gait diagnosis with computer-averaged electromyographic profiles. *Arch Phys Med Rehabil* 65:393–398, 1984.

Pediatric orthoses

Care of a child needing an orthosis requires the cooperation not only of the child but also of the parents and/or the extended family. All involved must have a strong understanding of the purpose of the orthosis in order to ensure success and follow-through. Everyone must be aware of the treatment program. Excellent lines of communication are needed between the orthotist and all other members of the treating team. Differing goals and expectations for an orthosis must be resolved. Funding issues and authorization for sophisticated and custom-made devices must be clearly defined and understood.

The orthotist must be prepared to exercise a great heal of patience. The child, his/her family members, and the treatment team must have a clear understanding of the potential for an orthosis and/or assistive device to satisfy the treatment goals for an affected area. Its purpose is to improve function and assist in disease management. Children are not "miniature adults." Many fine adjustments, tinkering, and customizing may be necessary. An orthotic device is not a cure for a disease but an aid for improved function and prevention of deformity.

Improved understanding of the disease has resulted from advances in molecular genetics and gene localization. It helps patients and their families cope with the medical issues and emotional responses. Genetic information, if available, can explain in clearer terms the inheritance, clinical manifestations, course, and prognosis of specific disease entities. Other disorders may occur without an understanding of the cause. Because the orthosis is not a cure, emphasis must be placed on functional goals. The treatment team can plan to use and develop resources, including orthoses and assistive devices, in a more beneficial and cost-effective fashion. One example of addressing functional goals is the custom-made thoracolumbosacral orthosis or containment body jacket, modified to accommodate ventilation equipment, which helps support the spine of a chid with type I spinal muscular atrophy (SMA) and allows him/her to be placed in a vertical position and to sit as early as possible. Another example is use of a supramalleolar orthosis in the hypotonic child to provide subtalar stabilization for improved balance in stance.

A reliable body of information derives from gait and motion studies. Understanding the subtle, more precise observations that are possible only through careful study of motion tapes may provide improved understanding of a problem and lead to improved orthotic prescription.

Since the last edition of this atlas, new techniques have been developed for contracture control. We have entered an era when the safe use of local injectable medications to decrease muscle spasticity has allowed the clinician to delay surgical intervention. Orthoses now can be more effective, but surgery may continue to be used often as definitive treatment.

Advances in materials resulting in orthoses that are lighter in weight while retaining their strength have led to greater compliance and acceptance. Improved understanding of deformities has led to surgical techniques resulting in better and more accurate correction of limb-length inequalities, rotational malalignment, and angular deformities in the extremities. Twister cables are rarely indicated. Another advance has been the use of craniofacial orthoses, using the benefits derived from chemical developments in plastic composition and manufacture.

Orthotic management of conditions resulting from childhood pathologies remains an inherent part of coordinated team management.

John D. Hsu

Section

Pediatric orthoses

Chapter

35

Congenital and acquired disorders

Keith Gabriel

Key Points

- Facilitation of normal growth and development is a common goal in the management of congenital and acquired disorders.
- Orthoses traditionally have been used for many conditions, either in preparation for definitive surgery or for maintenance of correction gained through surgery.
- Orthoses have been used to support a limb while awaiting expected improvement with growth. Sometimes the orthosis itself is the definitive management of the condition. Long-term reviews and prospective outcome studies of the use of these orthoses are conspicuously lacking. Opportunities abound for future important research.

Pediatrics is distinguished by the fact that the child is constantly growing and developing. *Growth* is an increase in physical measurements. *Development* is the acquisition and refinement of skills that follow a constant sequence, although at a rate that shows a wide range of normal variation.[67]

Orthoses and assistive devices have become important tools in the habilitation and rehabilitation of children with congenital and acquired disorders of the limbs. These devices can serve several purposes. An orthosis may directly facilitate and improve function of a limb. An orthosis may support one limb or segment so that the individual can concentrate on tasks involving a different part of the body. Unique to pediatrics is the opportunity to mold and guide the growing and developing body.

Goals of treatment interventions for children should include maximizing function, facilitating the attainment of specific skills, and encouraging the development of emotional maturity and self-reliance.[3] Unfortunately, even though orthoses are commonly included in these treatment interventions, little or no evidence-based literature actually documents the effectiveness of these devices in many conditions.

Congenital foot deformities

In humans, the feet serve a primary role as a weight-bearing surface for upright stance and ambulation. This function is affected not only by primary structural changes in the foot itself but also by deformities of other parts of the lower limb. This section discusses congenital foot deformities that may or may not occur in isolation. Information in this section inevitably will overlap with that pertaining to other more general pediatric diagnoses, such as myelomeningocele and cerebral palsy, covered in other chapters of this text.

Normal function of the foot in gait requires that the foot be flexible during swing phase and early stance phase, but that it converts to a rigid lever arm prior to toe-off. In general, maintenance of flexibility of the child's foot is of paramount importance in treatment of these disorders. Orthoses provide stability for the foot and ankle during function and can help to maintain available flexibility. In selected circumstances, orthoses may accomplish gradual improvement in both alignment and flexibility with growth.

Metatarsus adductus

Intoeing is one of the most frequent concerns that families have about their children. In the infant, the cause of intoeing often is metatarsus adductus (MA).

In MA, the forefoot is adducted with respect to the hindfoot. The cosmetic appearance of the foot has been described as kidney or bean shaped. Most often the anatomical site of deformity is the tarsometatarsal joints, with lesser degrees of

451

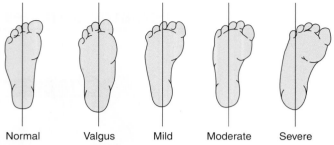

Normal   Valgus   Mild   Moderate   Severe

Fig. 35-1 Heel bisector method defines the relationship of the heel to the forefoot. *Normal*—bisecting between the second and third toes. *Valgus*—bisecting between the great and second toes. *Mild MA*—bisecting the third toe. *Moderate MA*—bisecting between the third and fourth toes. *Severe MA*—bisecting between the fourth and fifth toes. (Adapted from Bleck EE: *Dev Med Child Neurol* 24:545,1982.)

adduction through the transtarsal joints. The medial cuneiform–first metatarsal articulation often is oblique, and autopsy findings reported by Reiman and Werner[80] noted alterations in the size and shape of the first cuneiform. Usually no significant bowing of the metatarsals themselves is seen.

The subtalar joint, and therefore the heel, may be in various degrees of varus or valgus but most frequently is near neutral. Some authors use heel position to make a distinction between typical MA and metatarsus varus.[77,97] If the heel is resistant in valgus, the condition may be skewfoot (see section on skewfoot). Significant or rigid heel varus raises the possibility that the deformity is a clubfoot. A key differential between MA and clubfoot is ankle motion. In clubfoot, the calcaneus is resistant in equinus and the foot as a unit cannot be passively dorsiflexed normally at the ankle. The hindfoot in MA can be manipulated through a full range of dorsiflexion and plantarflexion at the ankle joint.

The exact etiology of MA is unknown, but the condition usually is attributed to intrauterine positioning. Although the incidence has been reported as 1:1,000, most practitioners argue that MA is much more frequent.[107] Bilateral involvement is present in over 50% of cases, and a positive family history is found in 10% to 15% of patients.[77] An initial report of association with hip dysplasia[50] has not been reproduced in other studies.[62]

The severity of MA is variable in terms of degree of deformity and flexibility of the foot. Radiographic classification of severity[12] has been criticized because of significant variability.[23] If a permanent image is desired, an impression of the weight-bearing foot can be made by having the child stand on a photocopying machine.[92] A clinical classification system proposed by Bleck[14] uses the heel bisector to describe the appearance (Fig. 35-1) and flexibility (Table 35-1) found at physical examination. Another simple assessment of flexibility[24] suggests that a type 1 foot actively corrects with stroking or tickling the lateral foot, a type 2 foot corrects only with passive stretching, and a type 3 foot cannot be passively corrected.

A long-term study by Farsetti et al.[36] confirmed that classification based on flexibility at the time of diagnosis is valid. Feet with mild or moderate deformity that were passively correctable did well untreated. Those with rigid MA responded well to correctly performed serial manipulation and plaster casting. These authors advise treatment as soon

Table 35-1 Clinical classification system for metatarsus adductus

Type	Presentation
I	Flexible, with abduction beyond the midline of the heel bisector
II	Partly flexible, with abduction only to the midline
III	Inflexible, rigid with no abduction possible

as the deformity is diagnosed and found not to be passively correctable. Bleck's large study of MA also emphasized that patient age at initiation of treatment was the best predictor of good outcome.[14]

Treatment of MA is based on severity, flexibility, and patient age. For infants younger than 6 months, feet that actively correct or that passively correct past the midline generally do well with observation and stretching. A typical regimen includes stretching of foot four to six times each day, 10 repetitions each time, with the forefoot held in the corrective position for no less than 6 seconds per repetition. Parents or caretakers should be taught to support the child's heel during this stretching, to prevent spurious correction through the subtalar joint with creation of heel valgus.

For infants and toddlers, treatment of the more rigid MA usually begins with serial manipulation and casting. Long leg casts are most often recommended,[77] with the knee flexed, the forefoot abducted, and the foot somewhat externally rotated. Katz et al.[56] believe that below-knee casts are just as effective. Casts are changed at 2-week intervals or more frequently, and with each cast change an attempt is made to manipulate the foot into an overcorrected position. Goals include correction of the static deformity and improvement of midfoot flexibility.

Once the foot can be easily brought to an overcorrected position, whether through stretching of the moderate deformity or through serial casting of the more rigid deformity, then various types of shoe modifications and orthoses may be useful in maintaining desired alignment. No evidence-based literature documents whether any particular bracing technique is superior.

In one popular method, the foot is braced with specially constructed shoes, commonly referred to as *orthopedic* or *corrective shoes*. The *last*, in this case meaning the basic shape of the sole of the shoe, determines the type of forces that are directed to the foot. *Reverse last shoes* (Fig. 35-2), also known as *tarsal pronator shoes*, turn outward at the midfoot to maintain the abducted position achieved by either surgical or manipulative correction. *Straight last shoes* accomplish that same goal to a lesser degree. Another useful commercial product is the Bebax shoe (Fig. 35-3),[4] which is designed with an adjustable multidirectional hinge between the hindfoot and forefoot sections. This setup allows progressive adjustment of position as the deformity becomes more flexible. Several authors have advised against joining the shoes with the Denis-Browne bar for treatment of MA. Addition of the bar results in a tendency to produce correction through the subtalar joint, leading to heel valgus and flatfoot.[12,77]

The Wheaton brace (Fig. 35-4), a plastic knee–ankle–foot orthosis (KAFO) or ankle–foot orthosis (AFO) with an extended medial sidewall to prevent forefoot adduction, is

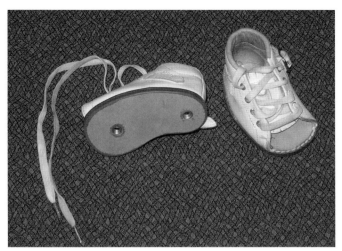

Fig. 35-2 Reverse last or "tarsal pronator" shoe is designed to brace the forefoot into abduction with respect to the hindfoot. The high-top design, along with the ankle strap, helps to keep the shoe in place.

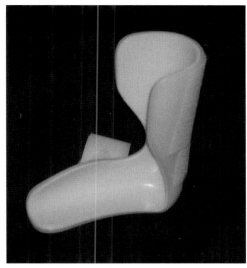

Fig. 35-4 Wheaton AFO is designed to maintain forefoot abduction. A KAFO design also is available.

frequently used. This polypropylene KAFO/AFO is manufactured with an outward flare shape to the foot section, much like the shape of a reverse last shoe.

Rarely, surgery is indicated for more severe cases and for older children with delayed diagnosis. Many procedures are available, and discussion of specific operations is beyond the scope of this chapter. Maintenance casts, orthoses, or special shoes are commonly advised following surgical correction. These devices are similar to the devices described earlier.

Long-term studies of MA in adulthood are scarce. Farsetti et al.[36] reported few adult complaints. Most pediatric orthopedists continue to observe the flexible deformities and treat the more severe rigid feet with serial casting, followed by bracing in straight last or reverse last shoes.

Skewfoot

Skewfoot is an uncommon deformity, and it is especially uncommon in the newborn.[68,72] The etiology is unknown.

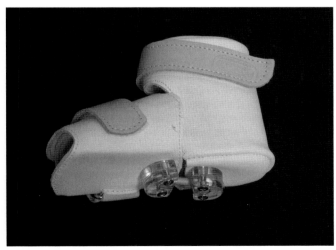

Fig. 35-3 Bebax "boot" is designed with an adjustable turnbuckle between the hindfoot and forefoot sections so that position and bracing forces can be adjusted.

The deformity presents generally as MA with heel valgus. On closer inspection, an almost "corkscrew" alignment of the foot is seen. The forefoot is in adduction with some degree of supination, while the hindfoot is in abduction with significant valgus. A key finding is lateral displacement of the navicular on the talus. Unfortunately the navicular does not ossify before age 3 to 6 years, so this displacement is radiographically silent in the infant or toddler. Berg[12] described simple and complex types of skewfoot, based on whether or not the calcaneocuboid joint was similarly displaced.

Treatment ranges from serial casting to surgical correction. Although Berg[12] believes that milder forms of skewfoot can be corrected with serial casting, Peterson,[72] in a review of the world literature, reported that all authors found nonoperative treatment to be unsuccessful. It has been suggested that a skewfoot results from improper manipulation and casting of MA.[77] Virtually all of the shoe modifications and orthoses used for treatment of simple MA have the potential to worsen heel valgus. No specific corrective orthosis is available for skewfoot. A foot orthosis (FO) can be custom molded to accommodate the foot shape for pain relief.

Clubfoot

Clubfoot, more properly called *congenital talipes equinovarus*, is easily recognized because the cosmetic appearance resembles a club on the end of the leg. The disorder is highly variable with regard to severity, rigidity, and response to treatment.

The incidence of clubfoot is different among geographic and ethnic groups, ranging from 0.64 to 6.8 per 1,000 live births.[7] About 70% of clubfoot occurs in males, and the right foot is more frequently affected. The condition is bilateral in about 50% of cases.

The etiology remains unknown in most instances. Familial associations are observed, but the genetic relationships are not determined. Clubfoot is quite common in some conditions, such as spina bifida, diastrophic dwarfism, arthrogryposis, and amniotic band syndrome. Clubfoot associated with these syndromes tends to be resistant to both nonoperative and surgical treatment.

Physical examination includes equinus and varus of the hindfoot, with adduction and supination through the midfoot. This combination brings the medial side of the great toe and first metatarsal adjacent to the medial distal tibia. A transverse crease is almost always present across the midfoot in the medial longitudinal arch. The appearance of the heel may be misleading, and it is important to palpate the actual location of the tuberosity of the calcaneus. Frequently the heel pad is "empty" and the ankle equinus has positioned the tip of the calcaneus more proximally, against the distal fibula. This resistant equinus deformity through the ankle distinguishes clubfoot from severe MA or skewfoot. Relative underdevelopment of the calf musculature and some shortening of the limb are almost always present with clubfoot. The family must be aware of these associations so that they are not subsequently identified as complications of treatment.

The pathoanatomy of clubfoot includes contracture and shortening of soft tissues, such as the tendons and ligaments; subluxation of joints, such as the subtalar and talonavicular articulations; and actual deformity of the bones, especially the talus. Whether one of these components is primary or causative to the clubfoot has not been proven. However, I believe that knowledge of hindfoot subluxation facilitates our understanding of soft-tissue contractures and bone deformity. The subtalar joint is subluxated, with the calcaneus displaced into varus beneath the talus. Simultaneously and inseparably, the calcaneus has rotated around an axis defined by the interosseous talocalcaneal ligament, bringing the tuberosity of the calcaneus laterally toward the lateral malleolus and the anterior end of the calcaneus medially toward the medial malleolus. The navicular is subluxated medially on the talar head, which brings the navicular immediately adjacent to the tip of the medial malleolus. The cuboid is displaced medially to a variable degree. As indicated, the ankle is in equinus. Further plantarflexion through the midfoot and forefoot creates an overall cavus condition. With the developing cartilage anlage of the foot displaced in this fashion, the talar neck is foreshortened and medially deviated, and the calcaneocuboid and medial cuneiform–first metatarsal joints are oblique medially. Posterior, medial, and plantar soft tissues are contracted.

Various orthoses are used for treatment of clubfoot. Most often, the orthosis is used as a holding device after correction by nonoperative or surgical methods. Typically a more restrictive orthosis is used initially on a full-time schedule. Once the child begins to crawl and/or walk, different bracing regimens for daytime and sleeping can be prescribed.

Scarpa in 1803 gave the first detailed description of an orthosis for treatment of clubfoot. The device was an AFO with metal upright bars and cuffs at the proximal calf and the malleoli, with a cup gripping the hindfoot. The orthosis produced a pronation and an abduction moment at the forefoot.

Straight last and reverse last shoes are the most commonly used orthoses for treatment of clubfoot. As discussed in the section on MA, the effectiveness of these shoes depends on the ability of the relatively stiff heel counter to control the hindfoot while the material of the medial side of the toe box pushes against the first ray of the forefoot. A high-top

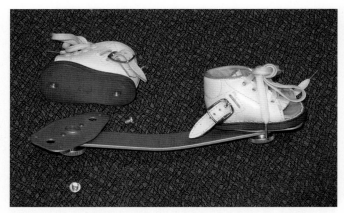

Fig. 35-5 Contemporary commercial Denis-Browne bar has adjustable footplates that attach to shoes using screw lugs in the shoe sole. This Denis-Browne bar has been bent, center downward, to provide additional valgus and dorsiflexion through the child's ankle.

design, often augmented with a strap over the dorsum of the ankle, is almost mandatory to minimize the number of times the child removes the shoe. The Bebax shoe is adjustable through the midfoot according to the amount of abduction force desired.

Denis Browne[20] described his special splint for treatment of clubfoot in 1934. Treatment consisted of taping the feet onto a bar to maintain the position obtained by manipulation. Modern commercial Denis-Browne bars have adjustable footplates with screw attachments designed to match threaded plugs in the soles of certain "corrective" shoes (Fig. 35-5). The Fillauer bar is a variation on this theme, with adjustable metal clamps designed to grasp the sole of the patient's shoe (Fig. 35-6). Typically the devices are adjusted to keep the feet externally rotated, augmenting the forefoot abduction forces provided by the shoes and adding an external rotation stretching force at the ankles. The bar can frequently be bent, center downward and away from the patient, to include a valgus moment at the hindfoot. With the footplates strongly rotated externally, this downward central bend adds some ankle dorsiflexion. In contrast to the caution given in the section on MA, application of corrective forces through the subtalar and ankle joints is desirable in patients with clubfoot. The length of the bar should approximate the width of the child's pelvis. A cost-effective variation of this combined shoes-and-bar orthosis, constructed of basic and readily

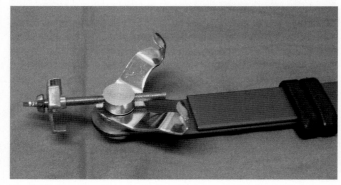

Fig. 35-6 Close-up view shows the clamping mechanism for attaching shoes of various sizes to a Fillauer bar. This Fillauer bar is adjustable for length, using the clamps shown at the right.

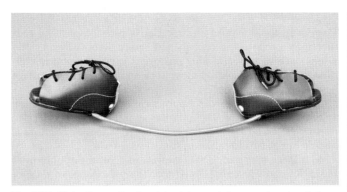

Fig. 35-7 Abduction orthosis advised for maintenance bracing following clubfoot correction using the Ponseti method can be constructed of very simple materials that are locally available.

available materials, has been designed for use in underserved and financially less able regions (Fig. 35-7).

AFOs and KAFOs have been adapted for use in treatment of clubfoot. They are similar to the molded braces described for the treatment of MA. The foot section incorporates an outward flare and an extended medial sidewall to ensure abduction through the midfoot. Valgus and external rotation shaping can be added to the orthosis as appropriate.

Enthusiasm for comprehensive surgical release and realignment of the clubfoot has waned with the reviews of surgically treated patients published in the 1990s and more recently noted disappointing outcomes.[5,29,55] The majority of current treatments emphasize nonoperative techniques, with limited operative interventions reserved for resistant or recurrent deformity. These techniques aim to provide painless foot function through the life of the patient with less regard to cosmesis or radiographic parameters. The French method of comprehensive physical therapy and taping and the Ponseti method of serial manipulations and holding casts both seem effective for restoration of a flexible plantigrade foot in most cases.

The initial stage of the French method relies on daily manipulation of the clubfoot by trained physiotherapists.[11,81] Between therapy sessions, foot position is generally maintained by taping. In this sense, the "orthosis" consists solely of the tape. The first English-language description of this program suggested using a Denis-Browne splint between therapy sessions for the first 2 or 3 weeks,[11] but subsequent reports presented in detail the technique for application of nonelastic and elastic tape and discouraged rigid bracing. In the early 1990s, continuous passive motion, provided with a specially designed machine appropriate to infants, was incorporated into the French method. At about the third month, when the foot is reasonably well corrected, continuous passive motion is discontinued and the family assumes responsibility for continuing the physical therapy and taping. When the child reaches an appropriate age to cooperate, active therapy exercises are added. No special shoes or molded orthoses are recommended. Treatment ends at about age 3 years, with monitoring to completion of growth.

In contrast, the Ponseti regimen[75] emphasizes the use of maintenance orthoses. This method of clubfoot treatment begins with serial manipulations and application of holding casts. The manipulations must be performed in a specific way,

initially maintaining the forefoot in supination to facilitate correction of the cavus component of the deformity. The forefoot is abducted in supination, with counterpressure over the dorsolateral head of the talus. The calcaneus must not be grasped or pushed so that movement of the calcaneus through the subtalar joint is not restricted. Rather, repositioning of the calcaneus occurs simultaneously and spontaneously as the talonavicular joint is reduced. Satisfactory overcorrection of the cavus, adductus, and varus usually is accomplished between cast numbers three and six, at which time residual ankle equinus is assessed. A percutaneous heel cord release is frequently done at this stage, followed by another 3 weeks of cast immobilization. Maintenance of correction requires strict adherence to a bracing program. Ponseti advises using an abduction orthosis consisting of straight last shoes attached to the Denis-Browne bar, with the footplates set at 70 degrees out-toe, and with the bar bent to encourage hindfoot valgus and about 15 degrees of ankle dorsiflexion. This appliance is worn on a full-time basis for 3 months, or until the child is learning to crawl. Night bracing is continued to age 3 or 4 years. Ponseti strongly states that an AFO is not effective for maintaining correction.[76] Although few outcome studies are available, published long-term results of the Ponseti method seem encouraging. More specifically addressing the use of orthoses, several authors have observed a very high recurrence rate in patients whose families did not adhere to the bracing recommendations.[31,99]

Congenital vertical talus

Congenital vertical talus (CVT) is a rare deformity that goes by many names, including congenital convex pes valgus, rocker-bottom foot, and Persian slipper foot. Physical examination reveals that the heel is in fixed equinus, with the forefoot dorsiflexed and everted. The arch is convex, and the head of the talus is prominent medially in the sole. Overall, the foot has a rocker-bottom appearance, and it is rigid and uncorrectable. A true CVT cannot be passively reduced with simple manipulation. If the talonavicular joint can be readily reduced and the ankle can be readily manipulated out of equinus, the deformity probably is either a calcaneovalgus positional deformity or the "oblique talus" of a severe flatfoot.

The etiology of CVT is unknown. Candidate genes have been suggested for some families.[28,89] Associations have been made with chromosomal disorders[100,101] such as trisomy 13, 14, 15, and 18 as well as neuromuscular disorders such as spina bifida, arthrogryposis, and sacral agenesis.

The important defining characteristic of the pathoanatomy is a fixed dorsolateral dislocation of the navicular onto the neck of the talus. In this situation, the sustentaculum tali and spring ligament are incompetent, such that the head of the talus rotates plantarward. The subtalar joint subluxates, with the calcaneus displaced laterally into valgus. Concomitant dorsal subluxation of the calcaneocuboid joint may be present. The ankle is resistant in equinus.

Radiographic confirmation of this diagnosis requires a lateral view of the foot in maximum plantarflexion.[61] The navicular will not be ossified in the infant, so direct visualization of the talonavicular relationship is not possible. However, in true CVT a line drawn through the long axis of the talus will project plantarward to the ossific nucleus of the cuboid.

Treatment of CVT begins with passive manipulation and holding casts, which stretch the soft tissues. Traditionally, actual realignment of the bones by closed means was not expected. This deformity almost always was thought to require surgical correction. A casting regimen pioneered by Dobbs et al.[30] advises gradual reduction of the talonavicular joint by manipulations suggestive of a "reverse Ponseti" method. This regimen minimizes surgery, requiring only pin fixation of the talonavicular articulation with percutaneous heel cord release.

Orthoses usually are advised after surgery to passively maintain correction. No literature supports the use of one orthosis over another. FO, supramalleolar orthosis (SMO), and AFO designs that incorporate support of the medial longitudinal arch are acceptable.

Calcaneovalgus foot

This positional variation is a frequent finding among newborns and must be differentiated from CVT. The incidence of calcaneovalgus probably is much greater than the reported 1:1,000 live births,[106,108] as it ordinarily resolves spontaneously and therefore may never attract medical attention. It is common in the firstborn of young mothers and is thought to be the result of intrauterine packing. No inheritance patterns are known.

The forefoot is abducted and dorsiflexed with the dorsum lying against the anterior leg, and the heel is in calcaneus with valgus. In severe cases, the ankle cannot readily be plantarflexed much beyond neutral. Overall, however, the foot is flexible. The heel and forefoot can be passively corrected into varus, and the entire foot can be moved as a unit into plantarflexion/dorsiflexion through the ankle joint. This flexibility and the position of the heel in calcaneus rather than equinus distinguish calcaneovalgus from congenital vertical talus. Radiographs are not ordinarily necessary, but the maximum plantarflexion lateral view can be reassuring.

Kite[60] pointed out the association of external rotation contractures of the hips with calcaneovalgus foot. Wetzenstein[106] noted the association with flexible flatfoot in later life. Congenital posteromedial bowing of the tibia is sometimes associated. It initially can cause some diagnostic confusion because a normal foot can have the cosmetic appearance of calcaneovalgus when significant posteromedial bowing is present.

Treatment of the calcaneovalgus foot begins with passive stretching. If the ankle cannot be easily plantarflexed beyond neutral, retention taping, casting, or bracing is indicated. A molded AFO with ankle positioned in plantarflexion and the foot in adduction is often used. No literature supports one orthosis over another.

Flatfoot

"The term flat foot is commonly used to describe a nebulous mixture of anatomical variations as well as a small core of pathological conditions."[83] Unfortunately, not all authors make any rigorous distinction between normal variations and the pathological condition, which leads to confusion in the literature regarding this subject.

Flatfoot posture

Flatfoot in the newborn and toddler is physiologic. The toddler may pronate the foot to gain more stability, especially when learning to walk. This posture is very common in children and is considered by most to be an anatomical variant of ligamentous laxity that does not need treatment.[94]

The critical age for development of the longitudinal arch appears to be 6 years. The arch has some natural tendency to improve even beyond that age, as the prevalence of flatfoot is higher in 6-year-olds than in the 10-year-olds.[79,83,94,103]

In a large study of 2,300 children in a rural population of India, Rao and Joseph[79] noted that the prevalence of flatfoot was higher in the shod foot and was quite low in the unshod foot. Their study suggests that closed-toe shoes inhibit the development of the arch more than open-toed shoes or slippers. A study of 1,846 mature individuals by Sachithanandam and Joseph[84] showed that the prevalence of flatfoot was less in persons who began wearing shoes only after age 16 years. In a study of 1,851 Congolese children, Echarri and Forriol[33] showed that development of the medial arch of the foot is influenced by three factors: age, gender, and wearing shoes. This report is contrary to Kelsey's earlier observation that the type of footwear does not influence the occurrence of flatfoot.[57]

Flexible flatfoot

"Flexible flatfoot" describes the very common situation in which the foot has a normal longitudinal arch and normal heel alignment when suspended and not bearing weight but then collapses into a flat pronated posture with heel valgus during stance. Sometimes the flatfoot posture arises primarily through the arch itself, with pronounced flexibility and sag through the naviculocuneiform and tarsometatarsal joints. Usually there is instability through the subtalar and talonavicular joints, with the talus oriented more vertically than normally and with the calcaneus oriented in valgus. The flexibility often can be demonstrated by passively dorsiflexing the great toe,[49] which should improve the height of the arch. Additionally, if heel valgus and flattening of the arch correct to slight heel varus with a normal arch during tiptoe stance, the child probably has a flexible flatfoot.

Heel cord contracture occasionally is seen with flexible flatfoot. It may be a primary cause of the foot posture or may develop secondary to the persistent pronated, valgus heel position.

Treatment of asymptomatic flexible flatfoot is controversial.[87,93] No evidence convincingly shows that early treatment will lead to the eventual development of a stable longitudinal arch.[40,71,105] Many adults have flexible flatfoot without pain and without functional impairment.[43,94] Overall, there is agreement that treatment may be beneficial in symptomatic flatfoot, if only to relieve pain.

A large variety of orthoses are available to cushion the foot, support the longitudinal arch, support beneath the sustentaculum tali, support the transverse metatarsal arch, and resist heel valgus in an attempt to relieve foot pain and improve foot posture. Aharonson et al.[1] used a footprint apparatus to help measure the amount of abnormal pressure being applied through the middle weight-bearing area of the foot. Their method demonstrated that introduction of a wedge of proper height under the medial portion of the

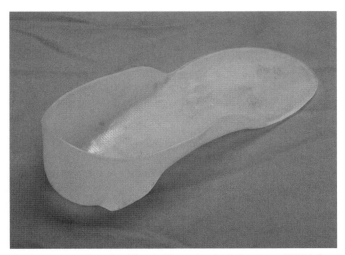

Fig. 35-8 University of California Biomechanics Laboratory (UCBL) foot orthosis.

heel brought about optimal correction of the hindfoot valgus and restored the normal longitudinal arch. Others have suggested use of the Blake inverted FP with various modifications and suggested the medial heel skive technique to enhance the pronation controlling features of FOs.[59] Helfet[45] recommended a heel cup. Jay et al.[53] developed a dynamic stabilizing innersole system that offsets the calcaneus into varus within a heel cup, thereby controlling hyperpronation. The custom-molded University of California Biomechanics Laboratory (UCBL) orthosis[48] incorporates a sustentaculum tali mold to directly resist collapse through the subtalar joint and a heel cup to control hindfoot valgus. Medial posting is added as needed. This orthosis extends distally beneath the metatarsals, so support for the transverse metatarsal arch can be added (Fig. 35-8).

A general approach to treatment of symptomatic flexible flatfoot should include passive Achilles tendon stretching exercises if the heel cords are tight. Initial orthotic intervention may be a semirigid arch support if heel valgus is not excessive. The materials from which the orthosis is constructed can be adjusted for more or less rigidity as desired. If heel valgus is significant, then a heel seat cup, with or without medial posting, can be very effective. In many cases, all components of the flexible flatfoot must be addressed simultaneously with the UCBL orthosis. To reiterate, these interventions are intended primarily to relieve pain. No evidence reported in the literature indicates that provision of an orthosis will assure the development of a permanent medial longitudinal arch.

Concepts for surgical management include tightening and raising the medial side of the foot, calcaneal osteotomies to realign the heel or lengthen the lateral side of the foot, and subtalar arthrodesis or arthroereisis to limit talocalcaneal instability. A description of surgical treatment is beyond the scope of this discussion.

Rigid flatfoot

The rigid flatfoot has no longitudinal arch when the foot is suspended, and the foot lacks normal flexibility on physical examination. This condition is uncommon in children and should prompt a search for an underlying systemic diagnosis or intrinsic pathologic condition, such as inflammatory arthritis, occult fractures, tumors, and abnormal tarsal bones including tarsal coalition. A thorough neurologic examination is an indispensable part of the evaluation, especially if the rigid flatfoot is unilateral.

Treatment of rigid flatfoot depends on the underlying diagnosis, and orthoses may or may not be a part of that treatment. In general, any orthosis is not expected to correct a rigid deformity. Use of orthoses therefore falls into the category of cushioning or accommodating the foot shape to relieve pain.

Tarsal coalition

Tarsal coalition is a frequent cause of rigid hindfoot, with or without flatfoot posture. The reported prevalence ranges from approximately 2% to as high as 6%.[44,46,95] Tarsal coalition is sometimes entirely asymptomatic, so the prevalence may be higher than reported. An autosomal dominant transmission has been postulated,[64] and at least one genetic defect has been isolated.[27] Associations with congenital and genetic conditions are common. There is no race preference.

The coalition involves partial or complete fusion of the tarsals. It may be fibrous, cartilaginous, or bony. The most common coalitions occur between calcaneus and navicular or between talus and calcaneus. Presumably the coalition begins in fetal life as a fibrous or cartilaginous connection and becomes symptomatic later as ossification of the affected bones occurs. Evidence for this process includes usual onset of symptoms at 8 to 12 years for calcaneonavicular coalitions and 12 to 16 years for talocalcaneal coalitions.[54,85]

Symptoms are highly variable but typically include activity-related midfoot pain. Tarsal coalition should be suspected whenever an adolescent experiences repeated ankle sprains.

The diagnosis is suggested when restriction of subtalar motion is found on physical examination. Typically the only flexibility comes through the joints surrounding the abnormal coalition itself and is very limited.

Localization of the specific coalition requires imaging. A lateral plain radiograph of the foot may show many clues, such as relative shortening of the neck of the talus, osteophytes at the talonavicular joint, or "anteater nose" elongation of the anterior process of the calcaneus.[69] The 45-degree oblique view of the foot usually is diagnostic for calcaneonavicular coalition. Talocalcaneal coalitions are more difficult to detect, and computerized tomography is recommended.[74] Magnetic resonance imaging will demonstrate possible fibrous coalitions.[35]

Results of nonoperative management of symptomatic tarsal coalition have been mixed. Initial treatment is aimed at alleviating pain. Nonsteroidal antiinflammatory drugs and injections of steroid and local anesthetic into the sinus tarsi are frequently advised. No orthosis will directly affect the coalition itself, but orthoses or casts can be used to minimize subtalar motion. For minor symptoms, a simple medial arch support or a medial heel wedge may suffice. Pain relief and modest improvement of position sometimes are possible with injection of the subtalar joint, manipulation of the foot under anesthesia, and immobilization in a short leg walking cast with the foot in neutral position for 3 to 6 weeks. Prolonged splintage for up to 6 months with a carefully molded FO is then advised. The FO should start by exerting only a mild inversional pressure against the deformity, to be increased as the patient is able to tolerate more pressure.[98] No outcome studies have documented the long-term effectiveness of orthoses in this condition.

The main indication for surgery is persistent pain. The type of surgery depends on the specific coalition, the age of the patient, and the absence or presence of degenerative changes in the tarsal joints. Full explanation of operative treatment is beyond the scope of this chapter.

Accessory navicular

Accessory bones are common in the foot. Symptomatic accessory navicular (AN) bone is a frequent finding, with a greater incidence in females. The AN lies on the medial plantar border of the navicular bone. It may be separate from the main navicular, may connect to the navicular by a synchondrosis, or may be fused to the navicular.[41] A portion of the posterior tibialis tendon inserts into the AN.

Asymptomatic AN may be mistaken for flatfoot, as the prominence of the AN fills the medial arch. Symptomatic AN is most often due to repetitive stress in young athletes. Pain at the AN itself may be accompanied by an element of posterior tibial tendinitis.

Nonoperative treatment is the mainstay and generally includes activity restrictions until symptoms are controlled. Cast immobilization is sometimes indicated for relief of especially acute symptoms. Orthoses are commonly prescribed as the patient gradually resumes activity. A soft navicular cookie or a heel seat cup with medial wedge may reduce the pull of the posterior tibialis. Rigid arch supports tend to exacerbate symptoms by increasing pressure on the AN. Treatment of the individual patient is empirical, and no literature supports the use of one orthosis over another. For chronic pain symptoms not relieved by orthoses, a simple excision of the ossicle can be curative.[10]

Cavus (and cavovarus) deformity

Cavus deformity is characterized by an excessively high arch resulting from a varus deformity of the hindfoot and a plantarflexed equinus deformity of the forefoot, especially the first metatarsal. This deformity almost always is secondary to an underlying neurologic dysfunction in the spinal axis or the peripheral nerves. Care must be taken to ensure accurate diagnosis of potential underlying causes.

Shoe modifications and orthoses are rarely effective in modifying the deformity. The cavus is invariably rigid and progresses according to the underlying neurologic condition. Additionally, sensory deficits often are present and limit any bracing opportunities.

The usefulness of orthoses is limited to accommodation of the deformity for relief of pain and protection of the soft tissues. An AFO prevent recurrent ankle sprains. Plantar callosities and symptoms due to abnormal pressure may be relieved by use of an arch support or metatarsal pad.[2] Rocker modifications of the shoe sole can be helpful substitutes for loss of ankle and midfoot motion. They are customized to the individual patient for relief of symptoms and preservation of function. No meaningful outcome studies of orthotic management are available.

Kohler disorder

Kohler disorder of the tarsal navicular is an uncommon but characteristic source of medial midfoot pain in children 4 to 7 years old. The etiology is unknown but presumably is related to a combination of mechanical stress at the time of ossification and vascular compromise with elements of avascular necrosis. Radiographic changes in the tarsal navicular mimic the avascular, fragmentation, and regeneration phases of Legg-Calvé-Perthes disorder of the hip. The condition is self-limited. Final healing almost always includes some minor diminution of the size of the navicular compared with the uninvolved contralateral side.

Only nonoperative treatment is indicated, with activity restrictions and selective use of cast immobilization being recommended.[16] Various orthoses have been suggested in an attempt to relieve pain and keep these young patients active, but no literature supports one orthosis over another. In general, the approach is support of the arch and decrease of stresses across the posterior tibialis and tarsal navicular. Soft and semirigid arch supports can be tried, as can heel seat cups, all with the goal of relieving pain. Rigid appliances may not be tolerated. No outcome studies suggest that any treatment method will affect the ultimate size or shape of the reossified tarsal navicular.

Bunion (hallux valgus)

Bunions in the child or adolescent are quite different than the same condition in middle-aged adults, both in etiology and in treatment. In young persons, a positive family history is frequent (about 60%). Bilaterality is the rule. The condition is nine times more common in females than in males, and it presents psychosocial problems for many. The etiology is somewhat controversial and includes various conditions such as metatarsus primus varus, ligamentous laxity, hypermobile forefoot, pronation of the foot, pes planus, structural anomalies of the first metatarsal head, overtreatment of MA, and excessively long metatarsals. Although ill-fitting shoes do not cause hallux valgus, they can aggravate bunion formation from pressure over the medial side of the first metatarsal head.

Evaluation of the patient should include a general medical history and physical examination, seeking evidence of generalized ligament laxity with or without associated genetic conditions. Directed examination of the foot usually shows a swelling over the medial aspect of the great toe metatarsophalangeal joint; but heavy callous formation, joint rigidity, and inflammation of the adult bunion are seldom seen in children. Flexible flatfoot and the widened forefoot of metatarsus primus varus are common in young people. Pronation of the great toe and overlapping of the second toe are less frequent than in affected adults.

Nonoperative treatment usually is directed to relief of shoe pressure on the first metatarsophalangeal joint. Shoe recommendations include a more roomy toe box, but most fashion-conscious adolescents likely will not wear shoes very different from those of their peers. FOs directed toward control of any associated flexible flatfoot can be helpful in relieving symptoms, but no outcome studies show whether these orthoses might change the natural history of the disorder. Similarly, use of nighttime hallux valgus splints

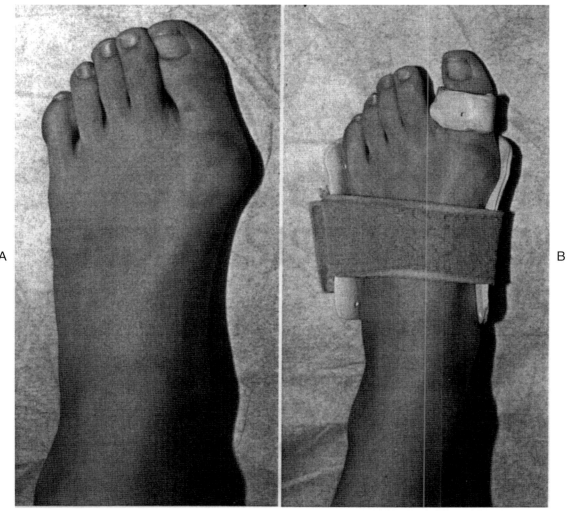

Fig. 35-9 A, Foot with hallux valgus and bunion deformity. **B,** Groiso splint demonstrating a medially directed force at the great toe and an improved foot shape.

seems to help maintain flexibility and relieve pain (Fig. 35-9). Groiso[42] presented a series of patients in which a custom-molded splint was effective in delaying or stopping the progression of deviation of the great toe and sometimes even completely corrected the deformity.

More than 200 surgical procedures for treatment of hallux valgus have been described. Most authors recommend conservative management until skeletal maturity because of the high risk of recurrence in growing children.[6,39,88,91] A possible exception is the double osteotomy of the first metatarsal advocated by Peterson and Newman.[73] Full discussion of operative treatment is beyond the scope of this chapter.

Freiberg infraction

In 1914 Freiberg used the term *infraction* to describe this painful condition of the metatarsal head, indicating that he believed the etiology was trauma.[38] The cause actually is unknown, but trauma, repetitive stress, and vascular compromise all have been proposed.

The condition presents as pain and swelling directly at the involved joint, most classically at the second metatarsophalangeal joint. The other metatarsals are involved less frequently. Symptoms usually begin in adolescence, more often in females.

Radiographically, Freiberg infraction includes mixed sclerotic and lucent changes in the involved metatarsal head, with flattening of the articular surface. Most often the process is self-limited, healing with a satisfactory joint surface. Occasionally Freiberg infraction progresses to subchondral bone collapse, arthritis, and osteophyte formation, resulting in a painful rigid metatarsophalangeal joint.

Nonoperative treatment attempts to redistribute weight across the forefoot and limit stresses across the involved metatarsal head. Metatarsal pads and a variety of FOs and shoe sole modifications can be effective for pain relief, but no comparative studies document any effect on the ultimate outcome.

Operative treatments are many, depending on the stage and severity of the disorder. Antegrade drilling of the avascular segment early during the course may promote ingrowth of new blood supply. Metatarsal osteotomy may relieve weight-bearing stresses. Cheilectomy and joint debridement are sometimes indicated to improve range of motion, and resection arthroplasty may serve as a salvage procedure.

Complete description of surgical options is beyond the scope of this discussion.

Foot gear/shoes

Determining which type of shoe is best for a child must take into account the demands of the modern environment along with the growth and development of the foot and the child. Numerous studies suggest that forefoot deformities such as hallux valgus and progressive narrowing of the exterior portion of the foot are more frequent in the shod foot.[34,47] A normal arch will develop without the wearing of shoes.[94] In a prominent comparative study of shod and unshod feet in a Chinese population in 1953, Sim-Fook and Hodgson[90] found that the unrestricted foot in its natural form was mobile and flexible without static deformities, whereas the foot restricted by use of stockings and shoes was altered and had static deformities, leading to patient complaints. It may be appropriate to state that, whenever possible, wearing of shoes should be avoided in childhood to preserve and strengthen natural functions of the feet. A normal foot does not need support from a shoe. However, the foot does require protection from lacerations, punctures, and inclement weather. The commercial shoe is the standard means of providing this protection. Well-made shoes serve this function while minimizing the inevitable foot changes. Merchandising "corrective shoes" is harmful to the child, is expensive for the family, and discredits the medical profession.[32]

Suggestions for a good shoe:

1. Proper fit cannot be overemphasized. The shoe should simulate as closely as possible the shape of the foot it covers. The shoe should fit snugly around the heel, allow adequate width across the ball of the foot, and have at least 5 to 7 mm between the end of the shoe and the longest toe.[52] Pedorthists currently measure the length and width of a child's foot using a Ritz stick, with the child standing and bearing weight on both feet. The study by Wenger et al.[104] emphasizes that growing children should have their shoe size checked frequently.
2. Proper material is important. Porous materials should be used because they permit aeration of the foot and reduce irritable dermatological conditions of the foot. Leather is one of the finest materials for good shoemaking because of its flexibility, porosity, and ability to absorb moisture.[52] Canvas also works well.
3. Soft soles are fine.
4. Heel height should be low or moderate. The cosmetic benefits of high-heeled shoes should not be directed to children.
5. Arch supports are not necessary.

Bowleg and knock-knee

Bowleg (genu varum) and knock-knee (genu valgum) are common in infants and children and most often are a part of normal development. The normal sequence initially includes lateral tibial bowing in early infancy. Later in infancy, physiological bowing involves both the femur and the tibia. Many children have concomitant internal tibial torsion at the infant/toddler stage. The bowing and internal tibial torsion are cosmetically additive, making the lower limb posture appear extreme, especially to concerned parents. The bowing gradually changes to knock-knee between 18 months and 3 years of age. This valgus in turn decreases to 5 or 6 degrees by about 7 years of age.[86]

Evaluation should include a comprehensive history, focusing on family growth patterns and diet. The physical examination should include height and weight percentiles, joint laxity assessment, and rotational profile. Assessment of the angular alignment, especially for serial documentation, is best done with the patient standing and the patellae aligned straight ahead. The thigh–leg (femoral-tibial) angle, normally less than 20 degrees, should be recorded. For genu varum, the intercondylar distance at the knees is measured while the child stands with medial malleoli touching together at the ankles. For genu valgum, the ankle intermalleolar distance while knees touch is measured. These distances remain less than 10 cm in most normal children. Significant differences from the expected physiological alignment pattern are cause for concern, as are asymmetry, stature below the fifth percentile, and other musculoskeletal abnormalities.

Anteroposterior standing radiographs of the lower limbs are indicated when there is suspicion of pathologic processes. Radiographic characteristics of normal physiological variations should include symmetrical deformity, present in both the femoral and tibial segments, equally distributed at the proximal and distal ends of each long bone. Ossification centers should be normal for age. Physeal plates should be of normal thickness with smooth borders. The diaphyseal cortex of the femur and tibia on the concave side should be thickened in comparison to the convex cortices.

Physiological bowleg and knock-knee represent, by definition, normal growth. Treatment interventions are generally not indicated. The key element in management is recognition of pathology that does need direct treatment. Reassessment of the patient at 4- to 6-month intervals often is necessary to ensure that alignment is progressing according to the expected pattern. Severe bowleg observed in infants, especially those who are overweight and who are early walkers, may subsequently prove to be the precursor to tibia vara (Blount disease). Recognition and treatment of that special situation are discussed in the following section.

Tibia vara (Blount disease)

Blount's classic review of tibia vara was published in 1937.[15] Tibia vara characteristically presents as a progressive bowing deformity, resulting from disordered growth of the proximal medial physis and metaphysis of the tibia.[63] Infantile (early-onset) and adolescent (late-onset) forms are described. Only the infantile type is discussed here; orthotic management for adolescent tibia vara is ineffective.

Children with tibia vara initially present with bowlegs that do not spontaneously improve within the expected physiological envelope. Most children are obese, and many are early walkers. Frequent associated findings include ligament laxity, a lateral thrust at the knee in stance, and a palpable "beak" at the proximal medial tibia. The occurrence is greater in children of African descent. Tibia vara is rare in many parts of the world. Left untreated, the deformity progresses to include growth arrest of the proximal medial tibia and lateral knee instability. A corresponding deformity of the distal femur may develop.

Radiographically, infantile tibia vara progresses through a series of stages that generally correspond to patient age, as described by Langenskiold and Riska.[63] The diagnosis cannot be confirmed without radiographic signs of fragmentation of the metaphysis and failure of further development of the proximal tibial epiphysis. These radiographic findings are seldom present before age 18 to 24 months.

The metaphyseal–diaphyseal angle of the proximal tibia[65] is useful for distinguishing between physiological bowing and tibia vara in young toddlers before Langenskiold changes are apparent. This radiographic measurement has been refined in several studies[17,37] and has been used to evaluate the deformity of the distal femur.[66] When the metaphyseal–diaphyseal angle of the proximal tibia is greater than 16 degrees, there is a 95% chance that the deformity will progress to obvious tibia vara.

Treatment depends on the age of the patient and the radiographic stage of the disease. Orthoses are recommended for treatment of patients younger than 3 years.[78,82,109] This approximately corresponds to radiographic stages I and II of Langenskiold[63] and includes children whose radiographs show a tibial metaphyseal–diaphyseal angle greater than 16 degrees varus even without obvious Langenskiold changes. Physeal damage at this point is generally reversible.

Bracing aims to provide a force at the medial side of the proximal thigh and medial malleolus with an opposing lateral support at the knee. Control of flexion of the knee and rotation of the leg is desirable. Sometimes pressure pads are mounted on swivels so that they rotate with the skin, which increases patient toleration of the orthosis. A classic Blount brace, an A-frame brace, or a specifically constructed KAFO can be used. Good results with an elastic Blount KAFO introduced by Supan and Mazur[96] (Fig. 35-10) have

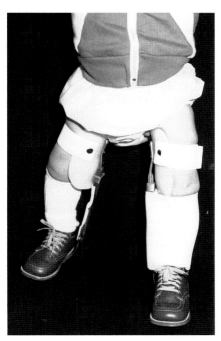

Fig. 35-10 KAFO orthoses designed for cases of severe bowleg and early-onset tibia vara (Blount disorder). Here the elastic strap on the child's right has been removed to show construction of the upright.

been reported.[78,82] The design consists of a medial thigh cuff that extends past the medial tibial plateau, a single medial upright with drop-locking knee joints from which an elastic strap wraps around the upper calf, and tibial growth extensions attached to a shoe or footplate through a free-motion ankle joint.

Beginning at about age 3 years or when a physeal bar has presented on the medial aspect of the proximal tibia (Langenskiold stage III), treatment invariably requires surgery. Multiple surgeries usually are required to correct the angular, rotational, and length problems.

Tibial bowing

Lateral tibial bowing

Lateral tibial bowing is a normal physiological variation during the first year of life. It reaches its maximum angulation between 18 and 36 months, in association with physiological bowing of the entire lower extremity. Treatment is observation to differentiate this condition from pathologic conditions, especially infantile tibia vara.

Anterior bowing

Anterior bowing of the tibia may be associated with an absent or hypoplastic fibula. Dimpling of the skin of the anterior leg usually identifies more fibular involvement. This condition is commonly called either *fibular hemimelia* or *postaxial hemimelia* and includes a spectrum of abnormalities of the lateral aspect of the limb. International Organization for Standardization (ISO) terminology incorporates a description of the components, which can be quite variable. The main problem here is tibial shortening, which may require correction by a contralateral epiphyseodesis or a limb-lengthening procedure. No specific orthotic recommendations are available.

Posteromedial bowing

Posteromedial bowing is associated with a calcaneus or calcaneovalgus foot deformity, triceps weakness, extension contracture of the ankle, and anisomelia.[26,70] Spontaneous improvement of the angulation occurs with growth, and operative correction should be delayed. Limb shortening is a problem and often is progressive.

Initial treatment is nonoperative and generally consists of passive stretching to relax the tight anterolateral soft tissues at the ankle. Casting and bracing with custom-molded AFOs are sometimes recommended, but no outcome studies or significant published series document the effectiveness of these treatments.

Anterolateral bowing

Anterolateral bowing of the tibia virtually always represents the mildest expression of pseudarthrosis of the tibia.[18] As such, it should be considered a precursor to frank pseudarthrosis. Anterolateral bowing, with or without pseudarthrosis, is associated with neurofibromatosis in more than 50% of patients.[25,102] One notable exception to these generalizations is the anterolateral bowing associated with duplication of the great toe, which seems to have a more benign natural history.[19]

As soon as this condition is recognized, support of the limb with a cast or orthosis is indicated to prevent the fracture that may never heal. For the young infant, orthotic management begins with a nonarticulated plastic KAFO. As the infant begins to stand and walk, the addition of an anterior molded panel to create a total contact orthosis is recommended. The older infant and young child are treated with an articulated KAFO, whereas a high AFO may suffice in the older child.

Although initial brace management is universally recommended, no literature documents that bracing will either correct the deformity or prevent fracture over the long term. In most cases, fracture progresses to frank pseudarthrosis, and subsequent surgical management can be difficult and frustrating. At the very least, it seems prudent to brace this deformity, even if bracing serves only to delay the inevitable until associated diagnoses are clarified and the child is large enough, thus facilitating surgery.

Upper extremity deformities

The functional imperatives for the upper limb are different than those for the lower limb. Manual dexterity is a primary goal in the treatment of congenital and acquired conditions of the upper limb. For congenital disorders, hand and finger function often is better without than with orthotic support. Orthoses are generally used very early in the overall management algorithm, to obtain or to maintain position of the hand in space. Over the long term, surgical releases or realignment procedures supplant orthoses. Long-term bracing is not common.

Radial dysplasia (radial clubhand)

Radial dysplasia is a failure of longitudinal formation of the preaxial side of the upper limb. The thumb, radial side of the carpus, and radius may be hypoplastic or completely absent, and the soft-tissue deficiency parallels the skeletal deficiency. The degree of involvement ranges from thumb hypoplasia with normal carpus and radius to complete absence of the radius. Radial dysplasia has been classified by Bayne and Klug,[9] as further modified by James et al.[51]

An injury to the apical ectodermal ridge during upper limb development probably causes radial dysplasia. Although many factors have been postulated, the actual insult leading to the developmental failure is not known. The condition is rare, occurring in 1:30,000 to 1:100,000 infants.[9] It is commonly associated with other syndromes and malformations, such as thrombocytopenia absent radius (TAR), Holt-Oram syndrome, and the VACTERL association (vertebral anomalies, imperforate anus, cardiovascular anomalies, tracheoesophageal fistula, renal anomalies, and limb bud failures). The inheritance mirrors those various conditions. Isolated radial aplasia generally is sporadic.

Treatment options address the maldirected and unstable wrist, the digital weakness, and the lack of thumb opposition. Most children with this deformity function well, although the cosmesis of the hand at approximately a right angle to the forearm is unsettling. Considerable discussion and counseling are necessary before determining whether the child should be treated surgically, because function through a wrist that is radially deviated but flexible may be better than that with a centralized but stiff wrist.

Management of radial dysplasia usually begins shortly after birth and includes occupational therapy and splinting or serial casting. The initial goals include stretching of the contracted radial soft tissues and passive centralization of the wrist. Various orthoses have been designed.[21,58] The most commonly used orthosis is an orthoplast or similar thermal-labile plastic splint that can be successively adjusted into more ulnar deviation as the child grows. No long-term studies or outcome studies recommend one specific orthosis in preference to another.

Surgical management of the various components of this disorder is common but is beyond the scope of this discussion.

Ulnar dysplasia (ulnar clubhand)

Ulnar longitudinal deficiency is less common than radial dysplasia, with an estimated incidence of 1:100,000 infants.[13] Most cases are sporadic. However, as with radial dysplasia, the condition may occur with other identified inheritable syndromes. Classification systems based on deficiencies in the elbow and forearm[8] or on the hand malformations[22] are available.

Ulnar dysplasia is not associated with major nervous system abnormalities. Children with this condition typically have normal intelligence and generally adapt and function well. Early occupational therapy, augmented with serial casting or splinting, is variably advised. No long-term studies support the use of any particular orthosis.

Summary

A variety of the more common congenital and acquired nontraumatic deformities of the extremities in children have been discussed. Facilitation of normal growth and development is a common goal in the management of these congenital and acquired disorders. Orthoses traditionally have been used in many conditions, either in preparation for definitive surgery or for maintenance of correction gained through surgery. Orthoses have been used to support a limb while awaiting expected improvement with growth. Sometimes the orthosis is itself the definitive management of the condition. Long-term reviews and prospective outcome studies of the use of these orthoses are conspicuously lacking. Opportunities abound for future important research.

References

1. Aharonson Z, Arcan M, Steinback TV: Foot-ground pressure pattern of flexible flatfoot in children, with and without correction of calcaneovalgus, *Clin Orthop Relat Res* 278:177–182, 1992.
2. Alexander IJ, Johnson KA: Assessment and management of pes cavus in Charcot-Marie-Tooth disease, *Clin Orthop Relat Res* 246:273–281, 1989.
3. Alexander MA: Orthotics, adapted seating, and assistive devices. In Molnar G, editor: *Pediatric rehabilitation: rehabilitation medicine library*, Baltimore, 1985, Williams & Wilkins.
4. Allen WD, Weiner DS, Riley PM: The treatment of rigid metatarsus adductovarus with the use of a new hinged adjustable shoe orthosis, *Foot Ankle* 14:450–454, 1993.
5. Aronson J, Puskarich CL: Deformity and disability from treated clubfoot, *J Pediatr Orthop* 10:642–647, 1990.
6. Ball J, Sullivan JA: Treatment of the juvenile bunion by Mitchell osteotomy, *Orthopaedics* 8:1249–1252, 1985.
7. Barker S, Chesney D, Miedzybrodzka Z, Maffulli N: Genetics and epidemiology of idiopathic congenital talipes equinovarus, *J Pediatr Orthop* 23:265–272, 2003.

8. Bayne LG: Ulnar club hand (ulnar deficiencies). In Green DP, editor: *Operative hand surgery*, ed 3, New York, 1993, Churchill Livingstone.

9. Bayne LG, Klug MS: Long-term review of the surgical treatment of radial deficiencies, *J Hand Surg Am* 12:169–179, 1987.

10. Bennett GL, Weiner DS, Leighley B: Surgical treatment of symptomatic accessory tarsal navicular, *J Pediatr Orthop* 10:445–449, 1990.

11. Bensahel H, Guillaume A, Czukonyi Z, Desgrippes Y: Results of physical therapy for idiopathic clubfoot: a long-term follow-up study, *J Pediatr Orthop* 10:189–192, 1990.

12. Berg EE: A reappraisal of metatarsus adductus and skewfoot, *J Bone Joint Surg Am* 68:1185–1196, 1986.

13. Birch-Jensen A: *Congenital deformities of the upper extremities*, Copenhagen, 1950, Ejnar Munksgaard Forlag.

14. Bleck EE: Metatarsus adductus: classification and relationship to outcomes of treatment, *J Pediatr Orthop* 3:2–9, 1983.

15. Blount WP: Tibia vara, osteochondrosis deformans tibiae, *J Bone Joint Surg* 19:1, 1937.

16. Borges JLP, Guille JT, Bowen JR: Kohler's bone disease of the tarsal navicular, *J Pediatr Orthop* 15:596–598, 1995.

17. Bowen RE, Dorey FJ, Moseley CF: Relative tibial and femoral varus as a predictor of progression of varus deformities of the lower limbs in young children, *J Pediatr Orthop* 22:105–111, 2002.

18. Boyd HB: Pathology and natural history of congenital pseudarthrosis of the tibia, *Clin Orthop Relat Res* 166:5–13, 1982.

19. Bressers MMFM, Castelein RM: Anterolateral tibial bowing and duplication of the hallux: a rare but distinct entity with good prognosis, *J Pediatr Orthop B* 10:153–157, 2001.

20. Browne D: Talipes equinovarus, *Lancet* 2:969–974, 1934.

21. Butts DE, Goldberg MJ: Congenital absence of the radius: the occupational therapist and a new orthosis, *Am J Occup Ther* 31:95–100, 1977.

22. Cole RJ, Manske PR: Classification of ulnar deficiency according to the thumb and first web, *J Hand Surg Am* 22:479–488, 1997.

23. Cook DA, Breed AL, Cook T, et al: Observer variability in the radiographic measurement and classification of metatarsus adductus, *J Pediatr Orthop* 12:86–89, 1992.

24. Crawford AH, Gabriel KR: Foot and ankle problems, *Orthop Clin North Am* 18:649–666, 1987.

25. Crawford AH, Schorry EK: Neurofibromatosis update, *J Pediatr Orthop* 26:413–423, 2006.

26. De Maio F, Corsi A, Roggini M, et al: Congenital unilateral posteromedial bowing of the tibia and fibula: insights regarding pathogenesis from prenatal pathology. A case report, *J Bone Joint Surg Am* 87:1601–1605, 2005.

27. Dixon ME, Armstrong P, Stevens DB, Bamshad M: Identical mutations in NOG can cause either tarsal/carpal coalition syndrome or proximal symphalangism, *Genet Med* 3:349–353, 2001.

28. Dobbs MB, Gurnett CA, Robarg J, et al: Variable hand and foot abnormalities in family with congenital vertical talus and CDMP-1 gene mutation, *J Orthop Res* 23:1490–1494, 2005.

29. Dobbs MB, Nunley R, Schoenecker PL: Long-term follow-up of patients with clubfoot treated with extensive soft-tissue release, *J Bone Joint Surg Am* 88:986–996, 2006.

30. Dobbs MB, Purcell DB, Nunley R, Morcuende JA: Early results of a new method of treatment for idiopathic congenital vertical talus, *J Bone Surg Am* 88:1192–1200, 2006.

31. Dobbs MB, Rudzki JR, Purcell DB, et al: Factors predictive of outcome after use of the Ponseti method for the treatment of idiopathic clubfeet, *J Bone Joint Surg Am* 86:22–27, 2004.

32. Driano AN, Staheli L, Staheli LT: Psychosocial development and corrective shoewear use in childhood [foot], *J Pediatr Orthop* 18:346–349, 1998.

33. Echarri JJ, Forriol F: The development in footprint morphology in 1851 Congolese children from urban and rural areas, and the relationship between this and wearing shoes, *J Pediatr Orthop B* 12:141–146, 2003.

34. Elmslie M: Prevention of foot deformities in children, *Lancet* 2:1260–1263, 1939.

35. Emery KH, Bisset GS, Johnson ND, Nunan PJ: Tarsal coalition: a blinded comparison of MRI and CT, *Pediatr Radiol* 28:612–616, 1998.

36. Farsetti P, Weinstein S, Ponseti IV: The long-term functional and radiographic outcomes of untreated and non-operatively treated metatarsus adductus, *J Bone Joint Surg Am* 76:257–265, 1994.

37. Feldman MD, Schoenecker PL: Use of the metaphyseal-diaphyseal angle in the evaluation of bowed legs, *J Bone Joint Surg Am* 75:1602–1609, 1993.

38. Freiberg A: Infraction of the second metatarsal bone: a typical injury, *Surg Gynecol Obstet* 19:191, 1914.

39. Geissele AE, Stanton RP: Surgical treatment of adolescent hallux valgus, *J Pediatr Orthop* 10:642–648, 1990.

40. Gould N, Moreland M, Alvarez R, et al: Development of the child's arch, *Foot Ankle* 9:241–245, 1989.

41. Grogan DP, Gasser SI, Ogden JA: The painful accessory navicular: a clinical and histopathological study, *Foot Ankle* 10:164–169, 1989.

42. Groiso JA: Juvenile hallux valgus. A conservative approach to treatment, *J Bone Joint Surg Am* 74:1367–1374, 1992.

43. Harris RI, Beath T: Hypermobile flat-foot with short tendo Achilles, *J Bone Joint Surg Am* 30:116–140, 1948.

44. Harris RI, Beath T: Etiology of peroneal spastic flatfoot, *J Bone Joint Surg Br* 30:624, 1948.

45. Helfet AJ: A new way of treating flat feet in children, *Lancet* 1:262–264, 1956.

46. Herschel H, Von Ronnen JR: The occurrence of calcaneonavicular synosteosis in pes valgus contractus, *J Bone Joint Surg Am* 32:280–282, 1950.

47. Hoffman P: Conclusions drawn from a comparative study of the feet of barefooted and shoe-wearing peoples, *Am J Orthop Surg* 3:105–136, 1905.

48. Inman VT: UC-BL dual-axis ankle-control system and UC-BL shoe insert: biomechanical considerations. In: *Biomechanics Laboratory, University of California, San Francisco and Berkeley, Technical Report 56*, San Francisco, 1969, The Laboratory.

49. Jack EA: Naviculo-cuneiform fusion in the treatment of flat foot, *J Bone Joint Surg Br* 35:75–82, 1953.

50. Jacobs JE: Metatarsus varus and hip dysplasia, *Clin Orthop Relat Res* 16:203–213, 1960.

51. James MA, McCarroll HR Jr, Manske PR: The spectrum of radial longitudinal deficiency: a modified classification, *J Hand Surg Am* 24:1145–1155, 1999.

52. Janisse DJ: The art and science of fitting shoes, *Foot Ankle* 13:257–262, 1992.

53. Jay RM, Schoenhaus HD, Seymour C, Gamble S: The Dynamic Stabilizing Innersole System (DSIS): the management of hyperpronation in children, *J Foot Ankle Surg* 34:124–131, 1995.

54. Jayakumar S, Cowell HR: Rigid flatfoot, *Clin Orthop Relat Res* 122:77–84, 1977.

55. Karol LA, Concha MC, Johnston CE: Gait analysis and muscle strength in children with surgically treated clubfeet, *J Pediatr Orthop* 17:790–795, 1997.

56. Katz K, David R, Soudry M: Below-knee plaster cast for the treatment of metatarsus adductus, *J Pediatr Orthop* 19:49–50, 2006.

57. Kelsey JLP: Disorders of the extremities. In Kelsey JLP, editor: *Epidemiology of musculoskeletal disorders*, New York, 1982, Oxford University Press.

58. Kennedy SM: Neoprene wrist brace for correction of radial club hand in children, *J Hand Ther* 9:387–390, 1996.

59. Kirby KA: The medial heel skive technique. Improving pronation control in foot orthoses, *J Am Podiatr Med Assoc* 82:177–188, 1992.

60. Kite JH: The treatment of flatfeet in small children, *Postgrad Med* 15:75–78, 1954.

61. Kumar SJ, Cowell HR, Ramsey PL: Vertical and oblique talus, *Instruct Course Lect* 31:235–251, 1982.

62. Kumar SJ, MacEwen GD: The incidence of hip dysplasia with metatarsus adductus, *Clin Orthop Relat Res* 164:234–235, 1982.

63. Langenskiold A, Riska EB: Tibia vara (osteochondrosis deformans tibiae): a survey of seventy-one cases, *J Bone Joint Surg Am* 46:1405–1420, 1964.

64. Leonard MA: The inheritance of tarsal coalition and its relationship to spastic flat foot, *J Bone Joint Surg Br* 56:520–526, 1974.

65. Levine AM, Drennan JC: Physiological bowing and tibia vara. The metaphyseal-diaphyseal angle in the measurement of bowleg deformities, *J Bone Joint Surg Am* 64:1158–1163, 1982.

66. McCarthy JJ, Betz RR, Kim A, et al: Early radiographic differentiation of infantile tibia vara from physiologic bowing using the femoral-tibial ratio, *J Pediatr Orthop* 21:545–548, 2001.

67. Molnar GE, Kaminer RK: Growth and development. In Molnar G, editor: *Pediatric rehabilitation: rehabilitation medicine library*, Baltimore, 1985, Williams & Wilkins.

68. Napiontek M: Skewfoot, *J Pediatr Orthop* 1:130–133, 2002.

69. Oestreich AE, Mize WA, Crawford AH, Morgan RC Jr: The "anteater nose": a direct sign of calcaneonavicular coalition on the lateral radiograph, *J Pediatr Orthop* 7:709–711, 1987.

70. Pappas AM: Congenital posteromedial bowing of the tibia and fibula, *J Pediatr Orthop* 4:525–531, 1984.

71. Penneau K, Lutter LD, Winter RD: Pes planus: radiographic changes with foot orthoses and shoes, *Foot Ankle* 2:299–303, 1982.

72. Peterson HA: Skewfoot (forefoot adduction with heel valgus), *J Pediatr Orthop* 6:24–30, 1986.

73. Peterson HA, Newman SR: Adolescent bunion deformity treated with double osteotomy and longitudinal pin fixation of the first ray, *J Pediatr Orthop* 13:80–84, 1993.

74. Pineda C, Resnick D, Greenway G: Diagnosis of tarsal coalition with computed tomography, *Clin Orthop Relat Res* 208:282–288, 1986.

75. Ponseti IV: Treatment. In Ponseti IV, editor: *Congenital clubfoot: fundamentals for treatment*, Oxford, 1996, Oxford University Press.

76. Ponseti IV: The Ponseti technique for correction of congenital clubfoot, *J Bone Joint Surg Am* 84:1889–1890, 2002.

77. Ponseti IV, Becker JR: Congenital metatarsus adductus: the results of treatment, *J Bone Joint Surg Am* 48:702–711, 1966.

78. Raney EM, Topoleski TA, Yaghoubian R, et al: Orthotic treatment of infantile tibia vara, *J Pediatr Orthop* 18:670–674, 1998.

79. Rao UB, Joseph B: The influence of footwear on the prevalence of flat foot: a survey of 2300 children, *J Bone Joint Surg Br* 74:525–527, 1992.

80. Reimann I, Werner HH: Congenital metatarsus varus. A suggestion for a possible mechanism and relation to other foot deformities, *Clin Orthop Relat Res* 110:223–226, 1975.

81. Richards BS, Johnston CE, Wilson H: Nonoperative clubfoot treatment using the French physical therapy method, *J Pediatr Orthop* 25:98–102, 2005.

82. Richards BS, Katz DE, Sims JB: Effectiveness of brace treatment in early infantile Blount's disease, *J Pediatr Orthop* 18:374–380, 1998.

83. Rose GK, Welton EA, Marshall T: The diagnosis of flat foot in the child, *J Bone Joint Surg Br* 67:71–78, 1985.

84. Sachithanandam V, Joseph B: The influence of footwear on the prevalence of flat foot. A survey of 1846 skeletally mature persons, *J Bone Joint Surg Br* 77:25–257, 1995.

85. Salomao O, Napoli MM, De Carvalho Junior AE, et al: Talocalcaneal coalition: diagnosis and surgical management, *Foot Ankle* 13:251–256, 1992.

86. Salenius P, Vankka E: The development of the tibiofemoral angle in children, *J Bone Joint Surg Am* 57:259–261, 1975.

87. Scheffler NM, Driggs GK, Kitchen BF, et al: Letters to the editor, *J Bone Joint Surg Am* 72:470–473, 1990.

88. Scranton PE, Zuckerman JD: Bunion surgery in adolescents: results of surgical treatment, *J Pediatr Orthop* 4:39–43, 1984.

89. Shrimpton AE, Levinsohn EM, Yozawitz JM, et al: A HOX gene mutation in a family with isolated congenital vertical talus and Charcot-Marie-Tooth disease, *Am J Hum Genet* 75:92–96, 2004.

90. Sim-Fook LR, Hodgson AR: A comparison of foot forms among the non-shoe and shoe-wearing Chinese population, *J Bone Joint Surg Am* 40:1058–1062, 1958.

91. Simmonds FA, Menelaus MB: Hallux valgus in adolescents, *J Bone Joint Surg Br* 42:761–768, 1960.

92. Smith JT, Bleck EE, Gamble JG, et al: Simple method of documenting metatarsus adductus, *J Pediatr Orthop* 11:679–680, 1991.

93. Smith MA: Flat feet in children, *BMJ* 301:942–943, 1990.

94. Staheli LT, Chew DE, Corbett M: The longitudinal arch. A survey of eight hundred and eighty-two feet in normal children and adults, *J Bone Joint Surg Am* 69:426–428, 1987.

95. Stormont DM, Peterson HA: The relative incidence of tarsal coalition, *Clin Orthop Relat Res* 181:28–36, 1983.

96. Supan TJ, Mazur JM: Orthotic correction of Blount's disease, *Clin Prosthet Orthot* 9:3–6, 1985.

97. Tachdjian MO, Congenital metatarsus varus. In Tachdjian MO, editor: Tachdjian's pediatric orthopaedics, vol IV, edition 2, Philadelphia, 1990, WB Saunders.

98. Tax HR: Regional orthopaedic problems of the lower extremity. In Tax HR, editor: *Podopediatrics*, ed 2, Baltimore, 1985, Williams & Wilkins.

99. Thacker MM, Scher DM, Sala DA, et al: Use of the foot abduction orthosis following Ponseti casts: is it essential?, *J Pediatr Orthop* 25:225–228, 2005.

100. Townes PL, Dehart GK Jr, Hecht R, et al: Trisomy 13-15 in a male infant, *J Pediatr* 60:528–532, 1962.

101. Uchida IA, Lesis AJ, Bowman JM, et al: A case of double trisomy: trisomy no. 18 and triple-X, *J Pediatr* 60:498–502, 1962.

102. Vitale MG, Guha A, Skaggs DL: Orthopaedic manifestations of neurofibromatosis in children: an update, *Clin Orthop Relat Res* 401:107–118, 2002.

103. Volpon JB: Footprint analysis during the growth period, *J Pediatr Orthop* 14:83–85, 1994.

104. Wenger DR, Mauldin D, Morgan D, et al: Foot growth rate in children age one to six years, *Foot Ankle* 3:207–210, 1983.

105. Wenger DR, Mauldin D, Speck G, et al: Corrective shoes and inserts as treatment for flexible flatfoot in infants and children, *J Bone Joint Surg Am* 71:800–810, 1989.

106. Wetzenstein H: The significance of congenital pes calcaneo-valgus in the origin of pes plano-valgus in childhood. Preliminary report, *Acta Orthop Scand* 30:64–72, 1960.

107. Wynne-Davies R: Family studies and the cause of congenital clubfoot, talipes equinovarus, talipes calcaneovalgus and metatarsus varus, *J Bone Joint Surg Br* 46:445–463, 1964.

108. Wynne-Davies R, Littlejohn A, Gormley J: Aetiology and interrelationship of some common skeletal deformities. (Talipes equinovarus and calcaneovalgus, metatarsus varus, congenital dislocation of the hip, and infantile idiopathic scoliosis), *J Med Genet* 19:321–328, 1982.

109. Zionts LE, Shean CJ: Brace treatment of early infantile tibia vara, *J Pediatr Orthop* 18:102–109, 1998.

Chapter

36

Pediatric hip orthoses

Shannon K. McClure and Laura L. Tosi

Key Points

- Success rates with the Pavlik harness are reported to be 90% to 100% for treatment of hip subluxation or dysplasia and 80% to 95% for treatment of hip dislocation.

- No outcome differences have been demonstrated in children with Legg-Calvé-Perthes disease whose management included no treatment, range-of-motion exercises, or bracing. Bracing may be useful as an adjunct to postoperative care after hip containment surgery.

- Hip orthoses typically are used to maintain abduction either postoperatively or after Botox injections in children with cerebral palsy. Hip orthoses can be helpful in controlling scissoring during ambulation.

- Use of bracing to the hip of children with lower extremity weakness or paralysis is controversial. However, a wide range of therapeutic options are available for children wishing independent mobility.

A large percentage of the pediatric orthopedic surgeon's practice involves treatment of hip pathology. Conditions that fall within this category include developmental dysplasia of the hip (DDH), Legg-Calvé-Perthes disease (LCP), cerebral palsy (CP), and lower limb weakness or paralysis associated with neuromuscular disorders, myelodysplasia, and spinal cord injury.

In patients with these conditions, the goal of treatment is to achieve the most desirable result using the least invasive procedure. Avoiding surgical intervention is desirable. Orthoses make possible the stabilization of joints, maintenance of joint range of motion, and, in the case of reciprocating gait orthoses (RGOs), assistance with coordination of multiple joint motions to allow for ambulation. For these reasons, orthoses are an attractive treatment option. In practice, however, few hip orthoses are used into adulthood.

This chapter describes commonly used hip orthoses, both past and present, and offers a brief review of the literature regarding their efficacy and safety. Hip orthoses are discussed as they relate to the most common childhood hip disorders.

Developmental dysplasia of the hip

DDH encompasses an array of hip pathologies, including hips that are stable but have dysplasia, hips that are subluxatable or dislocatable, and hips that are subluxated or dislocated. Dislocated hips can be further subdivided into those that can be reduced and those that are fixed (most often associated with other diagnoses such as arthrogryposis or myelodysplasia).

Successful treatment of DDH is based on an understanding of the natural history of the disease. There are four possible outcomes for abnormal neonatal hips: (1) they may normalize; (2) they may stabilize but have abnormal acetabular and/or femoral head development (dysplasia); (3) they may subluxate; or (4) they may dislocate.

Studies of the natural history of hip dysplasia indicate that radiographic evidence of residual hip dysplasia is associated with the development of degenerative joint disease.[5,13,28] Stulberg and Harris[42,43] reported that 48% of 130 patients with degenerative joint disease of the hip had evidence of primary acetabular dysplasia. True subluxation is more strongly associated with degenerative joint disease, with the degree of subluxation correlating with the age at onset of symptoms.[23,25] Symptoms of severe subluxation usually appear within the second decade of life.

The natural history of dislocated hips is dependent on whether the condition is unilateral or bilateral and on the presence or absence of a false acetabulum. In general, hips with a well-developed false acetabulum are more likely to be painful than are those without a false acetabulum. The pain is due to degenerative joint disease. Unilateral dislocations are more likely to be symptomatic than bilateral dislocations due in part to limb-length discrepancy, which leads to knee and back pathology. However, even bilateral dislocations are associated with back pain, probably because of hyperlordosis.[49,51,52]

The goals of DDH treatment in otherwise normal children are (1) to attain a concentric reduction of the hip, (2) to produce normal acetabular and femoral head development, (3) to avoid complications of treatment, including stiffness, infection, and avascular necrosis (AVN) of the femoral head, and (4) to avoid unnecessary patient and parental hardship (i.e., physical, emotional, financial).

Frejka pillow

In 1941, Bedrich Frejka introduced a soft abduction pillow for treatment of DDH in infants (Fig. 36-1).[34] He developed the device in response to the high rates of AVN associated with previous methods of treatment, which included Lorenz casting and various passive-abduction braces. The Frejka pillow was designed to maintain abduction; however, given the pillow's soft nature, infants could easily overcome the abduction pressure. The pillow subsequently was modified to create a firmer construct. The most recent version consists of a 9- × 9- × ¾-inch foam pillow that is placed around the child's buttocks, much like a diaper, and secured in place with a cloth harness and straps.

Even with this firmer construction, however, infants were not held in adequate abduction or flexion to allow the femoral head to be directed toward the triradiate cartilage. In addition to difficulties with attaining and maintaining reduction, the Frejka pillow developed a reputation for having high rates of AVN,[16,17] although the literature does not support this association.[4,45] Use of the Frejka pillow has essentially been abandoned in North America, although it is still used with reported good results in some areas of Europe.

Pavlik harness

Arnold Pavlik joined Frejka in practice in 1932.[34] The two men had a common interest in the treatment of hip dysplasia. Pavlik, noting the high rate of AVN with previous splints and the difficulty with maintaining hips in an acceptable position using the Frejka pillow, decided to design a new device (Fig. 36-2). His theory, as described in his classic article in 1957, was that with all previous devices, "the passive-mechanically reduced femoral head pushes against . . . obstacles in the acetabulum. Add to these circumstances the tension of the adductors and the passive-mechanically reduced femoral head cannot overcome these obstacles and damage to the head of the femur results."[37]

Pavlik suggested that the hip requires active motion in order to develop normally. His harness is designed to prevent only extension of the hips. By placing the hips in the "rider position," the device enables the adductors to relax with time and movement, allowing the head to spontaneously reduce. Once the head reduces, the harness maintains the reduction. Pavlik further argued that in cases where the acetabulum is filled with tissue, the constant motion of the hip (with associated redislocations and partial reductions) will create space for the head within the acetabulum. Furthermore, the motion prevents undue pressure on the head, thus preventing AVN.[37]

The Pavlik harness has two shoulder straps that cross in the back and are secured to a wide chest strap. Stirrups are suspended from the breast strap. When properly placed on

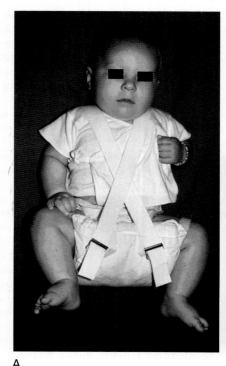
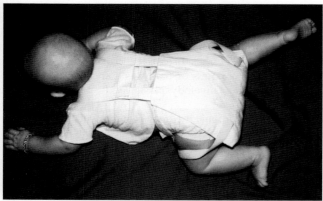

A B

Fig. 36-1 Frejka pillow. **A,** Anterior view. **B,** Posterior view.

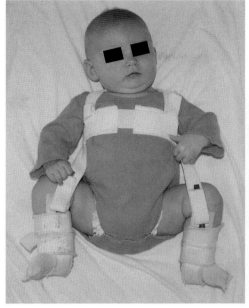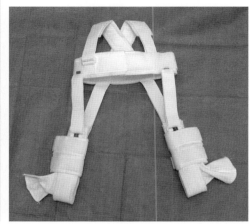

Fig. 36-2 Pavlik harness. **A,** Anterior view on patient. **B,** Posterior view.

the child, the chest strap is positioned at the nipple line, the anterior stirrup straps are located at the anterior axillary line, and the posterior straps overlie the scapulae. The anterior straps should maintain the hips in 90 to 110 degrees of flexion. Although it may seem that the posterior straps are designed to maintain wide abduction, this is distinctly counter to Pavlik's theory and design. The straps should be tensioned to maintain 20 to 30 degrees of abduction only, with the remaining abduction arising from gradual relaxation of the adductors.

The harness is indicated for patients with dysplastic, subluxated, or dislocated hips. Pavlik recommended its use for infants younger than 12 months[37]; however, others have decreased the upper age limit to 8 months.[12,33] Ultrasonography is used to determine the degree of dysplasia. Harcke's method of dynamic sonographic evaluation and Graf's static method are used to interpret the ultrasound scan and determine the need for treatment.

Once the harness has been placed, a radiography should be obtained to confirm appropriate positioning of the hip. The capital femoral epiphysis (or the metaphysis in the younger child in whom the head has not yet begun to ossify) should be directed toward the triradiate cartilage. The child then should be monitored weekly to confirm appropriate fit of the harness.

When used for treatment of dysplasia alone, the Pavlik harness should be worn 23 hours per day until acetabular and capital femoral epiphyseal development have normalized. Depending on the patient's age, either ultrasound or standard x-ray monitoring at 4- to 6-week intervals can be used to determine normalization. Once the hip has normalized, the child is weaned from the harness.

If the hip is dislocated upon initiation of the harness, the child should undergo weekly ultrasound evaluation until reduction is confirmed. If hip reduction cannot be documented within 3 weeks of beginning harness treatment, the harness should be abandoned because prolonged use of the harness without reduction can lead to significant complications. Most notably, persistent posterior dislocation maintained by the harness appears to erode the posterolateral acetabular wall,[23] a condition sometimes referred to as *Pavlik harness disease.* If the hip is found to reduce, a protocol similar to that described above, with full-time harness wear followed by gradual weaning once the hip is radiographically normal, is used.

Many researchers have attempted to identify risk factors for failure of Pavlik harness treatment.[11,12,25,48] The most commonly reported risk factors are bilaterally, absence of an Ortolani sign, age greater than 7 weeks at initiation of treatment, and less than 20% initial femoral head coverage as judged by ultrasound. Other risk factors are parental noncompliance and inappropriate use or application of the harness by the physician.

Complications associated with use of the Pavlik harness include Pavlik harness disease as well as skin irritation, femoral nerve palsy, inferior dislocation of the hip, and AVN of the femoral head.[8,9,22,24,32,38,44,46,47,53] Femoral nerve palsy and inferior dislocation of the hip have been associated with excessive flexion of the hip, and both have responded favorably to lengthening the anterior straps, which decreases the flexion. AVN is the most serious complication; long-term results in these hips are less favorable and less predictable. Reported rates of AVN vary from 0% to 27%, with higher rates reported for treatment of dislocated hips than treatment of subluxated or dysplastic hips. Most surgeons believe that the incidence of osteonecrosis likely will approach zero if the Pavlik harness is appropriately applied and monitored.

Success rates with the Pavlik harness are reported to be 90% to 100% for treatment of hip subluxation or dysplasia and 80% to 95% for treatment of dislocated hips.[8,9,12,32,37,38,44,47,53] These high rates of success, combined with the low rates of complication, make the Pavlik harness the gold standard for treatment of hip dysplasia and for the initial treatment of congenital hip dislocation.

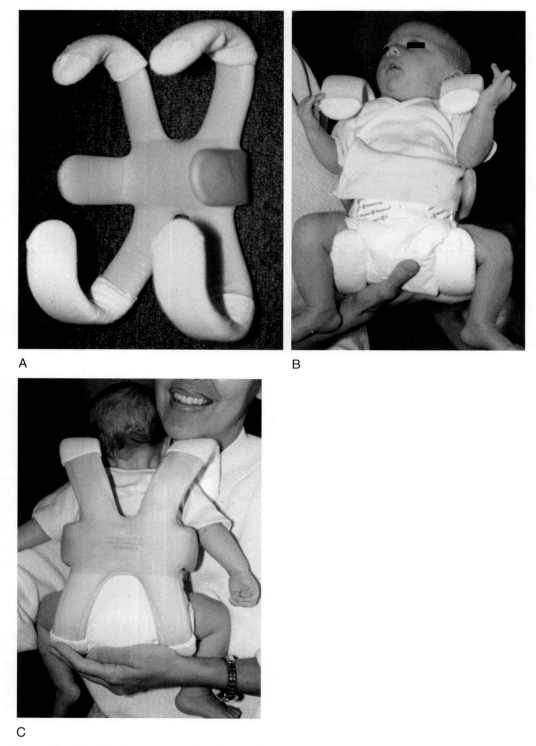

Fig. 36-3 A, Van Rosen orthosis. **B,** Anterior view on patient. **C,** Posterior view on patient.

Von Rosen orthosis

The Von Rosen orthosis is used in Scandinavian countries but is not frequently used in North America (Fig. 36-3). It is a passive restraining/positioning device. It is a malleable frame (originally metal but now plastic) with straps around the shoulders, waist, and thighs. The few available studies indicate very low rates of AVN but high rates of pressure ulcers with use of this device.[16,20]

Ilfeld orthosis

The Ilfeld orthosis is a passive positioning device that holds the hips in abduction but does not create significant hip

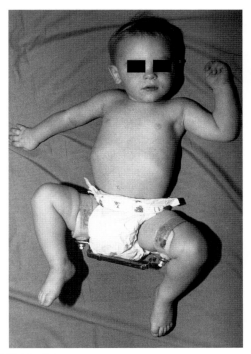

Fig. 36-4 Ilfeld splint.

flexion (Fig. 36-4). For this reason, it is more effective as a postoperative abduction device than for treatment of infantile hip dysplasia or dislocation. It consists of two thigh cuffs attached to an adjustable crossbar. This construct is attached to a waist strap to maintain positioning.

Plastazote hip abduction orthosis

Two different Plastazote hip abduction devices have been reported in the literature to successfully treat hip dysplasia and dislocation. Hedequist et al.[15] reported the successful use of an abduction brace in 13 of 15 patients with dislocated hips who had not responded to Pavlik treatment (Fig. 36-5). None of the children developed AVN. The authors suggest a 3- to 4-week trial in an abduction orthosis for children whose hips fail to reduce in a Pavlik harness. Using a somewhat different design, Eberle[7] reported his results on the use of an abduction orthosis in lieu of a Pavlik harness in 113 infants with 140 unstable hips (Fig. 36-6). Again, no instances of AVN occurred, and all but two hips had radiographic normalization without any further treatment. Both braces are made of a Plastazote foam that wraps around the legs and waist, maintaining the hips in approximately 70 to 90 degrees of flexion and wide abduction. Both allow free motion of the knees.

Legg-Calvé-Perthes disease

LCP disease is one of the most vexing problems faced by the pediatric orthopedist. The goal of treatment is to attain a congruous hip joint, ideally a Stulberg I or II. For this reason, the idea of containment, wherein the femoral head is maintained within the acetabulum and congruent remodeling is encouraged, is appealing. Multiple orthoses have been designed to hold the hip in abduction and to permit varying degrees of internal rotation and/or flexion, thus directing the head into

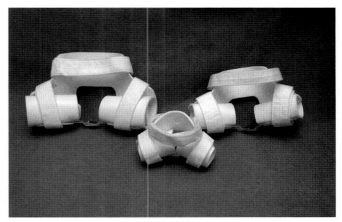

Fig. 36-5 Hinged Plastazote hip abduction orthosis.

the acetabulum. Although early reports on these devices were promising, subsequent reports were less favorable. Herring et al.[18,19] published their findings from a multicenter study that included 451 hips affected with LCP disease. These authors found no difference in outcome among hips that received no treatment, those treated with range-of-motion exercises, and those treated with bracing. Thus, although bracing may have a role after surgical containment, the current literature does not support the use of bracing alone for containment.

Toronto orthosis

Bobechko[2] introduced this ambulatory abduction orthosis in 1968 (Fig. 36-7). Two thigh cuffs are attached to a triangular frame, which in turn attaches to horizontal bars to which plates are attached. The hips are held in 45 degrees of abduction and are maintained in internal rotation by the fixed position of the shoes on the footplates. Hip and knee motion allow the child to ambulate with crutches.

Newington orthosis

Like the Toronto orthosis, the Newington orthosis is an ambulatory abduction orthosis that is used with crutches

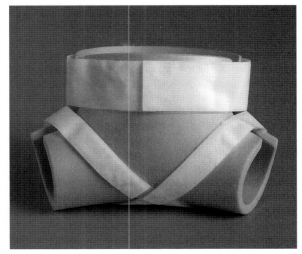

Fig. 36-6 Solid Plastazote hip abduction orthosis. (Courtesy Trulife.)

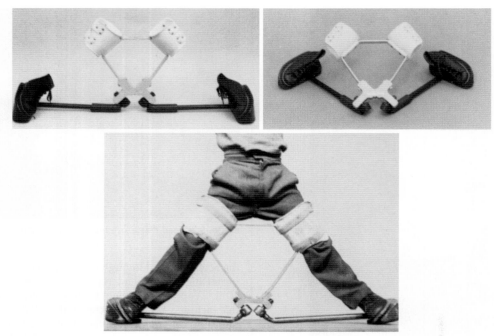

Fig. 36-7 Toronto orthosis.

(Fig. 36-8).[6] As in the Toronto orthosis, thigh cuffs are connected to a metal frame, but in the Newington orthosis the knees are held fixed in approximately 10 degrees of flexion. The shoes are attached to the footplates in a position that maintains the hips in relative internal rotation.

Atlanta Scottish Rite orthosis

Compared to the Toronto and Newington orthoses, the Atlanta Scottish Rite orthosis probably is the only device still in widespread use, typically for postoperative purposes rather than for nonsurgical containment.[30] It is occasionally used as an ambulatory abduction device in children

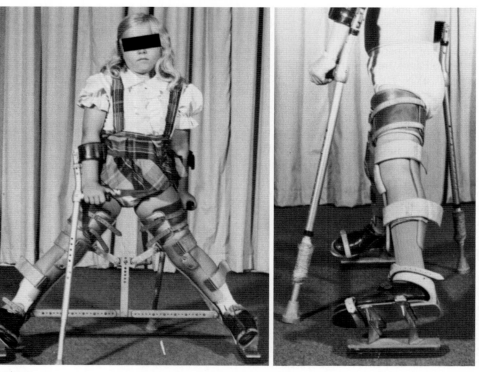

Fig. 36-8 Newington orthosis.

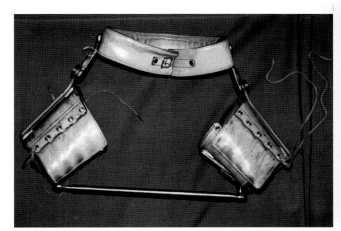

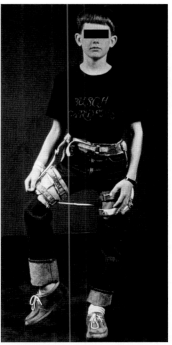

A   B

Fig. 36-9 Scottish Rite orthosis.

with DDH. The Scottish Rite orthosis, developed at the Scottish Rite Hospital in Atlanta, is far less cumbersome than Toronto and Newington orthoses. Another advantage of the Atlanta Scottish Rite orthosis is that it can be used without crutches.

The original orthosis had two thigh cuffs separated by an abduction bar (Fig. 36-9). Newer models offer stronger hinges that allow elimination of the abduction bar. Thigh cuffs are suspended from a waist band, which somewhat limits the tendency to widely abduct the unaffected leg while keeping the affected leg relatively adducted. Unlike the other orthoses, the Atlanta Scottish Rite orthosis has no extensions below the knee and thus has no rotational control.

Cerebral palsy

The increased muscle tone and muscular imbalance found in children with CP lead to limitations in hip range of motion and subluxations/dislocations of the hip. The goals of treating these hips are to (1) prevent painful hip subluxation/dislocation and (2) maintain or improve range of motion for ambulation, sitting balance, and hygiene.

Literature on the use of orthoses for treatment of CP is scant, probably because of the limited indications for their use in these patients.[36] Most commonly, they are used as a temporary adjunct to other treatment modalities, such as botulinum toxin type A (Botox) injections or surgical intervention.

Resting abduction orthoses

Nighttime abduction splinting theoretically is an attractive option for treating young children with early subluxation due to spastic quadriplegia or diplegia. By maintaining stretch on the hip adductors and flexors, these devices should enable patients to maintain, or even improve, range of motion. By positioning the hip in the central position within the acetabulum, the devices ideally should promote normal acetabular growth. Unfortunately, children with CP often have poor sleep patterns, and these braces frequently further disrupt sleep, so they often are abandoned.

One of the simplest forms of resting splints is a foam wedge, which can be held in place by hook-and-loop straps (Fig. 36-10). The wedge is inexpensive and easy to replace. A variant on this theme was reported by Hankinson and Morton[10] in 2002. Their technique incorporates the entire mattress system into the brace. Specifically, a modular mattress with incorporated abduction pads maintains the hips in abduction even when the child lies on his or her side. In their study, 5 of the 11 patients who used the system chose to continue its use.

A new product, the Hope 1 orthosis by Ultraflex, is custom fitted. Its advantage is that the amount of hip abduction can be precisely set and adjusted over time (Fig. 36-11).

SWASH orthosis

The SWASH (standing, walking, and sitting hip) orthosis is designed to allow the wearer to transition from sitting or crawling to standing or walking (Fig. 36-12). By providing variable hip abduction according to the degree of flexion or extension, it maintains the hips in abduction while the child is seated and holds the legs almost parallel while the child is standing. The brace not only positions the hips in abduction, providing maximal coverage to the femoral head, but also helps with sitting balance and preventing scissoring with ambulation. The SWASH orthosis is contraindicated in children with dislocated hips or with hips having greater than 20 degree flexion contractures. It also is contraindicated

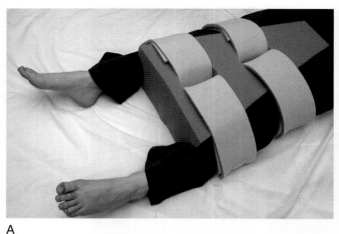
A

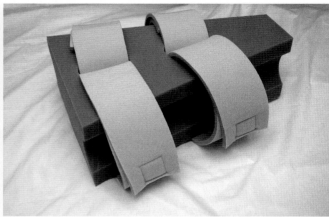
B

Fig. 36-10 Foam hip abduction pillow.

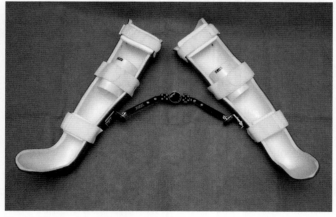

Fig. 36-11 Hope 1 abduction orthosis.

when lower extremity alignment results in excessive external foot progression angles.

Few reports in the literature support or oppose use of this brace. A single study of 39 patients, 20 of whom underwent physical therapy alone and 19 of whom underwent Botox followed by SWASH bracing, showed no statistical difference in gross motor function at 1 year.[3]

Torsional deformities

Use of orthoses for control of internal tibial torsion and excess femoral anteversion has essentially disappeared. However, "twister cables" remain a lightweight solution for controlling hip and foot rotation in the young child with lower extremity weakness, particularly spina bifida (Fig. 36-13).

Lower extremity weakness or paralysis

The impetus to improve orthotics that would assist children with paraplegia in walking developed in the 1970s, about a decade after development of the Spitz-Holter valve for treatment of hydrocephalus led to markedly improved survival rates in children with myelomeningocele.

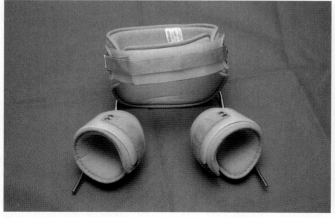
A

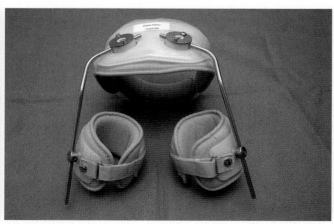
B

Fig. 36-12 SWASH orthosis.

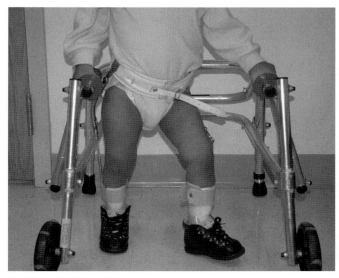

Fig. 36-13 Twister cable.

Unfortunately, efforts to improve mobility in these children using orthopedic surgery had not been generally successful. As a result, many centers sought improved bracing for enhanced ambulation. Two centers—the Orthotic Research and Locomotor Assessment Unit (ORLAU) in New South Wales and the Ontario Crippled Children's Center (now the Bloorview Hugh MacMillan Center) in Toronto—provided clinical services and developed more effective walking rehabilitation technologies, in the belief that such assistance would enable these children to achieve greater independence and improved quality of life. At that time, the benefits of erect posture and independent ambulation were thought to be myriad. For example, researchers believed that the force of gravity would result in improved pulmonary function and pulmonary toilet, improved bladder emptying, and increased bone mass. Improved orthoses would free the upper extremities for use and allow independent mobilization. The emotional and motivational benefits also were believed to be significant.

Mazur and Kyle[29] called this philosophy into question. They noted that most children who require significant bracing, such as a parapodium, hip–knee–ankle–foot orthosis (HKAFO), or RGO, give up walking by the time they reach adolescence, opting for a wheelchair as a more energy-efficient means of mobility. The cost of physical therapy, orthotics, and, frequently, surgery to reduce contractures far exceeds the cost of a wheelchair. Finally, the time commitment required for therapy, as well as for donning and doffing the braces, impedes socialization and education skills. Liptak et al.[26] found only limited differences in outcomes between patients who use orthotics and those who do not. For example, children who use wheelchairs have more sacral pressure sores, whereas parapodium users have more foot and skin sores.

In response, other investigators, particularly John Stallard[40] from the ORLAU, have argued that long-term outcomes indicate that children who ambulate achieve higher levels of independent functioning and suffer fewer costly pressure sores. Unfortunately, most brace studies use velocity or energy needed to walk rather than more functional

outcomes, such as ease of getting around, as primary outcome measures. Randomized controlled studies of this issue are needed.

At the same time, however, the incidence of spina bifida has decreased dramatically as a result of multiple factors, including prenatal screening and the use of folate in food. Two "new" populations have taken advantage of the technologies originally developed for children with spina bifida. First, an increasing number of patients with muscular dystrophy are surviving longer as a result of steroid treatment. Keeping these patients fit and free of contractures is an important goal. The second population is individuals who have suffered spinal cord injuries. Devices that may assist all individuals with lower extremity weakness are described below.

Lycra garments

Lycra-based orthotic undergarments (TheraTogs) are designed to provide dynamic splinting to control abnormal tone, stabilize posture, and improve function in individuals with neurological disorders such as CP and spina bifida (Fig. 36-14). The orientation of the fabric provides a gentle correctional force to the targeted body parts. Plastic boning on the posterior and lateral trunk provides extra support. The system emphasizes shortening underused, overlong muscles (rather than lengthening short muscles) and attempts to gradually change the user's movement and muscle-activation strategies. Lycra garments are popular among physiotherapists. Literature supporting their use is limited, but numerous studies are in progress.[1,21,39]

Standing frame orthoses

Vertical standers

Vertical standers are used for children who will never stand independently. Many rest on a stationary platform to improve stability. Several of the newer models include a sit-to-stand function, which makes lifting easier for caretakers and allows a child to spend a longer part of the day in the devices.

Standing braces

The standing brace (Variety Village Stander), a variant of the vertical stander, was designed at the Ontario Crippled Children's Center to allow independent standing and free use of the upper extremities for the very young child with good head control (Fig. 36-15). It also introduces a child to independent mobility using a walker and swiveling or hopping motions. It does not permit hip or knee flexion. The brace comes as a kit that consists of an unhinged upright frame with footplates, knee supports, and a chest/abdominal strap. It can be extended to accommodate growth

A-frame orthosis

The A-frame orthosis, similar to the standing frame, supports the patient in an erect posture. It has a pommel that provides for abduction of the hips and can support some of the patient's weight. The A-frame is indicated in children between the ages of 18 months and 4 years. With the A-frame, the hip positions of abduction and internal/external rotation can be controlled. This design is believed to be

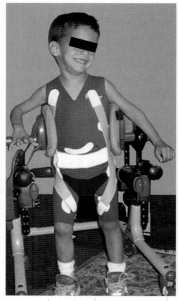
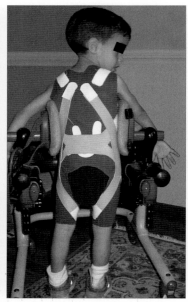

A B

Fig. 36-14 TheraTogs. (Courtesy TheraTogs.)

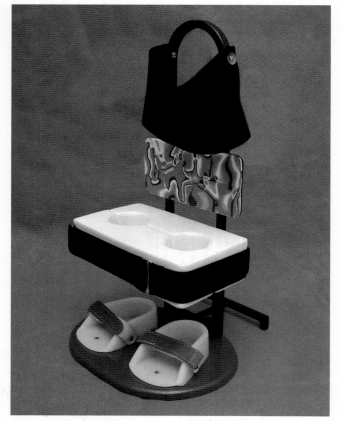

advantageous for children with conditions having a high incidence of hip subluxation and dysplasia.

Parapodium

The parapodium, which was developed in the early 1960s, enables children with spina bifida to stand without crutches for functional activities, leaving their upper limbs free (Fig. 36-16). It enables the child to sit or stand as well to change between these two positions. The original design included only hip locks; however, subsequent models include locking

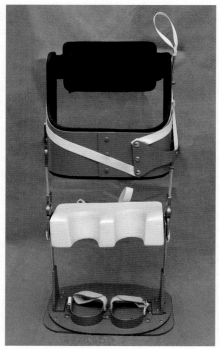

Fig. 36-15 Standing brace.

Fig. 36-16 Parapodium (rear view).

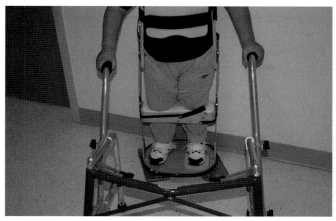
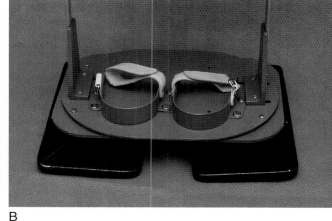

A B

Fig. 36-17 Swivel walker.

and unlocking joints at both the knee and hips, which allow the child to sit in a wheelchair as well as to stand.

The parapodium is indicated for children older than 3 years. It is worn over clothing. It provides an exoskeleton that consists of a spring-loaded shoe clamp, aluminum uprights, foam knee block, and back and chest panels. The hip and knee joints unlock with a lever to permit sitting. A four-bar linkage in the hip and a telescope bar allow patients to roll and ratchet themselves from the sitting to the standing position. The oval base plate (similar to that used in the standing frame) allows patients old enough to use crutches or a walker to propel themselves forward using a swivel-walk pattern.

Swivel walkers

Swivel walkers, first developed by the ORLAU, consist of a lightweight frame that provides an external skeleton attached to two swiveling foot pads (Fig. 36-17).[41] The pads are set at a slight camber that allows reciprocal forward motion as the child leans the trunk to the right and left. The device can be fitted to children as young as 1 year and requires very little strength to propel. Thus, it can be used by children with involvement of the upper limbs. The swivel walker is extremely durable and is easily adjusted for growth, thus amortizing its cost. One disadvantage is that it can be used only on flat, smooth surfaces (not uneven terrain or thick carpets). The device is heavy, and two to three people may be required to lift the child upright. Finally, movement in the swivel walker is slow. For these reasons, an RGO is generally preferred for individuals with good trunk and upper limb function. Although the swivel walker was designed for children with spina bifida, it has been used extensively in patients with disorders in which generalized weakness is problematic (e.g., spinal muscular atrophy, multiple sclerosis, and muscular dystrophy).

Hip–knee–ankle–foot orthoses

An HKAFO consists of a hip joint and pelvic band attached to a knee–ankle–foot orthosis (KAFO; Fig. 36-18). The hip joint can prevent abduction and adduction as well as hip rotation. Prior to the development of RGOs, HKAFOs were routinely

prescribed for a wide variety of disorders, including polio, myelomeningocele, and spinal cord injury. These braces allowed an upright posture, and children were able to ambulate using a pivot or swing-through gait.

Three types of hip joint brace typically are prescribed: (1) single-axis hip joint with lock, which allows only flexion and extension; (2) two-position lock hip joint, which can be locked at full extension or 90 degrees of flexion; and (3) double-axis hip joint, which has both a flexion–extension axis and an abduction–adduction axis. Unfortunately, these braces frequently are biomechanically insufficient because they cannot control the lumbar spine and pelvis, even when

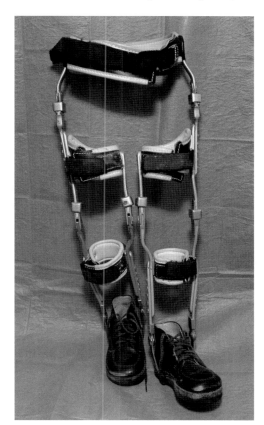

Fig. 36-18 HKAFO.

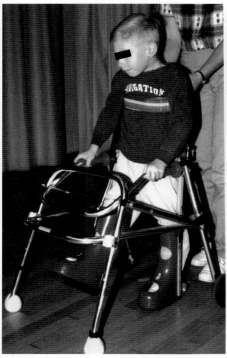
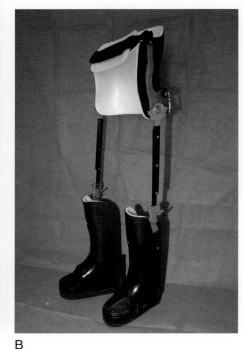

A   B

Fig. 36-19 Isocentric RGO.

the hip joints are locked. Thus, children with weak hip extensors tend to fall into a flexed, lordotic posture.

Although some HKAFOs still are made from metal and leather, the majority of contemporary designs are made of thermoplastic or laminated plastic and have metal hinge joints. Compared with metal orthoses, plastic devices offer comparable or greater support, are lighter in weight, distribute forces over a wider area, allow wearers to wear different pairs of shoes, and are more cosmetically pleasing. Pelvic bands complicate dressing after toileting unless the orthosis is worn under all clothing.

Hip guidance orthoses

The term *hip guidance orthosis* describes a brace with thrust-bearing hip joints that are connected by a rigid pelvic bar. The hip and knee joints can be unlocked for sitting. Several braces fall into this category.

Reciprocating gait orthosis

The RGO, designed by Motloch and modified by Yngve et al.,[55] was a major step forward in providing an energy-efficient gait and improved posture for children with lower extremity weakness. The RGO consists of bilateral KAFOs attached through hinges to a rigid pelvic band with a thoracic extension. A cable system couples hip flexion on one side to hip extension on the contralateral side and thus compensates for a lack of extensor power. The cable system also helps prevent forward pelvic tilt and lordosis. Strong upper extremities as well as assistive devices (crutches or a walker) usually are necessary for balance and control. The RGO provides a functional gait pattern and safe mobility over uneven terrain. It is compatible with wheelchair use. The RGO cannot

be used by a child with significant hip flexion contractures because the device interferes with the child's ability to initiate single-limb progression.

A study that compared energy expenditure for the RGO with swing-through crutch ambulation versus wheelchair ambulation found the two systems were nearly equal in energy requirements. No significant differences were noted in gait velocity with the RGO, and all patients achieved community ambulation status with the RGO.

The first RGO consisted of a cord-and-pulley modification to the bilateral HKAFOs of a young patient with spina bifida. The mechanical linkage translated hip flexion on one side into hip extension on the contralateral side. Numerous modifications subsequently have been made. The Louisiana State University (LSU) RGO consists of bilateral HKAFOs connected by a custom-molded thermoplastic pelvic girdle (or metal band) and dual cables cross-connected to thrust-bearing hip joints on the opposite side. A second device, the Fillauer horizontal cable system, replaced the LSU hooped cables with bilateral rocker arms linked to the hip joints and connected to each other at the corresponding ends by Teflon-coated cables. The advanced reciprocating gait orthosis (ARGO) uses a single low-friction, push–pull cable to effect reciprocal gait locomotion. The Isocentric reciprocating gait orthosis (IRGO) has become quite popular (Fig. 36-19).[54] It uses a centrally pivoting bar and tie rod arrangement in lieu of cables to link hip extension to contralateral hip flexion. The absence of cables reduces friction in the system by up to 300%.

Parawalker

The Parawalker (Fig. 36-20) was developed at the ORLAU in an effort to overcome the disadvantages of the swivel walker

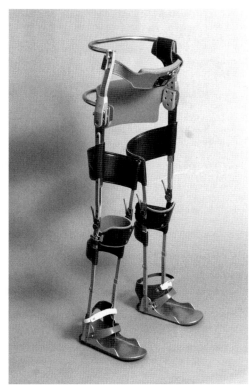

Fig. 36-20 Parawalker. (Courtesy ORLAU.)

and to allow patients with spinal cord lesions at the thoracic level to walk reciprocally with crutches.[27,35] The device consists of bilateral KAFOs with a ball-bearing hip joint and a body brace. Ambulation is performed through trunk motion transmitted to the lower extremities with hip flexion and extension via the brace. Hip flexion is restricted by a stop. Hip extension can be free or limited by a stop.

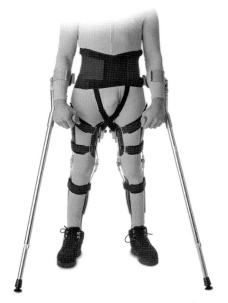

Fig. 36-21 UpandAbout Orthosis. (Courtesy Cascade.)

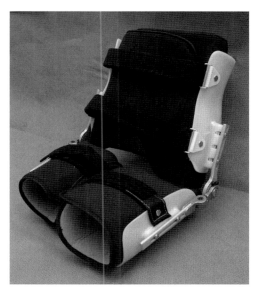

Fig. 36-22 Postoperative hip abduction orthosis.

Multiaxial subperineal hip joints

Some patients are "too good" for an RGO but "not good enough" to use a KAFO alone. The multiaxial subperineal hip joint (Center for Orthotics Design) and the UpandAbout System (Cascade; Fig. 36-21) use a medially mounted, single-axis hinge joint to link two KAFOs.[14] This is quite different from braces such as the RGO or the traditional HKAFO, which have laterally positioned hip joints. Patients who may benefit from this device include those with demonstrated spinal stability without significant deformity, controlled muscle spasm, less than 5 degrees of hip or knee flexion contracture, achievable neutral ankle position, mobility of the thoracolumbar spine into lateral flexion, good upper limb strength, and motivation. Reports of the effectiveness of this brace are limited; however, Middletown et al.[31] reported that 60% of all patients fitted with the brace had incorporated the orthosis into their lifestyles. According to Middletown et al., maintenance of joint mobility and psychological benefits were the most important outcomes of brace usage.

Postoperative hip orthoses

After hip reconstruction surgery in children with CP and spina bifida, hip spica casts have traditionally been applied and set at 30 degrees of unilateral hip abduction (combined 60-degree angle) and 30 degrees of hip flexion. Hip spicas have a number of disadvantages. They require considerable time to apply at the end of a lengthy surgery, they preclude visual inspection of surgical wounds during the postoperative period, and they can cause complications such as pressure sores. Other disadvantages of hip spicas are the need for intensive physiotherapy and, in most cases, hospital readmission to regain range of motion in hip and knee joints that stiffen from immobility in the cast.

A hip orthosis (Fig. 36-22) may overcome some of the complications associated with hip spica casts. The most suitable design includes a pelvic section connected to thigh cuffs with an orthotic joint that allows incremental adjustment of flexion and abduction that can be adjusted and locked in the selected position.

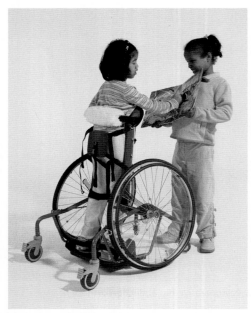

Fig. 36-23 Mobile prone stander. (Courtesy Rifton.)

Models now marketed include the Mapleleaf, designed at the Bloorview MacMillan Center in Toronto, for children ages 4 to 15 years; the Newport Jr Hip Orthosis (Orthomerica); and the Lil' Hip Hugger (Bolt Systems, Inc.)

Mobile standers

Stationary standers have been a part of the therapeutic arsenal for treatment of children and adults with disabilities for decades. Development of the mobile stander has allowed children with severe lower extremity weakness but good arm strength easy mobility and the opportunity to interact with peers at eye level (Fig. 36-23). In centers with adequate funding, the mobile stander has largely replaced the stationary stander for children with good cognitive function.

References

1. Blair E, Ballantyne J, Horsman S, et al: A study of a dynamic proximal stability splint in the management of children with cerebral palsy, *Dev Med Child Neurol* 37:544–554, 1995.
2. Bobechko W: The Toronto brace for Legg-Perthes disease, *Clin Orthop* 102:115–117, 1974.
3. Boyd RN, Dobson F, Parrott J, et al: The effect of botulinum toxin type A and a variable hip abduction orthosis on gross motor function: a randomized controlled trial, *Eur J Neurol* 8:109–119, 2001.
4. Burger BJ, Burger JD, Bos CF, et al: Frejka pillow and Becker device for congenital dislocation of the hip. Prospective 6-year study of 104 late-diagnosed cases, *Acta Orthop Scand* 64:305–311, 1993.
5. Cooperman DR, Wallensten R, Stulberg SD: Acetabular dysplasia in the adult, *Clin Orthop* 175:79–85, 1983.
6. Curtis BH, Gunther SF, Gossling HR, et al: Treatment for Legg-Perthes disease with the Newington ambulation-abduction brace, *J Bone Joint Surg* 56A:1135–1146, 1976.
7. Eberle CF: Plastazote abduction orthosis in the management of neonatal hip instability, *J Pediatr Orthop* 23:607–616, 2003.
8. Eidelman M, Katzman A, Freiman S, et al: Treatment of true developmental dysplasia of the hip using Pavlik's method, *J Pediatr Orthop* 12B:253–258, 2003.
9. Grill F, Bensahel H, Canadell J, et al: The Pavlik harness in the treatment of congenital dislocating hip: report on a multicenter study of the European Orthopaedic Society, *J Pediatr Orthop* 8:1–8, 1988.
10. Hankinson J, Morton RE: Use of a lying hip abduction system in children with bilateral cerebral palsy: a pilot study, *Dev Med Child Neurol* 44:177–180, 2002.
11. Harding MGB, Harcke HT, Bowen JR, et al: Management of dislocated hips with Pavlik harness treatment and ultrasound monitoring, *J Pediatr Orthop* 17:189–198, 1997.
12. Harris IE, Dickens R, Menelaus MB: Use of the Pavlik harness for hip displacements: when to abandon treatment, *Clin Orthop* 281:29–33, 1992.
13. Harris WH: Etiology of osteoarthritis of the hip, *Clin Orthop* 213:20–33, 1986.
14. Harvey LA, Davis GM, Smith MB: Energy expenditure during gait using the walkabout and isocentric reciprocal gait orthoses in persons with paraplegia, *Arch Phys Med Rehabil* 79:945–949, 1998.
15. Hedequist D, Kasser J, Emans J: Use of an abduction brace for developmental dysplasia of the hip after failure of Pavlik harness use, *J Pediatr Orthop* 23:175–177, 2003.
16. Heikkila E: Comparison of the Frejka pillow and Von Rosen splint in treatment of congenital dislocation of the hip, *J Pediatr Orthop* 8:20, 1988.
17. Herring JA: Conservative treatment of congenital dislocation of the hip in the newborn and infant, *Clin Orthop* 281:41–47, 1992.
18. Herring JA: Current concepts review. The treatment of Legg-Calve-Perthes disease. A critical review of the literature, *J Bone Joint Surg* 76A:448–458, 1994.
19. Herring JA, Kim HT, Browne R: Legg-Calve-Perthes disease. Part II: prospective multicenter study of the effect of treatment on outcome, *J Bone Joint Surg* 86A:2121–2134, 2004.
20. Hinderaker T, Rygh M, Uden A: The von Rosen splint compared with the Frejka pillow. A study of 408 neonatally unstable hips, *Acta Orthop Scand* 63:389–392, 1992.
21. Hylton N, Allen C: The development and use of SPIO Lycra compression bracing in children with neuromotor deficits, *Pediatr Rehabil* 1:109–116, 1997.
22. Iwasaki K: Treatment of congenital dislocation of the hip by the Pavlik harness: mechanism of reduction and usage, *J Bone Joint Surg* 65A:760–767, 1983.
23. Jones GT, Schoenecker PL, Dias LS: Developmental hip dysplasia potentiated by inappropriate use of the Pavlik harness, *J Pediatr Orthop* 12:722-726.
24. Kalamchi A, MacFarlane R III: The Pavlik harness: results in patients over three months of age, *J Pediatr Orthop* 2:3–8, 1982.
25. Lerman JA, Emans JB, Millis MB, et al: Early failure of Pavlik harness treatment for developmental hip dysplasia: clinical and ultrasound predictors, *J Pediatr Orthop* 21:348–353, 2001.
26. Liptak GS, Shurtleff DB, Bloss JW, et al: Mobility aids for children with high-level myelomeningocoele: parapodium versus wheelchair, *Dev Med Child Neurol* 34:787–796, 1992.
27. Major RE, Stallard J, Farmer SE: A review of 42 patients of 16 years and over using the ORLAU Parawalker, *Prosthet Orthot Int* 21:147–152, 1997.
28. Malvitz TA, Weinstein SL: Closed reduction for congenital dysplasia of the hip. Functional and radiographic results after an average of thirty years, *J Bone Joint Surg* 76A:1777–1792, 1994.
29. Mazur JM, Kyle S: Efficacy of bracing the lower limbs and ambulation training in children with myelomeningocoele, *Dev Med Child Neurol* 46:352–356, 2004.
30. Meehan PL, Angel D, Nelson JM: The Scottish Rite abduction orthosis for the treatment of Legg-Perthes disease: A radiographic analysis, *J Bone Joint Surg* 74A:2–12, 1992.
31. Middletown JW, Yeo JD, Blanch L: Clinical evaluation of a new orthosis, the "walkabout," the restoration of functional standing and short distance mobility in spinal paralyzed individuals, *Spinal Cord* 35:574–579, 1997.
32. Mubarak S, Garfin S, Vance R, et al: Pitfalls in the use of the Pavlik harness for treatment of congenital dysplasia, subluxation, and dislocation of the hip, *J Bone Joint Surg* 63A:1239–1248, 1981.
33. Mubarak SJ: Management of developmental dysplasia and dislocation of the hip. American Academy of Orthopaedic Surgeons 72nd Annual Meeting, Instructional Course Lecture, 2005.
34. Mubarak SJ, Bialik V: Pavlik: the man and his method, *J Pediatr Orthop* 23:342–346, 2003.
35. Patrick JH: Walking rehabilitation possibilities with the ORLAU parawalker, *Clin Rehab* 2:333–337, 1988.
36. Patrick JH, Roberts AP, Cole GF: Therapeutic choices in the locomotor management of the child with cerebral palsy: more luck than judgment? *Arch Dis Child* 85:275–279, 2001.

37. Pavlik A (translated by Leonard Peltier): The functional method of treatment using a harness with stirrups as the primary conservative therapy for infants with congenital dislocation of the hip, *Clin Orthop* 281:4-10, 1992.

38. Ramsey PL, Lasser S, MacEwen GD: Congenital dislocation of the hip: use of the Pavlik harness in the child during the first six months of life, *J Bone Joint Surg* 58A:1000–1004, 1976.

39. Rennie DJ, Attfield SF, Morton RE, et al: An evaluation of lycra garments in the lower limb using 3-D gait analysis and functional assessment (PEDI), *Gait Posture* 12:1–6, 2000.

40. Stallard J: Walking for the severely disabled: research and development, experience and clinical outcomes, *J Bone Joint Surg Br* 87:604–607, 2005.

41. Stallard J, Lomas B, Woollam P, et al: New technical advances in swivel walkers, *Prosthet Orthot Int* 27:132–138, 2003.

42. Stulberg SD, Cordell LD, Harris WH, et al: Unrecognized childhood hip disease: a major cause of idiopathic osteoarthritis of the hip. In Harris WH, editor: *The hip: proceedings of the third open scientific meeting of the Hip Society*, St. Louis, 1975, CV Mosby.

43. Stulberg SD, Harris WH: Acetabular dysplasia and development of osteoarthritis of the hip. In Cordell LD, Harris WH, Ramsey PL, MacEwen GD, editors: *The hip: Proceedings of the second open meeting of the Hip Society*. St Louis, 1974, CV Mosby.

44. Suzuki S, Yamamuro T: Avascular necrosis in patients treated with the Pavlik harness for congenital dislocation of the hip, *J Bone Joint Surg* 72A:1048–1055, 1990.

45. Tegnander A, Holen KJ, Anda S, et al: Good results after treatment with the Frejka pillow for hip dysplasia in newborns: a 3-year to 6-year follow-up study, *J Pediatr Orthop* 10B:173–179, 2001.

46. Tonnis D: An evaluation of conservative and operative methods in the treatment of congenital hip dislocation, *Clin Orthop* 119:76–88, 1976.

47. Ucar DH, Isiklar U, Kandemir U, et al: Treatment of developmental dysplasia of the hip with Pavlik harness: prospective study in Graf type IIc or more severe hips, *J Pediatr Orthop* 13B:70–74, 2004.

48. Viere RG, Birch JG, Herring JA, et al: Use of the Pavlik harness in congenital dislocation of the hip: an analysis of failures of treatment, *J Bone Joint Surg* 72A:238–244, 1990.

49. Wedge JH, Wasylenko MJ: The natural history of congenital disease of the hip, *J Bone Joint Surg* 61B:334–338, 1979.

50. Wedge JH, Wasylenko MJ: The natural history of congenital dislocation of the hip: a critical review, *Clin Orthop* 137:154–162, 1978.

51. Weinstein SL: Natural history and treatment options of childhood hip disorders, *Clin Orthop* 344:227–242, 1997.

52. Weinstein SL: Natural history of congenital hip dislocation (CDH) and hip dysplasia, *Clin Orthop* 225:62–76, 1987.

53. Weinstein SL, Mubarak SJ, Wenger DR: Developmental hip dysplasia and dislocation: part II, *Instr Course Lect* 53:531–542, 2004.

54. Winchester PK, Corollo JJ, Parekh RN, et al: A comparison of paraplegic gait performance using two types of reciprocating gait orthoses, *Prosthet Orthot Int* 17:101–106, 1993.

55. Yngve DA, Douglas R, Roberts JM: The reciprocating gait orthosis in myelomeningocoele, *J Pediatr Orthop* 4:304–310, 1984.

Chapter

37

Orthoses for the muscle disease patient

John D. Hsu

Key Points

- Orthoses for children with muscle disease can be lightweight because the devices need not supply structural rigidity to oppose high tone or spasticity.

- Spinal orthoses are containment devices and act as trunk support. They are not expected to prevent the progression of scoliosis.

- Mobile arm support may be useful for improving function in persons with severe proximal muscle weakness.

Patients with generalized, trunk, and extremity muscle weakness have a neuromuscular disorder originating in the motor unit. Muscle weakness can result from a disease originating in the motor neurone, the peripheral nerve, the neuromuscular junction, or the muscle tissue itself. Weakness in muscles originating in the muscle tissue is a primary disease of muscle, a *myopathy*. Muscle weakness secondary to a disorder in the motor unit proximal to the muscle causing muscle atrophy or deterioration is a *neuropathy. Muscle disease* can also be referred to as *motor unit disorder.*[15]

Today most of the conditions discussed—motor unit disorders—are considered genetic disorders in which a defect in the gene causes a structural abnormality of such magnitude that motor unit components and muscle cells are affected. Fortunately, scientific research has allowed development of methods and tools for identifying and precisely determining and/or localizing the area of defect.[34] Progress has been made but has not reached a level sufficient for permanent cure of diseases. Interest in the management of such cases is being reported from developing countries.[42] The genetic defect can be passed from one generation to the next. Children of such persons manifest problems earlier in life, so treatment, especially in the form of

supportive care, has become increasingly more important.[7,44,45] Heart transplantation can extend the life of neuromuscular patients.[39] Orthoses and modifications made to improve their use and efficiency have been emphasized by clinicians treating patients with progressive weakness and increasing disability. Lightweight materials (see Chapters 3 and 4), improved electronics, engineering advancements, and robotics (see Chapter 50) have led to the development of better tools and devices.

With better recognition of the disease and more accurate early diagnosis, treatment plans require review and modification. For example, after determining the orthopedic disabilities of a child with spinal muscular atrophy, Evans et al.[8] developed the principles for generalized management of orthopedic problems. Current literature suggests that unilateral hip subluxation should be managed operatively[52]; thus, continued review of the topic and of the disease are important. Evidence-based studies are underway, and useful information can be obtained from available and upcoming clinical studies.[43]

The problem

When a patient has muscle weakness, whether in the trunk, proximal part of the body, or distal extremities, orthoses can be used for support. Depending on the underlying condition, weakness can be generalized or regional, unilateral or bilateral, asymmetrical or symmetrical. Contractures result from weakness around a joint and occur because the extent of the disorder within, or the rate of muscle deterioration between, antagonist or agonist muscle groups is not be the same. Contractures can be influenced by positioning and gravity. The affected part (e.g., the spine or an extremity) may be pulled into a specific direction without significant resistance. When this condition persists over a long period, a fixed contracture can develop. Contractures can result from muscle cell death and fibrosis. For patients with muscle disease, orthoses are designed to support and maintain correction rather than work against a deforming force. In motor unit disorders, there is no increase in muscle tone, so spasticity is *not* present. Orthoses for this population can be lightweight because there is no requirement for structural rigidity to oppose high tone.

Clinical aspects and diagnosis

Identification of the underlying neuromuscular disorder is an extremely important aspect of the overall planning of treatment and bracing. Many motor unit disorders are associated with a genetic defect.[2,5] Knowledge of the family history is important and can help establish the diagnosis. The workup should include information about the time of onset of weakness, its clinical course, and a discussion of progression or stability of the disease process. The diseases that progress slowly or remain stable lend themselves to successful use of orthoses. Diseases that change may require frequent modifications, adjustments, or replacement of orthoses. Areas of weakness must be identified and muscle strength testing recorded using methods developed for manual muscle testing.[20] Can a pattern be identified? Is the weakness proximal, distal, or central, or does it affect only a specific area, such as the face, neck muscles, or scapular supporting musculature? Is the weakness focal, caused by parasites of an obstructive vascular disorder? Laboratory studies that determine the activity of enzymes such as creatinine phosphokinase (CPK), which reflects muscle tissue breakdown, provide useful support for the clinical impression. CPK is highly elevated in rapidly progressive muscle disorders with significant muscle tissue breakdown, such as Duchenne pseudohypertrophic muscular dystrophy (DMD), and generally are not elevated in stable conditions such as spinal muscular atrophy and congenital myopathies. Many genetic studies using blood studies have been developed[19] and provide accurate information on the nature of the underlying disorder. Other diagnostic tests frequently relied upon include electromyography, nerve conduction studies, ultrasonography, and muscle imaging.[29] Muscle biopsy, including histochemical and biochemical studies, and testing for dystrophin, the presence of which rules out DMD, may provide a more definitive answer. Once the diagnosis is established, prognosis and the clinical course of the neuromuscular disorder can be better evaluated. This allows for treatment planning to manage the patient's immediate and/or long-term problems and determine the extent and need for orthotic care.

Team approach

Long-term disability with loss of function is associated with most motor unit disorders. Polymyositis with severe generalized muscle weakness initially can be treated with steroids and immunosuppressant medications.[28] Improvement in muscle strength and function are expected with successful treatment, leading to control of the acute process. Neuropathies and myopathies require long-term management not only from the medical standpoint but also for overall care and maintenance of function. The treatment team must include *physicians* who have special knowledge of neuromuscular diagnosis and can understand the course of neuromuscular disorders and the disabilities they cause. Expertise in orthopedics, neurology, genetics, laboratory medicine, physical medicine, pulmonary medicine, pediatrics, and geriatrics may be needed to manage neuromuscular disorders. *Physical therapists* and *occupational therapists* must understand muscle grading and the affected patient's functional abilities together with available self-care aids, gait analysis data, mobility devices, and possible environmental adaptations. *Psychologists, liaison nurses, social workers, recreational therapists,* and *community workers and leaders* support the patient and family's needs and help the school and community understand the disabled person's special problems and concerns. They also interact with the community and special agencies that provide services to assist the disabled person. Governmental programs through schools, disabled workshops, and community centers may be available to help the disabled child's development and educational programs. The *certified orthotist* who is knowledgeable about support of weakened limbs and trunk is of utmost importance to the team because of special experience and training in the design, measurement, construction, fitting, maintenance, and repair of supportive and assistive devices or equipment.[27a]

Spinal orthoses

Spinal deformities are frequently seen in neuromuscular patients, whose spines require support. The orthoses used are generally considered *containment devices* (Fig. 37-1). They have been developed in many centers treating neuromuscular patients by adapting orthoses developed for control of idiopathic and acquired scoliosis.[3,10,24,46,50] For children with weak neck muscles, outriggers must be added to support the head.[37] Principles developed for the use of orthoses in the treatment of patients with idiopathic scoliosis cannot be directly applied to patients with neuromuscular scoliosis because these patients have weakness of the supportive musculature of the spine and spinal column collapse.[27,33]

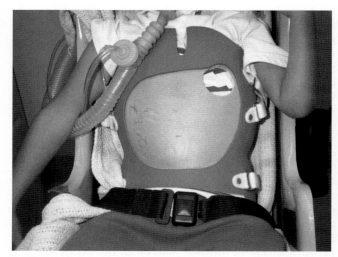

Fig. 37-1 TLSO for a respirator-dependent neuromuscular patient. Note that the main body of the body jacket is composed of fairly stiff material that contains the spine. The anterior aspect is made of softer material, and appropriate cutouts are made to accommodate ventilator and monitoring equipment.

When spinal orthoses are prescribed, special circumstances may be encountered. Provisions may be necessary when bracing the following patients:

A. Ambulatory patient who needs to continue walking
B. Person with weakened respiratory musculature or a tracheostomy
C. Person with rapid spinal collapse, which requires holding of the spine
D. Very young patient

It is important to know the natural history of spinal collapse in the neuromuscular condition being treated.[13,22,24,27,31] In the ambulatory person, recognizing the spinal curve pattern and its flexibility becomes important. Encumbering the spine with a corset can interfere with balancing and walking. In a patient with a progressive disease, such as DMD, frequent reassessments of the spine in the seated position should be performed at least every 6 months. A spinal curvature, if present, must be followed closely, with clinical examinations as frequently as every 3 months. If there is doubt about the nature and degree of the spinal curvature, an X-ray examination in the sitting position should be performed. If the curve progresses, it can become fixed and difficult to correct. Thus, a curve less than 35 degrees can be supported using a lightweight body jacket (thoracolumbosacral orthosis [TLSO]), especially in patients with very slowly progressive conditions, such as spinal muscular atrophy and congenital muscular dystrophy. When spinal collapse progresses to the degree where sitting becomes difficult and the arms and hands are supporting the trunk, pressure sores can occur, especially in the elbow, which bears the brunt of the body weight. Spinal fusion is definitely indicated whenever possible.[32]

Respiratory function tests, including vital capacity, should be performed when the body jacket is used. In patients in whom respiratory musculature has become weakened to such an extent that respiratory excursion may be even more limited upon application of resistance, large anterior cutouts are used. In patients with a tracheostomy, provisions should be made for easy attachment of a ventilator whenever it may become necessary to use.

It is important to follow the spinal curve clinically and radiographically even though support is provided externally by a TLSO or internally via spinal fusion and instrumentation.[9,35,40] In the growing child, posterior spinal fusion can cause arrest of posterior growth centers, resulting in severe lordosis. This presents difficulty in sitting because the head and neck tilt back into increasingly greater extension with age. Modification of the wheelchair or outrigger for support of the head is needed. This lordosis, which results from the "crankshaft phenomenon," must to be recognized and prevented. Use of an "expanding" rod and surgical implantation of a rod without spinal fusion are important areas of innovation and development. If successful, many of the growing problems of the spine with increasing spinal deformity can be controlled until definitive spinal fusion can be established without significant growth disturbances.[47]

Spinal fusions that are incomplete, too short, or made on growing spines can result in further progression of scoliosis, know as *falling off* or the *crankshaft phenomenon*. The results of such surgical corrections can take the form of deformities and bony prominences, such as a protuberant rib cage, and pain. These cases present special challenges to the orthotist making special customized supports[6,36,37] and devices that allow for continued comfortable seating, maintenance of function, and independence.

Lower extremity orthoses for the ambulatory patient

Orthoses are used in the ambulatory patient to provide support to the limb at the knee and ankle. The weakened lower extremity with functional muscles can be stabilized at the knee joint or ankle joint using orthotic support. Depending on the strength of the proximal musculature and the ability to stabilize the knee using voluntary knee control, a knee–ankle–foot orthosis (KAFO) or ankle–foot orthosis (AFO) can be selected.[33] Studies of gait disorders and posture changes may assist the clinician and orthotist in recognizing orthotic needs.[14,23,41]

If joint contractures or muscle imbalance is present, surgical release of tightened joint structures is indicated. In the walking child with DMD and fixed knee joint contractures less than 20 degrees, a distal iliotibial band and other posterior soft tissue releases to correct the knee to a fully extended position may allow for bracing so that the child can stand either independently in the orthosis or with the help of a standing table.[38,46]

Foot and ankle contractures require assessment. In DMD and Becker muscular dystrophy, equinovarus deformity is expected.[11,12] In spinal muscular atrophy, the feet of patients frequently tend to evert.[26] Fixed contractures may require surgical release.[17] Dynamic deformities can be corrected by tendon releases or transfers.[11,16,25,33,49] When ankle motion is sufficient to allow for a plantigrade foot, orthoses can help support the weakened and unstable joint.

Knee–ankle–foot orthosis

A KAFO can be prescribed for a patient with neuromuscular disease to continue standing and walking even with weakened quadriceps muscles (Fig. 37-2). KAFOs will not be successful if the patient has hip flexion contracture more than 35 degrees. Knee flexion contractures must be corrected as close to neutral as possible by serial casting or surgical releases so that the knee can be locked into extension by the brace. Ankle and foot deformities must be addressed, surgically if necessary. Special locks must be incorporated into orthoses such that a patient with weakened upper extremity musculature and hand function can lock and release the knee lock from an extended position.

KAFOs for the growing child present a special challenge to the orthotist. Constant adjustments to growth must be made by changing the size of the plastic components, the length of the supporting bars, and the position of the knee and ankle joints. The child must be seen whenever tightness in the brace occurs. Because many children "sit" on the proximal edge of their KAFOs, reexamination on a periodic basis is needed because of growth. For good results, the brace must fit almost perfectly. Aluminum and steel components can be lengthened easily, but carbon fiber composite upright components that become too short must be replaced by longer components.

Because the patient has muscle weakness caused by the inherent disorder and does not require control of abnormal

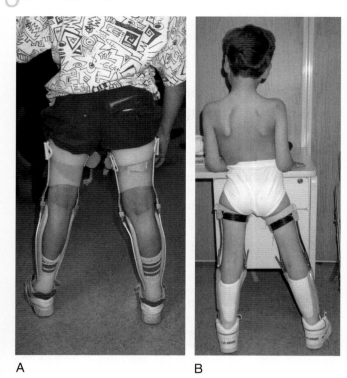

A   **B**

Fig. 37-2 A, KAFO with aluminum uprights and molded plastic thigh and pretibial components. **B**, KAFO incorporating lightweight carbon fiber composite support.

muscle pull or abnormal muscle forces owing to spasticity, lower extremity braces can made as lightweight as possible.[1] Their function is to support rather than correct for deforming forces or hold forcefully.

Ankle–foot orthosis

When ankle dorsiflexors are weak or ineffective, an AFO can be used to support the foot and ankle to achieve a stable brace, whereas maintenance of upright posture and mobility may be due to normal proximal hip musculature and good quadriceps strength. In the ambulatory patient, AFOs can allow the limb to continue to function, preventing the formation of a fixed equinus contracture at the ankle and supporting the foot for walking. In the nonambulatory or wheelchair dependent person, AFOs are used for positioning devices to keep the foot and ankle supported so that wheelchair foot rests can be used and fatigue is prevented.[17]

The most appropriate AFO for the neuromuscular patient should be manufactured of the most lightweight material possible. It should simulate the assistive function of normal musculature. This involves giving the patient up to 15 degrees of dorsiflexion while creating ground reaction forces to stabilize the patient's ankle and knee. Today, AFOs can be made with carbon fiber rods that enable the brace to support these loads without buckling, unlike molded plastic AFOs. Additionally, they allow tailoring of brace stiffness based on the weight, strength, and gait of the patient.[47]

An example of a vertebrace AFO designed by the Rancho Los Amigos National Rehabilitation Center's Rehabilitation Engineering center is shown in Figure 37-3.[30]

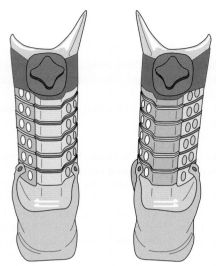

Fig. 37-3 Posterior view of orthoses fitted into shoes for an ambulatory person.

Most AFOs for neuromuscular patients are designed and made to be fitted inside a store-bought shoe. For these patients, the traditional double upright brace permanently connected by joint to the shoe is preferable (Fig. 37-4).

Muscle imbalance must be periodically reassessed when an AFO is used. If there is active muscle pull for the foot and ankle to be in varus or valgus, callosities or skin breakdown can form at the bottom of the foot, at the orthosis–skin interface, and along trim lines. This is especially relevant in patients with sensory impairment in addition to muscle weakness, such as those with Charcot-Marie-Tooth disease. Rebalancing the foot either surgically or by using dynamic devices, including hinging the orthoses at the ankle in the correct plane, can provide pressure relief.[11]

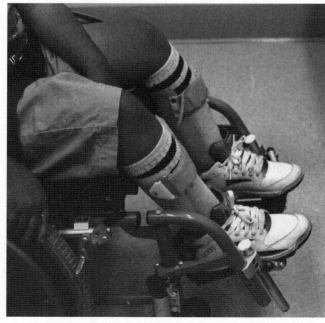

Fig. 37-4 Positioning AFOs used by a wheelchair-dependent patient with Duchenne muscular dystrophy.

Ambulatory AFOs may support the leg sufficiently to allow for short-distance walking.

Upper extremity orthoses

Orthoses for the upper extremity are used to provide support and prevent contractures. They are seldom used to control limb positioning or to prevent excessive forces or movement. A patient should undergo a manual muscle test to determine available and remaining muscle function. A functional assessment is of utmost importance before prescription for an orthosis can be considered. Contractures may be present and acceptable as long as function can be improved. Surgical releases are seldom necessary except for extreme conditions where a clenched fist or hand prevents use of the fingers or makes the remaining musculature pull so inefficiently that the muscles are nonfunctional.[18] For example, in a severely contracted DMD hand in which finger movement and hygiene have been severely compromised, release of finger flexors via a sublimus to profundus transfer operation may be indicated.[51] The hand, which can now clench over a knob to control wheelchair movement, allows the patient more freedom.

Controversy exists regarding the use of orthoses for the wrist and hand of a person with proximal interphalangeal and distal interphalangeal joint contractures due to intrinsic and extrinsic weakness. These contractures should be minimized by a preventive program of splinting and stretching. Static splinting is useful for maintaining range. Dynamic splinting is rarely used by neuromuscular patients with hand weakness and contractures because patients can readily compensate with substitute motions and activities rather than accept an encumbering and possibly unsightly device.

Mobile arm supports

The function of persons with proximal weakness can often be improved with the use of a mobile arm support (MAS). The MAS supports the weight of the arm, reducing the gravity loads on the shoulder and elbow. When the MAS is properly adjusted, gravity can be harnessed to assist selected movements, enabling easier movement and positioning of the hand and fingers. When applied at the appropriate time and with proper adjustments, increased functional capacity can be achieved even in patients with advanced muscular dystrophy.[4] The MAS can assist a person to reach areas on the tabletop as well as vertically, allowing them to perform activities such as feeding, light hygiene/grooming, operation of keyboards or communication devices, and participation in vocational/avocational activities.

Important indicators for successful MAS use include sitting stability with or without supporting device and elbow flexor strength of at least "poor" or grade 2/5. Continued use is dependent upon improved function in desired activities with MAS use and family support.[4,48]

Specific benefits of the MAS are seen in select candidates in the immediately postspinal fusion period. These patients now sit more erectly and often have difficulty using their compensatory motions to reach hand to mouth and face; the MAS has been found to assist in this motion.[48]

Interest has grown in improving the standard MAS, which was developed in the 1950s during the polio epidemic. In the late 1990s, the Rancho Los Amigos Rehabilitation Engineering Program began to develop a new MAS system, called the "MultiLink." The new design features address shortcomings of the standard MAS, which were identified through clinician and user surveys.[21] Design features of the new MAS include the following:

A. Quick and easy adjustments to the forearm support pivot and MAS working height allow device use in a variety of activities. The MAS can be easily stabilized so that the user can continue its wear when reclining or operating wheelchair controls, including traveling up/down inclines.
B. Narrower profile and improved appearance allow better doorway clearance and obstacle avoidance. The black anodized system with "high-tech" look is less obstructive, is more appealing, and is accepted by most patients and families.
C. The wheelchair mount is versatile and can accommodate a wide variety of new wheelchair designs on the market.

An example of MAS design and use is shown in Figure 37-5.

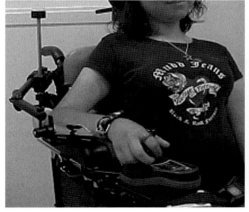 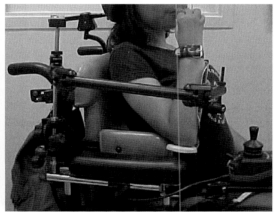

A   B

Fig. 37-5 MultiLink mobile arm support. **A,** Resting and wheelchair driving position. **B,** Position used for hygiene and feeding.

Acknowledgments

I thank Eunice Sumi, research therapist, and Pierre Leung, research engineer, for updated information on mobile arm supports and for supplying Figure 37-5. Ronan Reynolds, research engineer, supplied information on the vertebrace (ankle–foot) orthoses. All were affiliated with the Rancho Los Amigos National Rehabilitation Center, Los Amigos Research and Education Institute, Inc.

References

1. Barnett SL, Bagley AM, Skinner HB: Ankle weight effect on gait: orthotic implications, *Orthopedics* 16:1127–1131, 1993.
2. Bruns GAP: Assigning genes to chromosomes: family studies, somatic cell hybridization, chromosome sorting, in situ hybridization, translocations. In Rowland LP, et al., editor: *Molecular genetics of brain, nerve, and muscle*, New York, 1989, Oxford University Press.
3. Carlson JM, Winter R: The "Gillette" sitting support orthosis, *Orthot Prosthet* 32:35–45, 1978.
4. Chyatte SB, Long C II, Vignos PJ Jr: Balanced forearm orthosis in muscular dystrophy, *Arch Phys Med* 46:633–636, 1965.
5. de Goede C, Kelsey A, Kingston H, Tomlin P, Hughes M: Muscle biopsy without centrally located nuclei in a male child with mild X-linked myotubular myopathy, *Dev Med Child Neurol* 47:835–837, 2005.
6. Drennen JC, Renshaw TS, Curtis BH: The thoracic suspension orthosis, *Clin Orthop Relat Res* 139:33–39, 1979.
7. Dubowitz V: Therapeutic possibilities in muscular dystrophy: the hope versus the hype, *Neuromusc Dis* 12:113–116, 2002.
8. Evans GA, Drennan JC, Russman BS: Functional classification and orthopaedic management of spinal muscular atrophy, *J Bone Joint Surg* 63B:516–522, 1981.
9. Galasko CSB, Delaney C, Morris P: Spinal stabilization in Duchenne muscular dystrophy, *J Bone Joint Surg* 74B:210–214, 1992.
10. Gibson DA, Wilkins KE: The management of spinal deformities in Duchenne muscular dystrophy: a new concept of spinal bracing, *Clin Orthop Relat Res* 108:41–51, 1975.
11. Hsu JD: Orthopaedic care for children and adolescents with Charcot-Marie-Tooth disease. In Lovelace RE, Shapiro HK, editors: *Charcot-Marie-Tooth disorders: pathophysiology, molecular genetics and therapy*, New York, 1990, Wiley-Liss.
12. Hsu JD: Management of foot deformity in Duchenne's pseudohypertrophic muscular dystrophy, *Orthop Clin North Am* 7:979–984, 1976.
13. Hsu JD: The natural history of spine curvature in the nonambulatory Duchenne muscular dystrophy patient, *Spine* 8:771–775, 1983.
14. Hsu JD, Furumasu J: Gait and posture changes in the Duchenne muscular dystrophy child, *Clin Orthop Relat Res* 228:122–125, 1993.
15. Hsu JD, Gilgoff IS: Muscular dystrophy and neurogenic atrophy. In Nickel VL, Botte MJ, editors: *Orthopaedic rehabilitation*, ed 2, New York, 1992, Churchill-Livingstone.
16. Hsu JD, Hoffer MM: Posterior tibial tendon transfer anteriorly through the interosseous membrane: a modification of the technique, *Clin Orthop Relat Res* 131:202–204, 1978.
17. Hsu JD, Jackson R: Treatment of symptomatic foot and ankle deformities in the nonambulatory neuromuscular patient, *Foot Ankle* 5:238–244, 1985.
18. Hsu JD, Taylor D: Upper extremity deformities in Duchenne muscular dystrophy patients. In Fredricks S, Brody GS, editors: *Symposium on the neurologic aspects of plastic surgery*, St. Louis, 1978, CV Mosby.
19. Kaplan JC: Neuromuscular disorders: gene location, *Neuromusc Dis* 16:64–90, 2005.
20. Kendall HO, Kendall FP, Wadsworth GE: *Muscle testing and function*, Baltimore, 1971, Williams & Wilkins.
21. Landsberger S, Leung P, Vargas V, et al: Mobile arm supports: history, application and work in progress, *Top Spinal Cord Inj Rehabil* 11:74–94, 2005.
22. Lord J et al: Scoliosis associated with Duchenne muscular dystrophy, *Arch Phys Med Rehabil* 71:13–17, 1990.
23. Melkonian GJ, Cristofaro RL, Perry J, Hsu JD: Dynamic gait electromyography study in Duchenne muscular dystrophy (DMD) patients, *Foot Ankle* 1:78–83, 1980.
24. Merlini L, Granata C, Bonfiglioli S, Marini ML, Cervellati S, Savini R: Scoliosis in spinal muscular atrophy: natural history and management, *Dev Med Child Neurol* 31:501–508, 1989.
25. Miller GM, Hsu JD, Hoffer MM, Rentfro R: Posterior tibial tendon transfer: a review of the literature and analysis of 74 procedures, *J Pediatr Orthop* 2:363–370, 1982.
26. Moosa A, Dubowitz V: Spinal muscular atrophy in childhood, *Arch Dis Child* 48:386–388, 1973.
27. Murphy NA, Firth S, Jorgensen T, Young PC: Spinal surgery in children with idiopathic and neuromuscular scoliosis. What's the difference, *J Pediatr Orthop* 26:216–220, 2006.
27a. Nickel VL: Orthopedic rehabilitation: challenges and opportunities, *Bull Hosp Joint Dis* 29:1–21, 1968.
28. Norris Te: Rheumatoid arthritis and related disorders. In Taylor RB, editor: *Family medicine: principles and practice*, ed 4, New York, 1993, Springer Verlag.
29. Reimers CD, Fischer P, Pontgratz DE: Histopathological basis of muscle imaging. In Fleckenstein JL, Crues JV III, Reimers CD, editors: *Muscle imaging in health and disease*, New York, 1996, Springer.
30. Reynolds R, Weber R, Mulroy S, et al: Dual action posterior strut ankle foot orthosis: a tunable brace, In: *Proceedings 11th World Congress ISPO, Hong Kong*, August 2004.
31. Rideau Y, Glorion B, Delaubier A, Tarlé O, Bach J: The treatment of scoliosis in Duchenne muscular dystrophy, *Muscle Nerve* 7:281–286, 1984.
32. Robin GC, Brief LP: Scoliosis in childhood muscular dystrophy, *J Bone Joint Surg* 53A:466–476, 1971.
33. Rochelle J, Bowen JR, Ray S: Pediatric foot deformities in progressive neuromuscular disease, *Contemp Orthop* 8:41–50, 1984.
34. Russman BS: Development of an interest in spinal atrophy and disabilities, *Dev Med Child Neurol* 47:579, 2005.
35. Seeger BR, Sutherland ADA, Clark MS: Orthotic management of scoliosis in Duchenne muscular dystrophy, *Arch Phys Med Rehabil* 65:83–86, 1984.
36. Siegel IM, Silverman O, Silverman M: The Chicago insert: an approach to wheelchair seating for the maintenance of spinal posture in Duchenne muscular dystrophy, *Orthot Prosthet* 35:27–29, 1981.
37. Silverstein F, Siebens AA: Head-control-system for severely paralyzed patient, *Arch Phys Med Rehabil* 64:604–605, 1983.
38. Spencer GE Jr: Orthopaedic considerations in the management of muscular dystrophy, *Curr Pract Orthop Surg* 5:279–293, 1973.
39. Srinivasan R, Hornyak JE, Badenhop DT, Koch LG: Cardiac rehabilitation after heart transplantation in a patient with Becker's muscular dystrophy. A case report, *Arch Phys Med Rehabil* 86:2059–2061, 2005.
40. Sussman MD: Treatment of scoliosis in Duchenne muscular dystrophy, *Dev Med Child Neurol* 27:522–531, 1985.
41. Sutherland DH: *Gait disorders in childhood and adolescence*, Baltimore, 1984, Williams & Wilkins.
42. Thong M-K, Bazlin R, Wong K-T: Diagnosis and management of Duchenne muscular dystrophy in a developing country over a 10-year period, *Dev Med Child Neurol* 47:474–477, 2005.
43. Tovey D, Bognolo G: Levels of evidence and the orthopaedic surgeon, *J Bone Joint Surg* 87B:1591–1592, 2005.
44. Urtizberea JA: Therapies in muscular dystrophy: current concepts and future prospects, *Eur Neurol* 43:127–132, 2000.
45. Venance SL, Koopman WT, Miskie BA, Hegele RA, Hahn AF: Rigid spine muscular dystrophy due to SEPN1 mutation presenting as cor pulmonale, *Neurology* 64:395–396, 2005.
46. Vignos PJ Jr, Spencer GE Jr, Archibald KC: Management of progressive muscular dystrophy of childhood, *JAMA* 184:89–96, 1963.
47. Wilke H-J, Kluger P, Naumann T, Kron T, Claes LE, Puhl W: In situ rigidity of a new sliding rod for management of the growing spine in Duchenne muscular dystrophy, *Spine* 21:1957–1961, 1996.
48. Yasuda YL, Bowman K, Hsu JD: Mobile arm supports: criteria for successful use in muscle disease patients, *Arch Phys Med Rehabil* 47:253–256, 1986.
49. Yeap JS, Birch R, Singh D: Long-term results of tibialis posterior tendon transfer for drop-foot, *Int Orthop* 25:114–118, 2001.
50. Young A, Johnson D, O'Gorman E, Macmillan T, Chase AP: A new spinal brace for use in Duchenne muscular dystrophy, *Dev Med Child Neurol* 26:808–813, 1984.
51. Yu W, Schweigel JF: Flexor digitorum sublimus to profundus tendon transfer for flexion deformities of the hand and wrist in spastic paralysis, *J Bone Joint Surg* 55B:664, 1973.
52. Zenios M, Sampath J, Cole C, Khan T, Galasko CSB: Operative treatment for hip subluxation in spinal muscular atrophy, *J Bone Joint Surg* 87B:1541–1544, 2005.

Chapter

38

Orthoses for cerebral palsy

Tom F. Novacheck

Key Points

- Proper lever arm alignment promotes function.
- Optimal care of individuals with cerebral palsy is achieved using a multidisciplinary approach.
- A segmental analysis of the lower extremities helps to assure proper segmental function
- Avoiding crouch and excessive knee stress are important long-term goals.
- Understanding the different function of one- versus two-joint muscles is crucial.

Pathophysiology

Cerebral palsy (CP) is, by definition, a static encephalopathy with onset before maturation of the central nervous system. Although most cases are present at birth, most experts include injury to the brain before age 3 in the diagnostic grouping of CP. In general, anoxic events lead to quadriplegia. Prematurity resulting in periventricular leukomalacia results in diplegic CP. Vascular events such as intrauterine strokes cause hemiplegia.

Regardless of the type of CP, it is the central control system that is damaged. The neurological lesion may produce different tone abnormalities. In a patient with pure spasticity, only the pyramidal system is damaged. In a patient with athetoid CP, only the extrapyramidal system is involved. Both systems are injured when a mixed pattern is seen. The central nervous system lesion affects the musculoskeletal system. Primary abnormalities include the following[8]:

- Loss of selective motor control
- Dependence on primitive reflex patterns for movement

- Abnormal muscle tone
- Relative imbalance between muscle agonists and antagonists across joints
- Deficient equilibrium reactions
- Weakness

These primary abnormalities cause secondary growth disorders of the musculoskeletal system as the neurological impairments occur early during growth and development. Normal bone growth occurs only if the bones are subjected to typical development stresses. Children who are unable to walk, run, and play at typical ages with typical movement patterns are likely to develop bone and joint deformities. Infantile bony alignment is markedly different than typical adult alignment. Normal developmental remodeling of fetal femoral anteversion and internal tibial torsion is unlikely in the absence of typical growth stresses. Development of normal foot alignment and function is in jeopardy if muscle function is abnormal or if the stresses on the foot are excessive due to spasticity or abnormal weight-bearing positions. Longitudinal bone growth occurs at the physes present at both ends of long bones. Much of that growth probably occurs while the child is resting. Muscle growth, on the other hand, is driven by stretch. Normally that stretch occurs when a child, whose bones have grown during sleep, gets up and starts to run and play. Ziv et al.[31] showed that in order for normal muscle growth to occur, 2 to 4 hours of stretch per day is necessary. In addition, they showed that the muscles of spastic mice do not grow in response to stretch at the typical rate. The combination of this lack of response and the lack of "normal play" leads to secondary musculotendinous contractures.

Gait dysfunction in individuals with CP occurs as a result of these primary and secondary abnormalities, which rarely occur in isolation. Rather, they are multiple and consist of primary effects (due to the damage to the central nervous system), secondary deformities (from abnormal bone/muscle growth), and tertiary compensations (individual coping responses to minimize the gait inefficiency resulting from the primary and secondary abnormalities). Tertiary abnormalities are coping responses to restore lost attributes of normal gait[19] and include the following:

- Stability in stance
- Clearance in swing
- Appropriate prepositioning of the foot for initial contact
- Adequate step length
- Energy conservation

One example of a tertiary gait compensation is circumduction to compensate for clearance problems caused by cospasticity of the rectus femoris and hamstrings. This produces the stiff knee gait so common in patients with CP. Another example is premature plantarflexion in stance phase (typically referred to as *vaulting*), which is present in a child with hemiplegic CP to compensate for a lack of clearance on the hemiplegic side caused by either a drop foot in swing (tibialis anterior dysfunction) or rectus femoris spasticity. Too often, the "difficult to identify" vaulting is misinterpreted as a part of the pathology and is not recognized as compensation on the nonaffected side. As such, orthotic or surgical management may be prescribed, resulting in a detrimental effect on the child's function. Because primary, secondary, and tertiary abnormalities occur at all levels in the lower extremity, the management of gait dysfunction in children with CP truly is complex and was (and continues to be) the driving force for the development of computerized gait analysis laboratories.

Neurological conditions create greater distal than proximal dysfunction. The weakness and loss of motor control that can occur in individuals with CP typically are worse at the foot and ankle than at the hip. The unstable foot induces additional alignment abnormalities at the hip and knee. This explains why orthotic management is primarily directed toward compensating for foot and ankle dysfunction to improve walking function. These issues are addressed in the treatment sections of this chapter.

It is primarily the two-joint muscles (e.g., psoas, rectus femoris, hamstrings, and gastrocnemius) that are affected by excessive tone caused by CP. With time and growth, these muscles become contracted. It is interesting that the one-joint

muscles (e.g., gluteus maximus, vasti, and soleus) typically are too long due to the chronic effects of walking in crouch. The crouch position of excessive hip and knee flexion in conjunction with either excessive ankle dorsiflexion or midfoot breakdown puts these muscles in a position of excessive elongation as they cross the joints. These are also the muscles that are primarily responsible for our ability to maintain upright posture.[29] Upright posture requires good antigravity function of the one-joint muscles responsible for supporting body weight. Weakness and excessive elongation of these muscles in conjunction with spasticity of the two-joint muscles is primarily responsible for crouch gait. The management of ambulatory dysfunction in CP in the vast majority of cases is geared toward the treatment of crouch. The long-term consequences of crouch are excessive joint stress and gait inefficiency. This combination leads to decreasing ambulatory function in adolescence and adulthood due to joint pain and excessive energy costs.[13,27] The frequency of these problems in adulthood is disturbingly high[16] and ultimately is the reason why treatment of these problems in children and adults is so important.

To understand and treat physical function deficits requires a basic understanding of mechanics. A *lever arm* or *moment arm* is defined as the distance from a point to a force that is perpendicular to the line of action of that force. The force (measured in Newtons) times the length of the lever arm (in meters) is equal to the moment that acts around the center of rotation (in Newton-meters). In general, the length of the bone serves as the lever, and the joint at the end of that bone serves as the center of rotation or fulcrum. The magnitude and direction of the moment depends upon the point of action of the applied force (Fig. 38-1).

Moments are perhaps understood most easily if one thinks of a see-saw in which the mass of the larger individual times his or her distance from the fulcrum is equal to that of the smaller individual times her or his distance from the fulcrum (Fig. 38-2).

The principle is the same in walking. External moments produced by the ground reaction and inertial forces plus weights of the lower extremity segments are resisted by internal moments produced by the action of muscles, tendons, and/or ligaments (Fig. 38-3).

Lever-arm dysfunction is a term originally coined to describe the particular orthopedic deformities that arise in an ambulatory child with CP. However, the condition is common to any traumatic or neuromuscular problem that produces

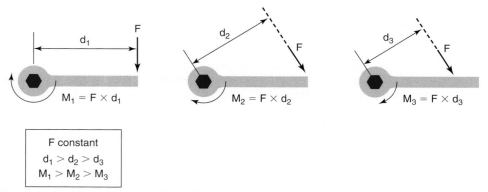

$M_1 = F \times d_1$ $M_2 = F \times d_2$ $M_3 = F \times d_3$

F constant
$d_1 > d_2 > d_3$
$M_1 > M_2 > M_3$

Fig. 38-1 Moments and lever arms. The magnitude of a moment (M) is the product of force (F) times the length of the lever arm (d). A lever arm is defined as the perpendicular distance between the force and the center of rotation. A change in either the position or the orientation of the applied force will cause a change in the magnitude of the moment. To create the largest moment, the force must be perpendicular to the lever.

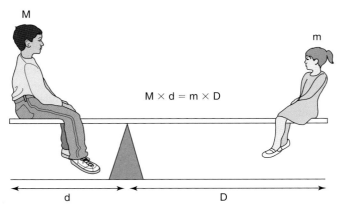

Fig. 38-2 Easily understood example of moments, shown as the relationship between an adult and a child on a teeter-totter. The larger mass of the adult sitting closer to the pivot point (fulcrum) balances the smaller mass of the child sitting further away.

alteration of the bony skeleton. Lever-arm dysfunction, then, describes a general class of bone modeling, remodeling, and/or traumatic deformities that includes hip subluxation, torsional and angular deformities of long bones, and/or foot deformities. Because the muscles and/or ground reaction forces must act on skeletal levers to produce locomotion, abnormalities of these lever-arm systems greatly interfere with the child's ability to walk.[8,9]

In a condition such as CP, the muscle and/or ground reaction forces are neither appropriate nor adequate because of muscle contractures, poor selective motor control, and/or abnormality of the bony lever arms. The five distinct types of lever arm deformity are (1) short lever arm, (2) flexible lever arm, (3) malrotated lever arm, (4) abnormal pivot or action point, and/or (5) positional lever-arm dysfunction (Table 38-1). A comprehensive discussion of lever-arm

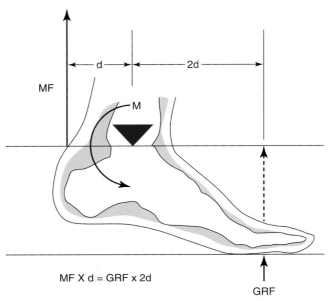

$$MF \times d = GRF \times 2d$$

Fig. 38-3 Relationship between the external moment produced by the ground reaction force (GRF) and the internal moment produced by the muscles. Both forces act on a skeletal lever around the fulcrum (joint center). In this illustration, the lever arm of the GRF is twice as long as that of the ankle plantarflexors. As a result, the magnitude of the muscle force would be twice that of the GRF.

Table 38-1 Examples of lever arm dysfunction

Type	Deformity
Short lever arm	Coxa valga
Flexible lever arm	Pes valgus
Malrotated lever arm	External tibial torsion
Abnormal pivot or action point	Hip subluxation/dislocation
Positional lever-arm dysfunction	Erect vs crouch gait

dysfunction is beyond the scope of this chapter, but a common example of lever-arm dysfunction that is seen in spastic diplegia will serve to illustrate the problem.

In normal gait during the second half of the stance phase, stability of the knee is maintained without quadriceps action by a mechanism termed the *plantarflexion/knee-extension couple* (Box 38-1). That is, the action of the soleus at the ankle restrains forward motion of the tibia over the foot and in so doing maintains the ground reaction force in front of the knee. The result is that the ground reaction force acting on the lever arm of the

---

BOX 38-1
PlantarFlexion/Knee-Extension Couple

A moment in the musculoskeletal system is the product of the muscle force times the length of the lever arm on which the muscle force is applied. Joint moments are necessary to provide for stance phase stabilization and propulsion. Stance phase stabilization is necessary because joints are inherently unstable. Without ligament and muscle function, the joints would collapse under the force of gravity. To maintain an upright posture (antigravity position), the hip, knee, and ankle joints are stabilized primarily under the influence of the hip extensors, vasti, and gastrocsoleus. To initiate and maintain walking, propulsive muscle forces are necessary to propel the body and the lower extremity body segments. Winter[29] showed that 50% of the moment production to maintain upright standing posture is supplied by the gastrocsoleus. The soleus typically is thought of as an ankle plantarflexor. However, when the foot is in a plantigrade position during second rocker, the soleus is active and works eccentrically to restrain the forward movement of the tibia. Therefore, it functions as a knee extensor. This is known as the *plantarflexion/knee-extension couple*. This normal coupling requires normal foot function, structure, and alignment, and normal gastrocsoleus activation and strength. Pathology can adversely affect any or all of these. Consequently, coupling frequently is excessive or insufficient. The knee may be driven into hyperextension during midstance by a well-aligned foot in the presence of gastrocsoleus spasticity or contracture. Unfortunately, the insufficient plantarflexion/knee-extension couple is common and contributes to crouch gait. Appropriate surgery and/or orthotic management can be effective in treating this deficiency. Likewise, inappropriate surgery and/or bracing not only are ineffective but also can cause iatrogenic worsening. These concepts are illustrated in specific examples in the section on orthotic management.

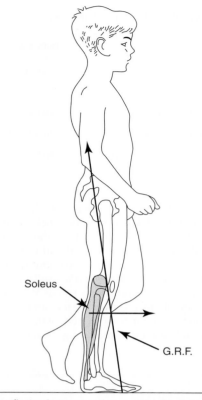

Soleus

G.R.F.

Fig. 38-4 Plantarflexion/knee-extension couple. During midstance in typical gait, the soleus resists ankle dorsiflexion and slows the forward movement of the lower leg (tibia). As a result, the GRF acting on the lever arm of the foot generates an extension moment on the knee that stabilizes the knee in an extended position without muscular activation of the larger muscle mass of the quadriceps (which would consume more energy to accomplish the same task). This extension moment is referred to as the *plantarflexion/knee-extension couple*.

forefoot produces an extension moment at the knee, which in turn maintains the joint in extension without the aid of the quadriceps (Fig. 38-4). However, the typical child with spastic diplegia frequently has femoral anteversion in conjunction with pes valgus and/or external tibial torsion. The plane of the foot often is as much as 40 degrees external to the plane of the knee. In addition, a valgus foot is an ineffective lever because it is supple rather than rigid. As a result, even if the magnitude of the ground reaction force were normal, because the lever arm is supple and maldirected, the magnitude of the extension moment can be greatly reduced (Fig. 38-5). Fortunately, lever-arm dysfunction usually is correctable with appropriate orthopedic surgery and/or bracing.

Many children with CP have weak ankle plantarflexors (gastrocnemius and soleus). Typically the ankle plantarflexors restrict dorsiflexion and tibial advancement in second rocker (midstance phase of the gait cycle) and act like a spring, providing power for push-off in third rocker (just before toe-off).

When the plantarflexors fail to function adequately in midstance, excessive dorsiflexion results and is accompanied by excessive knee flexion, or *crouch gait*. When the activity of the gastrocnemius is inadequate, insufficient power for push-off results in decreased clearance in swing, reduced step length, and decreased walking speed. Therefore, plantarflexor dysfunction leads to both stance phase (supportive) and swing phase (propulsive) deficiencies.

Evaluation of foot deformity is challenging (see Box 38-2). Two common foot deformity types exist in children with CP. In patients with hemiplegia, the *equinovarus* foot deformity is most common and may be associated with pes cavus. In individuals with diplegic and quadriplegic CP, the dominant foot deformity is *equinovalgus*. Although the etiology of this foot deformity is not completely certain, it most likely is related to equinus of the hindfoot (primarily gastrocnemius contracture and spasticity) leading to excessive forefoot weight-bearing early in a child's development when the structure of the foot's longitudinal arch is incompletely developed. Up until about age 6 years, pes planus is typical. With typical development, the arch forms and develops. In the case of neuromuscular pathology, this process may not occur, and equinovalgus foot deformity with midfoot instability can develop. With time, a forefoot varus deformity is not uncommon (Fig. 38-6). Treatment of this complex foot deformity type may require management of not only hindfoot equinus but also midfoot instability and forefoot varus.

Historical perspective

The history of orthotic management for treatment of fractures with closed reduction and splinting dates back to Hippocrates, but the recorded history for treatment of neuromuscular conditions is shorter. Ambrose Paré described shoe modifications for talipes equinovarus in the 16th century. Winthrop Morgan Phelps, an American orthopedic surgeon in the early 20th century, was primarily interested in the management of CP. Although he was an orthopedic surgeon, he advocated bracing rather than surgery as the primary method of controlling deformities in children with CP. His braces were constructed primarily from leather and metal.

The introduction of plastics after World War II revolutionized the world of orthotics. Thermoplastics remain the mainstay for fabrication of orthotics to this day. Although plastics are better than metal and leather, the search continues for strong, durable, and lightweight materials that may have even better structural characteristics.

Current issues

- Materials
- Understanding of gait function
- Understanding of foot deformity
- Variation in goals (short-term functional vs long-term joint preservation)

Current research

Motion analysis laboratories have been used over the past 15 to 20 years to objectively evaluate the effects of ankle–foot orthoses (AFOs) on gait function in children with CP. Numerous studies have reported significant improvements in linear parameters of velocity, step and stride length, and single-limb stance support time when children with CP are tested while wearing their AFOs.[1,2,7,14,20,22,28] These improvements indicate substantial functional improvement. In addition, net oxygen can be reduced 6% to 9% when children with CP are tested while wearing their AFOs.[15] Hainsworth et al.[10] reported that range of motion and gait deteriorated when

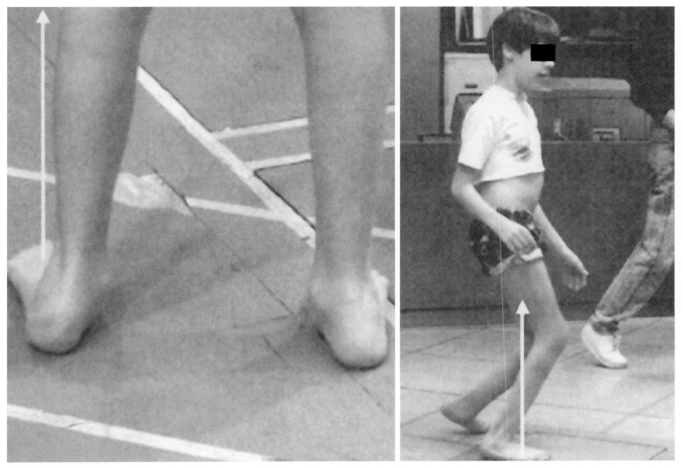

Fig. 38-5 Flexible lever arm dysfunction. **A,** During terminal stance, the arch typically stiffens due to tension created in the plantar fascia as it winches around the metatarsal heads during metatarsophalangeal joint extension. The heel moves into relative varus and the arch lifts. The rigidity of the foot renders it an effective lever for the ankle plantarflexors to generate push-off power. The midfoot instability associated with pes valgus allows the hindfoot to remain in valgus while the forefoot persists in a position of abduction and varus throughout stance. As a result, the foot is externally rotated to the knee axis. The lever arm is both maldirected and an ineffective lever arm, like a crowbar made of rubber. **B,** Typical pes valgus secondary to spastic diplegia. The normal plantarflexion/knee-extension couple is disrupted because the GRF is behind the knee axis in midstance. The entire task of sustaining an upright position with lower extremity extension falls to the hip and knee extensors. Unfortunately, as body size increases with age, the strength and power in these two muscle groups are not enough to assume this burden, and crouch gait develops.

AFOs were not worn by 12 children between 3 and 7 years old with CP.

In addition to global functional improvements, AFOs have been shown to improve abnormal gait parameters specific to ankle joint function.[1,21] Abel et al.[1] saw a reduction of abnormal power burst in midstance and an increase in late-stance ankle moment indicating improved ability to support body weight in a more appropriate alignment at the ankle in patients with either equinus or pes planovalgus.

Consistent and substantial changes in kinematics or kinetics at the pelvis, hip, or knee have not been identified. Despite improvements in parameters of global function and specific parameters of ankle function, little effect of AFOs on proximal joints of the lower limb have been noted.[1,2,5,18,20,21] Gait function is enhanced without significant changes noted at the proximal joints. Such improvements are more commonly seen in paralytic conditions such as myelomeningocele and poliomyelitis.

The question as to whether specific AFO designs lead to identifiable differences has received some attention. In a retrospective review of 115 patients with CP, White

et al.[28] found that gait improvements were independent of specific AFO design. A variety of styles provided similar results. Buckon et al.[2] showed that various configurations of AFOs (solid, hinged, and posterior leaf spring [PLS]) all normalized ankle kinematics in stance, increased step/stride length, decreased cadence, and decreased energy cost of walking. As expected, articulated AFOs resulted in greater ankle dorsiflexion in terminal stance than did solid AFOs, and preswing plantarflexion power was preserved.[2] There is no evidence that tone-reducing features incorporated in the footplate of a standard AFO provide additional benefit in gait parameters.[5] Romkes and Brunner[22] showed that hinged AFOs are superior to dynamic AFOs (supramalleolar) in improving gait parameters in children with hemiplegic CP. Lam et al.[14] found that the dynamic AFO did not reduce muscle overactivity as well as the AFO did. Despite this finding, the dynamic AFO was equally effective at correcting equinus in stance and swing and less restrictive of ankle movement. The authors noted that because the device is lighter and less bulky, compliance was improved. It is well known that children in general will choose the

The foot should be examined in non-weightbearing to determine segmental alignment of the forefoot to the hindfoot in the subtalar joint neutral position. The patient is prone with the foot over the end of the examining table. For examination of the right foot, the left thumb and index finger of the examiner are placed around the talonavicular joint medially and laterally (Fig. 38-6). The examiner's right thumb and index finger grasp the necks of the 4th and 5th metatarsals. The forefoot is then pronated and supinated until the examiner feels that the navicular is "reduced" in line with the head of the talus. The head of the talus is equally covered medially and laterally by the navicular. The forefoot is then loaded with slight dorsiflexion pressure on the necks of the 4th and 5th metatarsals to mimic weightbearing. In the subtalar joint neutral position, the alignment of the hindfoot relative to the tibia and the forefoot relative to the hindfoot can be assessed to identify deformities that may influence foot position and foot motion in weightbearing. Identification of subtalar neutral position also provides insight into the presence or absence of atypical tibial torsion and aids in the crucial differentiation between tibial torsion and foot deformity.

It is also important to assess flexibility of the foot. The foot should be flexible to function as a mobile adapter in first and second rocker, yet not excessively flexible so that it can function appropriately as a stable lever arm for the ankle plantarflexors in second and third rocker.

lightest, smallest, and least restrictive style brace, even in the absence of significant differences in gait parameters or energy expenditure.[24]

Some orthopedists are concerned that a hinged AFO with free dorsiflexion could have adverse effects on crouch. The hinged AFO controls the spastic and/or contracted gastrocnemius at the ankle, but the abnormal two-joint muscle pulls the knee into flexion. In other words, the hinged AFO allows crouch. Despite the beneficial effect of the hinged AFO on maintaining ankle power generation,[21] the authors raised concern about greater ankle dorsiflexion in terminal stance with articulated compared to solid AFOs. They warned that hinged AFOs should be considered only for "children who do not have a preexisting tendency to crouch." Buckon et al.[2] did note that some children with greater involvement had worsening of knee extensor moment, excessive ankle dorsiflexion, and greater energy cost with a hinged AFO. On the other hand, Radtka et al.[20] did not see the same adverse effects at the knee with the hinged AFO. The patients in that study may have had lesser involvement.[20]

Many children with neurological dysfunction have deficits of ankle plantarflexion function both for stance phase stability and for propulsion of the limb into swing. It would be desirable to use an AFO that is stiff enough to provide support in midstance yet flexible enough to allow energy return in third rocker, or push-off. Theoretically, that is the goal of the PLS AFO. It is often prescribed for this purpose and can be fabricated in a variety of designs. Current designs seem to succeed in achieving the first goal but not the second. Although the PLS AFO did improve footdrop in swing and increased power absorption in midstance, it did not augment push-off

power in terminal stance.[18] It is flexible enough to allow dorsiflexion but has no effect on knee kinematics. These authors concluded that "the name 'posterior leaf spring' is misleading in terms of the function of this AFO during gait in persons with CP, as this brace does not augment power-generating capabilities at the ankle." This issue is evaluated further in a discussion of stiffness testing of energy-storing orthotics later in this chapter.

Treatment recommendations

If we are going to treat CP well, we must understand the pathological mechanisms causing the gait abnormalities. The primary problems of deficient selective motor control, abnormalities of balance, and abnormal central nervous system tone drive the secondary abnormalities of inadequate muscle growth and bony deformity. The secondary abnormalities are amenable to treatment, whereas the primary abnormalities of CP, with the exception of spasticity, are difficult to alter. Consequently, we must learn to analyze the pathology and determine which portions of it can be corrected and which cannot.

Inadequate muscle growth can be treated by a variety of means, including any or all of the following: (1) passive stretch, (2) night splinting, (3) physical therapy, (4) botulinum toxin, (5) phenol or alcohol injections, (6) orthopedic lengthening, and/or (7) spasticity reduction. Bone deformity (lever-arm dysfunction) is best corrected by orthopedic surgery, but modest joint deformities are amenable to bracing.

Abnormal muscle tone is a primary problem and as such is more difficult to remedy. Minor degrees of tone abnormality may not be functionally limiting. They can and should be accepted. More severe, pure spasticity probably is best addressed by selective dorsal rhizotomy, provided the child meets the criteria for the procedure (pure spasticity, good selective motor control, adequate underlying muscle strength, age 4–7 years, and diagnosis of diplegic CP due to prematurity). Children with hypertonia, who do not meet the selection criteria for selective dorsal rhizotomy, currently are being treated at our center with the intrathecal baclofen pump. In general, extrapyramidal tone is not amenable to treatment, although oral pharmacological agents can be tried.

Deficits of selective motor control and abnormal balance mechanisms are permanent disabilities. Appropriate physical therapy should be used to maximize function, but currently these problems have no remedy. As such, they are the limiting factors of all types of treatment.

In order to apply the knowledge of CP gait pathology to guide treatment, the following management principles of ambulatory disability in CP can be useful.

1. Reduce spasticity
2. Correct contractures
3. Simplify the control system
4. Preserve power generators
5. Correct lever-arm dysfunction

The first two broadly guide treatment decision-making at all ages (although different treatment methods would be used to accomplish each of these goals at different ages). The last three are applied when planning orthopedic surgery.

Spasticity management and correction of contractures can be addressed in many different ways (physical therapy,

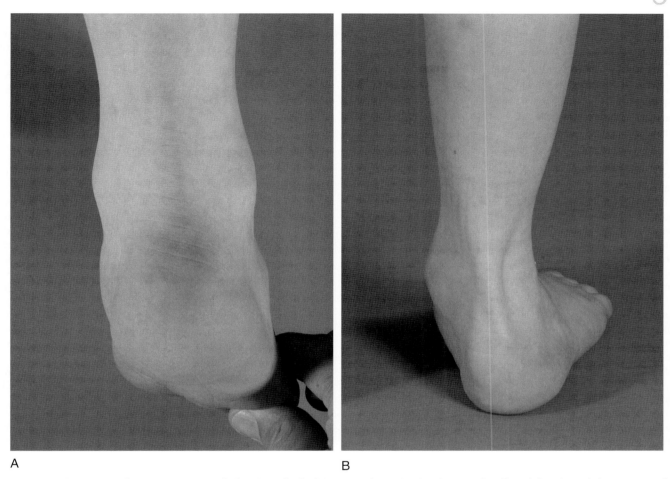

A   B

Fig. 38-6 Forefoot varus deformity. **A**, Non–weight-bearing subtalar joint neutral examination shows no hindfoot deformity and the presence of a forefoot varus deformity. **B**, Same foot in weight-bearing examination shows collapse into hindfoot valgus and pes planus.

orthotics, botulinum toxin injections, oral spastolytics, selective dorsal rhizotomy, intrathecal baclofen, and/or tendon lengthening). In practice, choosing among these options depends largely on the child's age. Global spasticity management is often the method of choice for children between the ages 4 and 7 years, whereas botulinum toxin injection and/or stretching casts are better choices for younger children and/or adolescents in the midst of their growth spurt. Little definitive scientific evidence compares the efficacy of each of these methods at different ages. The overall management scheme for decision-making as represented on the flowchart is based largely on clinical experience and knowledge of the pathomechanics of CP. If careful quantitative assessment and evaluation of outcomes are used as a routine part of the treatment program, optimal methods of achieving specific treatment objectives should become apparent.

Significant lever-arm dysfunction should be managed regardless of age. Consider, for example, the unstable talipes equinovalgus foot that is so common in children with spastic diplegia. Remember that moment-generating capability is dependent on both the ability to generate muscle force and the presence of an intact lever arm, emphasizing the importance of correcting pes valgus (lever-arm dysfunction). Controlling midfoot instability is the hallmark of managing

this deformity. In milder cases and younger patients, orthotic management incorporating accentuated arch support, an extended lateral border to prevent forefoot abduction, and medial internal forefoot posting of forefoot varus may successfully restore proper alignment of the forefoot relative to the ankle and knee. If not controlled, muscle force generation by the ankle plantarflexors does not lead to full ankle plantarflexion moment generation. Instead, external rotational moments are created by the ankle plantarflexors, and torsional deformities (particularly external tibial torsion) can result.

Whereas physical therapy and orthoses are appropriate for very young children with milder deformity, they typically are not adequate for older children, and surgical intervention is necessary. Numerous surgical options are available for this type of foot deformity. Choosing the appropriate surgical procedure(s) remains complicated, but the goals remain the same: restore functional alignment and maintain appropriate mobility. Improving braceability may be a reasonable goal.

Plantarflexor moment insufficiency can be a debilitating cause of crouch gait at any age. For young children, botulinum toxin injection to the gastrocnemius in conjunction with a well-fitting, solid AFO to maintain foot alignment and stability may be appropriate.

For older children with crouch gait, careful assessment should be made for bony deformities such as external tibial torsion, distal tibial valgus, pes valgus, femoral anteversion, knee flexion contracture, and/or patella alta (usually associated with knee extensor lag/insufficiency). In addition, crouch gait can be due to soleus weakness. Consequently, physical therapy to strengthen the soleus should be considered. A floor reaction AFO can be used if weakness remains an insurmountable problem.

Methods of treatment in the age of spasticity management are different than when tendon lengthenings alone were performed. Decreased spasticity allows the child to have greater range of motion, less spastic response to stretch, and better potential to develop and use voluntary muscle activity during gait. Consequently, orthotic needs are different. Frequently, less rigid PLS AFOs can be used. Spasticity hinders strengthening programs for children with CP, and insufficient muscle strength can be a major cause of ongoing disability. As a result of spasticity reduction, physical therapy for strengthening may now be more beneficial than in the past.

Remembering that moment-generating capability is the key to good musculoskeletal function will allow the treating physician to identify not only muscle strength deficiencies but also lever-arm dysfunction. Knee extensor lag and plantarflexor moment insufficiency both can be debilitating causes of crouch, especially in the adolescent.

Surgical management can improve the effectiveness of orthoses, decrease their complexity, decrease the risk of orthotic complications, or eliminate the need for orthoses altogether. For equinus, gastrocnemius Botox injection or gastrocnemius lengthening is commonly performed. Midfoot hypermobility associated with equinovalgus foot deformity is treated by os calcis lengthening, talonavicular reefing, or talonavicular arthrodesis. These procedures can be performed in isolation or in various combinations. In the past, subtalar arthrodeses and triple arthrodeses were more commonly performed but now are reserved for end-stage, severe deformities. Tendon transfers for this foot deformity type are not commonly performed because no clear evidence of benefit has been shown.

Tendon transfer or lengthening surgery is used for equinovarus feet. Frost intramuscular lengthening of the posterior tibialis, split posterior tibial tendon transfer, and split anterior tibialis tendon transfer typically are performed in combination with management of equinus as outlined above. Plantar fascial release may be required to manage pes cavus. Fixed adduction deformity may require lateral column shortening procedures such as os calcis or cuboid subtraction osteotomies. Forefoot deformities (especially plantarflexed first ray) are also common with this type of foot deformity.

Orthotic management

For practical purposes, hip–knee–ankle–foot orthoses are almost never used to manage ambulatory problems in individuals with CP. They are useful at rest to maintain proper alignment in children with total body involvement in an effort to prevent contracture and progressive hip subluxation.

Similarly, knee–ankle–foot orthoses (KAFOs) can be used at rest to maintain musculotendinous length of the hamstrings and gastrocnemius and prevent the development of knee flexion contracture. KAFOs were used more widely in the past to assist with walking function. They are cumbersome and have been shown to increase the energy cost of walking. The appropriate combination of surgery, rehabilitation, and below-knee bracing almost always can simplify the problems that adversely affect walking function and thereby eliminate the need to consider a KAFO. Fixed joint contractures may prevent normal excursion of the joint while walking. They can cause many abnormalities, including crouch gait and short step length. The orthotist should recognize when an otherwise appropriate orthoses cannot achieve its desired affect because of a hip or knee contracture (especially floor reaction AFOs).

For each of the AFO designs discussed in subsequent sections, the foot section is considered separately. The previous discussion regarding foot deformity types should be considered a guideline to assist with decision-making in this regard. If the goal of the orthosis is to assist with the dynamic function of walking, then the orthotist first must be able to assess alignment and to fabricate an orthosis that will be well tolerated and restore alignment. The orthotist must recognize when this goal is not possible. Possible causes include rigid uncorrectable foot deformity, tibial malrotation (external tibial torsion is the most common), and distal tibial valgus deformity. Although the latter is recognized as a fairly common deformity in myelomeningocele, it also can occur in patients with CP. It is more likely to be missed in patients with CP because it is less well documented.

An unrecognized coronal plane forefoot (varus or valgus) deformity is a frequent cause of orthotic intolerance or failure to provide adequate function. Foot deformity management has evolved over the past 10 years at Gillette Children's Specialty Healthcare due to improved recognition and understanding of these deformities. As a result, both orthotic and surgical treatments have been modified, leading to more effective restoration of foot function as an effective lever arm for the ankle plantarflexors. Surgically, this includes plantarflexion osteotomies of the first cuneiform or first metatarsal to correct forefoot varus deformity (likewise the plantarflexed first ray common with pes cavus is treated with dorsiflexion osteotomies at the base of the first metatarsal or through the first cuneiform). Orthotically, a footplate can be incorporated to compensate for the forefoot deformity using internal forefoot posting. The floor is "brought up to the foot" (Fig. 38-7). The mold is taken in its natural non–weight-bearing position in subtalar joint neutral position. The footplate incorporates midfoot control with forefoot posting. This footplate can be used as a foot orthosis (FO) alone or incorporated into a University of California Biomechanics Lab (UCBL) orthosis, supramalleolar orthosis (SMO), or AFO.

UCBL orthoses and SMOs are commonly used for treatment of CP (Fig. 38-8). Both can control varus or valgus deformities of the hindfoot and compensate for forefoot deformities. The longer lever arm of the SMO allows its application to more significant hindfoot and midfoot deformities. Both provide arch support and hindfoot varus/valgus control. Careful identification of fixed forefoot deformities and incorporation of appropriate forefoot posting lead to orthoses that are better able to achieve the functional goal of restoring proper lever arm alignment. The SMO occasionally lessens footdrop in swing to some

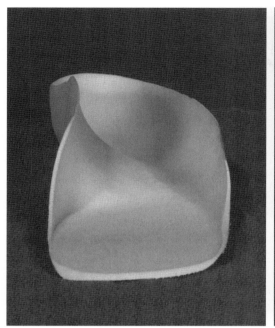

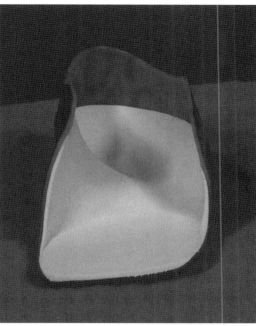

Fig. 38-7 "Total contact footplate." Figure depicts the most common design, which incorporates an arch mold that extends distally on the medial side of the forefoot under the metatarsals to compensate for a forefoot varus deformity and avoid the midfoot collapse and hindfoot valgus that would result in a weight-bearing position (see Fig. 38-6). An extended lateral border is necessary to contain the foot and avoid lateralization (abduction). Of note, opposite foot deformities, such as plantarflexed first ray with pes cavus, also can be managed using a footplate fabricated using the same steps with opposite design features.

degree even though it does not passively control sagittal plane ankle joint alignment.

Hinged AFOs (Fig. 38-9) are commonly prescribed for children with CP. They are frequently favored by physical therapists and physiatrists for children at young ages. The flexibility of the ankle joint allows the ankle mobility required for functional activities such as rising to a standing position, transitioning from one position to another, and stair climbing. Many variations are possible. The joint range of motion may be unrestricted. The hinge can be made from various materials with the theoretical advantage of providing a springlike return to its resting, neutral position (although this remains clinically unproven at this time). Plantarflexion and/or dorsiflexion stops can be added to achieve different effects. The plantarflexion stop can prevent footdrop in swing. Unfortunately, as children become older and larger, the hinged AFO with plantarflexion stop may be inappropriate and can contribute to crouch. Hinged AFOs are safer to use

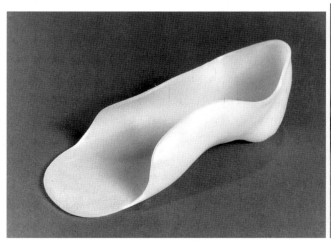

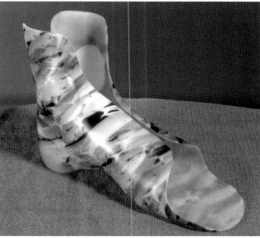

A   B

Fig. 38-8 **A**, University of California Biomechanics Lab (UCBL) orthosis. **B**, Supramalleolar orthosis (SMO). Both orthoses provide hindfoot control, an arch mold, and medial/lateral borders for forefoot motion control. Toe plate length and medial/lateral borders are variable, depending on patient needs. The longer lever arms of the SMO capturing the malleoli allow the device to be used for greater hindfoot varus/valgus control. Both can lead to improvements in foot progression angle and shorten excessive stance phase times.

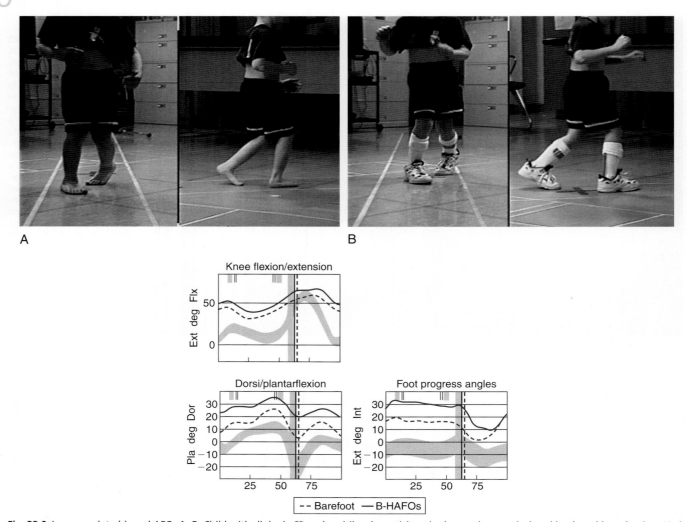

Fig. 38-9 Inappropriate hinged AFO. **A, B,** Child with diplegic CP and multilevel spasticity who has undergone isolated heel cord lengthening. He is walking in crouch with excessive ankle dorsiflexion. The hinged AFO with free dorsiflexion that was prescribed is contraindicated. **C,** Kinematic data show that crouch and excessive ankle dorsiflexion both are worse in the AFO (solid line) than barefoot (dashed). Gray bands indicate normal values. All graphs represent one gait cycle beginning and ending at initial contact. The vertical line in the second half of the gait cycle represents toe-off. The time before the toe-off line is stance phase and after is swing phase. Lever-arm deformity and joint malposition result in intoeing gait, which also is worse when tested with the orthoses. Surgical management will be required before this child can be an appropriate candidate for management with orthoses (likely a stiff PLS or floor reaction AFO).

for treatment of hemiplegia because children with this condition are less likely to go into crouch. In children with hemiplegia the soleus and the gastrocnemius are more commonly affected. This AFO design effectively treats the soleus and prevents contracture. In crouch, the one-joint soleus muscle actually becomes excessively elongated. Care must be taken to avoid sacrificing long-term function for short-term functional goals in children with diplegia and quadriplegia by using this brace to maintain a plantigrade foot at the expense of increased knee flexion contributing to progressive crouch. If the gastrocnemius is contracted and this style brace effectively prevents plantarflexion beyond neutral, the contracted gastrocnemius will pull the knee into flexion. Consequently, the action of the gastrocnemius is restricted to knee flexion,

which becomes progressively easier to accomplish as the plantarflexion/knee-extension couple becomes increasingly impaired. The hinged AFO with plantarflexion stop may be a safe choice for young children, but as children age, better methods than the hinged AFO can achieve functionally good results.

The PLS AFO is a one-piece AFO consisting of a calf cuff that tapers to a band of various widths and flexibility behind the ankle (the "leaf") and widens back out to capture the heel and extend to the tip of the toes. The material used and the arc of the leaf affect the stiffness of the AFO (Fig. 38-10). The flexibility of the brace depends upon the thickness of the material (usually plastic), radius of curvature of the leaf, and stiffness characteristics of the material used.[4,17,25]

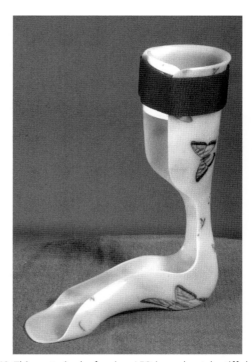

Fig. 38-10 This posterior leaf spring AFO is moderately stiff due to the thickness of the plastic as well as the radius of curvature and width of the leaf. This is an AFO design commonly used at our institution following lower extremity surgery to provide a relatively high level of stance phase support while the patient regains strength postoperatively. As strength and motor control are regained, the leaf can be trimmed to allow more flexibility. If muscle function is sufficient to avoid crouch, the portion of the orthosis above the ankle can be removed completely.

Initially, the primary indication for the leaf spring AFO was preventing drop foot in swing phase and ensuring appropriate prepositioning of the foot for initial contact. The very lightweight dynamic AFO is appropriate in children for whom a footdrop in swing is still the primary indication. Use of PLS AFOs has expanded to treat stance phase second rocker deficiencies as they can control dynamic equinus in stance. Elimination of premature heel rise avoids energy-inefficient midstance power generation and improves stability in stance. The "appropriate" stiffness of the leaf remains an intriguing and challenging question. Little science for guiding either the prescriber or the orthotist is available, but devices to test the stiffness characteristics of AFOs are being developed.[3] At Gillete Children's Specialty Healthcare, we are beginning to evaluate various leaf spring designs, degrees of stiffness, and materials. The differences in ankle joint function between second and third rocker lie at the root of this challenge. Some materials and designs are intended to facilitate the storage of energy, that is, the ability to capture the energy that develops as the device bends into

dorsiflexion, store it until the limb is starting to unload in terminal stance, and then return that energy for push-off. Newer PLS designs (Chevron, spiral, and carbon fiber) have been created that have a greater capacity for energy storage than the single-layer PLS AFO.[30]

In the future, we hope that the stiffness of the brace can be individualized to meet the needs of the patient properly resisting ankle dorsiflexion in second rocker and returning the energy for push-off in third rocker. Currently, the orthotist uses his or her expertise to adapt the stiffness of the AFO through design and material variables to comply with the physician's prescription. Several studies have addressed the contributions of stiff AFOs to the gait of patients who are plantarflexor deficient.[6,12,26] To date there is no way for the physician or orthotist to quantify the amount of stiffness required by a particular child to compensate for the abnormal second and third rockers in gait. Calculating the amount of energy storage that is appropriate to improve an individual's gait is even more challenging. Improvements in the design of orthotic testing devices will help answer these needs.

Following the previous discussion of PLS designs, the reader should recognize that the solid AFO (Fig. 38-11) is simply a PLS design that is so stiff that the ankle joint does not move with use. Indications are for increasingly severe spasticity and weakness typically accompanied by worsening motor control. Controlling alignment and providing stability are the primary goals. Functional deficits are severe enough that ankle motion cannot be allowed because stability would be sacrificed.

The floor reaction AFO (Fig. 38-12) is a rear-entry brace that has the maximal potential to restore the plantarflexion/knee-extension couple.[23] One of its primary uses is for completely incompetent plantarflexor function, such as previous overlengthening of the heel cord. Contraindications include fixed hip and knee contractures that prevent upright walking alignment and the presence of either tibial torsion or uncorrected foot deformity that adversely affects the alignment of the foot relative to the knee.[11] If knee extensor function is deficient (typically associated with patella alta), the floor reaction AFO can be used to minimize or eliminate crouch and relieve stress on the knee.

Best practice

- multidisciplinary approach including

  - Spasticity management
  - Orthopedic correction of lever-arm dysfunction
  - Physical therapy to maximize muscle function
  - Orthosis prescription and fitting to compensate for residual deficiencies

- Careful evaluation and control of foot deformity
- Orthosis prescription to improve plantarflexion/knee-extension couple
- Improved materials for orthosis fabrication (energy storing)
- Improved testing of stiffness characteristics to optimize orthosis prescription

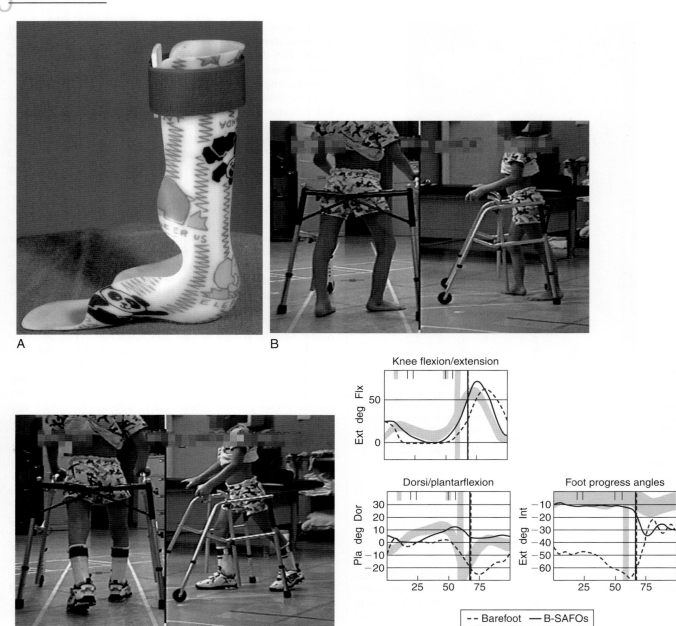

Fig. 38-11 A, of Solid AFO allows no ankle joint motion and is appropriate for use in this child whose strength and motor control distally are poor and whose balance mechanisms are impaired **(B, C). D,** Data for the right side are shown and document the dramatic improvement in external foot progression angle, equinus position in stance, and drop foot in swing. The knee is protected from hyperextension in stance and moves more appropriately during swing phase. This patient has insufficient strength to be a candidate for a less restrictive brace to aid in functional walking ability.

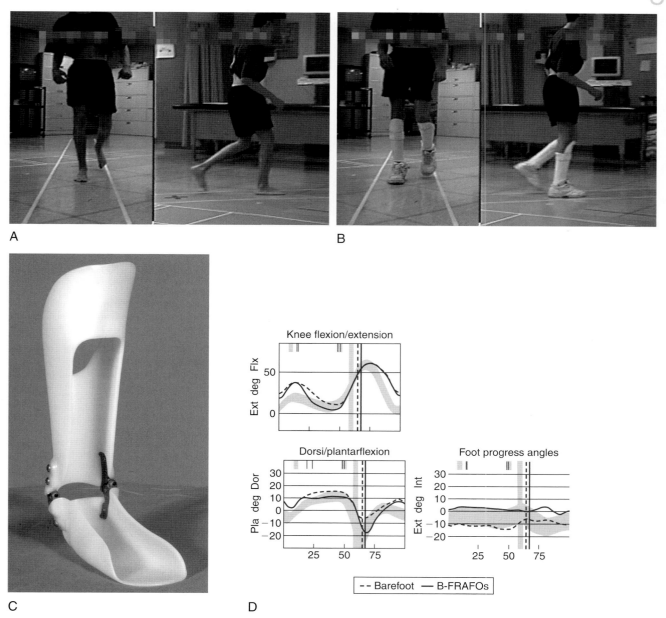

Fig. 38-12 A 15-year-old boy with diplegic CP had been developing anterior knee pain and slight worsening of crouch related to periadolescent growth **(A)**. He previously had undergone selective dorsal rhizotomy (SDR) and lower extremity surgery to correct bone malalignment. He had insufficient plantarflexion/knee-extension couple due to ankle plantarflexor weakness (2+/5). As a result, ankle dorsiflexion in midstance was excessive. Increased knee extension moment was measured (not shown), resulting in anterior knee pain. He was a good candidate for this orthosis because he had good bone alignment (out-of-brace foot progression angle is normal) and spasticity was minimal (normal range of knee motion in swing phase) **(B)**. **C,** Floor reacton AFO. Ankle dorsiflexion was blocked at 10 degrees (normal functional range), preventing excessive forward movement of the tibia over the plantigrade foot **(D)**. He no longer is in crouch in midstance as a result of the effect of the orthosis. There is little change in foot progression angle as anatomical and functional alignment in the transverse plane are good. Knee pain resolved as a result of the second rocker ankle restraint provided by the orthosis. At skeletal maturity, he was weaned out of this brace and now is wearing only UCBL orthoses without significant knee pain.

References

1. Abel M, Juhl GA, Vaughan CL, Damiano DL: Gait assessment of fixed ankle-foot orthoses in children with spastic diplegia, *Arch Phys Med Rehabil* 79:126–133, 1998.

2. Buckon C, Thomas SS, Jakobson-Huston S, et al: Comparison of three ankle-foot orthosis configurations for children with spastic diplegia, *Dev Med Child Neurol* 46:590–598, 2004.

3. Cappa P, Patane F, Pierro MM: A novel device to evaluate the stiffness of ankle foot orthosis devices, *J Biomech Eng* 125:913–917, 2003.

4. Convery P, Grieg RJ, Ross RS, Sockalingham S: A three center study of the variability of ankle foot orthoses due to the fabrication and grade of polypropylene, *Prosthet Orthot Int* 28:175–182, 2004.

5. Crenshaw S, Herzog R, Castagno P, et al: The efficacy of tone-reducing features in orthotics on the gait of children with spastic diplegic cerebral palsy, *J Pediatr Orthop* 20:210–216, 2000.

6. Duffy C, Graham HK, Cosgrove AP: The influence of ankle foot orthoses on gait and energy expenditure in spina bifida, *J Pediatr Orthop* 20:356–361, 2000.

7. Dursun E, Dursun N, Alican D: Ankle-foot orthoses: effect on gait in children with cerebral palsy, *Disabil Rehabil* 24:345–347, 2002.

8. Gage J: *The treatment of gait problems in cerebral palsy*, London, 2004, MacKeith Press.

9. Gage J, Schwartz MH: Dynamic deformities and lever-arm considerations. In Paley D, editor: *Principles of deformity correction*, Berlin, 2002, Springer-Verlag.

10. Hainsworth F, Harrison MJ, Sheldon TA, Roussounis SH: A preliminary evaluation of ankle orthoses in the management of children with cerebral palsy, *Dev Med Child Neurol* 39:243–247, 1997.

11. Harrington E, Lin RS, Gage JR: Use of the anterior floor reaction orthosis in patients with cerebral palsy, *Orthot Prosthet* 38:34–42, 1984.

12. Hullin M, Robb LE, Loudon IR: Ankle-foot orthosis function in low-level myelomeningocele, *J Pediatr Orthop* 12:518–521, 1992.

13. Koop S, Stout J, Starr R, Drinken W: Oxygen consumption during walking in normal children and children with cerebral palsy, *Dev Med Child Neurol* 31(suppl 59):6, 1989 (abstract).

14. Lam W, Leong JCY, Li YH, et al: Biomechanical and electromyographic evaluation of ankle foot orthosis and dynamic ankle foot orthosis in spastic cerebral palsy, *Gait Posture* 22:189–197, 2005.

15. Maltais D, Bar-Or O, Galea V, Pierrynowski M: Use of orthoses lowers the cost of walking in children with spastic cerebral palsy, *Med Sci Sports Exerc* 33:320–325, 2001.

16. Murphy K, Molnar GE, Lankasky K: Medical and functional status of adults with cerebral palsy, *Dev Med Child Neurol* 38:1075–1084, 1995.

17. Nagaya M Shoehorn-type ankle-foot orthoses: prediction of flexibility, *Arch Phy Med Rehabil* 78:82–84, 1997.

18. Ounpuu S, Bell KJ, Davis RB, DeLuca PA: An evaluation of the posterior leaf spring orthosis using joint kinematics and kinetics, *J Pediatr Orthop* 16:384–388, 1996.

19. Perry J: The gait cycle. In Willoughby C, editor: *Gait analysis: normal and pathological function*, New Jersey, 1992, McGraw-Hill (Slack, Inc.).

20. Radtka S, Skinner SR, Johanson ME: A comparison of gait with solid and hinged ankle-foot orthoses in children with spastic diplegic cerebral palsy, *Gait Posture* 21:303–310, 2005.

21. Rethlefsen S, Kay R, Dennis S, et al: The effects of fixed and articulated ankle-foot orthoses on gait patterns in subjects with cerebral palsy, *J Pediatr Orthop* 19:470–474, 1999.

22. Romkes J, Brunner R: Comparison of a dynamic and a hinged ankle-foot orthosis by gait analysis in patients with hemiplegic cerebral palsy, *Gait Posture* 15:18–24, 2002.

23. Saltiel J: A one-piece, laminated, knee locking, short leg brace, *Orthot Prosthet* 23:68–75, 1969.

24. Smiley S, Jacobsen FS, Mielke C, et al: A comparison of the effects of solid, articulated, and posterior leaf-spring ankle-foot orthoses and shoes alone on gait and energy expenditure in children with spastic diplegic cerebral palsy, *Orthopedics* 25:411–415, 2002.

25. Sumiya T, Suzuki Y, Kasahara T: Stiffness control in posterior-type plastic ankle-foot orthoses: affect of trimline. Part 1: a device for measuring ankle moment, *Prosthet Orthot Int* 20:129–131, 1996.

26. Thompson J, Ounpuu S, Davis RB, DeLuca PA: The effects of ankle-foot orthoses on the ankle and knee in persons with myelomeningocele and evaluation using three-dimensional gait analysis, *J Pediatr Orthop* 19:27–33, 1999.

27. Waters R, Mulroy S: The energy expenditure of normal and pathologic gait, *Gait Posture* 9:207–231, 1999.

28. White H, Jenkins J, Neace WP, et al: Clinically prescribed orthoses demonstrate an increase in velocity of gait in children with cerebral palsy: a retrospective study, *Dev Med Child Neurol* 44:227–232, 2002.

29. Winter D: Balance and posture in human gait. In Winter D: *The biomechanics and motor control of human gait: normal, elderly, and pathological*, Ontario, 1991, University of Waterloo Press.

30. Wolf S, Knie I, Retting O, et al: Carbon fiber spring AFOs for active push-off, Annual Gait & Clinical Motion Analysis Society Meeting, Portland, Oregon, 2005.

31. Ziv I, Blackburn N, Rang M, Koreska J: Muscle growth in normal and spastic mice, *Dev Med Child Neurol* 26:94–99, 1984.

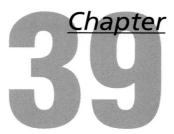

Chapter

39

Orthoses for myelomeningocele

Bryan S. Malas and John F. Sarwark

Key Points

- The degree to which orthotic management is implemented for myelomeningocele is largely based on the patient's neurological status and remaining motor function

- Orthotic treatment for myelomeningocele should begin early in the child's life with attention towards proper joint position, range of motion, and developmental milestones

- Determination for mobility should focus on function and activities of daily living. In some instances multiple mobility options provide the greatest opportunity for maximum function

- It is important to maintain continuous follow-up throughout the child's life to ensure that orthotic management is still viable and appropriate

- The multidisciplinary team approach remains the cornerstone for comprehensive care for myelomeningocele

Myelomeningocele is a neural tube defect and a major birth defect. It is an embryological abnormality that results in a myriad of complex neuromuscular problems. Children with spina bifida can be classified according to the level of neurological involvement or functional impairment. Myelomeningocele occurs in approximately 0.4 per 1,000 live births.[69] The incidence of myelomeningocele is slightly higher in females than males, at a ratio of 1.3:1. With a high prevalence of Chiari II malformation and hydrocephalus, myelomeningocele is characterized by a variation of motor impairments, ranging from minimal muscle weakness to complete paralysis. Spasticity may be present.[37] Musculoskeletal deformity and sensory deficits are common and, depending on the level of involvement, can adversely affect the child's abilities and functioning in the

community. Folic acid is important in preventing this birth defect. Reports indicate that folic acid intake in the preconception period can prevent up to 85% of spina bifida cases.[48] This success rate underscores the need to develop worldwide programs that will effectively manage and eradicate this neural tube defect.

Because of the complexity of this major birth defect, orthotic management is critical for the child's function and is a challenging endeavor for the orthotist. Successful orthotic treatment is based on a comprehensive understanding of the disease and on reasonable expectations for the goals of orthotic care as identified by the medical team. These goals and expectations must be clearly defined for the families so that they may appreciate the degree to which orthotic treatment can or cannot be successful. Success is predicated on a number of clinical issues that may include one or all of the following: (1) level of neurological involvement; (2) degree of musculoskeletal deformity; (3) sensory impairment; (4) acquired obesity; (5) existing muscle strength; (6) visual and motor perception impairment; (7) patient motivation; and (8) family support.[2,11,13,58] Consideration of these issues will result in more predictable outcomes for patient developmental milestones; postural control; mobility; age-specific function; protection of the insensate foot; and management of musculoskeletal deformities.

For the child with spina bifida, the capacity and degree to which function and ambulation can be achieved are based on their level of motor function and functional mobility.[2,18,28,40,63] Contractures, limited sitting balance, and obesity are factors that may adversely affect the child's ability to walk with or without orthoses. These factors in addition to the child's motor function level can strongly influence how effectively orthotic management improves functional ambulation. Early patient examination and orthotic intervention are important first steps if future ambulation is to be achieved.

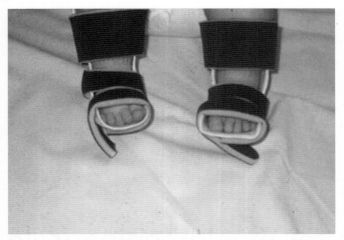

Fig. 39-1 Early orthotic intervention promotes proper joint alignment and muscle balance as the child grows, both of which are prerequisites for walking to be achieved.

Specific issues that warrant particular attention include (1) hip disorders (e.g., dislocation, subluxation, contractures), (2) knee flexion/extension contractures, and (3) foot/ankle deformities (e.g., equinovarus, clubfoot). In these cases, the orthotic goal(s) should be preventing deformity and maintaining proper joint alignment in order to achieve appropriate muscle balance during development. Achievement of these goals can facilitate the initiation of proper weight bearing and future ambulation (Fig. 39-1).

To understand the specific functional needs of the myelomeningocele population, the intact motor levels of function and their specific orthotic interventions must be identified. Each level of motor function requires a different orthotic prescription. A review of these levels of function and the corresponding orthotic intervention will provide an important contextual framework for the clinician.

Thoracic/high lumbar level

Lesions at motor levels designated as thoracic/high lumbar reveal a significant compromise of muscle strength to the lower limbs and some weakness of the upper limbs.[25] In addition, this patient population is likely to have hydrocephalus, Arnold-Chiari malformation, and often develops scoliosis, hip dislocation, and contractures of the hip and knee.[59] As a result of the higher-level lesion, the attributes of normal kinematic gait not only are compromised for the foot and knee but are dramatically compromised at the hip and pelvis compared to lower-level lesions. This is evident by the magnitude of compensatory motion during gait resulting from specific muscle deficits involving the hip joint.[67] For this lesion level, motor activity of the knee, ankle complex, hip extensors, and hip abductors typically exhibits muscle grade ≤ 2 on a five-point scale. Some sparing at the hip is evident for hip flexors and hip adductors exhibiting muscle grade ≥ 3. Some level of community ambulation can be achieved up to early adolescence with appropriate orthotic management; however, the ability for community ambulation quickly declines in adulthood as energy cost becomes too high for meaningful ambulation.[12] Functional ambulation in this group is further compromised as spinal deformity and contractures of the lower extremity become more clinically significant.[3]

The goal of mobility is important, but the manner of mobility for this level of myelomeningocele remains controversial. At the center of the controversy is a divide between assisted standing/ambulation through orthotic management (i.e., standing frame, parapodium, hip–knee–ankle–foot orthosis [HKAFO], reciprocating gait orthosis [RGO]) and use of mobility aids such as wheelchairs. Advocates for orthotic management have described physiological and psychological benefits with regard to upright standing and ambulation, including cardiac and pulmonary function, bowel and bladder function, issues related to the musculoskeletal system, and greater independence at a later age.[8,41,54] In an investigation of children with spina bifida by Mazur et al.,[36] children who had received orthotic management at an early age to facilitate ambulation exhibited fewer fractures and pressure sores compared to children who did not ambulate and receive orthotic management at an early age. However, proponents of wheelchair use have found that individuals are more energy efficient when using a wheelchair compared to orthotic management.[1] Liptak et al.[29] found no significant difference between early ambulators and wheelchair users in the areas of (1) severity of hip flexion contractures, (2) degree of urinary tract complications, (3) frequency of decubitus ulcers,[1] and (4) activities of daily living (ADLs). Because evidence suggests that both standing and wheelchair use can be beneficial, it is more paramount that mobility not be relegated to a strict choice between these two methods of mobility.[31] Mobility programs that incorporate advising on multiple options allow the family and child to determine which mobility option is most functional for the task or activity at hand. Many are less likely to give up ambulation completely.[6]

Orthotic management

Orthotic management for children with thoracic/high lumbar lesions strives to achieve age-specific goals consistent with sitting balance, standing, ambulation, and independent function. When standing and some level of ambulation are the goals for these children, then certain orthotic design requirements must be fulfilled in order to achieve effective management. According to Rose,[54] stabilization and alignment across the hip, knee, and ankle are essential for standing and ambulation in an orthosis. Acceptable forms of ambulation include swing through, swing to, swivel, and reciprocal, and are based in part on proper orthotic design and assistive device application. Orthoses for this population have unique design characteristics that, when applied correctly and to the right candidate, can offer greater functional capacity.

Standing frame

A child 12 to 24 months old with a thoracic/high lumbar lesion, good head control, and good sitting balance may be a candidate for a standing frame.[7,39] The standing frame promotes standing activities that are consistent with normal development (e.g., postural control, trunk strength, balance,

---

[1]Patients in a standing program had a higher incidence of skin breakdown in the lower limbs, whereas children using a wheelchair showed a higher incidence of skin breakdown over the sacrum.

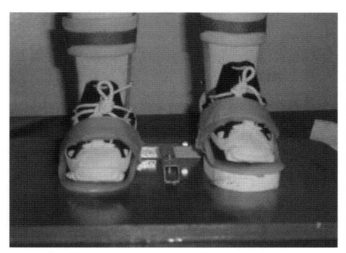

Fig. 39-2 When using a standing frame or parapodium, overall management should include consideration of proper foot and ankle position and accommodation for any leg-length discrepancy.

and righting reactions) and allows for free use of the upper extremities. Stabilization in the standing frame occurs through four-point stabilization across the hip and knee joints.[55] In conjunction with the standing frame, control should be considered for the foot and ankle complex, which can be managed effectively with bilateral solid ankle–foot orthoses (AFOs). This design can offer sagittal control of the ankle joint and coronal control of the subtalar joint in order to maintain appropriate antagonist–agonist muscle balance and foster a better base of support (Fig. 39-2).[10]

Parapodium

Designed by Motloch,[43] the parapodium uses many of the same design principles and force applications observed with the standing frame but has the additional capability to allow for sitting. Moreover, the parapodium supporting base can be modified to include a swivel component for an alternative means of forward ambulation for the child. The parapodium is a modular system that provides upright stability across the hip, knee, and, to a lesser degree, the foot and ankle complex. As in the case of the standing frame, if additional foot and ankle control is warranted, bilateral solid AFOs should be considered along with the parapodium. The parapodium itself has an aluminum alloy baseplate with the ability to support the feet and increase the base of support. Attached to the baseplate are shin and thigh tube sections that can rotate about a vertical axis.[61] Integrity of the vertical tubes is maintained by knee and pelvic bearing brackets that allow for appropriate joint alignment and stable upright standing. Housed within the vertical tubes are mechanical hip and knee joints whose axes, when parallel to the frontal plane, allow the joints to unlock for sitting. This position allows the child to sit while stability is maintained across the aforementioned anatomical joints.

Ambulation is possible with the addition of the swivel walker.[60] The swivel walker can be attached distally and underneath the supporting base of the parapodium. Ambulation occurs with the patient in an erect posture as he or she rocks laterally from side to side. The center of mass of the system is positioned just anterior to the swivel

bearing in order to foster easier forward progression for the child. Although beneficial, the swivel walker is used less frequently now because of the availability of alternative reciprocal designs. According to Stallard,[61] several indications for the swivel walker include younger children who have initiated upright posture, patients with upper limb weakness in whom assistive devices are not an option, and patients with limited mobility who require free upper limbs for function.

Hip–knee–ankle–foot orthosis

The HKAFO functions as either a fixed and/or dynamic orthosis. The orthosis has a pelvic band that is attached bilaterally to a knee–ankle–foot orthosis (KAFO) via left and right mechanical hip joints. For patients who lack motor function about and distal to the hip joint, it may be necessary to hold motion across the hip, knee, and ankle in order to provide stability during standing and mobilization.[22] Swing-through and swing-to gait patterns may be obstructed in some patients when hip motion is restricted in conjunction with a longer vertical pelvic interface. Dynamic HKAFOs are likely to be used in their more sophisticated form, the RGO. In both cases ideal motor function should, at a minimum, include hip flexor strength in order to initiate step ability for ambulation (i.e., swing-through, reciprocal). To achieve forward mobility, some form of assistive device is required.

Reciprocating gait orthosis

The RGO provides a means for reciprocal ambulation in individuals with marked lower extremity muscle weakness. The RGO design at a minimum requires active hip flexion to facilitate extension of the contralateral limb and ultimately drive the reciprocal gait pattern.[71] The dynamic capability of the RGO occurs via the hip joints. The hip joints can function independently from one another or, with a more sophisticated design, the mechanical hip joints work in unison via a cable or central posterior pivot point. Irrespective of the design, a comprehensive evaluation of the patient is critical to determining the likelihood of RGO utilization and ambulation. When motivation and family support are low, access to therapy is difficult, donning/doffing is problematic, and routine travel for appointments is not possible, consistent evidence suggests that the child probably will not continue wearing and using the RGO.[19,51] The medical team should consider these issues when evaluating children as candidates for an RGO.

Clinical factors are no less important and should be included in the overall assessment of the child to determine the appropriateness of the RGO. Considerations for RGO use include (1) upper limb strength,[33] (2) hip and knee flexion contractures less then 30 degrees, (3) active hip flexor strength, (4) no obesity, and (5) no significant spinal deformity. These factors are assessed in order to determine the likelihood of successful management with the RGO. In a study by Stallard et al.,[62] 34% of patients with myelomeningocele and a complete lesion level at or above L1 were able to attain community ambulatory status. Another study reported that children with mild spinal deformities, hip dislocation, and hip/knee contractures less then 30 degrees were able to function within an RGO.[16] Other studies have compared velocity in the RGO to other HKAFO designs and found that velocity increased more when the RGO was used compared to the HKAFO.[35,38,71] The results from these

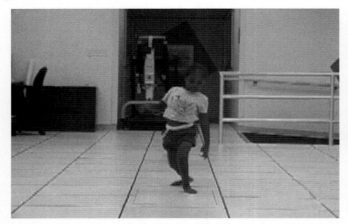

Fig. 39-3 Proper determination of the cause of knee malalignment in the coronal plane is necessary for appropriate orthotic treatment. This patient exhibits a triplanar deformity that is hyperpronatory in nature.

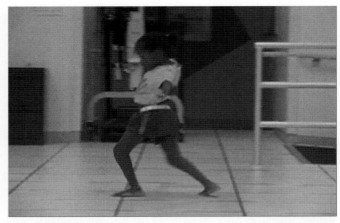

Fig. 39-4 Absent gastro-soleus motor function can have a profound effect on gait. This child has absent gastro-soleus bilaterally and as a result exhibits a crouch gait pattern. The gait pattern characteristically exhibits excessive foot and ankle pronation, ankle dorsiflexion, knee flexion, and hip flexion.

studies suggest that, under the right circumstances, RGOs can facilitate better functional mobility. With a comprehensive evaluation of the patient, the likelihood is greater that decisions will be made and tailored to the specific individual in order to effectively meet the needs of that patient.

Low lumbar level

A child with a lower lumbar lesion typically exhibits a functional level consistent with active hip flexors, hip adductors, knee extensors, and knee flexors. Motor deficits include hip extensors, hip abductors, and ankle plantarflexors and dorsiflexors. The resulting gait pattern is a combination of gait deviations that extend from the foot and ankle complex up to and including the trunk. Gait deviations typically include a posterior trunk lean throughout swing and stance, excessive pelvic rotation and obliquity, exaggerated stance phase hip abduction (lateral trunk lean), increased hip and knee flexion, and increased stance phase dorsiflexion.[14]

Hip extensor weakness is evident in gait with the appearance of a posterior trunk lean and increased anterior pelvic tilt. Posterior trunk lean is necessary for the child's stability at the hip as he or she provides an externally generated hip extension moment in an effort to reduce the demand on the already deficient hip extensors. This deficiency also results in a loss of sagittal pelvic control that ultimately presents as an exaggerated anterior pelvic tilt during ambulation.[70] The hip extensor weakness and unopposed action of the hip flexors lead to further hip flexion contractures, increased hip flexion in terminal stance, and diminished step length during gait. Also evident is deficient hip abductor strength and the associated lateral trunk lean. This lateral trunk lean to the ipsilateral side is a necessary action in order to decrease the external hip adduction moment, an event that normally requires subsequent hip abductor strength that, in this case, is not present.

As with lateral trunk lean, frontal plane assessment typically reveals a valgus stress at the knee in the stance phase limb. Several factors identified as contributing to this valgus stress are lateral trunk lean, closed-chain hyperpronation (internal hip rotation, increased knee flexion, ankle dorsiflexion, hindfoot valgus), and medial tibial torsion (Fig. 39-3).[20]

Excessive pelvic rotation remains a likely gait characteristic when combined hip flexion contractures and a crouch gait pattern are present. With the hip joint in a flexed position throughout stance, the child cannot generate forward momentum, and he or she will compensate with forward pelvic rotation when the ipsilateral limb is in swing phase.

During normal walking, plantarflexor activity progressively increases from loading response to peak activity at terminal stance. As the center of pressure propagates anteriorly along the plantar aspect of the foot, an external dorsiflexion moment progressively increases as ground reaction force moves further in front of the ankle joint axis. To oppose this external dorsiflexion moment, an internal moment is generated through eccentric plantarflexor activity. A child with a low lumbar lesion will exhibit weakness of the plantarflexors. As a result of this weakness, the soleus is unable to oppose the external dorsiflexion moment and the tibia is allowed to progress anteriorly, ultimately leading to excessive dorsiflexion, knee flexion, and hip flexion in stance phase (Fig. 39-4). Temporospatial data suggest a 60% decrease in walking velocity compared to normal.[68] Orthotic management for this functional level varies from solid polymer AFOs to KAFOs.

High sacral level

The child with a high sacral level lesion will have increased strength around the hip complex compared to the lower lumbar level. In this case, hip flexors and extensors, abductors and adductors, and knee extensors and flexors are active. Although active, hip extensors and hip abductors still exhibit weakness and similar gait deviations, such as posterior trunk lean, increased lordosis, increased anterior pelvic tilt, and lateral trunk lean. Dorsiflexor strength may vary among children; however, absent plantarflexor strength remains remarkable. The most common orthotic management in this population is the use of bilateral AFOs independent of external support such as assistive devices. As this group transitions from childhood to adulthood, evidence indicates that 98% of the population will continue to function as community ambulators.[57]

Low sacral level

Muscle weakness around the foot and ankle complex is typical for this level of lesion, but actual muscle strength is variable. Because of the variability, assessment should focus on functional issues related to fatigability of the affected muscle groups. Gait analysis that assesses prolonged walking is a better indicator of the child's actual gait pattern during ADLs and provides the information necessary to determine appropriate orthotic management.[66] For this population, orthotic management ranges from no orthotic management to bilateral solid AFOs.

Ankle–foot orthosis

Levels of function for which an AFO is indicated in the myelomeningocele population typically involve some compromise of gastroc-soleus strength. Effective orthotic management must address issues related to an overall gait presentation that is hyperpronated and high in O_2 cost. Proper orthotic selection is either a solid polymer AFO or a floor reaction polymer AFO. No study has compared design differences and effectiveness in this patient population. In both cases, several design considerations are necessary for effective orthotic treatment and include a rigid footplate and dorsiflexion stop. A solid ankle design with the capacity to stop forward tibial translation (dorsiflexion stop) in stance phase is essential to limiting the predominant crouch pattern of gait (Fig. 39-5). Key design features should include (1) trim lines anterior to the medial/lateral malleoli, (2) reinforcement around the ankle (e.g., carbon fiber, plastic corrugation), and (3) use of polypropylene plastic. All design features should ensure that the orthosis will not fail in the loaded and unload planes around the ankle in stance phase and allow a persistent crouch gait pattern.[24] Total-contact polymer systems and key design features will limit hyperpronation at the foot and ankle complex and indirectly limit valgus stress presentation at the knee. This is true if the valgus stress results from hyperpronation rather than lateral trunk lean during ambulation (Fig. 39-6). However, valgus stress secondary to a true coronal

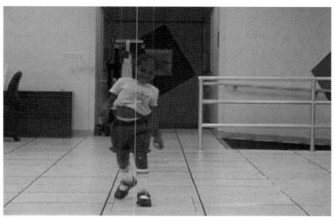

Fig. 39-6 Valgus stress at the knee can be addressed with a solid AFO, which limits the hyperpronatory forces that can contribute to valgus stress. In this patient, the valgus stress has been reduced as a result of orthotic intervention. Valgus stress that is persistent may be a result of weak abductors and concomitant lateral trunk lean in stance phase.

plane valgum at the knee will not respond well to AFO orthotic management. These key design features not only can address issues around the ankle but also can help limit excessive knee flexion if combined with a full rigid footplate and appropriate proximal trim line. The full-length footplate will allow the center of pressure along the plantar aspect of the orthosis to propagate anteriorly during gait and, coupled with the anteroproximal trim line of the AFO, facilitate a knee extension moment.[42] Knee flexion can be further augmented with an AFO that is sagittally aligned in several degrees of plantarflexion. It is important to avoid setting AFOs at 90 degrees sagittally with no consideration for shoe heel height, because relative dorsiflexion in the shoe may reach as high as 15 degrees and foster continued knee flexion in stance.[17,64] This knee extension moment can be effective with a foot progression angle less than 20 degrees[66] and usually secondary to excessive medial tibial torsion. Limitation of ankle plantarflexion is essential because dorsiflexion weakness is common and usually is most remarkable from initial contact to loading response. Inclusion of the plantarflexion stop can facilitate a better first rocker and initial contact for the child's gait pattern.

The orthotic practitioner should be aware that children with this presentation may exhibit an increased anterior pelvic tilt and a marked increase of lumbar lordosis when solid AFO designs are used in the presence of hip flexion contractures. In such cases, the AFO creates a knee extension moment in the presence of a hip flexion contracture in which the child must bring his or her center of mass more posterior in order to continue fostering necessary hip extension moment due to hip extensor muscle weakness. Therefore, careful attention should be focused on sagittal alignment that does not induce more lordosis than is necessary for hip stability.

Ankle–foot orthosis: floor reaction

The alternative design to the solid polymer AFO is the floor reaction AFO. Key design features include trim lines anterior to the malleoli bilaterally, ankle reinforcement, and a full-length rigid footplate. Unique to the floor reaction design is

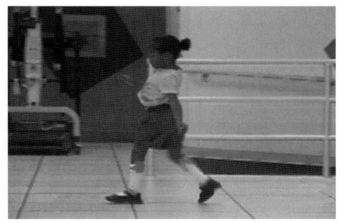

Fig. 39-5 Solid polymer AFOs can have a dramatic effect and improve gait kinematics in the sagittal plane. For this child, the crouch gait pattern has been reduced, as evidenced by the upright presentation during gait. Critical to the effectiveness of the solid AFO are the material and the design of the orthosis, which has the ability to stop dorsiflexion during the stance portion of gait.

the rigid anterior section that extends across the proximal anterior third of the tibia and terminates either midpatella or just distal to the patella.[56] The ultimate goal of this particular design is to facilitate more effective knee extension moment than provided by a solid AFO design.

Knee–ankle–foot orthosis

Knee instability can be present in a child with a lumbar-level lesion and may vary depending on the level of neurological insult. The patient with neurological variance and asymmetrical muscle strength bilaterally will require thorough evaluation. Deformity of the knee can present as excessive knee extension, knee flexion, valgus deformity (real or apparent), and/or rotational deformity.[9] When AFOs and assistive devices no longer can address the deformities related to the knee, increased orthotic management and use of KAFOs are necessary. For knee deformities in this population, material selection and KAFO design should be determined based on the patient's functional needs and skin integrity. In a patient with evidence of skin breakdown, a total-contact polymer design should be considered. Conversely, the patient with proximal skin irritation secondary to a total-contact system that limits aeration to the skin may require a hybrid design, that is, conventional components proximally (i.e., proximal and distal thigh band) and polymer AFO design distally. Depending on the knee deformity, specific features of the components should be considered to address deformity, improve function, and increase comfort.

The child may use excessive knee extension as a coping mechanism for quadriceps weakness, performing an exaggerated anterior trunk lean during stance phase to facilitate a knee extension moment that will stabilize the knee in stance phase.[50] The orthotic design may warrant some or complete limitation of motion with emphasis on reducing extension deformity while providing stability in stance phase. Excessive knee flexion usually results from knee flexion contractures secondary to muscle imbalance and may require a dial lock with ring lock and associated ball-bearing retainer. When coronal deformity at the knee is not rectified by either a solid AFO (i.e., closed-chained hyperpronation

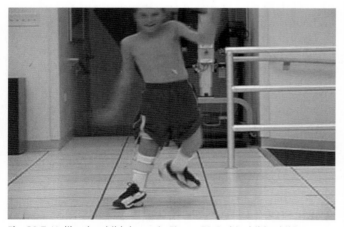

Fig. 39-7 Unlike the child shown in Figure 39-6, this child exhibits a true coronal plane valgus deformity at the knee and as a result cannot be treated effectively with a solid AFO. In this case, the child can benefit from a polymer KAFO that crosses the knee joint and effectively manages the genu valgum.

secondary to absent or weak plantarflexors) or crutches (i.e., limit lateral trunk lean secondary to absent or weak hip abductors), the child most likely is a candidate for a bilateral polymer KAFOs (Fig. 39-7). Particular attention should be paid to the integrity of the orthosis just proximal to the ankle and to the area where the mechanical knee joint interfaces with the proximal and distal sidebars. Because the deformity usually is not limited to pure coronal deformity but transverse deformity as well, these areas are frequently subjected to high levels of stress. If the force can overcome these design features, the material will fail and not adequately address the valgus presentation at the knee. Reinforcement of the ankle section (with corrugation or carbon fiber) and increased diameter of bar stock may help decrease the chance of material failure. Consideration should be given to extending the medial aspect of the AFO section more proximally (valgum extension) and the medial aspect of the thigh component more distally to better manage the coronal deformity through either accommodation or correction.[9,27]

Supramalleolar orthosis/foot orthosis

For lesions at the lower sacral level, the likely clinical presentation is deformities related to the foot. Surrounding muscles of the foot–ankle complex may exhibit some weakness that becomes progressively more apparent with onset of fatigue. When additional subtalar joint alignment cannot be properly managed with a foot orthosis and/or University of California Biomechanics Lab orthosis and an AFO is not warranted, an SMO is the appropriate choice for orthotic intervention. With the proximal trim line located just above the medial and lateral malleoli, the SMO offers an extended lever for controlling excessive subtalar motion that is detrimental to functional gait. In addition to hindfoot control, the SMO can control and influence midfoot and forefoot motion. The typical polypropylene design may include instrinsic and extrinsic posting of the orthosis.

For individuals in whom muscle fatigability is less of an issue than foot alignment and kinematic issues, foot orthoses are the most likely orthotic requirement. In many cases, multiple orthotic goals can be addressed and include improved weight-bearing distribution, increased shock attenuation, joint motion control, and proper joint alignment. As a result, orthotic management of the foot should focus on a combination of materials that address all areas of concern rather than categorization of orthotic designs as rigid, semirigid, or soft. Multidurometer designs such as Microcel puff, PPT, and cork offer the best solution for management of the foot. Careful attention should be paid to individuals susceptible to ulceration in the presence of diminished or absent protective sensation. In theses case, routine follow-up and patient education are equally important to overall patient care.

Spinal deformity

Spinal deformities in the child with myelomeningocele characteristically include scoliosis and/or kyphosis (developmental or congenital), with prevalence rates of 50% to 70% for scoliosis[20] and 8% to 15% for kyphosis.[34] The level of neuromuscular impairment (high to low) remains the prevailing cause of scoliosis in children with myelomeningocele.[21]

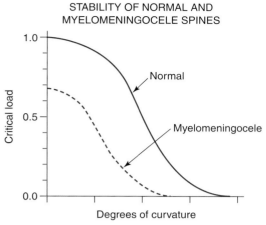

STABILITY OF NORMAL AND
MYELOMENINGOCELE SPINES

Fig. 39-8 Critical load is shown as a function of curve magnitude. The reduced stability of the myelomeningocele spine for all degrees of curvature can be compared with the normal spine. Reduced stability is due to loss of many of the stabilizing elements of the spine. (From Bunch WH, Patwardhan AG: *Scoliosis making clinical decisions*, St. Louis, 1989, CV Mosby.)

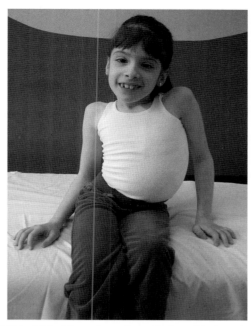

Fig. 39-9 This child with myelomeningocele is unable to ambulate and presents with scoliosis. Because of the scoliosis, the child must rely on her upper limbs to maintain stable sitting balance. As a result, the child's activities of daily living can be hindered throughout the day as she attempts to maintain proper sitting balance through use of her hands.

Although both conditions can be present, scoliosis deformities secondary to neuromuscular compromise are more common than are congenital anomalies.[30] The incidence of scoliosis appears to be most dependent on age and neurological lesion levels,[45,52] with the level of dysraphism strongly correlated to the prevalence of scoliosis (high to low).[46]

Clinical presentation

The neuromuscular (paralytic) curve usually is long and C-shaped with decompensation and, in the nonambulatory population, is evidenced by marked pelvic obliquity and problems with seating balance. Intraabdominal crowding secondary to large curve magnitudes may adversely affect gastrointestinal function as well as elevate the position of the diaphragm, ultimately hampering pulmonary function. The absence or malposition of the lamina and facets can adversely affect spinal stability and is compounded by the presence of surrounding muscle paralysis and the resulting asymmetrical muscle action.[52] Approximately 20% of patients have congenital vertebral anomalies classified as failure of formation (hemivertebra, wedged vertebra), failure of segmentation (bar vertebra), or a combination of both.[5] Loss of these stabilizing elements can lead to a reduction in the load-carrying capacity of the spine.[49] In other words, a patient with a larger curve magnitude will have proportionally less spinal stability and a greater likelihood of curve progression (Fig. 39-8). Although curve progression can occur as a result of spinal instability, it is important to note that when progressive loss of neurological function (tethered cord) is present, the spinal deformity likely will progress regardless of spinal stability.[5]

Nonoperative management

The presence of bony and neurological deficits adds to the complexity of orthotic management of spinal deformity secondary to myelomeningocele. Attention to detail is essential if complications are to be prevented and success achieved.

The main goals of orthotic management in this population include (1) delaying fusion until sufficient skeletal maturity is achieved in order to prevent growth disparity between internal organs and trunk growth and (2) preventing progression in patients with curves between 20 and 40 degrees.[53] During this period of orthotic management, additional considerations are improving pulmonary function, seating balance, postural positioning, and use of the upper extremities for ADLs rather than for maintenance of sitting balance (Figs. 39-9 and 39-10).[26] Although much of the literature suggests that orthotic management of curves greater than 40 degrees does not alter curve progression, some evidence suggests orthotic treatment of curve magnitudes less then 40 degrees may alter curve progression. In a study by Muller and Nordwall,[44] 14 patients with myelomeningocele initiated orthotic management after documented progression was determined (mean progression 5 degrees per year). At the conclusion of the study, two patients had yet to complete orthotic management, 11 had completed orthotic treatment, and one patient had a curve that progressed despite orthotic management and required surgery. Prior to orthotic management, the 11 patients had a mean curve magnitude of 35.7 degrees (25–43 degrees). At the conclusion of treatment (mean treatment 2.5 years), the out of orthosis mean curve value was 29.6 degrees. At mean follow-up of 3.2 years after treatment, all 11 curves had remained stable, with a mean curve magnitude of 28.4 degrees, and did not require surgery. These results are consistent with the literature reporting that curve flexibility, age of the child, and curves ≤ 30 degrees are ideal parameters for orthotic treatment.[28]

Of additional importance are variables that may preclude successful orthotic treatment and thus warrant careful consideration. Obesity in the presence of a spinal deformity may

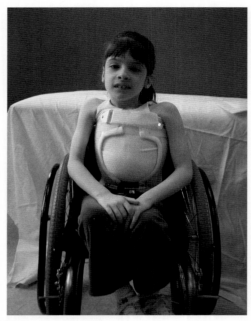

Fig. 39-10 The same patient as shown in Figure 39-9 is now wearing a TLSO. The TLSO can reduce the curve magnitude while creating a "hands-free" environment for activities of daily living because sitting balance is improved.

require treatment other than orthotic management. If the goal is to improve postural position or seating balance or to promote upper-limb ADL function (rather than supporting the patient in a seating system with the upper limbs), then orthotic treatment may be of benefit. However, if the intention is to achieve significant curve correction, a high level of caution is necessary because application of force sufficient to achieve correction may not be tolerated by the patient and should be considered contraindicated. The possibility of skin breakdown is another major concern and may be compounded by the presence of insensate skin. Careful and routine follow-up should be an integral part of any comprehensive orthotic treatment plan. Equally important is the ability to differentiate between direct orthotic failure and perceived failure of orthotic treatment in the presence of physiological or fitting complications.[5] For example, scoliosis in the presence of neurological deterioration (e.g., tethered cord syndrome) may progress regardless of orthotic treatment and should be identified as the primary source of progression rather than the orthosis. Inadequate orthotic fit or improper doffing should be identified and may warrant refabrication or better donning protocols rather than complete abandonment of orthotic treatment. Such factors should be routinely reviewed to determine the appropriateness of orthotic management.

Orthosis

Based on the overall clinical presentation of this population, the polymer thoracolumbosacral orthosis (TLSO) is considered the most appropriate. In a study by Gavin et al. (unpublished data), low-density polyethylene appeared to be the most appropriate material. The same study suggested that a low-density polyethylene TLSO provides the best immobilization at a lower cost to pulmonary function compared to other more rigid TLSO systems. Although this study included only normal subjects, some application to the

myelomeningocele population may be possible. Of additional significance is the design of the TLSO. Whereas circumferential designs with an anterior opening can be more difficult to don and doff compared to bivalve systems, overall fit and skin problems appear to be less of an issue with the TLSO.[53] At this time, the most appropriate design remains questionable and requires further investigation.

Patients in this population may have deficient sensorimotor and righting responses.[28] Because such deficiencies preclude the children from actively withdrawing from transverse stimuli created by the TLSO, they require application of a more passive force to address and reduce curve magnitudes. As a result, in many cases the traditional "three-point pressure system" has been replaced by a different approach that focuses on lateral bending toward the convexity of the curve and puts the iliotibial band on stretch during the impression technique.[5]

During rectification of the positive cast, consideration should include buildups for bony prominences, as occurs at the inferior costal margin, or a spinal gibbus. Care should be taken when removing material from the abdominal region anteriorly, because aggressive modifications may lead to gastrointestinal discomfort or may cause undue pressure on the urinary tract system.[44] Final fitting of the orthosis should include comprehensive patient and family education regarding donning/doffing procedures, routine skin assessment, adequate monitoring of growth changes that may adversely affect device function, and instruction on the appropriate sequence for tightening straps/closures.

The child with myelomeningocele who presents with a secondary spinal deformity requires careful and meticulous assessment in order to properly identify reasonable and appropriate orthotic goals. When orthotic goals (and limitations) are clearly defined, the impression process, design features, and orthotic outcome have a greater opportunity to realistically address the needs of the patient and family.

Postoperative management

Although new surgical techniques, instrumentation, and use of prophylactic antibiotics have helped to improve surgical outcomes, complications still can occur in the form of pseudoarthroses, hardware failure, and infection. These complications appear to have a higher incidence in the myelomeningocele population compared to surgical intervention for other pathologies associated with spinal deformity.[15] For the child or adolescent who has undergone surgery of the spine and requires orthotic management, a new set of issues must be considered for management to be successful. Accommodation of surgical alignment is the goal in order to provide optimal protection for the surgical construct and bone–construct interface. In addition, the orthosis is a vehicle to limit motion and allow for biological healing. Knowledge of the susceptibility of the surgical instrumentation to failure secondary to planar motion and the length of the fusion is necessary for proper selection of orthotic design. Design features should not encourage flexion that may decrease load sharing between the spine and instrumentation and conversely increase mechanical loading of the instrumentation.

Typically a polymer TLSO is indicated for this population and may warrant the addition of over-the-shoulder straps for fusion/instrumentation that extends superior to T3 and a thigh extension for fusion/instrumentation that extends to and includes the lumbosacral junction.[32,47] A bivalve TLSO design may be the most appropriate for this population because patients most likely will be recumbent after surgery, and donning and doffing movement may be limited because the patient can perform only a series of half log rolls. The bivalve design not only facilitates donning/doffing for families but allows for early mobilization of the patient and may reduce the complications associated with prolonged immobilization in a recumbent position. As with nonoperative management of spinal deformities, routine skin assessment is critical and especially necessary after initial fit of the orthosis. Volume changes of the patient's abdominal region occur frequently after surgery and may warrant several modifications to the orthosis during the first several weeks after surgery in order to ensure that optimal fit is maintained.

Younger children with larger curves who may not respond well to nonoperative orthotic management can be treated surgically with a short anterior spinal fusion and anterior instrumentation across the curve apex. In these cases, a combination of surgery and postoperative orthotic treatment can temporarily improve spinal alignment and preserve some spinal growth until more definitive surgery can be performed.[31]

Whether nonoperative or postoperative management is warranted, the orthotist should remain in close communication with the physician and family for the duration of orthotic treatment. Routine family follow-up should be an essential part of overall orthotic treatment if objectives are to be maintained and complications minimized.

Conclusion

Because of the complex nature of myelomeningoceles, careful attention to a child's clinical presentation and to his or her overall functional needs and goals is necessary if orthotic treatment is to be successful. A team approach, proper patient/family education, routine assessment, and early intervention all are essential for successful orthotic treatment but will go only as far as the orthotic practitioner can implement routine, competent, comprehensive orthotic care. Proper patient assessment, impression/measurements, and design selection; observation of relevant biomechanical principles; proper orthotic fitting/function; patient/family education; and routine follow-up all are requirements for providing comprehensive orthotic care that ultimately meets the needs of the patient and family. When such care is implemented and expectations are made clear to the patient and family, there is a much greater likelihood that goals will be met and family/patient satisfaction achieved.

References

1. Agree JC, Findley TW, McNally MC, et al: Physical activity capacity in children with myelomeningocele, *Arch Phys Med Rehabil* 68:372–377, 1987.
2. Asher M, Loson J: Factors affecting the ambulatory status of patients with spina bifida cystica, *J Bone Joint Surg Am* 65:350–356, 1983.
3. Banta JV, Hamada JS: Natural history of the kyphotic deformity in myelomeningocele, *J Bone Joint Surg* 58A:279, 1976.
4. Bartonek A, Saraste H, Knutson LM: Comparison of different systems to classify the neurological level of lesion in patients with myelomeningocele, *Dev Med Child Neurol* 41:796–805, 1999.
5. Bunch WH, Patwardhan AG: *Scoliosis making clinical decisions*, St Louis, 1989, CV Mosby.
6. Butler C: Augmentative mobility: why we do it? *Phys Med Rehabil Clin North Am* 2:801–813, 1991.
7. Campbell JH: Outcome study: uhe progression of spinal deformity in paraplegic children fitted with reciprocating gait orthoses, *JPO J Prosthet Orthot* 11:79, 1999.
8. Carroll N: The orthotic management of the spina bifida child, *Clin Orthop* 102:108–114, 1974.
9. Condie DN, Lamb J: Knee-ankle-foot orthoses. In Bowker P, Condie DN, Bader DL, Pratt DJ, editors: *Biomechanical basis of orthotic management*, Oxford, 1993, WA Wallace.
10. Condie DN, Meadows CB: Ankle foot orthoses. In Bowker P, Condie DN, Bader DL, Pratt DJ, editors: *Biomechanical basis of orthotic management*, Oxford, 1993, WA Wallace.
11. De Souza LJ, Carroll N: Ambulation of the braced myelomeningocele patient, *J Bone Joint Surg* 58:1112–1118, 1976.
12. Dias LS: Expected long-term walking ability. In Sarwark JF, Lubicky JP, editors: *Caring for the child with spina bifida*, Rosemont, Ill, 2001, AAOP.
13. Duckworth T, Yamashita T, Franks CI, et al: Somatosensory evoked cortical responses in children with spina bifida, *Dev Med Child Neurol* 18:19–24, 1976.
14. Duffy CM, Hill AE, Cosgrove AP, Corry IS, Mollan RA, Graham HK: Three-dimensional gait analysis in spina bifida, *J Pediatr Orthop* 16:786–791, 1996.
15. Geiger F, Parsch D, Carstens C: Complications of scoliosis surgery in children with myelomeningocele, *J Eur Spine* 8:22–26, 1999.
16. Gerritsma-Bleeker CL, Heeg M, Vos-Niel H: Ambulation with the reciprocating-gait orthosis: experience in 15 children with myelomeningocele or paraplegia, *Acta Orthop Scand* 68:470–473, 1997.
17. Glancy J, Lindseth RE: The polypropylene solid-ankle orthosis, *Orthot Prosthet* 26:14–26, 1972.
18. Graham HK, Harvey A, Rodda J, Nattrass GR, Pirpiris M: The functional mobility scale, *J Pediatr Orthop* 24:514–520, 2004.
19. Guidera KJ, Smith S, Raney E: Use of the reciprocating gait orthosis in myelodysplasia, *J Pediatr Orthop* 13:341–348, 1993.
20. Gupta RT, Vankoski S, Novak RA: Trunk kinematics and the influence on valgus knee stress in persons with high sacral level myelomeningocele, *J Pediatr Orthop* 25:89–94, 2005.
21. Hall PV, Lindseth RE, Campbell RL, et al: Myelodysplasia and developmental scoliosis: a manifestation of syringomyelia, *Spine* 1:48–56, 1976.
22. Herzog EG, Sharrard WJW: Calipers and braces with Dundee hip lock, *Clin Orthop Relat Res* 46:239, 1966.
23. Kelp-Lenane C, Butler-Figlioli S: Physical therapy intervention. In Sarwark JF, Lubicky JP, editors: *Caring for the child with spina bifida*, Rosemont, Ill, 2001, AAOP.
24. Klassion B, Convery P, Raschke S: Test apparatus for the measurement of the flexibility of ankle-foot orthoses in planes other than the loaded plane, *Prosthet Orthot Int* 22:45–53, 1998.
25. Latcha CM, Freeling MC, Powell NJ: A comparison of the grip strength of children with myelomeningocele to that of children without disability, *Am J Occup Ther* 47:498–503, 1993.
26. Letts M, Rathbone D, Yamashita T, et al: Soft Boston orthosis in management of neuromuscular scoliosis: a preliminary report, *J Pediatr Orthop* 12:470–474, 1992.
27. Lin RS, Moore TJ: Orthoses for postpolio syndrome. In Goldberg B, Hsu JD, editors: *Atlas of orthoses and assistive devices*, ed 3, St. Louis, 1997, Mosby.
28. Lindseth RE: Myelomeningocele spine. In Weinstein SL, editor: *The pediatric spine: principles and practice*, New York, 1994, Raven Press.
29. Liptak GS, Shurtleeff DB, Bloss JW, et al: Mobility aids for children with high-level myelomeningocele: parapodium versus wheelchair, *Dev Med Child Neurol* 34:787–796, 1992.
30. Lubicky JP: Spinal deformity in myelomeningocele. In Bridwell KH, Dewald RL, editors: *The textbook of spinal surgery*, ed 2, Philadelphia, 1997, Lippincott-Raven.
31. Lubicky JP: The surgical treatment of spinal deformities in myelomeningocele. In Sarwark JF, Lubicky JP, editors: *Caring for the child with spina bifida*, Rosemont, Ill, 2001, AAOP.
32. Lumsden RM, Morris JM: An in vivo study of axial rotation and immobilization at the lumbosacral joint, *J Bone Joint Surg* 50:1591–1602, 1968.
33. Major RE, Stallard J, Rose GK: The dynamics of walking using the hip guidance orthosis (HGO) with crutches, *Prosthet Orthot Int* 5:19–22, 1981.
34. Martin J, Kumar SJ, Guille JT, et al: Congenital kyphosis in myelomeningocele: results following operative and non-operative treatment, *J Pediatr Orthop* 14:323–328, 1994.
35. Mazur JH, Cummings RJ: Reciprocal biped walking in thoracic level spina bifida patients: is it cost effective? *Florida Orthop Soc J* 8:14–17, 1990.
36. Mazur JM, Shurtleff D, Menelaus M, Colliver J: Orthopaedic management of high-level spina bifida, *J Bone Joint Surg* 71A:56–61, 1989.

37. Mazur JM, Stillwell A, Menelaus M: The significance of spasticity in the upper and lower limbs in myelomeningocele, *J Bone Joint Surg Br* 68:213–217, 1986.

38. McCall RE, Douglass R, Rightor N: Surgical treatment in patients with myelodysplasia before using the LSU reciprocation-gait system, *Orthopedics* 6:843–848, 1983.

39. McDonald CM: Mobility issues and prescribing mobility aids for children with myelomeningocele. In Sarwark JF, Lubicky JP, editors: *Caring for the child with spina bifida*, Rosemont, Ill, 2001, AAOP.

40. McDonald CM, Jaffe KM, Mosca VS, et al: Ambulatory outcome of children with myelomeningocele, *J Bone Joint Surg Br* 68:213–217, 1986.

41. Menelaus MBD: Progress in the management of the paralytic hip in myelomeningocele, *Orthop Clin North Am* 11:17–30, 1987.

42. Michael JW: Lower limb orthoses. In Goldberg B, Hsu JD, editors: *Atlas of orthoses and assistive devices*, ed 3, St. Louis, 1997, Mosby.

43. Motloch W: The parapodium: an orthotic device for neuromuscular disorders. *Artif Limbs* 15:36–47, 1971.

44. Muller BA, Nordwall A: Brace treatment of scoliosis in children with myelomeningocele, *Spine* 19:151–155, 1994.

45. Muller BE, Nordwall A: Prevalence of scoliosis in myelomeningocele in western Sweden, *Spine* 17:1097–1102, 1992.

46. Muller BA, Nordwall A, Oden A: Progression of scoliosis in children with myelomeningocele, *Spine* 19:147–150, 1994.

47. Norton PL, Brown T: The immobilization efficiency of the back braces; their effect on the posture and motion of the lumbosacral spine, *J Bone Joint Surg* 39A:111–139, 1957.

48. Oakley GP Jr: Folic acid-preventable spina bifida and anencephaly, *JAMA* 269:1292–1293, 1993.

49. Patwardhan AG, Bunch WH, Meade KP, et al: A biomechanical analog of curve progression and orthotic stabilization in idiopathic scoliosis, *J Biomech* 19:103, 1986.

50. Perry J: *Gait analysis: normal and pathological function*, Thorofare, NJ, 1992, Slack.

51. Phillips DL, Field RE, Broughton NS, Menelaus MB: Reciprocating orthoses for children with myelomeningocele: a comparison of two types, *J Bone Joint Surg Br* 77:110–113, 1995.

52. Piggott H: The natural history of scoliosis in myelodysplasia, *J Bone Joint Surg* 62B:54–59, 1980.

53. Richards BS: Nonsurgical management of the myelomeningocele spine. In Sarwark JF, Lubicky JP, editors: *Caring for the child with spina bifida*, Rosemont, Ill, 2001, AAOP.

54. Rose GK: Surgical/orthotic management of spina bifida. In Murdoch G, editor: *The advance of orthotics*, London, 1976, Edward Arnold.

55. Rose GK, Henshaw JT: A swivel walker for paraplegics: medical and technical considerations, *Biomed Eng* 7:410–425, 1972.

56. Saltiel J: A one-piece laminated knee locking short leg brace, *Orthot Prosthet* 23:68–75, 1969.

57. Selber P, Dias L: Sacral level myelomeningocele: long term outcomes in adults, *J Pediatric Orthop* 18:423–427, 1998.

58. Sharrard WJW: The segmental innervation of the lower limb muscles in man, *Ann R Coll Surg Engl* 35:106–122, 1964.

59. Shurtleff DB, Menelaus MB, Staheli LT: Natural history of flexion deformity of the hip in myelodysplasia, *J Pediatr Orthop* 6:666–673, 1986.

60. Speilrein RE: An engineering approach to ambulation without the use of external power sources, of severely handicapped individuals, *J Inst Eng Aust* Dec: 326–333, 1963.

61. Stallard J: Hip Knee Ankle foot orthoses. In Bowker P, Condie DN, Bader DL, Pratt DJ, editors: *Biomechanical basis of orthotic management*, Oxford, 1993, WA Wallace.

62. Stallard J, Major RE, Butler PB: Theo orthotic ambulation performance of paraplegic myelomeningocele children using the ORLAU Parawalker treatment system, *Clin Rehabil* 5:111–114, 1991.

63. Stillwell A, Menelaus MB: Walking ability in mature patients with spina bifida, *J Pediatr Orthop* 3:184–190, 1983.

64. Tyo JH, Koch RD: Procedures for obtaining casts for ankle-foot orthoses, *Orthot Prosthet* 32:12–20, 1978.

65. Vankoski SJ, Kelp-Lenane C: Gait patterns in children with myelomeningocele. In Sarwark JF, Lubicky JP, editors: *Caring for the child with spina bifida*, Rosemont, 2001, AAOP.

66. Vankoski SJ, Michaud S, Dias L: External tibial torsion and the effectiveness of the solid ankle-foot orthoses, *J Pediatr Orthop* 20:349–355, 2000.

67. Vankowski SJ, Moore CA, Statler KD, Sarwark JF, Dias LS: Abstract: the influence of external support on pelvic and kinematic parameters in childhood community ambulators with low lumbar level myelomeningocele: don't throw away the crutches, *Dev Med Child Neurol* 37(suppl 73):5–6, 1995.

68. Vankoski SJ, Sarwark JF, Moore C, et al: Characteristic pelvic, hip, and knee kinematic patterns in children with lumbosacral myelomeningocele, *Gait Posture* 3:51–57, 1995.

69. Windham GC, Edmonds LD: Current trends in the incidence of neural tube defects, *Pediatrics* 70:333–337, 1982.

70. Winter DA: Kinematics and kinetic patterns in human gait: variability and compensating effects, *Hum Mov Sci* 3:51–76, 1984.

71. Yngve DA, Douglas R, Roberts JM: The reciprocating gait orthosis in myelomeningocele, *J Pediatr Orthop* 4:304–310, 1984.

Chapter

40

Cranial remolding orthoses

Deanna J. Fish and Dulcey Lima

Key Points

- Infant skull deformities can be the result of intrinsic changes as in craniosynostosis or extrinsic factors such as postnatal positioning or prenatal restriction.
- The three main head-shape deformities in young babies are deformational plagiocephaly, deformational brachycephaly, and deformational scaphocephaly.
- Cranial remolding orthoses are a time-specific treatment intervention used after 3 months and preferably prior to 12 months of age because active skull growth is required for remolding the cranium.
- Cranial remolding orthoses are considered Class II medical devices by the FDA and may only be manufactured by FDA-cleared facilities.
- The goal of treatment is to normalize the skull into a more symmetrical and well-proportioned shape.
- Orthotic intervention is indicated if the head shape deformity is moderate to severe and if conservative repositioning efforts are not effective.
- Clinical documentation includes anthropometric measurements at the beginning and end of the treatment program.
- A variety of cranial remolding designs are available, and it has not been proven that one design is more effective than the others.
- Effective materials include copolymer with dense foam liner, surlyn, and duraplex.
- The treatment program is generally 3 to 6 months.
- Cranial remolding orthoses may also be used postoperatively to maintain and/or improve the surgical correction.
- Despite a growing number of case reports, no controlled studies on the use of cranial remolding orthoses have been published.

The term *plagiocephaly* derives from the Greek *plagios*, meaning oblique, and *cephalo*, referencing the head.[16] Plagiocephaly has been used in the medical literature to refer to both synostotic (i.e., craniosynostosis) and nonsynostotic (i.e., deformational) conditions.

The terms *deformational plagiocephaly, deformational brachycephaly,* and *deformational scaphocephaly* refer to cranial deformities that are recognized in infancy and develop from both prenatal and postnatal factors. They are the primary focus of this chapter. These deformities are documented as deviations in proportion and/or symmetry of the neurocranium (i.e., skull), and often are accompanied by misalignment of the bones of the viscerocranium (i.e., face). Postoperative orthotic treatment programs for synostotic conditions are discussed here; however, protective cranial orthoses for developmental disabilities and seizure disorders are beyond the scope of this chapter. Cranial remolding orthoses have been used for many years to direct cranial growth patterns during infancy and produce greater symmetry and/or proportion of the skull. The time-sensitive nature of effective treatment requires early identification and intervention from health care professionals.

Pathophysiology

The pathogenesis of cranial deformities arises from three primary causes: (1) abnormalities in brain shape or development, (2) abnormalities in bone or suture development, and (3) prenatal and postnatal deforming forces.[7,12] Abnormalities in brain shape or development include conditions such as microcephaly, macrocephaly, and in utero cerebrovascular accident. Craniosynostosis involves premature fusion of one or more cranial sutures, and genetic disorders such as Apert syndrome and Crouzon syndrome produce

Table 40-1 Common clinical observations and classification of skull deformities

Deformational Plagiocephaly	Deformational Brachycephaly	Deformational Scaphocephaly
Asymmetry of the neurocranium and viscerocranium: • Unilateral occipital flattening • Ipsilateral anterior ear progression • Ipsilateral forehead bossing • Contralateral forehead depression • Contralateral occipital bossing • Facial asymmetry • Congenital muscular torticollis	Disproportion of the neurocranium and viscerocranium: • Bilateral occipital flattening • Bilateral forehead bossing • Increased height of cranial vault • Associated weakness of neck musculature	Disproportion of the neurocranium and viscerocranium: • Bilateral parietal flattening • Anterior forehead bossing • Posterior occipital bossing • Associated weakness of neck musculature

significant alterations in bone and suture development. The largest group of patients seen for orthotic cranial remolding procedures presents with cranial deformities secondary to prenatal and postnatal deforming forces.

Cranial deformities often begin with restrictive in utero environments. Fetal constraint may be due to multiple births, a large fetus, first pregnancies, or sustained abnormal positioning secondary to conditions such as oligohydramnios, breech positioning, or early descent into the maternal pelvis. Vaginal deliveries produce significant distortion of the fetal cranium as it passes through the birth canal, and prolonged labor and difficult deliveries exacerbate the deforming forces. Cesarean deliveries may be performed due to cephalopelvic disproportion, sustained abnormal positioning, or a developing medical crisis in the fetus or mother. Any of these situations creates deforming forces that act on the developing fetal skull.[5,6,32]

Premature infants are extremely susceptible to cranial deformation due to the increased plasticity of the underdeveloped cranial structures. Extended periods of lying on the side and back in neonatal intensive care units may exacerbate cranial deformation. Term infants are also subject to postnatal forces that act on the cranial structures during supine positioning, which became the sleeping position recommended by the American Academy of Pediatrics (AAP) in 1992.[1] The 1992 implementation of the "Back to Sleep" program was extremely successful in decreasing the incidence of sudden infant death syndrome; however, a corresponding increase in cranial deformities has been well documented.[2,22] Another variable is the influence of congenital muscular torticollis and neck muscle asymmetry, a common finding in young infants, specifically those with deformational plagiocephaly.[6,11,13,19,43] Unilateral neck involvement results in sustained head positioning that produces asymmetrical loading on developing cranial structures. Structural anomalies, such as cervical hemivertebrae, also contribute to skull deformity.

Ultimately, any combination of the following factors may produce or exacerbate cranial deformation: deforming forces in utero, deforming forces during the birth process, sustained supine positioning in compliance with the AAP Back to Sleep program, sustained supine positioning in neonatal intensive care units, sustained supine positioning during normal daily infant/caregiver routines, torticollis, and lack of education and information provided to caregivers relative to the importance of supervised prone positioning. In general, cranial distortion in the newborn is common and often resolves within the first 12 weeks of life if external forces acting on the skull

are consistently altered. A cranial deformity usually is considered for orthotic intervention when the infant's abnormal skull proportion and/or symmetry remains or fails to improve despite early intervention of repositioning and/or therapeutic efforts during the first 3 months after birth (Table 40-1).[2,6,13,32,37]

Three common presentations of cranial deformation are identified and treated with cranial remolding orthoses. Common clinical observations and classifications of skull deformities are detailed in Table 40-1, although many variations of the patterns of deformation exist. Deformational plagiocephaly is the most common cranial anomaly and presents with asymmetry of the right and left sides of the skull and face. Unilateral occipital flattening produces varying degrees of ipsilateral anterior ear displacement, ipsilateral forehead bossing, contralateral forehead flattening, and contralateral posterior occipital bossing. Facial structures are commonly affected, as evidenced by altered alignment of the eyes, cheeks, nose, mouth, and chin.

Deformational (symmetrical) brachycephaly and deformational scaphocephaly are less common and present with primary disruptions in cranial proportion (Fig. 40-1). Deformational symmetrical brachycephaly is clinically identified by central occipital flattening, increased cranial width, decreased cranial length, increased cranial vault height, and increased forehead bossing. A large number of infants have

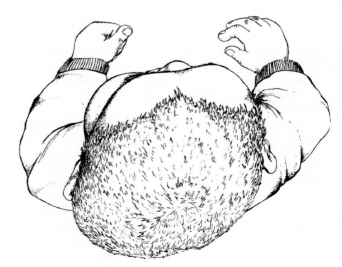

Fig. 40-1 Deformational plagiocephaly. (Courtesy Orthomerica Products, Inc.)

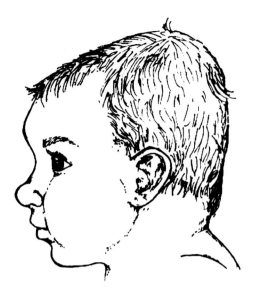

Fig. 40-2 Deformational brachycephaly. (Courtesy Orthomerica Products, Inc.)

characteristics common to both plagiocephaly and brachycephaly and present with an asymmetrical brachycephalic head shape deformity. These infants require a complex treatment approach that addresses the asymmetry and disproportion. Deformational scaphocephaly presents with bilateral parietal flattening, increased cranial length, decreased cranial width, and occipital and anterior forehead protrusion or bossing. Secondary asymmetry of varying degrees may accompany either of these deformities (Figs. 40-2 and 40-3)

Evaluation of cranial deformity includes consideration of the following elements:

- Degree of asymmetry
- Degree of disproportion
- Plasticity of bony structures
- Amount of translation of bony plates
- Cellular disruptions and alterations in suture development
- Soft-tissue involvement and/or contributions from neck musculature
- Genetic predisposition
- Effect of neurocranial structures and alterations on adjacent viscerocranial structures

Historical perspective

History has shown many different applications of *intentional cranial deformation*. Different cultures applied a variety of measures to alter the shape of the infant skull. Boards, vines, cloth bandages, and even the weight of stones were applied to the head of the infant to create a culturally desired cranial shape. Even these primitive cultures recognized that early and sustained application of these intentional and specific forces would produce long-standing changes in cranial shape. Globally, skulls were elongated, flattened, rounded,

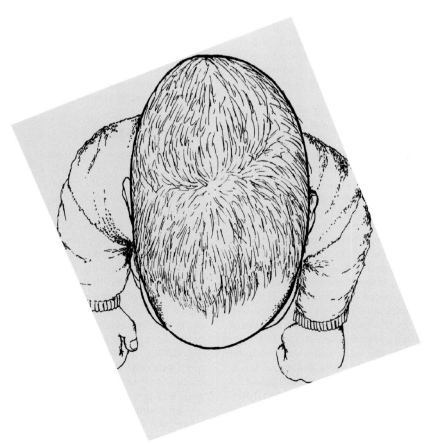

Fig. 40-3 Deformational scaphocephaly. (Courtesy Orthomerica Products, Inc.)

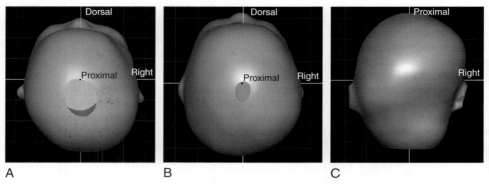

Fig. 40-4 A, Vertex view of left deformational plagiocephaly. **B**, Vertex view of right lambdoid synostosis. **C**, Posterior view of right lambdoid synostosis. (Courtesy Hanger Prosthetics & Orthotics.)

widened, or contoured for a variety of reasons,[33] yet all cultures opted for symmetrical distortion to meet some form of societal norm or distinction.

In 1979, Clarren et al.[6] were the first to report on deformational plagiocephaly and orthotic treatment as a result of their experiences at the Dysmorphology Clinic of the University of Washington in Seattle. At that time, most infants who presented with dysmorphology or craniofacial clinics were diagnosed and surgically treated for many different congenital or hereditary disorders of the developing brain, bone, or suture(s). Cranial remolding orthoses were being used postoperatively to provide both protection and continued reshaping of the skull once the growth impedance of the fused suture was removed. Infants diagnosed with deformational plagiocephaly, brachycephaly, and scaphocephaly were the exception. Clarren et al. reported on 10 infants diagnosed with nonsynostotic plagiocephaly who were treated with cranial remolding orthoses. The treatment concept was based on knowledge of *intentional cranial deformation* and understanding of resistive forces and directed growth within the confines of a symmetrical orthosis.

In the early to mid-1990s, the significant increase in the number of infants who presented with asymmetrical and disproportional skull deformities coincided with the AAP Back to Sleep program.[2,22] Craniofacial clinics experienced an overwhelming increase in the number of pediatric referrals. These specialty clinics were burdened by a large number of infants referred for suspected craniosynostosis when, in fact, they had deformational skull anomalies and were not actually surgical candidates. Particular confusion existed over the diagnosis of deformational plagiocephaly versus unilateral lambdoid synostosis, a relatively rare condition. Huang et al.[18] outlined specific anatomical features found during clinical evaluation that distinguished deformational plagiocephaly from synostotic plagiocephaly. Evaluation from the vertex view reveals asymmetry and unilateral occipital flattening in both conditions. In this same view, deformational plagiocephaly presents with a parallelogram shape and anterior advancement of the ear on the same side as the occipital flattening. In contrast, from the vertex view, unilateral lambdoid synostosis presents with a trapezoid shape and posterior displacement of the ear on the same side as the occipital flattening. Other distinguishing features have been discussed in detail previously (Fig. 40-4).[18]

Initially, definitive diagnostic criteria included x-ray, magnetic resonance imaging (MRI), or computed tomography (CT) scans evaluated by craniofacial specialists and were required for confirmation of deformational cranial involvement rather than synostotic processes. Since the landmark article by Huang et al. and by other investigators on the differentiation between craniosynostosis and deformational plagiocephaly, these diagnostic tests have been replaced by clinical evaluation procedures. Pediatricians and other health care providers now are better equipped to screen infants for these conditions and to refer parents to specialists when the history and clinical features suggest a synostotic deformity.

With the increased numbers of infants requiring orthotic treatment for deformational skull anomalies, nonsurgical treatment programs, including orthotic management with cranial remolding orthoses, have been developed and refined. These treatment programs are based on previous efforts in postoperative applications and the concept of *intentional cranial reformation*. Cranial remolding orthoses are designed to improve cranial proportion and/or symmetry in infants diagnosed with nonsynostotic cranial deformities with application of early and sustained resistive forces encountered during periods of rapid cranial growth.

Current issues

The natural history of untreated deformational skull deformities has not been thoroughly studied. A study conducted at the Children's Healthcare of Atlanta found that infants treated with cranial remolding orthoses showed significant improvement in symmetry measures, whereas the majority of untreated infants with deformational plagiocephaly showed changes in parameters related only to growth, not symmetry.[37] The impact on the functional competence of adjacent structures relating to hearing, vision, balance, mandibular symmetry, and brain development has only recently been addressed with more rigorous scientific investigation.[23,25,30,34] Many infants still remain undiagnosed and untreated, and those who receive treatment reveal the benefits of individual case presentation without the advantage of collaborative randomization for the advancement of medical science. Many questions regarding the natural history and spontaneous resolution will remain unanswered until a double-blind study with a larger sample size is conducted.

Early identification of skull deformities should be undertaken by a variety of health care professionals in contact with this young patient population. Referral to experienced team members is appropriate, and definitive diagnosis is largely the result of clinical evaluation. Specific features and distinctions of synostotic and nonsynostotic cranial deformities are well documented. Clinical diagnosis by experienced medical personnel limits additional and costly diagnostic procedures. Timely referral to therapy and/or orthotic evaluation is beneficial to the infant.

Clinical documentation includes a series of anthropometric measurements of the infant skull. These measures are used to justify the need for treatment as well as support the efficacy of the treatment program (see section on treatment recommendations). Reported outcomes support the use of cranial remolding orthoses for improving cranial proportion and/or symmetry in infants 3 to 18 months old. Greater results are noted in younger infants, and recommendations for completing treatment by age 12 months are based on well-documented cranial growth patterns. Significant and rapid circumferential cranial growth occurs in the first 6 months after birth and drops off significantly after age 12 months. Infants older than 12 months still may benefit from orthotic remolding procedures; however, the length of the orthotic treatment program is increased and results are not as favorable. Graham et al.[13] found that early diagnosis was critical and that delay may lead to incomplete or ineffective correction. Reduced correction in older babies likely is due to the increase in skull thickness with each passing month and greater difficulty with compliance because of the infant's improving dexterity and ability to remove the orthosis.

Current research

A systematic review of the literature reveals much agreement on the need for orthotic treatment of moderate and severe skull deformities.[2,6,13,14,32,37] Unfortunately, the medical literature reveals an abundance of case studies, case series, and expert opinion. A critical review of the medical literature by Rekate[39] in 1998 noted the following: confusion in terminology and definition; difficulty in determining the incidence of deformational plagiocephaly; contribution of both prenatal and postnatal factors to skull deformities; and three primary treatment options, including observation and repositioning, mechanical intervention, and surgery. A review by Lima[27] in 2004 reiterated the lack of consistent terminology and definition. Difficulty in establishing the incidence of skull deformities in young infants remained, although many citations suggested common risk factors and early intervention.[27] Of the 22 studies evaluated, most presented comparative or case-control studies; no randomized controlled trials were reported. A review by Bialocerkowski et al.[4] in 2005 reported that only 16 articles met inclusion criteria (12 case studies and four comparative studies). Based on these publications, it was not possible to draw conclusions regarding the effectiveness of nontreatment, repositioning, and/or orthotic intervention because of poor methodology and potential bias of the researchers.[4] More recent studies by Graham et al.[13,14] comparing orthotic management to repositioning for management of deformational plagiocephaly and brachycephaly use larger and more equivalent severity groups. The lack of randomized controlled trials hinders medical advancement and treatment criteria and should be addressed in a collaborative effort by medical professionals involved in the care of these infants (Fig. 40-5).

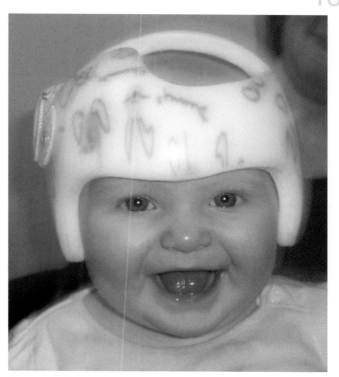

Fig. 40-5 Infant wearing a cranial remolding orthosis. (Courtesy Orthomerica Products, Inc.)

A 2004 consensus conference sponsored by the American Academy of Orthotists and Prosthetists revealed much agreement among convened experts on orthotic treatment protocols for infants with deformational plagiocephaly, brachycephaly, and scaphocephaly. The conference findings indicated that early identification of head shape deformities is the responsibility of all health care professionals treating this young pediatric population. Clinical evaluation and diagnosis usually are possible without costly procedures such as x-ray, MRI, or CT scan unless craniosynostosis is suspected. Once deformational head shape problems are diagnosed, aggressive repositioning should be initiated as the first course of action. Additional therapy evaluation may be required for infants exhibiting neck involvement and/or developmental delay. Repositioning and therapy programs should be implemented in the first 3 to 4 months after birth. After age 4 months, infants whose head shapes do not improve or demonstrate progression in the cranial deformity should be referred for orthotic management. Continued therapy for torticollis and/or developmental delay may be necessary during and after completion of the orthotic remolding process.[21] This type of expert opinion and consensus provides a strong foundation for future structured scientific investigation.

Treatment recommendations

Early identification of cranial deformities in young infants creates the opportunity for altering external forces that act on the skull and may exacerbate deformation or prevent symmetrical and proportional skull growth. Health care professionals, such as obstetricians, pediatricians, nurses, therapists, and family practitioners, should inspect the infant's head

Table 40-2 Anthropometric measurements, cranial landmarks, and calculations used for documentation of cranial deformities

Anthropometric Measurements	Cranial Landmarks
Cranial circumference	Taken at the equator
Cranial width	Euryon to euryon (eu − eu)
Cranial length	Glabella to opisthocranion (g − op)
Cranial vault, right and left	Frontozygomaticus to contralateral euryon
Orbitotragial depth (upper face), right and left	Exocanthion to tragion (ex − t)
Cranial base (lower face), right and left	Subnasion to tragion (sn − t)
Additional measures	**Calculations**[a]
Cephalic index (CI)	CI = Cranial width ÷ Cranial length
Cranial vault asymmetry (CVA)	CVA = Cranial vault (R) − Cranial vault (L)
Cranial vault asymmetry index (CVAI)	CVAI = [Cranial vault (R) − Cranial vault (L)] ÷ Cranial vault (R)
Orbitotragial depth asymmetry (OTDA)	OTDA = Orbitotragial depth (R) − Orbitotragial depth (L)
Cranial base asymmetry (CBA)	CBA = Cranial base (R) − Cranial base (L)

[a]*All calculations expressed in positive values.*

from the front, sides, back, and top during all clinic encounters. When infants with asymmetrical and/or disproportionate cranial development are identified, caregivers should be provided with educational materials and instruction on effective repositioning techniques. These techniques include supervised "tummy time" as well as strategic positioning during diapering, feeding, carrying, and handling. Limitations on time spent in car seats, carriers, and swings are imposed, and care is taken to position nursery furniture relative to bright areas that attract the infant's attention.[36] Purposeful and intentional efforts to alter the infant's position in the first 3 months of life serve to better distribute external forces acting on the developing infant skull.

Anthropometric skull measurements establish a baseline for clinical documentation of improvement or progression of the skull deformity. Common clinical measurements include cranial circumference, cranial width, cranial length, cranial vault, orbitotragial depth, and cranial base measurements. Other calculations of cranial vault asymmetry, orbitotragial depth asymmetry, and cranial base asymmetry can be made and ratios expressed for the cephalic index and cranial vault asymmetry index.[9,24,31,41] Table 40-2 lists specific anthropometric measurements, cranial landmarks, and calculations used for documentation, assessment, and comparison of cranial deformities.

Understanding normative values relative to cranial development is important in the early identification and intervention of skull deformities. Cranial circumference measurements document cranial growth patterns of the developing brain and skull and have been standardized for both boys and girls (Fig. 40-6).[8] Such cranial growth charts reveal approximately 2 cm of circumferential growth per month in the first 3 months, 1 cm of circumferential growth per month between 4 and 6 months, and approximately 0.5 cm of circumferential growth between 6 and 12 months. After age 12 months, cranial growth slows significantly. This information reinforces the need for early intervention for repositioning, therapy, and orthotic programs in the early months after birth. Waiting for spontaneous resolution of skull deformities reduces the window of opportunity for intervention with repositioning and limits the effectiveness of orthotic intervention.

Cranial width and length are used to calculate a proportional relationship, specifically the cephalic index. On average, cranial width is approximately 78% of the cranial length.[8] Infants with deformational brachycephaly have an increased cephalic index due to a very wide and short skull deformity. Infants with deformational scaphocephaly have a lower cephalic index due to a very long and narrow skull deformity. Deformational plagiocephaly tends to present with slightly higher than average cephalic index values. Table 40-3 lists cephalic index values for infants up to age 6 months.[8] Studies have documented increases in the cephalic index since initiation of the Back to Sleep program, but no new anthropological data on large numbers of infants have been reported.[14] Although a higher cephalic index has been documented in infants who sleep in a supine position than in infants who sleep in a prone position,[17] no study has shown that supine sleeping infants have the associated deformities of steep cranial vault and frontal bossing so often apparent in infants diagnosed with deformational brachycephaly. It is possible that the associated deformities result from a combination of nighttime and daytime supine positioning acting on the developing skull.

Cranial vault asymmetry, orbitotragial depth asymmetry, and cranial base asymmetry measures report differences in symmetry between the right and left sides of the skull and face. A perfectly symmetrical skull and face would reveal no differences between the right and left side measures. Most individuals have slight asymmetry; therefore, asymmetry in and of itself is not abnormal or indicative of deformity. Rather, it is the degree of asymmetry (and/or disproportion) that determines deformation, and standards have not yet been determined. As reported by Loveday and de Chalain,[29] the

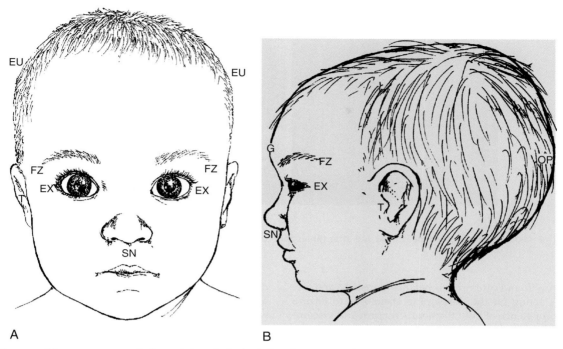

Fig. 40-6 Anthropometric measurements. **A**, Frontal view. **B**, Sagittal view. (Courtesy Orthomerica Products, Inc.)

cranial vault asymmetry index (CVAI) represents a relative value that allows comparison of asymmetry between skulls of different sizes or between the same skull over time as growth occurs. CVAI >3.5% was reported to represent "significant asymmetry." Ultimately, linear measurements may fail to represent the complexity of a three-dimensional deformity but are helpful in quantifying and comparing specific aspects of cranial deformation over time. Hutchison et al.[19] used a 6% difference between oblique cranial vault measurements and 94% cephalic index as measurements that determined a "case" in their study of 200 infants in New Zealand.

By infant age 3 months, focused repositioning efforts may produce significant changes to the overall symmetry and proportion of the skull and may prevent the need for additional medical treatments. Continued cranial deformation, developmental delay, and/or weakness or tightness of the neck musculature determine the need for additional therapy and orthotic evaluation. Therapy evaluation and treatment programs are indicated whenever the infant presents with generalized hypotonicity, developmental delay, asymmetry of nuchal folds, persistent positional preference, and/or when limitations in active and passive neck range of motion are noted.[10] Orthotic evaluation can be performed at any time to establish baseline measurements. Orthotic treatment programs are indicated after age 3 months when the infant's skull deformity fails to improve with repositioning and/or therapy efforts or progresses in severity despite efforts at intervention.

Orthotic management

Disruptions in cranial symmetry and/or proportion result from the application of external forces acting on developing cranial structures. Deformation of the infant skull occurs in response to the amount, direction, mode, and frequency of the forces applied. The mechanical function of adjacent structures, such as the temporomandibular joint or orbital alignment, also may be affected.[22] Orthotic modeling

Table 40-3 Cephalic indices for infants up to age 6 months[31]

Sex	Age	−2 SD	−1 SD	Mean	+1 SD	+2 SD
Male	16 days to 6 months	63.7	68.7	73.7	78.7	83.7
	6 to 12 months	64.8	71.4	78.0	84.6	91.2
Female	16 days to 6 months	63.9	68.6	73.3	78.0	82.7
	6 to 12 months	69.5	74.0	78.5	83.0	87.5

−SD is below the standard deviation mean.
+SD is above the standard deviation mean.

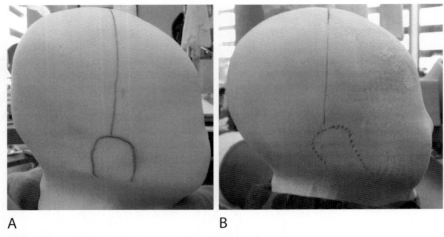

Fig. 40-7 Positive model of infant's head, before **(A)** and after **(B)** rectification procedures.

presumes growth and attempts to balance the static and dynamic forces acting on the developing structures to ensure functional competence of both the neurocranium and viscerocranium. General pediatric modeling considerations for the pediatric population include the following:

- Time of onset of condition
- Duration of deforming forces
- Degree of severity
- Degree of correctability
- Diagnosis/etiology
- Remaining growth of physiological structures
- Overall health of physiological structures
- Developmental level

Effective patient management begins with a thorough patient history and discussion with caregivers. Useful clinical information includes both prenatal and postnatal factors. Birth history includes information pertaining to gestational age, weight, length, fetal positioning, delivery, other or associated medical conditions, skin sensitivity, head shape at birth, and age when head deformity was first noted. Developmental observations include preferred sleeping positioning, repositioning efforts by caregivers, and acquisition of developmental milestones. Physical examination of the infant's face and skull includes visual observation from all angles as well as manual palpation of cranial sutures. Digital photographs and anthropometric measurements establish baseline measurements for future comparison and document asymmetrical and displaced skull and facial features as well as nonvertical orientation of the head relative to the trunk. Neck musculature and range of motion are evaluated, and consideration of referrals for therapy is made for patients showing weakness or limited range of motion. Discussions with caregivers should include an overview of the orthotic treatment program, determination of treatment goals and expectations, importance of supervised prone positioning, casting or scanning process, fitting and follow-up schedule, orthotic cleaning regimen, wearing schedule, signs indicating the need for adjustments, and situations requiring removal of the cranial remolding orthosis. These topics are reinforced during each visit.[9]

The casting or scanning procedure provides a representative model of the infant's head, and all efforts are made to decrease the stress to the infant and caregiver. A typical casting procedure takes 15 to 30 minutes and involves the application of plaster splints over stockinette on the infant's head. Once the plaster has cured, the cast is removed to produce an accurate negative model of the infant's head. Scanning procedures typically take 1 to 5 minutes for preparation and scanning and result in a digital representation of the infant's head. Both procedures have been used consistently to obtain an accurate model with identifiable anatomical landmarks necessary for rectification and fabrication of the custom cranial remolding orthosis.[40]

Rectification procedures of the positive plaster model and digital image are done with the same goal: to create a new model with greater symmetry and/or proportion than currently exists (Fig. 40-7). Areas of flattening are expanded to allow for planned and directed growth, and areas of bossing are maintained to resist continued growth. Various orthotic styles use slightly different rectification techniques, but the basic theory is the same: to resist growth in undesired areas and directions and promote growth in desired areas and directions.[35]

Cranial remolding orthoses have been inappropriately referred to as either *active* (or *dynamic*) or *passive*. In reality, most cranial remolding orthoses are passive, and the "active" part of the treatment program is the ongoing growth of the infant's brain and skull and the extent to which the orthotist is involved in directing head growth. The orthotist monitors and directs growth throughout the treatment program by the strategic addition or removal of lining material or strategic contouring of the rigid plastic shell. One specific design for scaphocephalic head deformities uses a bivalve orthosis with attachment bands of varying durometers to apply a continuous force to the anterior and posterior regions of the skull. This particular "dynamic" orthosis was designed to apply active and strategic forces to the skull rather than to resist forces encountered through normal brain and skull growth.[38]

A variety of plastics and lining materials are used to create cranial remolding orthoses (Fig. 40-8).[42] Other design variations include trim lines, strapping, construction of the inner liner, and rectification specifications. Ultimately, these design variations focus on regional development and experience; they have not been studied to determine whether use of

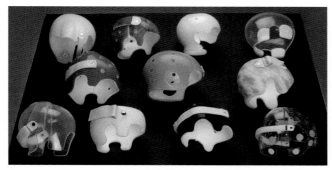

Fig. 40-8 Different design variations for cranial remolding orthoses. (Photograph taken at the American Academy of Orthotists and Prosthetists Consensus Conference on Plagiocephaly.)

specific materials results in positive or negative treatment outcomes. All cranial remolding orthoses operate on the basic premise of directed growth, and all have the potential to create improvements in symmetry and/or proportion when the following factors are present: effective fit of the orthosis, treatment provided during periods of cranial growth, compliance with wearing schedules, and age- and design-appropriate follow-up visits with the orthotist.

Orthotic treatment programs last from 3 to 6 months. Many individual factors affect the length of the treatment program and the results of treatment. Factors include but are not limited to biomechanics of skull growth, neuromotor maturation, chronological age at initiation of treatment, severity of deformity, type of cranial deformity, presence or absence of congenital muscular torticollis or other neck weakness or asymmetry, and cranial growth patterns. During the orthotic treatment program, consistent follow-up visits are scheduled to ensure proper fit and function of the orthosis, document changes in anthropometric measurements, perform necessary adjustments and modifications to the orthosis, verify compliance and understanding of the treatment program, and provide guidance and support to caregivers. Termination of treatment is considered by the entire medical team and caregivers when an acceptable level of improvement in symmetry and/or proportion has been obtained. The infant's developmental level also is considered, as regression of the deformity may occur in infants who are unable to reposition themselves by

rolling and/or lack independent sitting skills. Weaning from the cranial remolding orthosis may be immediate or implemented over a short period of time, depending on factors such as developmental level, fit of the orthosis, and regional medical practices. In all cases, follow-up is required to evaluate acceptable cranial growth patterns and dimensions and document the maintenance of orthotic outcomes (Figs. 40-9 and 40-10).

Cranial remolding orthoses used to maintain and enhance surgical procedures are created using similar processes. The infant is scanned or casted about 5 days after surgery to allow for reduction of swelling and initial healing of the suture site. Surgical procedures vary, and preoperative and postoperative orthotic requirements change relative to the type of surgery performed. Cranial vault restorations involve surgical remodeling and reshaping of the infant's skull. Preoperative and postoperative head shapes vary considerably, and partial or complete correction of skull symmetry and/or proportion relates to the severity of the initial head deformity.[3] Endoscopic procedures usually involve removal of the affected suture without extensive remodeling or reshaping of the infant's skull. Cranial remolding orthoses are especially indicated after such procedures to further direct growth of the skull. Postoperative cranial remolding orthoses also are protective, preventing inadvertent trauma to the skull (Fig. 40-11). Regardless of the specific surgical technique, many surgeons use a cranial remolding orthosis to discourage growth along specific suture lines and to maintain or improve the corrected head shape.[15]

Best practices

General recommendations for "best practices" are largely based on clinical experience and expert consensus and may not be well-supported in the medical literature. Scientific evidence for this patient population is sparse, and recommendations should be used as the basis for future medical research.

- *Cranial remolding orthoses should be considered in the medical management of infants with deformational plagiocephaly, brachycephaly, and scaphocephaly.* Cranial remolding orthoses have been used and documented

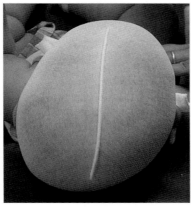
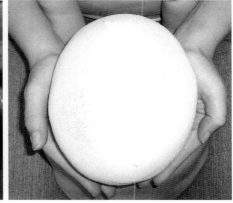

A   B

Fig. 40-9 Pretreatment **(A)** and posttreatment **(B)** views of infant diagnosed with deformational plagiocephaly. (Courtesy SCOPe and Orthomerica Products, Inc.)

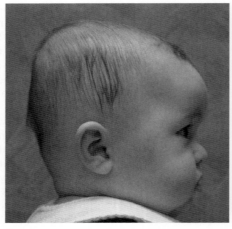
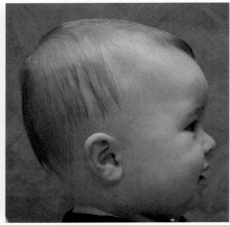

A　　　　　　　　　　　　　　　　　　　　　　B

Fig. 40-10 Pretreatment **(A)** and posttreatment **(B)** views of infant diagnosed with deformational brachycephaly. (Courtesy Tandem O&P and Orthomerica Products, Inc.)

in the medical literature since 1979 to produce improvement in cranial symmetry and/or proportion.[2,6,13,14,26,29,31,32]

- *Repositioning and therapy techniques should be started in the first 3 months after birth.* Early intervention has the potential to prevent the development and/or progression of skull deformities when initiated early and performed on a consistent basis.[2,6,13,14,26,29,31,32] Repositioning efforts are not effective in older infants as they begin to acquire and refine motor skills. Therapy for developmental delay and congenital muscular torticollis may continue during and after the orthotic treatment program.

- *Referrals for orthotic evaluation should be made by allied health care providers for infants with asymmetrical and/or disproportional skull deformities.* Health care providers in maternity wards, primary care offices, pediatric practices, therapy offices, and other health care facilities should be aware of their role in the prevention and early identification of infant skull deformities.[21,36]

- *Qualified orthotists should be included in the team management of infants with deformational plagiocephaly,* brachycephaly, *and scaphocephaly.* Orthotists assist in the clinical evaluation, provide documentation of anthropometric measurements, perform casting or scanning procedures, recommend orthotic design specifications, and provide a thorough and comprehensive orthotic treatment program.[21]

- *Therapists and orthotists should be aware of the relationship among conditions such as developmental delay, torticollis, and deformational skull deformities and make appropriate referrals.* Delayed acquisition of motor skills results in extended periods of supine positioning and continuous deforming forces acting on the skull if the infant is unable to lift the head, roll, or sit independently. A high incidence of congenital muscular torticollis has been documented in infants with deformational plagiocephaly. In such cases, concurrent therapy and orthotic treatment programs are likely to produce the best results.[10,11,13]

- *Most cranial remolding orthoses are based upon the same biomechanical principles of "directed growth."* Many different design variations have been developed, but no study has been performed to show superior outcomes of one design over another.

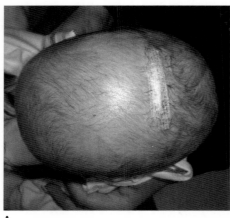
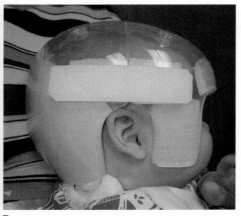

A　　　　　　　　　　　　　　　　　　　　　　B

Fig. 40-11 Infant diagnosed with craniosynostosis. Postoperative vertex view of suture **(A)** and wearing cranial remolding orthosis **(B)**. (Courtesy Hanger Prosthetics & Orthotics.)

- *Orthotists and other allied health care professionals should be aware of the risk factors for skull deformities.* Factors include but are not limited to in utero constraint, large gestational size, multiple births, premature births, difficult deliveries or birth trauma, sustained supine positioning, congenital muscular torticollis, generalized hypotonicity, developmental delay, and cervical abnormalities.[19,24,43]

- *The recommended age for treatment with a cranial remolding orthosis is between 4 and 8 months.*[26] There is general agreement that improved outcomes are obtained by early intervention,[2,13,43] although studies reported in the literature all used different ages to differentiate between the groups. Teichgraeber[41] found that when 6 months was used as the cutoff, no significant difference between the results was observed in infants treated earlier or later than 6 months. Because cranial remolding procedures depend on active growth patterns, early initiation prior to 8 or 9 months and completion of the orthotic program by 12 months of age seems appropriate for the best clinical outcomes. Older infants may still benefit from orthotic care, but the treatment period is longer and correction may not be as complete.

- *Clinical evaluation procedures are more commonly used than x-ray, CT, or MRI scan to provide a definitive diagnosis of deformational plagiocephaly, brachycephaly, and scaphocephaly.* Experienced health care professionals are often able to make a differential diagnosis of deformational plagiocephaly by completing a clinical examination, history, and physical examination of the infant. Routine skull x-ray films are obtained at some centers, and most often the diagnosis of deformational plagiocephaly is made without the additional expense, anesthesia, and radiation associated with more invasive procedures. Infants without a clear diagnosis of deformational involvement or those with suspected craniosynostosis are referred for high-resolution CT scan with surface reformations.[23]

- *Attempts to classify head deformities as mild, moderate, or severe have not been supported in the scientific literature.* These qualitative descriptors poorly define or differentiate severity of skull deformity. Further scientific research is needed to identify not only the severity but also the incidence, natural history, and potential long-term consequences in this patient population.[20]

- *Documentation and maintenance of complete clinical records are important.* It is the responsibility of all medical team members to maintain thorough and complete patient records regarding history, anthropometric measurements, repositioning efforts, therapy programs, orthotic design, clinical notes, and treatment outcomes.[9]

- *Cranial remolding orthoses have been classified as type II medical devices by the FDA since 1998.* This classification requires special 510(k) clearance, ongoing regulation, and scrutiny of these devices, and only facilities with this clearance are allowed to manufacture cranial remolding orthoses. Once cleared by the FDA, device manufacturers must comply with additional requirements, which include registration of the manufacturing facility, development of quality control systems, documented procedures to ensure the highest standards of manufacturing, and routine audits by the FDA.[28]

Supporting evidence

As noted, the scientific research regarding this patient population is limited. Many descriptive studies exist but, no randomized control trial proving the efficacy of cranial remolding orthoses has been reported. The studies listed in Table 40-4 reported the efficacy of cranial remolding orthoses in the management and treatment of infants diagnosed with deformational plagiocephaly, brachycephaly, and scaphocephaly.[27]

Table 40-4 Efficacy of cranial remolding orthoses[23]

Authors	Year	Level of Evidence	Population	Intervention	Outcomes Measured
Clarren et al.[6]	1979	VI	10 infants with deformational plagiocephaly	Cranial remolding orthosis	Visual assessment
Clarren[5a]	1981	V	25 infants with deformational plagiocephaly	Cranial remolding orthosis	Cranial vault asymmetry
Pattisapu et al.[34a]	1989	VI	24 infants with deformational plagiocephaly	Repositioning and/or cranial remolding orthosis	Qualitative assessment by family
Ripley et al.[39a]	1994	V	72 infants with deformational plagiocephaly	Cranial remolding orthosis	Cranial vault asymmetry, cranial base asymmetry, orbitotragial depth asymmetry
Pomatto et al.[34a]	1994	VI	3 infants (triplets) with deformational plagiocephaly	Cranial remolding orthosis	Cranial vault asymmetry, cranial base asymmetry, orbitotragial depth asymmetry

Continued

Table 40-4 Efficacy of cranial remolding orthoses[23] *(Continued)*

Authors	Year	Level of Evidence	Population	Intervention	Outcomes Measured
Argenta et al.[2]	1996	III	51 infants with deformational plagiocephaly	Repositioning or soft prefabricated helmet	Visual assessment
Loveday and de Chalain[29]	1996	III	74 infants with deformational plagiocephaly	Repositioning or cranial remolding orthosis	Two-dimensional cranial tracings, cephalic index, cranial vault asymmetry, cranial vault asymmetry index
Pollack et al.[37a]	1997	III	69 infants with deformational plagiocephaly	Repositioning or cranial remolding orthosis	Qualitative assessment by family
Littlefield et al.[28a]	1997	V	285 infants with deformational plagiocephaly	Cranial remolding orthosis	Cranial vault asymmetry, cranial base asymmetry, orbitotragial depth asymmetry
Moss[31]	1997	III	72 infants with deformational plagiocephaly	Cranial remolding orthosis or nontreatment	Cranial vault asymmetry, cranial base asymmetry, orbitotragial depth asymmetry
Kelly et al.[23a]	1999	V	504 infants with deformational plagiocephaly	Cranial remolding orthosis	Cranial vault asymmetry, cranial base asymmetry, orbitotragial depth asymmetry, cranial circumference, cranial width, cranial length, influence of age, impact of initial severity on length of treatment and correction
Kelly et al.[24]	1999	V	258 infants with deformational plagiocephaly	Cranial remolding orthosis	Age at initiation of treatment, total treatment time, overall asymmetry
Mulliken et al.[32]	1999	III	114 infants	Repositioning or cranial remolding orthosis	Cranial vault asymmetry, correction, and age at initiation of treatment
Littlefield et al.[28b]	2000	VI	4 infants with deformational plagiocephaly	Cranial remolding orthosis	Cranial vault asymmetry, cranial base asymmetry, orbitotragial depth asymmetry, cranial circumference
Vles et al.[44]	2000	III	105 infants with deformational plagiocephaly	Cranial remolding orthosis or nontreatment	Qualitative assessment by family
Terpenning[42]	2001	V	12 infants with deformational plagiocephaly	Cranial remolding orthosis	Cranial vault asymmetry, cranial base asymmetry, orbitotragial depth asymmetry
Teichgraeber et al.[41]	2002	III	125 infants with deformational plagiocephaly	Cranial remolding orthosis	Series of 18 anthropometric measurements
Teichgraeber et al.[41]	2002	III	23 infants with deformational brachycephaly and 71 infants with deformational plagiocephaly	Cranial remolding orthosis	Cephalic index, cranial vault asymmetry
Bruner et al.[4a]	2004	III	34 infants with deformational plagiocephaly	Cranial remolding orthosis	CT scans were compared and volumes calculated for each quadrant
Graham et al.[13] (repositioning vs orthotic therapy)	2005	III	176 infants treated with repositioning and 159 infants treated with orthotic intervention	Repositioning and cranial remolding orthosis	Cranial diagonal differences
Graham et al.[14] (deformational brachycephaly)	2005	III	193 infants with abnormal head shapes	Repositioning and cranial remolding orthosis	Cranial index

Conclusion

Although cranial remolding orthoses have been documented in the literature since 1979, until recently the majority of infants with head shape deformities were seen by orthotists in large university medical centers with craniofacial programs. With the increased incidence of deformational plagiocephaly and other head shape deformities since 1992, many more referrals have been made to orthotists who practice outside large medical institutions. Craniofacial specialists still refer infants for cranial remolding orthoses, but now pediatricians practicing in the community also refer infants to orthotists for treatment.

Orthotists need to recognize their role in educating caregivers about the value of alternate positioning as the first intervention for improving head shape symmetry and proportion. When these strategies fail to improve the head shape to an acceptable level, the orthotist should intervene on a timely basis and attempt to complete orthotic management before the infant is 12 months of age. Orthotic intervention in the first year exploits this period of active, infant head growth and maximizes the potential for improved symmetry and proportion. Orthotic management of this patient population requires precise documentation of the head shape before and after treatment and provides an opportunity for concentrated research and study. The escalating number of infants seen yearly for orthotic intervention is evidence that a great deal of work is needed to prevent the deformity and to manage these infants with excellent clinical care.

References

1. AAP Task Force on Infant Positioning and SIDS: Positioning and SIDS, *Pediatrics* 89:1120, 1992.
2. Argenta LC, David LR, Wilson JA, et al: An increase in infant cranial deformity with supine sleeping position, *J Craniofac Surg* 7:5–11, 1996.
3. Barringer WJ: The use of postoperative cranial orthoses in the management of craniosynostosis, *J Prosthet Orthot* 16:S56–S58, 2004.
4. Bialocerkowski AE, Vladusic SL, Howell SM: Conservative interventions for positional plagiocephaly: a systematic review, *Dev Med Child Neurol* 47:563–570, 2005.
4a. Bruner TW, David LR, Gage HD, Argenta LC: Objective outcome analysis of soft shell helmet therapy in the treatment of deformational plagiocephaly, *J Craniofac Surg* 15(4):643–650.
5. Bruneteau RJ, Mulliken JB: Frontal plagiocephaly: synostotic, compensational or deformational, *Plast Reconstr Surg* 89:21–30, 1992.
5a. Clarren SK: Plagiocephaly and torticollis: etiology, natural history, and helmet treatment, *J Pediatr* 98:92–95, 1981.
6. Clarren SK, Smith DW, Hanson JW: Helmet treatment for plagiocephaly and congenital muscular torticollis, *J Pediatr* 94:43–46, 1979.
7. Cohen M, editor: *Craniosynostosis: diagnosis, evaluation, and management*, New York, 1986, Raven Press.
8. Dekaban AS: Tables of cranial and orbital measurements, cranial volume, and derived indexes in males and females from 7 days to 20 years of age, *Ann Neurol* 2:485–491, 1977.
9. Fish DJ: Clinical evaluation processes and procedures for the orthotic treatment of infants with deformational plagiocephaly, *J Prosthet Orthot* 16(4):S24–S27, 2004.
10. Freed SS, Coulter-O'Berry C: Identification and treatment of congenital muscular torticollis in infants, *J Prosthet Orthot* 16:S18–S23, 2004.
11. Golden KA, Beals SP, Littlefield TR, et al: Sternocleidomastoid imbalance versus congenital muscular torticollis: their relationship to positional plagiocephaly, *Cleft Palate Craniofac J* 36:256–261, 1999.
12. In Graham JM, editor: *Smith's recognizable patterns of human deformation*, ed 2, Philadelphia, 1988, WB Saunders.
13. Graham JM, Gomez M, Halberg A, et al: Management of deformational plagiocephaly: repositioning versus orthotic therapy, *J Pediatr* 146:258–262, 2005.
14. Graham JM, Kreutzman J, Earl D, Halberg A, Samayoa C, Guo X: Deformational brachycephaly in supine-sleeping infants, *J Pediatr* 146:253–257, 2005.
15. Higuera S, Hollier H, Stevens PM, Stal S: A preliminary investigation of postoperative molding to improve the result of cranial vault remodeling, *JPO J Pract Orthod* 17(4):125–128, 2005.
16. http://medical-dictionary.com/dictionaryresults.php.
17. Huang CS, Cheng HC, Lin WY, Liou JW, Chen YR: Skull morphology affected by different sleep positions in infancy, *Cleft Palate Craniofac J* 32(5):413–419, 1995.
18. Huang MH, Mouradian WE, Cohen SR, et al: The differential diagnosis of abnormal head shapes: separating craniosynostosis from positional deformities and normal variants, *Cleft Palate Craniofac J* 103:371–380, 1998.
19. Hutchison BL, Thompson JM, Mitchell E: The determinants of nonsynostotic plagiocephaly: a case controlled study, *Pediatrics* 112:e316, 2003.
20. Hylton-Plank L: The presentation of deformational plagiocephaly, *J Prosthet Orthot* 16(4):S28–S30, 2004.
21. Journal of Prosthetics and Orthotics: Orthotic treatment of deformational plagiocephaly, brachycephaly and scaphocephaly, *J Prosthet Orthot* 16: 4(suppl), 2004.
22. Kane AA, Lo LJ, Vannier MW, et al: Mandibular dysmorphology in unicoronal synostosis and plagiocephaly without synostosis, *Cleft Palate Craniofac J* 33:418–423, 1996.
23. Kane AA, Mitchell LE, Craven KP, Marsh JL: Observations on a recent increase in plagiocephaly without synostosis, *Pediatrics* 97:877–885, 1996.
23a. Kelly KM, Littlefield TR, Pomatto JK: Importance of early recognition and treatment of deformational plagiocephaly with orthotic cranioplasty, *Cleft Palate Craniofac J* 36:127–130, 1999.
24. Kelly KM, Littlefield TR, Pomatto JK, et al: Cranial growth unrestricted during treatment of deformational plagiocephaly, *Pediatr Neurosurg* 30:193–199, 1999.
25. Kordestani RK, Patel S, Bard D, Gurwitch R, Panchal J: Neurodevelopmental delays in children with deformational plagiocephaly, *Plast Reconstr Surg* 117:207, 2006.
26. Larsen J: Orthotic treatment protocols for plagiocephaly, *J Prosthet Orthot* 16:S31–S34, 2004.
27. Lima D: The management of deformational plagiocephaly: a review of the literature, *J Prosthet Orthot* 16:S9–S13, 2004.
28. Littlefield TR: FDA regulation of cranial remolding devices, *J Prosthet Orthot* 16:S35–S37, 2004.
28a. Littlefield TR, Pomatto JK, Beals SP, et al: Efficacy and stability of dynamic orthotic cranioplasty: an eight year investigation. In Whitaker LA, editor: *Craniofacial Surgery VII*, Bologna, Italy, 1997, Monduzzi Editore, 109–111.
28b. Littlefield TR, Pomatto JK, Kelly KM: Dynamic orthotic cranioplasty: treatment of the older infant, *Neurosurg Focus* 9:1–4, 2000.
29. Loveday BP, de Chalain TB: Active counterpositioning or orthotic device to treat positional plagiocephaly? *J Craniofac Surg* 12:308–313, 2001.
30. Miller R, Clarren S: Long-term developmental outcomes in patients with deformational plagiocephaly, *Pediatrics* 105:1–5, 2000.
31. Moss SD: Nonsurgical, nonorthotic treatment of occipital plagiocephaly: what is the natural history of the misshapen neonatal head? *J Neurosurg* 87:667–670, 1997.
32. Mulliken JB, Vander Woude DL, Hansen M, et al: Analysis of posterior plagiocephaly: deformational versus synostotic, *Plast Reconstr Surg* 103:371–380, 1999.
33. Nichter L, Persing J, Horowitz J, et al: External cranioplasty: historical perspectives, *Plast Reconstr Surg* 77:325–332, 1986.
34. Panchal J, Amirsheybani H, Gurwitch R, et al: Neurodevelopment in children with single-suture craniosynostosis and plagiocephaly without synostosis, *Plast Reconstr Surg* 108:1492, 2001.
34a. Pattisapu JV, Walker ML, Myers GG, Cheever J: Use of helmets for positional molding, *Concepts Pediatr Neurosurg* 9:278–284, 1989.
35. Peethambaran A: The orthotic management of infants with plagiocephaly: modification procedures of the positive model, *JPO J Pract Orthod* 16:S42–S45, 2004.
36. Persing J, James H, Swanson J, Kattwinkel J: Prevention and management of positional skull deformities in infants, *Pediatrics* 112:199–202, 2003.
37. Plank LH, Giavedoni B, Lombardo JR, Geil MD, Reisner A: Comparison of infant head shape changes in deformational plagiocephaly following treatment with a cranial remolding orthosis using a noninvasive laser shape digitizer, *J Craniofac Surg* 17:1084–1091, 2006.
37a. Pollack IF, Losken HW, Fasick P: Diagnosis and management of posterior plagiocephaly, *Pediatrics* 99:180–185, 1997.

38. Pomatto J, Beals S, Joganic E: Preliminary results and new treatment protocol for cranial banding following endoscopic-assisted craniectomy for sagittal synostosis, *J Craniofac Surg* 9:47–49, 2001.

38a. Pomatto JK, Littlefield TR, Manwaring K, et al: Etiology of positional plagiocephaly in triplets using a dynamic orthotic cranioplasty device: report of three cases, *Neurosurg Focus* 2:e2, 1994.

39. Rekate HL: Occipital plagiocephaly: a critical review of the literature, *J Neurosurg* 89:24–30, 1998.

39a. Ripley CE, Pomatto JK, Beals SP, et al: Treatment of positional plagiocephaly with dynamic orthotic cranioplasty, *J Craniofac Surg* 5:150–159, 1999.

40. Sorensen AJ, Phillips MR: Obtaining a positive model for craniofacial deformities: an empiric review of casting procedures, *J Prosthet Orthot* 16:S39–S41, 2004.

41. Teichgraeber JF, Ault JK, Baumgartner J, et al: Deformational posterior plagiocephaly: diagnosis and treatment, *Cleft Palate Craniofac J* 39:582–586, 2002.

42. Terpenning JF: Orthotic cranioplasty: material and design considerations, *J Prosthet Orthot* 16:S46–S49, 2004.

43. van Vlimmeren LE, vander Graaf Y, Boere-Boonekamp MM, et al: Risk factors for deformational plagiocephaly at birth and at 7 weeks of age: a prospective cohort study, *Pediatrics* 119:e408–e418, 2007.

44. Vles JS, Colla C, Weber JW, Belus E, Wilmink J, Kingma H: Helmet versus nonhelmet treatment in nonsynostotic positional posterior plagiocephaly, *J Craniofac Surg*, 11(6):572–574.

Section
6
Assistive devices

Assistive devices encompass a wide range of items that enhance or facilitate function or the ability to participate in activities. Whereas orthotic devices are applied to the body to stabilize and facilitate movement, assistive devices are an extension of the body, and allow for control over the environment. Such devices may compensate for an impairment or facilitate an activity. They increase independent control of users to manipulate their surroundings at will.

Assistive devices are used in rehabilitation to promote the process of compensation and restoration of function. Physical disability that impairs mobility, activities of daily living, and communication can be affected by the timely introduction of a device that allows for participation. The World Health Organization (WHO) model of International Classification of Function, Disability, and Health (ICF) shifts from a negative perspective of impairment and handicap to an activity-based participation model (Fig. 1). Improving the ability to perform a task not only changes the person's self-perception but also contributes to changes in society's perception of the person with a disability as someone who contributes, both of which facilitate inclusion.

This section takes each functional sphere and discusses many of the increasing numbers of assistive devices, from the simple stick cane to the more complex and future oriented robotics. Experts in the areas of assistive technology provide the basis of compensation, the biomechanical science for use, and the presentation of equipment. Devices used in activities of daily life, sports and recreation, mobility aids, seating and positioning systems, environmental controls, and robotics are included in the realm of assistive devices.

This section is important for the professional involved with patients with physical disability, to have at their fingertips for problem solving but also to help provide rationale for medical necessity to secure support and funding. The application of such devices depends on creative and knowledgeable team members, motivated users, and funding to achieve the goals. Appropriate fitting, training, and follow-up are required for optimal utilization of a device. The device provided should make sense within the context of the person's environment and activities of interest. The ideal device is efficient to use, easy to store or carry, is not cumbersome, and is cost effective. If a device is perfect but not used, the device fails both the individual and society.

Many devices are standard and have not changed over several decades because they are ideal in simplicity and effectiveness. Newer devices, such as robotics and computers, are allowing more complex controls over the world around us. Keeping up with new technology as it improves in efficiency and user friendliness is necessary to provide clients with access to devices that best suit their needs.

The best of technology and materials can promote improvement in function so that more people with disabilities can be involved in vocation and recreational activity. Facilitating these goals contributes to the overall goals of rehabilitation, which are to achieve the highest levels of quality of life and participation possible, regardless of impairment. This is, after all, what we all seek.

Shubhra Mukherjee, Deborah J. Gaebler-Spira, and John R. Fisk

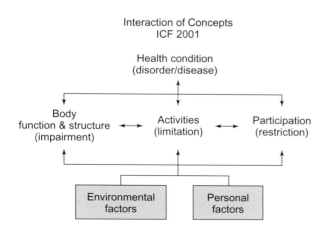

Fig. 1 WHO ICF model of function.

Appropriate technologies for assistive devices in low-income countries

Anna Lindström

Key Points

- Low-income countries deliver assistive technology differently due to cost, availability, and infrastructure issues. Special considerations are discussed.

- The terms *assistive technology* and *appropriate technology* are introduced as well as basic information on conditions in low-income countries, including cost issues.

- Production of assistive devices can be easy, but the distribution of devices is much more difficult.

- Training of professionals for local production is important and can be accomplished by alternative methods by national associations of professional groups.

- Community-based rehabilitation, accessibility, and universal design are discussed.

Assistive technology

"There are people with disabilities in all parts of the world and at all levels in every society. The number of persons with disabilities in the world is large and is growing."

These are the first sentences of the United Nations (UN) Standard Rules on the Equalization of Opportunities for Persons with Disabilities, which were adopted by the UN General Assembly in 1993.[7] Disabilities may affect all of us if we live long enough, no matter where we live. We all may need some assistive devices, depending on different life situations. There will always be a need for professionals for the production and provision of assistive technology all over the world, especially in low-income countries that do not have the means and resources to import expensive assistive technology for its population in need.

According to Rule 4 on support services and assistive technology of the UN Standard Rules on the Equalization of Opportunities for Persons with Disabilities: "States should ensure that development and supply of support services, including assistive devices for persons with disabilities, to assist them to increase their level of independence in their daily living and to exercise their rights."[7] The rule does not say how this should be done, but the rule clearly indicates it is the responsibility of each government. Even though many national and international nongovernmental organizations perform much of this work, it is essential to remember the responsibility and coordination of the national government.

Assistive technology is a term that is more extensive than the previous term *technical aids*. *Assistive devices* are the specific products used by individuals. As such, these terms are used when describing this field of work. The term *technical aids* should not be used because of confusion with the illness AIDS/HIV (acquired immunodeficiency syndrome/human immunodeficiency virus).

The human rights issue for people with disabilities has been discussed more during recent years. As a result of the UN's work on the International Convention on the Rights of Persons with Disabilities, the convention was adopted by the UN General Assembly in 2006.[8] It stresses the importance of assistive technology, including assistive devices, for people with disabilities as well as information and communication technologies, giving priority to technologies available at an affordable cost.

Access to devices is important for people with all types of disabilities. The ultimate aim of services in society should be to ensure that every person in need has access to assistive technology in order to have a better quality of life. For many persons with disabilities, assistive technology is a prerequisite for participation in the community. It is a tool in a process leading to equalization, participation, and independence, enabling individuals to participate in education and/or work, move between different places, dress and eat by themselves, communicate with other people, express their own thoughts and wishes, and otherwise enjoy life.[15]

Assistive devices give a freedom that we all would like to have, the freedom and the control over our lives. Assistive technology can provide a way to live independently and actively as well as to live safely and securely.

The earlier view that assistive devices only should compensate for a disability has been replaced by a view that the product also should give life quality and facilitate equal living conditions.

Appropriate technology

The term *appropriate technology* is more difficult to define. Should not all kinds of technology for people with disabilities be appropriate? Appropriate technology normally means that assistive devices should be produced locally by locally available material and tools. However, socioeconomic and cultural aspects also are involved.

The product must be affordable to most people and thus be appropriate to the people concerned. The cost for the country is another essential financial aspect. An imported product is costly for the country, and the money spent then cannot be used within the country. In addition, importing a product does not provide job opportunities in the country.

The cultural aspect is important so that the product is convenient to the people's traditions. A wheelchair is not always suitable for indoor use in Asia, where everyone usually sits on the floor or squats when performing household work and during family talks. A low trolley may be better in these situations.

The International Society for Prosthetics and Orthotics (ISPO) held a Consensus Conference on Appropriate Prosthetic Technology for Developing Countries in Phnom Penh, Cambodia, in 1995 and later declared the following at a meeting in Wuhan, China, in 1996[4]:

- Appropriate technology is a system that provides proper fit and alignment based on sound biomechanical principles, which suit the needs of the individual and can be sustained by the country at the most economical and affordable price.
- An appropriate technology should meet the physical needs of people with disabilities within their environment and economic situation.
- Local production of components from locally available materials should be encouraged.
- Use of different methods, procedures, and materials should be investigated, tested, and evaluated.
- Experiences related to appropriate technologies and use of materials should be properly documented and made available to others.

The UN Standard Rules on the Equalization of Opportunities for Persons with Disabilities also states in Rule 4 on support services that "States should recognize that all persons with disabilities who need assistive devices should have access to them as appropriate, including financial accessibility. This may mean that assistive devices and equipment should be provided free of charge or at such a low price that persons with disabilities or their families can afford to buy them."[7]

Low-income countries

Approximately 600 million people worldwide experience some form of disability. Eighty percent live in low-income countries; most of them are poor and do not have access to basic health services, including rehabilitation facilities.[11] The number of people with disabilities is increasing. War injuries, land mines, HIV/AIDS, malnutrition, chronic diseases, substance abuse, accidents, environmental damage, population growth, and medical advances that preserve and prolong life all have contributed to this increase. These trends are creating a great demand for rehabilitation services, including assistive technology, and improved accessibility in society.

In low-income countries, only 2% to 5% of the population in need can access the necessary rehabilitation services. One of the most neglected areas in rehabilitation is access to, and provision of, assistive devices to disabled and elderly people. In many low-income countries, assistive devices are accessible only through private services, which are inaccessible to the majority of people with disabilities because of high costs. The World Health Organization (WHO) estimates that only 5% to 15% of persons needing assistive devices have access to them.[11]

People with disabilities who have access to appropriate rehabilitation services can rise out of poverty and meet their basic needs, but the absence of such services contributes to a larger impoverished group. People with disabilities often belong to the poorest of the poor because they have no salary from employment and often do not have families to use as a protective net. Poverty-related illnesses, such as polio, leprosy, and lack of iodine, lead to disabilities such as mobility and intellectual impairments. Blindness is caused by a lack of vitamin A. Loss of hearing acuity and deafness are caused by chronic ear infections that are not treated properly.

Assistive devices play an important role in enhancing mobility and functionality and reducing dependency. Most people with disabilities and older people need assistive devices, particularly for mobility, hearing, and low vision. By 2020, more than one billion people 60 years and older will be living in the world; 700 million will be living in developing countries.

Elderly people face the risk of being affected by different age-related diseases. They will need assistive devices for dementia; impaired mobility, vision, or hearing; or general frailness. Elderly people often have several impairments at the same time, which make both the life situation and the care more difficult. Combinations of problems with mobility, sight, hearing, and cognition, that is, learning and understanding, result in more people with multiple disabilities. Elderly persons need more time to learn how to use assistive devices and learn how to take care of themselves in a new way.

The number of facilities that produce assistive devices in low-income countries is far from satisfactory. Where available, services are centralized, production is low, device quality is poor, and the number of trained personnel is insufficient.

If money is available to buy assistive devices, there are no problems. However, if money is lacking, there are problems with the production of devices and the distribution of devices to individuals. No firm can afford to produce many devices that are not sold.

Assistive devices alone cannot solve all problems. Other issues exist, such as accessibility, equal opportunities and human rights, and poverty alleviation, but assistive devices can result in change. Assistive technology will make people with disabilities visible and active contributors to society.

Issue of costs in low-income countries

Rule 4 on support services of the UN Standard Rules on the Equalization of Opportunities for Persons with Disabilities specifies where the responsibility lies with regard to the development, production, and provision of assistive devices[7]:

1. States should ensure the provision of assistive devices and equipment, personal assistance and interpreter services, according to the needs of persons with disabilities, as important measures to achieve the equalization of opportunities.
2. States should support the development, production, distribution, and servicing of assistive devices and equipment and the dissemination of knowledge about them.

However, this is not really the case in low-income countries where some governments follow Rule 4 but others do not. In the latter case, people with disabilities and their families suffer the consequences.

In some countries, private money is used to buy products or government systems are used to facilitate purchasing. However, in many countries these systems are not in place or do not function efficiently. Following are some questions and problems associated not only with technical issues but also with the distribution system, where most of the difficulties lie.

For people with disabilities, assistive devices are necessary for activities of daily life, such as attending school, supporting a family, working on a job, and living integrated in society. In Europe and North America, devices normally are produced in factories and at high cost. In many cases the cost is offset by insurance (private or public) and often is subsidized by society (i.e., by the federal/national government). In contrast, people with disabilities in Sweden find it difficult to buy assistive devices without the assistance of the general social insurance program.

Donor agencies can be asked to provide products, that is, devices can be imported from other countries at high cost. However, meeting the needs of all persons requiring devices in this manner is unrealistic in the long run and probably would be possible for only a small percentage of persons.

Second-hand equipment is an option, with only the costs of transportation from other countries to be considered. Such equipment may be adequate for urgent situations, for specific cases at hospitals, and for short-term solutions; however, much of the second-hand equipment in hospital storage is in need of repairs and maintenance, so it is not really a good alternative.

Repair of second-hand equipment is not always possible because spare parts are not available or are too expensive and must be obtained from the donor country. In addition, people with knowledge of how to repair the devices are needed. For example, wheelchairs often are not in good condition when they are received; they break easily and fall apart because they cannot withstand the difficult terrain in rough, sandy, and perhaps rural areas. In these locations, locally produced tricycles for outdoor use are more suitable and can be used for longer trips.

Donations that overload the market with free products can make survival of existing local workshops difficult. When the donation period is complete, local manufacturers will be needed but may no longer exist because they dissolved due to bankruptcy.

The situation can be solved by local production in the country or region concerned. Local production provides continuity and facilitates repairs and maintenance. Local labor can be used, and money is kept within the country.

People with disabilities are often employed in the workshops. Advantages include good job opportunities for people with disabilities, and persons with disabilities using their own experiences to develop better processes for production and serving as good role models for other disabled persons.

For many workshops producing specialized mobility devices such as wheelchairs and orthopedic equipment, the main problem is the market. The products often are too expensive for the individuals who need them. Difficulties with service delivery must be solved. Sometimes the government can buy the products and sell them at subsidized prices or distribute them free of charge. Sometimes local organizations with international support can place orders at the workshops. In a good working situation, workshops would concentrate on producing devices rather than searching for funds for poor clients. Local organizations would assess the needs of persons with disabilities and decide how much they can pay, and international support would be used for subsidies.

Production of assistive devices

Walking devices: These products are the most common devices produced locally using local materials that may differ from region to region. Walking devices include walking sticks, crutches, and framed walkers. Local materials available often are wood, metal tubes, and plastic items.[10]

Four-wheeled walkers: These devices provide users with stability for moving indoors safely and walking outdoors for longer distances. They are beneficial in allowing users to decide where to go and what to do, make contacts with others, and avoid isolation. They provide users with the ability to move around the neighborhood, and the feelings of safety and independence with device use are good for self-esteem. Maintaining personal contacts within the social network is important for mental health.

One in three people 65 years and older suffers a fall each year, with the resultant high costs of treatment (e.g., hip operations) and human suffering. Walkers are a good example of thinking in cost–benefit terms. Many walkers can be distributed as a preventative measure at the cost of one hip fracture operation. They are easily produced locally, which is another good example of a cost–benefit factor for the country concerned.

Wheelchairs: Information on wheelchairs is given in Chapter 45. A guide on manual wheelchairs by Hotchkiss et al.[3] is available.

Hearing aids: These devices are not easily produced by low-income countries. Very few countries in the world produce hearing aids. Without good hearing aids, people become essentially deaf and isolated. Often many hard of hearing persons are considered deaf because obtaining hearing aids is not possible due to a money shortage. Ongoing access to batteries is essential for long-term use of hearing aids but is costly for users. New developments in solar cell energy to be used instead of batteries will reduce the costs for battery products in the future.[12,13]

Low-vision aids: Devices in the form of strong eyeglasses and optical magnifiers are essential for people with low vision. Some of these products can be produced locally but others cannot. Good lighting is essential for persons with low vision and for elderly persons. The eye of a 60-year-old person requires three times more light than the eye of a 20-year-old person. To delay aging-related problems, eyeglasses provided at the right time and with the correct prescription strength are important. For blind people, white canes are essential for moving around and for orientation. These products can easily be produced locally.

Products used for hygiene and dressing: Such products can be produced locally using different plastic materials.

Many other forms of assistive devices can be locally produced (either at the community or the national level), such as seating equipment geared specifically for children and communication devices that incorporate pictures and symbols for people with intellectual or learning disabilities. When means and resources are not available, sophisticated items can be produced in simple versions that can function well in specific situation.[10]

The future may bring new information and communication technologies to persons in low-income countries requiring these technologies. Information and communication technologies are playing a larger role in society today, offering new opportunities and choices for individuals, improving public services, and facilitating communication among people regardless of disability. Possibilities include finding information on schools and educational resources, working life, culture, and public information as well as providing communication in ways not previously available.

Training professionals for local production

Training (both basic professional training and continuing education) of technicians who work at the local production level is important. Training courses, seminars, and information are necessary to develop competence in order to maximize the production of assistive devices. Training involves both technical and management issues as well as financial information for the workshops and centers producing devices. Employers should ensure that courses and seminars are available so that worker competence can be developed, but often this is not possible in low-income countries.

In many countries, associations of technicians are both trade union organizations and professional associations. Much knowledge is distributed to professionals via these organizations.

In west and central Africa, a network of professional technicians from 17 countries—the African Federation of Orthopaedic Technicians (FATO, from the organization's French name)—has been developed to provide training and information to professionals in the field of locally produced orthopedic devices (orthoses, prostheses, and orthopedic footwear). Today FATO has 215 members of an estimated 300 technicians in these countries and includes orthopedic technicians, assistant technicians, and orthopedic shoemakers.[1,6]

The population in the countries of west and central Africa is approximately 250 million, of whom approximately 24 million have disabilities. Of these, at least 2.5 million may need orthopedic devices or mobility devices such as walking aids and wheelchairs. The few technicians who are available benefit from being involved in an international network through which they can exchange experiences and develop competence, instead of being isolated in their own workshops in their own country. It was important to create a framework of dialogue, competence, and experience sharing among the African countries as well as with other countries around the world. FATO started in the French-speaking countries but now has reached some of the English-speaking countries in Africa and has established links with the International Society for Prosthetics and Orthotics.

Reasons for creating national associations of technicians and a regional federation are as follows:

- Technicians can become isolated in their workshops, which are far from each other and located in different countries. Few technicians are available for discussing professional problems. Technicians have difficulty receiving word on new developments.
- No further education is available in the countries. Budgets do not include this kind of education or competence training. Without ongoing knowledge, no improvements can be made in device production.
- Books and journals in the professional field are not easily accessible.
- Technicians may not receive proper recognition of their professional diploma. Sometimes they are regarded as only craftsmen in the production of assistive technology.
- The few technicians available are always occupied, so they have no time to adapt knowledge to their local socioeconomic situation or to investigate new development ideas that can be adapted to make better products for local conditions.
- Technicians need an outlet where they can get together to solve problems and develop channels for professional cooperation.

FATO has developed national and regional activities in order to:

- Train leaders and members of national associations
- Create a web site and newsletter for distribution of information

- Create a database with information about experts in the region
- Organize field visits and workshops/seminars for additional training

FATO can serve as a model for similar activities in other countries or regions in the field of professional training for local production of assistive technology and not only in the field of orthopedic devices. The main result would be providing knowledge that can be used to improve assistive technology for people with disabilities in accordance to situations in particular regions.

Community-based rehabilitation

Community-based rehabilitation (CBR) is a strategy developed by the WHO for improving disability services in low-income countries. The WHO manual "Training in the community for people with disabilities" has been the main source of information since its publication in 1989.[2] In 2004 the WHO, the International Labour Organization (ILO), and the United Nations Educational, Scientific, and Cultural Organization (UNESCO) published the joint position paper "CBR: A Strategy for Rehabilitation, Equalization of Opportunities, Poverty Reduction and Social Inclusion of People with Disabilities."[14] The WHO is in the process of compiling more material for the CBR guidelines to be published in 2008.[15] The guidelines will cover the fields of health (including assistive devices), education, livelihood, empowerment, and social issues.

CBR utilizes the resources available in the community, giving power to the people there—people with disabilities and their families. The community is involved in planning, decision making, and follow-up of rehabilitation. As much as possible, local resources are used for rehabilitation services, including social, educational, and vocational integration in the community. CBR includes production of assistive devices by local people.[5]

Accessibility

An accessible society can exist only if assistive technology also exists, because accessibility and assistive technologies are closely linked. Legislation is needed. It is wise to build correctly from the beginning. It is important to involve people with disabilities and to listen to their experiences and opinions about good accessibility. These persons are the best reference group and pressure group on decision makers to improve services for people with disabilities.

Societies have many barriers for people with disabilities, such as inaccessible buildings, transportation systems, and telecommunications. Adapting old inaccessible technology is costly, but ensuring that new buildings, trains, buses, and telecommunication systems are accessible does not involve much extra cost. It is a matter of how interested we are in making life accessible for people with disabilities.

Today accessibility means more than providing access to buildings and the physical environment by installing ramps, elevators, and wide doors for people with mobility impairments who use walking aids or wheelchairs. Just as important is making the environment accessible for people with low vision and blindness by providing information in Braille;

for persons with hearing loss by providing hearing loops in public places; for deaf persons by providing access to interpreters; and for people with cognitive disabilities by providing assistance in different ways for them to understand and orientate themselves better.

Universal design

Universal design, design for all, and *inclusive design* are new terms meaning that all needs should be covered from the beginning in order to decrease costs for adaptation later. Good design for people with disabilities often is good design for everybody. Simple and flexible adaptations permit more people to use the same product or service and at the same time are of benefit to other users. An example is the curb cuts and ramps that were introduced for use by people in wheelchairs. However, they also are used by people with bicycles, baby carriages, wheeled luggage, and delivery carts.

The Center for Universal Design in the United States gives the following definition for universal design: "Design of products and environments to be usable by all people, to the greatest extent possible, without the need for adaptation or specialized design."[9] The intent of universal design is to simplify life for everyone by making products, communications, and built environment more usable by as many people as possible at little or no extra cost. Universal design benefits people of all ages and abilities. Universal design should also cover services, not only products. Services from public authorities can be designed to meet the needs of people with disabilities.

The future

All people with disabilities, even those with severe and multiple disabilities, can develop their abilities. Assistive devices can be the tools for achieving good personal development.

The objective of a positive policy on assistive devices for people with disabilities is to create a society that enables people with disabilities to become fully active members of society. This is important from both the public economy perspective at a national level as well as the human perspective at an individual level.

CBR is a tool for providing rehabilitation to people with disabilities in low-income countries. It also is a tool for empowering the communities to improve living conditions for people with disabilities living in the community.

The UN Standard Rules on the Equalization of Opportunities for Persons with Disabilities are still an important instrument for national governments and the world community. The rules and the UN Convention on the Rights of Persons with Disabilities ensure that people with disabilities have equal rights and full participation in society. Rehabilitation and services for people with disabilities, including access to assistive devices, are now included among the human rights for all citizens. It is a challenge for all of us to fulfil the dream of a society for all its citizens.

References

1. FATO, African Federation of Orthopaedic Technicians, Ouagadougou, Burkina Faso, Available at *www.fatoafrique.org*.
2. Helander E, Mendis P, Nelson G, Goerdt A: *Training in the community for people with disabilities*, Geneva, Switzerland, 1989, World Health Organization.

3. Hotchkiss R, Crisp M, Wilhelmsson B: *Manual wheelchairs: a guide*, Vällingby, Sweden, 1986, Swedish Handicap Institute.

4. ISPO, International Society for Prosthetics and Orthotics: *The Wuhan Declaration on Appropriate Technology*, Copenhagen, Denmark, 1996, ISPO, Available at *www.ispo.ws*.

5. Lindström A, Eklund A: Community-based rehabilitation (CBR), *OrthoLetter ISPO/WHO* 6:5–22, 1996.

6. Lindström A: FATO: a regional federation for prosthetics and orthotics professionals, *OrthoLetter ISPO/WHO*, 10:1–3, 2002.

7. *United Nations Standard Rules on the Equalization of Opportunities for Persons with Disabilities*, New York, 1993, Available at *www.un.org/esa/socdev/enable/dissre00.htm*.

8. *United Nations Convention on the Rights for Persons with Disabilities*, New York, 2006, Available at *www.un.org/esa/socdev/enable*.

9. *Universal design definition*, Raleigh, NC, 2006, Center for Universal Design, Available at *www.design.ncsu.edu/cud/about_ud/about_ud.htm*.

10. Werner D: *Disabled village children*, Palo Alto CA, 1988, Hesperian Foundation.

11. *WHO Disability and Rehabilitation Team (DAR)*, Geneva, Switzerland, 2006, World Health Organization, Available at *www.who.int/disabilities*.

12. *WHO guidelines on hearing aids and hearing services in developing countries*, Geneva, Switzerland, 2004, World Health Organization, Available at *www.who.int/pbd/deafness/en/hearing_aid_guide_en.pdf*.

13. *WHO fact sheet no. 300 on deafness and hearing impairment*, Geneva, Switzerland, 2006, World Health Organization, Available at *www.who.int/mediacentre/factsheets/fs300/en/*.

14. *WHO CBR: A strategy for rehabilitation, equalization of opportunities, poverty reduction and social inclusion of people with disabilities (joint position paper 2004)*, Geneva, Switzerland, 2004, World Health Organization, Available at *www.who.int/disabilities/publications/cbr/en/index.html*.

15. *WHO CBR guidelines*, Geneva, Switzerland, 2008, World Health Organization, Available at *www.who.int/disabilities/cbr/activities/en/index.html*.

Chapter 42

Canes, crutches, and walkers

Joan E. Edelstein

Key Points

- Assistive devices may improve balance, assist propulsion, reduce load on one or both lower limbs, transmit sensory cues through the hand(s), enable the user to obtain the physiological benefits of upright posture and maneuver in places inaccessible by wheelchair, and notify passersby that the user requires special considerations.

- Canes can be described according to the design of the handle, shaft, and bottom.

- Crutches are available in four types: underarm, triceps, forearm (Lofstrand), and platform.

- Walkers are frames that provide bilateral support without the need to control two canes or crutches. They are described according to the design of the base, uprights, and proximal portion.

- The device must fit properly to enable the user to walk with the least effort and the greatest comfort.

- Complications in the hand, arm, shoulder, or axilla are not uncommon with the use of crutches and canes.

Assistive devices for ambulation have historical precedents, having been used since the Neolithic period. Whether necessitated by injury or disease or by the need to traverse rocky, hilly terrain, early people devised supports to enable them to get about, to sidestep starvation, and to evade predators. An ancient Egypt carving on the entrance portal of Hirkouf's tomb dating to the Sixth Dynasty (2830 BCE) depicts a figure leaning on a crutch-like staff (Fig. 42-1).[38,70] The contemporary bishop's staff, royal scepter, academic mace, and the walking stick used to climb The Great Wall in China are modern versions of the basic support.

The crutch remained a simple T design until approximately 1800, when use of the saw enabled modifications, such as splitting the staff, spreading the two halves, and inserting a cross-piece for the hand. The cane or walking stick was essential to the wardrobe of the stylish eighteenth- and nineteenth-century physician.[44]

New materials and designs, greater knowledge of biomechanics and pathology, and changing demographics and social mores have led to a myriad of cane, crutch, and walker designs. The expansion of the geriatric segment of the population gives assistive devices greater visibility. For all ages, the mandate of the Americans with Disabilities Act has prompted developers to use ingenuity to create appliances fostering easier access by people with disabilities. No longer is it a rarity to see someone in a shopping mall using a walker. Mobility-related assistive technology can be obtained through Medicare's durable medical equipment benefit.[136] Nevertheless, a national sample of 3,485 older Americans showed that income and insurance affect the use of canes and other assistive devices.[78] Assistive technology can enable many people to continue or resume ambulatory function at the maximum level possible.[59]

Assistive devices serve one or more functions:

- Improve balance
- Assist propulsion
- Reduce load on one or both lower limbs
- Transmit sensory cues through the hand(s)
- Enable the individual with paralysis to obtain the physiological benefits of upright posture and to maneuver in places inaccessible to a wheelchair
- Notify passersby that the user requires special considerations, such as additional time when crossing streets or taking a seat on the bus[17]

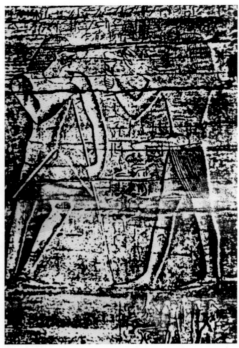

Fig. 42-1 Carving on the entrance portal of Hirkouf's tomb on the Isle of Elephantine, Egypt, Sixth Dynasty (2830 BCE).(From Epstein S: *Ann Med Hist* 9:304, 1937.)

Canes

Canes are made of many sturdy materials, such as walnut, oak, and other woods; metal, especially aluminum; and plastics, such as acrylics (e.g., Lucite) as well as fiberglass and carbon fiber. Canes are made in virtually every color of the rainbow and may display fanciful patterns.

Unlike the walking stick, which usually is a straight shaft, perhaps topped by an ornamental knob, the cane used in rehabilitation has a handle. A broad array of manufactured handles is available. The basic crook handle enables the person to hang the cane over the forearm or the back of a chair. One ergonomically shaped handle (available at *www.CanesCanada.com*) is designed to contact more of the hand, thus contributing to the user's comfort. The handle is made for right and left hand use. The Right-Grip (available at *www.fetterman-crutches.com*) has a contoured handle designed to keep the wrist in neutral posture rather than in dorsiflexion.

Cane shafts may be solid, height adjustable, or folding. The folding shaft makes storage more convenient; an adult-size cane can be folded to approximately 30.5 cm (1 foot). The SuperCane (Momentum Medical Corp., Idaho Falls, ID) has an offset shaft with a higher hand grip to be used when the patient walks and a lower hand grip that enables the person to start the standing maneuver while seated. A novel cane has a shaft containing a weight-measuring system and a feedback mechanism in the handle; the cane informs the user by vibration or lights as to the amount of weight borne, useful for those who need to limit loading on an affected leg.[37]

The base of the cane usually is the distal end of the shaft and terminates in a rubber tip. A spring-loaded tip absorbs shock at initial contact. The AbleTripod (available at

www.abletripodcane.com) has a flexible triangular tip that maintains floor contact at a wide range of shaft angles; the tip also absorbs shock. Retractable metal tips or spikes increase stability when the user walks on ice or snow.

Other base designs include the standard or wide-based quadruped (quad), which features a distal rectangle supporting four tips intended to increase the base of support.[59] Patients with hemiplegia may not find the four-footed cane any more advantageous than a standard cane with a single tip.[84] The Pilot rolling cane (available at *www.FullLifeProducts.com*) has an L-shaped base fitted with three casters that provide the user with the support of a quad cane without the need to lift the cane with each step. The cane also has a brake control in the handle for maximum stability. The Pilot step-up cane has a broad base with a flip-up platform that allows patients to maneuver over curbs and stairs without losing cane support. The user pushes a button on the handle to flip open the hinged platform; this enable the patient to step half the distance of the conventional 8-inch step. With the step retracted, the cane functions as a standard quad cane. The cane also has a second handle part way down the shaft that facilitates rising from toilets and other seats. The side walker/cane (available at *www.tfihealthcare.com*) has four widely spaced rubber tips that increase stability, especially when used unilaterally by a patient with hemiplegia.

The marketplace also has several novel cane-like designs intended for adults with lower-limb amputation. They enable the user to ambulate without a prosthesis. The Ed Walker (available at *www.theedwalker.com*) has a bicycle seat mounted on top of a vertical shaft. Jutting laterally is a second curved shaft, which has a platform for the amputation limb and terminates in a cane handle.[28] The iWalkFree (available at *www.fetterman-crutches.com*) has a platform on a vertical shaft that supports the transtibial amputation limb or an injured lower leg. The wearer supports weight through the thigh and knee. Both devices have a stationary base. The Roll-A-Bout (available at *www.roll-a-bout.com*) terminates in four 8-inch wheels. This folding device has a cushioned platform for the lower leg and a handle that the user holds while propelling with the opposite foot.

A major class of canes is long canes with the lower portion of the shaft colored red. These canes are used by people with visual impairment.[58,85,99,109] The shaft transmits to the user vibratory impulses regarding the terrain, while the red tip signals passersby not to impede the user.

Most patients use a single cane, usually on the side opposite the affected lower limb. However, some people walk with a pair of canes, particularly those who wear bilateral transfemoral prostheses. The cane offers balance or light support as well as sensory feedback from the walking surface.

Crutches

Crutches are of four major types (Figs. 42-2 and 42-3)[59]:

- Underarm
- Triceps
- Forearm (Lofstrand)
- Platform

Underarm crutches, sometimes called *axillary crutches*, are made of wood, aluminum, and titanium in sizes made to fit children and adults. Metal crutches have spring-loaded

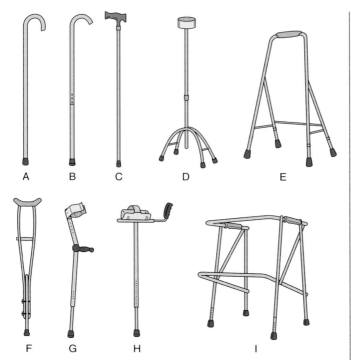

Fig. 42-2 A, C-handle or crook-top cane. **B,** Adjustable aluminum cane. **C,** Functional grip cane. **D,** Adjustable wide-base quad cane. **E,** Hemiwalker. **F,** Adjustable wooden axillary crutch. **G,** Adjustable aluminum Lofstrand crutch. **H,** Forearm support or platform support. **I,** Walker or walkerette. (From DeLisa DA, editor: *Rehabilitation medicine:principles and practice*, ed 2, Philadelphia, 1993, JB Lippincott.)

detents that facilitate adjustment of hand grip height and overall length. The top of the crutch is erroneously termed the axillary piece. The axilla should never be used as a support area because superficial nerves and blood vessels may be compressed by direct pressure from the axillary piece. The top is often covered with sponge rubber to increase friction and cushion stress against the user's chest. One design has a top resembling a shepherd's crook more than twice the length of the basic top; this design offers more support area on the chest. The Easy Strutter Functional Orthosis (available at *www.icanwalk.com*) has a crutch top that includes, in addition to the underarm piece, a cushioned strap over the shoulder to distribute weight over a broad, pressure tolerant area. The crutch has two parallel struts that terminate in a broad, spring-loaded shock-absorbing base. When three-point gait with axillary crutches was compared with performance with the Easy Strutter Functional Orthosis, the latter crutches imposed less stress on the palms. Subjects reported feeling more secure on level surfaces and stairs with the new crutches.[93]

The crutch handle should have a resilient cover to cushion compressive stress on the palm. Whether the handle is cylindrical or wide, the palmar load distribution is similar.[107]

Although the traditional shaft bifurcates partway up from the base, streamlined single shaft canes are widely available. The usual crutch tip is rubber; however, many cane tips can be used on crutches. The Safe Walk (available at *www.sailmarket.com/ticrutch*) has two distal shafts both ending with rubber tips; one tip is always on the ground regardless of angle of the

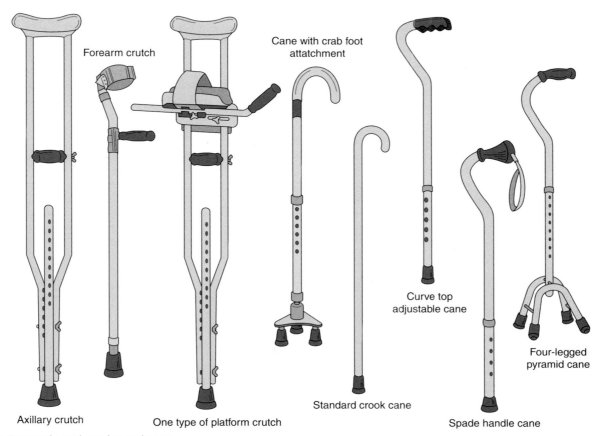

Fig. 42-3 Commonly used crutches and canes.

Forearm crutch

Cane with crab foot attachment

Curve top adjustable cane

Four-legged pyramid cane

Axillary crutch

One type of platform crutch

Standard crook cane

Spade handle cane

crutch.. A spring-loaded mechanism at the distal end of the shaft absorbs considerable impact shock.[96]

Triceps (Warm Springs) crutches are made of aluminum. They were developed at the Roosevelt Institute for Rehabilitation (Warm Springs, GA) during the twentieth-century poliomyelitis epidemic. The crutch has two posterior bands intended to keep the elbow extended, mimicking the action of the triceps muscle.

Forearm (Lofstrand) crutches are made of aluminum or titanium with a vinyl-covered steel forearm cuff. They have adjustable length and cuff positions. European model cuffs are streamlined. They are sold in a wide variety of colors and can be ordered in a collapsible model for convenient storage. One innovation is a forearm crutch made of compliant composite plastic with an S curve in the shaft; the crutch design and material contribute to shock absorption.[112]

A variation of the rigid cuff is a leather cuff, also known as the *Kenny armband*. It was named after Sister Kenny, a pioneering clinician who treated patients with poliomyelitis. The armband is less restrictive than the rigid cuff and is used by some people with poliomyelitis and some patients with cerebral palsy.

Platform crutches provide a trough that permits forearm weight bearing for those who cannot tolerate weight transmission through the hand.

Crutches, regardless of design, are ordinarily used in pairs.

Walkers

Walkers are frames that provide bilateral support without the need to control two canes or crutches.

A variety of walkers are manufactured and are described based on their design[59]:

- Base: Four tips, two tips and two wheels, four wheels, three wheels
- Uprights: Rigid, folding, reciprocating, stair climbing
- Proximal portion: Hand grips, platform

Most walkers are made of aluminum. The simplest model has four legs, each ending in a rubber tip to improve traction. Four-tip walkers provide maximum stability but must be lifted with each step. They are especially appropriate for high-friction surfaces, such as carpet, gravel, and grass. Walker uprights may be height adjustable. The Rising Star SuperWalker (Momentum Medical Corp.) has offset uprights with upper and lower handles that aid the user in rising from a chair. Walkers with wheels can be pushed forward to provide moderate stability; they are more suitable for smooth surfaces, such as linoleum.

Many walkers with two front wheels and two crutch tips are available. The Red Dot walker (available at *www.sunrise medical.com*) is a folding walker with two front-swivel 5-inch wheels and rear glide brakes. The Strider group of walkers (available at *www.sammonspreston.com*) has adjustable wheels and handles. Two-wheeled walkers may have tennis balls or other glides on the rear uprights to smooth ambulation. The WalkAbout has an upper portion that encircles the user.[135] It also has a built-in seat and a basket. Other walkers with seats include the folding steel Merry Walker (available at *www.mer rywalker.com*), Dura Walker (available at *www.duralife-usa.com*) made of polyvinylchloride, and the folding steel U-Step

(available at *www.ustep.com*), which has a padded seat, hand brakes, and an optional laser light intended to encourage patients with Parkinson disease to step forward. A walker can have a reciprocating mechanism to accommodate stepping more easily. The Universal Stair Climbing Walker (available at *www.tfihealthcare.com*) facilitates ascending and descending steps.

Three-wheeled walkers have three angled uprights each ending in a wheel—an example is the Rollator (available at *www.sammonspreston.com*)—are easier to maneuver in narrow corridors. Basic wheeled and four-tip walkers are manufactured in wide size to suit obese patients.

Adaptations can be made to many walkers. For example, the child with cerebral palsy may walk with better posture using a walker fitted with a hip guard. Direct-forming plastic can be used to make a walker handle more conforming so as to prevent some of the complications in the hand.

Reverse walkers for children with cerebral palsy may facilitate hip and knee extension, allowing them to walk with less energy and a better faster gait. Some walkers for young patients allow hands-free ambulation. These appliances may provide mobility for children who are unable to support the trunk over the pelvis. Examples are the Mulholland Walkabout Gait Trainer (available at *www.mulholland.com*), Pony walker (available at *www.gtkrehab.com.au*), Rifton gait trainer (available at *www.Rifton.com*), and SMART Walker (available at *www.llop.com*). The SMART walker consists of a trunk–hip–knee–ankle orthosis worn with high-quarter, extra-depth laced-to-toe shoes. The orthosis is attached to a square-wheeled frame that has a steering mechanism designed to reduce neuropathic forces that cause scissoring and internal rotation.

Still under development is a robotic walker, the Veterans Affairs Personal Adaptive Mobility Aid (VA-PAMAID).[101] Laboratory testing of the motorized device confirms durability and ease of use by elderly adults and those with visual impairment.

Measuring assistive devices

Whatever the device, the clinician must ensure that it fits properly.[103,106,125] Correct height of the device and proper positioning of the handle or cuff enable the user to walk with the least effort and the greatest comfort.

Device height should be measured with accessories, such as a rubber tip, hand cushion, and top pad, in place. The patient should wear the type of shoes that will be worn when using the device. The guidelines may need to be altered to suit a given person, with particular consideration to the individual's body proportions, joint mobility, and motor power. Measurement also is influenced by the type of gait pattern used.

Canes

Ordinarily, the single cane is held in the hand opposite the involved lower limb. First, remove the rubber tip by twisting on the shaft, not the handle. The patient stands with the elbow slightly flexed, no more than 30 degrees. Place the cane so that the end is 5 to 10 cm lateral and 15 cm anterior to the foot. The top of the handle should be at the wrist crease[31,65,73,86] or the greater trochanter.[110] After adjusting cane height, replace the rubber tip.

Canes that are too long cause the user to lean forward. Too short a cane imposes undue stress on the lumbosacral region. Shorter canes, however, enabled healthy subjects to perceive ground touch more accurately than with longer canes, suggesting that individuals with visual impairment will walk more safely with a slight decrease in cane length.[114]

Underarm crutches

Measure underarm crutches with the patient standing in a secure environment, such as between parallel bars. Each crutch should extend from a point approximately 4 to 5 cm (two finger breadths) below the axilla to a point on the floor 5 cm lateral and 15 cm anterior to the distal foot.[95] Hand piece placement should enable the patient to have a 30-degree resting elbow flexion angle.[100] Less flexion is suitable for the individual who walks by alternating foot steps.

In an alternative method used to determine crutch height, subtract 40 cm from the patient's height[16] or make the crutch equal to 77% of the subject's height.[14] When the person is supine, the crutch extends from 5 cm below the axilla to 5 to 7.5 cm from the lateral border of the heel.[110] In the sitting position, the patient can abduct both arms to shoulder level and extend the elbows. Crutch length is the distance from the tip of the middle finger to the tip of the olecranon process of the opposite arm.[88] An adjustable measuring crutch also can be used.[119]

Forearm crutches

The patient should stand with the crutch hand piece adjusted to provide 15 to 30 degrees of elbow flexion; more acute elbow flexion is required for gait patterns that require the user to lift both feet from the floor simultaneously. The crutch should contact the floor 5 to 10 cm lateral and 15 cm anterior to the toes. The cuff should lie on the proximal third of the forearm, approximately 2.5 to 4 cm below the olecranon process.[110] A double-blinded repeated measures study of healthy subjects demonstrated that crutch length within 2.5 cm of the recommended length did not affect respiratory exchange ratio, walking speed, or perceived exertion.[87]

Triceps crutches

The upper cuff should contact the proximal third of the arm, approximately 5 cm below the anterior fold of the axilla. The lower cuff should lie 1 to 4 cm below the olecranon process to avoid bony contact yet provide adequate stability to the arm.[110]

Platform crutches

If the crutch has a forearm platform, it should be angled so that the user has maximum comfort and control of the crutch; ordinarily the forearm rests on the platform at a 90-degree angle to the upper arm. Measuring may be facilitated with use of special devices[4] or variations on the techniques described.

Crutches that are too short compel the user to lean forward, whereas crutches that are too long force the shoulders up and risk compression of the radial nerve[22,98,105] or suprascapular nerve.[111] Even properly adjusted crutches, when used incorrectly, cause some patients to experience redness, pain, and abrasion of the lateral chest; tenderness over the medial aspect of the arm; cramping of the triceps; bruising of the medial epicondyle; shoulder pain; and ulnar neuropathy.

Walkers

Most people prefer having the walker adjusted so that each handle lies at the ulnar styloid when they stand erect with the elbow flexed 15 degrees.[49]

Gait patterns

Foot sequence determines the way an individual uses assistive devices.[19,72,110] Selection of gait pattern(s) depends on the patient's ability to move the feet reciprocally, tolerate full load on each leg, lift the body off the floor by pressing on the hands, and maintain balance. A gait pattern may be altered if the environment is crowded or the floor is slippery or sloping.

Alternating (reciprocal) gait pattern

Most people move reciprocally, one foot at a time, alternating with the walking aid. Alternating gaits are relatively stable and less stressful on the cardiovascular system and the upper limbs, but movement may be slow.

Four-point gait

Using two canes or crutches, the patient advances the right aid, then the left foot, then the left aid, followed by the right foot.

Two-point gait

With two aids, the patient advances the right aid and the left foot, followed by the left aid and the right foot. Anticipating two-point crutch-assisted functional electrical stimulation, one study investigated stability indices for each gait position and found that slow walking does not impose static instability.[7]

Three-point gait

With two aids, usually crutches, the patient advances both aids together with the affected limb, then advances the unaffected foot. The three-point gait reduces load on the affected leg. If subjects have difficulty in restricting weight bearing, shifting the center of gravity toward the uninvolved side reduces load on the affected limb.[69]

Cane gait

The cane usually is held on the side opposite the affected leg. The patient advances the cane and the affected foot, then moves the unaffected foot.

Walker gait

The patient advances the walker. The standard walker should be placed so that all four tips touch the floor simultaneously; walkers with two, three, or four wheels should be wheeled forward slightly. Then the user steps forward with one foot, following with the other foot. For the reverse walker, leg motion is almost simultaneous with advancement of the walker.

Swinging (simultaneous) gait patterns

These patterns require rhythmic use of a pair of axillary or forearm crutches to eliminate load from both feet by forceful shoulder depression and elbow extension. A walker is sometimes used for the drag-to or swing-to gaits.

Drag-to gait

Both crutches are advanced, either individually or together, followed by dragging both feet on the floor landing on an imaginary line just behind the crutches.

Swing-to gait

Both crutches are advanced individually or together, followed by swinging the feet slightly off the floor to an imaginary line just behind the crutches.

Swing-through gait

Both crutches are advanced together, followed by swinging the feet beyond the line of the crutches.[104] The swing-through gait is the fastest mode of crutch ambulation but requires the most floor space. The patient must be able to support the trunk and lower limbs long enough to allow the legs to swing from behind to a position in front of the crutches. In addition, the person must have confident balance when the posteriorly placed crutches are out of sight.

Kinetic and kinematic considerations

The duration and amount of force applied by patients to an assistive device vary considerably,[15] depending on whether the appliance is used primarily for balance or for unloading the lower limbs. Most individuals keep the cane on the floor during stance phase on the disabled limb, particularly those with a fractured pelvis or arthritis of the knee. In contrast, persons with paralysis agitans contact the floor with the cane just before stance on the more disabled limb, using the cane in a manner similar to that of individuals with visual impairment.

Subjects with arthritis had greater pain relief with contralateral cane use.[24] Survey of those individuals with rheumatoid and osteoarthritis disclosed that 30% of respondents did not use prescribed assistive devices; those who were older or had greater pain or disability were more apt to use devices.[124] These results were confirmed by a large-scale survey of older adults; those in poorer health or who had more severe disability were more likely to use equipment than rely on personal assistance. Equipment use maintains the user's self-sufficiency.[129] Among elderly fallers, cane use was not as effective as stepping backward when individuals were subjected to external perturbations on the chest.[48]

Kinematic studies of patients with hemiparesis confirmed that a cane held on the uninvolved side reduced mediolateral and anteroposterior sway, regardless of whether a standard or a four-footed cane was used.[84] Patients with hemiparesis lifted the cane only during the double-support phase of gait. Canes, particularly quad canes, reduced sway among subjects with hemiparesis.[66] Comparison of adults with and without peripheral neuropathy demonstrated that canes improved balance[6] and increased hip and knee excursion during gait.[64] Other research showed that cane use reduced erector spinae and tibialis anterior activity[23] and provided both support and braking function.[26] The type of cane did not result in significant differences in amount of load applied by subjects.[122]

A force transducer in the device can register the applied load.[21,26,35,36,46,94] Some investigators used a force plate to register loads on the cane or crutch.[116,134] Individuals with bone and joint disabilities applied significantly more force to the cane than did patients with neuropathies. A single cane can support approximately one quarter of the body weight, whereas a forearm crutch can bear almost half of the body weight. When greater weight relief is required, the patient needs a pair of canes or crutches.

A cane reduces force throughout the hip, particularly when the cane is held in the contralateral hand,[1,20,21,35,36,81,90] which reduces abductor muscle pull. Blount,[20] in his classic treatise "Don't Throw Away the Cane," demonstrated how a cane reduces stress. Some individuals prefer to hold the cane in the ipsilateral hand, using the device to reduce foot contact force.[17] A few people insist on using the cane in the dominant hand, regardless of the side of pathology. Biomechanical modeling of cane use confirmed that the cane increases stability.[120]

Research with healthy subjects demonstrated that a contralateral cane reduces medial force on the knee more effectively, whereas ipsilateral cane use is more effective for minimizing lateral force.[74] A cane was shown to sustain 25% of body weight compared with a wheeled walker, which unloaded one limb by as much as 50%.[138] Cane use affects lower limb muscle activity, with reduced contraction of contralateral hip abductors and increased medial hamstring activity; gastrocnemius and quadriceps activity was reduced, regardless of which hand held the cane.[127] Canes also caused reduction in upper limb muscle activity among healthy subjects.[27]

Biomechanical study indicated the high force that subjects can sustain on crutches.[113] They can support up to 80% of body weight and require a significant increase in energy expenditure, mostly because of the vertical rise of the body used to clear the ground during swing-to or swing-through gait.[67,104] Comparison of healthy subjects with patients having paraplegia showed that the latter had a longer crutch stance-phase duration and higher moment of force at the shoulders when ambulating at similar speeds.[92] Subjects with incomplete spinal cord injury had higher shoulder force and walked with longer strides than when using a front-wheeled walker.[50a]

Several investigators have studied the swing-through gait.[131] Using forearm crutches to perform the three-point gait, subjects sustained an average vertical force to the unimpaired leg of 1.32 times body weight, 16% higher than during normal walking.[116] Patients with tibial fractures exhibited higher medially than anteroposteriorly directed force.[94] With axillary crutches and the same gait pattern, subjects applied 44% of body weight to the arms.[46]

Investigations of disabled and nondisabled subjects using the swing-through gait indicated that the vertical excursion of the shoulders is greater than that of the hip and that, lacking the normal shock-absorbing function of the lower limbs, the person who uses crutches absorbs the shock of ground contact with the crutch tips and the upper limbs. Because the shoulder girdle has limited capacity to absorb shock, the swinging gaits impose high loads on the lower limbs[94]; conventional crutches do not absorb shock adequately.[96] Children may lack the necessary arm adductor strength to anchor the axillary piece of the crutch against the chest. The swing-through gait pattern with axillary crutches imposed dynamic loads at the hands from 1.14 to 3.36 times body weight and horizontal loads at the chest of 3% to 11% of body weight.[116]

Individuals with severely limited walking ability are more apt to use walkers than other assistive devices. Although walkers provide considerable stability, they do not eliminate the risk of falling.[25] With a four-wheeled walker, elderly individuals were able to walk somewhat faster and negotiate sidewalk cracks more easily than with a four-tip walker, which has no wheels.[33,34] Less attention is needed to maneuver a rolling walker compared with a standard model.[137] However, wheeled walkers are more difficult to maneuver on carpets[60] and, being relatively bulky, are more difficult to put in a car. Children with cerebral palsy did not exhibit significant differences in step length, cadence, or velocity when walking with a wheeled walker (Rollator) having vertical handles compared with a wheeled walker having horizontal handles.[68] Nondisabled children using a standard forward walker and then a two-wheeled posterior walker had a longer stride time with the posterior control walker and greater anterior trunk lean with the standard forward walker. Similar results were obtained with a four-wheeled posterior walker.[68] Disabled children had more upright posture and faster gait with posterior walkers compared with anterior walkers.[47,71]

Research with instrumented walkers demonstrates their unloading efficacy.[8,39] Meta-analysis of investigations of walker use confirms that walkers and canes increase balance and mobility, but they may impose more force on the upper limbs.[13] Among healthy subjects using walkers, rectus femoris and biceps femoris activity is correlated with the amount of weight bearing sustained by the device.[57] Walker-assisted gait is associated with more vertical support but slower gait and more forwardly flexed posture than with forearm crutches.[82] A drawback of walkers is that they may interfere with compensatory stepping when subjects are jostled.[12]

Subjects with recent lower-limb amputations are more likely to use a two-wheeled walker than a four-tip one; fewer individuals used one or two canes, a pair of crutches, or a four-wheeled walker.[62]

Instrumented crutches measure loads borne by the upper limbs.[102] Electromyographic investigation of healthy adults who used underarm crutches showed less activity of lower limb extensors than flexors; similar results were obtained when the ED walker was used.[28] Bilateral crutch use was associated with greater gait symmetry and more favorable time and distance factors, except when subjects used the three-point gait. With a single crutch or cane, gait kinematics were asymmetrical.[79]

Adults with hip arthroplasty who used forearm crutches took longer strides and had a more symmetrical gait, but they walked with lower cadence than when walking without crutches. Crutch use also was associated with less gluteus medius, quadriceps, and erector spinae activity on the affected side and less vastus medialis activity on the unaffected side.[115] Other subjects with arthritis had faster gait when using crutches, although upper limb force was higher.[29] Children with spina bifida had less pelvic motion with forearm crutches than without them, although pelvic displacement still was excessive.[126]

Physiological factors

Light touch on canes and other assistive devices enables patients with poor balance control to improve stability. Sensory input to the upper limb through fingertip contact on the device reduces postural sway.[57a] These haptic cues aid postural control in sighted and in blind individuals, particularly when the cane is held in a slanted, rather than a vertical, position. In addition, cane use resulted in decreased head motion of sighted subjects, suggesting that head movement control is linked to postural control through gaze stabilization reflexes.[57b]

Ambulating with assistive devices imposes physiologic stresses on the client, as indicated by heart rate and energy expenditure higher than resting values for those with disability as well as nondisabled persons.

Heart rate

Nondisabled adults using axillary crutches to perform the three-point gait had significantly higher heart rates than during normal walking; an average subject with a pulse rate limit of 130 beats/min sustained equal stress whether crutch walking at 60 m/min or running at 134 m/min. Heart rate increase and oxygen consumption were less with axillary crutches than with a standard or wheeled walker for nondisabled subjects performing the three-point gait.[53] Heart rates of healthy subjects who received preambulatory training with arm ergometry or free weights and pushups did not differ from heart rates of subjects who practiced the three-point gait with axillary crutches; all had elevated heart rates.[18] Compared with nondisabled adults, patients who use forearm crutches to relieve one lower limb of all weight have a significantly higher heart rate,[50] as do elderly women using a walker.[10] Among various designs of crutches, the triceps version is associated with less increase in heart rate than Sure-Gait and Ortho Crutches.

Energy expenditure

Energy demand based on oxygen utilization can be expressed as rate (i.e., consumption per time) or cost (i.e., consumption per distance). The three-point gait performed by patients with lower limb disorders required oxygen uptake as much as one third greater than for normal walking and a heart rate more than 50% higher.[56,130] Consequently, elderly patients using a cane or crutches reduced their walking velocity to maintain tolerable energy expenditure. The four-tip walker was associated with higher oxygen consumption per distance than the wheeled walker.[42] Energy demand is particularly high with the swing-through gait because of muscular demands in the upper limbs needed to lift the trunk and legs to initiate body-swing phase and then provide stability while the patient swings through the line of the crutches.[104,121] Walking speed affects metabolic cost, with patients using more energy when crutch walking at faster velocities[131] except when subjects are required to walk so slowly that rhythm is disturbed.[43]

Crutch design appears to have little effect on energy expenditure. Nondisabled adults using Ortho axillary crutches to perform the three-point gait initially used less oxygen and had lower heart rates than with standard axillary crutches; however, differences disappeared after subjects walked an average of 11.5 minutes.[52] Oxygen consumption and heart rate among nondisabled young adults were not affected by the type of crutch (axillary or forearm) used.[32,41] Most investigators found that walking with axillary crutches with a curved bottom (Sure-Gait) did not decrease the physiologic stress of crutch walking among nondisabled adults[5,91,118] and orthopedic patients.[11] However, some research suggests that the curved crutch bottom was associated with a 9% lower oxygen uptake; efficiency was attributed to the reduced height of vertical displacement.[45] The triceps crutch seems to exact a slightly lower metabolic cost, followed by the forearm crutch and the axillary crutch when used for the swing-through gait.[108,117]

Subjects with spinal cord injury ambulate more slowly and less efficiently,[55] whether they use a walker or crutches, as compared with nondisabled adults, although performance was somewhat less impaired with crutches.[123]

Benefits of assistive devices

Research confirms that many patients benefit from assistive technology. Those with stroke had longer stance time on the affected leg and walked faster with a cane than without one[51]; they also had greater stability[66] and less sway.[75] Cane use reduced sway among those with vestibular disorders.[89] People with Parkinson disease did not benefit markedly in terms of gait velocity or initiating gait when using a walker; however, the deficit was somewhat less with a wheeled walker.[30] Canes lower the stress on the tibia.[83] More adults with postpoliomyelitis used a cane, crutch, or walker (57%) than a wheelchair (21%).[63] Community-dwelling older adults are apt to use a cane to prevent falls.[3] A randomized controlled trial of elderly community dwellers showed that use of assistive technology reduced health care cost.[77]

Complications of assistive devices

Complications are not uncommon with use of crutches and canes. Problems can occur in the hand, arm, shoulder, or axilla. Injury to the ulnar,[128] median,[61,132] and suprascapular[111] nerves occasionally occurs. Adaptations to crutch grips, such as the ergonomically designed hand piece of the Right Grip forearm crutch (available at *www.fetter man-crutches.com*), may reduce the incidence of compression injury to the radial palmar nerve,[54] wrist osteoarthritis,[133] and stress to the ulna.[2] Other complications with improperly fitted or used underarm crutches are axillary artery thrombosis[40,80] and compression of the radial nerve.[9,22,105]

Some patients may refuse use of a cane, thinking that it is a sign of disability or senility. Adults who use a cane even though they deny gait difficulty are apt to be less active than age-mates who do not use assistive devices.[97] Hospitalized older adults who required a cane or walker at the time of discharge had more functional decline than those who could walk without assistance.[76]

Conclusion

Assistive devices improve mobility and participation in the community for many who have deficient balance, strength, motor control, or visual processing. Introduction of an assistive device should be considered an enabling process that compensates for various impairments, rather than a defeat. New materials and better understanding of patients' needs, goals, and potentials together with more precise evaluation of outcome allow the health care team to prescribe the most appropriate assistive device for each patient and train individuals to use the device optimally.

References

1. Ajemian S, Thon D, Clare P et al: Cane-assisted gait biomechanics and electromyography after total hip arthroplasty, *Arch Phys Med Rehabil* 85:1966–1971, 2004.
2. Amin A, Singh V, Saifuddin A, Briggs TW: Ulnar stress reaction from crutch use following amputation for tibial osteosarcoma, *Skel Radiol* 33:541–544, 2004.
3. Aminzadeh F, Edwards N: Exploring seniors' views on the use of assistive devices in fall prevention, *Public Health Nurs* 15:297–304, 1998.
4. Ang EJ, Goh JC, Bos K et al: Biofeedback device for patients on axillary crutches, *Arch Phys Med Rehabil* 70:644–646, 1989.
5. Annesley AI, Almada-Norfleet M, Arnall DA, Cornwall MW: Energy expenditure of ambulation using the Sure-Gait crutch and the standard axillary crutch, *Phys Ther* 70:18–23, 1990.
6. Ashton-Miller JA, Yeh MW, Richardson JK, Galloway J: A cane reduces loss of balance in patients with peripheral neuropathy: results from a challenging unipedal balance test, *Arch Phys Med Rehabil* 77:446–452, 1996.
7. Babic J, Karcnik T, Bajd T: Stability analysis of four-point walking, *Gait Posture* 14:56–60, 2001.
8. Bachschmidt RA, Harris GF, Simoneau GG: Walker-assisted gait in rehabilitation: a study of biomechanics and instrumentation, *IEEE Trans Neural Syst Rehabil Eng* 9:96–105, 2001.
9. Ball NA, Stempien LM, Pasupuleti DV, Wertsch JJ: Radial nerve palsy: a complication of walker usage, *Arch Phys Med Rehabil* 70:236, 1989.
10. Baruch IM, Mossberg KA: Heart-rate response of elderly women to non-weight-bearing ambulation with a walker, *Phys Ther* 63:1782–1787, 1983.
11. Basford JR, Rhetta HL, Schleusner MP: Clinical evaluation of the rocker bottom crutch, *Orthopaedics* 13:457–460, 1990.
12. Bateni H, Heung E, Zettel J et al: Can use of walkers or canes impede lateral compensatory stepping movements? *Gait Posture* 20:74–83, 2004.
13. Bateni H, Maki BE: Assistive devices for balance and mobility: benefits, demands, and adverse consequences, *Arch Phys Med Rehabil* 86:134–145, 2005.
14. Bauer DM, Finch DC, McGough KP et al: A comparative analysis of several crutch-length-estimation techniques, *Phys Ther* 71:294–300, 1991.
15. Baxter ML, Allington RO, Koepke GH: Weight distribution variables in the use of crutches and canes, *Phys Ther* 49:360–365, 1969.
16. Beckwith JM: Analysis of methods of teaching axillary crutch measurement, *Phys Ther* 45:1060–1065, 1965.
17. Bennett L, Murray MP, Murphy EF, Sowell TT: Locomotion assistance through cane impulse, *Bull Prosthet Res* 10:38–47, 1979.
18. Bhambani YN, Clarkson HM, Gomes PS: Axillary crutch walking: effects of three training programs, *Arch Phys Med Rehabil* 71:484–489, 1990.
19. Biering-Sorensen F, Hansen RB, Biering-Sorensen J: Mobility aids and transport possibilities 10–45 years after spinal cord injury, *Spinal Cord* 42:699–706, 2004.
20. Blount WP: Don't throw away the cane, *J Bone Joint Surg* 18A:695–708, 1956.
21. Brand RA, Crowninshield RD: The effect of cane use on hip contact force, *Clin Orthop* 147:181–184, 1980.
22. Brooks AL, Fowler SB: Axillary artery thrombosis after prolonged use of crutches, *J Bone Joint Surg* 46A:863–864, 1964.
23. Buurke JH, Mermens JH, Erren-Wolters CV, Nene AV: The effect of walking aids on muscle activation patterns during walking in stroke patients, *Gait Posture* 22:164–170, 2005.
24. Chan GN, Smith AW, Kirtley C, Tsang WW: Changes in knee moments with contralateral versus ipsilateral cane usage in females with knee osteoarthritis, *Clin Biomech* 20:396–401, 2005.

25. Charron P, Kirby RL, MacLeod DA: Epidemiology of walker-related accidents in the United States, *Am J Phys Med Rehabil* 74:237–239, 1995.

26. Chen CL, Chen HC, Wong MK et al: Temporal stride and force analysis of cane-assisted gait in people with hemiplegic stroke, *Arch Phys Med Rehabil* 82:43–48, 2001.

27. Chiou-Tan FY, Magee KN, Krouskop TA: Comparison of upper limb muscle activity in four walking canes: a preliminary study, *J Rehabil Res Dev* 36:94–99, 1999.

28. Clark BC, Manini TM, Ordway NR et al: Leg muscle activity during walking with assistive devices at varying levels of weight bearing, *Arch Phys Med Rehabil* 85:1555–1560, 2004.

29. Crosbie WJ, Nicol AC: Aided gait in rheumatoid arthritis following knee arthroplasty, *Arch Phys Med Rehabil* 71:299–303, 1990.

30. Cubo E, Moore CG, Leurgans S, Goetz CG: Wheeled and standard walkers in Parkinson's disease patients with gait freezing, *Parkinsonism Relat Disord* 10:9–14, 2003.

31. Dean E, Ross J: Relationships among cane fitting, function, and falls, *Phys Ther* 73:494–500, 1993.

32. Dounis E, Rose GK, Wilson RS, Steventon R: A comparison of efficiency of three types of crutches using oxygen consumption, *Rheumatol Rehabil* 19:252–255, 1980.

33. Eblen C, Koeneman J: A multidimensional evaluation of a four-wheeled walker, *Assist Technol* 3:32–37, 1991.

34. Eblen C, Koeneman JB: A longitudinal evaluation of a four-wheeled walker: effects of experience, *Top Geriatr Rehabil* 8:65–72, 1993.

35. Edwards BG: Contralateral and ipsilateral cane usage by patients with total knee or hip replacement, *Arch Phys Med Rehabil* 67:734–740, 1986.

36. Ely DD, Smidt GL: Effect of cane on variables of gait for patients with hip disorders, *Phys Ther* 57:507–512, 1977.

37. Engel J, Amir A, Messer E, Caspi I: Walking cane designed to assist partial weight bearing, *Arch Phys Med Rehabil* 64:386–388, 1983.

38. Epstein S: Art, history and the crutch, *Ann Med Hist* 9:304, 1937.

39. Fast A, Wang FS, Adrezin RS et al: The instrumented walker: usage patterns and forces, *Arch Phys Med Rehabil* 76:484–491, 1995.

40. Feldman DR, Vujic I, McKay D et al: Crutch-induced axillary artery injury, *Cardiovas Intervent Radiol* 18:296–299, 1995.

41. Fisher SV, Patterson RP: Energy cost of ambulation with crutches, *Arch Phys Med Rehabil* 62:250–256, 1981.

42. Foley MP, Prax B, Crowell R, Boone T: Effects of assistive devices on cardiorespiratory demands in older adults, *Phys Ther* 76:1313–1319, 1996.

43. Ghosh AK, Tibarewala DN, Dasgupta SR et al: Metabolic cost of walking at different speeds with axillary crutches, *Ergonomics* 23:571–577, 1980.

44. Gibbs D: When a cane was the necessary complement of a physician, *J Roy Coll Phys Lond* 33:85–89, 1999.

45. Gillespie FC, Fisher J, Williams CS et al: A physiologic assessment of the rolling crutch, *Ergonomics* 26:341–347, 1983.

46. Goh JC, Toh SL, Bose K: Biomechanical study on axillary crutches during single leg swing through gait, *Prosthet Orthot Int* 10:89–95, 1986.

47. Greiner BM, Czerniecki JM, Deitz JC: Gait parameters of children with spastic diplegia: a comparison of effects of posterior and anterior walkers, *Arch Phys Med Rehabil* 74:381–385, 1993.

48. Hall CD, Jensen JL: The effect of cane use on the compensatory step following posterior perturbations, *Clin Biomech* 19:678–687, 2004.

49. Hall J, Clarke AK, Harrison R: Guidelines for prescription of walking frames, *Physiotherapy* 76:118–120, 1990.

50. Hall J, Elvins DM, Burke SJ et al: Heart rate evaluation of axillary and elbow crutches, *J Med Eng Technol* 15:232–238, 1991.

50a. Haubert LL, Gutierrez DD, Newsam CJ et al: A comparison of shoulder joint forces during ambulation with crutches versus a walker in persons with incomplete spinal cord injury, *Arch Phys Med Rehabil* 87:63–70, 2006.

51. Hess S, Jahnke MT, Schaffrin A et al: Immediate effects of therapeutic facilitation on the gait of hemiparetic patients as compared with walking with and without a cane, *Electroencephalogr Clin Neurophysiol* 109:515–522, 1998.

52. Hinton CA, Cullen KE: Energy expenditure during ambulation with Ortho crutches and axillary crutches, *Phys Ther* 62:813–819, 1982.

53. Holder CG, Haskvitz EM, Weltman A: The effects of assistive devices on the oxygen cost, cardiovascular stress, and perception of nonweight-bearing ambulation, *J Orthop Sports Phys Ther* 18:537–541, 1993.

54. Hug U, Burg D, Baldi SV, Meyer VE: Compression neuropathy of the radial palmar thumb nerve, *Chir Main* 23:49–51, 2004.

55. IJzerman MJ, Baardman G, van't Hof MA et al: Validity and reproducibility of crutch force and heart rate measurements to assess energy expenditure of paraplegic gait, *Arch Phys Med Rehabil* 80:1017–1923, 1999.

56. Imms FJ, MacDonald IC, Prestige SP: Energy expenditure during walking in patients recovering from fractures of the leg, *Scand J Rehabil Med* 8:1–9, 1976.

57. Ishikura T: Biomechanical analysis of weight bearing force and muscle activation levels in the lower extremities during gait with a walker, *Acta Med Okayama* 55:73–82, 2001.

57a. Jeka JJ: Light touch contact as a balance aid, *Phys Ther* 77:476–487, 1997.

57b. Jeka JJ, Easton RD, Bentzen BL, Lackner JR: Haptic cues for orientation and postural control in sighted and blind individuals, *Percept Psychophys* 58:409–423, 1996.

58. Johnson JT, Johnson BF, Blasch BB, de l'Aune WD: Gait and long cane kinematics: a comparison of slighted and visually impaired subjects, *J Orthop Sports Phys Ther* 27:162–166, 1998.

59. Joyce BM, Kirby RL: Canes, crutches and walkers, *Am Fam Pract* 43:535–542, 1991.

60. Karpman RR: Problems and pitfalls with assistive devices, *Top Geriatr Rehabil* 8:1–5, 1992.

61. Kellner WS, Felsenthal G, Anderson JM et al: Carpal tunnel syndrome in the nonparetic hands of hemiplegics: stress-induced by ambulatory assistive devices, *Orthop Rev* 15:608–611, 1986.

62. Kirby RL, Tsai HY, Graham MM: Ambulation aid use during the rehabilitation of people with lower limb amputations, *Assist Technol* 14:112–117, 2002.

63. Kling C, Persson A, Gardulf A: The ADL ability and use of technical aids in persons with late effects of polio, *Am J Occup Ther* 56:457–461, 2002.

64. Kuan TS, Tsou JY, Su FC: Hemiplegic gait of stroke patients: the effect on using a cane, *Arch Phys Med Rehabil* 80:777–784, 1999.

65. Kumar R, Roe MC, Scremin OU: Methods to estimate the proper length of a cane, *Arch Phys Med Rehabil* 76:1173–1175, 1995.

66. Laufer Y: Effects of one-point and four-point canes on balance and weight distribution in patients with hemiparesis, *Clin Rehabil* 16:141–148, 2002.

67. LeBlanc MA, Carlson LE, Nauenberg T: A quantitative comparison of four experimental axillary crutches, *J Prosthet Orthot* 5:40–48, 1993.

68. Levangie PK, Guihan MF, Meyer P, Stuhr K: Effects of altering handle position of a rolling walker on gait in children with cerebral palsy, *Phys Ther* 69:130–134, 1989.

69. Li S, Armstrong CW, Cipriani D: Three-point gait crutch walking: variability in ground reaction force during weight bearing, *Arch Phys Med Rehabil* 82:86–92, 2001.

70. Loebl WY, Nunn JF: Staffs as walking aids in ancient Egypt and Palestine, *J Roy Soc Med* 90:450–454, 1997.

71. Logan L, Byers-Kinkley K, Ciccone C: Anterior vs. posterior walkers: a gait analysis study, *Dev Med Child Neurol* 32:044–1048, 1990.

72. Lovett RW: The tripod method of walking with crutches, *JAMA* 74:1306–1308, 1920.

73. Lu CL, Yu B, Basford JR et al: Influences of cane length on the stability of stroke patients, *J Rehabil Res Dev* 34:91–100, 1997.

74. Lyu SR, Ogata K, Hoshiko I: Effects of a cane on floor reaction force and center of force during gait, *Clin Orthop Relat Res* 375:313–319, 2000.

75. Maeda A, Nakamura K, Higuchi S et al: Postural sway during cane use by patients with stroke, *Am J Phys Med Rehabil* 80:903–908, 2001.

76. Mahoney JE, Sager MA, Jalaluddin M: Use of an ambulation assistive device predicts functional decline associated with hospitalization, *J Gerontol A Biol Sci Med Sci* 54:M83–M88, 1999.

77. Mann WC, Ottenbacher KJ, Fraas L et al: Effectiveness of assistive technology and environmental interventions in maintaining independence and reducing home care costs for the frail elderly: a randomized controlled trial, *Arch Fam Med* 8:210–217, 1999.

78. Mathieson KM, Kronenfeld JJ, Keith VM: Maintaining functional independence in elderly adults: the roles of health status and financial resources in predicting home modifications and use of mobility equipment, *Gerontologist* 42:24–31, 2002.

79. McDonough AL, Razza-Doherty M: Some biomechanical aspects of crutch and cane walking: the relationship between forward rate of progression, symmetry, and efficiency—a case report, *Clin Podiatr Med Surg* 5:677–693, 1988.

80. McFall B, Arya N, Soong C et al: Crutch induced axillary artery injury, *Ulster Med J* 73:50–52, 2004.

81. McGibbon CA, Krebs DE, Mann RW: In vivo hip pressures during cane and load-carrying gait, *Arthritis Care Res* 10:300–307, 1997.

82. Melis EH, Torres-Moreno R, Barbeau H, Lemaire ED: Analysis of assisted-gait characteristics in persons with incomplete spinal cord injury, *Spinal Cord* 37:430–439, 1999.

83. Mendelson S, Milgrom C, Firestone A et al: Effect of cane use on tibial strain and strain rates, *Am J Phys Med Rehabil* 77:333–338, 1998.

84. Milczarek JJ, Kirby RL, Harrison ER et al: Standard and four-footed canes, their effect on the standing balance of patients with hemiparesis, *Arch Phys Med Rehabil* 74:281–285, 1993.

85. Mount J, Howard PD, Dalla Palu AL et al: Postures and repetitive movements during use of a long cane by individuals with visual impairment, *J Orthop Sports Phys Ther* 31:375–383, 2001.

86. Mulley GP: Walking sticks, *BMJ* 296:475–476, 1988.

87. Mullis R, Dent RM: Crutch length: effect on energy cost and activity intensity in non-weight-bearing ambulation, *Arch Phys Med Rehabil* 81:569–572, 2000.

88. Najdeski P: Crutch measurement from the sitting position, *Phys Ther* 57:826–827, 1977.

89. Nandapalan V, Smith CA, Jones AS, Lesser TH: Objective measurement of the benefit of walking sticks on peripheral vestibular balance disorders, using the Sway Weigh balance platform, *J Laryngol Otol* 109:836–840, 1995.

90. Neumann DA: An electromyographic study of the hip abductor muscles as subjects with a hip prosthesis walked with different methods of using a cane and carrying a load, *Phys Ther* 79:1163–1173, 1999.

91. Nielsen DH, Harris JM, Minton YM et al: Energy cost, exercise intensity, and gait efficiency of standard versus rocker-bottom axillary crutch walking, *Phys Ther* 70:487–493, 1990.

92. Noreau L, Richards CL, Comeau F, Tardif D: Biomechanical analysis of swing-through gait in paraplegic and non-disabled individuals, *J Biomech* 28:689–700, 1995.

93. Nyland J, Bernasek T, Markee B, Dundore C: Comparison of the Easy Strutter Functional Orthosis System™ and axillary crutches during modified 3-point gait, *J Rehabil Res Dev* 41:195–206, 2004.

94. Opila KA, Nicol AC, Paul JP: Forces and impulses during aided gait, *Arch Phys Med Rehabil* 68:715–722, 1987.

95. Pardo RD, Deathe AB, Winter DA: Walker user risk index: a method for quantifying stability in walker users, *Am J Phys Med Rehabil* 72:301–305, 1993.

96. Parziale JR, Daniels JD: The mechanical performance of ambulation using spring-loaded axillary crutches: a preliminary report, *Am J Phys Med* 68:193–195, 1989.

97. Pine Z, Gurland B, Chren MM: Use of a cane for ambulation: marker and mitigator of impairment in older people who report no difficulty walking, *J Am Geriatr Soc* 50:263–268, 2002.

98. Platt H: Occlusion of the axillary artery due to pressure by a crutch, *Arch Surg* 20:314–316, 1930.

99. Ramsey VK, Blasch BB, Kita A, Johnson BF: A biomechanical evaluation of visually impaired persons' gait and long-cane mechanics, *J Rehabil Res Dev* 36:323–332, 1999.

100. Reisman M, Burkett RG, Simon SK, Norkin C: Elbow moments and forces at the hands during swing through axillary crutch gait, *Phys Ther* 65:601–605, 1985.

101. Rentschler AJ, Cooper RA, Blasch B, Boninger ML: Intelligent walkers for the elderly: performance and safety testing of VA-PAMAID robotic walker, *J Rehabil Res Dev* 40:423–431, 2003.

102. Requejo PS, Wahl DP, Bontrager EL et al: Upper extremity kinetics during Lofstrand crutch-assisted gait, *Med Eng Phys* 27:19–29, 2005.

103. Ross DE: Relationships among cane fitting, function, and falls, *Phys Ther* 73:494, 1993.

104. Rovic JS, Childress DS: Pendular model of paraplegic swing-through crutch ambulation, *J Rehabil Res Dev* 25:1–16, 1988.

105. Rudin LN, Levine L: Bilateral compression of radial nerve (crutch paralysis), *Phys Ther Rev* 31:229, 1951.

106. Sainsbury R, Mulley GP: Walking sticks used by the elderly, *BMJ* 284:1751, 1982.

107. Sala DA, Leva LM, Kummer FJ, Grant AD: Crutch handle design: effect on palmar loads during ambulation, *Arch Phys Med Rehabil* 79:1473–1476, 1998.

108. Sankarankutty M, Stallard J, Rose GK: The relative efficiency of "swing-through" gait on axillary, elbow and Canadian crutches compared to normal walking, *J Biomed Eng* 1:55–57, 1979.

109. Schellingerhout R, Bongers RM, van Grinsven R et al: Improving obstacle detection by redesign of walking canes for blind persons, *Ergonomics* 44:513–526, 2001.

110. Schmitz TJ: Preambulation and gait training. In O'Sullivan SB, Schmitz TJ, editors: *Physical rehabilitation: assessment and treatment*, ed 4, Philadelphia, 2001, FA Davis.

111. Shabes D, Scheiber M: Suprascapular neuropathy related to the use of crutches, *Am J Phys Med* 65:298–299, 1986.

112. Shortell D, Kucer J, Neeley WL, LeBlanc M: The design of a compliant composite crutch, *J Rehabil Res Dev* 38:23–32, 2001.

113. Shoup TE, Fletcher LS, Merrill BK: Biomechanics of crutch ambulation, *J Biomech* 7:11–19, 1974.

114. Sidaway B, Champagne A, Daigle K et al: The effect of cane length on the haptic perception of height, *Disabil Rehabil* 26:157–161, 2004.

115. Sonntag D, Uhlenbrock D, Bardeleben A et al: Gait with and without forearm crutches in patients with total hip arthroplasty, *Int J Rehabil Res* 23:233–243, 2000.

116. Stallard J, Dounis E, Major RE, Rose GK: One leg swing through gait using two crutches: an analysis of the ground reaction forces and gait phases, *Acta Orthop Scand* 51:71–77, 1980.

117. Stallard J, Sankarankutty M, Rose GK: A comparison of axillary, elbow and Canadian crutches, *Rheumatol Rehabil* 17:237–239, 1978.

118. Stevenson CA: Assessment of ambulation using Sure-Gait and standard axillary crutches, *Phys Ther* 71:S28, 1991 (abstract).

119. Tagawa TT: Adjustable measuring crutch, *Phys Ther* 43:113–114, 1963.

120. Tagawa Y, Shiba N, Matsuo S, Yamashita T: Analysis of human abnormal walking using a multi-body model: joint models for abnormal walking and walking aids to reduce compensatory action, *J Biomech* 33:1405–1414, 2000.

121. Thys H, Willems PA, Snels P: Energy cost, mechanical work and muscular efficiency in swing-through gait with elbow crutches, *J Biomech* 29:1473–1482, 1996.

122. Tyson SF: The support taken through walking aids during hemiplegic gait, *Clin Rehabil* 12:395–401, 1998.

123. Ulkar B, Yavuzer G, Buner R, Ergin S: Energy expenditure of the paraplegic gait: comparison between different walking aids and normal subjects, *Int J Rehabil Res* 26:213–217, 2003.

124. Van der Esch M, Heijmans M, Dekker J: Factors contributing to possession and use of walking aids among persons with rheumatoid arthritis and osteoarthritis, *Arthritis Rheum* 49:838–842, 2003.

125. Van Hook FW, Demonbreun D, Weiss BD: Ambulatory devices for chronic gait disorders in the elderly, *Am Fam Physician* 67:1717–1724, 2003.

126. Vankowski S, Moore C, Statler KD et al: The influence of forearm crutches on pelvic and hip kinematics in children with myelomeningocele: don't throw away the crutches, *Dev Med Child Neurol* 39:614–619, 1997.

127. Vargo MM, Robinson LR, Nicholas JJ: Contralateral v ipsilateral cane use: effects on muscles crossing the knee joint, *Am J Phys Med Rehabil* 71:170–176, 1992.

128. Veerendrakumar M, Taly AB, Nagaraja D: Ulnar nerve palsy due to axillary crutch, *Neurol India* 49:67–70, 2001.

129. Verbrugge LM, Sevak P: Use, type and efficacy of assistance for disability, *J Gerontol B Psychol Sci Soc Sci* 57:S366–S379, 2002.

130. Waters RL, Campbell J, Perry J: Energy cost of three-point crutch ambulation in fracture patients, *J Orthop Trauma* 1:170–173, 1987.

131. Wells RP: Kinematics and energy variations of swing-through crutch gait, *J Biomech* 12:579–585, 1979.

132. Werner R, Waring W, Davidoff G: Risk factors for median mononeuropathy of the wrist in post poliomyelitis patients, *Arch Phys Med Rehabil* 70:464–467, 1989.

133. Werner RA, Waring W, Maynard F: Osteoarthritis of the hand and wrist in the post poliomyelitis population, *Arch Phys Med Rehabil* 73:1069–1072, 1992.

134. Wilson JF, Gilbert JA: Dynamic body forces on axillary crutch walkers during swing-through gait, *Am J Phys Med* 61:85–92, 1982.

135. Wolfe RR, Jordan D, Wolfe JL: The WalkAbout: a new solution for preventing falls in the elderly and disabled, *Arch Phys Med Rehabil* 85:2067–2069, 2004.

136. Wolff JL, Agree EM, Kasper JD: Wheelchairs, walkers, and canes: what does Medicare pay for, and who benefits?, *Health Aff* 24:1140–1149, 2005.

137. Wright DI, Kemp TI: The dual-task methodology and assessing the attentional demands of ambulation with walking devices, *Phys Ther* 72:306–315, 1992.

138. Youdas JW, Kotajarvi BJ, Padgett DJ, Kaufman KR: Partial weight-bearing gait using conventional assistive devices, *Arch Phys Med Rehabil* 86:394–398, 2005.

Wheelchair mobility for disabled children and adults

Susan Johnson Taylor

Key Points

- Assess mobility and cognition of patient. Incorporate prognosis of condition to ensure flexibility of equipment when necessary.
- Determine needs based on mobility efficiency, daily requirements, and environment.
- Assess how the device will affect daily activities and functional skills to assist with appropriate technology match.
- Teach skills with powered and manual wheelchairs to ensure safe and functional mobility.

Pathophysiology

Mobility is the ability to move oneself from one place to another. The need to move oneself at will is as basic as breathing. Persons with physical disabilities that impede functional mobility often require a wheelchair to augment or replace the function of walking. The National Center for Health Statistics reports that more than 1.3 million people in the United States use manual wheelchairs, with more than 160,000 using powered devices such as powered wheelchairs and scooters.[17] When a person has a physical disability that impedes or prevents walking, a variety of methods, including orthotics, walkers, and crutches, can be used to augment or facilitate mobility. Wheelchairs are considered for a variety of patients, including persons who are unable to walk other than very short distances, whose physical abilities change from day to day or week to week, or who are unable to be mobile without the use of a wheelchair. The first two categories (can walk sometimes and under some circumstances) pose the most challenges to wheelchair evaluation in terms of when to

and when not to recommend wheelchairs. Remember that the purpose of mobility is to move from one place to another in the most efficient manner possible. Mobility is not the same as exercise; the person with inefficient mobility should be able to move about at will and still have the energy to accomplish tasks once he or she arrives at the destination. The choice to use a wheelchair need not negate aided or unaided walking. The mobility method should fit the activity.[30] For example, walking around the house or classroom may be functional, but grocery shopping or playing on the playground might require wheeled mobility.

Historical perspective

Historically, the ability to apply appropriate powered and manual wheelchair technology is young. The first folding manual wheelchair was produced in the United States by Herbert Everest and Harry Jennings in 1933.[33] This relatively heavy, steel, chromed wheelchair remained the basic style of the manual wheelchair until the late 1970s. The turmoil of the late 1960s and early 1970s produced the disability right's movements and independent living centers around the country. People with increasingly serious disabilities, including congenital problems such as spina bifida and acquired conditions such as traumatic brain injuries and spinal cord injuries, were surviving when before they had not. Because of consumer demand in the late 1970s and early 1980s, manual wheelchairs were designed and manufactured that provided choices and custom fitting with individual needs and preferences in mind. Marilyn Hamilton, who has paraplegia as the result of a hang gliding accident, led the way in the development of these types of manual wheelchairs.[33] Crude powered wheelchairs initially produced in the 1950s required good upper extremity skills to operate them. During the Vietnam war era, research was performed to develop access to powered wheelchairs for those who did not have upper extremity movement.[33] It was not until the flexibility of electronics that resulted from the development of microcomputers that access and control of powered wheelchairs became possible for clients with very severe physical disabilities. Twenty-five years later, health professionals are able to accommodate a variety of physical and functional needs.

Current issues

Twenty-five to thirty years ago, the variety of wheelchair technology available to assist persons with physical disabilities was limited. Today, a plethora of powered and manual wheelchair technology is available. The challenge for clinicians and wheelchair suppliers is matching client need to specific wheelchair technologies and components. This requires knowledge of clients' diagnoses and the implications of those diagnoses, their functional and activities of daily living (ADL) needs, and the environments in which they need to function.

Current research

Much of the current research involves manual wheelchair technology, how it should be applied, and factors that contribute to overuse injuries in adults. One of the factors that provided the impetus for some of this research is the large population of adults who are aging with an acquired disability. Studies have primarily retrospectively looked at individuals with spinal cord injury. A conclusion common to these studies is that upper extremity pain is a significant problem that potentially interferes with ADLs, and that manual wheelchair propulsion is one of the culprits. Pentland and Twomey[23,24] demonstrated an association between duration of injury, not necessarily chronological age, and shoulder pain. Waters and Sie[32] found that 46% of persons with tetraplegia and 36% of persons with paraplegia experience shoulder pain. They point out that even a small amount of pain and loss of shoulder range of motion can have a profound impact on a person's ability to carry out ADLs. Curtis et al.[11] noted that one of the most painful activities reported was wheeling up hills.

These and other studies performed in the last decade encouraged researchers take a critical look at the contribution of manual wheelchairs and how they are set up to an individual's upper extremity problems. A growing body of research assesses the relationship of the location of the rear wheel, forces at the hand rim, and how these forces translate through the wrist, elbow, and shoulder. For example, Boninger et al.[3] evaluated the effect of an appropriately set forward axle on 40 wheelchair users. They found lower peak forces, less rapid loading of the push rim, and fewer strokes necessary to get to the same speed as wheelchairs that did not have a forward axle.[3]

Some studies focus on quality of life, that is, they review the impact of mobility on clients' lives. In one such study, Davies et al.[12] studied 51 individuals in the United Kingdom (North West London) who had just been provided with powered wheelchairs. Diagnoses for this group included multiple sclerosis, muscular dystrophy, cerebral palsy, spinal cord injury, and cerebrovascular accident. The researchers found that mobility and perceived quality of life improved, and pain and discomfort were reduced.[12]

Treatment recommendations
Evaluation for manual and powered mobility

Although the development of manual and powered wheelchair technologies has seen rapid advances, the focus must be on the consumers and their needs and abilities. A poor match between consumer and technology at best will lead to abandonment of the technology and at worst will cause harm. For example, a manual wheelchair that is too difficult to disassemble for transport may not be used. A powered wheelchair prescribed to someone who is unable to safely operate it could result in a dangerous accident. As with any other clinical intervention, prescription of a powered or manual wheelchair begins with an evaluation. Specific areas must be evaluated and considered. Interwoven with the individual's needs and wants is medical necessity.[18] Most manual and powered wheelchairs are prescriptive devices, paid for by third-party payers. What will be approved through each payer (public or private insurers) varies as to what is considered medically necessary.

The accepted clinical team for a manual or powered mobility evaluation generally consists of a clinician and a rehabilitation technology supplier.[22] It is the responsibility of the evaluators to obtain and coordinate all medical, therapeutic, and other information relevant to the client's needs and abilities. It is taken for granted that the mobility evaluation will be performed once a seating evaluation has been completed. Only when the client's seated positioning needs are understood can an evaluation for wheeled mobility can take place. This is true whether the evaluation is for dependent or independent mobility. Dependent mobility involves caregivers moving the client in the wheelchair; independent mobility involves the client primarily moving himself or herself. Overall, the wheelchair mobility evaluation process comprises evaluation, trial of equipment, specific recommendations, funding process, and training (of the client and caregiver). Although no validated evaluations are available for wheelchair mobility, certain factors and areas must be considered[4]: physical considerations, cognitive and perceptual motor considerations, ADL and functional skills, environmental and transportation needs, and technology tolerance.

Physical considerations
Prognosis of condition

The first area that must be understood is the client's diagnosis and its characteristics and ramifications. Factors such as rate of disease progression and severity of weakness and spasticity may impact the prescription. A more quickly progressive disease process may lead toward recommendations for mobility that is modular, flexible, and changeable. A client who has no sensation or has poor ability to perform a pressure relief requires consideration for technology that provides a mechanical pressure relief.

Strength, posture, and stability

During an independent mobility evaluation, the clinician assesses the client's physical skills as they relate to movements necessary for propelling a manual wheelchair or accessing the controls of a powered wheelchair. The assessment may include strength and coordination of movements. Movements necessary for propulsion of a manual wheelchair typically include use of both upper extremities, one upper and one lower extremity, or both lower extremities. These movements should have sufficient strength and coordination that allow the client to move the manual wheelchair about the environments in which he or she needs to function. Additionally, the movements should not have a deleterious effect on the client's posture or stability. For example, a client with spastic quadriplegic cerebral palsy may have a kyphotic posture that is exacerbated by the motions of propelling with the upper extremities. A client with weak upper extremities, such as a client with C5-6 tetraplegia, may have to overuse available musculature, resulting in undesirable compensatory movements. The clinician and client need to balance the use of a manual wheelchair with the long-term effects of propelling full time.

Power mobility access

Movements or actions necessary to operate a powered chair are varied due to the wide array of powered chair access methods. It may involve a movement at a single site, such as hand function with a joystick, or multiple sites, such as using single switches by a client who is more severely physically involved. The movements used must allow for consistent and safe operation of the powered wheelchair.

Cognitive and perceptual motor considerations

A primary concern in the choice of method of wheelchair mobility is safety. Problem-solving ability in the environments in which clients will function must be assessed. Accommodations may allow a client with cognitive deficits to be provided with independent powered or manual mobility. A client with a consistent caregiver who can provide structure and supervision could be considered. There is no substitute for actually assessing the client in various environments in the type of wheelchair being considered. Safety must be the final outcome.

Another scenario is evaluation of a child for wheelchair mobility. Children require supervision commensurate with their age and developmental level, no matter what their method of mobility. The wheelchair mobility evaluation is performed with the expected outcomes in line with the child's developmental level. The child should be able to demonstrate "go" and "stop" and some cause/effect.

Clinical decision making about whether to provide independent mobility in either of these scenarios, especially power, depends on several factors. The availability of long-term, consistent training is among the most important. As with any other skill, consistent training is necessary. Training can come from a therapist, parent, or other person who can provide guided supervision. The therapist can provide a treatment plan or ideas for exposing the client to the environments in which he or she needs to function. A trial with a well-fitted "loaner" power mobility device may help determine the client's ability to operate and safely function in such a device, if such ability is in question.

Neurologic diagnoses such as stroke, multiple sclerosis, and cerebral palsy can result in visual field disturbances, such as field cuts or difficulty judging distances. Some clients may be able to compensate for these perceptual motor problems. Evaluating the client in a wheelchair is needed to actually see his or her response to moving through the environment.

Activities of daily living and functional skills

The clinician must have an understanding of ADL and functional skills that are performed in the wheelchair to ensure that the structural stability, dimensions, and components of the wheelchair match the client's needs. For example, the client may have a marginal ability to transfer based on the seat height of the wheelchair. Another client may dress in the wheelchair and require strong back posts to support this activity. Components such as oxygen containers, feeding bags, and ventilators must be safely incorporated onto the wheelchair base, without compromising safety or stability.

Environment and transportation

The wheelchair must fit into the client's current environments and method(s) of transportation. When evaluating a client who is new to wheeled mobility or who is considering a wheelchair that is different from what he or she currently uses, certain measurements need to be obtained. With an existing wheelchair, the minimum measurements taken should be the overall width and length of the chair and the height from the floor to the seat tubes/seat pan. The client's home should be measured and, where applicable, the client's adapted vehicle should be measured for width, length, and turning radii.

The types of environments in which the client functions should be ascertained. When possible, it is highly recommended that the wheelchair being prescribed be tried in the client's home, vehicle, workplace, and other relevant locations. Wheelchair types and component selections are made according to how the wheelchair will be used. This can help overprescribing and underprescribing. For example, a client who wants to use the wheelchair only in an indoor environment does not need a wheelchair base designed to handle rough terrain. A lightweight chair may be needed if the chair must be lifted into a car by the user.

Technology tolerance

Powered and manual mobility technology can be complex. The ability to use and maintain powered and manual mobility successfully must be assessed. Just because technology *can* be applied to a situation does not mean that it *should*. Some clients/caregivers can handle complex powered wheelchair systems, whereas others seem to have trouble just remembering to charge the wheelchair. The client and caregiver must be motivated to carry through with training, maintenance, and follow-up; otherwise, abandonment of the technology is likely.

The application and prescription of technology is discussed in the section on orthotic management.

Orthotic management

Understanding manual and powered wheelchair technology, the levels of technology, and how and why the technology adjusts is essential to successful prescription and training. Over a 10-year time period, an American National Standards Institute (ANSI) and Rehabilitation Engineering and Assistive Technology Society of North America (RESNA) committee has developed standards and methods by which manual and powered wheelchairs are tested. These standards are voluntary for manufacturers and provide objective data by which wheelchairs can be compared.[5] Some standards apply to powered and manual wheelchairs, and some apply to one or the other. Examples of tests include Determination of Static Stability and Determination of Overall Dimensions, Weight, and Turning Space.[6] Another area of standards work is in Wheelchair Transportation Safety. Standards have been developed to guide the industry and consumers toward safe wheelchair transportation practices. Information on obtaining these standards or interpreting them clinically can be obtained at the web sites of RESNA (*www.resna.org*) and ANSI (*www.ansi.org*).

Manual wheelchairs

Manual mobility technology can be broadly divided into two categories: wheelchairs that are meant for dependent mobility, and those that are designed for independent mobility.

Dependent manual wheelchairs

Although dependent manual wheelchairs are primarily designed to be pushed by a caregiver, is it possible for the client to have access to the rear wheels of several of these types of chairs. Even though it is possible for the client to propel some of these chairs, the propulsion would be for only short distances because of the weight of the chair and/or the rear wheel location. Manual upright bases include standard wheelchairs (US Medicare K0001-K0003), transport wheelchairs, and stroller bases. These wheelchairs are primarily designed to be pushed by a caregiver and easily stored for transport. Some upright wheelchairs have a limited amount of adjustment for seat to floor height for foot propulsion.

Manual tilt-in-space and/or recline wheelchairs usually are used by clients who cannot maintain an upright position for long periods, who require a caregiver to perform pressure reliefs for them, and/or who do not have the physical control to sit against gravity. Recline wheelchairs can be folded for transport (although they are heavy), but maintaining client positioning is more difficult. Tilt-in-space wheelchairs usually are rigid and do not fold, but they allow for maintenance of the client's body position while his or her position in space is changed. Figure 43-1 shows examples of a tilt and a recline manual chair. Some models, especially in sizes meant for small children, can tilt and can be folded for transport. Some tilt-in-space bases offer an adjustable rear axle to allow some degree of independent movement. It is possible to have both tilt and recline in the same base. This is indicated when the client has little available hip flexion, the client requires both tilt and recline in order to have a full pressure relief, or the client requires care (e.g., perineal care) while in the wheelchair, to limit the number of transfers over the course of a day.

When looking at a manual wheelchair base for a child or a patient with a changing condition, adjustability for growth and change is important, including changes in seat width, seat depth, seat height, and back cane angle. Figure 43-2 shows close-ups of an angle adjustable back and seat depth adjustment. A client discharged after a traumatic brain injury who has poor physical skills and an inability to sit upright against gravity may need a base that allows for improvements in function. Perhaps a tilt-in-space chair with an adjustable rear axle would suit poor physical skills now but would allow a measure of independence later.

When recommending manual mobility for children whose physical skills may improve, one must look at a wheelchair base that offers the possibility for self-propulsion later. For example, many stroller bases are meant for dependent mobility only. If the child has an increase in function but third party payers will not consider another base yet, the child would be stuck in a dependent base with no way to move at will.

Independent manual wheelchairs

Independent manual wheelchairs are lightweight, semiadjustable (Medicare K0004), or ultralightweight fully adjustable (K0005). Ultralightweight wheelchairs are further divided into *rigid frames* and *folding frames* (Fig. 43-3). The advantage of rigid frames is that they provide durability; they provide

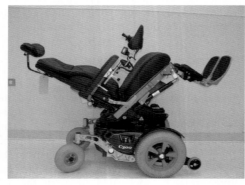

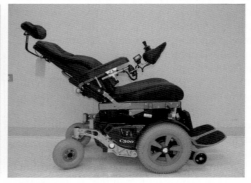

A   B

Fig. 43-1 Example of tilting **(A)** and reclining **(B)** chairs.

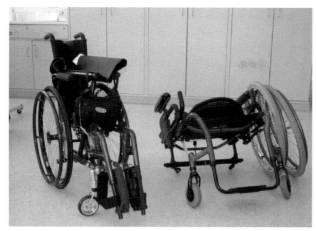

Fig. 43-2 Folding frame *(left)* and rigid frame *(right)* wheelchairs.

efficient propulsion because of fewer moving parts than a folding frame; they are lighter in weight; and they have the possibility of a shorter frame length. The disadvantage is that they do not fold for transport. For a wheelchair to be transported in a standard vehicle, usually the rear wheels must be removed and the back folded down. Folding frames offer the advantage of easier storage in a vehicle. It also is easier to change the size because of the cross frame design, although pediatric rigid frame chairs often come with built-in growth in the cross bars. Keep in mind that anything removable or adjustable in a wheelchair increases the weight of the wheelchair.

Adjustability of the wheelchair relates to the ability of the clinician and supplier to adjust the wheelchair to maximize the performance and seated stability of the client. Components such as tire type also have an impact on performance. Details of these adjustments and components will be explained. Typically, with the client sitting in a relaxed position, his or her fingertips should touch the middle of the axle of the wheel.[31] Having to reach too far rearward puts the shoulders into too much extension, setting them up for future orthopedic problems.[31] Adjustability and components include the following:

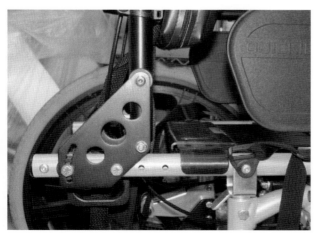

Fig. 43-3 Close-up of angle adjustable back and back depth adjustment.

> **CENTER OF GRAVITY**
> - Need to adjust back angle first, as this will affect client's center of gravity.
> - Moving the axle forward makes the chair less stable, but provides better wheel access.
> - Moving the axle rearward is more stable, but access to rear wheels more compromised.

Fig. 43-4 Axle adjustability for center of gravity.

- Axle adjustability, which controls:
  - Center of gravity of the client relative to the axle (forward and rearward movement of the axle; Fig. 43-4)
  - Rear seat height adjustment (up and down movement of the axle; Fig. 43-5)
  - Wheelbase width (moving the wheels closer to or farther away from the frame) (Fig. 43-6)
- Camber (Fig. 43-7)
- Casters (Fig. 43-8)
- Rear wheels and tires (Fig. 43-9)

Some rigid frame wheelchairs do not use an axle plate to provide adjustability. Instead they use a camber tube, which provides center of gravity adjustment and predetermined camber and wheelbase width (at the time of evaluation). Rear seat height adjustment usually is not controlled by the camber tube. Some wheelchairs adjust the rear seat height by moving the seat tubes up and down along the rear of the frame. Casters, rear wheels, and tires have an effect on performance and maneuverability.

Ultralightweight wheelchairs that are completely custom made have little, if any, adjustability. These wheelchairs usually are prescribed for individuals who have been using a wheelchair for an extended period and know the positions and postures with which they are comfortable. Because these

> **SEAT HEIGHT**
> - Adjusts rear seat height.
> - Will bring rear wheel farther up toward the client (increased elbow flexion and shoulder extension), or farther down way from the person.

Fig. 43-5 Axle adjustability for seat height.

> **WHEELBASE WIDTH**
> - "Sleeving in" brings the wheels closer to the user and decreases overall width.
> - "Sleeving out" brings the wheels farther away to accommodate the user's hips or armrests. Necessary when adding camber. Increases overall width.

Fig. 43-6 Axle adjustability for wheelbase width.

CAMBER

- Top part of wheel comes closer to person, bottom part goes out.
- Fairly easily changed with washers.
- Provides lateral stability, easier turning, more efficient push stroke.
- Increases overall width—varies according to how many degrees of camber.

Fig. 43-7 Axle adjustability for camber.

CASTERS

- Includes the wheel, fork and stem bolt.
- Determines front seat height and maneuverability (longer the fork, bigger the turning radius and vice versa)
- The larger the caster size (and wider even if smaller diameter) the better able to handle obstacles.
- Caster housing must be perpendicular to the ground.
- Some chairs have caster housing adjustability; "leading position," more anteriorly stable, but increases overall wheelbase length; opposite for "trailing" position.

Fig. 43-8 Casters.

REAR WHEELS AND TIRES

- Typically 20-26" in diameter. Size chosen relates to client's arm length relative to the wheel, as well as rear seat height (.i.e., smaller wheels for foot propellers to get set height of chair low).
- Wider tires, increased rolling resistance, but better on outdoor terrain.
- Air tires offer better shock absorbancy, but solid tires require no maintenance.
- Wheels can have spokes of different materials, or molded plastic or "mag" wheels. Spokes lighter by about 2 pounds or more.
- Specialized handrims can be added to provide extra friction or alternate means of gripping for those with decreased hand function or wrist problems.

Fig. 43-9 Rear wheels and tires.

wheelchairs are so custom made, care must be taken to ensure that the client is measured for the wheelchair according to the specific manufacturer's guidelines.[2]

Powered mobility

Powered mobility consists of powered wheelchairs, add-on power, and power assist devices for manual wheelchairs and scooters (power operated vehicles).

Powered wheelchairs

Powered wheelchair bases that are commonly used in rehabilitation settings are discussed here. Powered wheelchairs

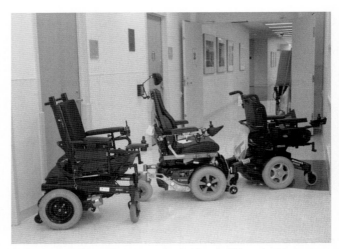

Fig. 43-10 Turning radius. Rear wheel drive *(left)* has the largest turning radius, front wheel drive *(middle)* has a midrange turning radius, and mid/center wheel drive *(right)* has the smallest radius.

are composed of the *base* of the chair, the *electronics*, and the *input method*(s) used to drive the wheelchair.

Bases Powered wheelchair bases come in rear wheel drive, mid/center wheel drive, and front wheel drive. Turning radii and driving styles vary in each base. The smallest turning radius is found with the mid/center wheel drive, then the front wheel drive, and finally the rear wheel drive (Fig. 43-10). The radius varies somewhat among manufacturers, so it is important to consult the manufacturer's literature and actually examine the bases, as some of them have "center of gravity" adjustments similar to manual wheelchairs. Powered wheelchair bases vary widely in their uses and characteristics. It is important to understand the conditions for which each type of base is meant. Using the wheelchair in a manner for which it is not designed can quickly wear out or break the wheelchair. For example, some powered wheelchair bases are meant primarily for indoor use and light outdoor use, whereas others are designed to withstand rough outdoor conditions. Fig. 43-11 shows an example

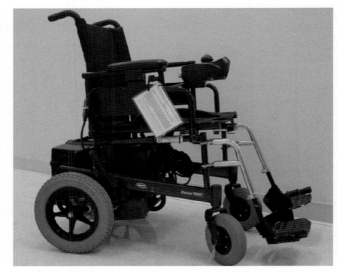

Fig. 43-11 Light-duty powered wheelchair.

of a light-duty wheelchair. Some powered bases can accept powered seating, such as powered tilt, powered recline, or powered seat elevator, whereas some cannot. For example, a "light-duty" wheelchair cannot be interfaced with powered seating.

Electronics Electronics vary with each powered wheelchair type. The controller is the part of the wheelchair that acts as the "brain," dictating the driving characteristics of the wheelchair as well as what types of input devices can be used. The client activates the input device, such as a joystick, the joystick operates the controller, and the controller operates the motors, which drive the wheelchair. Electronics of every powered wheelchair used in rehabilitation are, to some extent, programmable. Thus, the controller can be programmed to make the motors react commensurate with the client's physical, cognitive, and perceptual motor skills. At the low end, as in light-duty wheelchairs, the electronics are minimally adjustable and suit clients who are minimally physically involved. The types of parameters that can be programmed are outlined in Fig. 43-12.[19] Remember that each manufacturer lists these parameters with different terminology. Each manufacturer also has different parameters that can be adjusted other than those listed. It is recommended that the clinician and rehabilitation technology supplier consult each manufacturer's guide or use the manufacturer's representative to properly program each powered wheelchair. This is an absolutely essential part of evaluation and training. For example, a client may need fast acceleration set to provide an immediate reaction, but only up to a slow speed. Most wheelchairs have multiple speed channels or settings through which the client can toggle. All of the channels should be checked and programmed according to the client's needs.

Input methods The input method is how the client drives and controls the wheelchair. A wide array of input devices are available. Evaluators should never evaluate or train a client on an input device that they themselves have never driven. The must understand the cognitive, physical, and perceptual motor skills involved to be able to properly match their client to an appropriate input device. Input devices can be divided into those that are *proportional* and those that are *digital*. Either can be driven in *momentary* or *latched* mode. Momentary means that the wheelchair drives as long as the client is contacting the input device. Latched

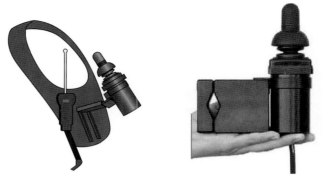

Fig. 43-13 Examples of joysticks. Bib mount for under chin *(left)* and for hand control *(right)*.

is like cruise control in a car; the chair drives until the driver actively stops it.

Proportional controls provide a range of direction and speed within 360 degrees. How large the 360-degree area can often be programmed. The controls typically are joysticks but can be devices such as touch pads. They can be placed anywhere the client has movement within that range and can be graded to allow for control of direction and speed. Joysticks (Fig. 43-13) are primarily operated by the hand but can be placed in other places, such as under the chin, behind the head, and under the foot. Proportional controls require the least complicated electronics, resulting in fewer parts to maintain.

Digital controls provide an on/off style of control, much like a light switch. There is no range of speed and direction, as with a proportional control, so the wheelchair will immediately drive exactly as programmed. With digital controls, there is one switch for each direction. Switches can include push switches, proximity switches, and pneumatic switches. These controls are used by clients who do not possess the ability to grade movements (e.g., athetoid cerebral palsy), have useful movements at various locations of their bodies (e.g., muscular dystrophy), or who are very physically limited (e.g., C3 tetraplegia). These controls require more electronic components as well as mounting systems. Digital controls are more often driven in latched. For example, if a client is using a sip and puff control, the command for the forward direction is a hard puff. If the control was not latched, the client would have to continually puff to make the chair go forward. Forward and reverse are the only directions that can be latched. Once latched in forward, the left and right directions remain momentary. When a client is driving in latched, a safety "kill" switch must be mounted where the client can consistently access in case of an emergency.

The input method can be used for functions other than driving. It also can be used to operate powered seating functions and, in some cases, other assistive technology devices such as an environmental control unit. This requires a display box to show the client which function he or she is in. A switch is also needed to change functions. Depending on the number of functions and the input method, the control can be cognitively complex.

Add-on power and power assist devices

Add-on power devices interface with a manual wheelchair. This allows the client to have a manual wheelchair that can be

---

BASIC CONTROLLER PARAMETERS

- ACCELERATION- How fast the chair ramps up to the programmed top speed in each of the directions:
  - Forward
  - Turning
- DECELERATION- How fast the chair comes to a stop once input device no longer contacted in each direction:
  - Forward
  - Turning
- SPEED- How fast the chair is allowed to go in each direction:
  - Forward
  - Reverse
  - Turning

Fig. 43-12 Basic controller parameters.

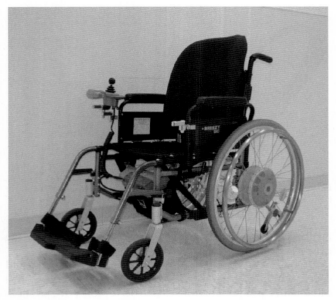

Fig. 43-14 E-fix add-on device.

scooters are available but are meant for outdoor use because of their large size and turning radius.

Best practice

ANSI/RESNA wheelchair standards provide manufacturing standards. Studies have been conducted using these standards. Funding has made it difficult to obtain more expensive ultralightweight manual wheelchairs in some cases. For example, Medicare has very stringent guidelines about who qualifies for this type of wheelchair.[14] Studies at the University of Pittsburgh found that ultralightweight wheelchairs were 10 times less costly to operate than depot wheelchairs and four times less costly to operate than lightweight wheelchairs over their lifetime.[7] Other studies found that 20% of "depot" (standard) wheelchairs, 30% of lightweight wheelchairs, and 80% of ultralightweight wheelchairs passed the minimum standards.[14] Evaluators should be aware of how models and manufacturers fare in these tests and whether the manufacturers of the wheelchairs they are recommending are compliant with the standards.

Another area of standards that has seen rapid development is wheelchair transportation safety. The standard WC-19 is voluntary for manufacturers. Currently 12 manufacturers and 48 models of wheelchairs are compliant with this standard. This standard provides four crash-tested securement points for effective wheelchair tiedown; testing to nominal 30 mph frontal crash; and crash-tested anchor pints on the wheelchair frame to which crash tested pelvic belts can be added.[16]

Few validated tools are used for manual or powered wheelchair evaluation or training. One tool, called the SmartWheel, is commercially available for objective evaluation of wheelchair setup for maximal propulsion performance.[29] This tool was developed by Dr. Rory Cooper and associates at the Human Engineering Research Labs in Pittsburgh, Pennsylvania.[8] The SmartWheel measures forces and torques applied to the pushrim. It is mounted to the user's wheelchair or to an evaluation wheelchair. Information gathered includes average speed, average stroke length, average propulsion force, and efficiency. The standard protocol for gathering this information includes performing a figure-of-eight on tile, a straight line on tile, a straight line on carpet, and a straight line on an Americans with Disabilities Act (ADA)-compliant ramp. A user's group is compiling this and other information from clinical investigations using the Smart Wheel.[13]

The Wheelchair Skills Program (*www.wheelchairskillsprogram.ca*) of Dalhousie University in Nova Scotia is a validated program designed to provide testing and training of manual wheelchair skills for both clients and caregivers. This program was created by Dr. R.L. Kirby, who has been a long-time researcher in the area of wheelchair safety. This web site provides published evidence related to the program, a list of publications (many related to wheelchair safety), and detailed images (still and movies) and written information for the development of manual wheelchair skills.

Mobility plays a critical role in functional independence as well as a fundamental role in rehabilitative medicine. Approximately 68% of manual wheelchair users report some type of upper extremity pain,[15,28] with the incidence of shoulder pain generally being the highest.[9,10,28] Research suggests that the relatively high joint moments at the shoulder during propulsion change significantly based on speed of

transported without an adapted vehicle. The client can use the manual wheelchair without the power add-on parts. Fig. 43-14 shows the E-fix (Frank Mobility, Oakdale, PA) add-on device. This device can only be operated through a joystick and has minimally adjustable electronics. Because the base is a manual wheelchair, it is meant for indoor and non-challenging outdoor terrain.

Push rim activated power devices add on to manual wheelchair bases. Their purpose is to augment the client's propelling to reduce the amount of force and effort required. They were developed in response to research on damage to upper extremities caused by long-term propelling. Additionally, the devices enable clients with weak upper extremities to propel in a more functional manner, especially in more challenging areas, such as areas with ramps. The disadvantage of these devices is that they are heavy (the motor is contained in the hubs of the wheels), and clients who currently transfer their own wheelchair into their vehicle may not be able to or may have difficulty with transferring the wheels. On the other hand, as with the power add-on, the manual wheelchair can be used without the device by removing the power assist wheels and using the regular wheels.

These devices can be used on almost any manual wheelchair. It is best to consult with each manufacturer.

Scooters (power operated vehicles)

Scooters provide mobility for clients who have good to normal upper extremity control and have the ability to sit against gravity. The advantage of scooters are that they are narrower than powered wheelchairs and are more conducive to carrying things because a basket can be added to the front of these vehicles. Additionally, they usually come with a swivel seat and powered seat elevator, which often can assist with transfers and other ADLs. Although they are more narrow, their turning radii tend to be bigger than with most powered wheelchairs. Their three-wheel design makes them potentially unstable on uneven surfaces. Four-wheel propulsion, ramp inclination, and pushrim diameters.[26–28] Although joint moments at both the shoulder and elbow are nearly double those at the wrist, complaints of wrist pain are equally common.[26] This finding suggests that mechanisms other than joint moment magnitude are indicators of overuse injury. Ergonomic research has revealed that neither isometric strength nor job demand alone is a sensitive predictor of job-related injury.[28] Study has shown that injury is more likely when a required task is performed at or near the defined maximal exertion.[28] Baley et al.[1] found that the most common etiology of shoulder pain is chronic rotator cuff impingement with subacromial bursitis. A relationship between time since injury and upper extremity complaints was reported. Complaints increased from 50% after 5 years to almost 100% after 20 years. The study concluded that upper extremity pain was a consequence of increased stresses placed on joints as a result of their use for weight bearing and mobility. Kinetic wheelchair propulsion studies have shown that the highest superiorly directed shoulder joint reaction forces were experienced by subjects with tetraplegia during contact with the pushrim.[20] This vertical force must be counterbalanced by increased action of the muscles that depress the humeral head to prevent impingement.[21] Strength testing showed that subjects with tetraplegia have reduced strength in the rotator cuff muscle group than do subjects with paraplegia.[21,25] Although persons with tetraplegia have reduced strength, they do not demonstrate significantly altered patterns of shoulder and elbow motions during propulsion.[21] Therefore, persons with tetraplegia may have higher incidences of shoulder pathology because of the alterations in patterns of shoulder muscle activity.[21]

Sabick et al.[28] found that the internal moments required by propulsion were greatest in shoulder flexion and elbow extension. The most common shoulder injuries are muscle and tendon pathologies; however, other bony disorders, such as degenerative arthritis and osteonecrosis, exist because these structures generate and/or transmit loads across the joint. An increase in muscle force will cause compression of articulating bones at joints; therefore, structures most commonly injured are most directly impacted because of their need to generate larger joint moments.[28]

In summary, choosing the method of wheeled mobility requires a deep understanding of the client's cognition, function ability, daily activities, and utilization pattern. The environment in which the device will be used, the options for distance transportation, and the cost must be considered. An intensive team consultative process is vital for determining the best device for each person's needs.

Acknowledgment

Special thanks to Erin Elizabeth Taylor, BSBE, for assistance in research and data compilation.

References

1. Bayley JC, Cochran TP, Sledge CB: The weight-bearing shoulder. The impingement syndrome in paraplegics, *J Bone Joint Surg Am* 69:676–678, 1987.
2. Betz K: Welded for wheeling: custom ultralights prescribed with confidence. In: *Proceedings of the 21st International Seating Symposium*, Orlando, Florida, February 2005, pp. 61–64.
3. Boninger ML, Baldwin M, Cooper R, Koontz A, Chan L: Manual wheelchair push rim biomechanics and axle position, *Arch Phys Med Rehabil* 81:513–608, 2000.
4. Brighton C: Rules of the road, *Rehabil Manage* April:18-21, 2003.
5. Cook A, Hussey S: *Assistive technology: principles and practice*, St. Louis, 1995, Mosby, p. 558.
6. Cook A, Hussey S: *Assistive technology: principles and practice*, St. Louis, 1995, Mosby, p. 559.
7. Cooper RA, Robertson RN, Lawrence B, et al: Life cycle analysis of depot vs rehabilitation model wheelchairs, *J Rehabil Res Dev* 33:45–55, 1996.
8. Cooper RA, Robertson RN, VanSickle DP, Boninger ML: Kinematics, upper limb biomechanics and wheelchairs: methods for determining 3 dimensional wheelchair and pushrim forces and moments: a technical note, *J Rehabil Res Dev* 34:162, 1997.
9. Curtis KA, Black K: Shoulder pain in female wheelchair basketball players, *J Orthop Sports Phys Ther* 29:225–231, 1999.
10. Curtis KA, Drysdale GA, Lanza RD, Kolber M, Vitolo RS, West R: Shoulder pain in wheelchair users with tetraplegia and paraplegia, *Arch Phys Med Rehabil* 80:453–457, 1999.
11. Curtis KA, Drysdale GA, Lanza RD, Kolber M, Vitolo RS, West R: Shoulder pain in wheelchair users with tetraplegia and paraplegia, *Arch Phys Med Rehabil* 80:453–457, 1999.
12. Davies A, DeSouza L, Frank A: Changes in the quality of life in severely disabled people following provision of powered indoor/outdoor chairs, *Disabil Rehabil* 25:286–290, 2003.
13. DiGiovine C, Koontz A: Development of and use of a standard clinical protocol for the assessment of wheelchair propulsion biomechanics. In: *Proceedings of the 21st International Seating Symposium*, Orlando, Florida, February 2005, p. 77.
14. Fitzgerald SG, Cooper RA, Boninger ML, Rentschler AJ: Comparison of fatigue life for three different types of manual wheelchairs, *Arch Phys Med Rehabil* 82:1484–1488, 2001.
15. Gellman H, Chandler DR, Petrasek J, Sie I, Adkins R, Waters RL: Carpal tunnel syndrome in paraplegic patients, *J Bone Joint Surg Am* 70:517–519, 1988.
16. Hobson D, VanRoosmalen L, Buning ME: Review of standards, principles and best practice of automotive safety for wheelchair seated passengers. In: Proceedings of the 21st International Seating Symposium, Orlando, Florida, February 2005, p. 55.
17. Jones ML, Sanford JA: People with mobility impairments in the US today and in 2010, *Assist Technol* 8:43–45, 1996.
18. Kreutz D, Taylor SJ: Wheelchair mobility. In Olson D, Dureyter F, editors: *A clinician's guide to assistive technology*, St. Louis, 2002, Mosby, p. 311.
19. Kreutz D, Taylor SJ: Wheelchair mobility. In Olson D, Dureyter F, editors: *A clinician's guide to assistive technology*, St. Louis, 2002, Mosby, p. 317.
20. Kulig K, Newsam CJ, Mulroy SJ, et al: The effect of level of spinal cord injury on shoulder joint kinetics during manual wheelchair propulsion, *Clin Biomech* 16:744–751, 2001.
21. Mulroy SJ, Farrokhi S, Newman CJ, Perry J: Effects of spinal cord injury level on the activity of shoulder muscles during wheelchair propulsion: an electromyographic study, *Arch Phys Med Rehabil* 85:925–933, 2004.
22. National Registry of Rehabilitation Technology Suppliers: NRRTS.org
23. Pentland W, Twomey L: Upper limb function in persons with long term paraplegia and implications for independence: part 1, *Paraplegia* 32:211–218, 1994.
24. Pentland W, Twomey L: Upper limb function in persons with long term paraplegia and implications for independence: part 2, *Paraplegia* 32:219–224, 1994.
25. Powers C, Newsam C, Gronley JK, Fontaine C, Perry J: Isometric shoulder torques in patients with spinal cord injury, *Arch Phys Med Rehabil* 75:761–765, 1994.
26. Robertson RN, Boninger ML, Cooper RA, Shimada SD: Pushrim forces and joint kinetics during wheelchair propulsion, *Arch Phys Med Rehabil* 77:856–864, 1996.
27. Rodgers MM, Gayle GW, Figoni SF, Kobayashi M, Lieh J, Glaser RM: Biomechanics of wheelchair propulsion during fatigue, *Arch Phys Med Rehabil* 75:85–93, 1994.
28. Sabick MB, Katajarri BR, An KN: A new method to quantify demand on the upper extremities during manual wheelchair propulsion, *Arch Phys Med Rehabil* 85:1151–1159, 2004.
29. SmartWheel: Three Rivers Holding, LLC, Mesa, AZ, *www.3rivers.com*.
30. Taylor SJ, Kreutz DJ: Powered mobility evaluation and technology, *Top Spinal Cord Injury Rehabil* 1:24, 1995.
31. Vanderwoude LHV, Veeger DJ, Rozendal RH, Sargeant TJ: Seat height in handrim propulsion, *J Rehabil Res Dev* 26:31–50, 1989.
32. Waters LH, Sie RL: Upper extremity changes in SCI contrasted to common aging in the musculoskeletal system, *Top Spinal Cord Rehabil* 6:61–68, 2001.
33. Wilson B: The evolution of wheelchairs, *Top Spinal Cord Injury Rehabil* 1:45–53, 1995.

Chapter

44

Seating and positioning for disabled children and adults

Jan Furumasu

Key Points

- The pelvis is key to seating and positioning.
- Points of control rely on a three-point system.
- Support is best with dispersed forces using large surface areas.
- Deformity is best accommodated rather than trying to correct.
- Support should not restrict daily activities.

People with disabilities are living longer, and their number is growing. In 2003, 34.3 million people (12.1% of the population) in the United States (noninstitutionalized) had physical limitations in activities due to a chronic condition. An estimated 1.6 million are wheelchair users. Baby boomers are coming of age and are acquiring disabling conditions. By the year 2030, the number of elderly will double to 71.5 million. Medical technology has improved the rate of survival for children and adults with disabilities and their long-term management. Long-term debility is a major risk factor for pressure ulcers. Improvement in the survival rate has increased the number of persons at risk for pressure sores. An estimated five million people in the United States have chronic wounds. From 1.1 to 1.8 million people develop new ulcers each year, and the financial cost and emotional burden are heavy.[4,49] The two groups at highest risk are the elderly and persons with spinal cord injury (SCI).[3,19] Advances in seating and mobility have made a difference in controlling deformities, preventing pressure sores, and expanding the individual's potential in life, ensuring participation socially, educationally, and vocationally. Proper seating is like an

external orthosis, important for support, comfort, and pressure relief in sitting.[18] Better anatomical alignment of the pelvis and trunk enhances physiological functions, such as swallowing and cardiopulmonary function, and affects upper extremity function. Postural supports enhance functional movement by decreasing the influence of abnormal tone and reflexes, thereby improving postural alignment and potential access to technologies, such as powered mobility, communication devices, and computers (Fig. 44-1). The seating system should be as dynamic as possible to allow for growth changes in a child or if a decline in function is anticipated. The seating system must be user friendly for the person in the wheelchair and for the caregiver. The user, family, and caregivers play a key role and must be interviewed extensively regarding the user's medical and functional needs, environmental considerations, and lifestyle issues.

The best prescription involves an evaluation process by a team of professionals knowledgeable in the medical issues. The evaluation should identify physical abilities and limitations, predict functional capabilities, identify problems with existing seating, and set goals to match the user's needs with the seating technology. The end result will be the recommendation of a useful and functional system.

Evaluation process for seating and mobility systems

A seating and mobility system evaluation should address all aspects of a person's medical and personal lifestyle issues. The following categories should be assessed thoroughly.

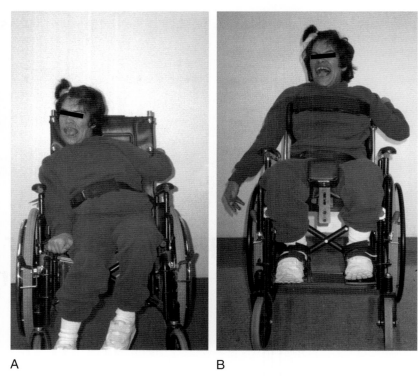

A   B

Fig. 44-1 A, Young woman before evaluation of seating system. **B,** Same woman with seating system that provides support and alignment, increasing functional abilities.

Medical History: All medical diagnoses (primary and secondary) are important to identify and document as well as whether the disability is stable, progressive, or fluctuates. Pertinent history that will have an impact on mobility and positioning needs includes history of pressure sores, spasticity management, medications, orthotic use, and sitting tolerance. A detailed interview regarding pressure sore development, management, and successful treatment is important in preventing recurrence. Prior and future surgical interventions, such as spinal fusion, muscle releases, and amputations will affect seating decisions. Prior equipment use and identification of previous problems is helpful in justifying future seating intervention.

Physical Assessment: Physical assessment includes the person's range of motion, skeletal alignment or posture, motor strength or motor control of the head, trunk and extremities, sitting balance, sensation, interfering tone, or reflexes. Is the muscle tone low or hypotonic? Does the client have hypertonicity, which may require more aggressive seating components to control tonic movement?

Range of Motion: Range of motion of the joints and spine assesses whether postural supports can correct or must accommodate perceived deformities. Flexibility and asymmetries of the hip and pelvis and hamstring tightness are critical areas of assessment. Evaluating asymmetries in hip flexion, scoliosis, and pelvic obliquities and determining whether the deformities are fixed or flexible is important to determining successful solutions. Seating starts from the pelvis and hips, so assessment of pelvic obliquity, scoliosis, tight hamstrings, and hip muscles is critical for ensuring proper positioning.

Reflex-Influenced Posturing: Is reflex-influenced posturing interfering with the patient's functional potential for maintaining the sitting position? For example, two influential primitive reflexes active in seated posture are the *tonic labyrinthine reflex*, which causes extension of the head, trunk, and extremities as the body tilts backward or reclines, and *asymmetrical tonic neck reflexes*, which cause rotation of head, trunk and pelvis and potentially a windswept deformity. At times, this reflex posturing is functionally used to extend the upper extremity in order to drive a power wheelchair or point to a communication device. Persons with athetosis or dyskinetic-type movement disorders may use reflex posturing for stability in order to use their extremities purposefully. The seating device may help inhibit unwanted movements and permit functional movements.[6]

Muscle Strength: Evaluation of muscle strength assesses functional potential with, and the need for, appropriate postural supports. The need for adequate support for sitting balance and pressure distribution versus adequate freedom of movement must be balanced. Overseating can discourage functional potential. For example, a high back on a person with functional low-level tetraplegia would eliminate his or her ability to balance the upper body or to hook the arm over the push handle of a lower back in order to increase forward reach with the opposite arm. Evaluating muscle strength helps determine whether posturing is compensatory for muscle paralysis, weakness, or imbalance. Clients with Duchenne muscular dystrophy have proximal muscle weakness and are able to increase their upper extremity reach by leaning forward and to the side. Restricting trunk motion limits their ability to compensate for proximal weakness in order to reach with and use the distal strength in their hands.

Evaluation of Protective Sensation: Evaluation of protective sensation and assessing for red areas or potential pressure areas helps to determine the appropriate seating surface. History of scar tissue or previous pressure sore intervention can predict areas of high risk. Aging affects the elasticity of the skin and increases risk of damage from shearing, pressure, heat, and moisture.

Functional assessment

Everything the person presently can accomplish from the seating system should be addressed in the functional component of the evaluation. This includes all areas of *mobility-related activities of daily living*: self-mobility, ability to stand and ambulate, transfer, manage the bladder, and drive a vehicle. New seating and mobility systems should not interfere with any previously independent abilities. For example, some persons with tetraplegia need to open the seat to back angle by reclining the back of the wheelchair in order to empty their bladder. Replacing the power back recline with a tilt-in-space system may affect bladder function by not allowing the person to empty the bladder as previously accomplished. Swingaway trunk supports allow trunk movement but lock in for stability when needed. Environmental accessibility, including school or work sites, and the person's recreational activities must be explored.

Transportation: Issues related to safe transportation of the person as a driver or passenger include tiedown (securing the wheelchair in a vehicle while the person is seated in it), wheelchair seat height, breakdown of the wheelchair for loading into a car, or overall length of the mobility base on van lifts.

Cognitive Status/Behavioral Assessment: Cognitive status/behavioral assessment includes memory skills, problem-solving abilities, ability to comprehend, concrete versus abstract reasoning, destructive behavior, motivation, and safety judgment. For example, clients who are agitated or have destructive tendencies require seating that is protective and durable so that body parts are not accidentally injured against hardware.

Visual/Perceptual Ability: Individuals who cannot separate head movement from eye movement can compensate for visual field cuts by head posturing or trunk movement. Compromises in seating supports are necessary to compensate for visual impairments. The position of the head and upper body in space affects visual field.

Other considerations include cosmesis, financial constraints, caregiver management, and changes that may occur due to physical, cognitive, or medical reasons.

The outcome of evaluation of a person's seating needs focuses on one of three areas in a framework for seating and positioning decision making categorized by Cook and Hussey[9]: technologies for postural control (typically for the child or client with cerebral palsy), technologies for pressure control, for those at high risk (e.g., population with SCI), or technologies for comfort (for the elderly or patient with amyotrophic lateral sclerosis).

Seating alignment

Ideal sitting alignment is different for an able-bodied person than for a disabled person, and depends on the individual's abilities. Sitting is dynamic; it is a continuous process of postural changes whether the position is task oriented or one of rest. For the able-bodied person, a sitting posture with an anterior pelvic tilt and decreased lumbar flexion is the most

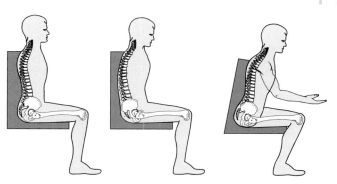

Fig. 44-2 Three dynamic postures of sitting: upright with slight anterior pelvis, posterior pelvis, and forward trunk or position of readiness.

favorable posture.[17,18,40] Generally three postures of sitting alignment are assumed (Fig. 44-2). Ideally, an upright, symmetrically balanced trunk over a stable pelvis allows better upper extremity reach, head control, and visual field. However, in the sitting position, the pelvis tends to roll back into a posterior tilt because the hips are flexed and the hamstrings pull the pelvis back; the tilt is accentuated when the knees are extended.[50] The line of gravity is posterior to the ischial tuberosities. This posture is adopted as a position of rest by an able-bodied person and as a position of stability by a wheelchair user with tetraplegia. The second sitting position is achieved by activating the back extensors to tilt the pelvis anteriorly into lumbar lordosis. As the pelvis rolls anteriorly, the line of gravity falls directly through the ischial tuberosities.[15] This posture usually is assumed by a person with muscular disease as it is functionally advantageous because of weakness that is greater proximally than distally.[16] The third seated posture is a forward sitting posture that has been described by Kangas[25] and Adrian and Cooper[1] as a functional task position or position of readiness. In this position, the trunk is forward and the line of gravity shifts toward the direction of activity. The trunk flexes forward in a position of anticipation. The arms and trunk are naturally brought forward into the visual field, and the feet are shifted backward behind the knees and bear more weight.

Outcome studies of seating and positioning for function

A number of studies reported on how seating affects functional activities, upper extremity function, head control, and visual field.[24,33,36] The components of a seating system can provide support to align the body, normalize tone, prevent deformities, and clearly influence upper extremity movement. In one study, the sitting surface was explored to better determine the capacity to maintain balance and posture as a prerequisite for activities of daily living. The center of pressure of reaching was determined to be significantly greater on a generically contoured sitting surface than on a flat foam surface or a 3-inch Roho seat cushion.[2] The effect of different backrest heights and types of cushions were investigated in the SCI population to determine the relationship between posture and upper extremity reaching. The posture adopted by the user and the American Spinal

Outcome Studies for Seating and Positioning

1. Normalization or decreased influence of abnormal tone and reflexes in clients with cerebral palsy.
2. Improved physiological functions including vocalizations, swallowing, vital capacity, and oral motor function.
3. Improved upper extremity reach in clients with spinal cord injuries.
4. Upper extremity function can be influenced by changes of positioning in space or of the sitting surface.
5. The sitting surface affects the comfort and function.
6. Prevention of pressure sores.

Fig. 44-3 Outcomes of studies of seating and positioning.

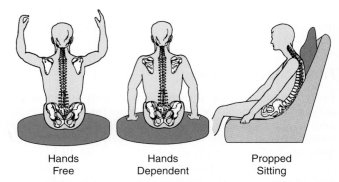

Hands Free Hands Dependent Propped Sitting

Fig. 44-4 Classification of sitting ability grouped according to the amount of trunk control present and the amount of support needed in a seating system.

Injury Association (ASIA) score were significant, and no evidence indicated that the type of cushion or back height affected reach.[48]

Improvements in autonomic functioning, including respiratory, oral intake and digestion in children with cerebral palsy was found following adjustments in seating systems with improvement of the trunk, neck and head alignment.[7] Hulme[23] found positive perceived changes in social interaction, positioning, tracking, grasping, and self-feeding skills. Nwaobi[37] found that the vital capacity in children with cerebral palsy improved with positioning in a seating system versus a sling type wheelchair. Improvements in speech intelligibility were documented in children with cerebral palsy using adapted seating versus without.[34]

Reports on the effects of seating on upper extremity function are conflicting. In a 1986 study of children with cerebral palsy, different amounts of hip flexion were found to affect upper extremity function.[36] Another study found that children with cerebral palsy were able to activate and release a switch the fastest when they were in an anterior 15-degree tilt or in the position of readiness versus 0, 15, or 30 degrees of tilt back.[35] However, McPherson et al.[31] found no significant differences in the quality of upper extremity movement in subjects with cerebral palsy in four different positions. Seeger et al.[45] also did not find any improvement (Fig. 44-3).

Seating assessment

Hands-on evaluation should be performed with the person either sitting or supine on the mat. Critical assessment of whether deformities are dynamic or fixed is more accurate when the patient is supine. Depending on the person's disability, a mat assessment is not always mandatory. The three main determinations of the hands-on evaluation are as follows:

1. Person's ability to sit
2. Pattern of deformity while the patient is in the sitting position
3. Deformity is fixed or flexible

Classifications and description of sitting ability

The ability to sit independently is one factor that determines the type or amount of seating support needed. Hoffer[21] classified a person's ability to sit according to the amount of trunk control present. His classifications were modified by Tredwell and Roxborough in 1991 to include generalizations regarding the type of seating needed (Fig 44-4):

Hands-Free Sitting Ability: Maintains independent sitting for long periods without using hands for support. Demonstrates good trunk balance and the ability to weight shift. In general, a person needs a simple seating system designed primarily for pelvic stability, comfort, and mobility (e.g., person with paraplegia).

Hand-Dependent Sitting Ability: Requires either one or both hands for support. Trunk control and balance are generally poor. Trunk supports are needed to allow use of hands for functional activities. Providing a more stable base of pelvic support may change a hand-dependent sitter to a hand-free sitter.

Propped Sitting Ability: Because of severe physical involvement or structural deformity, the person is unable to sit without total body support. Trunk and head control are very limited. Total support of the trunk, head, and extremities is needed, as for a person who demonstrates total body involvement with cerebral palsy, has a severe muscle disease, or has a high-level tetraplegia.

Patterns of deformity

The position of the pelvis influences the alignment of the trunk and therefore of the shoulders, upper extremities, and head. The three common patterns of postural malalignment are as follows[28]:

Symmetrically Slouched: This position begins with a posterior pelvic tilt. The trunk collapses into a C curve, and the shoulders are protracted with the head forward. The most common cause of a posterior pelvic tilt in persons with cerebral palsy is hamstring hypertonicity. For persons with tetraplegia, the symmetrically slouched position can be a position of stability in which they are able to raise their arms for balance and functional activities[28].

Lordotic Posture: This posture begins with an anterior pelvic tilt. The pelvic tilt locks the lumbar facets into extension, mechanically providing spinal stability. Hyperlordosis typically is observed in patients with Duchenne muscular dystrophy prior to spine fusion because of proximal weakness and an imbalance in strength between the abdominals and back extensors.

Asymmetrical or Windswept Posture: This posture is one of the most difficult deformities to control and to treat. The windswept deformity is described as being windswept to the left if the left thigh is abducted and the right thigh is adducted. It is associated with a triad of deformities: dislocated or subluxed hip usually on the adducted side, pelvic obliquity, and scoliosis. A dislocated hip may be painful, severe scoliosis may compromise cardiopulmonary function, and the increase in pelvic obliquity increases the risk for pressure sores.[12,41] The person may try to offload the painful hip, which worsens the position and pressure distribution.

The relationship among windswept hips, pelvic obliquity/hip dislocation, and scoliosis was first described by Letts in 1984 in children with cerebral palsy. "Acquired and preventable Special Seating will **NOT** prevent a contracted hip from dislocating." However, Letts did advocate abduction of the lower extremities to 25 degrees and not just neutral to decrease abnormal muscle activity.[27] Increased abduction also results in good approximation of the head of the femur into the acetabulum, which promotes bony joint development in children. Therefore, flexion and abduction of the hip are recommended to prevent extensor and adductor posturing in children with cerebral palsy who are at risk for development of the windblown syndrome. Without adequate fixation of the pelvis, however, this position may be difficult to obtain.

High complication rates have been documented in patients with severe neuromuscular scoliosis: 81% by Loinstein[30] in 1984 and 48% by Boachi[8] in 1989. They believed that the high risk of surgery outweighs the benefits, so comfortable seating is the treatment of choice. Table 44-1 lists possible causes and equipment solutions for postural alignment problems.

Severity of the deformity (fixed vs flexible)

Rang et al.[41] categorized severity of the deformity into to three stages: (a) flexible or preventable deformities, (b) deformities amenable to surgical correction that must be maintained, and (c) deformities that are fixed and are not surgically correctable. Evaluating whether deformities are fixed or flexible is important for determining the type of seating components needed. For example, many flexible deformities can be supported by adjustable positioning components, whereas fixed deformities may require more customized solutions.

Biomechanical principles of seating

As a general guideline, providing proximal stability will enhance distal function. Alignment of the pelvis and trunk affects the upper extremities and head, which in turn affect the visual field. The following biomechanical principles should be considered when determining a person's seating prescription.

Assessing for seat to back angle

Seat to back angle is important in maintaining pelvic positioning. Muscle tone and range of motion are assessed together to determine the seat to back angle. The popliteal angle, or how far the knee will extend with the hip flexed to 90 degrees,

must be determined to address dynamic range limitations affecting foot placement (Fig. 44-5).[41]

Hip flexion range should be carefully checked for asymmetry. At least 90 degrees of hip flexion is ideal. If hip flexion in one hip is less than 90 degrees, an asymmetrical seat or cushion will be needed. The hip with less flexion (e.g., 70 degrees of flexion as a result of heterotrophic ossification) should be accommodated by cutting a trough in the cushion to allow the femur to extend. The opposite hip with adequate flexion range (90 degrees) keeps the pelvis from sliding into a posterior tilt. The amount of extensor tone should be assessed as the hips and knees are flexed. Hypertonicity of the hamstrings can pull the pelvis into a posterior tilt, causing the hips to slide down. Stabilizing the pelvis by flexing the hips and knees, sometimes more than 90 degrees, decreases the influence of extensor posturing (Fig. 44-6).

The pelvis is the key!

The influence of pelvic stability on alignment and function cannot be overemphasized. Stabilizing the pelvis influences trunk alignment and balance. The three main points of control are (a) support beneath the pelvis, capturing the ischial tuberosities to prevent a posterior tilt, incorporated into the seat or seat cushion; (b) posterior support (lumbosacral back support); and (c) anterior support, such as that provided by a hip belt.

The following are seating considerations that improve pelvic position.

An *antithrust seat* maintains an upright pelvis by preventing the ischial tuberosities from sliding forward (Fig. 44-7). The ischial tuberosities are blocked from sliding forward by a dense block of foam raised up to support the thighs. If pressure relief is a concern, then the pelvis must be incorporated in a softer medium or suspended (see section on pressure relief). This "positioning" can be achieved within the wheelchair frame by *"squeezing" the frame.* Increased hip flexion with the back rest perpendicular to the floor, sometimes referred to as "squeeze" or "bucket" in a wheelchair frame, has been demonstrated to increase upper extremity vertical reach. The low back supports the pelvis upright, and the increased hip flexion (14 degrees of seat angulation) prevents the pelvis from sliding into a posterior tilt. This positioning of the frame decreases shoulder protraction and forward head posture, and decreases posterior pelvic tilt in persons with paraplegias and low-level tetraplegia (Fig. 44-8). The standard wheelchair configuration demonstrates an increase in posterior pelvic tilt in such individuals.[18]

Pelvic rotation must be evaluated with seat depth. If the pelvis is rotated forward, a longer sitting surface under the thigh of the forward anterior superior iliac spine (ASIS) is needed for adequate support. Likewise, the depth should be cut back on the side of the backwardly rotated pelvis to prevent the pelvis from being pulled into posterior tilt (Fig. 44-9). *Posterior support of the pelvis* begins with a solid back or adjustable lumbosacral support. A firm support behind the posterior iliac spine will prevent the pelvis from tilting back. Providing support of the posterior pelvis separate from the upper torso has been a challenge for manufacturers of seating systems. The "biangular back" consists of two components. The lower component supports the pelvis in an upright position, and the upper component adjusts

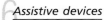

Table 44-1 Causes and equipment for patterns of deformities

Problem	Cause	Equipment Solutions
Slouched posture		
Posterior pelvic tilt	Sling upholstery	Three-point control: solid seat, firm back, and pelvic/hip seat belt
		Rigid anterior pelvic support: subasis bar, knee blocks
	Inappropriate seat depth	Measure from PSIS to popliteal, include fixed kyphosis
Hip/knee extension	Extensor tone (hip and knee)	Antithrust seat
		Increase hip angle >90 degrees
		Increase knee angle >90 degrees (foot placement behind knee)
	Hip extension contracture	Accommodate seat cushion to unilateral contracture
Thoracic kyphosis	Trunk weakness/paralysis	Unilateral split seat or leg trough, to maintain trunk upright
	Fixed deformity	Recline back, tilt back in spine
		Lower back height, accommodate in back cushion
Shoulder protraction	Spasticity/weakness	Firm back with lumbar/thoracic extension
	Back height too high	Appropriate back height
		Accommodate with molded back
		Shoulder straps pulling up and back
Forward head posture	Weakness	Occipital support with capital extension
	Spasticity	Head band (stationary or dynamic) attached to head rest
	Reflex posturing if too reclined	Recline back or tilt back to seat angle
Rotational/oblique posture		
Pelvic obliquity/pelvic rotation	Sling seat	Firm seat
	Scoliosis	Lateral hip guides
	Hip dislocation	Flexible: build up under low side for even pressure
	Asymmetrical hip ROM	Fixed: build up under high side, relieve pressure under low side
		Custom-molded seat
		Off-set cut-out in cushion
		Accommodate seat depth for leg length discrepancy
		Anterior pelvic belt
		Two-piece sub-ASIS bar
Hip problems	Sling seat	Firm seat with medial thigh support
Hip adducted—internal rotation	Adductor tone	Medical thigh support
Hip abduction—external rotation	Hypotonia	Lateral thigh/knee stabilizers
	Fixed deformity	Accommodate
Windswept hips	Pelvic rotation	Three-point control: hip guides, medial, and lateral thigh support
Adducted thigh with abducted thigh	Dislocated hip	Build up for lack of thigh support
	Scoliosis	Custom-molded seat
Thoracic scoliosis	Pelvic obliquity and rotation	Three-point control: pelvic/trunk supports
Flexible	Weakness	Deep contoured back or trunk supports

Table 44-1 Causes and equipment for patterns of deformities *(Continued)*

Problem	Cause	Equipment Solutions
	Spasticity	Rotational deformity: curved supports
Fixed	Asymmetric tone/muscle strength	Custom-molded back or adjustable-tension back upholstery to accommodate to rib hump deformity
Asymmetric head posture	Scoliosis	Appropriate support of pelvis, trunk, and shoulder girdle
	Fluctuating tone	
	Reflex posturing	Head and neck support. Support of occiput to mastoid process or over the ear to the temple for lateral control
	Weakness	
	Visual compensation	Stationary or dynamic headband
Lordotic posture		
Anterior pelvic tilt	Muscle imbalance	Placement of belt across ASIS
Hip flexion	Abdominal weakness	Wedge seat/cushion to accommodate if fixed
Thoracic lordosis	Contractures	Tilt in space manual or power frame, adjustable seat angle
		Anterior chest support: molded chest plate, wide Velcro strap
Retracted shoulders	Spasticity	Appropriate pelvic/trunk positioning with chest support
	Posturing for trunk weakness	Shoulder wedges
Extended head posture	Spasticity	Neck ring
	Weakness	Occipital support

to align the upper torso over the pelvis instead of being pitched forward if the back were straight.

Anterior support, usually a crucially placed seatbelt, is the third point in controlling the pelvis. The angle of pull, between 45 and 90 degrees, depends on the position of the pelvis and the amount of support needed. Preventing hip adduction assists in decreasing extensor tone. Clients who demonstrate increased extensor tone benefit from abduction of the hip, using a medial thigh stabilizer or abductor to position the thighs past midline to stabilize the pelvis anteriorly. The medial stabilizer should never be used against the groin but used only to position the thighs from midline to wider.

Three points of control

To control deformities, opposing forces are applied around the joint center (Fig. 44-10). To support a scoliosis, offset trunk and lateral hip supports are needed. Likewise, for

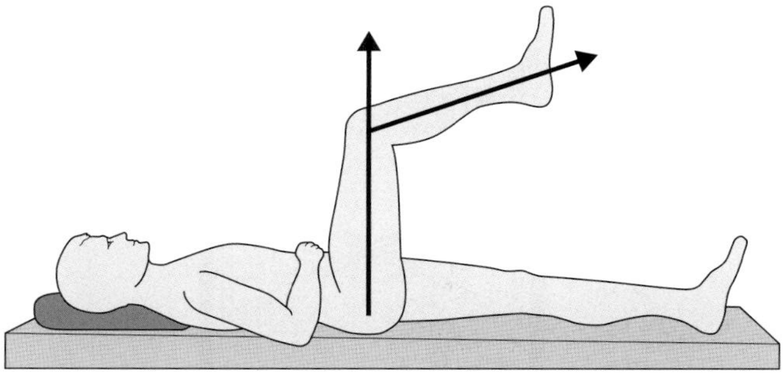

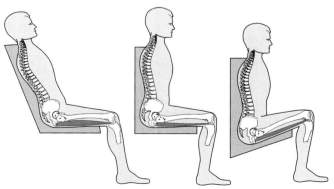

Fig. 44-5 Evaluation of popliteal angle to determine hamstring tightness with 90 degrees of hip flexion.

Fig. 44-6 Assessment of hip flexion, tone, and trunk control to determine seat to back angle.

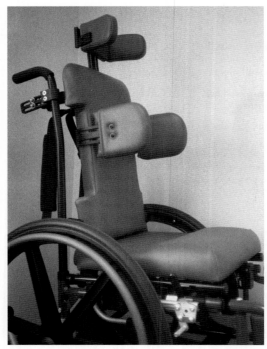

Fig. 44-7 Antithrust seat prevents ischial tuberosities from sliding forward and maintains pelvic positioning.

controlling a kyphosis or lordosis in the sagittal plane, an anterior support of the shoulder girdle and pelvis is needed. Seating supports have been documented to improve flexible scoliosis in 35% of children with cerebral palsy using a three-point force system configuration compared to no support and only a two-point lateral support system.[22]

Control Forces as Far Away from Joint as Possible: Less force is needed distally. Scoliosis or windswept hip deformities are best controlled with maximum lever length and a three-point control system.

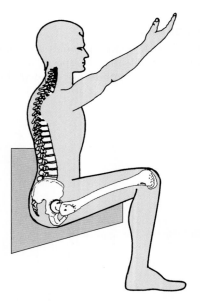

Fig. 44-8 Squeezing a frame maintains pelvic positioning, improving upper extremity reach.

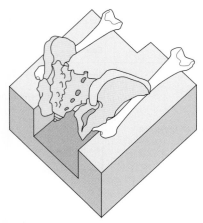

Fig. 44-9 Accommodation of seat depth because of pelvic rotation, leg–length discrepancy, or hip dislocation.

Firm versus Flexible Supports: Firm supports hold posture better than do flexible supports. For example, sling seat upholstery does not provide as much support as a rigid seat.

Increased Surface Contact to Disperse Pressure: To optimize pressure distribution, the contact surface area should be increased to disperse the pressures over a larger area. For example, a contoured seating system distributes sitting pressures better than a planar seating system.

Accommodation versus Correction of Deformity

Fixed deformities as well as "functional posturing" must be accommodated. For example, to accommodate a fixed pelvic obliquity with the right side down, the cushion must be built up on the left and/or relieved under the right to distribute the weight-bearing pressures as evenly as possible. Another example is a child who must turn his head because of a visual field deficit. This posturing should not be "corrected" or prevented if it is the child's way of compensating.

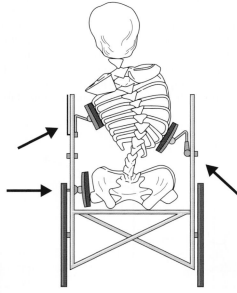

Fig. 44-10 Opposing forces of a three-point control system to control a deformity.

Positioning in space

Position in space affects a person's trunk balance and control. In an upright position, trunk movement forward and laterally can be balanced with minimal muscle activity. This is especially important for people with muscle diseases. Children with cerebral palsy may be more affected by the tonic labyrinthine reflex when they are reclined back, experiencing an increase in extensor tone and posturing overall.[32] However, once their trunk and head is positioned in a more upright posture, extensor tone is less influential and access to technology using their head or upper extremities may improve.[35] Nonetheless, for patients with poor trunk and head control, the back must be slightly reclined to assist with support. Upright positioning is critical for use of mouth sticks and mobile arm supports by the tetraplegic population. The anterior tilt of the seat forward assists with upper extremity function[24,35] and standing transfers. However, this position cannot be maintained because the back extensors fatigue and the pelvis begins to slide, so the positioning is available dynamically through tilt-in-space systems. Circumferential support provided by a thoracolumbosacral orthosis in the pediatric population allows children to sit upright without using their upper extremities to hold up their trunk, maximizing use of their upper extremities for function and allowing an upright posture for using their head, neck, and weak shoulder girdle.

Simulation

In order to accurately choose or predict the functional effect of a seating system, a trial of the system is important. Changing the position in space by holding the person manually is difficult. Using a simulation, tone fluctuations, upper extremity function, and head control can be observed by varying the position. The potential system can be "mocked up," or a simulator can be used to capture the posture in a molded system and allow the client to experience the positioning before it is finalized. Simulation of the supports begins at the pelvis, hips, and trunk and proceeds to the extremities. This anatomically systematic approach is followed to reevaluate the effect on the person's overall posture and control before proceeding to the next body segment in hopes of preventing "overseating." Measurements are taken to ensure an accurate fit.

The following measurements are needed as a "picture" of the person (Fig. 44-11):

Hip to top of head (A)
Hip to top of shoulder (B)
Seat depth (C)
Leg length–knee to heel (D)
Chest depth and width (E, F)
Hip width (trochanter to trochanter) (G)
Hip to underarm left and right (HL) (HR)

Types of seating systems

The severity of the deformity or the deforming forces influences the type of seating system. Flexible deformities usually can be held using modular planar or contoured systems. Fixed deformities usually must be accommodated with custom systems, either molded or an eclectic mix depending on the clients, needs.

Planar systems

Planar systems are flat positioning components that allow the user the freedom to move. Backs, seats, lateral trunk supports, lateral hip or thigh stabilizers, and medial thigh or abductors are composed of different foam interfaces on a wood or plastic base (Table 44-2). The pressure distribution is minimal. These systems are composed of modular components that are interchangeable between manufacturers, making for the best overall system. They are easily adjustable as the person grows or changes (Fig. 44-12).

Simple contoured systems

Commercially available systems provide basic generic contoured support of the pelvis and trunk. They offer increased contact of the body for more even distribution of pressures compared to planar systems. Therefore, they provide more support and stability and perhaps less freedom of movement for patients who would benefit, such as individuals with athetoid cerebral palsy. An antithrust seat is a contoured seat intended to prevent the pelvis from sliding forward. The difference between the comfort, pressure-relieving, and positioning seat cushions depends on the contour depth and the interface material.

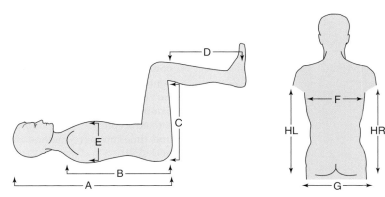

Fig. 44-11 Measurements needed for a seating system.

Table 44-2 Components of a seating system

Solid seat	Planar, contoured, antithrust, seat cushion incorporated into the surface
Solid back	Planar, contoured, biangular, molded surface interfaced to accommodate deformities
Medial thigh stabilizer (abductor, pommel)	Used to maintain thigh abduction or prevent adduction
Knee blocks	To prevent sliding out of a seat and allow repositioning by the user
Trunk supports	Straight for lateral stability and curved swing away for better support of rotational scoliosis
	Three-point control, trunk and pelvis for scoliosis
Shoulder retractors	Straps pulling up chest vest or harness needed for upper trunk stability to improve head control and not affect upper extremity function
Head supports	Neck ring to maintain head midline and support below occiput to prevent stimulation of the tonic labyrinthine reflex, which causes head extension with pressure under the occiput in the cerebral palsy patient
	Lateral head control asymmetric for asymmetric tonic neck reflex posturing
	Occipital support of capital extension
Foot rests	Placement important for stability and to prevent pulling of hamstrings. Solid footboard with straps or shoe holders allows feet to bear weight of lower legs, decreasing pressure on back of thighs

Custom-molded systems

Custom-molded systems are used by a limited population of patients with fixed deformities. The intimate contours of custom-molded systems accommodate fixed deformities, maximize pressure distribution, and provide good support for clients who exhibit poor central control. The technique typically requires a skilled therapist or a certified rehabilitation technology specialist and can be labor intensive.

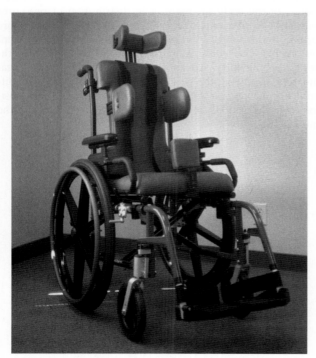

Fig. 44-12 Planar seating system with modular components.

Typically custom-molded seats and backs are limited to persons who cannot propel a manual wheelchair because the torso movement needed for propulsion may cause shearing to bony pelvic areas. However, recessing areas of bony prominences will decrease the effect of shearing. A study compared four materials used as an interface in areas recessed in molded seats. Seven participants, five with cerebral palsy, sat in molded seats with areas recessed under bony prominences. Pressure distribution was compared between two foam materials (Pudgee and Sunmate) and two gel interfaces (Floam and Flolite). Foams (particularly Sunmate) demonstrated better pressure distribution and lower peak pressures.[5] Heat retention is a disadvantage of conventional contoured seating systems because of the intimate contact and use of materials that do not breathe. Heat and moisture retention become factors for skin breakdown. Traditionally, custom-molded systems that provide intimate contact with body contours are better for postural control but are not suitable for clients at high risk for skin breakdown. The three most common methods for making custom-molded systems described by Hobson[20] in 1990 are as follows:

1. Hand-shaped foam method involves layering foam over a framework of Ethafoam wedges or foam wedges of different densities. For example, in an antithrust seat configuration, Sunmate foam is layered over a no. 5 contoured foam base. The process can involve hand carving foam to match the client's deformity, for example, cutting into a block of foam to accommodate a fixed kyphosis or rib hump. This can be a very labor- and time-intensive method that requires experience and skill.

2. Liquid foam in place consists of a direct pour around the client. Two chemicals and a catalyst are mixed, producing carbon dioxide gas and causing the

polyurethane foam to expand. The expanding foam envelops the client and sets within minutes. The foam is encased inside a plastic bag under a loose back cover. As with any custom molding, the client must sit in the exact position needed.

3. Vacuum consolidation involves using a simulator with a vacuum beaded bag. As the client sits in the optimal position, a mold is made by removing air. Two methods are used to produce the mold. One method is direct vacuum consolidation, in which a slow-acting glue is added to the beads and the mold slowly hardens. The second is an indirect method that involves either making a negative plaster cast of the mold (Contour-U) or digitizing the mold and sending the information to a central fabrication location. The advantage of the digitized method is no shipping of a bulky plaster mold is needed. Lemaire et al.[26] compared the cast simulator method with the computer-aided design/computed aided manufacturing (CAD/CAM) or computerized method and asked clients to rate their satisfaction. The clients had no difference in opinions regarding the two approaches; therefore, the researchers concluded the CAD/CAM method was as effective as the cast-molded method (Fig. 44-13).

Incorporating pressure relief into seating systems

Factors that cause pressure sores

1. *Pressure* under bony prominences (perpendicular stress) compromises blood flow, causing ischemia to the tissue. *Pressure* is defined as the perpendicular force divided by

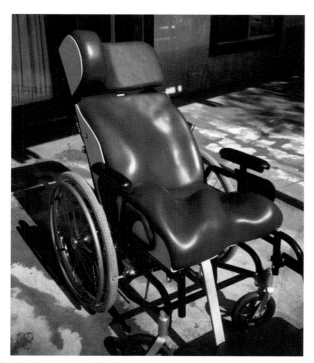

Fig. 44-13 Custom-molded seating system with negative cast mold seat and direct mold back.

the area over which it acts. Differences in circulatory tissue perfusion between persons with and those without SCI have been documented and demonstrate that tissue perfusion changes in persons with SCI significantly impaired the response to external pressure loads.[38] Pressures exceeding normal capillary pressures (32 mm Hg) can lead to tissue necrosis.[26] For individuals at high risk (SCI with insensate skin), maximum acceptable pressures recommended are ischial tuberosities 40 mm Hg, coccyx 0 mm Hg, trochanters 60 mm Hg, and sacrum < 20 mm Hg.[13,14] However, Reswick and Rogers[42] emphasize that no one maximum allowable pressure suits all individuals and that time is another variable. They recommend ischial pressures not exceed 30 to 60 mm Hg. Individuals who are thin and have poor muscle tone are at greater risk for tissue breakdown.

2. *Shearing* is the abrasive lateral (parallel stress) force that occurs when you move in your chair. Shearing forces occlude blood vessels at a deeper level than does friction (a component of shear), which contributes to pressure sores on a more superficial level.[9] Aging skin has less tolerance for friction and shear.

3. *Heat accumulation* causing an increase in skin temperature of 1°C is accompanied by a 10% increase in metabolic demands. Tissue already compromised by pressure is placed at further risk when heat builds up. Foam cushions have been found to increase skin temperature and gel or water cushions decrease skin temperature; however, gels increase the humidity between the seat and buttock interface.[9]

4. *Moisture* can cause skin maceration from lack of thermoregulation when there is poor air exchange.[46] Therefore, the skin is more susceptible to damage from pressure and shear. The environmental climate also has an effect: warmer, humid climates increase risk, so use of materials that release heat buildup and wick away moisture are important.

Issues in cushion selection

Client-centered factors include whether protective sensation is intact or absent, prominence of bony areas, ability to weight shift, stability provided, transfer ability, and trunk stability.

Cushion-centered factors include frictional properties of the cushion and cover, moisture and heat accumulation, overall cushion height, durability, maintenance, and fire retardancy.[13] Springle et al.[47] identified and described five properties of cushion material: density, stiffness, resilience, dampening, and envelopment.

Evaluation of pressures includes knowledge of the anatomy and relationship of bony prominences of the pelvis and the ability to palpate bony areas accurately to solve pressure problems. Palpation is the primary means of evaluation and may be done in combination with pressure mapping systems. Measurement of pressure has evolved from single-sensor measurement to a multiple matrix of sensors that continuously measure pressures.[9] Interpreting pressure mapping systems should not be done exclusive of palpating the anatomy for accurate interpretation of data; it adds only another piece of information to the problem-solving process.

Principles of pressure relief

Pressure or Weight Distribution: Method of evenly distributing pressure over the entire sitting surface. Cushions are made of materials that redistribute pressure from high areas such as the ischial tuberosities to areas of less pressure. The medium conforms to the individual's pelvis and by immersion evenly distributes the pressure; however, the tradeoff is a less stable base of support for the pelvis. Media such as air, water, and gel are sometimes used as an interface on a closed-cell foam base.

Air: Air cushions have good resilience and are lighter weight, but the disadvantage is that air pressures change with changing altitudes and over time may feel less stable than firmer media. They may decrease a person's stability and balance. The Varilite cushion, which has an adjustable air interface over a contoured base, provides the pelvis with a base of stability under the air interface. Because the buttocks are suspended in air, heat is dissipated more easily (Fig. 44-14).

Gel: Another medium that distributes pressure by immersion of the pelvis into a fluid or gel-like substance. Movement or shearing is reduced. Elastomeric gels have poor resilience, tend to be heavy, and increase the humidity at the seating interface; however, the gel lowers skin temperature and has good dampening. The Jay cushion is a solid contoured base with a pad of Flolite over the base. The Deep Contour has more Flolite and 1 inch of foam padding (Fig. 44-15).

Foam: Cushions are categorized by their structure as open-cell or closed-cell foam. Closed-cell foam does not absorb water. Depending on the density, open-cell foam has good ventilation and relatively good resilience, and depending on the stiffness, the foam has good envelopment. It loses resiliency over time and is affected by moisture. They insulate body heat, which may cause dampness and contribute to skin breakdown. In general, foam cushions are lighter weight and more economical but must be replaced every 6 to 12 months. Polyurethane and latex foams (Sunmate, T foams) compress slowly to a load and provide good envelopment. These types of foam are generally used in combination over denser foams for a softer interface that compresses to load more slowly.[47] Studies have demonstrated increased seating capacity, comfort, and function with polyurethane contoured cushions.[29,44,47]

Load Distribution: Cutout cushions help by redistributing the body weight normally borne by the ischial tuberosities to areas where higher pressures are tolerated, such as the

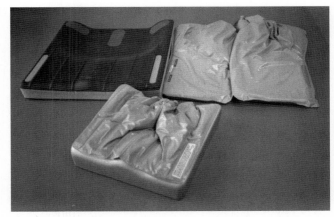

Fig. 44-15 Jay cushion with contoured base and Flolite interface.

posterior thighs and trochanters. The concept was first introduced by Reswick and Rogers[42,43] and has been used successfully for more than 30 years. Three inches of no. 5 density foam is laminated to 1 inch of no. 3 foam on top, and a rectangular shape is cut out to relieve pressure under the ischial tuberosities and coccyx. After study of 1,000 cadavers, the pelvis of a male was determined to be 1 inch narrower than the pelvis of a female; therefore, the cutout is 8 inches wide and 6 inches deep for a female pelvis and 7 inches wide and 5 inches deep for a male pelvis. The ischial tuberosities and coccyx are suspended (1 inch of no. 5 foam remains at the bottom of the cutout for stability), and the rest of the pelvis and lower extremities are enveloped in 1 inch of medium-density foam over the no. 5 foam (Fig. 44-16).[39]

Force/Load Isolation: This method of selective pressure relief under bony areas and redistribution of pressure to the soft tissues under the femurs has been used as the basic concept for a newer custom-molded cushion by Rides Design. The concept of custom molding the pelvis and recessing areas specifically under the ischial tuberosities is the orthotic principle of forced isolation as opposed to pressure distribution. A box 4 inches deep, which is the size of the wheelchair seat, is used to capture the impression of the pelvis. The negative mold captures contours of pelvis. Bony landmarks are identified to recess areas of the ischial tuberosities and coccyx,

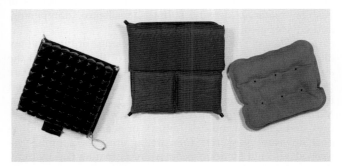

Fig. 44-14 Three types of air cushions: Roho, Varilite, and Bye-Bye Decubiti.

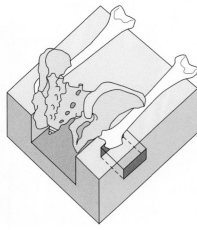

Fig. 44-16 Ischial tuberosities suspended in a cutout foam cushion with relief for trochanter.

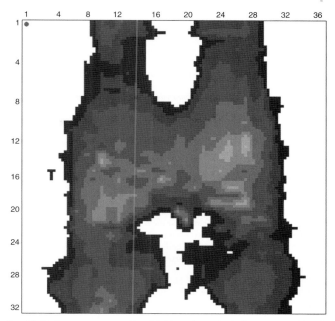

Fig. 44-19 Same person as Fig. 44-18 on force isolation-type cushion by Rides Design. Same concept as foam cushion, with cutout to offload pressure from ischial tuberosities and coccyx.

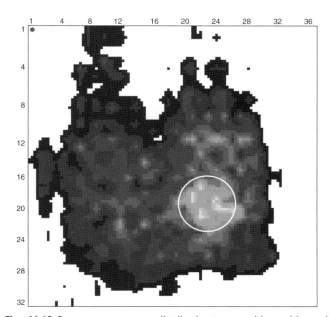

Fig. 44-17 Rides Design created from a mold with Brock composite foam material.

leaving room to avoid the effect of shear with functional movement. The mold is modified to further relieve areas of pressure but to capture the soft tissues surrounding the pelvis for suspension. The foam composite material used is lightweight, breathable, and waterproof. It allows air flow, so it does not retain heat or moisture. Outcomes with this newer cushion design and material are not yet determined (Figs. 44-17 to 44-19).[10,19]

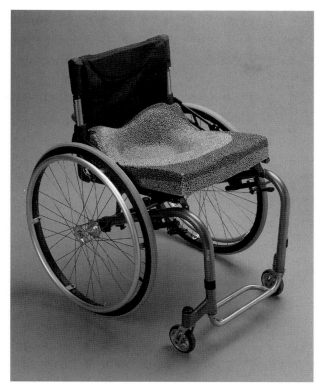

Fig. 44-18 Person on pressure distribution-type cushion with peak pressures under the right ischial tuberosity circled.

All postural deformities of the pelvis and hips must be evaluated with the client sitting on the cushion to determine if bottoming out is occurring due to obliquities or anatomical changes. Evaluation of whether a deformity is fixed or flexible determines if the modifications need to accommodate or to correct. Pelvic obliquity, if flexible, can be reduced by using an insert of denser foam on the low side or by increasing air pressure. If the obliquity is fixed, the insert of denser foam or the increase in air pressure should be on the high side to unweight the low side of the pelvis, thereby redistributing pressure from the lower ischial tuberosity.

References

1. Adrian MJ, Cooper JM: *Biomechanics of human movement*, Indianapolis, 1989, Benchmark Press.
2. Aissaoui R, Boucher C, Bourbonnais D et al: Effect of seat cushion on dynamic stability in sitting during a reaching task in wheelchair users with paraplegia, *Arch Phys Med Rehabil* 82:274–281, 2001.
3. Alblaza VJ, Fischer J: Wound care via telemedicine: the wave of the future. Available at: http://www.rubic.com/articles/articles1.html
4. American Hospital Association: Curative Health Services. Available at: http://www.curative.com.
5. Apatsidis DP, Solomonidis SE, Michael SM: Pressure distribution at the seating interface of custom-molded wheelchair seats: effect of various materials, *Arch Phys Med Rehabil* 83:1151–1156, 2002.
6. Bergen AF, Colangelo C: *Positioning the client with CNS deficits: the wheelchair and other adapted equipment*, Valhalla, NY, 1985, Valhalla Publications.
7. Bergen AF, Presperin J, Tallman T: *Positioning for function: wheelchairs and other assistive technologies*, Valhalla, NY, 1990, Valhalla Rehabilitation Publications.
8. Bodchie-Adjei O, Lonstein JE et al: Management of neuromuscular spine deformities with Luque segmental instrumentation, *J Bone Surg Am* 71(4):548–562, 1989.
9. In Cook AM, Hussey SM, editors: *Assistive technologies: principles and practice*, St. Louis, 1995, CV Mosby.
10. Corbett B: *21st century seating: new mobility life on wheels*, 2004, pp. 17–20. New Mobility.
11. Cron L, Springle S: Clinical evaluation of the hemiwheechair cushion, *Am J Occup Ther* 47:141–144, 1992.

565

12. Dummond D, Breed AL, Narechania R: Relationship of spine deformity and pelvic obliquity on sitting pressure distributions and decubitus ulceration, *J Pediatr Orthop* 5:396–402, 1985.

13. Edberg LE, Cerny K, Stauffer ES: Prevention and treatment of pressure sores, *Phys Ther* 53:246–252, 1973.

14. Ferguson-Pell MW: Seat cushion selection, *J Rehabil Res Dev* 2(suppl):49–73, 1990.

15. Frankel VH, Nordin M: *Basic biomechanics of the skeletal system*, Philadelphia, 1980, Lea & Febiger.

16. Furumasu J, Swank S: Functional activities in spinal muscular atrophy patients after spinal fusion, *Spine* 14:771–775, 1989.

17. Harrison DD, Harrison SO, Croft AC, Harrison DE, Troyanovich SJ: Sitting biomechanics part I: review of the literature, *J Manip Physiol Ther* 22:594–609, 1999.

18. Hastings JD, Fanucchi ER, Burns SP: Wheelchair configuration and postural alignment in persons with spinal cord injury, *Arch Phys Med Rehabil* 84:528–534, 2003.

19. Hetzel TR: Seating: the next generation, *Mobil Manage* 3:22–24, 2004.

20. Hobson DA: Seating and mobility for the severely disabled. In Smith RV, Leslie JH, editors: *Rehabilitation engineering*, Boca Raton, Fla, 1990, CRC Press.

21. Hoffer MM: Basic considerations and classifications of cerebral palsy. In: *American Academy of Orthopedic Surgeons: instructional course lectures, vol 25*, St. Louis, 1976, CV Mosby.

22. Holmes KJ, Michael SM, Thorpe SL, Solomonidis SE: Management of scoliosis with special seating for the non-ambulant spastic cerebral palsy population—a biomechanical study, *Clin Biomech* 18:480–487, 2003.

23. Hulme J, Poor R, Schulein M, Pezzino J: Perceived behavioral changes observed with adaptive seating devices and training programs for multihandicapped, developmentally disabled individuals, *Phys Ther* 63:203–208, 1982.

24. Hundertmark LH: Evaluating the adult with cerebral palsy for specialized adaptive seating, *Phys Ther* 65:209–212, 1985.

25. Kangas KM: Seating, positioning, and physical access. In Hussey SM, editor: *Developmental disabilities special interest sections newsletter, special issue on assistive technology*, Rockville, Md, 1991, American Occupational Therapy Association14:2–3..

26. Landis EM: Micro-injection studies of capillary blood pressure in human skin, *Heart* 15:209–228, 1930.

27. Lemaire ED, Upton D, Paialunga J, Martel G, Boucher J: Clinical analysis of a CAD/CAM system for custom seating. A comparison with hand-sculpting methods, *J Rehabil Res Dev* 33:311–320, 1996.

28. In Letts RM, editor: *Principles of seating the disabled, Boca Raton*, Fla, 1991, CRC Press.

29. Lim R, Sirett R, Conine T, Daechsel D: Clinical trials of foam cushions in the prevention of decubitus ulcers in elderly patients, *J Rehabil Res Dev* 33:311–320, 1988.

30. Lonstein JE, Beck K: Hip dislocation and subluxation in cerebral palsy, *J Pediatr Orthop* 6(5):521–526, 1986.

31. McPherson JJ, Schild R, Spaulding SJ, Barsamian P et al: Analysis of upper extremity movement in four sitting positions: a comparison of persons with and without cerebral palsy, *Am J Occup Ther* 45:123–129, 1991.

32. Minkle JL: Seating and mobility considerations for people with spinal cord injury, *Phys Ther* 80:701–709, 2004.

33. Myhr U, Wendlt L: Improvement of functional sitting position for children with cerebral palsy, *Dev Med Child Neurol* 33:246–250, 1991.

34. Nwaobi OM: Effects of body orientations in space on tonic muscle activity of patients with cerebral palsy, *Dev Med Child Neurol* 28:41–44, 1986.

35. Nwaobi OM: Effects of different seating orientations on upper extremity function in children with spastic and athetoid cerebral palsy. In: *Proceedings 10th Annual Conference Rehabilitation Technology*, 1987, pp. 264-265.

36. Nwaobi Om, Hobson D, Trefler E: Hip angle and upper extremity movement time in children with cerebral palsy. *Proceedings 8th Annual Conference Rehabilitation Technology*, 1986, pp. 39-41.

37. Nwaobi Om, Smith PD: Effects of adaptive seating on pulmonary function of children with cerebral palsy, *Dev Med Child Neurol* 28:351–354, 1986.

38. Patterson R, Crammer S, Fisher S, Engel R: The physiological response to repeated surface pressure loads in the able bodied and spinal cord injured. In: *Proceedings RESNA International Conference*, 1992, Arlington, VA: RESNA Press.

39. Peterson M, Adkins H: Measurement and redistribution of excessive pressures during wheelchair sitting, *Phys Ther* 62:990–994, 1982.

40. Pynt J, Higgs J, Mackey M: Seeking the optimal posture of the lumbar spine, *Physiother Theory Pract* 17:5–21, 2001.

41. Rang M, Douglas G, Bennet GC, Koreska J: Seating for children with cerebral palsy, *J Pediatr Orthop* 1:279, 1981.

42. Reswick JB, Roger JE: Experience at Rancho Los Amigos Hospital with devices and techniques to prevent pressure sores. In Kenedi RM, Cowden JM, Scales JT, editors: *Bedsore biomechanics*, Baltimore, 1976, University Park Press.

43. Rogers JE: Tissue trauma group, *Annu Rep Progr* 1973.

44. Rosenthal MJ, Felton RM, Hileman D, Freidman M et al: A wheelchair cushion designed to redistribute sites of sitting pressures, *Arch Phys Med Rehabil* 77:278–282, 1996.

45. Seeger BR, Caudrey DJ, O'Mara NA: Hand function in cerebral palsy: the effect of hip flexion angle, *Dev Med Chil Neurol* 26:601–606, 1984.

46. Seymour RJ, Lacefield WE: Wheelchair cushion effect on pressure and skin temperature, *Arch Phys Med Rehabil* 66:103–108, 1985.

47. Springle S, Chung KC, Brubaker CE: Factors affecting seat contour characteristics, *J Rehab Res Dev* 27:127–134, 1990.

48. Springle S, Wotten M, Sawacha Z, Theilman G: Relationships among cushion type, backrest height, seated posture, and reach of wheelchair users with spinal cord injury, *J Spinal Cord Med* 27:262, 2004.

49. Wu SY, Green A: *Projections of chronic illness prevalence and cost inflation, John Hopkins University Partnership for Solutions*, 2000, Washington, DC, Rand Corp.

50. In: Zacharkow D: Essential wheelchair modifications for proper sitting posture: *Wheelchair posture and pressure sores*, Springfeild, Ill, 1984, Charles C Thomas.

Chapter

45

Wheelchair prescription in international settings

David Constantine

Key Points

- Poverty and disability amplify each other.
- A wheelchair may provide greater access to basic human rights for a person with a mobility disability.
- Issues of financing and distribution of mobility aids require reexamination.
- Wheelchair design may require modification in low-income countries.
- Wheelchairs need to use local materials and construction without compromising biomechanical principles for support and safety.

Wheelchair provision in low-income countries

More than 20 million people worldwide are in desperate need of a wheelchair. Millions more require other mobility aids. The adverse effects of this basic lack of mobility are exaggerated by the fact that the majority of people with mobility disabilities in low-income countries come from the poorest sections of the community. Poor people with disabilities are caught in a vicious cycle of poverty and disability, each being both a cause and a consequence of the other.

Disabled people in low-income countries are disenfranchised, marginalized, and generally devoid of access to their most basic human rights. It is important to recognize that an appropriate wheelchair is merely a tool that provides people with mobility impairments greater opportunity to access their rights to an integrated lifestyle within their own communities, leading to greater independence and an improved quality of life.

Financing of mobility aids

Why the independent living model should replace the charity model

Many donors of wheelchairs operate under a charity model rather than an independent living model. Wheelchair users in low-income countries often cannot afford to pay for their own wheelchairs, so government agencies, development organizations, and charitable and religious institutions act as consumers instead. The usual market forces of consumer-based supply and demand are absent; as a result, end users are removed from the design, production, and selection processes and become passive recipients of charity rather than empowered consumers. When donors focus their attention on the product instead of the end users, the distribution of wheelchairs takes precedence over the socioeconomic integration of people with disabilities into their communities.

Why the social model should replace the medical model

The medical model defines mobility disability as a matter of impairment to be solved with wheelchairs. This common perspective of donors is flawed because disability is a problem of socioeconomic immobility as much as physical immobility. The issue is not simply that millions of people are physically immobilized, but that their immobility often prevents them

Table 45-1 Comparison of industrialized and low-income countries service model

Service Models	Industrialized Country	Low-Income Country
Beneficiary	Wheelchair user	Wheelchair user
Service	Occupational therapist Physiotherapist Rehabilitation engineer Clinical assistant	Few integrated services or professionally trained staff
Product	Commercial wheelchair manufacturer	Local workshop or donated wheelchairs

Table 45-2 Donation of recycled wheelchairs approach

Strengths	
Recycled	Discarded wheelchairs fit in the "anything is better than nothing" approach
Low cost	Recycled and refurbished fairly inexpensively (through volunteer programs)
Fast	Large quantities can be delivered quickly
Weaknesses	
Adjustability	Rarely adjustable to fit the individual Often incorrect size for children High risk of secondary complications due to poor fit
Suitability	Wheelchair designs from industrialized countries, designed for use in hospital or indoor settings, are not suitable for uneven or unpaved roads and sandy terrain No choice in wheelchair design for individual needs
Durability	Wheelchairs are unsuitable for harsh conditions and break easily Repairs are extremely expensive or not possible when replacement parts are not available locally
Sustainability	Working with a "charity" model approach Large influx of free donated wheelchairs can put local wheelchair producers out of business, eliminating the long-term source of wheelchairs for the community No follow-up or support for wheelchair users after distribution Health authorities do not take responsibility or make provisions for wheelchair services

from pursuing an education, marrying, having families, working to support themselves or their families, or otherwise participating in their communities. The social model advocates that disability must be seen as an ongoing part of life within local social, cultural, economic, and political contexts, and not as a medical emergency to be solved if only enough wheelchairs can be charitably given away to those in need. The technology is only part of the solution.

Why appropriate service models should replace the industrialized health service model

Wheelchair provision in low-income countries often is based on industrialized countries' service models, which are inappropriate and ineffective. Infrastructure systems, such as health professionals and commercial wheelchair manufacturers, are lacking, and the largely rural population in low-income countries is not served effectively by an institutional-type health service. As a result, many wheelchair users do not have access to official health care systems (Table 45-1).

Evaluation of wheelchair provision approaches

In order to provide comprehensive responsible service and appropriate long-lasting wheelchairs, the approach to provision must meet the following four criteria:

1. **Adjustability:** The wheelchair must be made to the measurements of the user or easily adjustable to fit the user. It must always come with a pressure relief cushion that can be maintained or replaced.
2. **Suitability:** The wheelchair design must reflect the terrain that the wheelchair user will push through. Wheelchairs must be available in a range of designs that will meet individual needs and ensure quality of life and independence.
3. **Durability:** The wheelchair must be well made, durable, and easily repaired. Replacement parts should be easily available.
4. **Sustainability:** The wheelchair should be supplied in a manner that provides wheelchairs to the community for the long term.

Wheelchair distribution methods

Four types of wheelchair provisions are discussed. The strengths and weaknesses of each approach are assessed, with consideration of the issues involved in providing wheelchairs to low-income countries.

Donation of recycled wheelchairs from industrialized countries

Many organizations, particularly in higher-income countries, have responded to the critical need for wheelchair distribution in low-income countries by refurbishing orthopedic hospital-style wheelchairs and delivering them overseas (Table 45-2).

Mass production and export of free wheelchairs to low-income countries

There are advantages to utilizing mass production and export of free wheelchairs if wheelchair designs and methods of distribution are carefully considered (Table 45-3). In the past, the process has been unsuccessful because of poor wheelchair designs and little consideration to the distribution system and the needs of the users.

Table 45-3 Mass production and export of free wheelchairs approach

Strengths	
Appropriate	Designs are sometimes appropriate
Low cost	Mass production helps to lower the price of wheelchairs
Large quantities	Large quantities can be delivered quickly
Weaknesses	
Adjustability	Wheelchairs are often not prescribed Expatriate staff are not based locally in the country and therefore are not available for review or follow-up (if wheelchairs are prescribed)
Suitability	Designs that are not appropriate often will not be suitable
Durability	Repairs are difficult because replacement parts usually are not available locally
Sustainability	Working with a "charity' model" approach Mass distribution of chairs is damaging to local producers "Ceremonies" that hand out wheelchairs free to users are demeaning and patronizing No follow-up or support for wheelchair users after distribution Health authorities do not take responsibility or make provisions for wheelchair services Considerable transportation costs used for this approach could have been spent on strengthening local production

Table 45-4 Local workshops approach

Strengths	
Adjustability	Individually fitted wheelchairs Can be custom built to suit a wider range of needs Follow-up service
Suitability	Needs of the individual are assessed to prescribe the most appropriate design Training in wheelchair use maximizes the user's mobility
Durability	Local staff can provide designs and adaptations that are appropriate to the local environment and the user's needs Repairs can be made because designs are made from local materials
Sustainability	Workshops can become more efficient and cost effective with design and technology advances and training Workshops are a source of employment and support the economy through the purchase of local materials and resources Local workshops potentially can integrate their services to join or establish a national rehabilitation system
Weaknesses	
Higher cost	Small workshops may not be able to take advantage of economies of scale; keeping costs down and quality high can be difficult
Suitability	Local producers often copy designs of imported wheelchairs because of limited training and information on appropriate designs
Sustainability	Small-scale operations lack economic stability Vulnerable to competition from free or very-low-cost wheelchair providers Funding scarcity due to inability of recipients to significantly contribute toward costs and lack of governmental or donor support for costs Very low production levels without regular sales or wheelchair financing systems

Local workshops

Local workshops in low-income countries have been providing a service to wheelchair users for many years (Table 45-4). They often are established by disabled persons organizations (DPOs) that have been frustrated by the lack of appropriate wheelchairs in their own communities.

Mass production and distribution of low-cost wheelchairs by local organizations in low-income countries

There is an important difference between mass producing wheelchairs for donation and mass producing wheelchairs for effective distribution through local partner groups (Table 45-5). Effective provision systems can be established in collaboration and consultation with local wheelchair producers and DPOs. This involves training personnel in assessment, educating users on seating and mobility skills, providing a range of wheelchairs with pressure relief cushions, and giving access to financing schemes for wheelchairs to ensure that the people most in need have access to a wheelchair.

Whichever approach is adopted, a comprehensive financing system is critical to ensure access to wheelchairs to people who cannot afford them. Giving away wheelchairs for free can lead to an attitude of "easy come, easy go" such that the wheelchairs are not looked after or maintained. Paying for at least a portion of the equipment creates a sense of ownership and places a value on the wheelchairs.

Wheelchair assessment and prescription

Most developing countries lack wheelchair services that offer individual assessment, wheelchair prescription, and basic instruction on how to use and maintain wheelchairs. This lack of services has negative consequences for wheelchair users:

- Many wheelchair users receive a wheelchair that does not fit them and is not appropriately adjusted. For people who use a wheelchair more than a few hours a day, a badly fitting wheelchair can lead to a range of physical problems, including postural deformities, shoulder pain, and pressure sores.

- Many wheelchair users receive no information or education on how to use or maintain their wheelchair. Without this information, the benefits of the wheelchair are greatly reduced. In this context, many wheelchair users who otherwise would be highly able are not aware that, with the right techniques, they

Table 45-5 Mass production of low-cost wheelchairs with local organizations approach

Strengths	
Adjustability	Provision of a range of appropriate and adjustable wheelchairs, individually prescribed and fitted by trained local staff who are available for follow-up and repairs
Suitability	Prescription process includes assessment of the user's needs in order to prescribe an appropriate wheelchair Training in wheelchair skills is an integral part of the service and can be provided by wheelchair users of the local DPO or workshop
Durability	Wheelchair designs that are appropriate for the environment are provided Local production ensures that repairs can be made and that necessary materials are available locally and at reasonable cost
Sustainability	Importing appropriate low-cost wheelchairs can reduce service costs by removing the pressure of local wheelchair fabrication Local services can ensure effective distribution of suitable wheelchairs to match demand and identify individuals most in need Local services can maintain wheelchair provision by strengthening and integrating rehabilitation services and DPOs Potential to create an integrated national rehabilitation system
Weaknesses	
Sustainability	Transport costs and logistics must be funded and organized Funding is needed for capacity building local partners Close links with local DPOs and local workshops are essential to ensure effective provision

DPO, Disabled persons organization.

have the potential to propel themselves and to transfer independently.

- Wheelchair users tend to be ill informed about wheelchairs as a product, having little awareness of the range of wheelchairs and component options available in developed countries. In many cases, wheelchair users are grateful for what is, in reality, an inappropriate wheelchair for their lifestyle, disability, or physical context. The lack of information reduces the potential of wheelchair users as a group to actively lobby for better, more suitable products.

Creating opportunities for access to wheelchair services for users in developing countries is a challenging task. Many countries have limited rehabilitation services, severe shortages (or absence) of physical and occupational therapists, lack of government commitment and/or capacity to operate wheelchair services, and shortage of finances to sustain services. On the positive side, there is a growing recognition from development agencies, international nongovernmental organizations (INGOs), national nongovernmental organizations (NGOs), and DPOs that the provision of wheelchairs cannot be accomplished without addressing the individual needs of wheelchair users, which requires the development of wheelchair services that offer, at a minimum, wheelchair assessment, prescription, and basic instruction on wheelchair use.

Wheelchair design considerations for users

The majority of low-income countries have a severe shortage of trained rehabilitation staff and often have no professional therapists. Given the absence of professionals, the prescription provided in Table 45-6 is specifically designed for use by nonprofessional staff who may not be able to identify a specific disability but can recognize characteristics of a disability that will enable effective assessment and prescription.

Psychological issues for wheelchair users and wheelchair design

Disability in low-income countries is often seen in a negative light and in some traditional belief systems is seen to result from a curse. Many people regard wheelchair users as a burden, believing that people in wheelchairs cannot be independent and contribute to society. Because the appearance and performance of a wheelchair can have positive or negative effects on the psychological well-being of the user and on the reaction of other people, these factors must be considered in the design of appropriate products. A wheelchair that is big and bulky affects the user's appearance, making him or her "disappear" into the wheelchair. A wheelchair that is difficult to use or is uncomfortable or broken will not encourage the user to be independent or to feel good about himself or herself. A wheelchair that is well made, fits the user correctly, and meets the needs of the disability and the environment will enhance the user's appearance and independence, increasing his or her confidence and self-esteem. This in turn will generate a more positive reaction from other people toward the user, further increasing the user's confidence and self-esteem.

Appropriate manual wheelchair design for low-income countries

Many types of manual wheelchairs meet the physical and lifestyle needs of individual users in low-income countries. The main role of a wheelchair is to provide mobility. However, a wheelchair also is responsible for the user's comfort and posture.

Many different types of manual wheelchairs are available (Table 45-7), and most of them can be divided into the following groups:

Three-wheel wheelchairs
Four-wheel wheelchairs

Table 45-6 Prescription chart for wheelchair user characteristics

User Characteristic	Wheelchair Part	Why
Poor sitting balance	High backrest	Provides support and good sitting posture
Average sitting balance	Middle backrest	Provides some support but allows for some mobility
Good sitting balance	Low backrest	Provides less support but allows for much more mobility
Needs a lot of support in the back for sitting	Solid backrest	Long lasting; solid surface encourages good sitting posture
Needs support but a lightweight wheelchair to assist with mobility	Fabric backrest	Increasing tension may provide back support
Needs accommodating backrest		
Decreased skin sensation and at risk for developing pressure sores	Pressure relief cushion	Provides pressure relief for vulnerable areas of the body
Problems with bladder and/or bowel	Waterproof cover	Can easily wash and dry cover
		Can wipe down or wash cushion
Very active user with good sitting balance	Active wheel position	Wheelchair less stable so is easier to balance on back wheels, which allows for greater mobility and easier movement over obstacles and steps
Active user who needs equal amounts of stability and mobility	Middle wheel position	Allows wheelchair to be equally stable and mobile
User has sudden uncontrolled movements	Safe wheel position (posterior)	Makes the wheelchair very stable and less able to tip back
Bilateral amputee with less sitting balance		
First time user of wheelchair who is not confident with wheelchair mobility		
User lives in very hilly area		
User needs to use wheelchair on sandy, muddy terrain	Wide castor wheel	Wider wheel surface so wheels do not sink into the ground
User needs to use wheelchair on flat, concrete ground	Thin castor wheel	Narrow surface of wheel good for speed on hard surfaces
User needs to use chair on rough terrain	Large-diameter castor wheel	Large castor wheel can roll very easily over small obstacles (e.g., stones)
For standing transfers	Flip-up footrests	Allows user to stand up when transferring in and out of wheelchair
User had different leg lengths	Separate footrests	Allows for correct footrest height if legs are different lengths
User does not need to stand up to transfer	Rigid footrests	Footrests that do not need to fold out of the way are stronger
Feet fall backward off footrest	Calf strap/ankle strap	Protects feet from getting knocked and wounded
Feet fall forward off footrest	Foot strap	
Active user transfers using sideways transfer	Fixed curved armrest	Follows line of chair
Less active user transfers using sliding transfer	Short lever brakes	Do not interfere with transfers
	Removable armrest	Can remove armrest from wheelchair
	Short lever brakes	Interfere far less with transfers
For small spaces	24-inch wheels	Smaller turning circle
For working under desk/table		Wheelchair is lower to the ground
User lives in area where 24-inch wheels not available	26-inch wheels	Wheels are inexpensive and easily available
Need to transport the wheelchair often	Quick-release wheels	Wheels are easily removable from the frame
For sport activities	Camber	Wider base provides more stability required for active sports
Assistant needs to push wheelchair	High push handles	Protects assistant against back problems
Assistant needs to push wheelchair but high push handles get in the way of the user self-propelling	Adjustable push handles	Low height allows mobility for the user; high push handles allow assistant to push
User has difficulty with hand and arm function	Long lever brakes	Longer lever is easier to put on and off
User only able to use one arm (e.g., patient with stroke)	One-sided brakes	Both brakes activated from one side only
User is weak and condition likely will worsen	Resting armrests	Additional support for user with padding for comfort

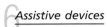
Table 45-7 Appropriate manual wheelchair designs and prescription

Type of Wheelchair	When Should This Wheelchair Be Prescribed?	Advantages	Disadvantages
Orthopedic	User needs a wheelchair for short periods in a hospital or institutional environment	High push handles for attendant propulsion	No postural adjustment No rear wheel adjustment Unsuitable for rough terrain Heavy
Three-wheel wheelchair: Two large rear wheels and single front castor wheel Front castor wheel often is large Usually footplates do not move out of the way for standing transfers	Good for rural environments: sand, mud, rough terrain, hilly area Good for going over obstacles and going down small steps or slopes	Very stable Provides smooth ride and good control over rough terrain (all three wheels stay in contact with the ground) Easy to navigate over or around obstacles Excellent stability when going down slopes (due to extended castor wheel) Negotiate steps without back wheel balancing due to frame length	Frame usually is quite long (problem in small spaces; more difficult to transport) Larger turning circle than compact four-wheel wheelchair Sometimes looks unusual in places where people are not accustomed to seeing them Central beam is located between the user's legs, which is not always popular Standing transfers are difficult due to position of the central beam
Four-wheel folding: Slung seat and backrest allow wheelchair to fold Usually has flip-up footplates Originally designed for short-term use in a hospital or urban environment	User needs to fold wheelchair for storage or transport Short-term use Use in urban area Flip-up footrests are needed Indoor use	Easy to store and transport Flip-up footrests make standing transfers easier	Not as durable as fixed-frame chairs due to more moving parts, which wear with time and use Slung seats can "stretch" and sag; difficult to retighten the fabric; once fabric stretches, seat no longer provides good postural support and pressure relief cushions do not work correctly Folding mechanism can be more complicated for local production Folding mechanism adds weight Worn folding mechanism can result in wheelchair instability
Four-wheel wheelchair: Two large rear wheels and two front castor wheels	Does not fold Strong frame is needed Indoor use Use in urban area	More compact than three-wheel wheelchair due to shorter wheel base Most models have a smaller turning circle than a three-wheel wheelchair	Four-wheel wheelchairs are not as stable as three-wheel wheelchairs or as easy to push over rough terrain

	Durability needed		
Child's wheelchair Three wheels (Note: Four-wheel wheelchairs also are available)	Small size to fit children properly Easy to push Use in rural area; good on sand, mud, rough terrain, hilly area Good for going over small obstacles and small steps	More suitable than an adult wheelchair for an active child Child can self-propel (child is more independent) Seat and backrest height can be lengthened as child grows	Child eventually will grow out of the wheelchair
Fixed-frame wheelchair: Does not fold Can be three-wheel or four-wheel design Many have a fold-down backrest and quick-release wheels	Active user needs a sturdy wheelchair Does not have a fold-down backrest and quick-release wheels, so is good for user who does not travel much	Stronger than cross-folding frame Provides reliable postural support and cushion pressure relief Can be quite light due to absence of a folding mechanism Performs better than folding frame for sports activities	Can be bulky and difficult to transport if wheelchair does not have fold-down backrest and quick-release wheels
Low rider	Domestic environment	Use in countries where daily activities (cooking, washing, food preparation) are carried out on the floor	Restricts user to low level, making it difficult to negotiate market situations and crowds Not good for traveling long distances
Supportive seating	Provides good postural support for children who cannot sit by themselves	Very good postural support for children with mild to severe cerebral palsy Wheelchair can be adjusted as the child grows	Usually more expensive than standard wheelchair Requires a high level of seating knowledge to give a good fit Not suitable for all disabilities More complex production process than for other wheelchairs
Sports wheelchair	Lightweight and stable Easy and quick to maneuver for sports activities Camber makes wheelchair turn quickly and gives stability	More suitable for sport than everyday use Allows user to participate in team/individual activities Enhances societal integration and fitness	Not suitable for daily use Few users can afford a second chair

Folding-frame wheelchairs
Fixed-frame wheelchairs

Table 45-7 lists the main wheelchair types, identifies who they should be prescribed for, and evaluates their advantages and disadvantages.

Specific wheelchair features important for low-income countries

Key features that make some wheelchairs more suitable for low-income countries than for other countries are the rear wheels, front castors, and cushions.

Types of wheels

24-inch wheels "Standard" wheelchairs from more industrialized countries usually are made with 24-inch wheels.

Advantages

- Wheelchairs with 24-inch wheels are slightly smaller and therefore are slightly lighter and more maneuverable.
- Wheelchairs with 24-inch wheels fit under tables and desks more readily than do wheelchairs with larger wheels.

Disadvantages

- 24-inch wheels are produced especially for wheelchairs but are not easily available in many countries, which can make wheel replacement difficult. A 26-inch or 28-inch wheel cannot be used on a wheelchair designed for a 24-inch wheel without making many alterations to the wheelchair frame.
- 24-inch wheels usually are more expensive than 26-inch or 28-inch wheels.

26- or 28-inch wheels Many wheelchairs are designed to use bicycle (26-inch) or cycle rickshaw (28-inch) wheels.

Advantages

- In most countries, 26-inch wheels are readily available. In countries where cycle rickshaws are used, 28-inch

wheels are readily available. Thus, wheels of this size can be repaired or replaced easily and inexpensively.
- Larger wheels are easier to push on rough terrain.

Disadvantages

- Wheelchairs with 26-inch or 28-inch wheels are slightly larger, making access within buildings more difficult.

Front castors

Front castors support the front of the wheelchair and enable the chair to turn smoothly.

Types Different types of castor wheels are available in all shapes and sizes to navigate different terrains. The two main types of castor wheel are as follows:

- Pneumatic, which provide a smooth ride but can be punctured; spare parts can be expensive and difficult to obtain
- Solid, which last a long time and usually are less expensive than pneumatic castors

Table 45-8 lists advantages and disadvantages of different wheel shapes and sizes.

Pressure relief cushions

The design of an appropriate wheelchair cushion is of major concern in the overall design of a wheelchair. A well-designed cushion can reduce the risk of pressure sores, which are one of the most common life-threatening complications occurring in people who use wheelchairs, particularly in low-income countries. The wheelchair and cushion act together to form a seating system that should have the following characteristics:

- Promote good posture
- Maximize the user's functional potential
- Provide adequate skin protection

To achieve the best distribution of pressure, the wheelchair and cushion must be considered together at the initial design stage.

A cushion will add up to 100 mm to the seat height, and this extra height must be taken into account when evaluating the following factors:

Table 45-8 Evaluation of wheelchair wheels

	Advantages	Disadvantages	Who/Where
Wide wheel	Travels most effectively over soft terrain (e.g., sand, mud)	Heavy	Large wide wheel is good for person living in rural area
Narrow wheel	Lightweight Travels well over hard smooth terrain	Digs into soft terrain	Large narrow wheel is good for person living in pot-holed urban area
Large wheel	Travels most effectively over rough terrain	Heavy Larger turning circle can make the whole wheelchair larger	Large wide wheel is good for person living in rural area
Small wheel	Lightweight Small wheels have a smaller turning circle, which makes the chair smaller	Can "stick" in potholes or bumps in the road that a large wheel would ride over, causing user to tip out of wheelchair	Used on sports wheelchairs For person who lives in well-maintained urban area or uses wheelchair indoors
	Fits under tables		

- Relationship between the user and the push rims
- Overall height of the wheelchair in relation to tables, desks and other furniture
- Altered position of the user's arms and lap when a cushion is used

Acknowledgments

This chapter was written with material and illustrations from selected Motivation publications and various training courses: Motivation "The Wheelchair Service Guide for Low-Income Countries"; Fit for Life prescription course and technical training course; Wheelchair Technologists Training Course, TATCOT, Tanzania; and donated wheelchair fact sheets.

Resource list

Motivation
Brockley Academy
Brockley Lane
Backwell, Bristol, United Kingdom BS48 4AQ
Phone: +44 (0)1275 454012; fax: +44 (0)1275 454019
E-mail: info@motiavation.org.uk
www.motivation.org.uk
www.motivationsrilanka.org
www.worldmade.info

Tanzanian Training Centre for Orthopaedic Technologists (TATCOT)
Mr. Shangali
PO Box 8690
Moshi, Tanzania
Phone: +255 27 275 3986/7; fax: +255 27 275 2038
E-mail: tatcot@eoltz.com
www.kcmc.ac.tz/TATCOT/Wheelchair%20Technology.htm

Whirlwind Wheelchairs International (WWI)
San Francisco State University
1600 Hollaway Avenue
San Francisco, CA 94132
Phone: +1 (415) 338-6277
www.whirlwindwheelchair.org

Communication devices and electronic aids to activities of daily living

Edward C. Hitchcock

Key Points

- Assistive devices can allow persons with a disability to participate in activities while decreasing dependence on caregivers.
- Assistive technology can help persons with a disability to live independently rather than in a long-term care facility.
- Physical impairments, including range of motion, muscle weakness, and pain limitations on physical activities, are the common indicators that an assistive device may be warranted.

Various forms of assistive devices and equipment have become part of the daily life of most, if not all, people with disabilities. These devices can allow persons with a disability to participate in activities that otherwise may not be available to them while decreasing dependence on caregivers. They can encourage participation in community or social activities that increase quality of life. They facilitate participation in vocational opportunities that allow for economic self-sufficiency. Assistive technology (AT) can help persons with a disability to live independently rather than in a long-term care facility. Patients who are independent with a given activity when using equipment (as opposed to requiring assistance) have been noted to experience higher levels of autonomy and self-sufficiency.[36] Two studies have found that equipment was the most efficacious method of reducing and resolving limitations[35] (over assistance from caregivers or other people). This chapter addresses equipment options for basic self-care through high-level community, leisure, or vocational pursuits.

Not everyone is an appropriate candidate for assistive devices. Frequently, equipment that is thought to be appropriate is issued (at considerable expense). It then remains unused unless several factors are identified and appropriately addressed.

Clinical team

Clients are generally evaluated by an occupational therapist working in concert with an interdisciplinary team. Equipment that is prescribed must complement and work with equipment prescribed by other disciplines. For example, if a physical therapist issues a walker to a client for ambulation, the occupational therapist can provide a walker basket to assist the client with carrying items during cooking or community activities. Medical status and prognosis provided by the physician have significant impact on technology needs. Nursing staff can provide valuable input on whether the client is using his or her equipment appropriately and independently. A case manager or social worker determines the discharge situation, which has a profound influence on equipment needs. Psychology services assist a client with adjustment to a disability and stress management or can assess a client's best method of learning.

Clients who have significant difficulty with verbal communication will benefit from *augmentative and alternative communication* (AAC) (as discussed later in the chapter). A speech and language pathologist who specializes in AAC can be a valuable member of the team to address this area. They also may play a significant role in remediation/compensation of cognitive deficits that can impact use of technology.

Evaluation

An evaluation will determine the client's needs. Physical deficits, including range of motion, muscle weakness, and pain limitations on physical activities, are among the most common indicators that an assistive device may be warranted. Range of motion is assessed through a visual assessment of available range. Strength and pain can be assessed through client report, a manual muscle test, or both. If clients have difficulty reaching the head, devices can ease processes such as hair care or donning a shirt, thus allowing more independence. Clients with difficulty reaching the feet can benefit from a variety of long-handled equipment. Clients with even minimal fine motor or perceptual deficits can benefit from a variety of options that allow for more efficient computer access.

Modifying factors for consideration

Goal areas for the client are the most important factors in using an assistive device. Clients must be motivated to use their device. Clients who self-initiate use of an assistive device will have better outcomes than persons who do not. Client who have a device that addresses a goal area that they have identified will generally use the devices for the long term. For example, a client who has goals to return to work will use a button hook for his dress shirt as opposed to a client who is not returning to work and wears an easier to don pullover shirt.

Cognitive, perceptual, and new learning abilities are critical to independent use of a device. If clients display poor learning ability, they may need to adopt compensatory strategies prior to training with an assistive device. Some technology can be used to supervise or allow clients with cognitive deficits to be more independent or require less supervision (as in the case of an emergency call system).

A client's psychosocial adjustment to long-term disability is an important factor in using assistive devices because assistive devices typically are a compensatory strategy for a long-term disability. The client who is unrealistic about his or her prognosis may not participate in goals involving the device but instead be fixed on doing things "the normal way." Mood, depression, anger control issues, and inability to persist with a difficult task can affect new learning and should be addressed.

There are exceptions for short-term disability. For example, most clients with range of motion precautions following a hip arthroplasty are open to the use of long-handled equipment for bathing and dressing. Some clients will accept the use of an assistive device "in the meantime" while their function remains impaired (if prognosis is unclear, as in motor hemiplegia resulting from a stroke).

It is useful with these clients to emphasize that use of an assistive device will not inhibit return of function. However, clients in these cases are generally not open to devices that require a significant investment to learn. They may be more inclined to have a caregiver perform any tasks that require a significant effort.

Aesthetics of the device and body image should be considered. A client with a significantly changed body image (as in the case of a burn survivor) may be confronted by an assistive device. The addition of a piece of equipment that he or she will need to use in daily life (and which may need to be carried with the client) may complicate the psychosocial adjustment. Some clients (especially teenagers or children) benefit from using stickers or designs to make the device "their own."

A client's "gadget tolerance" should be assessed. Some people with disabilities prefer not to work with devices in the first place, as with the general population. A client with poor gadget tolerance may avoid assistive devices. A client with significant premorbid experience with technology or gadgets will have both aptitude for learning a new device as well as fewer adjustment issues. This is particularly the case for more complex assistive devices used for the computer and environment. All devices should be easy to clean, store, and maintain.

These factors are important in a client's adjustment to a device. This is one place where a team approach, including counseling and sensitivity from therapists, will enhance a client's acceptance of the disability and/or the assistive device.

Funding issues

Funding should be considered for all assistive devices. Some devices are covered by commercial health insurance. Substantial effort may be required to write letters of medical necessity for higher-cost items or items that do not have a clear medical benefit. For items that have significant health implications, justification must be presented to the insurance company. Justification of financial benefit to the insurance company also may be needed. For example, an adapted telephone may be considered medically justified for security purposes, enabling clients to call 911 in an emergency, or for calling doctors for follow-up care. Likewise, client control of a hospital bed may be a medical and financial benefit by giving clients the ability to change their position to prevent costly medical complications from bedsores.

In general, AAC equipment and techniques are paid for by Medicare and Medicaid (government health insurance), with some limitations. Most (but not all) health insurance companies will follow their lead. An AAC will be funded by most insurance companies only if recommended by the physician and a speech language pathologist.

Worker's compensation usually proves to be a much better funder of most assistive devices. Although justifications may need to be provided, workmen's compensation will generally fund basic assistive devices through highly expensive and complex computer access programs (along with a computer to run the program), AACs, or electronic aids to daily living (EADLs) as described later in this chapter.

Clients who have vocational or educational goals may have funding available through their state Office of Rehabilitation Services (in the United States). Although the assistive devices or applications must be related to specific return to work or school goals, this agency can be a source of funding for computer access as well as modifications to a work environment that are not well funded by other payers.

For many lower-cost items, some clients will be required to pay out of pocket. Otherwise, alternative funding can be investigated. Some hospitals fund equipment from a charity care fund. Clients with certain diagnoses may be able to acquire funding through organizations dedicated to that diagnosis.

Pediatric clients may be eligible for benefits through a variety of charitable organizations. Some clients may belong to community groups or churches that maintain or can raise funds to meet some of these expenses. Some U.S. states maintain programs for clients with disabilities to purchase adaptive telephones. For higher-cost items, some clients may qualify for low-interest loans through state AT programs.

Equipment options

The following sections offer brief descriptions of some of the many commonly used devices. Most of the options are commercially available. However, for particular clients and abilities, creative modifications (necessity is the mother of invention) or investigation of similar devices (with slightly different features) may be needed. The first section addresses assistive devices for daily living skills, such as basic activities of daily living (ADL; dressing, bathing) and complex ADL (home management, cooking, and cleaning). The second section focuses on AT, which is normally powered in some fashion and has specific applications related to the computer, the home electronic environment, and/or communication ability.

An occupational therapist is versed in the use of many lower-technology options that assist with basic or complex ADL. Many larger rehabilitation hospitals have a number of these devices available for trial and resale. These hospitals may offer an ADL apartment that provides clients with an opportunity to trial these devices prior to purchase. Clients who do not have access to these services may be able to find more information on the Internet from vendors, suppliers, and other web sites dedicated to the consumer of assistive devices (see resource list[37]).

Basic self-care devices

Self-feeding

Feeding is one of the first activities clients will return to after the onset of disability. If grip is impaired, lighter-weight utensils or utensils with a built-up handle can benefit clients. Clients with an arthritic grip may benefit from these devices to decrease future negative impact on the joints and to reduce pain. Clients with quadriplegia due to spinal cord injury may lack isolated finger control or grip and may benefit from the use of a universal cuff to hold utensils. Many common splints for clients with spinal cord injury can be adapted with a specialized slot to hold utensils or other tools. Utensils with a swivel handle can allow clients with limited supination/pronation to obtain food or soup from a plate. A rocker knife can allow persons to use one hand to cut their food using a rocking motion that will not move the food as a "sawing" motion would. Clients who are unable to hold a standard cup because they lack isolated finger motion may benefit from use of a mug/cup with a T-shaped handle. A long straw or tubing attached to a gooseneck or other mount such as Loc-Line (gooseneck-type mount with a flexible straw inside) can be used for drinking.

Mobile arm supports (MAS) are used by persons with limitations in shoulder movement and for feeding. The MAS is a portable device that can attach to a wheelchair It helps with hand-to-mouth movements by assisting with raising the arm against gravity. Several adaptations with the MAS

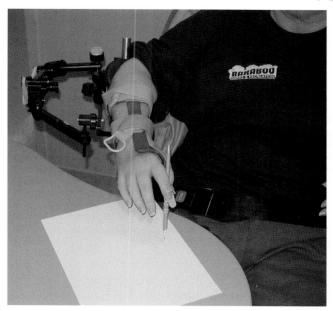

Fig. 46-1 A mobile arm support can be used to assist a client with limited upper extremities in self-feeding, writing, or grooming activities.

allow clients to more adequately obtain food with their utensil, raise the utensil to their mouth, and reach for a cup. Combined with the proper adaptive feeding devices and splints, many clients with quadriplegia or other upper extremity dysfunction require only setup with a MAS to feed themselves. Clients using a MAS will require minimal shoulder flexion/abduction and minimal elbow flexion to allow for successful use (Fig. 46-1).

Hygiene and grooming

Clients who cannot reach the face for hygiene and grooming may benefit from an MAS. A universal cuff or other wrist hand orthosis can be adapted to hold lipstick applicators, hair brushes, combs, and toothbrushes. Some people with limited shoulder motion (but intact grip) may benefit from use of a long-handled comb or brush. As with feeding, many clients will benefit from built-up handles or lightweight utensils. Clients with hemiplegia normally will have sufficient grip and range of motion in their uninvolved upper extremity to brush their dentures or apply shaving cream to a shaving brush when the device is stabilized with a suction cup. Although these items can be useful, they may require extra sink space and can be unreliable or break more easily. Thus, some clients may develop one-handed methods.

Upper extremity dressing

Most clients with significant bilateral upper extremity dysfunction probably are not able to participate physically (with orthoses or not) with their dressing. They can and should be active participants through direction of the task. However, those who have adequate function in one arm will benefit from adaptive methods to don their clothing. Hook-and-loop fasteners can be used in place of standard buttons or ties. An orthosis such as a button hook with a zipper pull can allow people to access buttons and zippers with one hand. It can benefit clients with impaired grip (Fig. 46-2).

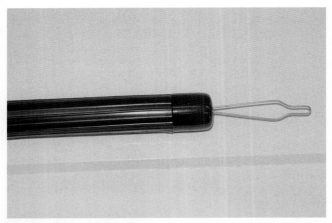

Fig. 46-2 A button hook can allow a person with limited pinch to independently button a shirt or other fasteners.

Lower extremity dressing

In clients with balance difficulties or weakness in the lower extremities, clothing management (pulling pants or a skirt up or down for dressing or toileting) can be accomplished using a walker or grab bar to stabilize their balance. Many clients will benefit from equipment to dress their lower extremities. A dressing stick can be used to start pants or a dress over the feet and pull the clothing item up to mid-thigh in clients with hip range of motion precautions following an arthroplasty. A sock aid and long-handled shoe horn can be used to allow clients to don socks/shoes. Elastic shoelaces or hook-and-loop straps can eliminate shoe tying. Clients may find donning pants or skirts with elastic waistbands easier than manipulating belts or fasteners.

Toileting/bathing

Many appliances are useful for toileting. Clients with limited reach may be able to use tongs for perineal cleansing. Similarly, clients with limited reach may benefit from a long-handled sponge or brush for washing their feet or other areas. Some people will consider using a bidet for cleaning themselves. An elevated toilet seat can allow standing or sitting with greater ease. Clients with limited mobility may benefit from use of a male urinal or a freshette (*www.freshet te.com*) for women. A bedside commode can facilitate clients toileting themselves in a timely manner as opposed to use of a standard toilet in another room.

Safety during bathing and toileting should always be addressed. Bathroom safety devices as addressed have been demonstrated to decrease the risk of falls and injuries in elderly people.[4] Bathtub transfers have been noted as one of the most difficult transfers for seniors. This can be an even greater challenge for persons with a mobility deficit due to disability. A well-placed grab bar or tub seat can help prevent potentially serious falls for all people but even more so for persons with a disability. Despite the safety advantages offered by access to bathing and toileting aids, these devices are woefully underutilized. Naik and Gill[28] found that only 54% of people with a disability related to their bathing had access to bathing aids that could facilitate function and enhance their safety.

Bathing using a shower chair or bench can allow more independence for clients with impaired transfers. A long shower hose attached to a hand-held shower will benefit these clients. People with decreased endurance will benefit from using a chair, especially while shampooing hair (as the energy expenditure of reaching overhead while standing may preclude shampooing for these clients.) Clients with decreased hand function will benefit from use of a shower mitt (washcloth sewn into or with a pouch to hold soap), liquid soap dispenser, soap on a rope, or suction soap holder.

Home/office work

Reading

Clients who are unable to hold a book or other reading material may benefit from a number of devices. A book holder with an elastic string can hold pages in place while other pages are being turned. Clients unable to reach a book holder may be able to use a mechanical page turner. These devices can be accessed by either switches or joysticks to activate a combination of rollers and a sticky substance to allow the page to be grabbed and turned. These devices usually are expensive and can be unreliable for certain kinds of books or magazines. If clients are unable to look down (i.e., cervical spine is immobilized), they may benefit from use of prism glasses, which reflect light at a 90-degree angle and allow clients to read a book in their lap. Clients with low vision may benefit from book magnifiers that use external screens or closed circuit television systems that allow for contrast of text on anything from books to bills to prescriptions labels. A number of books are available for reading on a computer (given consistent access to the computer as described later). Commercially available books frequently are available in electronic format designed for reading on a computer screen. Many books that are past their copyright are available for free downloading, and some web sites for downloading copyrighted books are designed for people with disabilities.[34]

Safety devices

For clients who are alone at any time, independent control of lighting is critical to preventing falls. Touch lamps or lights that are activated by sound can be used to improve lighting during a transfer. Halogen lamps or other extremely bright lights should be used in poorly lit areas. X-10 (smarthome) technology can activate overhead lights or other household appliances through a small console or wireless remote. Consideration should be given to removing scatter rugs or taping them down to prevent tripping.

Telephone access

A variety of telephones can assist persons with placing and receiving calls. Clients who cannot hold a standard telephone (because of impaired grip) can use a built-up handle or palm hook on the receiver. A speakerphone or a telephone with a headset can allow for access. Clients who have difficulty with hitting multiple buttons to dial in a timely manner can use speed dial functions. A cordless phone can be used by clients if access is needed from the bed or other areas. Cellular telephones are readily available for the same purpose. People who need more features than the readily available commercial options may benefit from other options discussed later in the chapter.

Call systems

Clients can use a variety of call systems. Clients who are nonverbal may benefit from use of a hand bell or other device. If clients need a device that will sound for farther distances, a wireless doorbell available at most hardware stores may work. Clients activate the button to sound a doorbell placed in a central location where the caregiver can hear it. If clients with limited upper extremity function cannot push the small button, then they may benefit from a personal pager.[7] This device allows larger buttons such as switches (see section on switches) to activate a pager. Some clients who can manipulate an intercom can call for assistance. An intercom can be latched on or a baby monitor can be used; however, many people prefer other options so that they do not have to listen to the client's activities (e.g., telephone conversations or television shows).

If clients are alone during the day, they need a system that allows them to summon assistance from outside the home. Clients who can operate a cordless phone can attach one to their wheelchair with hook-and-loop closure. If clients are at risk for falling while alone, a button worn as a pendant or wristwatch can be used to activate an emergency call system. A monitored emergency call system will contact a 24-hour monitoring service. The service will automatically receive the call along with previously provided information about the client's condition and contact numbers. Clients who can speak to the monitoring service (with the included speaker phone) can instruct the service to take appropriate action (call neighbor, call 911, etc.). If clients are unable to speak, the service will follow a prearranged plan. Some studies have found that use of an emergency call system can decrease utilization of hospital days and increase the amount of time that elderly persons can remain in the home (as opposed to a long-term care facility).[19] If clients are physically unable to push the pendant, alternate switches can be used (see section on switches).

A monitored service usually requires a monthly fee for the duration of service. For persons who require this service for a long period but the expense is a concern, a nonmonitored system can be purchased. When activated by a pendant similar to that used by the monitored system, the nonmonitored system will call a series of up to five numbers in succession. It will continue to call the numbers until an individual answers (the system will not activate for a voice mail service or answering machine). When the individual picks up the phone, a prerecorded message plays (usually indicating the person's name and address and that the person needs help). This system is dependent on someone answering the phone and taking the appropriate action. A speakerphone can be activated on some systems. 911 can be one of the numbers programmed, and all municipalities can track the location of someone calling and thus send emergency response providers.

Meal preparation

A variety of options allow clients to prepare their meal more efficiently. Stoves with dials on the front can be reached by persons in a wheelchair (as opposed to dials located above the stove). A wooden push–pull stick can be used to extend reach when pulling oven racks in and out of the oven. A rope or cord attached to a refrigerator door handle can be used to pull open the door. Clients who are ambulatory may benefit from

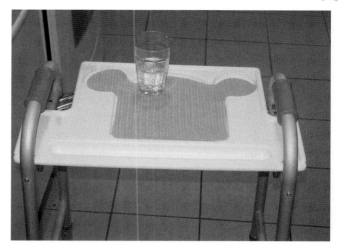

Fig. 46-3 A walker tray can allow a client using a walker to carry objects or containers during meal preparation or other activities.

a rolling cart that can be used to transport items from the stove or refrigerator to a countertop or dining table. Clients who already are using a walker can use a walker tray or basket (Fig. 46-3), although they must be educated to not overload the tray and possibly unbalance the walker. A variety of tools are available to assist persons having limited upper extremity function with food preparation. Cutting boards with a spike protruding up through it will hold food in place so that persons using one hand can cut or chop the food. Other cutting boards come with a variety of stabilizers to hold food in place (Fig. 46-4). A variety of jar openers allow persons with a weak grip to use stronger forearm pronators and supinators to open a tight lid.[27] Electric can openers, food processors, and blenders can reduce energy expenditure and time. Clients may prefer to use a microwave oven for food preparation given the decreased time and ease of use over a standard oven. People who have reduced sensation may need protective equipment to prevent burns from a stove or hot containers.

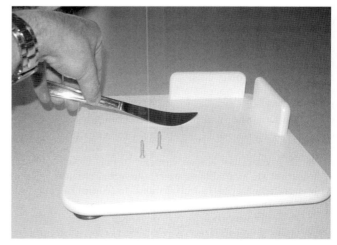

Fig. 46-4 A rocker knife combined with a spike cutting board can allow a person with use of one upper extremity to cut food.

Home maintenance

Clients may perform lighter household cleaning using common cleaning equipment. A long-handled dust brush and dust pan can be used by persons in a wheelchair or by ambulatory clients who have difficulty reaching the floor. Likewise, a sponge mop can be used for light mopping. A lighter-weight canister vacuum with an attached hose is easier to manipulate than an upright vacuum.

Home egress and outdoor options

Clients who are unable to access standard doors have options to make egress possible. Door handles with a lever shape, as opposed to the standard knob, are much easier to use by clients with limited hand function. Doorknob holders may allow persons with a weak grip to use their forearm muscles to turn a doorknob. Keys can be put onto a key holder that adds a longer lever arm and allows clients to use their forearm rotators as opposed to finger pinch for key turning. Power door openers can be installed in a home or office to allow a door to be opened or closed. These openers are available for inner and outer doors. Clients who use a wheelchair or have limited arm placement will benefit from a dowel or a reacher to push elevator buttons. A cellular telephone can be used for a variety of features, including calling for assistance or direction. Various devices can be combined with global positioning satellite (GPS) technology to determine location, both providing direction to clients or locating clients in an emergency.

Higher-technology options

For clients requiring higher-technology options (for access to telephone, computer, or household electronics) or clients who are unable to speak, many options are available. This section addresses options that are not readily available (such as call systems discussed earlier) or have been designed specifically for people with disabilities. These devices usually are referred to as assistive technology (AT).

EADLs are devices that allow clients to control common household electronics. Clients who are unable to access a standard remote control can operate electronic devices through a number of switch options (which can be activated by head, arm, leg or a variety of other motions) or speech recognition. These devices include a television, stereo system, telephone, lights, and/or fans. They also include options such as call systems, window blinds, power doors, and pet feeders. Computer access refers to options that can allow clients to control a computer. Options for physical impairment, cognitive impairment, and visual impairments are available to help clients access their computer. Clients who are unable to operate a keyboard or mouse may benefit from options such as speech recognition programs that allow for command and control of their computer as well as dictation of text. Clients with significant perceptual impairment can use auditory feedback or magnification options to make the computer screen appear larger. AAC refers to options that are available to assist nonverbal clients or clients with significant speech impairment to communicate with people in their environment. These options range from a simple communication board or single message device to a portable computerized device that can communicate multiple novel messages as well as provide access to a computer and the environment.

These options allow for vocational purposes, leisure pursuits, communication, and socialization. Clients with disabilities frequently do not have access to the same community resources or social opportunities that most others do; these options will allow for modified participation in these pursuits. The computer can be an equalizer for people with disabilities who are otherwise unable to participate in educational and vocational activities.

Clients who wish to pursue these options will benefit from an AT evaluation with a therapist who specializes in these services. AT is a specialized field that requires significant training to successfully match a piece of AT to a specific client's needs. The Rehabilitation Engineering Society of North America (RESNA) maintains an assistive technology practitioner (ATP) credential that requires practitioners to acquire a certain level of knowledge. However, many qualified practitioners do not seek this credential. Additionally, because AT includes knowledge of wheelchair seating and positioning, a consumer should interview practitioners about their experience related to computer access, EADLs, and AACs.

AT vendors can provide some knowledge and expertise to clients. Vendors of given pieces of AT will generally have a greater knowledge of their particular devices. However, they are committed to the sale of their pieces of technology and may not consider options available from other vendors. An AT clinician, familiar with the wide range of available technology, can provide an evaluation that will consider the best options available to a given client.

Involvement of the vendor of higher-technology products may be warranted during a trial period of a given device. If the device is computerized or electronically complex, troubleshooting, long-term device maintenance, and information related to the warranty are important to evaluate. If the device breaks down, how quickly will the vendor respond to fix the problem? Will the device need to be shipped to the manufacturer for evaluation and repair (thus leaving the client without access to a device that makes them independent)? Some vendors may make house calls to repair or troubleshoot a device. Different clients in different situations will have different tolerances for the various options available.

Referrals to ATPs in local areas are available through the RESNA web site, as are referrals to state AT projects that may be able to refer to qualified clinicians. As with other options, clients who have very specific and limited needs may be able to determine appropriate equipment by looking through catalogs or obtaining information from the Internet. Clients with more significant impairment or multiple needs usually will benefit from seeking an evaluation with a qualified practitioner.

Other team members who may be involved are rehabilitation engineers. Rehabilitation engineers have specific training in biomedical sciences that allows them to match, modify, or create technology to assist clients to perform a given task. A rehabilitation engineer may be involved in making custom devices that allow clients to access paperwork and multiple office documents through a motorized rotating shelf. They may be involved in working with a wheelchair modification that allows clients to more effectively transport a laptop or portable communication device. Ambulatory clients may benefit from a custom carrying case that will allow them access to a device while they are standing and walking. A cellular phone headset can be modified to allow clients with limited hand function to activate the speech recognition features to place or answer calls. Although some of these products are commercially available, a rehabilitation engineer may be able to provide the custom "tweaking" to make a device truly functional for a given client.

If a client has AAC needs, a speech and language pathologist will be involved in the assessment to determine appropriate devices and techniques. A speech therapist can determine a device or technique that is appropriate for the client's language level. For example, a child who has never developed language will have very different needs from an adult who has sustained a brain injury (and may have coexisting perceptual or cognitive deficits). The speech therapist can determine the most appropriate device or techniques (as described later in this chapter).

Clients who do not have access to a qualified practitioner or who wish to increase their knowledge can take advantage of various Internet resources. Most AT vendors maintain web sites devoted to their products, offering descriptions, technical specifications, and prices. Clinicians may benefit from resources available through RESNA or the American Occupational Therapy Association.

Closing The Gap is an organization that addresses AT needs and is designed for consumers and their caregivers. They have an online database of AT products and a large bulletin board system for exchange of ideas. The California State University at Northridge and Closing The Gap offer a yearly conference with presentations related to AT and large vendor exhibits. Abledata maintains a web site (*www.abledata.com*) that contains reviews, purchase options, and other information related to all types of assistive devices. It is notable for its inclusion of products related to leisure activities and a variety of articles related to consumer information for people with disabilities.

Training

Clients who pursue any of the moderately complex pieces of technology usually will benefit from training with the device. Depending on their aptitude for technology and the intuitiveness of a device, clients may require one training and orientation session for a simple electronic aid or several sessions to review and practice a speech recognition program for hands-free access to a computer. Training needs should be part of an evaluation, and prescription of a device should not be made without identifying who will perform training and follow-up. Vendors of a given product may be involved in this process but may not be appropriate if clients have significant cognitive or perceptual deficits that require a clinician's skill.

Training with complex equipment needs to address a variety of factors. Clients' previous experience with similar technology is very relevant. If clients have minimal previous experience with a computer, training in basic computer operation and functions must be provided. These clients may benefit from computer training available through local community colleges and programs (if accessible to them). Training may need to focus on limited tasks until mastery is achieved, before moving on to more complex or multiple operations. New learning ability should be evaluated to determine the best method for clients to acquire new knowledge. Many clients benefit from written and visual reminders of common functions to remind them when the trainer

is not present. Clients should expect to practice with a given device multiple times before they can demonstrate proficiency and maintain competency with the device over time.

A number of available products have either demonstration software or evaluation periods that can be used to determine if the products are beneficial to a given client. It is strongly recommended that clients take advantage of opportunity and spend the full evaluation product for several similar products to determine the best option for their situation. Additionally, various institutions, including state AT projects and large AT centers, have lending libraries that may be able to provide devices for evaluation. This opportunity will allow people with disabilities to trial a given option in their home environment.

Reliability and durability of given devices can be assessed through a trial period. The quality of technical support available or the ability of caregivers to troubleshoot a given device usually will be apparent during a rental or trial period. This should be given due consideration when evaluating if a device is appropriate for purchase.

Access

This section addresses various methods of accessing given devices. Access refers to a given method for controlling a computer, EADL, or AAC device. In this chapter, access is divided into three main sections: direct selection, switch access, and voice recognition.

Access for more complex cognitive tasks (e.g., computer use or communication) may require significant training for clients to allow them efficient use of the access. Efficient touch typists can type 40 words per minute (WPM), and they do not need to think about hitting the correct key. This access is subcognitive and allows typists to focus their conscious attention on what they are creating, as opposed to thinking about the process of hitting the correct key. This form of access is what clients using their computer or communication device need to strive for, such that they can concentrate on the message they are trying to communicate or the computer tasks they are performing. Significant practice may be required to accomplish this goal. For the same reason, the access method chosen should be the simplest possible to allow clients to make the access subcognitive.

Access needs to be as simple as possible given the capabilities of the client. Equipment abandonment is a significant issue particularly given the expense of equipment. Three participants in a study abandoned equipment that they perceived as too complicated to use.[8]

Direct selection

Direct selection refers to the ability to activate a single control with a single result. For example, pushing an "A" on a keyboard results in the letter "A" being typed into a document. Pushing "Power" on your TV remote results in the TV turning on. Direct selection can be accomplished by a finger motion or by devices such as a mouth stick, typing stick, or head pointer. If the motor ability for direct selection is present, it is the preferred method because of its great ease, speed, and cognitive simplicity.

Given that direct selection is motorically demanding, fatigue and positioning factors must be addressed. Clients who may be able to type using direct selection for 2 hour during a clinical evaluation may find that typing for 8 hours in a competitive employment situation is impossible. The same concept can apply even more for people using a mouth stick or typing stick, who may be required to type for long periods of time while using gross head or arm movement as opposed to isolated finger control.

Positioning must be evaluated. Many clients who can access a television remote or cordless telephone while sitting may not be able to activate them while lying supine in bed. Seeing the control while lying down while positioning the device for its own function (as in the case of a remote for a television) can be challenging.

Finally, prognosis must be addressed. Clients with a diagnosis of amyotrophic lateral sclerosis (ALS) or other degenerative diseases who may be able to accomplish direct selection at one point in their disease process should be cognizant that this ability may not always be present. They will benefit from a device that allows for multiple access methods.

Direct selection has an economic advantage over scanning and voice recognition devices. Normally it is among the least expensive options. In general, the price increases with device complexity.

Switch access

When motor function is not sufficient for direct selection, switch access can be considered. Switches can be combined with any single available motion to provide full access to a computer, EADL, or AAC device. A button switch can be combined with a gross arm or head motion. Light-touch switches, such as the Micro light switch, require only 0.4 oz of pressure.[32] Pneumatic switches can provide a stable switch for clients to use. Switches such as electromyelogram (EMG), proximity, or even brainwave switches can be considered if the motor skills available indicate it. Eye blink switches are available but can be very difficult to appropriately position.

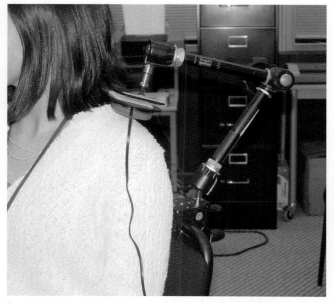

Fig. 46-5 Magic Arm positions a switch near a client's consistent motion site to allow him or her to consistently activate it. (Courtesy R.J. Cooper.)

Positioning of an eye blink switch such that it is not activated by natural eye blinks but is activated by an exaggerated eye blink or cheek twitch can be difficult. Clients with multiple caregivers may find it difficult to train all of their caregivers to appropriately position the switch. This is especially difficult if caregivers care for multiple clients.

Stability of a switch (such that it does not fall away from the control site) must be considered. Mounting arms such as a Magic Arm (Fig. 46-5) may allow for easy positioning of a switch if the client's position is changed.[1] A more stable or custom-made switch mount, such as the Daessy Stem system, can reduce the need for a caregiver to carefully position a switch.[14]

Aesthetic concerns for switches may be considerable. Switches positioned by the head or near the face may be undesirable to many clients. Most switches are available in multiple colors and may assuage this issue. Similar consideration should be given to mounting arms. Some clients prefer that their mounts be spray painted an appropriate color or positioned closer to existing frames on a chair.

Development of switch access

Children and/or adults with significant cognitive disabilities may require significant training to develop efficient switch access. Clients need to demonstrate proficiency in the following areas:

- Cause/effect related to a switch
- Ability to activate the switch
- Ability to release the switch in a timely manner
- Divided attention sufficient to attend to switch and device access

Various devices can be used to perform this training, including switch-accessible computer software, switch latch timers, and battery adapters to operate simple games or activities. If clients have significant communication difficulty, switch training can be prescribed in preparation for use of a high-end AAC device.

Scanning

Once a stable switch site has been developed, scanning may be investigated as an option for access to a device. The most common form of scanning is one switch or automatic scanning. With this method, a visual and/or auditory indicator moves between options available on a device (Fig. 46-6). (Options may include letters or prestored phrases or macros

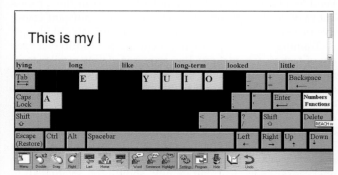

Fig. 46-6 REACH keyboard removes letters that will not follow a given letter after the first letter is typed. For example, after "L" is typed, Smart Keys removes "Q," "W," "R," and other letters that would never follow an "L."

on a computer or communication device, or functions available on an EADL.) When the desired option is indicated, clients activate the switch. The speed of the scan can be adjusted to slower rates during training. As client skills improve, increased speed will increase efficiency.

Two-switch step scanning or inverse scanning may offer access to clients who have difficulty with the cognitive/perceptual or motor demands of automatic scanning. In step scanning, clients activate one switch to move the indicator to the desired selection. Clients then activate the second switch to select the option. This process removes the need for timely switch activation (required by automatic scanning), which may be difficult for clients with significant spasticity. Step scanning also generally requires less cognitive ability and can be a precursor to automatic scanning. Step scanning is more fatiguing because it requires a greater number of switch activations. Inverse scanning consists of clients holding down a switch. As long as the switch is held down, the indicator moves between the given options. When the desired option is reached, clients release the switch to make the selection. This can be useful for clients with high tone. In these cases, the switch is positioned above the leg or arm. When the desired option is reached, they can relax, allowing gravity release of the switch. Inverse scanning combined with auditory feedback has been noted to be easier for clients with perceptual deficits.

Other methods of switch access are available. Some clients benefit from encoding over scanning. Encoding techniques, such as Morse code, may offer a relatively fast method of access to a device; two switch users have demonstrated the ability to type as fast as 20 to 25 WPM. Additionally Morse code has potential to be subcognitive.[26] However, this technique requires a significant learning investment to memorize the codes, and few devices offer Morse code. Computer programs such as EZ-Keys and AAC devices (DV4 and MT4) from DynaVox allow for Morse code access.

Clients with good vocal control may utilize speech or voice recognition for access to the computer or EADL. Speech recognition for the computer may provide highly efficient access for typing tasks or EADL. Voicing (for clients with significant speech deficits) also may be beneficial for certain computer tasks or EADL (as long as clients can produce a consistent utterance). Although voice recognition typically is the fastest method of access, it also can be the most cognitively demanding method. Additionally, the reliability of voice recognition during client voice fluctuations (with anxious clients or cases of laryngitis) should be considered.

Once the most efficient access method has been identified, clients can start to consider possible devices. The following section considers devices available for EADL, computer access, and AAC. Note that considerable overlap may exist between these areas. For example, many AAC devices allow for infrared control of household devices. Additionally, some computer access methods allow for AAC or EADL access. A trained AT clinician can parse out these benefits. An effort has been made to present a range of devices, but the following section is not meant to be exhaustive. Many devices that previously were available are no longer manufactured, and new devices are introduced each year. Consultation with an AT clinician with current knowledge of available devices is always recommended to determine the best option for clients with significant disability.

Electronic aids to daily living

A number of options are available for clients who desire to control household appliances. Telephones, infrared remote controls, and plug-in devices (e.g., lamps or fans) are available for use or modification for clients with disabilities. Client can control thermostats, window blinds, power doors, and pet feeders. Most electronic devices can be controlled through an EADL.

Studies have demonstrated multiple benefits to clients who use EADL. Clients with spinal cord injury who are successful with an EADL have demonstrated increased independence as well as decreased frustration while performing tasks.[31] This study demonstrated a significant and positive impact on the psychosocial well-being of these clients. Of note, the successful use of the EADL was achieved in operation of devices that were a high priority to clients, in accordance with the earlier discussion on the importance of involving the client's goals in the evaluation for an appropriate EADL. Nursing home staff have reported a decrease in their frustration following introduction of the EADL.[13]

Telephones

Speaker phones, cordless telephones, and cellular telephones controlled via switch and/or voice access are available. The RC 200 Speakerphone offers a variety of features that allow for telephone access. A switch-activated remote allows for answering the phone, as does a voice answering feature (if clients cannot use a given switch). If clients wish to place a call, the switch activates an automatic scan of up to 20 different phone numbers. The RC 200 can be combined with a headset to allow for private conversations or for use by clients with weaker voices who have difficulty being heard over a speaker phone. The SAJE Communicator allows clients to push a switch and then use spoken commands to operate a two-line telephone for business purposes or home use. Funding options for telephones may be available in some states in the United States that offer services for clients with disabilities to acquire and receive funding for adaptive telephones.

X-10 is technology that has been developed for home automation purposes. An X-10 signal can be sent from a transmitter to a receiver that is plugged into existing house electrical wiring. The transceiver then sends a signal over the existing AC wiring of the house. The signal is received by a module that has a household appliance, such as a lamp or fan, plugged into it. The module then either supplies or withdraws power to the device. Various handheld remotes can be used through direct selection to turn on or off multiple appliances. In addition to devices such as lamps and fans, window blinds, pet feeders, thermostats, and many other household features can be automated and controlled through an EADL by persons with a disability. A number of devices as well as a number of articles offering troubleshooting and tips for use are available from *www.Smarthome.com*.

Devices such as the Relax series allow clients to control infrared devices through automatic scanning (or step scanning available in the Relax 2 and Relax 3 models).[33] The Mini Relax offers access to one infrared device such as a television or stereo with limited functionality. This may allow persons with cognitive deficits to access a device as opposed to the more complex form of scanning in the

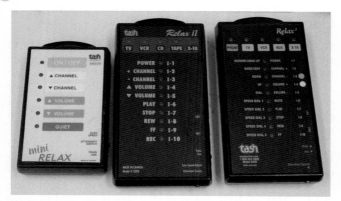

Fig. 46-7 Mini Relax, Relax 2, and Relax 3 from Tash, Inc.

Relax 2 and Relax 3 models. The Relax 2 allows for control of multiple infrared devices and the X-10. The Relax 3 adds access to a speakerphone with a directory of 40 different telephone numbers or five speed-dial numbers (Fig. 46-7).

The Gewa PROG is a small portable device (slightly larger than a deck of cards) that allows for direct selection or one- or two-switch activation of multiple infrared devices in addition to a speaker phone and X-10. It offers approximately 130 different infrared signals (compared to 30 or 40 for the Relax series), but it requires clients to navigate between different levels to access the signals while remembering which number or symbol is associated with which function. Thus the device is much more cognitively demanding. The Gewa Progress is manufactured by the same company and is based on a pocket PC. It also allows for use of symbols or words corresponding to given functions, thus eliminating the need to remember which keys perform what function (TV Power symbol will turn on the TV, as opposed to Key 5 on level 2 activating TV power as on the PROG).

A myriad of higher-end devices, such as the SAJE Powerhouse or Roommate, allow for voice activation of EADL features. Clients can use a switch to activate the SAJE and then give a voice command such as "TV Power" or "Call Bob." The Sicare is a portable unit that requires only voice commands to activate multiple devices, including the X-10 and a speaker phone. Although the Relax series and Gewa products have limitations on the number of devices supported, the SAJE series and the Sicare allow for control of almost unlimited home equipment. The SAJE series requires relatively clear speech from clients to match the voice modeling used. It also requires a computer running the Windows operating system (OS). Although the stability and reliability of computers have significantly increased, the device may be susceptible to computer viruses and other maladies that can befall computers. The Sicare requires a computer for training and setup but not daily operation. Because the Sicare requires that clients train their voice into the device, clients without a clear voice may be able to control the Sicare only as long as their vocalization is consistent from day to day.

Computer access
Computers can be accessed through a variety of methods. The cognitive and perceptual ability of a given client should be carefully considered for computer access trials. Most common computer tasks involve significant cognitive effort.

Learning an alternate access method (while learning tasks such as how to use e-mail) can make this process more challenging. Clients with cognitive impairments may benefit from several trials to determine if the time, effort, and expense are worthwhile.

Computers and the Internet can provide a method for isolated persons to gain peers and social supports. Residents of long-term care centers reported increased feelings of competence and autonomy following training in computer tasks.[24] Caregivers also will use the Internet to seek support.[22] One article describes a program that provided elderly and disabled people (who were unable to leave their homes) with computers. The participants were provided with computers, appropriate AT, and training that allowed them to join an online "community." At the end of 1 year, participants reported marked improvement in their satisfaction with social contact.[10] From a vocational or educational standpoint, successful computer use can allow clients to compete with peers in their studies or job. The computer has been called an "electronic curb cut" for students with disabilities in a postsecondary school setting.[15]

Some clients with significant cognitive impairment or younger children can benefit from computer access activities. Children enjoy age-appropriate computer games that are available through alternative access (via switch, joystick, or other access method). Single-switch computer games are available for clients to use for leisure purposes and/or for training switch access for use of more complex devices.

For more traditional computer tasks, a variety of alternatives are available. Clients may benefit from modifications or changes to their computer mouse, keyboard, or monitor. Specific modifications are discussed here.

Keyboard options
Software modifications to standard keyboards can enhance or allow access to a keyboard. Accessibility options such as filter keys or sticky keys are available in both the Windows OS and Macintosh OS. If clients have difficulty with multiple hits on a keyboard or holding down the keys too long, filter keys can be set to ignore repeated hits, slow down repeat rate, or require a key to be held down for a length of time. Sticky keys will allow one-finger or one-hand typists to tap a modifier key and then move on to the key to be modified (as opposed to holding both keys at the same time).

Clients with ataxia may benefit from a keyguard, which is a rigid plastic overlay that is custom sized to a particular keyboard. The plastic overlay allows clients to slide their finger into the intended key while avoiding accidental key presses of adjacent keys (Fig. 46-8).

Many clients may benefit from enlarged keyboards, or smaller keyboards, depending on their motor and perceptual ability. Clients with significant ataxia or clients with decreased vision may benefit from a larger keyboard with oversized keys, such as BigKeys. Clients with significant proximal range of motion limitations may benefit from a small keyboard, such as the Tash USB Mini keyboard (Fig. 46-9). A variety of ergonomic keyboards are available for clients who have overuse injuries.

One-handed keyboard options are available for both standard keyboards as well as alternate keyboards that are specifically designed for access by one hand. Five-finger typing tutors are available for people who are one-handed typists.

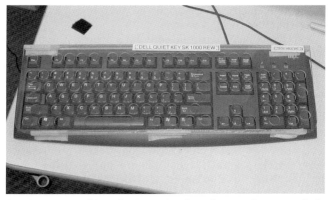

Fig. 46-8 Keyguard is a plastic overlay that allows a client to push the correct key while avoiding pressing adjacent unintended keys.

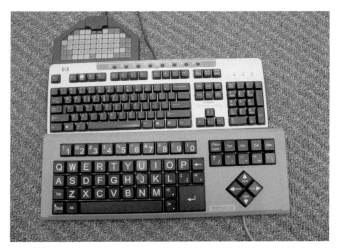

Fig. 46-9 From top to bottom, USB Mini Keyboard (Tash, Inc), standard computer keyboard, and BigKeys LX keyboard (Greystone Digital).

Keyboards such as the Half-QWERTY or the FrogPad allow all keys to be typed from one position as opposed to having to move the hand around the keyboard. The BAT keyboard allows for use of a chording system that allows all the keys in that area on a standard keyboard to be typed using a combination of seven keys. Clients who have efficient mouse access can use an onscreen keyboard, which is software that emulates the standard keyboard (Fig. 46-10).

Clients with keyboarding difficulty (or slowed typing) may benefit from abbreviation expansion, which allows persons to type a two- to three-letter code that then expands out to a longer preprogrammed phrase. Typing "AT" would expand to "Assistive Technology." Clients with a decreased keyboarding rate (< 7–8 WPM) may benefit from word prediction software. This software allows clients to type the first two to three letters of a word, such as "He." This produces a list of words that match those letters (Heat, Hello, Helicopter), which clients can pick from to finish typing the word. Word prediction can increase writing ability and self-esteem in clients with learning disabilities who are fast typists. Word prediction can decrease the number of keystrokes required to complete a word, but it is not helpful in increasing speed. Additionally, for many users, the increased cognitive load of using word prediction may offset any gains (Fig. 46-11).[5]

Mouse options

Many clients benefit from modifications to the computer OS that enhance or allow mouse access. Mouse speed and clicking options can be adjusted to benefit clients. Mouse Keys is an OS modification that uses the number pad to control the mouse. With this feature enabled, clients can move the mouse up by pressing the "8" key, down by pressing the "2" key, and so on. Left clicking and other click functions (including dragging) are available via the number pad.

Many computer functions that are frequently accessed through the mouse can be operated through keyboard shortcuts. For example, pressing "CTRL P" will print a document in

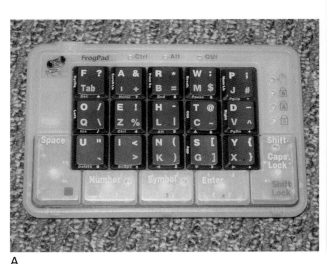

A

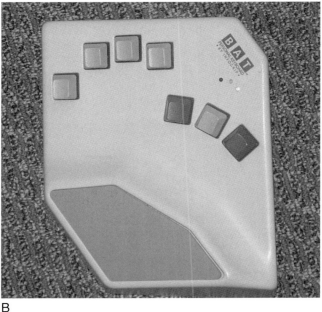

B

Fig. 46-10 One-handed keyboards. **A**, FrogPad. **B**, BAT keyboard.

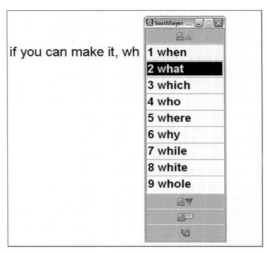

if you can make it, wh

1	when
2	what
3	which
4	who
5	where
6	why
7	while
8	white
9	whole

Fig. 46-11 Soothsayer word prediction software (Applied Human Factors) predicts words that start with the letters typed, in this case "wh."

most Microsoft Windows programs and will accomplish the task faster than locating the mouse, moving the mouse cursor, and then clicking on the appropriate icon or menu. Keyboard shortcut summaries are readily available on the Internet or by navigating through the menus of most programs.

Many clients may be able to move the mouse but have difficulty with efficient mouse clicks. Dwell software can be used to replace mouse clicking by allowing clients to hover their mouse on a target for a preset length of time, after which the software sends a click. Hardware modifications can be used to allow a switch external to the mouse to send mouse clicks.

Hardware options to replace a standard mouse are available. Trackballs are commercially available and can allow clients with finger impairment or absence to control mouse functions. Touch pads, joysticks, and other pointing devices can replace a standard mouse. Clients with upper extremity dysfunction may benefit from use of a head-operated mouse. This allows clients to wear a small reflective dot on the forehead or eyeglass frame (Fig. 46-12). The device tracks head motion and translates it into mouse motion. Mouse clicking is accomplished through dwell software or external switch. For clients with severe motor impairment (e.g., C1 complete spinal cord injury), an eye gaze or eye-controlled mouse may be used to translate eye movement into

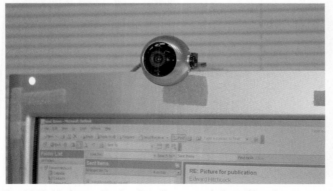

Fig. 46-12 Madentec Tracker Pro allows translation of head movement into cursor movement.

mouse movement. A click can be sent through either a "long" blink or dwell software.

For clients who are proficient with a switch, a number of hardware/software options are available that access to mouse and/or keyboard options through switch access. The aforementioned EZ-Keys can be accessed through one- or two-switch scanning or encoding (or a mouse). It offers a variety of keyboard setups, including frequency of use layouts (which move more commonly used keys such as the vowels closer to the beginning of the scanning layout). The REACH keyboard offers Smart Keys technology, which removes any keys from the scanning layout that are not used after typing the first letter.[6] For example, if a person types the word "Hello," REACH automatically removes most of the consonants, such as q, w, and l, because no words in the dictionary have the letter "h" followed by these letters. Thus, the scanning program scans more quickly to letters that do follow the letter "h." (This same feature can be beneficial to persons who use a mouse to access the REACH keyboard.)

Some options are available for people who do not benefit from switch or direct selection as described previously. Devices such as the Cyberlink can allow clients to access a computer through a combination of EMG signals from the forehead and eyes, as well as alpha and beta brainwaves.[11] The device allows for access through either a switch (combined with scanning) or control of a mouse cursor. The device allows for access even in persons with significantly limited motor control but can be difficult to acquire and use because of its cost and complexity.

Visual and perceptual dysfunction

If clients present with decreased vision or visual perceptual skills, a number of OS changes, software packages, or hardware changes can enhance or allow access. Some clients benefit from increased font and icon sizes that are adjusted through the OS. Microsoft Windows and Macintosh offer one-step options for increasing contrast and font size for the overall OS. Magnification options are readily available to allow persons with low vision to read or see text on the monitor. Finally, some clients benefit from a larger monitor that allows for larger images.

Clients with more severely impaired vision can utilize both magnification and auditory feedback to navigate and use the computer. Commercially available packages such as ZoomText (Fig. 46-13) offer powerful magnification options as well as options to enlarge mouse and caret cursors.[2] An auditory feedback feature allows for readback of text on Internet pages or on the screen as well as allowing for typing feedback. Tools such as Desktop Finder and Web Finder can help clients with decreased vision to navigate visually complex environments on the computer.

Clients who are blind can use a screen reader to access a computer through auditory feedback. JAWS allows for access using the keyboard and auditory feedback to read back information on the screen.[16] Proficient users can surf the Internet, read and respond to e-mail, and use spreadsheets. The most recent version of the Macintosh OS (10.4 Panther) has a full-featured screen reader embedded in the OS.

Clients with learning disabilities or milder visual perceptual issues can use software designed for this purpose. Word prediction can assist people with spelling difficulties. Auditory feedback can assist clients who have better auditory

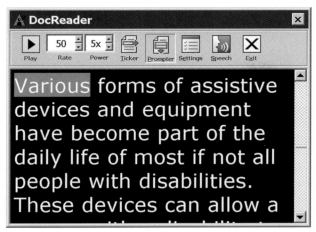

Fig. 46-13 ZoomText offers a variety of magnification options, visual enhancement to the mouse and cursor, and auditory feedback.

comprehension than reading comprehension. Visual highlighting and masking can allow clients to follow more effectively words that are being read. Some software suites offer integrated study tools, such as the ability to take voice or written notes (which are embedded in the document), and to highlight sections, and an integrated dictionary. Kurzweil 3000,[21] WYNN,[17] and a suite of products available from Premier Assistive Technology[29] allow this kind of functionality (Fig. 46-14).

Many clients can benefit from the use of speech recognition. Continuous speech recognition can be used to control the computer as well as dictate text at a rapid rate. Dragon Naturally Speaking is available for Windows and offers a variety of features, including hands-free control of the computer. Users can dictate letters, e-mail, numbers, or sentences into most Windows programs, including word processors and spreadsheets. Users with limited ability to use a mouse or keyboard can use Dragon to start or close programs, click on Internet links using their voice, or dictate into text fields or forms.

Dragon requires users to train a file that is customized to their voice. Over time, if the file is appropriately managed,

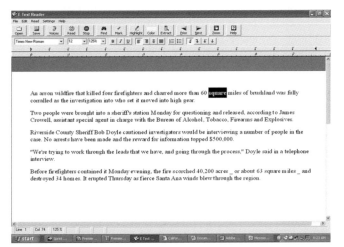

Fig. 46-14 In the E-Text Reader (Premier Assistive Technology), the highlight moves through the words to provide visual cues while a speech synthesizer reads the word out loud.

the recognition accuracy is improved. The ability to recognize that the computer has made an error (as opposed to a human error or environmental noise that is recognized as a word) and the ability to use the appropriate steps to correct the misrecognition are critical for successful use of the program. Many people who try the program and do not receive the training to use it or who lack the cognitive ability to learn and utilize the techniques will not be successful with the program.

Although speech recognition can require a significant cognitive and time investment, it has been successfully utilized for computer access by many people with disabilities. If clients do not have a standard voice pattern, some modifications can be made to the training to allow them to successfully utilize the program. If clients have coexisting visual or perceptual deficits, they may have better success with speech recognition using bundled products that allow for enhanced visual and/or auditory feedback. ZoomText, JAWS, and Keystone Screen Reader (for clients with reading difficulty) all can be integrated with Dragon to utilize the program more effectively.

The Windows Vista OS has speech recognition embedded in the OS. Some clients with learning disability that impairs their typing may benefit from the use of SpeakQ,[30] which bundles a speech recognition program with a word prediction program (WordQ). If clients are unable to spell a particular word, they can dictate the word or phrase, which will appear in a word prediction list. Auditory feedback is available to determine the correct spelling of the word and then insert it into their document. The program also provides usage examples to help users distinguish between confusing homophones such as "their" and "there."

Augmentative and alternative communication

Clients who have significant difficulty with their speech may benefit from AAC. The American Speech Language and Hearing Association defines augmentative communication as "An area of clinical practice that attempts to compensate (either temporarily or permanently) for the impairment and disability patterns of individuals with severe expressive communication disorders." Everyone uses AAC in addition to speech in the form of gestures, facial expressions, body language, and written words.

Assessment
An AAC assessment involves both an occupational therapist and speech language pathologist. There are no prerequisites to using AAC. The individual's receptive/expressive language skills, cognition, literacy skills, vision/hearing skills, and motor abilities all are assessed by the therapist team.

Low technology versus high technology
AAC involves low-technology and high-technology systems. Low-technology systems are noncomputerized systems, such as communication boards and books. High-technology systems are powered speech-generating devices. AAC can be accessed through direct selection, scanning, eye gaze, or other methods. Many of the higher-technology devices

allow for use of multiple access methods. AAC users usually depend on a combination of high- and low-technology communication methods.

Low technology The following are examples of low-technology AAC.

Communication boards Communication boards are fabricated by the speech language pathologist once the assessment is complete. Vocabulary on the boards can be represented by objects, pictures, photographs, tactile symbols, single words, phrases, sentences, or letters. The size, number, and organization of symbols will vary with the individual's needs and abilities. Often the therapist works with the client to obtain appropriate vocabulary for situations and activities in which the client participates. This allows the boards to be individualized to the user and environments in which he or she is involved.

Eye gaze boards For individuals unable to use direct selection with a board, eye gaze boards may be an option. Eye gaze boards have the center removed so that the communication partner can see where the user's eyes are focused. Vocabulary is positioned around the perimeters of the board. As with communication boards, vocabulary can be represented by objects, pictures, photographs, single words, phrases, sentences, or letters. Often, the user is told to focus the eyes on his or her selection for a count of three in order to ensure that the communication partner is accurately reading the user's eye gaze.

Letter boards Letter boards are provided to clients with adequate literacy skills. They be look like computer keyboards, referred to as the QWERTY layout, or they can be in alphabetical order, referred to as an AEIOU layout. The AEIOU layout is in alphabetical order, and all of the vowels are in the far lefthand column. Individuals who are unable to use their hands may use partner-assisted scanning. For this

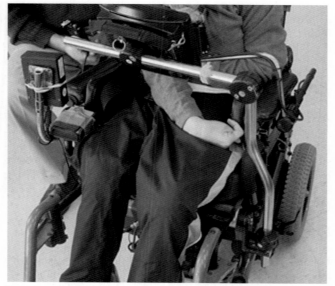

Fig. 46-15 Rigid mount (Daedalus Technologies) keeps an augmentative and alternative communication device safe and accessible to a client in a wheelchair. (Courtesy Daedalus Technologies.)

technique, the communication partner begins verbally scanning through each row ("Is it in the A row, E row, I row, O row, U row?") and asks the user to indicate a "yes" response (via eye blink, finger movement, vocalization, etc.) when the communication partner comes to the row that contains the first letter. The communication partner then proceeds to go through each letter in the row ("Is it A .B .C .D ") until the user again signals a "yes" response.

Modified ETRAN boards A modified ETRAN board is a technique used for spelling words and numbers that involves encoding accessed through eye gaze. The board consists of eight squares positioned around the open center of the board. Each square contains six letters and numbers that are color coded to match small colored squares placed at the extreme boarders of the board. To make a selection, the user first looks at the square in which the letter is located, then to the center, and finally to the colored square of the letter.

Many users will benefit from a single-message device or other auditory signal that allows them to call for attention and to indicate to an unfamiliar communication partner that they can use a board for more detailed communication.

High-technology devices Speech-generating devices can have digitized, synthesized, or both forms of speech output. Digitized speech output is natural speech that has been recorded onto the device. It is a close replica of speech when played back. Synthesized speech output is produced when the device converts text into speech based on intricate rules of pronunciation. It is not as natural as digitized speech; however, users are able to spell novel and unique messages and have them spoken aloud. Devices with both digitized and synthesized speech allow individuals with progressive diseases, such as ALS, to voice bank. Voice banking involves recording phrases (while the voice is intact) that can be loaded onto a communication device (at a later time). This allows the user to produce messages such as "I love you" in their own voice.

Devices can be text based with keyboards, symbol based, or both. Many people use a combination of both. The speech language pathologist will assess how users will have their vocabulary represented (e.g., photographs, picture symbols, words, etc.). They also will determine whether users require prestored messages ("I need to use the bathroom"), the ability to produce novel messages ("Excuse me, can you tell me which way to Clark Street?"), or a combination of both. All devices have the ability to be customized to fit the individual's needs. Prefabricated page sets come on many of the different devices. These page sets often are developed by speech language pathologists and are based on different language concepts. For example, some devices have symbols based on associations. An apple could indicate "red, fruit, eat, food, round or apple." Other devices have their vocabulary organized categorically and topically. In addition to how vocabulary is represented, it is important to determine how it is displayed. Speech-generating devices can have either static or dynamic screens. Static screens do not change. They remain permanent while the user is accessing their vocabulary. Dynamic screens change when a button is activated. Users can navigate between pages to locate vocabulary.

Access

AAC devices are available that can be accessed through direct selection, scanning, mouse alternatives, or switch alternatives. For clients who will benefit from access devices that only work with computers, a variety of software packages allow for AAC software to be accessed on a standard computer.

Combination of equipment

Most higher-level devices can be used in concert, or they may have features that eliminate the need for a separate computer or EADL. For example, many high-technology AAC devices include a method for sending signals to a computer for controls such as mouse movement and keyboard functions. Many also include the ability to send infrared signals to activate X-10 devices, televisions, and telephones. Likewise, computers can be loaded with speech-generating software and used for AAC purposes. However, battery life and the relative unreliability of a computer should be considered for AAC users who are dependent on the device for communication. In general, an AT therapist is needed to determine the best options for these kinds of cases.

Mounting of equipment

Consideration must be given to the mounting, transport, and access to any AT device. If clients are independent with their mobility in a wheelchair, then they should have access to their AT from any place. Most devices (assuming they are portable) can be mounted on a wheelchair. Lightweight devices (< 5 lb) can be mounted to devices such as a Magic Arm. Care should be taken to account for the weight of the activation force. Clients with a "heavy" hand or ataxic motion may easily exceed the 5-lb limit for a Magic Arm and may require a more durable mount. Additionally, many devices are heavier than the 5-lb limit to begin with, so the Magic Arm is most commonly used with switches.

Device mounts are generally mounted to the frame of the wheelchair with a removable pole that can hold a device in a position accessible to clients. If clients can independently transfer, they must be able to move the mount out of the way during their transfer. Some mounts can be swung out of the way to position the mount and the device to the left of clients such that the clients can transfer to their right side. Depending on ability, clients may be able to remove the pole and device to place them carefully aside before transferring (Fig. 46-15).

Care must be taken to avoid restricting the client's vision (i.e., their driving view) with their device as well as the casters and other features of the wheelchair. Although mounting can add considerable complexity to a prescription, it also allows clients to be functional in many environments.

Devices can be mounted for clients who are in bed. Custom-made longer poles can be attached to a hospital bed such that clients can see their device for access purposes. Some clients will benefit from use of an over-bed table or table that has been specifically designed for mounting of devices. Some clients benefit from a pole that allows the device to be tilted for them to see more effectively, especially when clients are supine.

Future of technology

Although many advances have been made over the last decades, more is still to come. Brain–computer interfaces have been the subject of several research studies. People with disabilities have been able to answer yes and no questions using electroencephalogram (EEG) readings.[25] Control of a television has been achieved by clients with SCI using EEG.[12] Other clients have been able to control a video game in real time (requiring timely activation of the switch in response to changing game conditions) using an EEG-based switch.[23] Given adequate training, four adults with ALS learned to use a brain–computer interface to control cursor movement.[20] Although these devices are not currently available commercially, it is hoped that they will enter the mainstream to be used by clients with disabilities such as end-stage ALS.

Braingate is a technology that currently is under clinical study. This system consists of a computer chip implanted directly on the cortex of a client with significant motor dysfunction. The chip allows the client to control a computer using his or her thoughts, which are translated into cursor movement on the screen. Although this device is under clinical study only, it may have great promise for people with significant motor disability to interface with a computer and use it in their daily life for communication, vocational purposes, or leisure activities.[18]

Some clients are able to work with functional near-infrared imaging (fNIR).[3] fNIR is a technique that picks up increased blood flow and oxygenation in the brain associated with neuronal activity. The Kokoro Gatari (currently available only in Japan through Hitachi) is an fNIR device that has been adapted for use by clients with ALS. Neuronal activity has been translated into one word answers such as "yes" to allow clients to communicate. This has significant application for clients with end-stage ALS or other clients with severe movement disorders who may not be able to access a given switch. A number of other brain–computer interfaces are under investigation, both invasive (such as BrainGate) and noninvasive (such as fNIR, functional magnetic resonance imaging, and magnetoencephalography).[9]

The efficiency and functionality of all the AT discussed here are expected to continue improving and playing valuable roles in allowing clients with a disability to participate fully in society.

Acknowledgments

Thanks to Erin Didde, MA, CCC-SLP/L, and Kim Eberhardt, MS, OTR/L, for contributions to this chapter.

Resource list

Adaptivation
2225 W. 50th Street, Suite 100
Sioux Falls, SD 57105
800-723-2783

Ai Squared
P.O. Box 669
Manchester Center, VT 05255
800-859-0270

Applied Human Factors, Inc.
P.O. Box 228
Helotes, TX 78023
888-243-0098

Brain Actuated Technologies, Inc
1350 President Street
Yellow Springs, OH 45387-1815

Daedalus Technologies, Inc.
2491 Vauxhall Place
Richmond, BC V6V 1Z5, Canada
604-270-4605

Freedom Scientific
1800 31st Court North
St. Petersburg, FL 33716-1805
800-444-4443

Greystone Digital Inc.
P.O. Box 1888
Huntersville NC 28078
800-249-5397

Infogrip Inc.
1794 East Main Street
Ventura, CA 93001
800-397-0921

Kurzweil Educational Systems, Inc.
100 Crosby Drive
Bedford, MA 01730-1402
800-894-5374

Premier Assistive Technology
1309 N. William Street
Joliet, IL 60435
815-927-7390

Quillsoft Ltd.
2416 Queen Street East
Toronto, Ontario M1N 1A2, Canada
866-629-6737

Sammons Preston Rolyan
270 Remington Boulevard, Suite C
Bolingbrook, IL 60440-3593
630-226-1300

Tash Inc.
3512 Mayland Court
Richmond VA 23233
800-463-5685

References

1. Adaptivation: see resource list.
2. Ai Squared: see resource list.
3. Al-Rawi PG: Near infrared spectroscopy in brain injury: today's perspective, *Acta Neurochir Suppl* 95:453–457, 2005.
4. Aminzadeh F, Edwards N, Lockett D, Nair R: Utilization of bathroom safety devices, patterns of bathing and toileting, and bathroom falls in a sample of community living older adults, *Technol Disabil* 13:95–103, 2000.
5. Anson D, Moist P, Przywara M, Wells H, Saylor H, Maxime H: The effects of word completion and word prediction on typing rates using on-screen keyboards, *Assist Technol* 18:146–154, 2004.
6. Applied Human Factors: see resource list.
7. Available from Adaptivation See resource list.
8. Bell P, Hinjosa J: Perception of the impact of assistive devices on daily life of three individuals with quadriplegia, *Assist Technol* 8:87–94, 1995.
9. Birbaumer N, Weber C, Neuper C, Buch E, Haapen K, Cohen L: Physiological regulation of thinking: brain-computer interface (BCI) research, *Progr Brain Res* 159:369–391, 2006.
10. Bradley N, Poppen W: Assistive technology, computers and internet may decrease sense of isolation for homebound elderly and disabled persons, *Technol Disabil* 15:19–25, 2003.
11. Brain Actuated Technologies, Inc.: see resource list.
12. Craig A, Moses P, Tran Y, McIsaac P, Kirkup L: The effectiveness of a hands-free environmental control system for the profoundly disabled, *Arch Phys Med Rehabil* 83:1455–1458, 2002.
13. Croser R, Garrett R, Seeger B, Davies P: Effectiveness of electronic aids to daily living: Increased independence and decreased frustration, *Austr Occup Ther J* 48:35–44, 2001.
14. Daedalus Technologies: see resource list.
15. Fichten C, Barile M, Asuncion J: Computer technologies and postsecondary students with disabilities: implications of recent research for rehabilitation psychologists, *Rehabil Psychol* 48:207–214, 2003.
16. Freedom Scientific: see resource list.
17. Freedom Scientific: see resource list.
18. Available at: *http://www.cyberkineticsinc.com/content/medicalproducts/braingate.jsp.*
19. Available at: *http://www.lifelinesys.com/pdf/publications/personalemergencyresponse.pdf.*
20. Kubler A, Nijboer F, Mellinger J, Vaughan TM, et al: Patients with ALS can use sensorimotor rhythms to operate a brain-computer interface, *Neurology* 64:1775–1777, 2005.
21. Kurzweil Educational Systems: see resource list.
22. Mann W, Belchior P, Tomita M, Kemp B: Computer use by middle-aged and older adults with disabilities, *Technol Disabil* 17:1–9, 2005.
23. Mason S, Bohringer R, Borisoff J, Birch G: Real time control of a video game with a direct brain computer interface, *J Clin Neurophysiol* 21:404–408, 2004.
24. McConatha D, McConatha J, Dermingny R: The use of interactive computer services to enhance the quality of life for long term residents, *Gerontologist* 4:553–559, 1994.
25. Miner LA, McFarland DJ, Wolpaw JR: Answering questions with an electroencephalogram-based brain-computer interface, *Arch Phys Med Rehabil* 79:1029–1033, 1998.
26. King TW: *Modern morse code in rehabilitation and education new applications in assistive technology,* Needham, Mass, 1999, Allyn & Bacon.
27. Sammons Preston; see resource list.
28. Naik A, Gill T: Underutilization of environmental adaptations for bathing in community living older persons, *J Am Geriatr Soc* 53:1497–1503, 2005.
29. Premier Assistive Technology: see resource list.
30. QuillSoft: see resource list.
31. Rigby P, Ryan S, Joos S, Cooper B, Jutai J, Steggles E: Impact of electronic aids to daily living on the lives of persons with cervical spinal cord injuries, *Assist Technol* 17:89–97, 2005.
32. Tash Inc.: see resource list.
33. Tash Inc.: see resource list.
34. The Gutenberg project offers many books in electronic format that are past copyright at *http://www.gutenberg.org/.* Bookshare is a service for people with disabilities that includes books still under copyright at *http://www.bookshare.org/.*
35. Verbrugge L, Sevak P: Use, type, and efficacy of assistance for disability, *J Gerontol B Psychol Sci Soc Sci* 57B:S366–S379, 2002.
36. Verbrugge LM, Rennert C, Madans J: The great efficacy of personal and equipment assistance in reducing disability, *Am J Public Health* 87:384–392, 1997.
37. *www.abledata.com* maintains an extensive web site devoted to cataloging assistive devices with reviews and other resources.

Assistive devices for recreation

Samuel Andrews, Joseph Gomez, Carol Huserik, and Jill Stelley Virden

Key Points
- Recreation and leisure planning can help a person through the adjustment period after he or she has sustained a disability.
- Therapeutic recreation when introduced early can aid with rehabilitation and lead to later activity enjoyment.
- Early consideration of recreational interests may lead to cost savings as equipment facilitating those interests is ordered.
- Social, mechanical, and environmental precautions must be exercised when planning recreational activities.
- A recreational therapist can assist in identifying specific activities that are suitable for a person with a disability and that address his or her interest and ability.

During the rehabilitation process, the person with a newly acquired disability goes through a difficult period of psychological and physiological readjustment. Through recreation and leisure planning, independence and quality of lifestyle can be restored regardless of the disability. Therapeutic recreation can help ease the traumatic adjustment process. The overall goal of therapeutic recreation is to assist and encourage each person to reach his or her fullest potential no matter how limited his or her abilities may be.

In patients who have experienced physical impairment, the goal is accomplished by introducing new activities in which they can successfully participate or by reintroducing activities they enjoyed prior to the injury. Patients and their families should be shown that the individuals still are capable of participating in the entire spectrum of recreational activities, with a few appropriate modifications. One focus of therapeutic recreation intervention is to promote self-acceptance and confidence by helping individuals develop skills and talents to compensate realistically for the disability. By using a functional practical approach, the therapist can offer community reentry and ideas for a leisure lifestyle of the patient's choice. Success is an essential part of the implemented program. A patient's involvement in recreation must provide a measure of success with a minimum of frustration. Enjoyment, fun, and accomplishment are obvious rewards for participating in recreation. This chapter applies to individuals who incur any form of disability regardless of severity. Often, severe disability is addressed. The reader is encouraged to understand the various adaptations and that the intervention process requirement may be simpler if the complexity is reduced from the examples given. Peterson and Gunn's *Therapeutic Recreation Program Design: Principles and Procedures* is the cornerstone reference for service delivery.[6] Coyle et al.[2] cite the many benefits of therapeutic recreation service.

Evaluation

Early evaluation of the patient is essential to obtain important information about the patient's leisure background and lifestyle. During the early evaluation, the therapeutic recreation specialist becomes acquainted with the patient and family, states the purpose of the intervention, and, when the time is appropriate, discusses what therapeutic recreation entails. In general, the patient with a relatively new injury and the patient's family are understandably preoccupied with the severity of the medical situation and are not receptive to much more than words of optimism and encouragement. This applies regardless of the severity.

Additional information can be obtained from the family at appropriate times. Often family members are willing to discuss which recreation, leisure, and sports activities the patient enjoyed prior to the injury.

Functional information should be gathered through Functional Independence Measure protocols (developed at State University of New York at Buffalo) in a coordinated effort with other treating disciplines.[8] The Leisure Competence Measure (developed at Parkwood Hospital and Oklahoma State University) also should be used to focus on leisure concerns.[3] The Leisure Competence Measure assesses leisure skills, attitudes, and preferences. These items in conjunction with the Functional Independence Measure can provide clear information on patient status and, more importantly, an indication of what should be addressed in a collaborative and cooperative interdisciplinary approach to developing an effective, efficient treatment program. It is important to understand that any measurement should be used as just that, and that the ultimate focus must be on an effective outcome well beyond discharge. Assessment modalities have been compiled in the three-volume series *Assessment Tools for Recreational Therapy.*[1] The authors present a vast array of assessment processes that can be of value in therapeutic recreation intervention.

Active intervention

As soon as the patient is medically stable and settled into the routine of daily therapies is typically the appropriate time for the therapeutic recreation specialist to begin working in earnest to implement leisure assessment modalities. Long-term (discharge and postdischarge) and short-term (main amount of time of patient's initial stay) goals can be established. Again, collaboration with other disciplines is imperative to implement fast and efficient use of staff. Physicians, nurses, other therapists, and counselors can provide information that will assist the therapeutic recreation specialist in determining the proper timing and intensity of therapeutic recreation intervention.

During the assessment, the exact role of therapeutic recreation should be reviewed with the patient and family so that they formulate realistic expectations of the recreation staff. Recreation has such broad and general meaning to people of varied backgrounds that it cannot be assumed that the patient and family will automatically understand the role of therapeutic recreation staff.

Early intervention with the patient is frequently and effectively enhanced by strong, active physician support. Initiating activity in conjunction with other therapy activities and/or appropriate nursing functions greatly enhances the relationship between the therapeutic recreation specialist and the patient and family. Examples include (1) coordinating with the physical therapists using a basketball to work on strength and endurance, along with eye–hand coordination, while exploring basketball and its required adaptations as a viable sports and recreational pursuit; and (2) nursing staff and therapeutic recreation specialists coordinating sitting tolerance, self-medication protocol, or implementation of meaningful activity designed to reduce unnecessary dependency on nurses.

Therapeutic recreation specialists should be adequately and properly trained, and any process essential to the general safety and comfort of the client should be implemented. Although other staff generally works with the patient when all the specialty support disciplines are more readily available, the therapeutic recreation specialist often works with the patient during times or in locations when or where those services are reduced or unavailable. This is not to say that the therapeutic recreation specialist should go beyond what is deemed reasonable by the attending physician, but that the therapeutic recreation specialist should perform in competent fashion those functions that family members are ordinarily expected to perform. This clearly enhances patient availability for therapeutic recreational activities and sessions. It also serves as a positive example, often encouraging family members to become proficient in those functions sooner.

The skill training phase of therapeutic recreation intervention includes four general components: values clarification, communication, use of adaptive techniques, and use of adaptive equipment. Values clarification is an important component because it provides the high quadriplegic with enhanced insight into the types of events and activities most important to him or her. He or she often can learn not only what aspects of his or her life are important but, more importantly, why. A clearer understanding of why certain events, thoughts, and activities are important greatly enhances the perception of needs. When needs are more clearly understood, then identifying and meeting those needs become easier. The therapist and the patient can set out to meet those needs rather than expend unwarranted time and energy trying to duplicate activities in which the patient was engaged before injury. The amount of time that the patient and the therapeutic recreation specialist spend together is limited, so it is essential to make most efficient use of that time. This becomes increasingly essential as the average time the patient spends in the health care facility steadily decreases.

It is important to review the communication and decision-making skills of the patient and family. This is not the time to make major changes in the patient's communication techniques with family and friends, and attempting to make major changes in the family's communication style with the patient is not practical. However, it is important to review with each the value of communicating needs beyond basic survival needs such that positive outcomes are enhanced.

All rehabilitation disciplines should strive to encourage all parties to clearly communicate their values and needs while maintaining the same parties open to hearing and understanding the values and needs of others. The recreational setting is an excellent medium in which to review and possibly refine such skills. It is a more realistic and practical setting with real issues in value judgment, community interaction, and interpersonal communication that constantly but naturally occur among family members and friends. For example, having an older child assist his or her hemiplegic parent into and out of the car gives both child and parent a "hands on" experience of the effort involved (which sometimes is less involved than feared).

Clearly sharing the patient's needs and desires with others through assertive behaviors and having realistic expectations of others (i.e., family and friends accompanying the patient) are extremely important tools for successful social and leisure encounters that will help the individual and family become less dependent on the health care system in the long run. Therapeutic recreation specialists should dedicate substantial time and effort in communication skill enhancement as well as decision-making training with the patient and, if possible, the family. A shopping trip is an excellent medium to practice effective options for requesting assistance while providing the

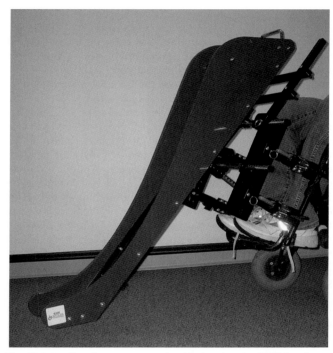

Fig. 47-1 Bowling from a power wheelchair using the IKAN bowler.

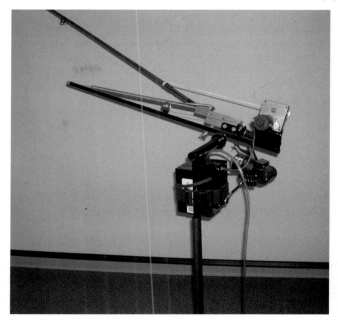

Fig. 47-2 Adaptive fishing device with pneumatic sip-and-puff controls for casting and reeling.

patient with the opportunity to exercise self-directed decisions. Dealing with a store clerk, cashier, waiter, and family in a public forum provides the essential components to practice vital interactions.

Adaptive techniques must be learned in place of typical methods of function. For example, the individual may need to learn to throw a ball or to draw with the hand and arm opposite the one used before the disability. The ability to use one hand instead of two to perform a motor task takes effort and innovation. Use of adaptive equipment also may be necessary. Adaptive swim strokes to compensate for imposed limitations can be appropriately implemented.

Skills in the use of adaptive equipment, whether durable medical equipment or less medically essential equipment, must be learned. A broad spectrum of equipment is available, such as a mouth-operated long bow trigger, a bowling adaptation that attaches directly to the patient's chair (Fig. 47-1),

a fishing device that casts and reels without requiring the use of hands (Fig. 47-2), and a pool cue modified for disabled use (Fig 47-3). The social/recreational experience is greatly enhanced as the individual learns and practices appropriate and effective use.

Equipment and resources

The individual with physical disability may or may not use a great deal of adaptive equipment. It is extremely important that the therapeutic recreation specialist work closely with other treating disciplines early during the process so that basic equipment meets as many recreational needs as possible. Examples of such considerations include prosthetic devices, such as arm prostheses designed to hold pottery tools; equipment enhancements, such as mechanical devices that cock a crossbow, and brackets and wheelchair superstructure for attaching bipod mounts for cameras or rifles; and appropriate

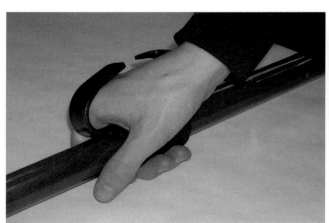

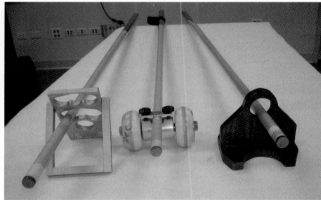

Fig. 47-3 Various modifications for billiards are available for individuals with a wide range of abilities.

tires and casters or crutches that allow the patient to properly negotiate anticipated terrains. Preplanning can reduce long-range costs to the disabled patient as well as to third-party payers. Each coordination of customizing equipment can reduce the need for additional specialized equipment, which represents additional bulk and increases the user's vulnerability to equipment malfunction.

Specialized equipment for recreational activity is often needed. It is important that no equipment be recommended until its practicality has been thoroughly investigated. Too often in their enthusiasm for the patient's success, the staff assists in acquiring specialized equipment without consideration of issues such as weight, size, storage, maintenance, and installation away from the rehabilitation setting. The danger of the unused equipment becoming a reminder of the disability to the patient must be carefully avoided.

Resource exploration is an essential component to any recommendation made by the therapeutic recreation specialist to the patient. As patient values and needs are explored, immediate consideration for resources that meet those needs and values should be made. Consideration for factors such as transportation resources (e.g., accessible bus, taxi, or personal vehicle), human assistance resources (e.g., service organizations, family, friends, community outdoor and/or recreation personnel), financial resources (costs of activities and possible adaptive costs), and accessibility to devices such as a specialized wheelchair, prosthetic leg, or cane should be given for both the short term (i.e., during the rehabilitation process) and the long term (subsequent to discharge). When resource planning for leisure activity after discharge, resources often break down even under the best of conditions. The therapeutic recreation specialist must be prepared to follow up to ensure that planned resources have been placed in effect.

The number of entities that exist solely to provide resource information is growing daily. Examples include *Sports 'n Spokes* magazine, *Disabled Outdoors* magazine, and *Easy Access to National Parks*.[7] *Access to Recreation* is a catalog devoted specifically to adaptive recreation equipment for the physically challenged. The Americans with Disabilities Act (ADA) has started to have an effect on fostering resources in communities across the United States. Organizations that address the assistive needs of individuals with disabilities are rapidly increasing in number. Examples include Flying Wheels (Owatonna, Minnesota), local chapters of the Multiple Sclerosis Society, Paralyzed Veterans of America (PVA), Outdoor Buddies (Denver, Colorado), Handicapped Scuba Association, National Sports Center for the Disabled (Winter Park, Colorado), the outdoor adventure organization POINT (Dallas, Texas), and an Assistive Technology Project in each state. Sharing information about these entities with the patient is imperative.

Precautions

A Certified Therapeutic Recreation Specialist (CTRS) and members of the other disciplines should teach precautionary considerations for leisure activity. Beyond the general safety and precautionary considerations for individuals with greater disability, three other categories play an important role in the success of leisure pursuits: social, mechanical, and environmental considerations.

From a *social* standpoint, certain considerations will enhance the disabled individual's recreational experience. One example is clear communication between the individual with a disability and other participants before a scheduled social event regarding the individual's physical requirements during the event and how he or she intends to handle them. This will prevent the need for the individual to continually ask for assistance from those who are unfamiliar with what may be required. The delicate topic of what is needed to assist with the individual's bowel and bladder issues should not be forgotten, but this often is easily remedied by having an attendant accommodate the individual's needs. Another example of a difficult social situation is one in which full consideration is not given to everyone who will be attending an event, for example, the noise made by adaptive equipment may be distracting to those in a theater watching a movie. Practical remedies include prearranging with theater management seating in an area adjacent to an exit so that the individual can quietly and quickly move to the lobby for less conspicuous attendance to personal needs. As a courtesy, persons seated nearby should be advised of possible unusual sounds or excessive noise or movement so that they can change their seats if they so choose. Remedies to these situations can create a more acceptable and, therefore, more satisfying recreational situation.

The second category concerns *mechanical* considerations. The therapeutic recreation specialist can provide a great deal of information on the use of backup mechanical equipment by demonstrating its use in recreational activities. One example of a simple mechanical adaptation for safety backup is a connection to a motor vehicle's the electrical system that provides auxiliary electricity for operating a ventilator, especially suctioning equipment, or the mechanical components of a wheelchair in case of power failure. Such a system might eliminate the need to carry extra batteries. Gel cell batteries used for powering equipment can make air travel much more convenient. These adaptations might remove some of the deterrents to the disabled patient leaving the comforts of home and participating in recreational activities.

The third category is *environmental* conditions. The therapeutic recreation specialist should spend educational time with the patient discussing the effect of various environmental conditions. Through close collaboration with physicians and nursing staff, information should be shared on the effects of conditions such as dust, heat, sun, cold, ice, altitude, and humidity. Again, the aim of such education is to give the individual the opportunity to enjoy the success of the activity rather than suffer negative consequences of preventable environmentally induced problems.

It is extremely important to identify individual needs when designing individual programs. The patient's interests, values, recreational needs, leisure resources, and capabilities must be taken into consideration so that realistic goals with a high probability of achievement can be set. Various diagnostic and profile assessments published by therapeutic recreation and psychological specialists can be used. A compilation of many of these instruments is available.[1]

Activities

Socially, an individual with a disability needs to nurture a sense of belonging, of being accepted by society. When a

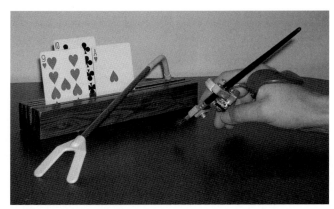

Fig. 47-4 Card holder, mouth stick, and implement holder.

person with a disability accomplishes a goal or successfully fills a role in society, he or she has an opportunity to build his or her self-image.

Enhancing a person's self-image can be achieved through a variety of activities, such as competitive and recreational sports, arts and crafts, gardening, and photography. All activities that can be accomplished using a head, mouth, or chin control should be explored. Keeping modifications as simple and practical as possible is important; the rule of thumb is to make the least elaborate modification as is necessary to complete the activity. This reduces the complexity of the activity and of any repairs needed to modifications of adaptive equipment.

Board games and card games can be easily modified. A mouth-stick device can be used to select or move the cards or game pieces. Individuals with upper extremity function can use an implement holder. The mouth stick and implement holder can be used to move cards, draw, paint, and write (Fig. 47-4). These games can be played with a friend, family member, or staff member. Cards from any type of table game can be arranged in a simply constructed cardholder.

Individuals with a wide range of functional abilities can participate in fishing. Commercially produced fishing rod holders can work well for individuals with use of only one hand or arm when the holders are placed in a convenient location for maximum use. A modification as simple as a built-up or extended handle on a reel may be all that is needed for a person to be an independent fisher (Fig. 47-5). A more sophisticated adaptive self-casting rod and reel apparatus is available (Fig. 47-2). This pneumatically controlled

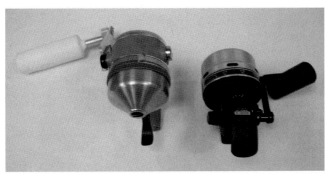

Fig. 47-5 Fishing reels with modified handles.

device allows an individual to independently cast and reel. The device can be attached to a wheelchair, dock, or boat. Many more options for fishing devices and other pieces of adaptive equipment are available at Don Krebs' *Access to Recreation* web site (*www.accesstr.com*).

Aquatic activities can provide an environment for socialization and independence. Radio-controlled sailing is one type of aquatic activity. A control is positioned so that the two radio-controlled joystick levers are within reach of the high quadriplegic's mouth, chin, or mouth stick. When the boat is in the water, the individual's level of disability becomes moot. Family members and friends can participate in this type of activity, and no previous sailing experience is required because the basic skills are quickly learned. This type of activity provides an avenue for competition through model yachting clubs across the United States that organize races featuring radio-controlled boats. In these races, the disability presents no disadvantages or handicaps to competition. Even with mouth controls, a high quadriplegic or double-arm amputee can compete on an equal basis with anyone. The same operational principles for the sailboats apply to radio-controlled cars, airplanes, gliders, and powerboats. Activities such as these lend themselves to valuable family interaction (especially with youngsters) and afford a wide spectrum of activity involvement.

Other aquatic activities can include rafting, sailing, kayaking, boating, canoeing, and scuba diving. These higher-risk activities are recommended only after much preliminary work to ensure appropriate safety conditions. Each situation presents its own safety considerations that should be researched and problem solved with the individual before the event is pursued. During inpatient rehabilitation, the recreational therapist can facilitate progressive aquatic experiences, beginning with basic water adjustment in a therapy pool environment. Community aquatic resources should be explored and visited as appropriate. Combining the therapist's expertise with that of the community contact will go a long way to ensure the patient's successful involvement in the activity.

Camping is another feasible activity for the individual with a disability. The individual can provide himself or herself the opportunity to be with family or friends away from the home or institutional environment. Although the individual may be dependent on others for care, he or she can be responsible for making decisions such as campsite selection, weather-related contingencies, campsite arrangement, and menu choices. Accessible campsites can be easily researched using the Internet. Many states offer a reduced cost annual entrance pass to state parks for certain disabled residents. The federal government offers the Golden Access Passport to individuals with permanent disability. This is a free, lifetime admission pass to national parks, monuments, historic sites, recreation areas, and national wildlife refuges that normally charge an entrance fee.

Gardening provides a range of opportunities for the person involved in rehabilitation and progressing to the home setting. Using horticultural therapy as a treatment modality increases the patient's endurance, strength, and mobility while he or she resumes an activity of interest. Raised beds, container gardening, and adapted tools make gardening from a wheelchair manageable and enjoyable. Individuals without use of their hands can design and direct the garden

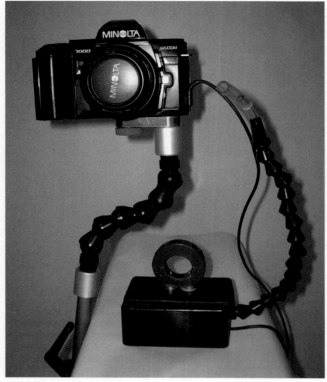

Fig. 47-6 Telescoping and articulated camera mount, and pneumatic sip-and-puff remote shutter control.

plan with the help of others and still enjoy the outcome of a productive, beautiful garden.

Music and theater arts serve as important therapeutic modalities as well as pleasurable activities. Coaching and cheering at athletic events should be considered opportunities for creativity, self-fulfillment, and expression. Creating or participating in skits, dances, talent shows, dramatic productions, athletic events, and other spectator events provides an opportunity to escape the physical confines of the wheelchair. The person may even be able to build lung capacity and strength while striving to sing or project the voice.

Another activity for major consideration is photography. Use of a bipod or camera strap as a stabilizer makes photography or videotaping viable. Great latitude for creativity and self-expression exists. Today's cameras have automatic features that meet individualized needs and easily accommodate the person's specific preference. For some patients, use of an adapted camera holder is all that is needed to help them hold the camera (Fig. 47-6). Patients with higher-level injuries

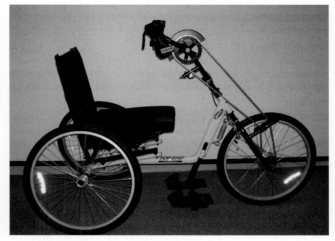

Fig. 47-8 Top End Excelerator hand cycle.

might benefit from the use of a bipod or suspension equipment that attaches to the electric wheelchair and places the camera in a desirable position (Fig. 47-7). Other adaptations to camera controls, such as manual focus and light aperture, can be made according to individual desires. Activity can easily be carried to the darkroom for additional creativity in photocomposition.

The field of exercise is available to many individuals through adapted programs. Rehabilitation centers across the nation realize the value of exercise options and equipment for people with disabilities during their stay in the rehabilitation setting and in their life after discharge. Hand cycles (Fig. 47-8), recumbent foot pedal bikes (Fig. 47-9), and the stationary Saratoga cycle (Fig. 47-10) are examples of equipment that is commercially available for exercise and recreation. Attachments are available for those who do not have sufficient grip to hold onto hand cranks (Fig. 47-11). With this equipment, the person can participate individually, competitively, and with family and friends.

The physical aspect is only one component of all activities. Mental, social, and emotional aspects of intervention also must be considered. Recreational outings offer a means of testing out self-image in public, and they can be times of

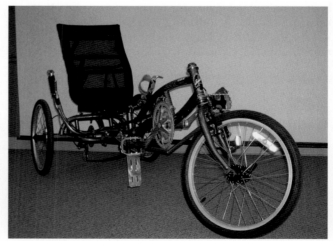

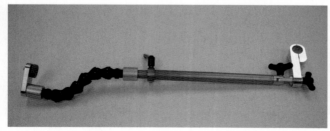

Fig. 47-7 Adapted camera holder.

Fig. 47-9 EZ3 USX recumbent foot pedal bike.

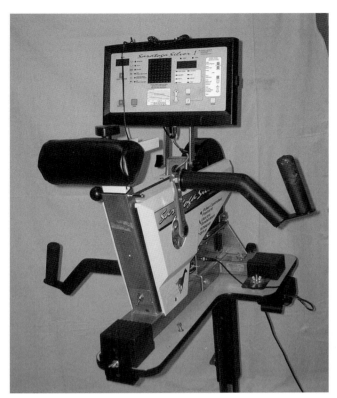

Fig. 47-10 Saratoga exercise hand cycle.

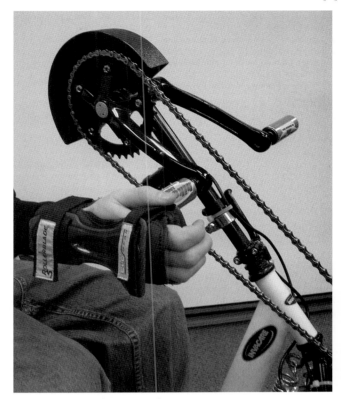

Fig. 47-11 Hand cycle grip attachment.

socialization and utilization of community resources and public transportation. A successful outing can encourage a person with a disability to try that or similar activities at a later time. Challenging outings can expose the person and his or her family and friends to situations that might be encountered at home. The person can begin to problem solve on his or her own or with others so that these challenges are less threatening later. As families are given more opportunities to problem solve, especially with the assistance of staff, the outings subsequent to discharge are less of a burden and are more "user friendly," thus enhancing the probability that the individual will go out into the community on a more frequent and likely healthier basis.

Activities once thought impractical, if not impossible, often are "doable" with appropriate planning and coordination with members of the other disciplines of the rehabilitation program. Adventuresome activities may include hand cycling, international travel, hot air ballooning, and big game hunting. These activities are popular and become less difficult to conduct with increased experience. A great deal of planning, ingenuity, safety consideration, and resource analysis are essential components to short-term and long-term success. The person with a disability should be involved in all of these aspects as well as personal care issues, such as skin care (i.e., padding), bowel and bladder function, and maintenance of hydration and body temperature.

Most devices can be adapted by consulting experts in rehabilitation engineering, therapeutic recreation, and adaptation at rehabilitation centers and community recreation centers. It is essential to keep modifications and adaptations simple, efficient, and user friendly. Store-bought materials often are effective and the most economical. Maddox[4] and Nesbitt[5]

provide extensive ideas and information based on practicality and success.

Conclusion

This chapter discussed experiences that have been demonstrated to be effective in therapeutic recreation intervention. Following a basic format of introduction and assessment, skill training, and resource exploration, therapeutic recreation intervention provides the individual with an increased opportunity to return to a healthy, active lifestyle. The individual and his or her family should use recreational skills and resources to add strong incentives for the individual to live in as healthy and as independent a condition as possible after all the effort, energy, and resources expended to return the individual to medical health. Most activities across the entire recreational spectrum can be adapted to the individual with a disability. It is the individual's decision whether the activity and its adaptation are meaningful and appropriate.

Once the patient is discharged, regular follow-up and re-evaluation are essential to ensure that appropriate leisure skills are commensurate to the desires and abilities of the individual as conditions in his or her life change. Referral to community resources is a most important transitional step from the health care facility to the community.

References

1. Burlingame J, Blascko TM: *Assessment tools for recreational therapy*, Seattle, 1990, Frontier Publishing.
2. Coyle C, Kinney W, Riley B, Shank J, editors: *Benefits of therapeutic recreation: a consensus view*, Philadelphia, 1991, Temple University.

3. Kloseck, et al: *Leisure competence measure*, Stillwater, Okla, 1992, Oklahoma State University.

4. Maddox S: *Spinal network*, Boulder, Colo, 1998, Sam Maddox, Publisher.

5. Nesbitt JA, editor: *The international directory of recreation-oriented assistive device sources*, Marina Del Rey, Calif, 1985, Lifeboat Press.

6. Peterson CA, Gunn SL: *Therapeutic recreation program design: principles and procedures*, Englewood Cliffs, NJ, 1984, Prentice-Hall.

7. Roth W, Tompane M: *Easy access to national parks*, San Francisco, 1992, Sierra Club Books.

8. *Uniform Data System for Medical Rehabilitation: functional independence measure*, Buffalo, NY 1997, State University of New York at Buffalo.

Chapter

48

Sports adaptations for the physically challenged athlete

*David F. Apple, Jr., Susan A. Skolnick, Patrick Matthew Edens,
Gregory D. Horneber, Joseph A. Metzger, and Kelly Mixon*

Key Points

- History of adaptive sports
- Strategies to adapt multiple community sporting activities
- Web-based resources for further information are provided

Recreation and sports are important components of an active lifestyle. This is no less true for individuals with physical disabilities. While a physical disability can impact participation, activities and equipment can be modified to meet the needs of the individual. While examining some of these adaptations, this chapter outlines a majority of the recreational and competitive sports that are available for individuals with physical disabilities.

Before 1950, few resources were available in the sporting world for people with physical disabilities. Largely through the efforts of Sir Ludwig Guttmann at the Stoke Mandeville Hospital outside of London, England, the sports movement for people with disabilities began as the annual wheelchair games. These games took on added significance when other countries joined the games, giving them an international flavor similar to the Olympics.

In 1960, the International Stoke Mandeville Games (which later came to be known as the Paralympic Games) were held in the Olympic host city of Rome, Italy, elevating these games to the equivalent of the Olympic Games. Since that time, national and international sports federations have been established for the majority of disabled sports. These federations hold national and international competitions to promote

excellence in their specific sport. Beginning with the 1988 Olympic Games in Seoul, Korea, the Paralympics have been held shortly after the summer and winter Olympics in the same host city and at the same venues.

Many of the sports discussed in this chapter are appropriate for athletes with various physical disabilities, and in many instances, little or no adaptive equipment is necessary. For sports that require adaptations, this chapter highlights the equipment and modifications that are available.

All-terrain vehicles

All-terrain vehicles (ATVs) are used for recreational enjoyment as well as a means to help access terrain that otherwise might be inaccessible. For individuals with decreased upper and/or lower extremity functioning who use a wheelchair for mobility, transferring onto an ATV can be somewhat of a challenge. A sliding board can help ease the transfer by bridging the gap between the wheelchair and ATV. Using a ramped platform for the wheelchair that is at the same height as the ATV is another technique that decreases the difficulty of the transfer.

The two main categories of ATVs that people with physical disabilities use are four-wheelers and utility vehicles. A four-wheeler should be driven only by someone who has the upper extremity functioning and trunk balance necessary to safely operate the vehicle. Under no circumstance should drivers ever strap themselves onto a four-wheeler. Individuals with decreased lower extremity functioning and sensation may need to select a four-wheeler that is automatic, and they may need to pad off the engine or the sides of the vehicle to protect their skin from the vehicle's heat.

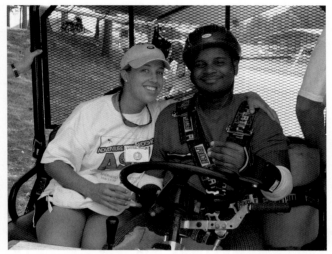

Fig. 48-1 All-terrain vehicle. Utility vehicle has a harness system, accelerator and brake hand control, tripod wrist grip, and added padding for trunk stability.

For utility vehicle users, seat belts are a standard feature and should be used by anyone with decreased balance and stability. A harness system similar to that used in racing cars can be added as extra support for individuals with little to no trunk balance. Foam padding can be placed between the individual, the vehicle, and the harness system to provide even greater stability. The foot accelerator and braking systems can be converted to a hand control system for individuals with decreased lower extremity functioning. For an individual with decreased grip, a grasping cuff can be used with the hand control system, and the steering wheel can be modified by adding a ball grip or a tripod wrist grip (Fig. 48-1).

Archery

A large selection of adaptive equipment is available that makes archery accessible to almost everyone. A tripod mounting system can be used to help stabilize and hold the bow. To assist with gripping the bow or the arrow and releasing the bowstring, archers who have decreased upper extremity functioning can use wrist and elbow supports, archery cuffs, quick-release cuffs, and mechanical trigger releases. Archers can use a self-retaining, draw-locking mechanism to draw the bowstring back and lock it in a fully drawn, ready-to-shoot position. For someone with an upper extremity amputation or little to no upper extremity functioning, a bite tab that is controlled with the archer's mouth can be used to draw the bowstring. A crossbow can be adapted for someone with limited upper extremity functioning. A trigger activator and shooting rest are the two main pieces of equipment necessary to adapt a crossbow. The specifics of this equipment are discussed in greater detail in the section on shooting.

Basketball

Basketball requires few adaptations to the equipment and rules. It is played by individuals who have a lower extremity physical disability that prevents them from running, jumping, and pivoting. Players use wheelchairs designed specifically for basketball. The wheelchairs are lightweight, have cambered wheels, and use pressured tires that allow for quick turns and easy maneuvering. Players also can use a body bracer that goes around their chair and waist to maintain balance, as well as leg straps above the knees to sustain proper leg positioning. Spoke guards can be used to protect both the spokes of the wheels and the players' hands.

Billiards

Several pieces of adaptive billiards equipment are available for individuals with decreased upper extremity functioning. Pool cuffs and grasping cuffs, which are secured to both the hand and the pool cue, can assist with gripping the pool cue (Fig. 48-2A). Prostheses can be used to hold a pool cue. Pool bridges can be used to help support and stabilize the tip of the pool cue. Generally, three types of bridges can be used: a standard pool bridge, a stationary bridge rest that sits on the pool table, and a mobile bridge that attaches to the tip of the pool cue (Fig. 48-2B).

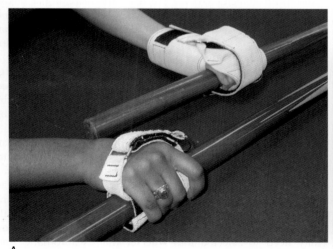
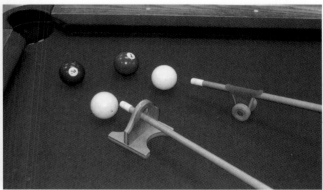

A   B

Fig. 48-2 Billiards. **A,** Pool cuff and grasping cuff. **B,** Stationary bridge rest and mobile bridge.

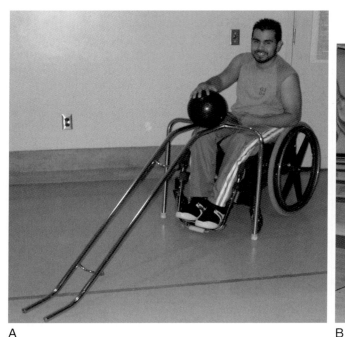 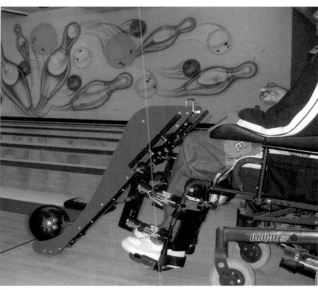

A   B

Fig. 48-3 Bowling. **A,** Standard bowling ramp. **B,** Bowling ramp that attaches to the wheelchair and allows the bowler to control the ball by driving and stopping the wheelchair.

Boating

With regard to boating, the main issues for individuals with a physical disability are access onto the boat and seating. Pontoon boats typically are the easiest boats to board because most can pull up evenly with a dock and have gates that provide access onto the boat. Boaters who use a wheelchair for mobility will be able to wheel onto the boat, as long as the gate is wide enough to accommodate the wheelchair. A ramp can be used to bridge any gap between the dock and the boat. With most other motorboats, boaters will need to transfer out of the wheelchair and into the boat, which can be difficult because the boat typically will not be positioned evenly with the dock. In such instances, boaters can transfer independently, use the assistance of other individuals, or modify the boat to include a hydraulic lift system that will lift them out of their wheelchairs and into the boat. Some boats can be modified to include a ramp that unfolds and allows easy roll-on and roll-off wheelchair access.

Once on a boat, if boaters choose to remain in their wheelchair, lock-down systems can be added to the floor of the boat to secure the wheelchair. If boaters choose to transfer into one of the boat's seats, seats with a high back and armrests can provide stability to boaters who have decreased balance. Boaters with decreased sensation from the waist down can benefit from sitting either on the cushion from their wheelchairs or on a boat seat that is well padded. For boaters who have decreased grip and want to drive a boat, a grasping cuff or T-bar mount can be used to work the throttle, and the steering wheel can be modified by adding a ball grip or a tripod wrist grip.

Bowling

Bowling can be adapted to meet the physical abilities of any bowler. A bowler who lacks the finger strength and/or

dexterity to completely grip a standard bowling ball can use a bowling ball with a spring-loaded handle or a bowling ball pusher. A bowler who is unable to bowl free-arm or use a ball pusher can use a bowling ramp. A standard bowling ramp can be placed in front of the lane, and the bowler releases the ball from the top of the ramp with a very light push (Fig. 48-3A). The spring-loaded handle bowling ball, the bowling ball pusher, and the standard bowling ramp all can be used from a seated or a standing position. A bowler who uses a wheelchair for mobility and has little to no upper extremity functioning can use a bowling ramp that attaches to his or her power wheelchair. The bowler controls the speed, direction, position, and timing of the release of the ball down the ramp by driving and stopping the wheelchair (Fig. 48-3B).

Cycling

Advances in technology have helped introduce adaptive cycling to individuals with various physical disabilities. Cyclists with visual impairments can use tandem bicycles with a sighted pilot; cyclists with amputations can use a standard bicycle customized to accommodate a prosthesis; and cyclists with balance difficulties can use a triwheeled bicycle. Cyclists who have a physical disability that limits lower extremity functioning can use a three-wheeled handcycle.

Handcycles are arm-operated bicycles with a wide, backed seat that accommodates and provides support for the cyclist's frame. Lateral supports can be added to the backrest to provide greater stability for a cyclist with decreased trunk control. Handcycles are equipped with multiple gears and hand brakes, and they are propelled by a crank system that is connected to the front fork. Tripod wrist cuffs, universal cuff style handles, grasping cuffs with hooks, and prostheses can be used to assist cyclists with grasping the crank handles.

All of these grasping devices allow for cyclists to move between the handles, gears, and brakes as needed.

The two main styles of handcycles are upright and recumbent. In an upright model, the cyclist is in a position similar to that created when sitting in a chair. In a recumbent model, the torso is more reclined, and the legs are extended out in front of the cyclist. Upright handcycles use a pivot steer system, whereas recumbent handcycles can have either a pivot steer or lean-to-steer system.

Equestrian sports

Horseback riding can be enjoyed as a therapeutic modality, a leisure activity, and a competitive sport by individuals with physical disabilities. Riders who cannot mount a horse by climbing up on it often use a ramped platform that positions them at the height of the horse's back. Many riders customize their saddles to meet their needs. Extra padding can be added to the saddle to guard against skin sores from pressure and shearing. Riders who need assistance with balance can attach a backrest to the saddle, and a bellyband can be used to secure their trunk to the backrest (Fig. 48-4). Stirrups can be customized and are important for maintaining balance and protecting a rider's legs from injury. For riders with decreased trunk control who cannot sit on a horse, carriage driving is another option. In carriage driving, a horse pulls a carriage that is designed to accommodate a wheelchair or an adaptive seat. Access to the carriage typically is gained through a ramp or a hydraulic lift on the back of the carriage, and the carriage has a built-in safety system that secures the wheelchair to the carriage. The reins and how the reins are held can be adapted to allow drivers with decreased grip to control the horse.

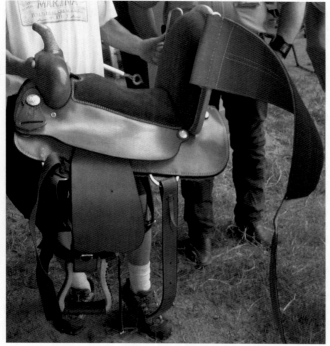

Fig. 48-4 Equestrian sports. Horseback riding saddle with backrest and bellyband.

Extreme sports

Extreme sports is a fast-growing recreation field due to the advancements of adaptive technology and the "can do" attitude of individuals with physical disabilities. Nature enthusiasts and thrill seekers are able to continue to enjoy the thrills of adventure-based activities such as camping, hiking, backpacking, mountain biking, rock climbing, high ropes courses, skydiving, paragliding, hang gliding, flying, whitewater rafting, and more. Organizations that provide these recreational and educational opportunities exist all over the world.

Outdoor areas such as campgrounds, beaches, and trails are becoming more accessible with the progression of the Americans with Disabilities Act (ADA). Wheelchair accessible tents are available. Trails are being designed and built with width, grade, cross-slope, and surface texture in mind to meet the needs of all trail users. Rig-shaw poles, all-terrain wheelchair tires, and the assistance of other individuals can enable hikers to access the roughest of terrains.

Off-road mountain biking can be enjoyed by cyclists with good trunk stability and upper extremity functioning. Downhill mountain biking, with the use of a harness system and/or adaptations for grip, can be enjoyed by individuals with decreased upper extremity functioning. Mountain bikes can be either three-wheeled (two wheels in the front and one in the back) or four-wheeled, and the rider can be positioned in a low profile or forward lean position. Mountain bikes can be equipped with a hand crank system for propulsion, a steering column, a brake system, a suspension system, all-terrain tires, a wide, backed seat that accommodates and provides support for the cyclist's frame, and lateral supports. The style and makeup of the bike depend on the type of mountain biking as well as the cyclist's physical abilities and personal preferences.

Rock climbing and high ropes courses can be enjoyed with minimal adaptive equipment or techniques. Climbers with upper or lower amputations can use or adapt their day-to-day prostheses, and climbers with visual impairments rely on the guidance from a sighted climber or instructor. A sling seat and pulley system enables a climber with little to no upper and lower extremity functioning to access a high ropes course. Climbers with decreased upper extremity strength and little-to-no lower extremity functioning can utilize a climbing ascender. Instead of using the rock face or climbing holds, climbers use an ascender to pull themselves up the rope. Grasping cuffs can be used with the ascender by someone with decreased hand function. A chest harness can assist someone with decreased trunk control, and climbing harnesses with wider straps can be used to prevent shearing. It is important for climbers with decreased circulation and sensation to protect their bodies with appropriate equipment and padding.

Paragliding, hang gliding, and skydiving can be done in tandem by someone with decreased lower extremity functioning, trunk control, and/or upper extremity functioning. Gliders and divers with visual impairments can communicate with a buddy through the use of headphones. Hand controls can be adapted and landing techniques modified to meet the needs of the individual taking to the air. Protective padding can be used to prevent injuries upon landing.

Flying, which includes planes, helicopters, and sailplanes, can be both recreational and vocational. Anyone can enjoy taking to the air as a passenger. Adaptations to flying controls and instruments can be made for those who want to pilot an aircraft. Foot controls can be converted to hand controls, and anyone has the option of learning to fly as long as they can manage the controls.

Whitewater rafting can be enjoyed safely with minimal adaptations. For water safety, rafters who require assistance rolling from a prone to supine position can use a type I personal flotation device. Rafters with decreased lower extremity functioning can attach flotation devices to their legs in order to prevent their lower extremities from hanging in the water should they be thrown from the raft. Rafters with decreased trunk balance can sit in the middle or the inside of the raft with adaptive seating. Rafters with an upper extremity amputation can use a prosthesis to hold a paddle, and paddles can be adapted with handholds to assist rafters with decreased grip in grasping the paddle. The specifics of this equipment are discussed in greater detail in the section on paddling sports.

Fencing

Wheelchair fencing is one of the oldest sports for people with physical disabilities. Fencers compete in foil, epee, and saber events. Each event has three classes, and the fencer's class is determined by functional abilities. All fencers must compete from a wheelchair. The wheelchair is secured into a fencing frame with a lock-down system that prevents any wheelchair movement while allowing the fencer freedom of movement in the upper body (Fig. 48-5). Fencers also can use a strap around their legs to assist with leg positioning. Fencers with decreased hand function can use a specialized glove or wrap to assist with holding their weapon. Other than a protective cover worn over the fencers' laps to protect their lower extremities from accidental contact, wheelchair fencers use the same protective gear worn by able-bodied fencers.

Fishing

Fishing is a sport in which anyone with a physical disability can participate. Adaptive equipment for fishing is readily available to individuals with decreased upper extremity functioning. Rod holders and grasping cuffs assist individuals with varying amounts of upper extremity functioning to hold and grasp a fishing rod. Rod holders either attach to a chair or fasten around the individual's waist and neck. Hand and arm cuffs assist with grasping the rod and, in many instances, make it easier to cast and reel using one or both upper extremities. Individuals with decreased trunk control can wear a body bracer around their trunk and chair to help maintain balance when casting and reeling.

Casting and reeling can be adapted in many ways for an individual with decreased finger function and strength. One example is adding a lever to the casting button, which can be depressed by the side of a hand. Another example is using a crank aid (a dowel rod and PVC pipe adapter in a universal hand cuff) to depress the button. Reeling can be adapted by building up the handle with tape, placing a foam ball over the handle, or using a crank aid to turn the handle. Individuals with little to no upper extremity functioning can benefit most from using an electric reel. With an electric reel system, the line can be cast by someone else and then the line can be reeled in by depressing a button or joystick with a finger, the side of a hand, the head, or the mouth/tongue.

Fitness

Exercise should be a part of everyone's life to help maintain function and good health. A variety of equipment is available for cardiovascular exercise as well as for strength training. Cardiovascular equipment provides the individual with an aerobic workout, and strength equipment provides the individual with muscle training. Many individuals with physical disabilities can use standard exercise equipment simply by transferring onto the equipment, removing a bench or chair to allow access from a wheelchair, using attachments that allow prostheses, wrist/ankle cuffs, or grasping cuffs to be attached, or choosing equipment that most meets their functional abilities (i.e., wrist weights or resistive exercise bands instead of hand weights, etc.). Individuals who are unable to use standard exercise equipment have a wide variety of adaptive equipment from which they can choose.

Adaptive cardiovascular equipment includes crank turn and push/pull arm ergometers, total body conditioning recumbent bikes and steppers, and total body conditioning standing gliders. These pieces of equipment allow for simultaneous movement in both the upper and/or lower extremities; as such, individuals can use their better functioning extremities to compensate for those with decreased functioning. Ergometers, bikes, steppers, and gliders come in various styles that allow for use either directly from a wheelchair or by transferring onto the equipment. Individuals can use prostheses, grasping cuffs, or adhesive wrap bandages to help grasp the equipment, and they can use straps or other equipment-specific accessories to help hold their lower extremities in place.

Adaptive strength equipment mainly consists of freestanding, multistation gyms that provide a variety of weight-training exercises that can be performed from a wheelchair. These systems allow for the individual to set the level of resistance, and the systems vary based on their use of power resistance rods, cable weight systems, or lever/slide weight systems. Wrist cuffs, grasping cuffs, tripod wrist grips, adhesive wrap bandages, and/or prostheses can be used to help grasp the equipment.

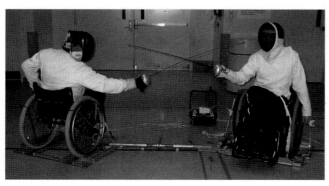

Fig. 48-5 Fencing. Wheelchair fencing frame.

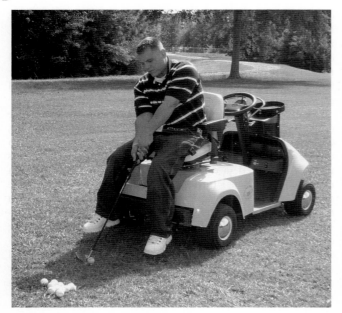

Fig. 48-6 Golf. Swivel-seat golf cart.

Golf

Implementation of the ADA on golf courses, coupled with advances in adaptive equipment, makes golf more accessible for individuals with physical disabilities. The ADA requires golf courses to be readily accessible to, and usable by, individuals with disabilities. Adaptive golf carts have assisted with increasing access. Adaptive carts can be equipped with a swivel seat that swings out to either the side or the back of the cart, which allows the golfer to remain seated while hitting the golf ball (Fig. 48-6), or the carts can be equipped with a power-assist swivel seat that brings the golfer to a standing position to hit the golf ball. Both types of carts are equipped with safety straps to assist the golfer with balance, leverage, and stability.

Golfers can adapt standard clubs in many ways to meet their needs, such as selecting lightweight clubs and club heads, modifying the bend in the shaft, building up the grip, or using a raised golf tee. Shorter clubs can be used if a golfer prefers to hit a ball one-handed from the side of a wheelchair. A number of pieces of adaptive equipment allow golfers with an upper extremity amputation to attach their prosthetic arm to a golf club, thereby enabling them to swing with both hands. Devices are available to help golfers tee-up and retrieve their ball.

Hunting

Hunting can be pursued by individuals of all abilities due to the wide range of adaptive equipment that is available. Mobility in the woods is one of the more common barriers, but it can be managed with all-terrain wheelchairs, all-terrain wheelchair tires, ATVs, or other modified vehicles (e.g., golf carts, pick-up trucks). To conceal themselves and their equipment, hunters can use ground blinds or camouflage netting, or they can position themselves in an elevation stand. Elevation stands include a box blind on hydraulic lifts that is wheelchair accessible and raises up to 20 ft in the air (Fig. 48-7A); a tree stand chair that climbs trees with the push of a button; a wheelchair platform or a fixed seat on a tripod or lean-to stand that raises up to 20 ft in the air with a manual or electric winch and cable system; and personally fabricated designs (Fig. 48-7B).

Information on adaptive shooting equipment for hunting is discussed in the sections on archery and shooting.

Ice hockey

The Paralympic version of ice hockey is known as ice sledge hockey. This fast-paced, highly physical sport follows regular ice hockey rules and is played by individuals who demonstrate good balance and upper extremity functioning. Instead of skates, players are seated on a two-bladed sledge that allows the puck to pass underneath while they propel

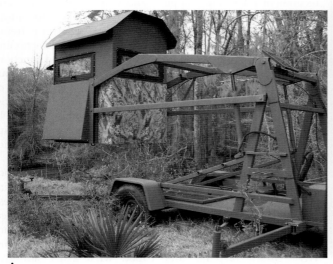

A

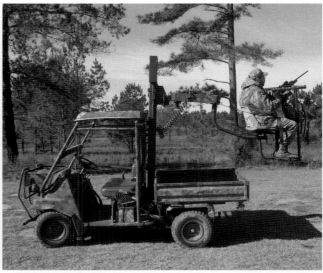

B

Fig. 48-7 Hunting. **A,** Wheelchair-accessible box blind on hydraulic lifts. **B,** Personally fabricated chair lift on an ATV.

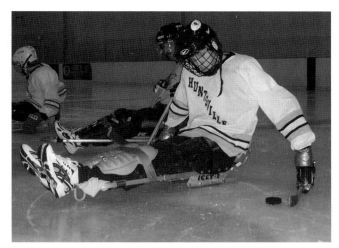

Fig. 48-8 Ice hockey. Two-bladed sledge and pick.

themselves across the ice by means of a special hockey stick (Fig. 48-8). These sticks (also known as picks) double as a mobility tool and a scoring device. On one end is a spike (similar to the toe pick of figure skates) that allows the players to maneuver across the ice; on the other end is a traditional hockey stick blade for puck control and shooting.

Paddling sports

Paddling encompasses canoeing, kayaking, rowing, and crew. In most instances, adaptations to standard equipment can be made for paddlers with a physical disability. Seating, body positioning, and paddling are the main areas that need to be considered. Standard removable paddling seat backs and seating systems can be added to a boat to assist with body positioning and trunk stability. If necessary, these seats can be modified to provide paddlers with even greater stability by adding lateral supports or placing foam padding between the paddler, the seat, and the boat.

Padding is very important for someone with decreased sensation, because it protects the skin from the bumps and rubbing that can occur with paddling. Any area of skin that is exposed and has the possibility of rubbing against something (e.g., the sides or bottom of the boat, the seat, etc.) should be padded. Paddlers can use a type of cushion that straps around the waist and legs and protects the buttocks area. Padding should be placed in such a way as to ensure that the paddler is able to exit the boat safely if the boat flips.

Paddlers with decreased upper extremity functioning and/or trunk control but who have full lower extremity functioning can use a system that allows them to paddle with their feet. The system supports a standard paddle that has been adapted with footholds. Paddlers with an upper extremity amputation can use their prosthesis to hold a paddle/oar. Paddlers with full grip in one upper extremity can use a one-handed paddle. Paddlers with decreased grip in both upper extremities can use grasping cuffs, adhesive bandage wraps, and/or inner tubing from a bicycle or wheelchair tire to assist with holding a paddle/oar. Once grasping cuffs and adhesive bandage wraps are attached to the paddle/oar and the paddler's hand, they become part of the paddler and are not quickly detachable. However, inner tubes can be tied or taped to the paddle/oar so that a tight fit is created when the

paddler's hand is slipped between the paddle/oar and the inner tube. This setup makes it relatively easy for paddlers to remove their hands from the paddle/oar if needed. In kayaking, hand paddles can be used by paddlers with decreased trunk control and/or upper extremity functioning.

Powerlifting

Powerlifting is the ultimate test of upper body strength, and it is a sport in which all disability groups compete. Lifters are classified by weight and gender. The regulation bench used in competition is designed for safety and function. Adjustable upright supports on both sides of the bench hold the bar horizontally and allow the bar to be appropriately positioned based on the lifter's physical needs. Adjustments to the bench, lifting requirements, and equipment can be made to meet the physical/anatomical needs of the lifter. The lifter's lower body can be strapped to the bench for safety. Spotters can assist the lifter with removing and returning the bar to the rack.

Power soccer

Power soccer is only for individuals who use a power wheelchair and who demonstrate control and safety of their wheelchairs. Power soccer is played on a regulation-size basketball court with an 18-inch soccer ball. A large guard is placed around the wheelchair and the player's feet and lower legs (Fig. 48-9). The guard is used to pass the soccer ball to another player, to shoot at the goal, and to protect the player from injury. A goal is scored when the ball is maneuvered over the goal line.

Quad rugby

Quad rugby is for individuals with quadriplegia who independently use a manual wheelchair. Rugby is played with a volleyball on a basketball court. Players use wheelchairs designed specifically for rugby. The wheelchairs are lightweight, have cambered wheels, use spoke guards to protect both the spokes of the wheels and the players' hands, and have front guards used for hitting into opponents and protecting the players' feet (Fig. 48-10). Body bracers can be used around the trunk/waist and the back of the chair to help maintain balance. Ankle straps can be used to help keep

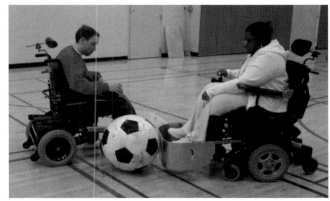

Fig. 48-9 Soccer ball and power wheelchairs with chair and foot guards.

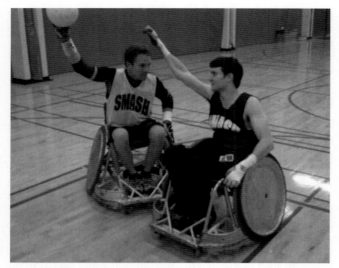

Fig. 48-10 Quad rugby. Rugby wheelchairs with front foot guards and spoke guards and player with a trunk/waist body bracer.

players' legs positioned within the chair when hitting into other players. A goal is scored when a player touches or crosses the opponent's goal line while maintaining possession of the ball.

Sailing

An extensive variety of adaptations are available for sailing, and several styles of boats are specifically designed to meet the needs of sailors with a physical disability. Adaptive equipment and styles of boats generally focus on seating systems, maximizing mobility in the cockpit, steering, and safety. Seating systems can be either fixed or mobile. In many instances, chest, seat, leg, and foot straps can be used to help stabilize the sailor. With a fixed seating system, the seat remains in the same position, and the sailor can perform only those functions that are within reach. With a mobile system, the sailor can switch sides of the boat and perform functions in a variety of locations. The most common types of mobile seating systems are seats that actually move across the boat and transfer benches that allow the sailor to move from one side to the other.

Adaptations to steering devices include collapsing tillers that allow movement from one side of the boat to the other; vertical control levers on both sides of the boat; wheel steering systems; replacement of stock tillers with T-bar mounts; electronic joystick steering systems; sip-and-puff mechanisms that control the rudder and trim the sails; automated systems for sail sheeting and bilge pumping; and hand pedal quick-release systems that control the tiller.

Safety features that can be considered when selecting a boat include strategically placed handholds and bars, multiple buoyancy compartments, and increased ballast ratio, vertical center of gravity, and keel stability.

Scuba diving

Individuals with a physical disability can pursue scuba diving with a small amount of additional dive training,

assistance, and equipment. Certification as a diver with a physical disability is required. In situations where a diver cannot perform specific physical performance standards of diving, a qualified dive buddy is required to assist the diver. Dive buddies may assist the diver with entering and exiting the water, mask clearing, equalization, and operating the buoyancy control device. Today's standard diving equipment can accommodate the needs of most divers with a physical disability.

Traditional jacket-style buoyancy control devices provide the best overall control for divers with a disability. Divers who require greater buoyancy control can use weight-integrated jackets and pneumatically assisted deflation devices. Divers with reduced respiratory ability or limited arm movement should use masks and snorkels with a purge valve for easy clearing and equalizing. Regulators should have an additional regulator (also known as an octopus) for buddy breathing. This allows the diver's hands to remain free for propulsion or carrying objects. Webbed neoprene hand fins can be used to increase arm power. Divers with adequate upper body strength can use underwater diver propulsion vehicles as an alternative to arm propulsion.

Divers can wear dive skins and wet suits to help protect their skin from abrasions and the sun as well as to assist with temperature regulation. Dive skins and wet suits can be modified with zippers and hook-and-loop strips to decrease the diver's difficulty in donning and doffing the suits. Hard-soled dive boots provide maximum protection for the diver's feet and additional flotation for the diver's legs. Fins are recommended for divers with decreased lower extremity functioning, as the fins assist with both propulsion and balance and provide protection for their feet. Divers can attach small weights to their ankles or the bottom of their scuba tanks if they find that the lower portion of their body has too much buoyancy.

Shooting

Shooting can be adapted to meet the needs of shooters with a wide variety of physical disabilities. Shooters who have decreased balance, decreased upper extremity functioning, or an upper extremity amputation primarily need adaptations related to supporting the firearm and pulling the trigger.

Sandbags, a bipod, tripod, shooting rail, or shooting rest can be used to help support the firearm. A shooting rest supports all or part of the weight of the gun and allows the shooter to take aim by maneuvering the gun both vertically and horizontally (Fig. 48-11A). Shooting rests are available that allow shooters with little or no arm function to independently control the maneuvering of the gun with a joystick mechanism and the firing of the gun through a sip-and-puff mechanism (Fig. 48-11B).

Trigger pull adaptations exist for individuals who have upper extremity functioning but not enough finger strength to pull the trigger. A mechanical trigger activator can be attached to the trigger guard (Fig. 48-11A), the trigger pull can be lightened by a gunsmith, or a hand/finger splint can be used. Shooters with visual impairments can use laser sights, PVC tube sites, or camera systems to aim at the target while a sighted partner directs them as to where they should aim.

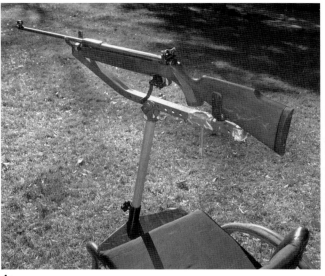

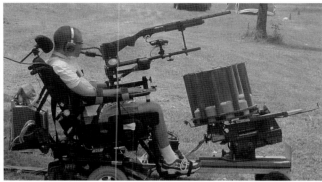

A   B

Fig. 48-11 Shooting. **A,** Swivel shooting rest and rifle adapted with a mechanical trigger activator. **B,** Sip-and-puff trigger activator with a joystick-operated shooting rest.

Snow skiing

Snow skiing is one of the most widely enjoyed winter sports for people with physical disabilities. Depending on the physical disability, conventional ski equipment with minor modifications can be used, or specially designed ski equipment may be needed. Outriggers, four-tracking, three-tracking, sit mono-skis, and sit bi-skis are the main adaptations available for skiers with physical disabilities.

Outriggers are forearm crutches with ski tips mounted on the bottom to aid the skier with balance, mobility, and turning; they adjust to fit the height of the skier. Outriggers are used in place of standard ski poles. Four-tracking is for a skier who has full use of all four extremities but has problems with balance. The skier uses two standard skis and outriggers, thus providing four points of contact on the snow for increased balance. The skis can be connected at the tips to provide even greater stability. Three-tracking is for a skier who has full use of one lower extremity and both upper extremities. The skier uses one standard ski and two outriggers, thus providing three points of contact on the snow for increased balance.

Skiers who cannot stand but who demonstrate good upper body balance, strength, and coordination can use a sit mono-ski. A mono-ski consists of a molded seat (also known as a bucket) mounted to a single ski, and two outriggers are used to assist with balance and turning (Fig. 48-12A). The sit bi-ski is similar to the mono-ski, except that the seat is attached to two shorter and wider skis, thus allowing for greater stability and assistance with balance than the mono-ski (Fig. 48-12B). Two outriggers are used to assist with balance and turning; in some instances, the outriggers are attached to the ski. Skiers with a visual impairment use standard skis and poles; however, a sighted instructor usually skis close behind and verbally guides the skier regarding direction and speed.

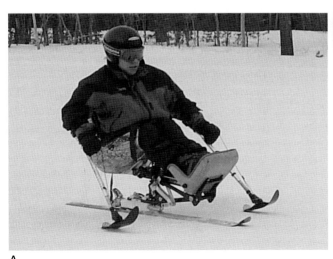

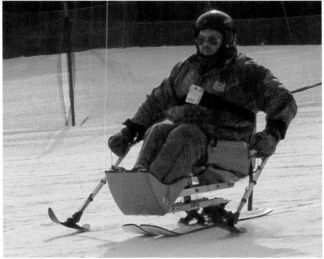

A   B

Fig. 48-12 Snow skiing. **A,** Sit mono-ski and outriggers. **B,** Sit bi-ski.

Softball

Wheelchair softball is played in manual wheelchairs, which must have footrests. The game follows the rules of 16-inch slow-pitch softball, and it is played on a level, smooth, hard surface. When batting, a player can use an assistive device called a block, which usually is made out of wood or metal piping. A block helps to stabilize and support the wheels of the chair while the player swings the bat with both hands. Players who do not use a block stabilize their chairs by placing one hand on their wheel while using the other hand to swing the bat. Players with decreased hand function can use approved gripping devices to modify the bat. When fielding a ball, players can use a softball glove; however, many choose not to based on the size and density of the softball. Players can use the wheels of their chairs for support and balance while fielding, catching, and throwing the ball.

Swimming

The ADA makes access to swimming pools easier for individuals with physical disabilities. Public swimming pools must have a means of entry into the pool, such as a chair lift, ramp, or transfer wall. Several assistive devices can assist with swimming and water exercise, such as a ski belt, inflatable neck collar, training paddles, and resistive/flotation weights.

Although assistive devices exist for the recreational swimmer, athletes are not allowed to wear prostheses or use assistive devices during competition. Swimmers are classified by functional ability, and competition exists for athletes with all types of physical disabilities. Competitive events include multiple distances in breaststroke, backstroke, freestyle, and butterfly.

Table tennis

On a competitive level, table tennis for players with physical disabilities is divided into different divisions using a functional classification system. Players who are able to stand follow standard table tennis rules, and few modifications to these rules are necessary for those who play from a wheelchair level. The table must allow wheelchair access without obstructing the player's legs. Players can use body bracers to assist with maintaining body positioning and balance. For players with limited grip, grasping cuffs or other strapping devices can be used to assist with gripping the racket.

Tennis

Wheelchair tennis integrates easily into able-bodied tennis. It is played on a standard tennis court, with no modifications to the court, balls, or racket. The only difference in wheelchair tennis is that the players are allowed two bounces of the ball, with the first bounce falling within the bounds of the court. Tennis chairs are used in competitive play, but they are not always necessary for recreational play. Tennis chairs are lightweight, have cambered wheels, and often have only three wheels (one centered in the front and two in the back), all of which allow for faster and easier mobility. Body bracers and straps can be used around the trunk, knees, and ankles to assist with balance and body positioning. Players who have decreased grip can play tennis by strapping or taping the racket to their hand.

Track and field

Track and field represents the largest sport for athletes with physical disabilities, both in terms of number of events and number of athletes. Events include track, jumps, throws, pentathlon, and marathon. Rules are very similar to able-bodied track and field events, with some adaptations to assist with safety and accessibility. For throwing events, the seated athlete throws from a fixed bench seat that is secured to the ground to prevent the bench from moving. The bench is equipped with rails for seating balance and leverage, and it is fully padded to protect the athlete's skin. For track and field athletes with a visual impairment, runners compete with a guide runner who is tethered at the wrist, and field athletes use acoustic devices or a sighted caller.

Prosthetic technology and wheelchair technology continue to improve. Prostheses and racing wheelchairs are custom fitted to the athlete, with the focus on speed and durability. They are designed to be lightweight, easy to maneuver, and very aerodynamic. Racing chairs consist of two large rear wheels, one smaller front wheel, an extra long wheel base between the front wheel and the rear wheels, and a small bucket seat over the two rear wheels (Fig. 48-13). Racing chairs are propelled by "punching" the back wheels, and they are steered through a compensator system that controls the front wheel. To protect their hands and to absorb the shock from propelling their chairs, racers wear padded gloves made from a formulated rubber that grips well both in wet and dry conditions (Fig. 48-13).

Water skiing

Water skiing is easily adapted to meet the needs of skiers with a physical disability. Skiers with a visual impairment use standard water ski equipment, but they may have a sighted skier ski alongside as a guide. Skiers with arm and/or leg amputations generally use standard water ski equipment as well, and they have the option to ski with a prosthesis. A sling or harness can be used to assist with holding the towrope. Skiers who are unable to stand use a sit ski.

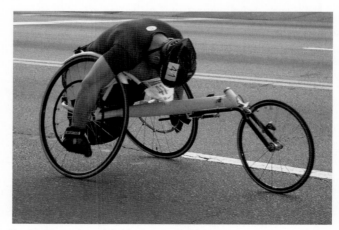

Fig. 48-13 Track and field. Racing wheelchair and padded propulsion gloves.

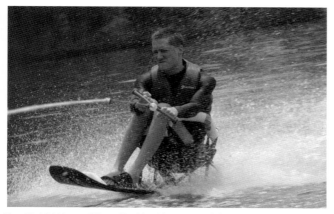

Fig. 48-14 Water skiing. Sit ski with cage and footplate.

A sit ski consists of several parts: a ski that is similar to a surfboard with a fin on the bottom to help steady the ski, a custom seating frame (also known as a cage) made of padded metal and a sling, and a footplate (Fig. 48-14). Both the cage and the footplate are mounted to the ski, and they adjust to fit the height of the skier. Skiers have the option of holding the towrope or attaching it to the ski. If the towrope is attached to the ski, a quick-release mechanism is used for safety. Additional adaptive equipment can be added to the sit ski to meet the needs of the skier. If a skier needs assistance with balance, outriggers can be attached to both sides of the ski, and a back support can be added to the cage. Different styles of sit skis are available for beginner, intermediate, and advanced recreational skiers as well as competition skiers. Competition skiing consists of events in slalom, tricks, and jumping, and each event has its own style of sit ski.

Conclusion

As with able-bodied sports and athletes, injury is always a potential risk. To minimize the risk, additional safety measures are incorporated into the modifications and equipment available to athletes with physical disabilities. As long as the equipment is used accordingly, athletes can reduce their risk for injury.

Although adaptive equipment is readily available, the cost is not always covered by health insurance. As with other durable medical equipment, athletes must check with their insurance companies to determine whether insurance will cover the cost of equipment. In many instances, athletes will incur out-of-pocket expenses for their adaptive sports equipment. Most equipment can be purchased commercially, or, in some cases, it can be made by the athlete.

Information on equipment, disabled sports opportunities, rules and regulations, and governing bodies can be easily obtained from the Internet. The Internet, the variety of available adaptive equipment, and the increasing number of community-based adaptive recreation organizations and programs have had a tremendous impact on opening up the world of disabled sports to interested athletes. Athletes with physical disabilities are able to participate both recreationally and competitively in sports and by so doing gain the physical, psychological, and emotional benefits that everyone needs for an active and healthy lifestyle.

Bibliography

Bike-on. Retrieved January 16, 2006. Available from *http://www.bike-on.com/newhandcycles/OneOffPage.htm*.

BlazeSports. Retrieved December 19, 2005. Available from *http://www.blazesports.com/DesktopDefault.aspx?tabid=120&tabindex=2*.

Flyability. Retrieved January 16, 2006. Available from *http://www.flyability.org.uk/About-Flyability.htm*.

International Paralympic Committee. Retrieved January 23, 2006. Available from *http://www.paralympic.org/release/Main_Sections_Menu/index.html*.

International Paralympic Committee. Retrieved January 23, 2006. Available from *http://www.paralympic.org/release/Main_Sections_Menu/Paralympic_Games/*.

International Paralympic Committee. Retrieved January 23, 2006. Available from *http://www.paralympic.org/release/Summer_Sports/*.

International Paralympic Committee. Retrieved January 23, 2006. Available from *http://www.paralympic.org/release/Winter_Sports/*.

International Sailing Federation. Retrieved January 23, 2006. Available from *http://sailing.org/default.asp?MenuID=0170GN`wzzCp20/HuCVrCBO43?HJUg/NHk6QAAKYQGfHafcoQ1NvaW6S1xy08vacdqfEGGAlk6xnz80FtRtM7NWy AR~Qb4K8Eič~SKAMUWhGtGHYoyLsjr*.

International Wheelchair Aviators. Retrieved January 24, 2006. Available from *http://www.wheelchairaviators.org/info.html*.

Maine Handicapped Skiing. Retrieved January 23, 2006. Available from *http://www.skimhs.org/what_we_do/adaptive_equipment_techniques/document_public*.

Manor Acre. Retrieved January 23, 2006. Available from *http://www.manoracre.com/driving.htm*.

National Wheelchair Softball Association. Retrieved January 2, 2006. Available from *http://www.wheelchairsoftball.org/aboutnwsa.htm*.

North American Riding for Handicapped Association. Retrieved December 8, 2005. Available from *http://www.narha.org/Driving/DrivingHomePage.asp*.

Northeast Passage. Retrieved January 24, 2006. Available from *http://www.nepassage.org/sportsDev.html*.

Pieces of Eight. Retrieved January 16, 2006. Available from *http://iml.jou.ufl.edu/projects/students/lane/Po8.htm*.

Sailing Web. Retrieved January 23, 2006. Available from *http://www.footeprint.com/sailingweb/boats.htm*.

USA Water Ski. Retrieved January 23, 2006. Available from *http://usawaterski.org/pages/divisions/WSDA/main.htm*.

U.S. Paralympics. Retrieved January 23, 2006. Available from *http://www.usolympicteam.com/paralympics/paralympic_games.html*.

U.S. Paralympics. Retrieved January 23, 2006. Available from *http://www.usolympicteam.com/paralympics/teams.html*.

US Sailing. Retrieved January 4, 2006. Available from *http://www.ussailing.org/swsn/technical-adapt.htm*.

United States Driving for the Disabled. Retrieved January 26, 2006. Available from *http://usdfd.org/carriages.htm*.

United States Handcycle Federation. Retrieved January 2, 2006. Available from *http://www.ushf.org/handcycling101.html*.

Chapter

49

Driving and related assistive devices

John Anschutz, Patricia P. Daviou, James Kennedy, and Michele Luther-Krug

Key Points

- Driver evaluations include clinical and on the road assessment.
- Driver training may be necessary following a driver evaluation.
- Fitting and orientation are essential to the success of using adaptive equipment.
- There are numerous assistive devices and driving techniques used in the field.
- Modifications to vehicles and controls are often required.
- Three case studies will be presented to illustrate how function impacts driving solutions.

Driving is a complex, multisensory task that requires physical skill and coordination as well as cognitive understanding of the rules and responsibilities that accompany it. Learning to drive is a challenge for everyone. To drive safely, everyone must learn the basic rules of the road and how to handle various driving situations. Primary and secondary controls allow safe maneuvering of the vehicle. A disability may impact the driver–control interface. When a person with a disability must use the primary and secondary controls differently, special modifications and training are necessary once the driver's ability has been assessed.

Primary controls include the steering wheel, accelerator, and brake. Secondary controls can be divided into two groups. The first group includes the ignition, shift, headlights, and any system that should be used while the vehicle is stationary. The second group, referred to as the driving systems group, includes the turn signal, horn, dimmer, wipers, and any system used while the vehicle is in motion. Many types and styles of primary and secondary controls can be matched to a client's abilities. Through driver evaluation, training, and appropriate modifications, a person with a disability may be able to be a safe and independent driver.

Generally, driver evaluations and driver training for people with disabilities are performed by a driver rehabilitation specialist (DRS) or certified driver rehabilitation specialist (CDRS). A DRS specializes in driver rehabilitation services for individuals with disabilities. The CDRS should have basic education in these skills. A CDRS is certified through the Association of Driver Rehabilitation Specialists (ADED; formerly the Association for Driver Educators for the Disabled) after passing a skills test. This certification indicates that the individual has basic knowledge, has fulfilled certain requirements, and is responsible for maintaining skills through continuing education.

Funding sources for driver evaluation and training are explored with the client during the intake procedure and preassessment. In many cases, traditional health insurance coverage for outpatient occupational therapy funds the clinical evaluation. The cost of on-the-road evaluation, training, and equipment may be funded through vocational rehabilitation services, state-funded trust funds, or other charitable organizations. If the disability was incurred as a result of a work injury or motor vehicle accident, insurance benefits may cover the driver rehabilitation and equipment costs if the client is approved by a referring physician.

Either a DRS or a CDRS can evaluate a client to determine whether the client is a candidate for driving. Once this determination has been made, a DRS or CDRS can recommend the type of adapted driving equipment that will best meet the client's needs. Choosing the appropriate vehicle to modify and installation of the adaptive equipment are done in partnership with a vehicle modifier who is a member of the National Mobility Equipment Dealers Association (NMEDA).

It is through the teamwork of this group of professionals that the needs of the client can best be met.

Driver evaluation

A comprehensive driver evaluation can be obtained by making a referral to a driver rehabilitation program. Most referrals are generated by the physician treating the individual with a disability or functional limitation. The driver rehabilitation program should include a multidisciplinary team with specialized training and certification in driver evaluation for people with disabilities. The comprehensive team includes a driver educator and/or occupational therapist with driver education credentials and access to assistive technology practitioners and wheelchair seating specialists. This team completes a clinical evaluation and an on-road evaluation to determine safe vehicle operation and potential risk management. The team prescribes the appropriate adaptive driving equipment for safe independent driving. Referrals are given for possible funding sources and qualified vendors who can install the prescribed modifications to the client's vehicle.

Clinical evaluation

A clinical evaluation of prerequisite skills for safe motor vehicle operation comprises several main skill components. Depending on the state, a DRS may have received licensure from the state's department of motor vehicles (DMV) and professional boards. A DRS with diverse experience in the treatment of persons with physical, visual, and psychological disabilities is best equipped to complete the clinical evaluation. The following are common areas that are evaluated during the clinical evaluation.

Medical history/driving history

The clinical evaluation starts with a thorough interview of the client's medical history and the etiology of the client's disability. The clinician carefully evaluates congenital, pathological, and traumatic conditions that may impact the physical function for driving. The DRS should inquire about the client's history of seizures and episode status if seizures have occurred, history of dizziness, and visual changes. The DRS must comply with each state's DMV rules as they relate to physical visual and psychological conditions. If there are areas of concern, the DRS should refer the patient to a specialist for the condition in question to gain possible clearance for driver training or to learn recommended driver restrictions.

The interview should include driving history, including past experience of operating motor vehicles, all-terrain vehicles, motorcycles, and heavy machinery. Understanding the client's driving history can give the DRS valuable insight as to which adaptive methods and equipment will best suit the client. The client's driving history also can help determine which clinical assessments should be administered during the driving evaluation.

Vision

A visual screening should be completed to ensure that the client meets the state's minimum requirements for distance acuity, contrast sensitivity, glare recovery, and peripheral vision. Ocular motor skills should be screened to determine ability to track, fixate, and perform saccadic eye movements necessary for visual search. Testing might include various scanning tests. Screening equipment should be chosen that is accepted and used by the state's DMV where applicable. Clients who do not meet the legal vision requirements should be referred to a vision specialist for evaluation.

Cognition/perception

The DRS should perform various standardized assessments to gauge simple, divided, and selective visual attention as well as the client's comprehension of multistep directions. The DRS should evaluate perceptual abilities that have a functional impact on driver performance, including visual closure, visual memory, figure ground, spatial relations, position in space, midline orientation, visual attention, and visual processing speed. Specific tests that evaluate these abilities include the Motor Free Visual Perceptual Test Version 2, Line Bisection Test, Trails Making B, Topographical Orientation, and Useful Field of View. It is important to assess perceptual skills so that functional outcomes that may affect safe vehicle operation, such as lane position, negotiation of curves, parking, merging and lane changes, ability to preplan, and problem solving ability in varied traffic levels, can be accommodated. Areas of concern with these skills may indicate a deficit in risk management skills as they relate to motor vehicle operation.

If compensation techniques cannot be used for these cognitive skill deficits, appropriate assistive technology devices might be used instead. Using assistive devices may require additional education and training in how they interface with vehicle operation. Persons who have difficulty with topographical orientation may benefit from technology such as navigational systems, global positioning satellite systems, and cell phones. Once these components are programmed, the DRS will carefully design a treatment plan that facilitates a gradual increase in complexity as the ability of the driver improves, as well as internalization of these compensatory driver behavioral skills. The on-the-road evaluation then can be appropriately tailored to enhance the evaluator's ability to assess if the driver is able to compensate for the cognitive/perceptual skill concerns identified in the clinical evaluation.

Physical/functional ability

Driving ability and safety depend on both cognitive and perceptual acuity, but the client's physical ability is equally important. Therefore, the DRS should assess the client's physical abilities during the clinical evaluation. The following physical systems should be observed during the clinical evaluation:

- Cervical motion
- Trunk balance
- Upper extremity and lower extremity range of motion
- Upper extremity and lower extremity tone
- Upper extremity and lower extremity strength
- Upper extremity and lower extremity sensation
- Upper extremity and lower extremity coordination
- Upper extremity and lower extremity motor planning
- Presence of pain
- Reaction time
- Endurance
- Presence of startle reflex

In addition, the DRS should assess the client's ability to transfer independently to the vehicle. If the client uses a mobility device, such as a scooter or a wheelchair, the DRS should assess the client's ability to load and unload his or her mobility device into a vehicle independently. All of these factors will influence the DRS's selection of method and any equipment to be used for the on-the-road evaluation. (Please refer to chart Fig.49-1 on function/mobility needs/vehicle for how these areas all must be considered when looking at driving). Physical function will also help determine the proper route and traffic level during the on-the-road evaluation.

On-the-road evaluation

Once the clinical evaluation has been completed and the client remains eligible for driver training, the client should be taken on the road for an on-the-road assessment by a qualified DRS. The clinical evaluation helps determine which vehicle and driving equipment, if needed, will be used for the driving portion of the evaluation. This on-the-road evaluation is dynamic and may include changes in equipment and configuration as more information is gathered during the on-the-road assessment. During the on-the-road evaluation, speed control is evaluated. Coordination of gas and brake, hill starts, range of speeds, stop locations, and following distance all should be tested. Steering is evaluated, including execution of turns, lane tracking, and lane corrections. Operation of secondary controls, ability to park, ability to change lanes, ability to follow the rules of the road, judgment, risk management, problem solving, and endurance are part of the evaluation. It is important to remember that the on-the-road portion of the evaluation must be graded to the ability of the driver. Assessment of the client's ability to drive in residential areas, on secondary roads, and on limited access highways will depend on the driver's ability. Further training may be a recommendation resulting from this evaluation.

Driver training

For most individuals, training will be required to master the skills for safe operation of adaptive driving equipment or methods. The process for training should be individualized for each client's skill level. A new driver will require an average of 40 hours of training, but an experienced driver may require only 5 to 10 hours of training. A DRS will determine the driver rehabilitation training plan upon completion of the initial driver evaluation.

The driver training process focuses on safe motor vehicle operation with or without adaptive driving aids, proper scanning techniques, and risk management skills. Educational videos, simulators, textbooks, and homework assignments often supplement behind-the-wheel training sessions. A skilled DRS develops formalized routes that will teach all skills required to pass the DMV state road test.

Traffic routes are an important component of the training process. Routes are graded from simple, low-traffic environments and to complex, high-traffic levels and expressway driving. If the client is unable to progress successfully through these routes to achieve full skill mastery, the treatment plan can be altered to allow driver training in a familiar area. This may result in recommendations for driving restrictions to a particular mile radius, time of day, speed limit, or roadway type.

High-technology driving systems (e.g., servo controls, discussed below) will require a minimum of 40 hours of training. This time will allow the DRS to develop a comprehensive vehicle modification prescription that will optimize the fit of the wheelchair mobility device with electronic primary and secondary controls. Wheelchair lock-downs, lift systems, and vehicle structural modifications, including lowered floor, raised roof and doors, and seat modifications, all will become specifications for the client's vehicle prescription. Once the client's vehicle is completed, a DRS will complete a fitting at the vehicle modifier's shop, and final training hours in the modified vehicle will be done after the fitting is completed.

Fitting and orientation

After the vehicle has been built, a fitting is performed while the driving equipment is being installed. Appropriate setup for the equipment is crucial for safety and best driving performance. For best results, a fitting and orientation should be done by the DRS who provided the training. This will ensure that modifications and equipment are installed and operate correctly based on the client's needs. The fitting process will vary depending on the complexity of the equipment. The fitting should be completed at the installer's shop so that adjustments can be made as needed. The fitting is a complex process that assesses how the client interfaces with the vehicle and the primary and secondary controls. The fitting should confirm that the driver has the ability to independently enter the vehicle and get into the driver's area. It is important to confirm that the client is able to load and unload his or her mobility device from the vehicle during the fitting.

Once the fitting is complete, a client orientation is done. During the orientation, the client drives the adapted vehicle on the road. Orientation is best completed on all types of roadways and in light to heavy traffic conditions. The orientation should confirm that the client can safely control the vehicle with the adaptive equipment and that the client is comfortable with the vehicle's handling. This moving, dynamic assessment may indicate that adjustments are needed. For this reason, the orientation will be completed at the vehicle modifier's shop so that any adjustments to the equipment can be done easily and quickly and so that the client can test the alteration. It is important to keep in mind that further training may be required to make the client comfortable and safe in the new vehicle. As with any driver, the client will need to grow accustomed to handling the vehicle and will need to develop defensive driving skills.

Assistive devices/adapted driving techniques

Although the client's diagnosis certainly influences the type of assistive technology that the client may need in order to drive, the client's functional ability often is the more influential factor in determining what kind of modifications and adaptive equipment are needed. It is the individual's physical, visual, and cognitive functions that help determine the appropriate adaptive driving equipment and driving techniques, and the on-the-road evaluation will verify these findings. For example, one client with cerebral palsy might

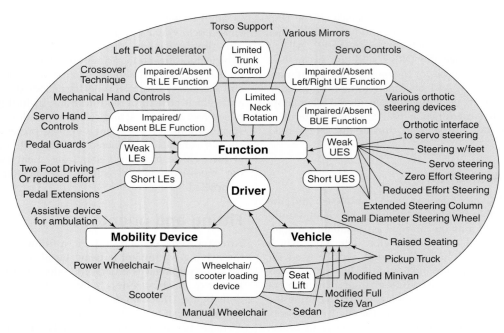

Fig. 49-1 Chart detailing safe interfacing of function and ability, mobility device, and vehicle is a crucial factor in creating safe independent drivers. (Courtesy Shepherd Center, Atlanta, GA.)

require hand controls, whereas another client with cerebral palsy might not require any equipment at all. For this reason, it is important that adaptive equipment operation is tested under both static and dynamic conditions. Safe interfacing of function and ability, mobility device, and vehicle is a crucial factor in creating a safe independent driver (Fig. 49-1).

The following is a reference list of common adaptive driving equipment and techniques.

Mirrors

Numerous mirrors can assist drivers with visual and cervical rotational limitations:

- Lane changer mirror
- Smart view mirror
- Panel mirror
- Forty-five–degree mirror
- Panoramic mirror

Torso support

A chest strap provides additional lateral and forward trunk support when sitting balance is impaired. A chest strap aids trunk stability during the execution of turns, on entrance ramps for interstates, on downhill grades, and for braking maneuvers. The strap is measured to fit the upper torso and is attached to the vehicle seat. The strap is put around the driver's torso once the client reaches the appropriate driving position.

Steering devices

Various orthotic steering devices assist the driver who will be steering with one hand. The individual's gross grasp function

will help determine which device will be most appropriate. Steering devices include the following:

- Spinner knob
- Quad grip with pin
- Tri-pin
- V-grip
- Upright quad spinner
- Flat spinner
- Amputee ring

Mechanical hand controls

Hand controls are used by individuals with impaired or absent lower extremity function. Hand controls include push brakes with four types of acceleration: right angle, pull, twist, and rocker type (Figs. 49-2 and 49-3).

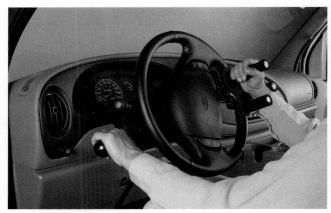

Fig. 49-2 Right-angle hand controls and tri-pin steering device. (Courtesy Mobility Products & Designs.)

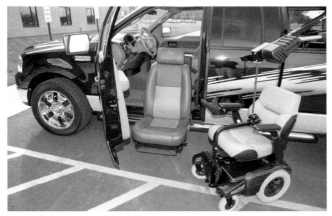

Fig. 49-3 Lift seat and wheelchair loading device. (Courtesy Ford Mobility.)

Servo hand controls

Servo hand control systems amplify force and motion and thereby compensate for reductions in force and motion application. This system can be operated electrically, hydraulically, or pneumatically. These hand controls are helpful for individuals who do not have the strength or range of motion to operate mechanical hand controls.

Pedal guards

Pedal guards prevent the driver's feet from accidentally hitting the accelerator or from becoming an obstruction under the accelerator or brake pedal when the feet are not being used. Pedal guards are removable and can allow an able-bodied family member to operate the vehicle with standard original equipment manufactured (OEM) foot pedals.

Pedal extensions

Pedal extensions can be attached to the brake or accelerator pedal to extend the height and width of the pedals.

Two-foot driving

Two-foot driving uses the left foot for the brake pedal and the right foot for the accelerator pedal. This method of accommodation can be used when the driver has limited ankle inversion and eversion but intact proprioception, dorsi flexion, and planter flexion. Reaction time often is improved with this technique, but this driving technique is not legal in all states.

Reduced-effort brake

Most cars manufactured today offer power assist to the brake function. In most cases the OEM brake system can be modified to provide for lower forces than those that are standard on the vehicle. The user of reduced-effort braking may be required to shift from using pressure-related sensory feedback to positional sensory feedback in order to properly regulate braking. Because of this shift in sensory feedback

systems, the user of this equipment may require several hours of additional training.

Left foot accelerator

A left foot accelerator can be used when the left leg must be used to operate both the brake and the accelerator. The left foot accelerator replaces the OEM pedals. Users should be aware that left foot accelerators can easily lead to accidents for people who are not aware that they are installed.

Crossover technique

When the right leg is impaired, the left leg can be used in a crossover technique. With this technique, the left leg is used to operate the OEM pedals of the vehicle. When exploring this option, left hip comfort, left leg length, and ability to position the right leg away from pedals should be considered.

Reduced-effort steering

For the person with limited upper extremity strength, reducing the amount of effort to steer may be necessary. The amount of effort required to turn the steering wheel can be reduced by 30% to 50% from the standard amount. Vehicles vary but generally require approximately 25 to 32 lb per inch of torque. Reduced-effort steering requires 14 to 20 lb per inch of torque to achieve the same effect.

Steering with feet

This system is designed for a driver with severely impaired or absent upper extremity function but intact lower extremity function. One foot is used to steer a small wheel located by the accelerator and brake pedals. The other foot is used to operate the OEM accelerator and brake pedal. Maximum reduced-effort steering normally is required for this system.

Zero-effort steering (maximum reduced-effort steering)

If reduced-effort steering cannot compensate for weak upper extremity strength, then zero-effort steering (as known as maximum reduced-effort steering) may be a viable option. Zero-effort steering requires 4 to 9 lb per inch of torque. However, the self-centering characteristic of the OEM steering wheel is removed with reduced-effort steering. Proper technique and training are required for new users of this system.

Small-diameter steering wheels

A small-diameter wheel can be used by a driver with limited range of motion, who is small in stature, or who is very obese. Reduced-effort steering or zero-effort steering is required when using a small-diameter steering wheel.

Servo steering

A servo system may be required for a driver with limited range of motion and limited strength. This type of system also might be useful for a driver who has only limited use of one arm. With servo controls, the range of motion required can be adjusted to the user's ability. Joystick driving or a small-diameter steering wheel are examples of servo steering.

Orthotic interface to servo steering

Orthotic devices can be customized to interface the user with the servo steering system (see case study 3).

Raised seating

Various power seats can provide the most appropriate position for safe driving. After-market power seat bases can be adjusted to increase seat height to accommodate a driver with short upper extremities. Seat height can be lowered to accommodate a driver with short lower extremities. Six-way and eight-way power seat bases allow greater forward or backward positioning as well as rotation to the cargo area for drivers with impaired mobility and limited ability to transfer. Users with more function may use a cushion to adjust their height to achieve optimum visibility rather than an electric power seat base.

Extended steering columns

Extended steering columns are used by individuals who are short in stature or who require positioning farther from the standard steering wheel because of body size. A reduced-diameter steering wheel with an extended steering column often is required.

Mobility devices

A mobility device should be chosen to meet the needs of the individual first and the appropriateness for driving second. It is important that the vehicle, mobility device, and necessary assistive technology all interface safely and that together all three facilitate optimum function. A wheelchair seating specialist and a DRS should collaborate to meet the wheelchair user's optimal functional and community mobility needs. As with all assistive technology, adequate trials with the various proposed equipment should be done.

Assistive devices for ambulation

Assistive devices for ambulation vary and include walkers, canes, ankle–foot orthoses, and lower extremity prostheses. When evaluating a client who uses an assistive ambulation device, it is important to consider these devices and how they impact independent driving. Sometimes people can drive with either an AFO or a prosthesis and sometimes they cannot. If a driver uses a walker or cane, the driver will need to be able to enter and exit the vehicle safely.

Scooter

Motorized scooters are often used for community mobility and occasionally will need to be transported in a motor vehicle. Some scooters can be taken apart and loaded into the back of a vehicle. Other scooters may need a scooter loading device to place them in the back of a vehicle. The scooter can never be occupied when it is being transported. A modified van often is the best vehicle for transporting a scooter.

Manual wheelchair

Manual wheelchairs can be either rigid or folding, that is, the wheelchair collapses into a more portable configuration. Important considerations are whether a wheelchair user can independently load, secure, and unload the wheelchair, as well as transfer from his or her wheelchair, with or without adaptive equipment. This ability may affect what type of equipment and vehicle are obtained.

Power wheelchair

Unlike the scooter, the power wheelchair can be transported while it is occupied by the client. Transporting a power wheelchair, whether or not it is occupied, generally requires a modified van. Sometimes people drive from their power wheelchair when they are not able to independently transfer into a seat in the driver's area. Whether or not occupied, the power wheelchair must be properly secured in the vehicle for safety.

Vehicles/Modifications

All drivers have selection criteria when choosing a vehicle. However, a person with a disability often must consider additional criteria before choosing his or her vehicle. It is crucial that the driver with a disability chooses the most appropriate vehicle based on the clinical and driver evaluations.

Sedan

A sedan can be used by a person with a disability with little or no modifications. If the sedan cannot be used, then a modified van might be required.

Pickup truck

Various wheelchair loading devices are available. Some are used to load wheelchairs into the inside of an extended cab; other loading devices are used to put the mobility device into the bed of a pickup truck. A lowered-floor pickup truck is available and can be driven by a wheelchair driver who can access the truck by a wheelchair platform lift. However, a tall driver might not be able to fit in the driver position in this vehicle because of the limited head room in the driver's area.

Modified minivan

The floors of some minivans can be lowered. This will increase the height of the door opening and the interior height, which will accommodate the overall height of a person sitting in a wheelchair. Because these vehicles already are low to the ground, a ramp is used to enter the vehicle rather than a lift. A crash-tested manual tie-down system or an automatic lock-down system will be required to secure the wheelchair occupant safely. Minivans are built like station wagons and therefore drive and wear like cars.

Modified full-size van

Some full-size vans can have their roofs and doors raised. In addition, the floors in full-size vans can be lowered. An automatic wheelchair platform lift for loading the wheelchair occupant into the vehicle is needed with modified full-size vans because the distance between the ground and the van's floor is increased. A crash-tested lock-down system will be required to secure the wheelchair occupant. Full-size vans are built like trucks and therefore drive and wear like trucks.

Wheelchair/scooter loading device

A wheelchair or scooter can be loaded mechanically into a vehicle in various ways. A car topper can lift a folding manual wheelchair and store the wheelchair in a covered carrier on top of a sedan once the driver has transferred into the driver's seat. Various loading devices can help load a wheelchair or scooter into the back, either inside or outside, of various vehicles depending on the lift. A vehicle modifier could help determine possible lift options.

Seat lift

Power seat lifts are available for sedans, trucks, and mini- and full-size vans. Seat lifts come in many styles and perform various functions. Generally, seat lifts are used to help the driver enter and exit the vehicle and to help the driver reach a functional driving position.

Modifications to secondary controls may be necessary and include the following:

- Ignition
- Electric shift
- Wipers
- Turn signals
- Horn
- Heater/air conditioning
- Power windows
- Door/lift controls
- Electric gear selector
- Headlight dimmer
- Electric parking brake
- Radio

Sometimes there can be simple solutions for adapting or modifying secondary control operations, such as a right-hand turn signal lever or a left-hand gear selector lever. A quad key holder or quad key turner provides leverage for someone with impaired hand function so that he or she can independently turn a key. A driver with more involved physical limitations might require higher-technology solutions, such as touch pad controls, single-switch scanning controls, and voice command systems to operate the secondary driving functions.

Special precautions

It is important that family, friends, and service technicians are aware that adaptive driving equipment has been installed in the vehicle. Due to the specialized training needed to operate a modified vehicle, no one who has not been properly trained should drive the adapted vehicle.

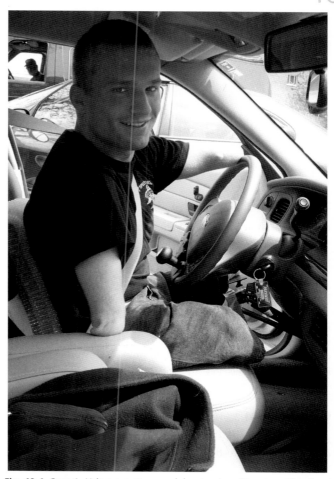

Fig. 49-4 Case 1. Using a custom pedal extension. (Courtesy Shepherd Center, Atlanta, GA.)

Case studies

Case 1

The client was born with transhumeral and transfemoral deformity. His arms terminate just below the elbow, and his legs end just below the knees. Only one modification was necessary to make this client a safe independent driver. Custom pedal extensions were made, which allow his legs to operate the gas and brake. He is able to steer using the standard steering wheel, and he operates the secondary controls, including turning the key in the ignition, without any adaptive equipment. (Figs. 49-4 and 49-5).

Case 2

The client's legs have been amputated. His right leg is amputated just above the knee, and his left leg is amputated just below the knee. After evaluation and training, this client is a safe and independent driver who uses his left leg with a prosthesis to operate a left foot accelerator and the OEM brake (Figs. 49-6 and 49-7).

Case 3

The client is a quadrilateral amputee with bilateral shoulder disarticulation and bilateral above knee amputation.

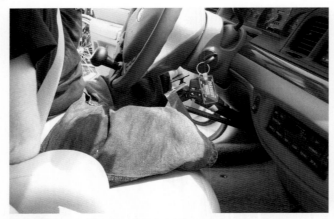

Fig. 49-5 Case 1. (Courtesy Shepherd Center, Atlanta, GA.)

A custom cuff orthotic was secured to a servo hand control. The client uses this modified hand control to operate the gas and brake by protracting and retracting his right shoulder (Figs. 49-8 and 49-9).

The client also slides his leg into a custom orthotic that interfaces with a servo steering system. The client then moves the control to the right or to the left to steer. The client also uses a touch pad system and mouth stick to access some of the secondary controls when the vehicle is stationary (Fig. 49-10).

Conclusion

A disability does not preclude driving. Through appropriate evaluations and testing with trained professionals, vehicle modifications by a certified professional, orientation, and proper training, many people with disabilities can drive safely and independently.

Resources

Organizations

Association for Driver Rehabilitation Specialists (ADED)
8601 Six Forks Road
Suite 400
Raleigh, NC 27615
www.aded.net

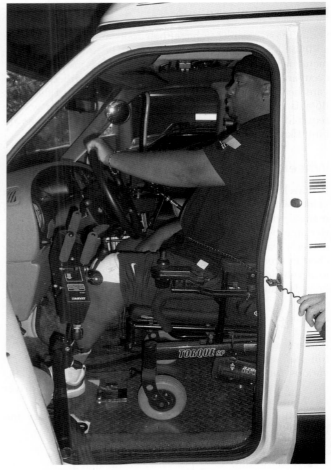

Fig. 49-7 Case 2. (Courtesy Shepherd Center, Atlanta, GA.)

American Occupational Therapy Association (AOTA)
4720 Montgomery Lane
PO Box 31220
Bethesda, MD 20824-1220
www.aota.org
National Highway Traffic Safety Administration (NHTSA)
400 Seventh Street SW
Washington, DC 20590
www.nhtsa.dot.gov

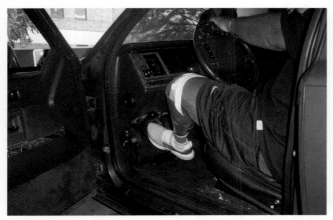

Fig. 49-6 Case 2. Using a left foot accelerator. (Courtesy Shepherd Center, Atlanta, GA.)

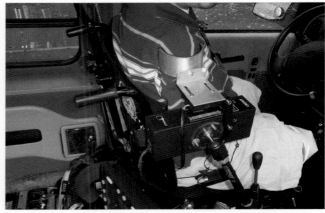

Fig. 49-8 Case 3. Using custom orthotics to interface with adaptive driving equipment. (Courtesy Shepherd Center, Atlanta, GA.)

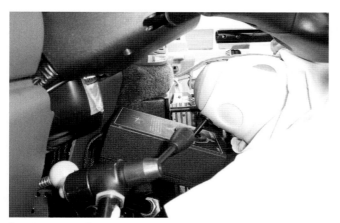

Fig. 49-9 Case 3. (Courtesy Shepherd Center, Atlanta, GA.)

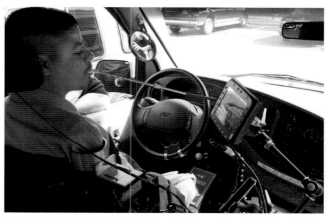

Fig. 49-10 Case 3. (Courtesy Shepherd Center, Atlanta, GA.)

National Mobility Equipment Dealers Association (NMEDA)
3327 West Bearss Avenue
Tampa, FL 33618
www.nmeda.org

Publications

Physicians Guide to Assessing and Counseling Older Drivers
American Medical Association/National Highway Traffic Safety Administration/US Department of Transportation, June 2003
American Medical Association
515 North State Street
Chicago, IL 60610

Digest of Motor Laws
AAA Traffic Safety Department
1000 AAA Drive
Heathrow, FL 32746-5063

Bibliography

Johnston J, Stocks SJ, Datta Chaudhuri M, Dey P: Driving after stroke: a study of recollection of advice and compliance with guidelines. *Int J Ther Rehabil* 11:355–358, 2004.

Mazer BL, Korner-Bitensky NA, Sofer S: Predicting ability to drive after stroke. *Arch Phys Med Rehabil* 79:743–750, 1998.

Miller GJ: Evaluating reaction time, threat recognition, and crash avoidance, Scientific/Technical Session 107-B.

Myers RS, Ball KK, Kalina TD, Roth DL, Goode KT: Relation of useful field of view and other screening tests to on-road driving performance. *Percept Mot Skills* 91:279–290, 2000.

Owsley C, Ball K, McGwin GJr, Sloane ME, Roenker DL, White MF, Overley ET: Visual processing impairment and risk of motor vehicle crash among older adults. Predicting future crash involvement in older drivers: who is at risk? *JAMA* 279:1083–1088, 1998.

Chapter

50

Robotic devices for rehabilitation of patients with spinal cord injury

Rüdiger Rupp and Hans Jürgen Gerner

Key Points

- The greatest impact of the application of robotics to rehabilitation likely will not be the devices themselves but the insights they provide into the principles of rehabilitation.

- Using robots to assist the rehabilitation process will provide more precise, objective, detailed data on what actually occurs in patients during recovery. This in turn will lead to a better understanding of the key biomechanical and neurological factors required for a successful rehabilitation process.

- A greater understanding of the underlying mechanisms of recovery will lead to better ideas of how technology can be beneficial in rehabilitation.

- New fields of applications of rehabilitation robots will lead to a better outcome for all people with disabling conditions as well as increased utility by the able-bodied population.

The incidence of spinal cord injury (SCI) in industrial countries is approximately 40 new cases per year per million population. In 2004 there were 1,800 new cases in Germany[15] and 11,000 in the United States.[32] The majority of SCIs are caused by trauma, but an increasing number are caused by nontraumatic injuries. Injuries of the spinal cord lead to variable losses in limb movement and sensation. Loss of function, such as walking, mobility, or hand movement for activities of daily living, creates dramatic changes in the lives of patients. In the past, almost every patient with SCI died within the first 5 years after sustaining the injury. However, increased understanding of the complications related to SCI and improved treatments during rehabilitation have changed

the life expectancy of patients.[32] Medical complications, if managed well, provide us the opportunity to maximize remaining motor function during rehabilitation using appropriate training methods or technical assistive devices.

Only 30% of patients have complete SCI.[32] In patients with incomplete SCI, some sensory and/or weak motor functions are preserved. Eighty percent of patients improve to a higher functional level within the first year after injury. The greatest extent of neurological recovery occurs within the first 6 months after injury and reaches a plateau 12 to 15 months after injury.[46]

According to this time line, three phases of primary rehabilitation with different therapeutic goals can be defined. The first phase, the *very acute stage*, begins at the date of injury and lasts for the first few weeks. This phase, which directly follows the lesion, is characterized by immobilization of patients due to cardiopulmonary problems and the consequences of spine stabilization surgery, which is performed in almost all patients in Europe and the United States. The very acute stage is followed by the *subacute stage*, which is the period from 2 to 6 months after the lesion. During this phase, clinicians and therapists aim at functional improvement of patients using gains in muscle strength resulting from spontaneous neurological recovery. The last stage during primary rehabilitation is the *chronic stage*. This phase consists of the period from 6 months after the injury and beyond when typically only minor neurological recovery occurs. Within this phase, preserved and permanent functional limitations of patients must be carefully analyzed in order to derive valid recommendations for surgical interventions, such as muscle–tendon transfers, or implementation of technical aids.

Although the goals may change during the three phases of primary rehabilitation, different technical systems in the form of robotic devices are used in the clinical environment to support patients and therapists through the entire rehabilitation period.

Robotics in therapeutic applications
Lower limb rehabilitation

Novel therapeutic methods for rehabilitation of the lower extremities in patients with SCI are based on recent neurophysiological findings. These findings suggest that the spinal cord is more than just a connection between the motor areas of the brain and the muscles of the lower extremities. Experiments performed mainly in cats by Grillner and Wallen[16] and in humans by Barbeau and Rossignol[2] show that the spinal cord contains functional networks of nerve cells. If adequately stimulated from afferent input sources, this neural network, called the *central pattern generator*, is capable of producing complex muscle activation sequences in terms of stepping movements. In contrast to spinalized cats, humans with complete SCI do not show locomotion-like intrinsic activity. Even if no autonomous spinal activity is present in patients with complete SCI, some rhythmic activity of spinal origin can be induced. Involuntary stepping movements in patients with incomplete SCI have been reported.[6] Dietz et al.[9] showed that the spinal cord below the site of lesion in completely paralyzed patients is able to adequately process information from peripheral sensors (forces or joint angles) and to transform this information into a functional muscle activation pattern.

Early mobilization of patients with SCI

If these principles of "spinal intelligence" are incorporated appropriately into the rehabilitation scheme, they can be successfully applied to reduce the initial problems of patients with SCI. During the very acute stage after injury, spinal reflexes are absent in most patients (spinal shock). Venous pooling occurs in the lower extremities, and the circulatory system is unstable. Together these symptoms are the cause for the extended period of immobilization. Standard therapy during this period consists of static verticalization of patients using a tilt table and application of passive movements of the legs by physiotherapists for about 10 minutes once per day. However, bedrest studies have shown that prolonged immobilization leads to quick loss of muscle mass, negative hemodynamic effects, and severe bone demineralization.[41]

In order to provide the clinical basis for an effective mobilization therapy at this very early stage of rehabilitation, two centers dedicated to the rehabilitation of SCI patients (Orthopedic University Hospital, Heidelberg, Germany and Balgrist University Hospital, Zurich, Switzerland) developed a novel robotic tilt table called the *Erigo*. This device moves the patient's legs in a manner comparable to the physiological gait pattern. In contrast to conventional devices that provide continuous passive motion, the Erigo achieves not only appropriate physiological kinematics in terms of adequate hip extension but also kinetics (loading/unloading of the foot sole) that are close to a normal gait. The importance of these factors as triggers for the central pattern generator has been shown in experiments in spinalized cats[11] and in

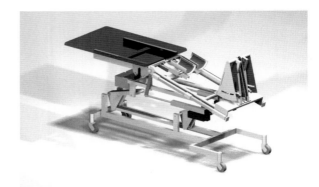

Fig. 50-1 Simplified overview of the basic components of the Erigo robotic stepping device.

humans.[10] A main design criterion of the device was the possibility of increasing the stepping frequency to a value comparable to that of normal walking.

Erigo device

The Erigo is based on a traditional tilt table (Fig. 50-1). The upper body part can be continuously tilted from the supine position up to 80 degrees. When the patient is lying on the tilt table, the patient's upper body is secured through a harness, with chest and shoulder fixed. Each thigh is fastened by a cuff to a linear drive mechanism that is controlled by a microcomputer. In order to generate hip extension according to the physiological principles, the upper body part of the device also can be tilted downward up to 20 degrees in relation to the leg part. The foot is fixed by a strap onto a proprietary footplate. For physiological loading of the foot, a special spring damper mechanism is integrated into the footplate. Load is applied to the foot sole during the stance phase (hip and knee extension) by clamping of a spring beneath the plate. When the hip and the knee are flexed, the spring is released from the plate, and no load is generated.[8] The overall load on the foot increases with the degree of tilting, as a greater percentage of the patient's body weight counteracts with the spring-damped footplate.

With these design principles, the Erigo combines the generation of a physiological load pattern with a continuously adjustable tilt and a stepping frequency up to one step cycle per second.

Clinical results of the Erigo

Early work suggests that blood pressure may stabilize with use of this device, leading to better postural adjustments and earlier onset of mobilization in wheelchair in rehabilitation.

To prove the hypothesis that this device leads to stabilization of the cardiovascular system, we initiated a clinical pilot study where we included six acutely injured patients with clinically complete injury of the cervical spinal cord (ASIA impairment scale A, lower extremity motor score 0) 4 weeks after injury and analyzed relative changes in blood pressure compared to baseline measurements recorded with patients in the initial resting position.[8] Baseline measurements were recorded in the horizontal position because patients could not tolerate 10 minutes of upright standing position without signs of presyncope, especially at the onset of study participation. With the automated movement therapy, blood pressure increased up to 5% even though

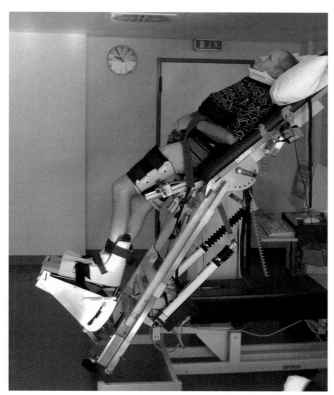

Fig. 50-2 Application of the Erigo device to a patient with a very high lesion (C3), complete spinal cord injury.

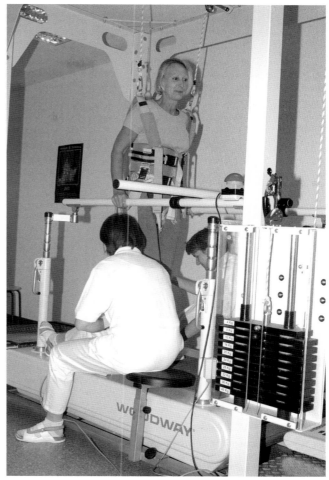

Fig. 50-3 Manually assisted treadmill training by an incomplete paraplegic patient. The counterweights (seen in the right lower corner) are attached to the patient's harness for body weight support.

patients were tilted to the 60-degree upright position after the baseline interval (Fig. 50-2). After stopping the movement in this position, mean arterial pressure decreased significantly (−30%), thus showing the direct effect of passive movement on the circulatory system in these patients.[8] From these results, this robotic stepping device seems to help reduce the negative side effects that occur during the early immobilization phase and shorten the time to functional training in a wheelchair. The Erigo device is commercially available (Hocoma, Volketswil, Switzerland).

Plasticity of neural structures

Experiments with spinalized cats with complete transection of the spinal cord in the thoracic region have shown the occurrence of training-induced reorganization of neural networks in the spinal cord. Lovely et al.[26] and Edgerton et al.[12] demonstrated that a spinalized cat that undergoes locomotor training walks much better than a cat without training. However, when locomotor training was stopped, the cat's walking function deteriorated. This finding leads to the conclusion that the structure of the neural network responsible for movement generation is highly flexible and that it can adapt to changes caused by injuries to the central nervous system. The described phenomenon is called *training-induced neural plasticity*. The plasticity is based on feedback of afferent signals coming from force and joint position sensors and increased afferent input to the spinal cord when a dedicated functional task, such as walking, is performed. The increased stimulation results in reorganization of axonal connections and leads to improvement of function.

Treadmill training with partial body weight support

The traditional method for mobilization of patients with restrictions in gait function during the subacute phase of rehabilitation is the use of parallel bars, where patients strut themselves on the bars with their arms and thereby are able to walk a few steps. This kind of mobilization is considered ineffective with respect to the principles of training-induced plasticity. Repetition of a dedicated movement leads to accelerated skill acquisition of a motor function.[13] This is the main reason why locomotor training on the treadmill has been established as a standard therapy for rehabilitation of neuromuscular gait disorders over the last 10 years.[18,47] Whereas patients can walk only a dozen steps in parallel bars, they can walk up to 20 times the distance on a treadmill. During treadmill training, patients are first secured in a harness and then attached to a counterweight, which ensures constant body weight support during all gait phases (Fig. 50-3). Initial support up to 60% of the body weight can be used; higher percentages appear to be less effective because of insufficient loading of the foot soles. The initial slow walking speed, which is chosen by the patient, is increased during the training course up to a normal walking speed.

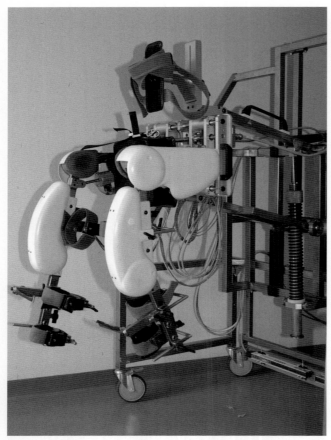

Fig. 50-4 Overview of the Lokomat robotic gait training device.

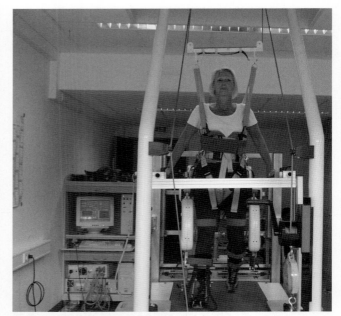

Fig. 50-5 Application of the Lokomat device.

Robot-assisted locomotion therapy

In general, patients with only a few residual functions at the beginning of the subacute rehabilitation phase and patients with severe spasticity are not able to walk independently, even with a high degree of body weight support. Their stepping movements must be manually assisted by one or two therapists, who stabilize the knee during stance phase and lift the foot during swing phase, and possibly by a third therapist, who stabilizes the trunk. This manual assistance is provided under ergonomically bad conditions; in some cases, a remarkable effort is required from the therapists to get the patient walking. This results in shorter training times and makes the quality of therapy highly dependent on the physical capacity of the therapists.

To overcome these limitations of manually assisted treadmill training, Colombo et al.[7] (ParaCare, University Hospital Balgrist, Zurich, Switzerland) developed the Lokomat motor-driven gait orthosis, which is commercially available in combination with a treadmill. The Lokomat consists of a steel frame, which can be adjusted to the patient's body properties, and a motorized bilateral hip and knee joint (Fig. 50-4). The Lokomat is fixed to the patient's thigh and shank by three cuffs of different sizes made of hook-and-loop material (Fig. 50-5). Joint movements are generated by linear spindles at walking speeds comparable to a normal gait (up to 3.5 km/h). With implementation of a recently released adaptive impedance control algorithm, the Lokomat can precisely produce the amount of force necessary to support the patient's preserved motor functions for achievement of a physiological gait pattern.[35]

A multicenter study of 20 chronic, incomplete SCI patients (injury for more than 2 years, stable neurological status) performed at four SCI centers (Schweizerisches Paraplegikerzentrum, Basel, Switzerland; Department of Physical Medicine and Rehabilitation, University of Illinois, Chicago, Illinois; Orthopaedic University Hospital, Heidelberg, Germany; and Balgrist University Hospital, Zurich, Switzerland) showed positive effects of a 4-week Lokomat training program (45-minute training session, 3–5 times per week). Patients who were able to walk with walking aids at the beginning of the training were able to walk almost two times faster and two times further after training. However, only two of the 20 patients were able to achieve significantly reduced dependency on their walking aids (walkers, crutches).[48]

Another robotic device, a commercially available gait trainer developed by Hesse group (Berlin, Germany), has shown beneficial effects in patients with stroke and in a few patients with subacute incomplete SCI.[19] However, our experience with the device revealed handling problems when training SCI patients with severe limitations of body and lower limb posture control. The basic design principle of the gait trainer, which generates walking movements only by motor-driven positioning of the foot, does not provide sufficient stabilization of the trunk and the legs and seems to be less effective in terms of physiological afferent stimulation of the spinal pattern generator.

Upper limb rehabilitation

Although the existence of a cervical spinal pattern generator in the upper extremities of humans has not yet been proved, the principles of training-induced plasticity by task-specific and goal-oriented repetition of movements are valid for therapy of neurological disorders of the upper extremities. This training has been used mainly in the rehabilitation of stroke patients, but a growing number of clinicians within the SCI community believe that a higher number of repetitive movements of the upper extremity would have a positive effect on hand and arm function in incomplete tetraplegic patients.

Several devices for application of robot-assisted motor therapy of the upper extremities have been developed and clinically tested during the last decade. Hogan et al.[21] introduced the MIT-MANUS, a two-degree-of-freedom robot that enables unrestricted movement of the shoulder and elbow joint by two-dimensional movements of the patient's hand in the horizontal plane. Impedance control intended to simulate manual guidance by an experienced therapist provides the robot with a soft compliant feel during movement and ensures that its intrinsic dynamics will minimally encumber the patient. A video screen displays the trajectories to be followed by patients. The same group recently developed a three-degree-of-freedom wrist manipulator for combined training of the arm and hand. For evaluation of the two-degree-of-freedom MIT-MANUS, the group conducted several randomized controlled trials with a large number of subjects having acute hemiparesis.[1,44,45] By the end of treatment, muscle strength in the trained shoulder and elbow in the group that used the robot was significantly larger than in the control group. The strength of the untrained wrist and hand did not differ between groups. Follow-up evaluations for up to 3 years in a subgroup of patients revealed sustained elbow and shoulder motor power gains in the upper limb compared with control individuals.

Another robotic device, the mirror-image motion enabler developed by Burgar et al.[4] (Stanford University, Palo Alto, CA, USA) consists of a commercial six-degree-of-freedom robot arm attached to a forearm splint. Because of the greater number of degrees of freedom compared to the MIT-MANUS, the forearm can be positioned within a larger range of positions and orientations in three-dimensional space. Four therapy modes can be implemented: passive, active-assisted, active-constrained, and bilateral. In the active-assisted mode, the patient initiates the movement and works together with the robot. Active-constrained movement is performed with the robot providing low resistance in the direction of the desired movement and springlike forces in all other directions. Lum et al.[27] conducted a randomized controlled trial with chronic hemiparetic subjects allocated to two groups. Subjects in the robot group practiced shoulder and elbow movements while assisted by the robot; subjects in the control group underwent neurodevelopmental therapy that targeted proximal upper limb function and negligible time of exposure to the robot in each session. Both groups were the same at the start of the study with respect to major clinical characteristics and outcome variables. The group that used the robot had greater improvements in the proximal movement portion of the applied functional test after 1 and 2 months of treatment. The group that used the robot also had larger gains in proximal arm strength and larger increases in extent of reach after 2 months of treatment. At 6-month follow-up, the two groups no longer differed in their functional test results; however, the group that used the robot had larger improvements in competence in daily activities.

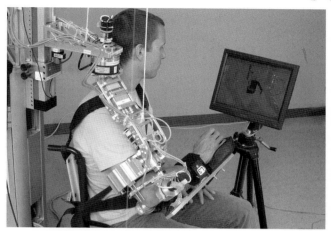

Fig. 50-6 ARMin rehabilitation robot designed specifically for the training demands of tetraplegic patients. (With permission.)

The MIT-MANUS and the mirror-image motion enabler robot were designed primarily for therapy for stroke patients. These patients normally have a stable trunk and do not require additional stabilization of the shoulder and torso. For application of an appropriate movement therapy to tetraplegic SCI patients in whom trunk stability often is missing and shoulder and elbow joint positions must be actively controlled, the ARMin robot (Fig. 50-6) is being developed by the Riener group[36] (Swiss Federal University of Technology; ETH, Zurich, Switzerland) and the Balgrist University Hospital (Zurich, Switzerland). The robot is fixed to the wall with the patient sitting beneath. The distal part is characterized by an exoskeletal structure, with the patient's arm placed inside an orthotic shell. The current version has four active degrees of freedom to allow elbow flexion/extension and spatial shoulder movements. Several multiple-axis force sensors and four position sensors enable the robot to work in different impedance control modes. The efficacy of the device still must be proved in clinical trials, which are scheduled for the near future.

Types of assistive rehabilitation robots

For the chronic stage of rehabilitation, during which no or little neurological recovery is expected, technical systems may compensate for substantial functional restrictions and assist patients. These systems apply to complete paraplegic patients with limited environmental mobility; however, these systems are of utmost importance to complete tetraplegic patients for whom missing hand or arm function results in constant dependence on caretakers. Huge efforts have been made over the last 20 years to build assistive robotic systems based on manipulator arms that provide the flexibility and usefulness of a human's upper extremity for persons with missing hand function.

Upper extremity assistive rehabilitation robots

Assistive rehabilitation robots can be classified into three categories. The *workstation-based system* consists of a manipulator

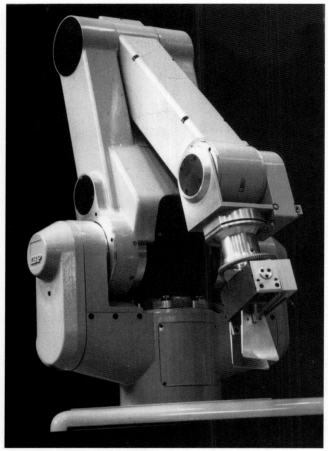

Fig. 50-7 Heidelberg manipulator, a historical workstation manipulator.

that is fixed to a single location. The workstation consists of the robot and typically a predefined environment. Because the environment in a workstation is structured, the robot can be programmed to perform complete movement tasks with a single user command.

The main alternative to a fixed-location robot is the *wheelchair-mounted manipulator*, which usually is mounted to the side of a powered wheelchair. The wheelchair-mounted arm has a greater degree of flexibility in that it can easily be moved around from place to place.

The third type of assistive rehabilitation robot is the *mobile robot*, which consists of a remotely controlled mobile platform that may have a robotic manipulator arm mounted onto it. This type of system is in the research and development stage. However, it has the greatest potential to affect the daily lives of elderly people, people with disabilities, and nonhandicapped persons who can use them as service robots.

Workstation-based manipulators

Work in the area of rehabilitation robotics using manipulators started in the mid 1970s. One of the earliest projects was the system designed by Paeslack and Roesler.[33] The purpose-designed, five-degree-of-freedom manipulator was placed in a specially adapted desktop environment (Fig. 50-7). Another early workstation system was developed by Seamone and Schmeisser.[39] The arm of this system was based around an electrically powered prosthetic arm mounted on a horizontal

track. Various pieces of equipment (e.g., telephone, book rest, disks) were laid out on the simple but cleverly designed workstation table and could be manipulated by the arm using preprogrammed commands. In France, the Spartacus robot was built around a large high-quality manipulator that originated in the nuclear industry.[24] With such a potentially powerful device, safety was a consideration, and early training of users was performed with the arm behind a clear screen. This project has been a starting point for multiple international and national projects.

Several generations of the desktop vocational assistive robot (DeVAR) workstation using an industrial robot have been developed. The DeVAR IV workstation is aimed at a vocational environment. The robot arm is mounted upside-down on an overhead track, which increases its working range.[17] The RT series produced by OxIM (Oxford, United Kingdom) is a type of robot that has been widely used in rehabilitation robotics and actively promoted by the manufacturers as suitable for rehabilitation applications. Boeing (Seattle, WA, USA) developed an early system based on the RTX robot, initially intended for use by one of the company's disabled programmers.[14] The Master project in France, a continuation of the Spartacus work, used an RTX robot in a workstation environment.[5] The manipulator was mounted at the back of the workstation, with shelving units on both sides that could be accessed by the arm. More recently, as part of the European TIDE funded RAID project, an RT200 robot was built into an extended workstation.[5] At the end of the RAID project, the workstation was commercialized by the manufacturers of the RT robots and the same workstation was commercialized into a similar system by Afma Robots in France.

The Regenesis workstation robot was developed at the Neil Squire Foundation (Vancouver, BC, Canada).[3] It consists of a six-degree-of-freedom manipulator mounted on a horizontal bar, which allows sideway movement over a bed or table. The system is commercially available.

All of the workstation-based robot systems discussed can be programmed to perform a number of manipulations in a structured environment. They offer ease of control because complex movements can be stored in the computer and called repeatedly by single user commands. However, superior control is gained at the expense of flexibility. Because the user may not have direct control over robot movements, any change in the environment has to be "taught" to the robot. Some workstation-based systems offer a combination of programmed and interactive modes of control, with varying levels of autonomy. However, this benefit is accompanied by increased complexity in controlling the robot because of the changing nature of the environment.

Even though the technical complexity of peripheral components around the manipulator differs among the systems, the flexibility of workstation-based rehabilitation robots still is limited, which in turn restricts the user's autonomy. From our experience, support for reintegration of SCI people into the work environment is considered low.

Feeding devices

Although robots are defined to be multifunctional, a device that is programmable for a specific task also can be defined as a rehabilitation robot. Feeding application is one area where robotic devices have been used more successfully than workstation manipulator systems. In 1987, as a Masters Research project, Topping set himself the task of helping his neighbor, a 12-year-old boy with spastic paraplegia, to feed himself. This was the beginning of the Rehab Robotics company, whose Handy 1 robot has sold more than any other rehabilitation robot.[42] The functionality of the device has been increased to include applying cosmetics, shaving, and painting. Other powered feeding devices are the Winsford Feeder (Winsford Products Inc., Pennington, NJ, USA), which has been on the market for 15 years, the Neater Eater (Neater Solutions Ltd., Buxton, UK), and the MySpoon (Secom, Tokyo, Japan). The commercial success of these devices is based on their simplicity, ease of use, and, most importantly, low cost. However, as with any technical aid, critical analysis of how often and how successfully these systems are used by patients in their domestic environment after discharge from the hospital is needed. Cost–benefit analysis for each setting is important, because many people still require one-on-one assistance for setup.

Wheelchair-mounted manipulators

Although use of robotics is intended to bring increased flexibility, the workstation approach itself is limited. A fixed-site robot arm can interact only with objects arranged around it (i.e., by an able-bodied person), a situation that does not represent real-life conditions encountered in daily life. Therefore, the idea of a mobile robot is attractive.

Among wheelchair-mounted manipulators, the MANUS is one of the success stories in rehabilitation robotics. It has been sold commercially by Exact Dynamics since 1990. It was developed in 1985 at the Hoensbroek Institute for Rehabilitation Research and TNO (Delft, The Netherlands).[25] Another interesting approach to the design of a wheelchair-mounted manipulator was developed by Hennequin and his Inventaid company. This manipulator was based around a novel pneumatic actuator, known as "Air Muscle." Simplicity (with implications of low cost, reliability, and easy maintenance) was one of the aims of the project, and the basic system involves no digital or microprocessor circuitry. The other wheelchair-mounted robot, now commercially available, is the Raptor arm (Rehabilitation Technologies Division, Applied Resources Corporation, Wharton, NJ, USA).[28] The Raptor is much simpler than the Manus. It has four degrees of freedom, a gripping device, and a less sophisticated user interface system. Although the Raptor has less functionality than the Manus, it is significantly less expensive. Based upon the Manus concept, the Graeser group[29] at the University of Bremen (Bremen, Germany) developed an "intelligent" wheelchair-mounted manipulator, the FRIEND II rehabilitation robot (Fig. 50-8). The FRIEND II system is equipped with a humanlike robotic arm with seven-joint kinematics, two interchangeable prosthetic grippers, force torque sensors, and stereo camera system. It also has several smart devices, such as a smart tray and a new control concept called the *kinematic configuration control*. This device represents the current state of the art for what is technically possible in the field of assistive rehabilitation robotics.

In order to make use of the spatial flexibility of wheelchair-mounted systems, robotic systems are mostly user controlled; that is, the user is provided with the option to send elementary movement commands to the robot arm. This option provides greater flexibility but requires a certain skill with the device and has a higher demand for support. Individual

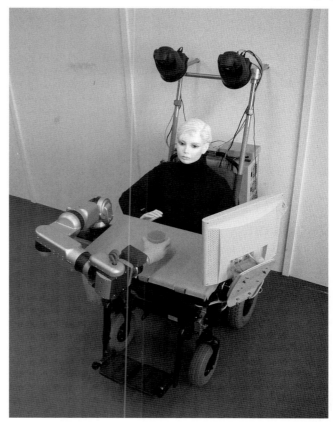

Fig. 50-8 FRIEND II system. A powered wheelchair serves as a mobile platform for the wheelchair-mounted manipulator and video processing system. (With permission.)

movements, which are controlled by a "keyboard" (like the MANUS), requires an extended number of preserved functions of the user's hands and fingers, thus limiting use of this system. In addition, speech control through elementary commands is arduous and strenuous because of the high degree of concentration required over an extended period of time. This applies especially to complex activities of daily living (e.g., pouring liquid into a glass). Automatic execution of such tasks would be highly desirable, but even in case of the highly sophisticated FRIEND II system, error-free quick operation with minimum effort from the user is not possible at the current stage of technology. Achieving this performance will be a crucial prerequisite for overall acceptance of these systems by severely disabled persons and is a big challenge for future research.

Robotic exoskeletons for the lower extremity

Whereas the manipulative systems for tetraplegic patients are not fixed to the patients, assistive robotic systems for mobility enhancement of paraplegic patients interact directly with the lower extremities of patients. Several groups worked to develop a driven-gait orthosis that would restore independent walking by SCI patients. In 1972, Hughes[20] developed a concept for a pneumatically driven exoskeleton. Hydraulically driven systems were later developed by Seireg and Grundman[40] and Miyamoto et al.[30] The first orthoses using direct-current drives were constructed by

Rabischong et al.[34] (Montpellier, France). Devices currently under development are the Berkeley lower extremity exoskeleton (BLEEX; Berkeley University, Berkeley, CA, USA) and the hybrid assistive limb (HAL) device (Tsukuba University, Tsukuba, Japan).[23] Although all of these powered orthoses are designed to extend the mobility range of patients in their natural environment, the power supply problem remains unsolved and calls into question the overall usefulness of these devices. Furthermore, because these devices cannot control upright balance of the body, additional support by crutches or parallel bars is required, which further restricts their beneficial application. Therefore, from the clinical point of view, these devices do not appear to offer an advantage over wheelchairs.

Discussion

Modern rehabilitation medicine mainly focuses on functional restitution by patients. Because the majority of SCI patients today have incomplete SCI, a major improvement of function can be achieved by activating and training preserved residual function. Recent neurophysiological findings have initiated the development of novel robotic devices for training motor control and supporting the patient rather than substituting for loss of function. Analysis of the most recent scientific literature (Medline search for "rehabilitation" and "robot") shows that this branch of rehabilitation robotics is a quickly developing field. Even at the current stage, many specialized SCI centers worldwide have integrated these devices into their overall rehabilitation programs.

Introduction of the Erigo device has opened new doors to physiological mobilization therapy at a very early stage for SCI patients as well as other patient groups. Positive circulatory effects in SCI patients with high cervical lesions have been shown.[8]

Locomotion training on a treadmill in combination with partial body weight support has been established over the last decade for rehabilitation of various gait disorders with neurological origins, including SCI. The possibility of extended repetition of stepping movements leads to faster relearning of walking due to training-induced plasticity of the central nervous system. The commercially available Lokomat system has overcome the limitations of reproducibility of movements and of the strenuous efforts required by therapists for manually assisted training. Using this robotic device, a therapeutically relevant extension of the training period is possible. Patients appreciate this kind of training because of the regularity of movements and the longer training sessions.[48] If novel drugs for spinal axonal regeneration become available for clinical use,[38] then robotic-assisted locomotion devices will become increasingly more important in enhancing neuroregenerative effects through adequate functional training.

Therapists may fear that robots will replace their manual work and that only a single therapist will be needed to supervise therapy performed by several robots at the same time. However, it must be emphasized that robotic training machines have been developed as an adjunctive tool to increase the intensity of therapy based on novel principles of motor rehabilitation and to offer this therapy to patients who are difficult to train manually.

Developments in the field of assistive rehabilitation robotics in the form of manipulators for severely paralyzed patients and exoskeletons for patients with gait disorders have paralleled the developments of industrial robotic applications. The 1980s opened with almost boundless optimism about the future of industrial robotics, with the potential value of this technology seen to be high. That early enthusiasm has been tempered by the experiences of the past decades. Although much progress has been made and increasingly more complex hardware and software components have been implemented into manipulative systems, robotic systems still are not in widespread clinical use.[43] Perhaps the introduction of novel control methods will quicken the process of clinical integration.[31] Many factors, including the aesthetic appearance of robotic systems, affect the user's decision on whether or not to use the device. Thus, careful analysis of user requirements concerning handling, price, complexity, and reliability are needed to determine the most important criteria for user acceptance. Another option is implantable neuroprostheses,[37] which have been introduced in the clinical environment as a serious alternative to external manipulators for functional restoration of upper extremity function.

Conclusion

Robotics provide insight into the principles of rehabilitation. Using robots to assist the rehabilitation process will provide more precise, objective, detailed data on what actually occurs in patients during recovery. This in turn will lead to a better understanding of the key biomechanical and neurological factors required for a successful rehabilitation process. A greater understanding of the underlying mechanisms of recovery will lead to better ideas of how technology can be beneficial in rehabilitation. New fields of applications of rehabilitation robots will lead to a better outcome for all people with disabling conditions as well as increased utility by the able-bodied population.

References

1. Aisen ML, Krebs HI, Hogan N, et al: The effect of robot assisted therapy and rehabilitative training on motor recovery following stroke, *Arch Neurol* 54:443–446, 1997.
2. Barbeau H, Rossignol S: Enhancement of locomotor recovery following spinal cord injury, *Curr Opin Neurol* 7:517–524, 1994.
3. Birch GE, Cameron W, Fengler M, et al: Regenesis robotic manipulator for persons with severe disabilities, *Eur Rev Biomed Tech* 12:320–323, 1990.
4. Burgar CG, Lum PS, Shor P, van der Loos HF: Development of robots for rehabilitation therapy: the Palo Alto VA/Stanford experience, *J Rehabil Res Dev* 37:663–673, 2000.
5. Busnel M, Cammoun R, Coulon-Lauture F, et al: The robotized workstation "MASTER" for users with tetraplegia: description and evaluation, *J Rehabil Res Dev* 36:217–229, 1999.
6. Calancie B, Needham-Shropshire B, Jacobs P, et al: Involuntary stepping after chronic spinal cord injury. Evidence for a central rhythm generator for locomotion in man, *Brain* 117:1143–1159, 1994.
7. Colombo G, Wirz M, Dietz V: Driven gait orthosis for improvement of locomotor training in paraplegic patients, *Spinal Cord* 39:252–255, 2001.
8. Colombo G, Schreier R, Plewa H, Rupp R: Novel tilt table with integrated robotic stepping mechanism: design principles and clinical application, *Proceedings IEEE 9th International Conference on Rehabilitation Robotics* 227–230, 2005.
9. Dietz V, Colombo G, Jensen L: Locomotor activity in spinal man, *Lancet* 344:1260–1263, 1994.
10. Dietz V, Colombo G, Müller R: Single joint perturbation during gait: neuronal control of movement trajectory, *Exp Brain Res* 158:308–316, 2004.
11. Duysens J, van de Crommert HWAA: Neural control of locomotion. Part 1: the central pattern generator from cats to humans (review), *Gait Posture* 7:131–141, 1998.

12. Edgerton VR, de Leon RD, Tillakaratne N, et al: Use-dependent plasticity in spinal stepping and standing. In Seil FJ, editor: *Advances in neurology: neuronal regeneration, reorganization and repair*, ed 7, Philadelphia, 1997, Lippincott-Raven.

13. Field-Fote EC: Spinal cord control of movement: implications for locomotor rehabilitation following spinal cord injury, *Phys Ther* 80:477–484, 2000.

14. Fu C: An independent vocational workstation for a quadriplegic, *Proceedings of the RESNA Conference* 182–184, 1986.

15. Gerner HJ: *Die die querschnittlähmung: erstversorgung, behandlungsstrategien, rehabilitation.* Oxford, 1992, Blackwell.

16. Grillner S, Wallen P: Central pattern generators for locomotion with special reference to vertebrates, *Annu Rev Neurosci* 8:233–261, 1985.

17. Hammel J, Hall K, Lees D, et al: Clinical evaluation of a desktop robotic assistant, *J Rehabil Res Dev* 26:1–16, 1989.

18. Hesse S, Bertelt C, Jahnke MT, et al: Treadmill training with partial body weight support compared with physiotherapy in nonambulatory hemiparetic patients, *Stroke* 26:976–981, 1995.

19. Hesse S, Werner C, Bardeleben A: Electromechanical gait training with functional electrical stimulation: case studies in spinal cord injury, *Spinal Cord* 42:346–352, 2004.

20. Hughes J: Powered lower limb orthotics in paraplegia, *Paraplegia* 9:191–193, 1972.

21. Hogan N, Krebs HI, Sharon A, Charnnarong J, inventors; Massachusetts Institute of Technology, assignee: *Interactive robotic therapist*, US patent 5,466,213, 1995.

22. Jones T: RAID–towards greater independence in the office and home environment, *Proceedings International Conference on Rehabilitation Robotics* 201-206, 1999.

23. Kiguchi K, Tanaka T, Fukuda T: Neuro-fuzzy control of a robotic exoskeleton with EMG signals, *IEEE Trans Fuzzy Syst* 12:481–490, 2004.

24. Kwee HH, Tramblay M, Barbier R, et al: First experimentation of the Spartacus telethesis in a clinical environment, *Paraplegia* 21:275, 1983.

25. Kwee H, Quaedackers J, van de Bool E, et al: Adapting the control of the MANUS manipulator for persons with cerebral palsy: an exploratory study, *Technol Disabil* 14:31–42, 2002.

26. Lovely RG, Gregor RJ, Roy RR, Edgerton VR: Weight-bearing hindlimb stepping in treadmill-exercised adult spinal cat, *Brain Res* 514:206–218, 1990.

27. Lum PS, Burgar CG, Shor PC, et al: Robot-assisted movement training compared with conventional therapy techniques for the rehabilitation of upper-limb motor function after stroke, *Arch Phys Med Rehabil* 83:952–959, 2002.

28. Mahoney R: The raptor wheelchair robot system, *Proceedings 7th International Conference on Rehabilitation Robotics* 135-141, 2001.

29. Martens C, Ruchel N, Lang O, et al: A FRIEND for assisting handicapped people, *IEEE Robot Automat Mag* 8:57–65, 2001.

30. Miyamoto H, Israel I, Miyamoto H, et al: Approach to a powered orthosis for paralyzed lower limbs, *Proceedings International Conference on Advanced Robotics* 451-458, 1985.

31. Müller-Putz GR, Scherer R, Pfurtscheller G, Rupp R: EEG-based neuroprosthesis control: a step towards clinical practice, *Neurosci Lett* 382:169–174, 2005.

32. NSCISC: *2004 Annual statistical report.* National Spinal Cord Injury Statistical Center, University of Alabama at Birmingham, 2004.

33. Paeslack V, Roesler H: Design and control of a manipulator for tetraplegics, *Mech Machine Theory* 12:413–423, 1977.

34. Rabischong E, Sgarbi F, Rabischong P, et al: Control and command of a six degrees of freedom active electrical orthosis for paraplegic patient, *Proceedings IEEE International Workshop on Intelligent Robots and Systems* 987–991, 1990.

35. Riener R, Lunenburger L, Jezernik S, et al: Patient-cooperative strategies for robot-aided treadmill training: first experimental results, *IEEE Trans Neural Syst Rehabil Eng* 13:380–394, 2005.

36. Riener R, Nef T, Colombo G: Robot-aided neurorehabilitation of the upper extremities, *Med Biol Eng Comput* 43:2–10, 2005.

37. Rupp R, Gerner HJ: Neuroprosthetics of the upper extremity: clinical application in spinal cord injury and future perspectives, *Biomed Tech (Berl)* 49:93–98, 2004.

38. Schwab ME: Nogo and axon regeneration, *Curr Opin Neurobiol* 14:118–124, 2004.

39. Seamone W, Schmeisser G: Early clinical evaluation of a robot arm/worktable system for spinal-cord-injured persons, *J Rehabil Res Dev* 22:38–57, 1985.

40. Seireg A, Grundman J: Design of a multi-task exoskeleton walking device. In Ghista D, editor: *Biomechanics of medical devices*, New York, 1981, Marcel Dekker.

41. Topp RF, Ditmyer MF, King KF, et al: The effect of bed rest and potential of prehabilitation on patients in the intensive care unit, *AACN Clin Issues* 13:263–276, 2002.

42. Topping M: An overview of the development of Handy 1, a rehabilitation robot to assist the severely disabled, *J Intell Robot Syst Theor Appl* 34:253–263, 2002.

43. Van der Loos FM: VA/Stanford Rehabilitation Research and Development Program: lessons learned in the application of robotics technology to the field of rehabilitation, *IEEE Trans Rehabil Eng* 3:46–55, 1995.

44. Volpe BT, Krebs HI, Hogan N, et al: Robot training enhanced motor outcome in patients with stroke maintained over 3 years, *Neurology* 53:1874–1876, 1999.

45. Volpe BT, Krebs HI, Hogan N: Is robot-aided sensorimotor training in stroke rehabilitation a realistic option? *Curr Opin Neurol* 14:745–752, 2001.

46. Waters RL, Adkins R, Yakura J, Sie I: Donal Munro Lecture: functional and neurologic recovery following acute SCI, *J Spinal Cord Med* 21:195–199, 1998.

47. Wernig A, Nanassy A, Müller S: Laufband (treadmill) therapy in incomplete paraplegia and tetraplegia, *J Neurotrauma* 16:719–726, 1999.

48. Wirz M, Dietz V, Zemon DH, et al: Effectiveness of an automated locomotor training in patients with a chronic incomplete spinal cord injury: a multicenter trial, *Arch Phys Med Rehabil* 86:672–680, 2005.

Future trends and research in orthoses

Alberto Esquenazi and Mukul C. Talaty

Key Points

- Advances in materials and other technologies will have a positive impact on orthotics in the future.
- Reduction in weight and improvement in the biomechanics of gait will greatly benefit users of orthotic devices.
- Future technologies, such as longer-lasting batteries and nanotechnology, should result in significant advances in orthotics.

Advances in the areas of materials, biomechanics, electronics, miniaturization, and bionics present great potential for improvement of orthoses. Judicious application of developing technology coupled with extension of our knowledge of how orthotics function and how best to match that function to patient needs should allow for improved orthotic outcomes. This chapter reviews some important advances in technology and speculates about some of the possibilities they present and trends to come.

Current devices

The large majority of orthoses currently used in clinical care are passive, energy-storing devices constructed of relatively rigid thermoplastics lined with soft foam. They contain springs and dampers that provide limited assist and control motion. Use of metal reinforcement can augment stiffness and thus support; however, this adds both weight and cost. More contemporary designs, which include lightweight, energy-storing composites such as carbon fiber, in orthotic construction have shown promising results in terms of patient acceptance and function;[5,10] however, these devices are nearly an order of magnitude more expensive and offer little opportunity for postfabrication modification. Traditional ankle–foot

orthoses (AFOs) can be fabricated with metal joints. These joints allow simple and much increased adjustment potential, but they increase weight, maintenance, and cost.

Stance control devices

In the past few years, electromechanical knee–ankle orthoses (KAFOs), known as *stance control devices*, have matured and established themselves, at least commercially. These devices automatically provide support during stance phase and allow knee flexion during swing phase, based on a few simple rules. For example, one device remains locked until contact sensors indicate the leg is in swing phase, and thus the knee is allowed to bend. Another device uses joint kinematics and kinetics to determine when to provide support and when to allow free knee motion. Generally, such selective control makes sense as an improvement over a permanently locked brace that disrupts the fluidity and biomechanics of walking at the cost of providing stance phase stability. How well patient function improves and how well this technology will be received remain to be seen.[7] With a sufficiently strong response and interest from patients, practitioners, and insurance companies, more complex control rules may be developed to ensure appropriate functioning across a range of activities and patient abilities. Optimization of control rules likely will take considerable efforts and trial and error; coding up the rules into the mechanics or electronics will be relatively simpler. Others have developed low- or no-power dampened devices to provide variable stiffness. One group uses an oil damper in which flow rate is mechanically controlled, thus allowing variable resistance.[13] Another group uses magnetorheological fluid to allow variation of resistance throughout stance phase.[1] Both of these applications provide some variability and flexibility, as do the stance control devices. The trick will be to determine precisely what control each patient needs and to implement that control in a practical and tolerable manner with minimal limitations or trade-offs. This concept of selective control is just another step toward restoring exactly the physiological function lost without providing any restrictions.

The concept of a "patient-tuned" orthosis that is manufactured to respond to the specific needs of a patient is intriguing. Stanhope and his group from the National Institutes of Health (NIH) have developed a preliminary technique for selecting optimal stiffness and set angle for a carbon graphite AFO. The brace can be manufactured using a special three-dimensional forming machine. Using traditional and advanced techniques in gait analysis, the researchers were able to demonstrate improved outcomes over less custom settings for the brace.

Powered devices

Improvement of human–machine interaction likely will result in devices that are an intimate extension of the body—structurally, neurologically, and dynamically.

Related advancements have centered on developing exoskeleton-powered devices that assist weakness by actuating motion rather than just providing support. Several groups have developed prototypes that do exactly this for knee (Yobotics, Cincinnati, OH, USA) or ankle actuation.[1,2] One device seems to have the capability of generating sufficient force outputs, but the device appears bulky and not sufficiently cosmetic to allow long-term use.[2] In addition, the reliance on pneumatic power makes it unclear whether the device can be adapted to a low-power, sustained-use, portable electronic device. One limiting factor to full-time use of powered devices is whether their energy requirements can be made sufficiently low or easy and quick to replenish. Also, the need for minimal bulk to achieve high patient compliance is opposed by the need for relatively larger-size actuators to provide sufficient forces.

Although knee orthoses seem to be the target for many of the new product developments, others have realized the potential to provide considerable system-wide control from the ankle and have chosen to focus on this region.[1,2,11] The latter group has quantified the effects of ankle support on control of knee stability and speculated that a smart device—one that matches the control required in a pathological gait—may be realizable from the ankle in many situations. AFOs are generally smaller, lighter, more invisible, and less expensive, making them popular choices. It seems reasonable that combinations of this approach with the myriad of new materials and controls being implemented will result in the most versatile and well-tolerated device.

Development of new materials, particularly new electrically controlled fluids (magnetorheological) and actuators that use ionic polymer–metal composites (IPMCs) and microelectromechanical system (MEMS) switches, have the potential to transform the orthotic industry with low-cost, high-performance components.[1,13] Electroactive polymers are essentially plastics that can serve as actuators (Fig. 51-1). They can be made to generate forces and displacements on the order of muscles and can do so with considerably less bulk than a typical electrical motor. Field-activated polymers can respond quickly and have high electromechanical coupling that can allow for overall efficiencies as high as 80%.

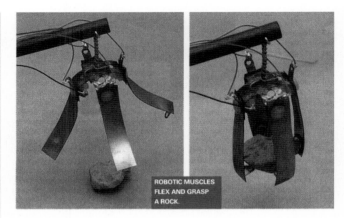

Fig. 51-1 Example of an electroactive polymer used as a gripper. (Courtesy NASA JPL-Caltech.)

Perhaps most significantly, they can exceed the peak power of natural muscle, allowing for devices of size and mass comparable to natural muscles. These devices will be able to stabilize a joint at the exact time necessary and allow free motion when no or minimal control is needed; all of this at a fraction of the weight of current braces. Commercial development for biomechanical use is under way. Such technology holds promise to supplement or entirely replace conventional passive materials used in braces today. In theory, utilizing the muscles already in place is another step in this direction. Functional electrical stimulation aims to do just this but has limitations.

Functional electrical stimulation systems

Historically, functional electrical stimulation has made possible the restoration of limited use to paralyzed muscles. This same technology can be used to provide an invisible or biological brace. Although this idea has been around since the early 1960s, implementation has evolved from single, hard-wired, preprogrammed surface stimulation units to multichannel, microcontroller-based, multisensor-keyed, fully implanted devices.[6] Although a surface electrode is convenient for treatment, it is difficult to use for stimulation of deep areas, and muscle response may change each time the electrode is placed on the skin.[6] In addition, patients often feel pain from the activation of sensory fibers. The percutaneous electrode can stimulate muscles selectively and in deep areas easily.[4] The response is stable and allows control of stimulation parameters with external devices. Electrode failure due to infection, breakage, and movement is a frequent problem. A combined implanted electrode and stimulator may prove to be better because it should have a smaller risk of infection and no problems related to movement. Such a device, the radiofrequency RF BION (developed by the Alfred Mann Foundation), is available in the United States (Fig. 51-2).[12] The BION has been used to relieve the chronic intractable pain from shoulder subluxation following stroke. Implanting the BION in the middle and posterior deltoid muscles reduced shoulder subluxation and restored function to the paralyzed muscles, with relief of shoulder pain. Pilot work has shown that this technology improves walking

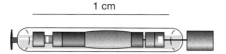

1 cm

Fig. 51-2 Implantable Bion. (Courtesy Alfred Mann Foundation.)

function in subjects with footdrop.[12] Stimulation of the deep peroneal nerve provided more selective control of muscle activation while improving swing phase clearance, walking speed, and physiological cost associated with walking. Implementation of natural sensors, such as recording from the sural nerve via an electrode, continues to streamline designs while maintaining high-fidelity sensory inputs to the system.[4] Finding the optimal control scheme is an area that would benefit from further research.[6]

Emerging technologies

New exciting opportunities in orthotic design are looming in the near future as the pace of technology change accelerates. Nanotechnology, tissue engineering, and computer science developments are areas where orthotic design, fabrication, and application will take place. Among products in research and development stages are smart fabrics that can serve as underpinning for wearable computers, miniature sensors, and even electrostatically controlled tissue interfaces that will eliminate use of external joints because the fabric can change its molecular structure when a small current is passed through. Sensors and software that facilitate stumble recovery and even prevent falls should become available and make walking safer.

Powered orthoses that can enhance the physiology of the musculoskeletal systems may become a reality. Exoskeleton systems that can unload a weak or painful limb and, in some scenarios, increase limb segment function beyond its physiological limitations are within reach. Power supply, computational speed, and heavy materials were the main problems in the past. Within the next decade, with developing and future

technologies the systems should become part of the available treatment armamentarium.[3]

Another area of work in progress is the development of higher-density power supplies. Attention to this issue is a requirement in view of current energy-consuming technologies. Such batteries will need to be lightweight, long lasting, and ideally environmentally friendly. Another option for development is recovery of energy generated during walking, for example, from heel impact, or by carrying a backpack load that converts mechanical energy to electricity while walking.[8,9]

References

1. Blaya J, Herr H: Adaptive control of a variable-impedance ankle-foot orthosis to assist drop-foot gait, *IEEE Trans Neural Syst Rehabil Eng* 12:24–31, 2004.
2. Ferris D, Czerniecki J, Hannaford B: An ankle-foot orthosis powered by artificial pneumatic muscles, *J Appl Biomech* 21:189–197, 2005.
3. Guizzo E, Goldstein N: The rise of the body bots, *IEEE Spectrum* 42:50–56, 2005.
4. Haugland MK, Sinkjær T: Cutaneous whole nerve recordings used for correction for foot drop in hemiplegic man, *IEEE Trans Biomed Eng* 3:307–317, 1995.
5. Heim M, Yaacobi E, Azaria M: A pilot study to determine the efficiency of lightweight carbon fiber orthoses in the management of patients suffering from post-poliomyelitis syndrome, *Clin Rehabil* 11:302–305, 1997.
6. Lyons GM, Sinkjaer T, Burridge JH, Wilcox DJ: A review of portable FES-based neural orthoses for the correction of drop foot, *IEEE Trans Neural Syst Rehabil Eng* 10:260–279, 2002.
7. McMillan AG, Kendrick K, Michael JW, Horton GW: Preliminary evidence for effectiveness of stance control orthoses, *J Prosthet Orthot* 16:6–13, 2004.
8. Rome LC, Flynn L, Goldman EM, Yoo TD: Generating electricity while walking with loads, *Science* 309:1725–1728, 2005.
9. Shenck MS, Paradiso JA: Energy scavenging with shoe mounted piezoelectrics, *IEEE Micro* 21:30–42, 2001.
10. Steinfeldt F, Seifert W, Gunther K: Modern carbon fiber orthoses in the management of polio patients: a critical evaluation of the functional aspects, *Z Orthop Ihre Grenzgeb* 141:357–361, 2003.
11. Talaty M: *Intersegmental dynamics analysis of the effect of an ankle foot brace on walking*, PhD thesis, Philadelphia, 2002, Drexel University.
12. Weber D, Stein R, Chan K, et al: BIONic WalkAide for correcting foot drop, *IEEE Trans Neural Syst Rehabil Eng* 13:242–246, 2005.
13. Yamamoto S, Hagiwara A, Mizobe T, Yokoyama O, Yasui T: Development of an ankle-foot orthosis with an oil damper, *Prosthet Orthot Int* 29:209–219, 2005.

Index

Page numbers followed by f indicate figures; t, tables; b, boxes. Special indicators are not listed when content is on multiple inclusive pages. Special indicators are listed separately from page content as appropriate.